Gerontological Nursing Competencies for Care

Second Edition

Edited by

Kristen L. Mauk, PhD, RN, CRRN-A, GCNS-BC

Professor of Nursing

Kreft Endowed Chair for the Advancement of Nursing Science

Valparaiso University

Health Care Consultant, Mauk Financial Solutions, LLC

Valparaiso, Indiana

JONES AND BARTLETT PUBLISHERS

Sudbury, Massachusetts

BOSTON TORONTO LONDON SINGAPORE

World Headquarters
Jones and Bartlett Publishers
40 Tall Pine Drive
Sudbury, MA 01776
978-443-5000
info@jbpub.com
www.jbpub.com

Jones and Bartlett Publishers
Canada
6339 Ormindale Way
Mississauga, Ontario L5V 1J2
Canada

Jones and Bartlett Publishers
International
Barb House, Barb Mews
London W6 7PA
United Kingdom

Jones and Bartlett's books and products are available through most bookstores and online booksellers. To contact Jones and Bartlett Publishers directly, call 800-832-0034, fax 978-443-8000, or visit our website, www.jbpub.com.

Substantial discounts on bulk quantities of Jones and Bartlett's publications are available to corporations, professional associations, and other qualified organizations. For details and specific discount information, contact the special sales department at Jones and Bartlett via the above contact information or send an email to specialsales@jbpub.com.

The authors, editor, and publisher have made every effort to provide accurate information. However, they are not responsible for errors, omissions, or for any outcomes related to the use of the contents of this book and take no responsibility for the use of the products and procedures described. Treatments and side effects described in this book may not be applicable to all people; likewise, some people may require a dose or experience a side effect that is not described herein. Drugs and medical devices are discussed that may have limited availability controlled by the Food and Drug Administration (FDA) for use only in a research study or clinical trial. Research, clinical practice, and government regulations often change the accepted standard in this field. When consideration is being given to use of any drug in the clinical setting, the health care provider or reader is responsible for determining FDA status of the drug, reading the package insert, and reviewing prescribing information for the most up-to-date recommendations on dose, precautions, and contraindications, and determining the appropriate usage for the product. This is especially important in the case of drugs that are new or seldom used.

Production Credits
Publisher: Kevin Sullivan
Aquisitions Editor: Emily Ekle
Aquisitions Editor: Amy Sibley
Associate Editor: Patricia Donnelly
Editorial Assistant: Rachel Shuster
Associate Production Editor: Amanda Clerkin
Senior Marketing Manager: Barb Bartoszek
V.P., Manufacturing and Inventory Control: Therese Connell
Composition: Auburn Associates, Inc.
Cover Design: Scott Moden
Cover Image: © Monkey Business Images/Shutterstock, Inc.
Printing and Binding: Malloy, Inc.
Cover Printing: Malloy, Inc.

Library of Congress Cataloging-in-Publication Data
Gerontological nursing : competencies for care / [edited by] Kristen L.
Mauk. — 2nd ed.
p. ; cm.
Includes bibliographical references and index.
ISBN-13: 978-0-7637-5580-5
ISBN-10: 0-7637-5580-X
1. Geriatric nursing. I. Mauk, Kristen L.
[DNLM: 1. Geriatric Nursing. 2. Aging—physiology. 3.
Aging—psychology. WY 152 G36967 2009]

RC954.G4746 2009
618.97'0231—dc22

2008040210

6048

Printed in the United States of America
13 12 11 10 10 9 8 7 6 5 4 3

Dedication

To Norman Volk
for his vision of the place that nursing will hold in the care of older adults,
his international leadership through the John A. Hartford Foundation,
and his far-reaching efforts to promote gerontological nursing

KLM

Contents

PREFACE

Although there are numerous excellent gerontological nursing texts on the market today, the approach to this book is unique in that it is based on an essential document from the American Association of Colleges of Nursing and the John A. Hartford Foundation Institute for Geriatric Nursing (July 2000) entitled *Older Adults: Recommended Baccalaureate Competencies and Curricular Guidelines for Geriatric Nursing Care.* This book is intended to be a basic baccalaureate-level gerontological nursing text, and it is structured to ensure that students will obtain the recommended competencies and knowledge necessary to provide excellent care to older adults. It can be used for a stand-alone course or in sections to be integrated throughout a nursing curriculum.

Using the recommended competencies as a guide, each chapter is written to assist students of gerontological nursing to acquire the essential knowledge and skills to provide excellent care for older adults. Competencies as set forth in the AACN/Hartford Foundation document are listed at the beginning of each chapter to help direct students' learning.

This book has several outstanding features. First, the framework, as described, is unique. In addition, the text is an edited work with a diverse authorship of 38 contributors from three countries who represent all areas of gerontological nursing, including management, education, quality assurance, clinical practice in a variety of settings, advanced practice roles, research, business, consulting, and academia. This second edition adds 10 new authors, with the vast majority of authors from the first edition continuing their work in the new edition. All chapters have been updated to include current resources and evidence-based clinical practice. Interdisciplinary collaboration of many chapters was accomplished by including nurse authors writing with colleagues whose backgrounds are in psychology, social work, pharmacy, gerontology, rehabilitation, biology, sociology, and business management.

For the second edition, comments and recommendations of instructors who used the text were carefully considered. In answer to requests, a new chapter was added on healthy aging, which is also a theme more heavily emphasized in the new edition. Photos and content portray older adults as actively aging. A new chapter with specific content on dementia, as requested by users of the first edition, has also been included. In addition, the book has a unique chapter on future trends that impact gerontological nursing.

The text has a user-friendly and comprehensive format. Several new features have been added to appeal to students. The following pedagogical features are used:

- Learning objectives
- Key terms list (with terms highlighted in chapter)
- Tables that summarize key points
- Boxes to highlight interesting information
- Web exploration and links
- Notable quotes from distinguished persons

- Pictures/diagrams/drawings
- Original photographs
- Research highlights with application to practice
- Critical thinking exercises
- Personal reflection exercises
- Case studies with questions
- Resource lists
- References (including Web sites)
- Recommended readings
- Glossary

Students will be delighted to have a glossary at the end of the text, as well as definitions of key terms within the text. The competencies recommended by the AACN/Hartford Foundation are threaded throughout the book. Students will also benefit from new online resources and educational materials available for free from the publisher.

Instructors will find the accompanying online instructor's manual to be a time-saving tool. It is designed to provide a complete curriculum for instructors and students, even for those who may lack a strong geriatric background. The instructor's manual suggests activities for learning and in-class exercises, and provides PowerPoint slides for lectures that coincide with student readings in the main text. A test bank is also provided. Most of the work for development of a gerontological nursing course or integration in portions into the curriculum has already been done for instructors.

This book is divided into sections that directly follow the AACN/Hartford Foundation Institute's Competencies document *Recommended Baccalaureate Competencies and Curricular Guidelines for Geriatric Nursing Care.** The 30 competencies shown here are those necessary to provide high-quality care to older adults and their families:

1. Recognize one's own and others' attitudes, values, and expectations about aging and their impact on care of older adults and their families. (Section 1)
2. Adopt the concept of individualized care as the standard of practice with older adults. (Section 1)
3. Communicate effectively, respectfully, and compassionately with older adults and their families. (Section 2)
4. Recognize that sensation and perception in older adults are mediated by functional, physical, cognitive, psychological, and social changes common in old age. (Section 2)
5. Incorporate into daily practice valid and reliable tools to assess the functional, physical, cognitive, psychological, social, and spiritual status of older adults. (Section 3)
6. Assess older adults' living environment with special awareness of the functional, physical, cognitive, psychological, and social changes common in old age. (Section 3)
7. Analyze the effectiveness of community resources in assisting older adults and their families to retain personal goals, maximize function, maintain independence, and live in the least restrictive environment. (Section 3)
8. Assess family knowledge of skills necessary to deliver care to older adults. (Section 3)
9. Adapt technical skills to meet the functional, physical, cognitive, psychological, social, and endurance capacities of older adults. (Section 3)
10. Individualize care and prevent morbidity and mortality associated with the use of physical and chemical restraints in older adults. (Section 3)
11. Prevent or reduce common risk factors that contribute to functional decline, impaired quality of life, and excess disability in older adults. (Section 4)
12. Establish and follow standards of care to recognize and report elder mistreatment. (Section 4)
13. Apply evidence-based standards to screen, immunize, and promote healthy activities in older adults. (Section 4)

14. Recognize and manage geriatric syndromes common to older adults. (Section 5)
15. Recognize the complex interaction of acute and chronic comorbid conditions common to older adults. (Section 5)
16. Use technology to enhance older adults' function, independence, and safety. (Section 6)
17. Facilitate communication as older adults transition across and between home, hospital, and nursing home, with a particular focus on the use of technology. (Section 6)
18. Assist older adults, families, and caregivers to understand and balance "everyday" autonomy and safety decisions. (Section 7)
19. Apply ethical and legal principles to the complex issues that arise in care of older adults. (Section 7)
20. Appreciate the influence of attitudes, roles, language, culture, race, religion, gender, and lifestyle on how families and assistive personnel provide long-term care to older adults. (Section 8)
21. Evaluate differing international models of geriatric care. (Section 9)
22. Analyze the impact of an aging society on the health care system. (Section 9)
23. Evaluate the influence of payer systems on access, availability, and affordability of health care for older adults. (Section 9)
24. Contrast the opportunities and constraints of supportive living arrangements on the function and independence of older adults and on their families. (Section 9)
25. Recognize the benefits of interdisciplinary team participation in care of older adults. (Section 10)
26. Evaluate the utility of complementary and integrative health care practices on health promotion and symptom management for older adults. (Section 10)
27. Facilitate older adults' active participation in all aspects of their own health care. (Section 11)
28. Involve, educate, and when appropriate, supervise family, friends, and assistive personnel in implementing best practices for older adults. (Section 11)
29. Ensure quality of care commensurate with older adults' vulnerability and frequency and intensity of care needs. (Section 11)
30. Promote the desirability of quality end-of-life care for older adults, including pain and symptom management, as essential, desirable, and integral components of nursing practice. (Section 12)

By using this text and the instructor's manual as a curricular guide, instructors should be able to ensure that nursing students will meet the essential competencies that are recommended for excellent care of older adults.

*From the AACN/John A. Hartford Foundation Institute. (2000). *Recommended baccalaureate competencies and curricular guidelines for geriatric nursing care*. New York: Author, pp. 3–4.

Acknowledgments

Many people contributed their time, expertise and support to see this work finished. Thank you especially to the chapter authors and reviewers for their invaluable contributions and commitment to gerontological nursing. Rachel Shuster from Jones and Bartlett was of great assistance in preparation of the manuscript, and a special thanks must be said to all the others from Jones and Bartlett who believed in this text from its inception and did an outstanding job of marketing the first edition. My deepest thanks to my colleagues in the College of Nursing at Valparaiso University who have continuously supported the integration of gerontological nursing into our curriculum—their tireless commitment to excellence is an inspiration to me. The continued international leadership of Norman Volk through the Hartford Foundation and his forward-thinking vision of the place that nursing will hold in the care of older adults, as well as Mathy Mezey's pioneering and lifelong efforts to promote gerontological nursing have guided the direction of the profession and been a source of encouragement throughout my career. Lastly, my deepest appreciation goes to my husband and children for their patience while this project was completed.

FOREWORD

With the overwhelming majority of patients in hospitals, home care, and nursing homes made up of people age 65 or over, care of older adults is clearly the "core business" of our health care system. The recently released (2008) Institute of Medicine (IOM) report *Retooling for an Aging America* underscores both the aging imperative and the need for a health workforce capable of delivering competent care to older adults.

Baccalaureate nursing education has led nursing in assuring a nurse workforce prepared to care for older adults. Major strides have been made in curriculum revisions to incorporate geriatric content and in the development of faculty prepared in geriatrics. Yet, despite substantial progress, much remains to be done. In 2003, only one-third of baccalaureate nursing programs had a required stand-alone course in geriatrics, and, although almost all programs indicated that they integrated geriatrics into the curriculum, the degree of integration was quite limited (Berman et al., 2005).

In 2000, the American Association of Colleges of Nursing (AACN) took a major step to ensure the infusion of gerontological nursing into the curriculum of baccalaureate nursing programs. In collaboration with the Hartford Foundation Institute for Geriatric Nursing at New York University, AACN developed the document *Older Adults: Recommended Baccalaureate Competencies and Curricular Guidelines for Geriatric Nursing Care*. Developed to parallel AACN's document *The Essentials of Baccalaureate Education for Professional Nursing Practice* (1998), the geriatric competencies provide baccalaureate nursing programs with a framework of how to structure curricula in order to ensure competencies in care of older adults for their graduates.

This second edition of *Gerontological Nursing: Competencies for Care* expands on its original intent to take the AACN gerontological competencies to the next logical step. As was the case in the first edition, it continues to provide faculty with a text and an instructor's manual to foster curricular implementation. The second edition, however, includes new content focused on interdisciplinary education and on healthy aging, topics highlighted in the IOM report.

Such a text is critical because in most baccalaureate programs there continues to be at best only one faculty member prepared in gerontological nursing. The unique approach adopted by this text can help gerontological nursing faculty transmit essential information to other faculty, thus helping to imbed the gerontological competencies throughout the curriculum. It also provides the structure for curriculum development and course content for those schools seeking to create free-standing required or elective courses in gerontological nursing.

Mathy Mezey, EdD, RN, FAAN
Professor and Director
The Hartford Institute for Geriatric Nursing
College of Nursing
New York University

References

Berman, A., Mezey, M., Kobayashi, M., Fulmer, T., Stanley, J., & Rosenfeld, P. (2005). Gerontological nursing content in baccalaureate nursing programs: Comparison of findings from 1997 and 2003. *Journal of Professional Nursing, 21*(5), 268–275.

Institute of Medicine. (2008). *Retooling for an aging America*. Washington, DC: National Academies Press.

Contributors

Patricia A. Areán, PhD
UCSF Department of Psychiatry
San Francisco, California

Liat Ayalon, PhD
Senior Lecturer
School of Social Work
Bar Ilan University, Israel

Teresa Cervantez Thompson, PhD, RN, CRRN-A
Dean and Professor
College of Nursing and Health
Madonna University
Livonia, Michigan

Creaque V. Charles, PharmD, CGP
Pharmacy Clinical Practice Specialist
Department of Geriatric Services
University of Texas Medical Branch
Galveston, Texas

Deborah Conley, MSN, APRN-CNS-BC, FNGNA
Gerontological Clinical Nurse Specialist
Nebraska Methodist Hospital
Assistant Professor of Nursing
Nebraska Methodist College
Omaha, Nebraska

Claudia M. Diebold, RN, MSN, CNE
College of Nursing
University of Kentucky

Deborah Dunn, EdD(c), MSN, GNP-BC, ACNS-BC
Associate Professor
College of Nursing and Health
Madonna University
Livonia, Michigan

Frances Fanning-Hardin, RN, MSN
Lecturer
College of Nursing
University of Kentucky

Leilani Feliciano, PhD
Clinical Psychology Fellow
Department of Psychiatry
University of California, San Francisco

Dawna S. Fish, RN, BSN, COS-C
Quality Assurance Supervisor
Great Lakes Home Health and Hospice
Jackson, Michigan

Sheila Grossman, PhD, FNP, APRN-BC
Professor and Director
Family Nurse Practitioner Program
School of Nursing
Fairfield University
Fairfield, Connecticut

Lorna Guse, PhD, RN
Associate Professor
Faculty of Nursing
University of Manitoba
Winnipeg, Manitoba, Canada

David Haber, PhD
Professor
Ball State University
Muncie, Indiana

Jennifer Hamrick-King, PhDc
Graduate Student
Graduate Center for Gerontology
College of Public Health
University of Kentucky
Lexington, Kentucky

Patricia Hanson, PhD, APRN, GNP
Professor
College of Nursing and Health
Madonna University
Livonia, Michigan

Sonya R. Hardin, PhD, RN, CCRN, ACNS-BC
Associate Professor
School of Nursing
University of North Carolina at Charlotte

Janice M. Heineman, PhD
Senior Research Associate
Institute for the Future of Aging Services
American Association of Homes and Services for the Aging
Washington, D.C.

Donald D. Kautz, PhD, RN, CNRN, CRRN-A
Assistant Professor of Nursing
University of North Carolina at Greensboro

Luana S. Krieger-Blake, MSW, LCSW
Social Worker
Hospice of Porter County
Visiting Nurse Association
Valparaiso, Indiana

Jean Lange, PhD, RN, CNL
Associate Professor
Fairfield University School of Nursing
Fairfield, Connecticut

Cheryl A. Lehman, PhD, RN, CRRN-A, BC
Associate Professor/Clinical
University of Texas Health Science Center
School of Nursing
San Antonio, Texas

Pamela A. Masters-Farrell, MSN, RN, CRRN
Clinical Educator-Rehabilitation
Rehab ClassWorks, LLC
Salt Lake City, Utah

James M. Mauk, BS, ChFC, CASL
President, Mauk Financial Solutions, LLC
Valparaiso, Indiana

Kristen L. Mauk, PhD, RN, CRRN-A, GCNS-BC
Professor of Nursing
Kreft Endowed Chair
Valparaiso University
Health Care Consultant
Mauk Financial Solutions, LLC
Valparaiso, Indiana

Joan Nelson, RN, MS, DNP
Assistant Professor
University of Colorado Denver
College of Nursing
Denver, Colorado

Carole A. Pepa, PhD, RN
Professor of Nursing
Valparaiso University
Valparaiso, Indiana

Linda L. Pierce, PhD, RN, CNS, CRRN, FAHA
Professor
College of Nursing
Medical University of Ohio

Andrea Poindexter, RN, MSN, APRN
Geriatric Nurse Practitioner
Department of Geriatric Services
University of Texas Medical Branch
Galveston, Texas

Beth Scaglione Sewell, PhD
Associate Professor
Valparaiso, Indiana

Christine E. Schwartzkopf, MSN, RN, CRRN
Nursing Instructor
Dayton VAMC
Dayton, Ohio

Jeanne St. Pierre, MN, RN, GCNS-BC
Gerontological Clinical Nurse Specialist
Ball Memorial Hospital
Muncie, Indiana

Victoria Steiner, PhD
Assistant Professor
College of Medicine
Medical University of Ohio at Toledo

Kathleen Stevens, PhD, RN, CRRN
Director of Nursing Education
Rehabilitation Institute of Chicago
Assistant Professor
Northwestern University, Feinberg School of Medicine
Chicago, Illinois

Marilyn Ter Maat, MSN, CRRN-A, NEA, BC, FNGNA
Rehabilitation Nurse Consultant
Windcrest, Texas

Prudence Twigg, PhDc, RN, ANP-BC, GNP-BC
Visiting Lecturer
Department of Family Health
Indiana University School of Nursing at Indianapolis
Gerontological Nurse Practitioner
Advanced Healthcare Associates
Indianapolis, Indiana

Ramesh C. Upadhyaya, RN, MSN, MBA, CRRN
University of North Carolina at Greensboro
Greensboro, North Carolina

Patricia Warring, RN, MSN, ACHPN
Clinical Nurse Specialist
VNA of Porter County
Valparaiso, Indiana

Contributors to the First Edition

I would also like to thank these contributors to the first edition whose fine work was built upon for the second edition.

Jennifer Cowley, RN, MSN
Norma G. Cuellar, DSN, RN, CCRN
Jan Coleman Gross, PhD, ARNP-C

Unit One

Core Knowledge

SECTION

1

CRITICAL THINKING
(Competencies 1, 2)

CHAPTER 1

Introduction to Gerontological Nursing

Jeanne St. Pierre, MN, RN, GCNS-BC
Deborah Conley, MSN, APRN-CNS-BC, FNGNA

LEARNING OBJECTIVES

At the end of this chapter, the reader will be able to:

- Define important terms related to nursing and the aging process.
- Outline significant landmarks that have influenced the development of gerontological nursing as a specialty.
- Identify several subfields of gerontological nursing.
- Develop the beginnings of a personal philosophy of aging.
- Describe the unique roles of the gerontological nurse.
- Discuss the scope and standards of practice in gerontological nursing.
- Examine core competencies in gerontological nursing.
- Contrast various settings in which nurses care for older adults.
- Distinguish the educational preparation, practice roles, and certification requirements of the various levels of gerontological nursing practice.

KEY TERMS

- Activities of daily living (ADLs)
- Ageism
- Assisted living facility
- Certification
- Continuing care retirement community
- Core competencies
- Financial gerontology
- Geriatrics
- Gerontological nursing
- Gerontological rehabilitation nursing
- Gerontology
- Geropharmacology
- Geropsychology
- Hospice
- Independent living
- Middle old
- Old old
- Rehabilitation
- Skilled care
- Social gerontology
- Subacute care
- Unlicensed assistive personnel (UAP)
- Young old

THE HISTORY OF GERONTOLOGICAL NURSING

The history and development of gerontological nursing is rich in diversity and experiences, as is the population it serves. There has never been a more opportune time than now to be a gerontological nurse. No matter where nurses practice, they will at some time in their career care for older adults. The health care movement is constantly increasing life expectancy; therefore, nurses must expect to care for relatively larger numbers of older people over the next decades. With the increasing numbers of acute and chronic health conditions experienced by elders, nurses are in key positions to provide disease prevention and health promotion, and to promote positive aging.

The *American Journal of Nursing,* the American Nurses Association (ANA), and the John A. Hartford Foundation Institute for Geriatric Nursing at New York University contributed significantly to the development of the specialty of gerontological nursing. The specialty was formally recognized in the early 1960s when the ANA recommended a specialty group for geriatric nurses and the formation of a geriatric nursing division, and convened the first national nursing meeting on geriatric nursing practice. The growth of the specialty soared over the next three decades. In the early 1970s, the ANA *Standards for Geriatric Practice* and the *Journal of Gerontological Nursing* were first published (in 1970 and 1975, respectively). Following the enactment of federal programs such as Medicare and Medicaid, rapid growth in the health care industry for elders occurred. In the 1970s, the Veterans Administration funded a number of Geriatric Research Education and Clinical Centers (GRECCs) at VA medical centers across the United States. Nurses were provided substantial educational opportunities to learn about the care of older veterans through the development of GRECCs. The Kellogg Foundation also funded numerous certificate nurse practitioner programs at colleges of nursing for nurses to become geriatric nurse practitioners. These were not master's in nursing–level programs, but provided needed nurses who were trained in geriatrics to meet the growing needs of an aging population.

Terminology used to describe nurses caring for elders has included geriatric nurses, gerontic nurses, and gerontological nurses. These terms all have various meanings; however, *gerontological nursing* provides an encompassing view of the care of older adults. In 1976, the ANA Geriatric Nursing Division changed its name to Gerontological Nursing Division and published the *Standards of Gerontological Nursing* (Ebersole & Touhy, 2006; Meiner & Lueckenotte, 2006).

The decade of the 1980s saw a substantial growth in gerontological nursing when the National Gerontological Nursing Association was established, along with the ANA statement on the *Scope and Standards of Gerontological Nursing Practice.* Increased numbers of nurses began to obtain master's and doctoral preparation in gerontology, and higher education established programs to prepare nurses as advanced practice nurses in the field (geriatric nurse practitioners and gerontological clinical nurse specialists). Thus, interest in theory to build nursing as a science grew and nurses were beginning to consider gerontological nursing research as an area of study. Implementation of five Robert Wood Johnson (RWJ) Foundation Teaching-Nursing Homes provided the opportunity for nursing faculty and nursing homes to collaborate to enhance care to institutionalized elders. An additional eight community-based RWJ grant–funded demonstration projects enabled older adults to remain in their homes and fostered cooperation between social service and health care agencies to partner in providing in-home care.

In the 1990s, the John A. Hartford Foundation Institute for Geriatric Nursing was established at the NYU Division of Nursing. It provided unprecedented momentum to improve nursing education and practice and increase nursing research in the care of older adults. In addition, it focused on geriatric public policy and consumer education. The Nurses Improving Care for Healthsystem Elders (NICHE) program gained a national reputation as the model of acute care for older adults.

The 21st century has provided a resurgency in gerontological care, as older adults are gaining full status and recognition by society. As the baby boomers enter the older age group in 2011, this cadre of individuals will not only expect but demand excellence in geriatric care. In 2003, the collaborative efforts of the John A. Hartford Institute for Geriatric Nursing, the American Academy of Nursing, and the American Association of Colleges of Nursing (AACN) led to the development of the Hartford Geriatric Nursing Initiative (HGNI). This initiative substantially increased the number of gerontological nurse scientists and the development of evidence-based gerontological nursing practice. Today, there are multiple professional journals, books, Web sites, and organizations dedicated to the nursing care of older adults. One of the newest journals to emerge in 2008 was the *Journal of Gerontological Nursing Research*.

The development of gerontological nursing as a specialty is attributed to a host of nursing pioneers. The majority of these nurses were from the United States; however, two key trailblazers were from England. Florence Nightingale and Doreen Norton provided early insights into the "care of the aged." Nightingale was truly the first geriatric nurse, because she accepted the nurse superintendent position in an English institution comparable to our current nursing homes. She cared for wealthy women's maids and helpers in an institution called the Care of Sick Gentlewomen in Distressed Circumstances (Wykle & McDonald, 1997). Doreen Norton summarized her thoughts on geriatric nursing in a 1956 speech at the annual conference of the Student Nurses Association in London. She later focused her career on care of the aged and wrote often about the unique and specific needs of elders and the nurses caring for them. She identified the advantages of learning geriatric care in basic nursing education as: 1) learning patience, tolerance, understanding, and basic nursing skills; 2) witnessing the terminal stages of disease and the importance of skilled nursing care at that time; 3) preparing for the future, because no matter where one works in nursing the aged will be a great part of the care; 4) recognizing the importance of appropriate **rehabilitation**, which calls upon all the skill that nurses possess; and 5) being aware of the need to undertake research in geriatric nursing (Norton, 1956).

LANDMARKS IN THE DEVELOPMENT OF GERONTOLOGICAL NURSING

Nurse scientists, educators, authors, and clinicians forged the way for the overall development of gerontological nursing as we know it today. Some of the most notable pioneers were Irene Burnside, Sister Rose Theresa Barr, Virginia Stone, Lucille Gress, Laurie Gunter, Doris Schwartz, Eleanor Pingrey, Terri Brower, Thelma Wells, Pricilla Ebersole, Patricia Hess, Mary Opal Wolanin, Cynthia Kelly, Florence Cellar, Neville Strumpf, Bernita Steffl, Edna Stilwell, Charlotte Eliopoulos, Lois Evans, Mathy Mezey, Terry Fulmer, Jeannie Kyser-Jones, Cornelia Beck, Meridean Maas, Kathleen Buckwalter, and Anne Leukenotte.

The following is a summary of significant landmarks in the development of gerontological nursing as a specialty:

1902 *American Journal of Nursing (AJN)* publishes first geriatric article by an MD

1904 *AJN* publishes first geriatric article by an RN

1925 *AJN* considers geriatric nursing as a potential specialty

Anonymous column entitled "Care of the Aged" appears in *AJN*

1950 First geriatric nursing textbook, *Geriatric Nursing* (Newton), published

First master's thesis in geriatric nursing completed by Eleanor Pingrey

Geriatrics becomes a specialization in nursing

1952 First geriatric nursing study published in *Nursing Research*

1961 ANA recommends specialty group for geriatric nurses

1962 ANA holds first National Nursing Meeting on Geriatric Nursing Practice

1966 ANA forms a geriatric nursing division

First Gerontological Clinical Nurse Specialist master's program begins at Duke University

1968 First RN (Gunter) presents at the International Congress of Gerontology

1970 ANA creates the *Standards of Practice for Geriatric Nursing*

1973 ANA offers the first generalist **certification** in gerontological nursing (74 nurses certified)

1975 First nursing journal for the care of older adults published: *Journal of Gerontological Nursing* by Slack, Inc.

First nursing conference held at the International Congress of Gerontology

1976 ANA Geriatric Nursing Division changes name to Gerontological Nursing Division

ANA publishes *Standards of Gerontological Nursing*

1977 Kellogg Foundation funds Geriatric Nurse Practitioner certificate education

First gerontological nursing track funded by the Division of Nursing at the University of Kansas

1979 First national conference on gerontological nursing sponsored by the *Journal of Gerontological Nursing*

1980 *AJN* publishes *Geriatric Nursing* journal

Education for Gerontic Nurses by Gunter and Estes suggests curricula for all levels of nursing education

ANA establishes Council of Long Term Care Nurses

1980 First Robert Wood Johnson (RWJ) Foundation grants for health-impaired elders given (eight in the United States)

1981 First International Conference on Gerontological Nursing sponsored by the International Council of Nursing (Los Angeles, California)

ANA Division of Gerontological Nursing publishes statement on scope of practice

John A. Hartford Foundation's Hospital Outcomes Program for the Elderly (HOPE) using a geriatric resource nurse (GRN) model developed at Yale University under the direction of Terry Fulmer

1982 Development of RWJF Teaching-Nursing Home Program (five programs in the United States)

1983 First endowed university chair in gerontological nursing (Florence Cellar Endowed Gerontological Nursing Chair) established at Case Western Reserve University

1984 National Gerontological Nursing Association (NGNA) established

ANA Division on Gerontological Nursing Practice becomes Council on Gerontological Nursing

1986 National Association for Directors of Nursing Administration in Long Term Care established

ANA publishes *Survey of Gerontological Nurses in Clinical Practice*

1987 ANA revises *Standards and Scope of Gerontological Nursing Practice*

1988 First PhD program in gerontological nursing established (Case Western Reserve University)

1989 ANA certification established for Clinical Specialist in Gerontological Nursing

1990 ANA establishes Division of Long Term Care within the Council of Gerontological Nursing

1992 Nurses Improving Care for Healthsystem Elders (NICHE) established at New York University (NYU) Division of Nursing based on the HOPE programs

1996 John A. Hartford Foundation Institute for Geriatric Nursing established at NYU Division of Nursing

NICHE administered through the John A. Hartford Foundation Institute for Geriatric Nursing

1998 ANA certification available for geriatric advanced practice nurses as geriatric nurse practitioners or gerontological clinical nurse specialists

2000 American Academy of Nursing, the John A. Hartford Foundation, and the NYU Division of Nursing develop the Building Academic Geriatric Nursing Capacity (BAGNC) program

2002 American Nurses Foundation (ANF) and ANA fund the Nurse Competence in Aging (NCA) joint venture with the John A. Hartford Foundation Institute for Geriatric Nursing

2003 The John A. Hartford Foundation Institute for Geriatric Nursing, the American Academy of Nursing, and the American Association of Colleges of Nursing (AACN) combine efforts to develop the Hartford Geriatric Nursing Initiative (HGNI)

John A. Hartford Foundation Institute for Geriatric Nursing at NYU awards Specialty Nursing Association Programs-in Geriatrics (SNAP-G) grants

2004 American Nurses Credentialing Center's *first* computerized generalist certification exam is for the gerontological nurse

2005 *Journal of Gerontological Nursing* celebrates 30 years

2007 NICHE program at John A. Hartford Foundation Institute for Geriatric Nursing at NYU receives additional funding from the Atlantic Philanthropies and U.S. Aging Program

2008 *Geriatric Nursing* journal celebrates 30 years

Journal of Gerontological Nursing Research emerges

ATTITUDES TOWARD AGING AND OLDER ADULTS

As a nursing student, you may have preconceived ideas about caring for older adults. Such ideas are influenced by your observations of family members, friends, neighbors, and the media, and your own experience with older adults. Perhaps you have a close relationship with your grandparents or you have noticed the aging of your own parents. For some of you, the aging process may have become noticeable when you look at yourself in the mirror. But for all of us, this universal phenomenon we call aging has some type of meaning, whether or not we have taken the time to consciously think about it.

The way you view aging and older adults is often a product of your environment and the experiences to which you have been exposed. Negative attitudes toward aging or older adults (**ageism**) often arise in the same way—from negative past experiences. Many of our attitudes and ideas about older adults may not be grounded in fact. Some of you may have already been exposed to ageism, which is often displayed in much the same way as sexism or racism—via attitudes and actions. This is one reason for studying the aging process—to examine the myths and realities, to separate fact from fiction, and to gain an appreciation for what older adults have to offer.

Population statistics show that the majority of your careers as nurses will include caring for older adults. As Mathy Mezey, director of the John A. Hartford Foundation Institute for Geriatric Nursing at NYU, stated, "The population of older Americans is exploding. Geriatric patients are not one subgroup of patients but rather the core business of health systems" (Mezey, 2005). Providing high-quality care to elders requires knowledge of the intricacies of the aging process as well as the unique syndromes and disease conditions that can accompany growing older.

As you read and study this book, you are encouraged to examine your own thoughts, values, feelings, and attitudes about growing older. Perhaps you already have a positive attitude toward caring for older adults. Build on that value, and consider devoting your time and efforts to the practice of gerontological nursing. If, however, you are reading this chapter with the idea that gerontological nursing is a less desirable field of nursing, or that only those nurses who cannot find jobs elsewhere work in nursing homes, or that working with older people would be an option of last resort, then you may need to re-examine these feelings. Armed with the facts and some positive experiences with older adults, you may change your mind.

Advocates for older adults, such as Nobel laureate Elie Wiesel, feel that older adults, as repositories of our collective memories, should be appreciated and respected. As the 1997 American Psychological Association's keynote convention speaker, Wiesel said, ". . . an old person represents wisdom and the promise of living a full life . . . the worst curse is to make him or her feel worthless" (American Psychological Association, 2008).

The older population is changing dramatically as the baby boomers (those born from 1946–1964) reach retirement age (as of 2011). Because this phenomenon is happening in many places around the globe (see Chapters 2 and 23), gerontology is the place to be! Caring for the largest number of older adults in history will present enormous opportunities. With the over-85 age group being the fastest growing, the complexity of caring for so many people with multiple physical and psychosocial changes will present a challenge for the most daring of nurses. Will you be ready?

The purpose of this book is to provide the essential information needed by students of gerontological nursing to provide quality care to older adults. In your study of this text, you will be presented with knowledge and insights from experienced professionals with expertise in various areas of gerontological nursing and geriatrics. Each chapter contains thought-provoking activities and questions for personal reflection. Case studies will help you to think about and apply the information. A glossary is included at the end of the chapter to help you master key terms, and plenty of tables and figures summarize key information. Web sites are included as a means of expanding your knowledge. Use this text as a guidebook for your study. Use all the resources available, including your instructors, to immerse yourself in the study of the aging process. By the end of this book, you will have learned about the essential competencies needed to provide excellent care to older adults.

DEFINITIONS

Gerontology is the broad term used to define the study of aging and/or the aged. This includes the biopsychosocial aspects of aging. Under the umbrella of gerontology are several subfields including geriatrics, social gerontology, geropsychology, geropharmacology, financial gerontology, gerontological nursing, and gerontological rehabilitation nursing, to name a few.

What is old and who defines old age? Interestingly, although "old" is often defined as over 65 years of age, this is an arbitrary number set by the

Social Security Administration. Today, the older age group is often divided into the **young old** (ages 65–74), the **middle old** (ages 75–84), and the **old old**, very old, or frail elderly (ages 85 and up). However, these numbers merely provide a guideline and do not actually define the various strata of the aging population. Among individuals, vast differences exist between biological and chronological aging, and between the physical, emotional, and social aspects of aging. How and at what rate a person ages depends upon a host of factors that will be discussed throughout this book. The aging population as well as theories and concepts related to aging are discussed further in Chapters 2 and 3.

Geriatrics is often used as a generic term relating to the aged, but specifically refers to medical care of the aged. For this reason, many nursing journals and texts have chosen to use the term *gerontological nursing* instead of geriatric nursing.

Social gerontology is concerned mainly with the social aspects of aging versus the biological or psychological. "Social gerontologists not only draw on research from all the social sciences—sociology, psychology, economics, and political science—they also seek to understand how the biological processes of aging influence the social aspects of aging" (Quadagno, 2005, p. 4). **Geropsychology** is a branch of psychology concerned with helping older persons and their families maintain wellbeing, overcome problems, and achieve maximum potential during later life. **Geropharmacology** is the study of pharmacology as it relates to older adults. The credential for a pharmacist certified in geropharmacology is CGP (certified geriatric pharmacist).

Financial gerontology is another emerging subfield that combines knowledge of financial planning and services with a special expertise in the needs of older adults. Cutler (2004) defines financial gerontology as "the intellectual intersection of two fields, gerontology and finance, each of which has practitioner and academic components" (p. 29). This field is further discussed in Chapter 25.

Gerontological rehabilitation nursing combines expertise in gerontological nursing with rehabilitation concepts and practice. Nurses working in gerontological rehabilitation often care for older adults with chronic illnesses and long-term functional limitations such as stroke, head injury, multiple sclerosis, Parkinson's disease, spinal cord injury, arthritis, joint replacements, and amputations. The purpose of gerontological rehabilitation nursing is to assist older adults to regain and maintain the highest level of function and independence possible while preventing complications and enhancing quality of life.

Gerontological nursing, then, falls within the discipline of nursing and the scope of nursing practice. It involves nurses advocating for the health of older persons at all levels of prevention. Gerontological nurses work with healthy elderly persons in their communities, acutely ill elders requiring hospitalization and treatment, and chronically ill or disabled elders in long-term care facilities, skilled care, home care, and hospice. The scope of practice for gerontological nursing includes all older adults from the time of "old age" until death. Gerontological nursing is guided by standards of practice that will be discussed later in this chapter. Several roles of the gerontological nurse will be discussed in the following sections.

ROLES OF THE GERONTOLOGICAL NURSE

Provider of Care

In the role of caregiver or provider of care, the gerontological nurse gives direct, hands-on care to older adults in a variety of settings. Older adults often present with atypical symptoms that complicate diagnosis and treatment. Thus, the nurse as a care provider should be educated about disease processes and syndromes commonly seen in the older population (see **Case Study 1-1**). This may include knowledge of risk factors, signs and symptoms, usual medical treatment, rehabilitation, and end-of-life care. Chapters 13, 14, and 15 cover management of common illnesses, diseases, and health conditions, imparting essential information for providing quality care.

Teacher

An essential part of all nursing is teaching. Gerontological nurses focus their teaching on modifiable risk factors and health promotion (see Chapters 9, 11, and 12). Many diseases and debilitating conditions of aging can be prevented through lifestyle

Case Study 1-1

Rose is a 52-year-old nursing student who has returned to school for her BSN after raising a family. She is the divorced mother of two grown children and has one young grandson. In addition to being a full-time student in an accelerated program, Rose also cares for her 85-year-old mother in her own home and occasionally helps provide childcare for her grandson while his parents work. Rose's mother has diabetes and is legally blind. Rose is taking a gerontology course this semester and finds herself going home quite upset after the first week of classes when attitudes toward aging were discussed. While sharing with the course instructor her feelings and surprising emotional discomfort, Rose is helped to identify that she is afraid of getting older and being unable to care for her ailing mother and herself. As a single woman, she is unsure that she can handle what lies ahead for her as she is beginning to feel the effects of aging herself.

Questions:

1. What can Rose do to become more comfortable with facing her own advancing age?
2. What factors may have influenced her discomfort with the course material?
3. Is there anything the instructor of the course might do to help Rose cope with the feelings she is having as she completes the required coursework?
4. There may be some activities that Rose can do in order to understand her feelings about aging better. Can you think of some such activities?
5. What is Rose's role as the caregiver in this situation? How may the role change over time?
6. How much does Rose's present home and living situation contribute to her fears and perceptions of aging?

modifications such as a healthy diet, smoking cessation, appropriate weight maintenance, increased physical activity, and stress management. Nurses have a responsibility to educate the older adult population about ways to decrease the risk of certain disorders such as heart disease, cancer, and stroke, the leading causes of death for this group. Nurses also may develop expertise in specialized areas and teach skills to other nurses in order to promote quality patient care among older adults.

Manager

Gerontological nurses act as managers during everyday practice as they balance the concerns of the patient, family, nursing, and the rest of the interdisciplinary team. Nurse managers must be skilled in leadership, time management, building relationships, communication, and managing change. Nurse managers may supervise other nursing personnel including licensed practical nurses (LPNs), certified nursing assistants (CNAs), technicians, nursing students, and other **unlicensed assistive personnel (UAP)**. The role of the gerontological nurse as manager and leader is further discussed in Chapter 23.

Advocate

As an advocate, the gerontological nurse acts on behalf of older adults to promote their best interests and strengthen their autonomy and decision making. Advocacy may take many forms, including active involvement at the political level or helping to explain medical or nursing procedures to family members on a unit level. Nurses may also advocate for patients through other activities such as helping family members choose the best nursing home for their loved one or listening to family members vent their frustrations about health problems encountered. Whatever the situation, gerontological nurses must remember that being an advocate does not mean making decisions for older adults, but empowering them to remain independent and retain dignity, even in difficult situations.

Research Consumer

The appropriate level of involvement for nurses at the baccalaureate level is that of research consumer. Gerontological nurses must remain abreast of current research literature, reading and putting into practice the results of reliable and valid studies. Using evidence-based practice, gerontological nurses can improve the quality of patient care in all settings. Although nurses with undergraduate degrees may be involved in research in some facilities, such as assisting with data collection or providing research ideas inspired by clinical problems, their basic preparation is aimed primarily at using research in practice. All nurses should read professional journals specific to their specialty and continue their education by attending seminars and workshops, participating in professional organizations, pursuing additional formal education or degrees, and obtaining certification. In being a research consumer, gerontological nurses can improve the quality of patient care in all settings.

Expanded roles of the gerontological nurse may also include counselor, case manager, coordinator of services, collaborator, geriatric care manager, and others. Several of these roles are discussed in Chapters 20, 23, and 25.

CERTIFICATION

To provide competent, current care to elders, nurses need to have gerontological nursing content in their basic undergraduate nursing curricula and are encouraged to become certified in gerontological nursing. Less than 1% of nurses in the United States are certified in gerontological nursing; however, more than 50% of the patients cared for are elders. Adults age 65 or older utilize 48–50% of the nation's total health care resources and represent approximately 38% of all admissions to hospitals (Stierle et al., 2006). Patients and their families are knowledgeable about quality health care and patient safety and want the most expert clinicians at the bedside. Certification provides reassurance to patients and their families that the nurses caring for them are highly skilled and possess expert knowledge in providing excellence in gerontological nursing care (Hartford Institute for Geriatric Nursing, 2008).

Nurse certification is a formal process by which a certifying agency validates a nurse's knowledge, skills, and competencies through a written examination in a specialty area of practice. There are two levels of certification: generalist and advanced practice level. Each has different eligibility standards. The American Nurses Credentialing Center (ANCC) is the certifying body for both levels of gerontological nursing practice.

Generalist Certification

The generalist in gerontological nursing has completed a basic entry-level program in nursing, which can be a diploma in nursing, or an associate or bachelor of science degree in nursing. Before meeting additional eligibility requirements to become certified in gerontological nursing, the applicant must be a licensed registered nurse for at least 2 years. ANCC offers the generalist computerized exam in gerontological nursing at over 300 computer-based testing sites across the country. This exam was the first one to become computerized, increasing the convenience of sitting for gerontological nursing certification.

Certified gerontological nurses utilize principles of gerontological nursing and gerontological competencies as they implement the nursing process with patients. Gerontological certified nurses:

- Assess, manage, and deliver health care that meets the needs of older adults
- Evaluate the effectiveness of their care
- Identify the strengths and limitations of their patients
- Maximize patient independence
- Involve patients and family members (American Nurses Credentialing Center [ANCC], 2008)

There are a number of compelling reasons for nurses to pursue gerontological nurse certification. Certified gerontological nurses:

- Experience a high degree of professional accomplishment and satisfaction
- Demonstrate a commitment to their profession
- Provide higher quality of care to older adults
- Act as resources for other nurses and interdisciplinary team members
- Demonstrate evidence-based gerontological nursing care
- Are recognized as national leaders in gerontological nursing care
- Create the potential for higher salaries and benefits
- Are actively recruited for employment at nursing faculty, in Magnet and NICHE designated hospitals, in long-term care facilities, in acute rehab, and in community health agencies (ANCC, 2008; Hartford Institute for Geriatric Nursing, 2008)

See the ANCC Web site (http://www.nursecredentialing.org) for eligibility requirements and information about gerontological nurse certification and recertification.

Advanced Certification

The ANCC offers two separate advanced practice certification exams in gerontological nursing: the clinical specialist in gerontological nursing (GCNS-BC) and the gerontological nurse practitioner (GNP-BC). There are different eligibility requirements for each exam. The ANCC Web site (http://www.nursecredentialing.org) provides eligibility requirements and information on certification and recertification. As with most certifications, minimum educational and practice requirements must be met and maintained. Both certifications are considered to signify expert clinicians; those certified must hold a minimum of a master's degree in nursing, which includes at least 500 hours of precepted clinical practice. Recertification mandates retaking the exam or submitting a portfolio that demonstrates that the candidate has met specific requirements.

Many states require advanced practice registered nurses (APRNs) to hold a separate license as an APRN. The advanced practice role encompasses education, consultation, research, case management, administration, and advocacy in the care of older adults. In addition, APRNs develop advanced knowledge of nursing theory, research, and clinical practice. The APRN is an expert in providing care for older adults, families, and groups in a variety of settings.

The gerontological clinical nurse specialist focuses on three spheres of influence: patient/family care, developing nurses, and impacting organizations and systems. Gerontological clinical nurse specialists (CNSs) play important roles in acute care by developing and implementing gerontological nursing evidence-based practice. In addition, some roles involve a collaborative practice or consultative role with hospitals or long-term care facilities and interdisciplinary teams. In some states, gerontological CNSs may obtain prescriptive authority and broaden their scope of practice. Gerontological CNSs have developed and managed clinics for common conditions in the older population such as incontinence, falls, wounds, or cognitive impairments. The ANCC describes the role of the gerontological CNS as follows:

> *The Clinical Nurse Specialist in Gerontological Nursing (GCNS) is a registered nurse prepared in a graduate level gerontological clinical nurse specialist program to provide advanced care for older adults, their families, and significant others. The GCNS has an expert understanding of the dynamics, pathophysiology, and psychosocial aspects of aging. The GCNS uses advanced diagnostic and assessment skills and nursing interventions to manage and improve patient care. Using theory and research, the GCNS's practice considers all influences on a patient's health status and the related psychosocial and behavioral problems arising from the patient's altered physiological condition. The GCNS practices in diverse settings and is actively engaged in education (e.g., patient, staff, students, and colleagues), case management, expert clinical practice, consultation, research, and administration. (ANCC, 2008)*

The gerontological nurse practitioner (GNP) practices in acute or long-term care settings and in collaborative practice with physicians who maintain large geriatric practices. GNPs make regular visits to nursing homes where patients in their collaborative practice reside. GNPs practice in rehabilitation facilities, working in outpatient clinics for rehabilitation patients after discharge or with specialty

TABLE 1-1 Web Sites for Test Content Outlines

http://www.nursecredentialing.org/NurseSpecialties/Gerontological.aspx
http://www.nursecredentialing.org/NurseSpecialties/GerontologicalCNS.aspx
http://www.nursecredentialing.org/NurseSpecialties/GerontologicalNP.aspx

BOX 1-1 Web Exploration

Explore the following Web sites for further information on certification and gerontological associations of interest to nurses.

Educational Web Sites

Hartford Geriatric Nursing Initiative, About HGNI
www.gerontologicalnursing.info

Hartford Geriatric Nursing Initiative, ConsultGeriRN.org
www.consultgeriRN.com

American Nurses Association (ANA)
www.nursingworld.org

Associations

U.S. Administration on Aging
www.aoa.dhhs.gov

American Geriatrics Society
www.americangeriatrics.org

American Nurses Credentialing Center (ANCC)
www.nursecredentialing.org

Gerontological Society of America
www.geron.org

Hospice and Palliative Nurses Association (HPNA)
www.hpna.org

John A. Hartford Foundation Institute for Geriatric Nursing
www.hartfordign.org

National Adult Day Services Association
www.nadsa.org

National Association of Geriatric Nursing Assistants (NAGNA)
www.culturechangenow.com/stories/nagna.html

National Association of Professional Geriatric Care Managers
www.caremanager.org

National Council on the Aging
www.ncoa.org/

National Gerontological Nursing Association
www.ngna.org

National Institute on Aging
www.nia.nih.gov

physicians, managing caseloads, and diagnosing and treating geriatric syndromes. The ANCC describes the role of the gerontological nurse practitioner as follows:

> *The Gerontological Nurse Practitioner (GNP) is a registered nurse prepared in a graduate level gerontological nurse practitioner program to provide a full range of health care services on the wellness-illness health care continuum at an advanced level to older adults. The GNP practice includes independent and interdependent decision making, and is directly accountable for clinical judgments. The graduate level preparation expands the GNP's role to include differential diagnosis and disease management, participation in and use of research, development and implementation of health policy, leadership, education, case management, and consultation. (ANCC, 2008, p. 1)*

SCOPE AND STANDARDS OF PRACTICE

The scope of nursing practice is defined by state regulation, but is also influenced by the unique needs of the population being served in a given setting. The needs of older adults are complex and multifaceted, and the focus of nursing care depends on the setting in which the nurse practices.

Gerontological nursing is practiced in accordance with standards developed by the profession of nursing. In 2001, the ANA Division of Gerontological Nursing Practice developed the second edition of the *Scope and Standards of Gerontological Nursing*

BOX 1-2 Additional Resources

American Nurses Credentialing Center (ANCC)
P.O. Box 791333
Baltimore, MD 21279-1333
202-651-7000
800-284-2378
www.nursecredentialing.com

John A. Hartford Foundation
55 East 59th Street
16th Floor
New York, NY 10022-1178
212-832-7788
E-mail: mail@jhartfound.org
www.hartfordign.org
www.jhartfound.org

Geriatric Nursing Review Syllabus: A Core Curriculum in Advanced Practice Geriatric Nursing (GNRS) (2003–2005)
Available from the American Geriatrics Society
1-800-334-1429 ext. 2529

Practice, in collaboration with the National Gerontological Nursing Association, the National Association of Directors of Nursing Administrators in Long Term Care, and the National Conference of Gerontological Nurse Practitioners. Standards are provided both for clinical care and for the professional role of the nurse. These standards include assessment, diagnosis, outcome identification, planning, implementation, and evaluation. The standards of professional gerontological nursing performance include quality of care, performance appraisals, education, collegiality, ethics, collaboration, research, and research utilization. Students should note that these are the basic standards for professional nursing, but here they are applied to the care of the older adult. Core competencies, discussed in the next section, provide specific guidelines for gerontological nursing care. A full description and copy of the scope and standards is available at www.nursingworld.org or www.ngna.org.

CORE COMPETENCIES

Specific **core competencies** have been identified for gerontological nursing in addition to general professional nursing preparation. These competencies are influenced by the level at which the nurse will function and the role expectations of the nurse. Core competencies provide a foundation of added knowledge and skills necessary for the nurse to implement in daily practice. For example, the gerontological nurse in advanced practice has expanded expertise and skills to fulfill specialized roles. Common bodies of assumptions, knowledge, skills, and attitudes that are essential for excellent clinical nursing practice with older adults have been developed and provide the basic foundation for all levels of gerontological nursing practice.

The American Association of Colleges of Nursing (AACN) and the John A. Hartford Foundation Institute for Geriatric Nursing gathered input from qualified gerontological nursing experts to publish *Older Adults: Recommended Baccalaureate Competencies and Curricular Guidelines for Geriatric Nursing Care* (2000). This document also provided the framework for this text. The core competencies set forth for gerontological nursing appear in **Table 1-2**. The purpose of this document specific to gerontological nursing was to use the AACN's *Essentials of Baccalaureate Education for Professional Nursing Practice* (1998) as a framework to help nurse educators integrate specific nursing content into their programs. The original AACN document suggested core competencies, knowledge, and role development for professional nurses. These appear in **Table 1-3**. The geriatric competencies in Table 1-2 correlate with and were derived from the suggestions in the more general AACN document in Table 1-3. By using these published documents as guides, nursing professors and others who educate in the area of gerontological nursing should be able to prepare students to be competent to provide excellent care to older adults.

CONTINUUM OF CARE

Gerontological nurses practice in a multitude of settings. Adults over age 65 comprise 48% of patients

TABLE 1-2 Competencies Necessary for Nurses to Provide High-Quality Care to Older Adults and Their Families

1. Recognize one's own and others' attitudes, values, and expectations about aging and their impact on care of older adults and their families.
2. Adopt the concept of individualized care as the standard of practice with older adults.
3. Communicate effectively, respectfully, and compassionately with older adults and their families.
4. Recognize that sensation and perception in older adults are mediated by functional, physical, cognitive, psychological, and social changes common in old age.
5. Incorporate into daily practice valid and reliable tools to assess the functional, physical, cognitive, psychological, social, and spiritual status of older adults.
6. Assess older adults' living environment with special awareness of the functional, physical, cognitive, psychological, and social changes common in old age.
7. Analyze the effectiveness of community resources in assisting older adults and their families to retain personal goals, maximize function, maintain independence, and live in the least restrictive environment.
8. Assess family knowledge of skills necessary to deliver care to older adults.
9. Adapt technical skills to meet the functional, physical, cognitive, psychological, social, and endurance capacities of older adults.
10. Individualize care and prevent morbidity and mortality associated with the use of physical and chemical restraints in older adults.
11. Prevent or reduce common risk factors that contribute to functional decline, impaired quality of life, and excess disability in older adults.
12. Establish and follow standards of care to recognize and report elder mistreatment.
13. Apply evidence-based standards to screen, immunize, and promote healthy activities in older adults.
14. Recognize and manage geriatric syndromes common to older adults.
15. Recognize the complex interaction of acute and chronic co-morbid conditions common to older adults.
16. Use technology to enhance older adults' function, independence, and safety.
17. Facilitate communication as older adults transition across and between home, hospital, and nursing home, with a particular focus on the use of technology.
18. Assist older adults, families, and caregivers to understand and balance "everyday" autonomy and safety decisions.
19. Apply ethical and legal principles to the complex issues that arise in care of older adults.
20. Appreciate the influence of attitudes, roles, language, culture, race, religion, gender, and lifestyle on how families and assistive personnel provide long-term care to older adults.
21. Evaluate differing international models of geriatric care.
22. Analyze the impact of an aging society on the health care system.
23. Evaluate the influence of payer systems on access, availability, and affordability of health care for older adults.
24. Contrast the opportunities and constraints of a supportive living arrangement on the function and independence of older adults and on their families.
25. Recognize the benefits of interdisciplinary team participation in care of older adults.
26. Evaluate the utility of complementary and integrative health care practices on health promotion and symptom management for older adults.
27. Facilitate older adults' active participation in all aspects of their own health care.

(continues)

TABLE 1-2 (continued)

28. Involve, educate, and when appropriate, supervise family, friends, and assistive personnel in implementing best practices for older adults.
29. Ensure quality of care commensurate with older adults' vulnerability and frequency and intensity of care needs.
30. Promote the desirability of quality end-of-life care for older adults, including pain and symptom management, as essential, desirable, and integral components of nursing practice.

SOURCE: American Association of Colleges of Nursing and the John A. Hartford Institute for Geriatric Nursing. (2000). *Older adults: Recommended baccalaureate competencies and curricular guidelines for geriatric nursing care*. Washington, DC: Author.

seen in the hospital, 80% of home care patients, and 90% of those in nursing homes (Mezey, 2005). A few of these settings will be discussed here. Some additional unique areas of employment are suggested in Chapter 23.

Because of the nature of the aging process, it is likely that older adults will enter and exit the health care system at many different points throughout old age. **Figure 1-1** presents the web of health care that often occurs when older adults enter the system due to illness or accident.

Settings of care can be described and titled in a variety of ways. Following is a brief description of some of the most common settings of care, employing commonly used nomenclature.

Acute Care Hospital

The acute care hospital is often the point of entry into the health care system for older adults. Nurses working in hospitals are likely to care for older adults even if they do not specialize in geriatrics, because about half of all patients in this setting are 65 years of age or older. In this setting, gerontological nurses focus on nursing care of acute problems, often involving exacerbations of cardiopulmonary conditions, cancer treatment, and orthopedic problems. All nursing units (with the exception of labor and delivery, postpartum, and pediatrics) in acute care hospitals admit older adults, so nurses may encounter elderly patients in critical care or rehabilitative services or anywhere in between. The goal of inpatient care will be to promote recovery and prevent complications.

Acute Rehabilitation

Rehabilitation may be found in various degrees in several settings, including the acute care hospital,

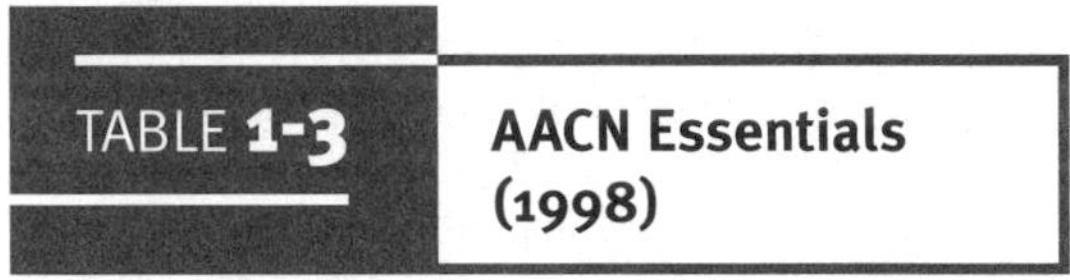

TABLE 1-3 AACN Essentials (1998)

Core Competencies
Critical thinking
Communication
Assessment
Technical skills

Core Knowledge
Health promotion, risk reduction, and disease prevention
Illness and disease management
Information and health care technologies
Ethics
Human diversity
Global health care
Health care systems and policy

Role Development
Provider of care
Designer/manager/coordinator of care
Member of a profession

SOURCE: American Association of Colleges of Nursing. (1998). *Essentials of baccalaureate education for professional nursing practice*. Washington, DC: Author.

FIGURE 1-1 The "web" of health care for older adults.

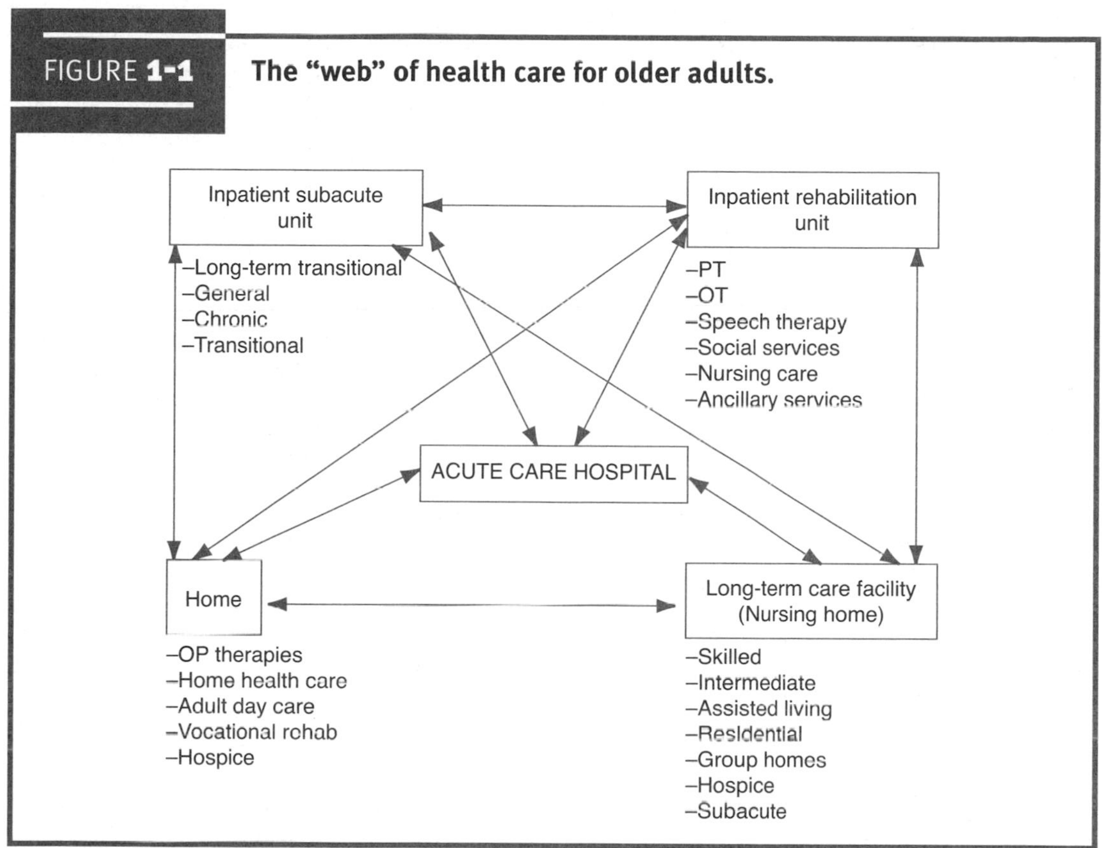

SOURCE: Easton, K. L., 1999, Gerontological Rehabilitation Nursing, p. 14. Philadelphia: W.B. Saunders. Used with permission.

subacute care or transitional care, and long-term care facilities (LTCFs). Regardless of the setting, rehabilitation is accomplished through the work of an interdisciplinary team that includes nurses, therapists, and physicians as well as other professional staff. The goals of rehabilitation are to maximize independence, promote maximal function, prevent complications, and promote quality of life within each person's strengths and limitations.

The level of intensity of acute rehabilitation is greater than for subacute or long-term care. For older adults to qualify for rehabilitation in the acute care hospital, they must be able to tolerate at least 3 hours of therapy per day. The interdisciplinary team will work together to set up mutually established goals with the patient. Inpatient rehabilitation in the acute setting is beneficial to help persons recovering from or adapting to such conditions as stroke, head trauma, neurological diseases, amputation, orthopedic surgery, and spinal cord injury.

Home Health Care

Independent-living older adults requiring a longer period of observation or care from nurses may be candidates for home health care services. Home health care is designed for those who are homebound due to severity of illness or immobility. Visiting nurse associations (VNAs) have long been known for their positive reputation in providing home health care. For reimbursement of allowable expenses, home health care services must be ordered by a physician and the person must be considered homebound. There has been record growth in the number of home health agencies in the past decade. People's desire to be cared for in familiar surroundings by their families, versus an institution, has fueled the need for more agencies.

Although physical, occupational, and speech therapies may be obtained through home care, as well as home health aide services, a nurse must open the case file and the individual must warrant some type of nursing services to qualify. The majority of home health care patients are elderly with a variety of nursing needs, such as wound care, intravenous therapy, management of newly diagnosed diabetes, and tube feedings.

Long-Term Care Facility

Traditionally referred to as nursing homes, long-term care facilities (LTCFs) provide support to persons of any age who have lost some or all of their capacity for self-care due to illness, disability, or dementia. Though not acutely ill, residents of LTCFs, like hospitalized patients, require 24-hour nursing care (SeniorHousingNet, 2008).

Registered nurses working in long-term care provide care planning and oversight of numerous residents, often directing and coordinating the care via licensed practical nurses and certified nursing assistants or other unlicensed assistive personnel (UAP). Nurses working in long-term care will be challenged to maintain the functional and nutritional status of residents, while preventing complications of impaired mobility such as pressure ulcers and falls. Dementia care is often a substantial part of the nursing care provided, as is managing residents' health conditions and medication regimens. Long-term care facilities often house specialty care units such as skilled nursing units and Alzheimer's care units, described in the next section.

Skilled Nursing Facilities

Skilled nursing facilities (SNFs), sometimes called subacute or transitional care, are for those patients requiring more intensive nursing care than provided in long-term care and are usually found as specially designated units within long-term care facilities or occasionally within hospitals (SeniorOutlook.com, 2008). SNF patients are often transferred from the hospital to continue their recovery from an acute episode and often require continued therapy (physical, occupational, and/or speech). Frequent patient assessments are needed for a limited time period for stabilization or completion of a treatment regimen. "Typical individuals seen in subacute care are those needing assistance as a result of non-healing wounds, chronic ventilator dependence, renal problems, intravenous therapy, and coma management and those with complex medical and/or rehabilitative needs, including pediatrics, orthopedics, and neurological. These units are designed to promote optimum outcomes in the least expensive cost setting" (Easton, 1999, p. 15).

Good assessment and communication skills are needed to care for these complex patients. The skilled care nurse should have knowledge of transfer techniques, prevention and assessment of swallowing problems, bowel and bladder management, and nutrition. The gerontological nurse working in skilled care must have expertise in preventing the hazards of immobility such as pressure ulcers and contractures. Gerontological nurses working in this setting would benefit from having a critical care background and rehabilitation experience as well.

Alzheimer's Care

A growing trend in LTCFs is to offer dedicated units for the care of persons with Alzheimer's disease and other dementing illnesses. Because of the high rate of Alzheimer's with advanced age, there is a growing need for units that provide nursing care for elders in the various stages of dementia. Often, family members can care for their loved ones at home during the early stages. However, due to impaired judgment that may pose safety issues, during middle and late stage dementia the older adult cannot be left alone. As memory loss progresses, home caregivers often feel overwhelmed and unable to provide the required care.

The goal of dementia care is to preserve the functional status of the demented person via supportive care that fosters self-worth and socialization even within the context of diminishing cognitive capacity. Alzheimer's units can be a great benefit to the community by having gerontological nursing staff with expertise in the management of this challenging disease. Nurses can help family members understand disease progression and assure them that their loved one is being well cared for even to the end of this ultimately fatal disease.

Hospice

Gerontological nurses may also choose to work in **hospice**, caring for dying persons and their families. Although many patients in hospice are not elderly, the majority of the dying are older. The concept of hospice is centered on holistic, interdisciplinary care that helps the dying person "live until they die." (See Chapter 24 for further discussion.) A number of team members who specialize in thanatology and palliative care work together to provide quality care for patients in their last months, weeks, days, and hours of life. Pain management and comfort care are the standards upon which treatment is based. Nurses and physicians work closely with social workers, chaplains, psychologists, and other hospice professionals to make death as comfortable and as easy a transition as possible.

Hospice care is found in a variety of facilities. Some hospices are stand-alone organizations with their own building. Home care often offers hospice, and certain nursing homes will offer a hospice unit or care within the skilled unit or from an outside hospice nurse. Clinical nurse specialists provide a great service as expert clinicians and consultants to the hospice team. Whatever the setting, hospice requires a great deal of patience, expertise, understanding, interdisciplinary communication, and compassion on the part of the gerontological nurse.

Respite Care

Caregiving for a dependent older adult can be a demanding task. Caregivers often need a break from caregiving to relieve stress and prevent burnout. Respite care provides time off for family members who care for someone who is ill, injured, frail, or demented. Respite care can be provided in an adult daycare center, in the home of the person being cared for, or in an **assisted living facility** or long-term care facility. Although there are different approaches to respite care, all have the same basic objective: to provide caregivers with temporary, intermittent, substitute care, allowing for relief from the daily responsibilities of caregiving.

Respite care is not covered by Medicaid or Medicare, but may be covered by long-term care insurance policies or by local social service agencies, with fees based on a sliding scale of financial need.

Continuing Care Retirement Community (CCRC)

Also referred to as a life care community, a **continuing care retirement community** (CCRC) provides a continuum of care from **independent living** to **skilled care** (the latter consisting of care typically provided by traditional nursing homes), all within a single campus, with levels of care adjusted to individual needs. Depending on the facility's contract, additional services are provided for an additional fee or are included in a lump-sum upfront payment. Older adults can move seamlessly among independent living, assisted living, skilled care, or long-term care as their conditions warrant. Some CCRCs include independent and assisted living, but provide home health services within the facility instead of moving the resident to a skilled unit. Nurses play a role in the care of CCRC residents as they progress from independent living to requiring skilled nursing care, but gerontological nurses may also function in the area of health promotion to help older adults maintain independence for as long as possible.

Assisted Living

As older persons continue to age, it is likely that common disorders associated with the aging process may interfere with their ability to care for themselves. Assisted living facilities (ALFs), a burgeoning option for older adults, provide an alternative for those older adults who do not feel safe living alone, who wish to live in a community setting, or who need some additional help with **activities of daily living (ADLs)**. The ALF may be connected with a long-term facility or care network, or may be free-standing. For those units that are part of a larger facility, residents who find themselves in need of greater assistance may then progress to the next level of care. The drawback of a free-standing facility is that older adults whose condition worsens and who need greater assistance may need to pay extra for that assistance, depending on the terms of their contract. Some may even need to find an alternate facility that provides a higher level of care than that provided by their ALF.

The typical resident in an assisted living facility has a private room or apartment (with a variety of designs available for different costs). All rooms will have some type of kitchen or kitchenette and private bathroom with shower. The rest of the space includes a bed or bedroom, living area, and closet space. Older adults who enter an ALF often sell their homes and plan to spend as long as possible living with minimal assistance.

Assisted living facilities generally provide healthy meals, planned activities, places to walk and exercise, and pleasant surroundings where adults can socialize with others in a safe and protected environment. Walking paths, aviaries, workout rooms, beauty salons, community gathering rooms, chapels, and game rooms are part of many assisted living facilities.

Foster Care or Group Homes

Foster care and/or group homes are for those older adults who can do most of their ADLs, but may have safety issues and require supervision with some activities such as dressing or taking medications. Foster or group homes generally offer more personalized supervision in a smaller, more family-like environment than a traditional nursing home and, depending on state regulations, may be licensed to provide such services. Some persons offering this service have a small number of elders inside their existing home, whereas others have purchased a larger dwelling for this purpose (see

FIGURE 1-2 **Assisted living facilities aid older people with activities of daily living.**

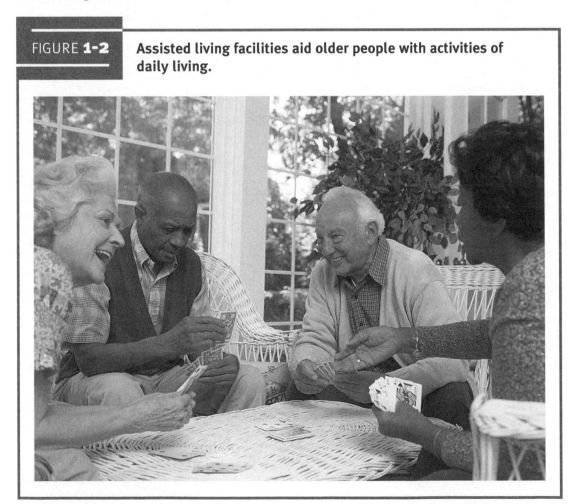

SOURCE: © Comstock Images/Alamy Images.

Figure 1-2). This type of setting provides an alternative to nursing home care for some older persons. Although nurses may own and operate a group home, there is no requirement that a person have a health care background to do so, nor is there a requirement that a nurse's services be available, so persons should take care to investigate the facility prior to placement of a loved one. Social workers can usually provide good information about local foster or group homes.

Green House Concept

Endorsed by the Centers for Medicare & Medicaid Services, the Green House model, as conceived by geriatrician Dr. William Thomas (Thomas, 2004), is becoming an increasingly popular alternative to traditional long-term care facilities. The first Green Houses were constructed in Tupelo, Mississippi, in 2003. Now that an intensive evaluation has documented their success, Thomas has teamed up with the Robert Wood Johnson Foundation to replace more than 100 nursing homes nationwide with clusters of small, cozy houses, each housing 8 to 10 residents in private rooms, with private bathrooms and an open kitchen.

The primary purpose of the model is to serve as a place where elders can receive assistance and support with activities of daily living and clinical care without that assistance becoming the focus of their existence. Caregivers in Green Houses are empowered to provide individualized care to older adults who retain control over daily activities, in short, creating an environment that is a home.

Adult Daycare

Adult daycare or day services provide another avenue for older adults who are unable to remain at home during the day without supervision. These services are often used by family members who are caring for older parents or loved ones in their own home, but who may work during the day and wish to have their relative safely cared for in their absence (see **Case Study 1-2**). This is an excellent alternative to institutionalization. "Adult day services are community-based group programs designed to meet the needs of functionally and/or cognitively impaired adults through an individual plan of care. These structured, comprehensive programs provide a variety of health, social, and other related support services in a protective setting

BOX 1-3 Research Highlight

Aim: This study described what caring meant for geriatric nurses.

Methods: Parse's phenomenology was used to survey 30 nurses in Taiwan who worked on medical-surgical units caring for older adults. The nurses were asked open-ended questions about the meaning of caring in providing care to the elderly.

Findings: The researcher concluded that, for geriatric nurses, the meaning of caring included several concepts: deliberation, concern, tolerance, sincerity, empathy, initiative, and dedication. The author suggests that caring for the elderly should be natural and not superficial in order for the elderly to feel cared for.

Application to practice. Geriatric nurses in this study demonstrated the meaning of caring in several distinct ways. Core moral and ethical values appeared in their descriptions of the meaning of caring for older adults. Nurses may improve their care of older adults by attending to these core concepts related to caring. Gerontological nursing education may benefit by including more about caring theory.

Source: Lui, Shwu Jiaun. (2004). What caring means to geriatric nurses. *Journal of Nursing Research, 12*(2), 143–152.

Case Study 1-2

The Brokowskis are a close-knit family of five whose grandfather, Papa B., has been living with them in their home since he was widowed 10 years prior. Papa B. is 88 years old and has recently been diagnosed with Alzheimer's disease in the early stage. The family is having increasing difficulty supervising Papa B. and feels it is no longer safe for him to be at home alone. Both parents in the family work, and the three children are in high school during the day. The family wishes to keep Papa B. at home, but do not know what possibilities there are in the community to help them.

Questions:

1. What services might the Brokowski family use to help them keep Papa B. at home? Do these services seem feasible at this time?
2. As Papa B.'s condition worsens with the progression of Alzheimer's disease, what other services discussed in this chapter might be necessary at various points in time?
3. What assessments would a nurse need to make in order to determine the best placement for Papa B.? Given the history of this family, what recommendations for the future might be made? Which interdisciplinary team member could provide additional information to the nurse and the family about community services?

during any part of a day, but less than 24-hour care" (National Adult Day Services Association, 2008).

Adult daycare programs may be sponsored by a variety of different organizations including churches, hospitals, health care systems, or the local YMCA. Centers provide socialization, planned outings, nutritional meals, and therapeutic activities that would appeal to older adults with moderate physical and/or mental decline. All functions are supervised by qualified personnel. Services are offered only during the day, often from 6 a.m. to 6 p.m. (or normal business hours) with an emphasis on recreation and some health promotion. Some programs offer weekend hours. Costs vary depending on the sponsoring agency.

SUMMARY

Gerontological nursing is a specialty practice that focuses on the unique needs of older adults and their families. It builds on the theories and foundations of nursing practice, with application of a growing body of literature generated by gerontological nursing scientists. Caring for older adults is influenced by many factors, one of which is recognizing one's own attitude about aging. It is important with the aging of today's population that all nurses should have basic gerontological nursing concepts and principles taught in their undergraduate programs. With the growth of the older population, more nurses specializing in gerontology will be needed. Gerontological nurses practice in almost all settings and there are emerging subfields of this specialty that offer promise of future roles for nurses who care for older adults. Nurses should explore the multiple career options in this exciting, creative, and innovative field of gerontological nursing.

Critical Thinking *Exercises*

1. Do this exercise with another student as a partner. Close your eyes. Picture yourself as an 85-year-old. Note your appearance, sights, sounds, and surroundings. Open your eyes and describe yourself at 85 to your partner. Then discuss how your mental image of yourself as an older person might have been influenced by your family history, grandparents, and perceptions about aging.
2. Go to a local card shop and browse. Look at the birthday cards that persons might buy for someone getting older. What do they say about society's attitudes toward aging? Do the cards you read point out any areas that we stereotype as problems with advancing age?
3. Complete this sentence: Older people are . . .
   List as many adjectives as you can think of. After making your list, identify how many are negative and how many are positive descriptors. Think about where your ideas came from as you did this exercise.
4. Check out the Web site at www.consultgerirn.org. How could you use this Web site to enhance your knowledge about the care of older adults? What services are available through the Web site?
5. Look at the list of competencies for gerontological nurses in Table 1-2. How many of these competencies do you feel you meet at this point? Make a conscious effort to develop these skills as you go through your career.
6. Visit a local nursing home that offers various levels of care. Call ahead of time to arrange a tour from a nurse and ask questions about the services they offer to older adults.

Personal **Reflections**

1. How do you feel about aging? Do you dread getting older, or look forward to it? Do you see advanced age as a challenge or something to fear?
2. Have you ever cared for an older adult? If so, what was that experience like? How do you feel about caring for older adults in your nursing practice?
3. What do you think about nurses who work in nursing homes? Have you ever considered a career in gerontology? What are the positives you can see about developing expertise in this field of nursing?
4. Have you ever seen ageism in practice? If so, think about that situation and how it could have been turned into a positive scenario. If not, how have the situations you have been in avoided discrimination against older adults?
5. Which of the settings for gerontological nursing practice appeal to you most at this time in your professional career? Is there any one setting that you can see yourself working in more than another? Do you think this will change as you progress in your career?

References

American Association of Colleges of Nursing. (1998). *The essentials of baccalaureate education for professional nursing practice.* Washington, DC: Author.

American Association of Colleges of Nursing & the John A. Hartford Foundation Institute for Geriatric Nursing. (2000). *Older adults: Recommended baccalaureate competencies and curricular guidelines for geriatric nursing care.* Washington, DC: Author.

American Nurses Association. (2001). *Scope and standards of gerontological nursing practice*. Washington, DC: American Nurses Publishing.

American Nurses Credentialing Center. (2008). *Clinical nurse specialist in gerontology*. Retrieved September 12, 2008, from http://www.nursecredentialing.org/Documents/Certification/Application/NursingSpecialty/GerontologicalCNS.aspx

American Psychological Association. (2008). *Why practitioners need information about working with older adults.* Retrieved July 3, 2008, from http://www.apa.org/pi/aging/practitioners/why.html

Cutler, N. E. (2004). Aging and finance 1991 to 2004. *Journal of Financial Service Professionals, 58*(1), 29–32.

Easton, K. L. (1999). *Gerontological rehabilitation nursing*. Philadelphia: WB Saunders.

Ebersole, P., & Touhy, T. (2006). *Geriatric nursing: Growth of a specialty*. New York: Springer.

Eliopoulos, C. (2005). *Gerontological nursing*. Philadelphia: Lippincott.

Hartford Institute for Geriatric Nursing. (2008). Retrieved May 9, 2008, from http://www.consultgerirn.org

Lui, S-J. (2004). What caring means to geriatric nurses. *Journal of Nursing Research, 12*(2), 143–152.

Meiner, S., & Lueckenotte, A. (2006). *Gerontologic nursing*. St. Louis, MO: Mosby.

Mezey, M. (2005). *About us.* Retrieved December 25, 2005 from http://www.geronurseonline.org

National Adult Day Services Association. (2008). Retrieved October 12, 2008, from http://www.nadsa.org/

Norton, D. (1956, July 6). The place of geriatric nursing in training. *Nursing Times*, 264.

Quadagno, J. (2005). *Understanding the older client*. Boston: McGraw-Hill.

SeniorHousingNet. (2008). *Finding senior housing and care*. Retrieved July 3, 2008, from http://www.seniorhousingnet.com/seniors

SeniorOutlook.com. (2008). *Glossary of senior housing terms*. Retrieved July 3, 2008, from http://www.senioroutlook.com/glossary.asp

Stierle, L. J., Mezey, M., Schumann, M. J., Esterson, J., Smolenski, M. C., Horsley, K. D., et al. (2006). Professional development. The Nurse Competence in Aging initiative: Encouraging expertise in the care of older adults. *American Journal of Nursing, 106*(9), 93–94, 96.

Thomas, W. (2004). *What are old people for? How elders will save the world.* Acton, MA: Vanderwyck & Burnham.

Wykle, M., & McDonald, P. (1997). The past, present and future of gerontological nursing. In Dimond M. et al. (Eds.), *A national agenda for geriatric education*. New York: Springer.

CHAPTER 2

The Aging Population

Cheryl A. Lehman, PhD, RN, CRRN-A
Andrea Poindexter, RN, MSN, APRN

LEARNING OBJECTIVES

At the end of this chapter, the reader will be able to:

- Review statistics related to aging in the United States.
- Describe social and economic issues related to aging in the United States.
- Discuss aging across different cultures.
- Recognize differences between aging in the 21st century and aging in the past.
- Critically evaluate successful aging.

KEY TERMS

- Baby boomers
- Centenarian
- Chronic disease
- Cohort
- Demographic tidal wave
- Elderly
- Foreign-born
- Graying of America
- Native-born
- Older adult
- Oldest old
- Pig in a python
- Seniors

U.S. society, and indeed, U.S. families, will be greatly challenged by the **graying of America** over the next few decades. A steadily growing aging population has the potential to affect social policy, societal resources, businesses, and communities, not to mention health care systems.

THE NUMBERS

About one in eight Americans is age 65 or older. This older population numbered 36.8 million in 2005, an increase of 3.2 million or 9.4% since 1995. In this same decade, 1995–2005, the number of Americans ages 45–64—who will reach 65 over the next two decades—increased by 40%. The 65 or over population will increase from 35 million in 2000 to 40 million in 2010 (a 15% increase) and then to 55 million in 2020 (a 36% increase for that decade). The **oldest old** (85+ years) is projected to increase from 4.2 million in 2000 to 6.1 million in 2010 (a 40% increase) and then to 7.3 million in 2020 (a 44% increase for that decade) (Administration on Aging, 2006a). By the mid-21st century, old people (those 65 or older) will outnumber young people for the first time in history (Winokur, 2005).

Why the Recent Increase in the Number of Older Adults?

The recent trend of increasing numbers of **older adults** in the United States is due to two main causes:

the increased life expectancy of our **seniors** and the fertility of the U.S. population at various points in time.

In 1935, when Social Security was enacted, the life expectancy for someone who was 65 years old was 12 years for males (or 77 years total) and 13 years for females (or 78 years total). This has risen to 16 and 19 years, respectively. By 2080, life expectancy for 65-year-olds is expected to have increased to 20 years and 23 years, respectively (Munnell, 2004). There is less of a racial difference in life expectancy than in other parameters of aging. In 2001, life expectancy at birth was 5.5 years higher for whites than for blacks, but at age 65, whites could expect to live for 2 years longer than blacks. For those who live to age 85, the life expectancy for black people is slightly higher than for whites (Federal Interagency Forum, 2004).

Changes in life expectancy throughout the 20th century were mainly due to improved sanitation, advances in medical care, and the implementation of preventive health services (Merck Institute of Aging and Health [MIAH], Centers for Disease Control and Prevention [CDC], & Gerontological Society of America [GSA], 2004). In the early 1900s, deaths were mostly due to infectious diseases and acute illnesses. The older population of today, however, must deal with challenges unfamiliar to their own parents. These are the challenges of dealing with **chronic disease** as well as funding for health care services. The average 75-year-old now has three chronic diseases and uses five prescription drugs (MIAH, CDC, & GSA, 2004). Modern treatments for diseases that used to kill older adults, such as myocardial infarction and stroke, as well as the improved technical procedures for health services such as transplants and intensive care, have contributed to the increased longevity of the population. Health care costs, including medication costs, have thus become a primary issue for many seniors. The repercussions of rising health care costs have been felt within the state and federal governments, as they seek to help support their senior citizens' health. Nearly 95% of health care expenditures for older Americans are for chronic diseases (MIAH, CDC, & GSA, 2004).

Fertility of the population also affects the number of older adults. The fertility rate in the United States has been steadily falling for the past 200 years. In 1800, the average woman had 7 children. By the end of World War II, this had decreased to 2.4 children. But after the war, from 1946 to 1964, the fertility rate increased to 3.5 children (Munnell, 2004). Of course, one could argue that some of these changes have less to do with fertility rate and more to do with the influence of other factors such as the acceptance and use of birth control as well as the changing values of different generations.

The growth of the older population slowed somewhat during the 1990s because of the relatively small number of babies born during the Great Depression of the 1930s. But the older population will explode between 2010 and 2030 when the **baby boomer** generation reaches age 65. This extremely large segment of the U.S. population, who were born between 1946 and 1964, will start turning 65 in 2011. This anticipated increase has been called both a **demographic tidal wave** (MIAH, CDC, & GSA, 2004) and a **pig in a python** (meaning a bulge in population moving slowly through time) (Munnell, 2004).

Beginning in 2012, nearly 10,000 Americans will turn 65 every day (MIAH, CDC, & GSA, 2004). By 2030, the older population will comprise 20% of the total population of the United States (which will be about 70 million people) (Federal Interagency Forum, 2004; MIAH, CDC, & GSA, 2004). This group of older adults will be the "healthiest, longest lived, best educated, most affluent in history" (Experience Corps, 2005). After 2030, the population of oldest old (those over 85 years) will grow the fastest. According to the Federal Interagency Forum (2004), the U.S. Census Bureau projects that the population of those 85 or older could grow from 4.2 million in 2000 to 21 million by 2050 (see **Figure 2-1**).

The Distribution of Seniors in the United States

The distribution of older Americans varies across the United States, due in part to patterns of migration after retirement. It is also due to birth and death rates in the various states and regions. In 2005, one-half of persons age 65 or older lived in nine states: California, Florida, New York, Illinois, Texas, Pennsylvania, Ohio, Michigan, and New Jersey. Persons 65+ constituted approximately 14% or more of the total population in eight states in 2005: Florida (16.8%), West Virginia (15.3%), Pennsylvania (15.2%), North Dakota (14.7%), Iowa (14.7%), Maine (14.6%), South Dakota (14.2%), and Rhode

FIGURE 2-1 Real and projected numbers of people 65+ in the United States, 1900–2050.

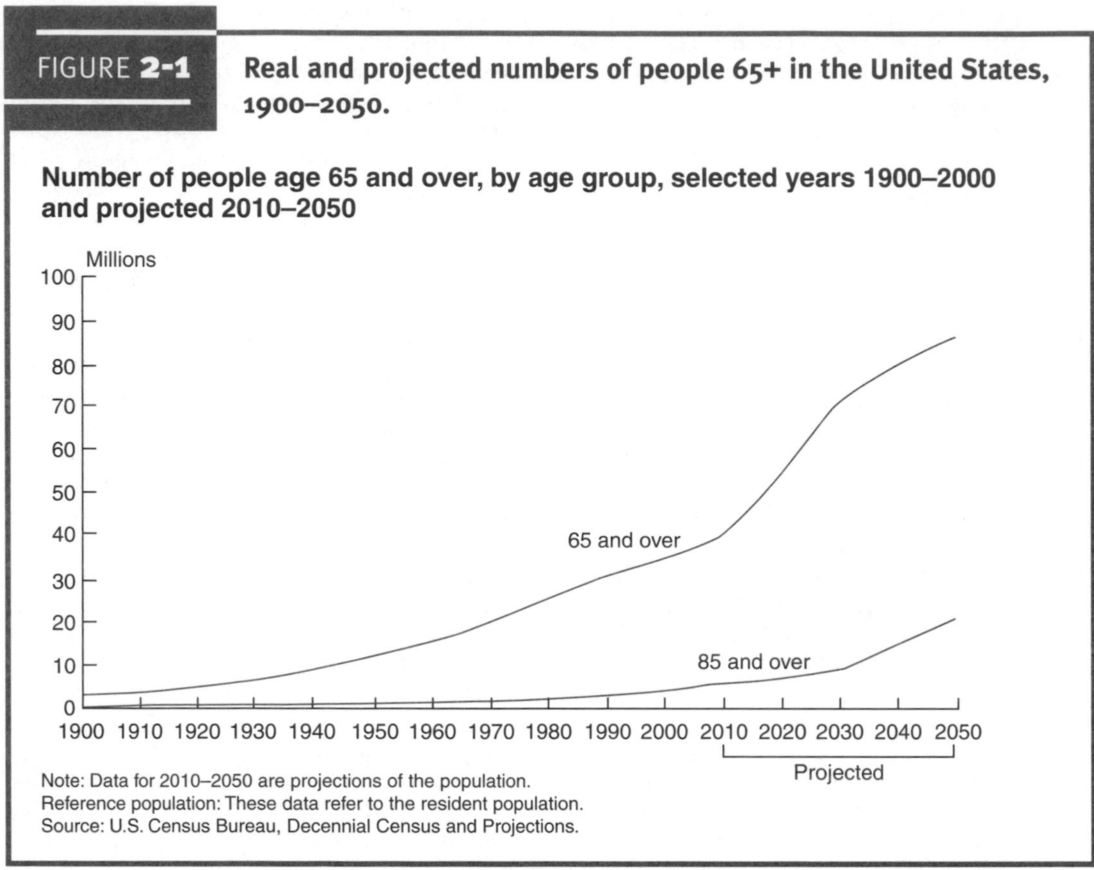

SOURCE: Federal Interagency Forum on Aging-Related Statistics. (May 2006). *Older Americans update 2006: Key indicators of well-being.* Washington, DC: U.S. Government Printing Office. Retrieved September 17, 2007, from http://www.agingstats.gov/Agingstatsdotnet/Main_Site/default.aspx

Island (13.9%). In 10 states, the 65+ population increased by 20% or more between 1995 and 2005: Nevada (56.6%), Alaska (47.5%), Arizona (31.4%), New Mexico (26.5%), Utah (24.1%), Colorado (23.3%), Delaware (22.9%), Idaho (22.8%), Georgia (20.8%), and South Carolina (20.6%). Most persons 65+ lived in metropolitan areas in 2005 (79.8%). About 50% of older persons lived in the suburbs, 29% lived in central cities, and 20% lived in nonmetropolitan areas (Administration on Aging, 2006a).

The **elderly** are less likely to change residence than other age groups. From 2004 to 2005 only 4.2% of older persons moved as opposed to 13.4% of the under-65 population. Most older movers (51.6%) stayed in the same county and 72.1% remained in the same state. Only 25.5% of the movers moved out of state (Administration on Aging, 2006a).

Issues of Gender

Women outnumber men in the United States, a trend that is expected to continue. In 2005, there were 21.4 million older women in the United States, compared to 15.4 million older men. This is a ratio of 139 women for every 100 men. The female to male sex ratio increases with age. For the age group 65–69, it is 115:100; for those 85+ it is 218:100 (with more than two females for every male). In 2003, a 65-year-old female could be expected to have an additional 19.8 years of life expectancy; for males it was 16.8 years (Administration on Aging, 2006a).

In 2005, 72% of older men were married, compared to 42% of women. Only 36.4% of women ages 75–84 were married; this dropped to 15.1% in the 85 or older age group. For men 85 or older, 58.3% were married. Four times as many women as men were widowed (8.6 million women; 2.1 million men). Divorce is more unusual in this age group. In 2005, 10% of older men and 11% of older women were divorced. A smaller proportion of older adults had never been married (Administration on Aging, 2006a).

Education

Level of education can affect the socioeconomic status of the older adult. **Figure 2-2** shows sources of income for groups of older adults. Those with more education tend to have more money, higher standards of living, and above-average health. The comparisons over the years are interesting. In 1950, 17% of the older adults in the United States had

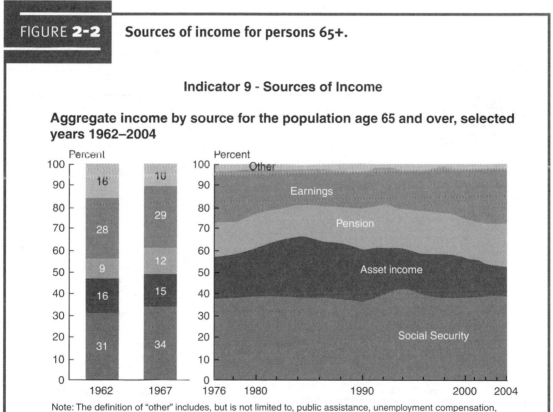

FIGURE **2-2** **Sources of income for persons 65+.**

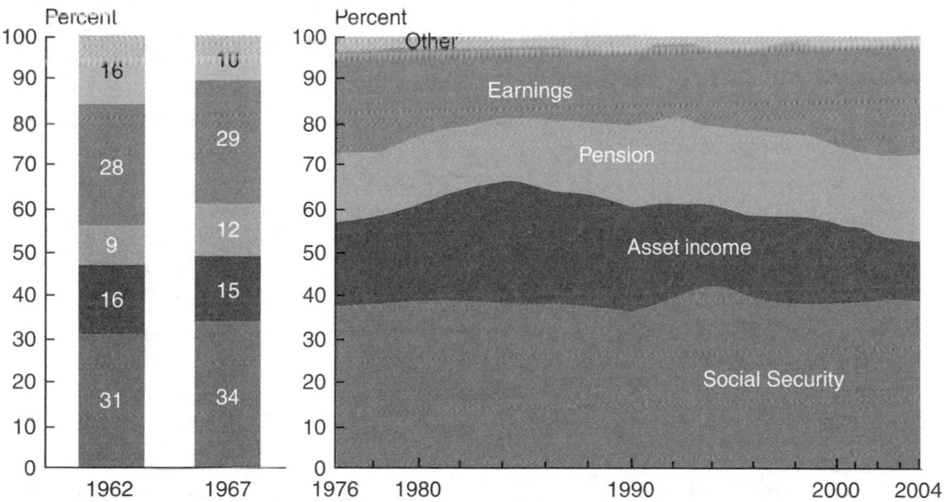

Note: The definition of "other" includes, but is not limited to, public assistance, unemployment compensation, workers' compensation, alimony, child support, and personal contributions.

Reference population: These data refer to the civilian noninstitutionalized population.

Source: Social Security Administration, 1963 Survey of the Aged, 1968 Survey of Demographic and Economic Characteristics of the Aged; U.S. Census Bureau, Current Population Survey, Annual Social and Economic Supplement, 1976–2004.

SOURCE: Federal Interagency Forum on Aging-Related Statistics. (May 2006). *Older Americans update 2006: Key indicators of well-being.* Washington, DC: U.S. Government Printing Office. Retrieved September 17, 2007, from http://www.agingstats.gov/Agingstatsdotnet/Main_Site/default.aspx

graduated from high school, and 3% had at least a bachelor's degree. In 2005, however, 74% of older adults had graduated from high school, while 19% of older adults had at least a bachelor's degree. Differences also exist in education between ethnic groups. In 2005, 79% of older non-Hispanic whites, 66% of older Asians, 54% of older blacks, and 40% of older Hispanics had completed high school (Administration on Aging, 2006a; Federal Interagency Forum, 2004).

Living Arrangements

Living arrangements of older adults are linked not only to income, but also to health status. Older people who live alone are more likely than their married counterparts to live in poverty. Over half of noninstitutionalized older adults lived with their spouse in 2005. In that year, older men were more likely to be living with a spouse than were older women (71.7% compared to 42%; see **Figure 2-3** for statistics through 2004). Only 30.2% of women age 75 or older lived with a spouse. Older women were twice as likely as older men to be living alone (38.4% compared to 19.2%). The likelihood of living alone increases with age: among women age 75 or older, 47.7% lived alone in 2005.

A total of about 1.57 million older adults lived in households with a child present in the house in 2005. Nearly one-half million of these were grandparents over 65 years of age with the primary responsibility for their grandchildren who lived with them (Administration on Aging, 2006a).

Although only a small percentage (4.5%) of older adults resided in nursing homes in 2000, the

FIGURE 2-3 Population 65 and over living alone, 1970–2004.

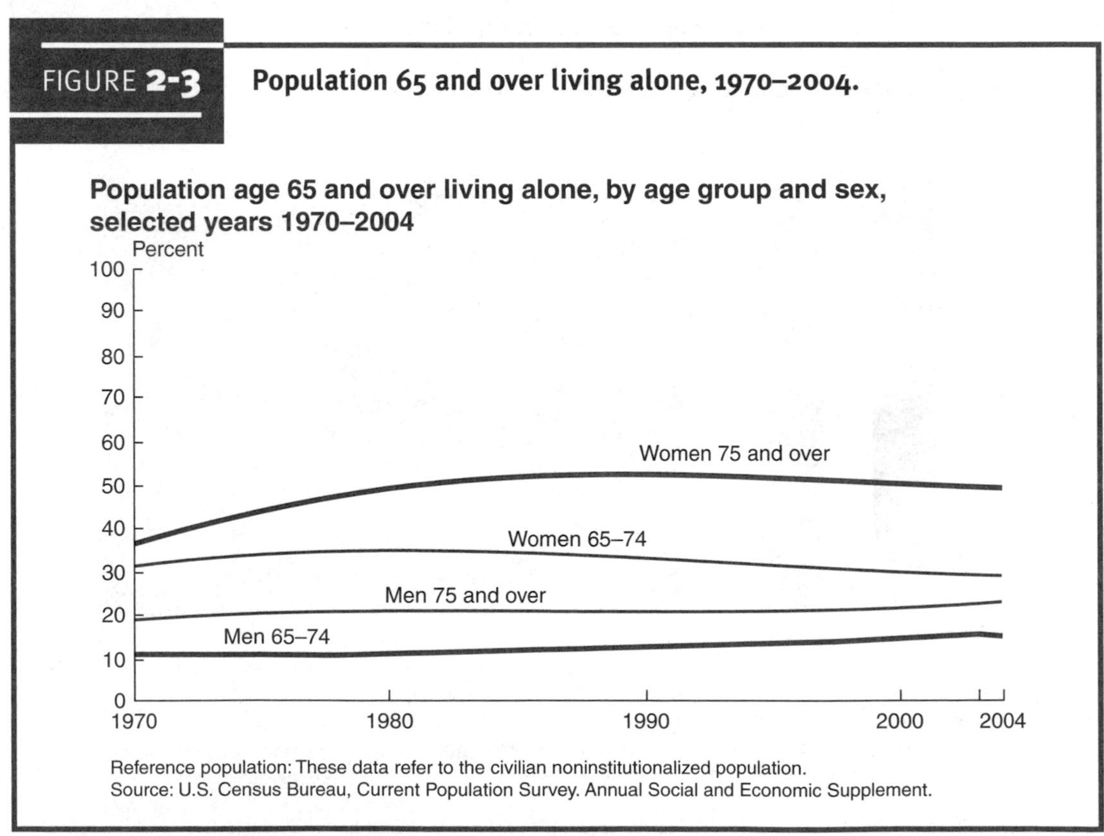

SOURCE: Federal Interagency Forum on Aging-Related Statistics. (May 2006). *Older Americans update 2006: Key indicators of well-being.* Washington, DC: U.S. Government Printing Office. Retrieved September 17, 2007, from http://www.agingstats.gov/Agingstatsdotnet/Main_Site/default.aspx

percentage increases with age. This ranges from 1.1% for persons ages 65–74, to 4.7% for persons ages 75–84, and to 18.2% for persons ages 85+. Another 5% of older adults lived in "senior housing" in 2000, which often offers supportive services to residents (Administration on Aging, 2006a).

Living arrangements, like education, also vary by race and ethnicity. In 2003, older Asian women were more likely than older women of other races to live with relatives other than a spouse. Older non-Hispanic white and older black females were more likely than others to live alone. Older black men lived alone three times as much as older Asian men. Older Asian men were more likely than other races and ethnicities to live with relatives other than a spouse. The state of living alone increases as age increases.

Older people who lived alone had higher poverty rates than those who lived with their spouse. In 2002, 16% of older men and 21% of older women who lived alone lived in poverty. Only 5% of older married men and women lived in poverty (Federal Interagency Forum, 2004).

Effects of Ethnicity

The growing aging population consists of a significantly increased proportion of minorities. Minority elders will make up 22% of the elderly population over the next 20 years (Ross, 2000). The diversity as well as the vast increase in number of this group provides a distinct challenge in meeting health care needs. The losses (spouses, friends, independence, levels of function, status in society) often encountered in aging coupled with low socioeconomic status and lifetime racial discriminations put this group at increased risk for poor outcomes (Markides & Miranda, 1997). An understanding of cultural diversity and the unique challenges it poses is needed to address health issues and promote wellness.

The older population in the United States is growing more racially and ethnically diverse as it ages. In 2003, 83% of U.S. older adults were non-Hispanic whites, 8% were black, 3% Asian, and 6% Hispanic (see **Table 2-1**). Between 2004 and 2030, the white population age 65 or older is projected to increase by

TABLE 2-1 U.S. Population Age 65+ by Race and Hispanic Origin, 2000

Total 65+	Numbers	Percentage
Non-Hispanic		
Black	2,787,427	8.0%
American Indian/Alaskan Native	124,797	0.4%
Native Hawaiian/Pacific Islander	19,085	0.1%
Asian	796,008	2.3%
Two or More Races	264,588	0.8%
Other Race	21,397	0.1%
Hispanic (any race)	1,733,591	5.0%
Total Minority	5,746,893	16.4%
White (Alone—Non-Hispanic)	29,244,860	83.6%
Total 65+	34,991,753	100.0%

DATA SET SOURCE: Administration on Aging. Census 2000 Summary File 1 (SF 1) 100-Percent Data *Retrieved from:* www.aoa.gov/prof/Statistics/minority_aging/facts_minority_aging.asp

74%, compared to an increase of 254% for older Hispanics; 147% for older African Americans; 143% for American Indians, Eskimos, and Aleuts; and 208% for Pacific Islanders (Administration on Aging, 2006a; Federal Interagency Forum, 2004).

African Americans

African American elders make up the largest cultural minority and are projected to increase from 3 million in 2004 to over 10.4 million by 2050. In 2004, African Americans comprised 8.2% of the older population. By 2050, this is expected to increase to 12%. The poverty rate for older African Americans was 24% in 2004, compared to 10% for the total elderly population. Households containing families headed by African Americans age 65 or older reported a median income of $26,282 in 2004, compared to $35,825 for all older households. The median personal income for African American men was $14,960, and $9,884 for African American women, compared to $21,102 for all elderly men and $12,080 for all elderly women (Administration on Aging, 2006b). There is also a great disparity in net worth between black and white households headed by older Americans. In 2003, net worth among older black households was estimated to be $26,300, compared to $215,000 among older white households (Federal Interagency Forum, 2006). The lack of economic resources and poor access to health care add to the increased incidence of disease with greater complications in this subgroup (see **Case Study 2-1**).

Higher rates of diabetes, hypertension, and chronic kidney disease are seen in African Americans (Ross, 2000). African Americans are twice as likely as whites to have diabetes (Illinois Department on Aging, 2001). African American men have higher incidences of lung and prostate cancer as compared to whites, and African Americans' overall risk to develop kidney disease is highest of the senior groups.

Among the most frequently occurring chronic conditions among African American elderly in 2002–2003 were hypertension (68%), arthritis (53%), heart disease (25%), diabetes (25%), sinusitis (15%), and cancer (11%). This generally compares negatively to the following figures for all older persons in the United States: hypertension (51%), arthritis (48%), heart disease (31%), diabetes (16%), sinusitis (14%), and cancer (21%) (Administration on Aging, 2006b).

Case Study 2-1

Mrs. Johnson is an 87-year-old African American female admitted to the hospital from her home. She is widowed and has no children. Her neighbors watch out for her, bringing her groceries and making sure that she's OK each day. Mrs. Johnson's neighbor, Mrs. Edwards, accompanies her to the hospital.

Mrs. Johnson is admitted for shortness of breath, attributed to nonadherence to her medication regimen for congestive heart failure. She is alert, oriented, and very pleasant.

Mrs. Edwards takes you aside and tells you that she is concerned about Mrs. Johnson's home situation.

Questions:

1. What might you suspect about Mrs. Johnson's financial situation?
2. What might you suspect about Mrs. Johnson's home situation?
3. How might these factors contribute to her hospital admission?
4. Based upon your suspicions, what questions might you ask Mrs. Johnson as you admit her to your unit?

African Americans often do not use routine preventive services at recommended rates and are less likely to have a regular provider of health care, opting instead for hospital outpatient departments, historically known for long waits and inconsistent providers (Markides & Miranda, 1997). The top five causes of death among African Americans are heart disease, cancer, stroke, diabetes, and unintentional accidents (Centers for Disease Control and Prevention [CDC], 2005). From these statistics, it is evident that preventive services have the potential to affect the longevity of this population.

Hispanics

The Hispanic population is the second largest and most rapidly growing ethnic minority in the United States (Hazuda & Espino, 1997). The over-65-year-old Hispanic population is the fastest growing segment of the total U.S. population. By 2028, the Hispanic population ages 65 or older is projected to be the largest racial/ethnic minority in this age group (Administration on Aging, 2006c). By 2050, Hispanic elderly will make up 16.4% of all U.S. elderly, adding up to 13.4 million Hispanics over the age of 65 (Administration on Aging, 2000). The Hispanic population in the United States consists of a diverse population from Mexico, Cuba, Puerto Rico, the Dominican Republic, and other countries of Central and South America. The poverty rate in 2004 for Hispanic elderly in the United States was nearly twice that of the total older population, 18.7% compared to 9.8% (Administration on Aging, 2006c).

The chronic diseases of cardiovascular disease, diabetes, cancer, and cerebrovascular disease are seen in significant numbers in the Hispanic population. Centers for Disease Control (CDC) data show Hispanics are less likely to obtain preventive services such as flu and pneumonia vaccines and mammograms as compared to whites (CDC, 2005). The age-adjusted rate of diabetes in this population is 44% higher than for non-Hispanic whites (Administration on Aging, 2006c). Hispanics also have higher rates of cervical, esophageal, gallbladder, and stomach cancer as compared to whites. Poverty levels, only slightly lower than for African American elderly, and language barriers are often impediments to accessing health care coverage and health care services (Ross, 2000). The top five causes of death among Hispanics are heart disease, cancer, stroke, chronic obstructive pulmonary disease (COPD), and pneumonia/influenza (Sahyoun, Lentzner, Hoyert, & Robinson, 2001).

In 2002, 72% of Hispanics age 60 or over lived in four states: California, Florida, New York, and Texas (Administration on Aging, 2003). Hispanics in general receive assistance in the home when functionally declining, versus in long-term facilities (Angel & Angel, 1997). Family members frequently act as their caregivers, and multigenerational families under one roof are common. On average, Hispanic families and households are larger than non-Hispanic families and households (Aranda & Miranda, 1997). Overall, the percentage of Hispanic elderly living alone is lower than that of the general population (Administration on Aging, 2006c). Older Hispanics are more likely to be married and to rely on family over friends when compared to white elderly.

Asians and Pacific Islanders

This subgroup actually is composed of 40 different ethnic groups with various economic, educational, and health profiles (Ross, 2000). Some identified ethnicities include Asian, Chinese, Filipino, Japanese, Pacific Islander, and Hawaiian. National data, however, do not necessarily discern between ethnicities, which complicates identifying demographics and patterns for each culture. The Asian American and Pacific Islander population has been the fastest growing racial/ethnic group in the United States recently, having increased 141% between 1970 and 1980 and 99% between 1980 and 1990 (Elo, 1997). According to the U.S. Bureau of the Census, projections for the years 2000–2050 include population increases for Asian Americans and Pacific Islanders from 2.4% to 6.5% of the U.S. population (Administration on Aging, 2000).

Life expectancy data have historically shown an advantage for the Asian American and Pacific Islander population. Census data from 1995 showed life expectancy at birth of Asian Americans and Pacific Islanders to be 79.3 years for males and 84.9 years for females, as compared to 73.6 and 80.1 for white males and females, respectively. Elo (1997) questions inconsistencies in the data due to the heterogeneity of the group. The evaluation of mortality data did place Chinese, Japanese, and Filipinos well below white Americans. As a whole, cancer and heart disease contribute less to all-cause mortality in the Asian American and Pacific Islander population than in whites. Cerebrovascular disease, however, is a more prominent cause of death for some subgroups of Asian Americans and Pacific Islanders (Elo). Discrepancies are seen in mortality causes depending on whether persons are native or foreign-born, pointing to the impact of acculturation in U.S. society. But overall, the top five causes of death among Asian Americans or Pacific Islanders are heart disease, cancer, stroke, pneumonia/influenza, and COPD (Sahyoun et al., 2001).

Kitano, Tazuko, and Kitano (1997) note the inconsistency of this minority group's use of community professional resources. Dependence on familial and informal ethnic resources is seen more often than use of traditional health resources.

Length of the family's time in this country (recent arrival vs. present for a century) impacts comfort and ease of resource use. Health care providers will need to address not only the diversity within this minority group, but also the time or extent of acculturation and assimilation within each subgroup.

American Indians and Alaskan Natives

The category of American Indians and Alaskan Natives represents 500 nations, tribes, bands, and native villages in which 150 languages are used (Kramer, 1997). Although the American Indians and Alaskan Natives make up a small percentage of the nation's elderly, they are one of the fastest growing groups of minority elderly, behind Asian and Hispanic groups (Chapleski, 1997). American Indians and Alaskan Natives over the age of 60 were 152,000 in number per the 2000 census (Administration on Aging, 2000). The over-75 years of age cohort of American Indians and Alaskan Natives is expected to double by the year 2050 (Chapleski, 1997). Two-thirds of American Indian and Alaskan Native elders live in 10 states. Historical and political developments forced the concentration of American Indians first onto reservations west of the Mississippi and then to more urban areas (Chapleski, 1997). Due to these relocation efforts, American Indians and Alaskan Natives are not necessarily in close proximity to Indian Health Services (IHS) facilities. Only 59% of this population actually lives in IHS areas (Chapleski, 1997). Although the majority of American Indians and Alaskan Natives live in rural areas, many have moved to urban areas.

Chronic disease prevalence in American Indians and Alaskan Natives increased significantly in the 20th century (see **Case Study 2-2**). The IHS made tremendous efforts to increase life expectancy from 51 years in 1940 to 71 years in 1980 through a reduction in infectious disease. Now, however, there is a tremendous prevalence of chronic disease due to dietary changes, sedentary lifestyles, and technology that is similar to Western society (Kramer, 1997). The leading causes of death for older American Indians and Alaskan Natives are heart disease, cancer, diabetes, stroke, and COPD (Sahyoun et al., 2001).

Diabetes is a serious threat to morbidity and mortality in the American Indian and Alaskan Native population. They are 2.5 times more likely to get diabetes as compared to same-age whites (Ross, 2000).

Case Study 2-2

Mr. Andrew Crow is a 67-year-old American Indian. He has been unemployed for the past 5 years. He lives on a reservation in Oklahoma with his wife and three teenaged children. Mr. Crow came to the health clinic for a routine checkup. You note that he is overweight.

Questions:

1. How should you focus your physical assessment?
2. What chronic diseases might Mr. Crow be at high risk for?
3. What are the implications for his family?
4. Develop a plan of care for Mr. Crow and his family members.

Complications of diabetes are also seen more frequently, with end-stage renal disease occurring 6.8 times more in American Indians and the number of nontraumatic lower extremity amputations far exceeding non–American Indian populations (Kramer, 1997). These high rates of disease and complications are seen in younger age cohorts as well.

Heart disease is the leading cause of death among American Indians and Alaskan Natives due to a rise in risk factors (obesity, diabetes, smoking, hypertension, high cholesterol, and sedentary lifestyle) (Kramer, 1997). Younger American Indians (in their 40s) experience a three to four times greater cardiovascular mortality than the general population. Hypertension prevalence in general is low, but when coupled with obesity and diabetes, long-term effects are devastating—end-stage renal disease, proliferative retinopathy, cerebrovascular disease, and myocardial infarction (Kramer, 1997).

Rheumatoid arthritis is seen in higher rates in American Indians as compared to Alaskan Natives and whites, with individual Indian tribes affected in larger numbers. Cancer is the third leading cause of death of American Indians. Survival rates are the lowest compared to any other U.S. population (Kramer, 1997). Lung cancer is most common.

The National Indian Council on Aging study of 1981 noted the health, functional, and social status of American Indian elders (Kramer, 1997). It was noted that 45-year-olds on reservations and 55-year-olds in urban areas were considered elders and matched criteria of white Americans at age 65 (Kramer, 1997). This shifts the necessity for health interventions and disease management to occur at a much younger age to impact the significant mortality and morbidity in the American Indian and Alaskan Native population.

Other Minorities

The Older Foreign-Born Population in the United States

The **foreign-born** are those people who are living in the United States who were not U.S. citizens at birth. As of 2000, the 65-year-old and older foreign-born population in the United States numbered 3.1 million. More than one-third of U.S. foreign-born immigrants are from Europe, a pattern that will change in the future according to immigration laws and world events. It is expected that, in the future, the older foreign-born will be more likely to come from Latin America or Asia (He, 2000).

Nearly 66% of the older foreign-born in the United States have lived here for more than 30 years. The older foreign-born are also twice as likely to be naturalized citizens as the foreign-born of all ages (see **Table 2-2**). Almost 50% of the older foreign-born have not completed high school (compared to 29% of **native-born** older Americans). Older foreign-born are more likely than native-born elders to live in family households, and their poverty rate is also higher than for native-born U.S. citizens. They are also less likely to have health coverage (He, 2000).

U.S. Veterans

Changes in the population of older Americans who are veterans of the armed services are also expected as the Vietnam-era cohort ages. In 2000, there were 9.8 million veterans age 65 or older in the United States—two of every three men 65 or older were veterans. More than 95% of these veterans were male. Between 1990 and 2000, the number of male veterans age 85 or older increased from 142,000 to 400,000 (**Figure 2-4**). There is a projected increase after 2010 as the Vietnam-era cohort ages. The number of veterans 85 or older is expected to increase steadily to a peak of 1.4 million in 2012 (Federal Interagency Forum, 2004). This increase in the number of veterans will challenge the U.S. Department of Veterans Affairs, which has traditionally supplied a major proportion of the health care that veterans receive.

Changes in the health care systems of the military are currently being seen as a direct result of the Iraq and Afghanistan wars. It is unknown how the numbers of wounded military personnel from these wars will affect the U.S. Department of Veterans Affairs in the short or in the long term. It can be anticipated, however, that the number of veterans with significant physical and emotional disabilities will increase and that their needs for health care will also increase as this newest cohort ages. The greater incidence of those with polytraumatic injuries and multiple limb amputation who have survived the advanced weapons of war today will pose an additional challenge to the health care system as they age. The impact on the health care system of the unusual deployment of older troops to Iraq and Afghanistan is also unknown.

The Aging Disabled Population

Advances in health care have increased the life span of persons with disability. These include those traumatically injured as well as those born with disability.

Traumatically injured persons are now more likely to receive expert emergency services at the time of their accident. Advances in intensive care services, surgical services, diagnostic services, and the knowledge and skills of health care workers have combined to prolong the lives of persons who used to die within days or months of their traumatic injuries. For the first time in history, persons with spinal cord injuries and brain injuries are living to become elderly. They are truly entering a time in their life that is unpredictable, because they are the first to reach these advanced ages. Unforeseen effects of aging in persons with spinal cord injury, for example, include shoulder injury (from repetitive movements related to wheelchair mobility) and increased risk of pressure ulcers.

Developmentally disabled individuals are another special aging group. Technological advances and improvements in health care are prolonging the lives of those with disabilities such as mental retardation. Twelve percent of persons with developmental disabilities are now 65 or older. This translates to between 200,000 and 500,000 people.

TABLE **2-2** **Age and Sex of the Population Aged 65 and Over by Citizenship Status: March 2000 (Numbers in thousands)**

		Total		Nativity/Citizenship							
				Native		Foreign-Born		Naturalized Citizen		Not a Citizen	
		Number	Percent	Number	Percent	Number	Percent	Number	Percent	Number	Percent
Total	Total	32,621	100.0	29,507	100.0	3,115	100.0	2,188	100.0	927	100.0
	65 to 74 years	17,796	54.6	16,019	54.3	1,778	57.1	1,195	54.6	582	62.8
	75 years and older	14,825	45.4	13,488	45.7	1,337	42.9	992	45.4	345	37.2
	– 75 to 84 years	11,685	35.8	10,721	36.3	965	31.0	695	31.8	269	29.1
	– 85 years and older	3,140	9.6	2,767	9.4	373	12.0	297	13.6	75	8.1
Male	Total	13,886	100.0	12,540	100.0	1,346	100.0	963	100.0	384	100.0
	65 to 74 years	8,049	58.0	7,251	57.8	799	59.3	543	56.4	256	66.7
	75 years and older	5,837	42.0	5,289	42.2	548	40.7	420	43.6	128	33.3
	– 75 to 84 years	4,796	34.5	4,390	35.0	406	30.1	299	31.0	107	27.9
	– 85 years and older	1,041	7.5	899	7.2	142	10.5	121	12.6	21	5.5
Female	Total	18,735	100.0	16,967	100.0	1,768	100.0	1,225	100.0	543	100.0
	65 to 74 years	9,747	52.0	8,768	51.7	979	55.4	652	53.3	327	60.1
	75 years and older	8,988	48.0	8,199	48.3	789	44.6	573	46.7	217	39.9
	– 75 to 84 years	6,889	36.8	6,331	37.3	559	31.6	396	32.3	163	29.9
	– 85 years and older	2,099	11.2	1,868	11.0	231	13.0	176	14.4	54	10.0

SOURCE: U.S. Census Bureau. Current Population Survey, March 2000. Internet Release Date: October 2, 2002.

FIGURE 2-4 **Male veterans 65+, 1990–2000.**

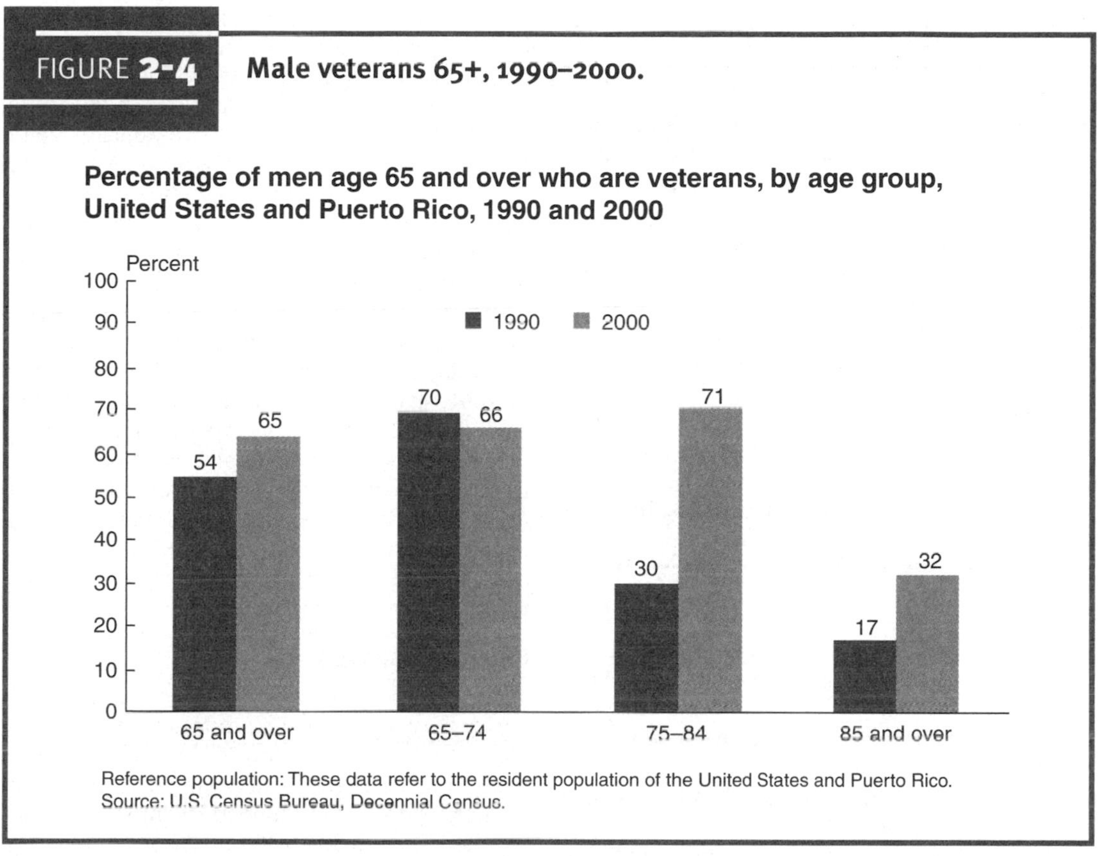

SOURCE: Federal Interagency Forum on Aging-Related Statistics. (May 2006). *Older Americans update 2006: Key indicators of well-being.* Washington, DC: U.S. Government Printing Office. Retrieved September 17, 2007, from http://www.agingstats.gov/Agingstatsdotnet/Main_Site/default.aspx

There are great implications for the U.S. health care system as this population continues to age, grow, and outlive their parents. Unforeseen secondary health problems are beginning to be seen in this older population, including obesity, chronic skin problems, and early aging (Connolly, 1998).

Elderly Inmates

One oft-forgotten segment of the elderly population in the United States is the prisoners. There are more than 55,000 inmates over the age of 55 in the United States and even more are growing old. It is anticipated that the number of inmates over age 55 could double every 5 years (Winokur, 2005). Bureau of Justice statistics note that in 2003 there were 208 male inmates age 55 or over per 100,000 U.S. population. Females 55+ accounted for 8 per 100,000. In 2003, inmates 55+ accounted for 5.9% of the federal prison population (see **Case Study 2-3**).

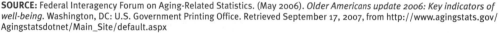

Elderly even has a different connotation in the world of jail cells. Due to the stresses of prison life and the earlier onset of age-related problems, "elderly" begins at age 50 or even earlier for those in prison (Schreiber, 1999). A 50-year-old inmate may have a physiological age that is 10–15 years older than his or her biological age, due to the use of illicit drugs, alcohol intake, and limited access to preventive care and health services. It can cost three times as much money to care for an older inmate, compared to a younger one. Inmates age 55 or older tend to have at least three chronic conditions, and up to 20% have a mental illness (Mitka, 2004).

Case Study 2-3

Mr. Everett is a 62-year-old inmate in a state penitentiary, admitted to your unit for hypertension, heart failure, and chest pain. He is accompanied by a prison guard, who watches your every move. The guard has handcuffed Mr. Everett to the bed.

This is the first prisoner that you've ever cared for. You are surprised about how old Mr. Everett looks. You complete your admission assessment and talk to him about the plans for his care.

Questions:

1. Why might this patient appear to be older than his stated age?
2. How could his social situation affect his plan of care, hospital stay, and recovery?

Aged inmates can require such complicated and costly procedures as dialysis three times weekly, special diets, and expensive medications. Adaptive equipment, such as walkers and wheelchairs, may also be needed for mobility. In 2003 in Texas, 1,159 inmates over the age of 65 required 24-hour skilled nursing care (McMahon, 2003).

Prisoners have been called the only population in the United States with a legal right to health care. Due to these legal rights, and the expanding aging prison population, combined with tight federal and state budgets, it is no wonder that some think that the U.S. prison system is overdue for a health care crisis (Mitka, 2004). Some states, like Texas, have developed separate facilities for their geriatric prisoners. Others have integrated telemedicine into their facilities or developed chronic care clinics. And some, recognizing the likelihood of inmates not only aging in place in prison but also dying of chronic disease while in prison, have implemented hospice programs for their dying, elderly prisoners.

MORTALITY AND MORBIDITY

Causes of Death

The leading cause of death for older adults in 2001 was diseases of the heart, followed by malignant neoplasms, cerebrovascular diseases, chronic lower respiratory diseases, influenza and pneumonia, and diabetes. Death rates for diseases of the heart and cerebrovascular diseases decreased by one-third from 1981 to 2001. Age-adjusted death rates for diabetes mellitus increased by 43% from 1981 to 2001, and death rates for chronic lower respiratory diseases increased by 62% during the same time period. Diseases of the heart and malignant neoplasms are the top two causes of death for people age 65 or older in the United States, regardless of race, gender, or ethnic origin. Race and ethnicity do play a part in other causes of death, however. In 2001, diabetes mellitus was the fifth leading cause of death among black men, the fourth among Hispanic men, and the sixth among white men and men of Asian or Pacific Islander origin. For women age 65 or older, diabetes mellitus was the fourth leading cause of death for Hispanics and blacks, and the seventh leading cause of death among whites (Federal Interagency Forum, 2004).

Chronic Diseases

The prevalence of chronic diseases increases with age. Four of the six leading causes of death among older Americans are chronic diseases such as heart disease, stroke, cancer, and diabetes. Older women report higher numbers of chronic diseases such as hypertension, asthma, chronic bronchitis, and arthritis, whereas men report more heart disease, cancer, diabetes, and emphysema. Ethnic and racial differences also exist in the prevalence of chronic diseases. Older blacks report higher levels of hypertension and diabetes than non-Hispanic whites, whereas Hispanics report higher levels of diabetes than non-Hispanic whites. Both diabetes and hypertension are increasing among older Americans (Federal Interagency Forum, 2004).

Sensory impairments and oral health problems become more frequent with aging. Early detection can prevent or postpone the physical, social, and emotional effects that these changes have on a senior's life. In 2002, nearly 50% of older men and nearly 33% of older women reported difficulty with hearing. Those age 85 or older reported more difficulty than those 65–74. Vision trouble affects about 18% of older adults. In 2002, of those people 65 or over who reported trouble with vision, 16%

reported ever having glaucoma, 16% reported ever having macular degeneration, and 44% reported having cataracts in the past 12 months. Thirty-eight percent of persons 85 years of age or older reported edentulism (lack of teeth). Poorer older adults were less likely to have teeth than those above the poverty threshold (46% compared to 27%) (Federal Interagency Forum, 2004). Glasses, hearing aids, and dentures can be difficult to obtain for financial reasons: They are expensive and they are not covered services under Medicare. Thus, many older adults may not possess these assistive devices, or may have out-of-date or ill-fitting devices, which can affect cognitive status (hearing aids and glasses), nutritional intake (dentures), and likelihood of falling (glasses).

Memory loss is not unusual in the older adult. Older men are more likely to experience moderate or severe memory impairment than older women. In 2002, 15% of men age 65 or older and 11% of women of the same age experienced moderate to severe memory impairment. At age 85 or older, nearly 33% of both women and men suffered from this impairment. In 2002, the proportion of people age 85 or older with moderate or severe memory impairment was 32% compared to 5% of people ages 65–69 (Federal Interagency Forum, 2004).

Many people feel that older age is highly correlated with disability. The age-adjusted proportion of people in the United States age 65 or older with chronic disabilities actually declined from 1984 to 1999. Due to the population growth, however, the actual numbers of older persons with chronic disabilities increased from 6.2 million in 1984 to 6.8 million in 1999. Older women reported more difficulties in physical functioning than older men. In 2003, 31% of older women reported that they were unable to perform at least one of five activities, compared to 18% of men (see **Figure 2-5**). Those age 85 or older had more physical limitations than those 65–74. Physical functioning is also somewhat related to race and ethnicity. Seventeen percent of non Hispanic white males were unable to perform at least one physical activity, compared to 26% of non-Hispanic blacks and 22% of Hispanics. For women, 30% of non-Hispanic whites were unable to perform at least one activity, compared to 36% of non-Hispanic blacks and 29% of Hispanics (Federal Interagency Forum, 2004).

Good Health in Aging?

Feeling depressed about aging and the aged? Although the statistics can sound grim, in actuality, aging is enjoyed by the vast majority of seniors. More than 72% of seniors report having good to excellent health (see **Figure 2-6** and **Table 2-3**). The number of seniors living in nursing homes declined from 5.2% in 1990 to 4.5% in 2000. Only 18.2% of those age 85 or older lived in nursing homes in 2000, compared to 24.5% in 1990. In 2000, 1 out of every 5,578 people was 100 years of age or older (U.S. Census Bureau, 2001). Older adults in the United States are, by and large, active and healthy.

THE HISTORY OF AGING IN THE UNITED STATES

Patterns of aging in the United States have changed throughout the years. From 1650 to 1850, older Americans made up less than 2% of the population (Fleming, Evans, & Chutka, 2003). Old age in those times was considered to start at 60 years of age. In colonial times, elders were greatly respected. They were given the best seats in church. Puritans taught youth how to behave toward their elders (Egendorf, 2002). By 1870, older adults made up 3% of the U.S. population, and only 0.37% were over the age of 80. Some older adults lived with nuclear families and were treated with great respect. Among the upper classes, the older adults tended to control the family's land and wealth, thus maintaining authority over the family. Poor people in those times often did not live to old age—old age was a privilege of the rich. The elderly poor were seen as a burden on society, so if old age was attained by a poor person, it was accompanied by derision and scorn from other citizens (Fleming et al., 2003).

Youth came to be increasingly valued during the American Revolution. Older adults declined in status. Fashion favored a youthful look, and clothing flattered the younger frame. Claimed ages in the census drifted downward, because people did not want to acknowledge their actual age. Terms such as "old fogey," "codger," and "geezer" came into being. Retirement from public office became mandatory at age 60 or 70 in many states (Egendorf, 2002; Fleming et al., 2003).

FIGURE 2-5 **Medicare enrollees with limited function, 1991 and 2003.**

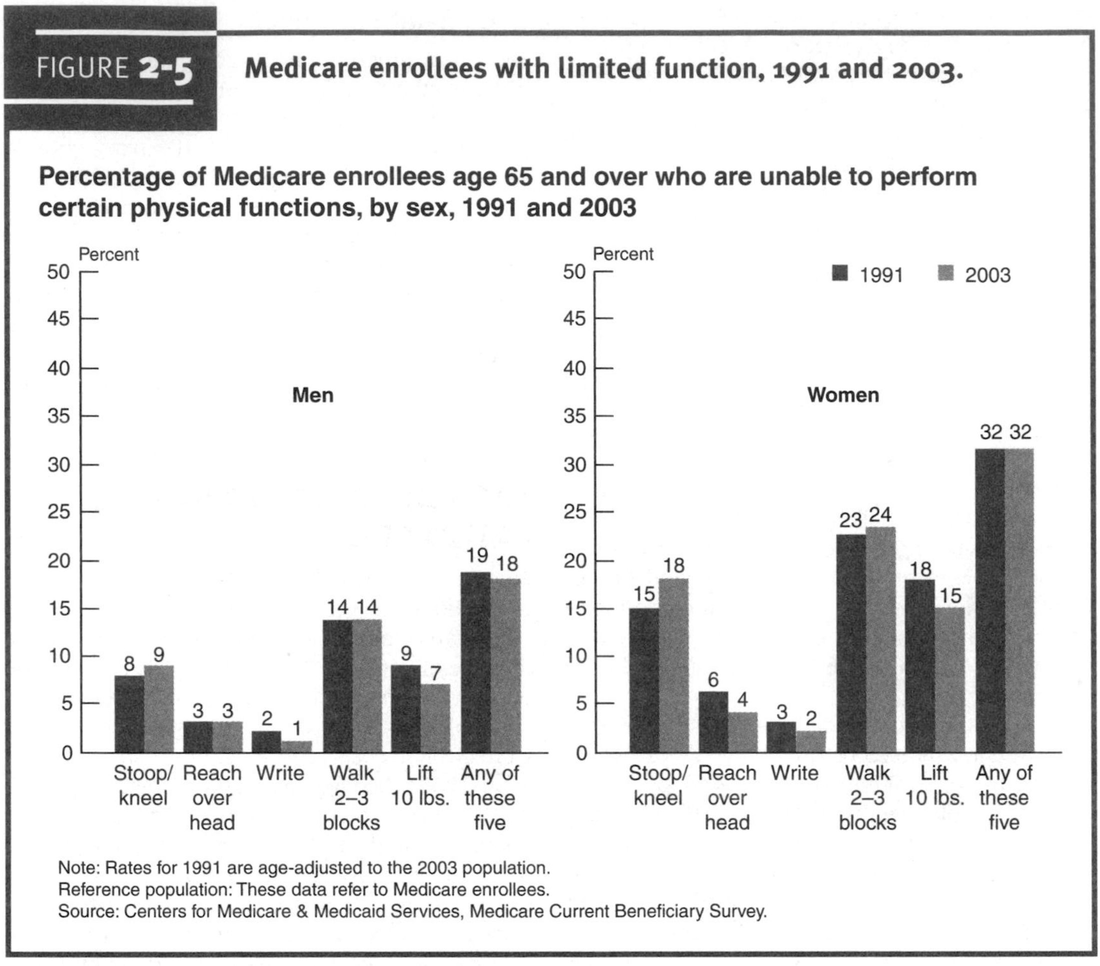

SOURCE: Federal Interagency Forum on Aging-Related Statistics. (May 2006). *Older Americans update 2006: Key indicators of well-being.* Washington, DC: U.S. Government Printing Office. Retrieved September 17, 2007, from http://www.agingstats.gov/Agingstatsdotnet/Main_Site/default.aspx

By the end of the 19th century, age stratification was prevalent in American life. Activities like school attendance, marriage, and retirement became based on age. By the start of the 20th century there were increasing numbers of older adults. Cultural focus shifted to business, medicine, and scientific advances. Older adults were devalued (Fleming et al., 2003).

Throughout history, old age has often been associated with lack of income and dependency on others. Poverty was greater in the southern states, especially among widows and blacks. Immigrants and blacks were the least prepared for the lack of income after retirement. Here is a quote from a former slave:

> *When my mother became old, she was sent to live in a lonely log-hut in the woods. Aged and worn out slaves, whether men or women, are commonly so treated. No care is taken of them, except, perhaps, that a little ground is cleared about the hut, on which the old slave, if able, may raise a little corn. As far as the owner is concerned, they live or die as it hap-*

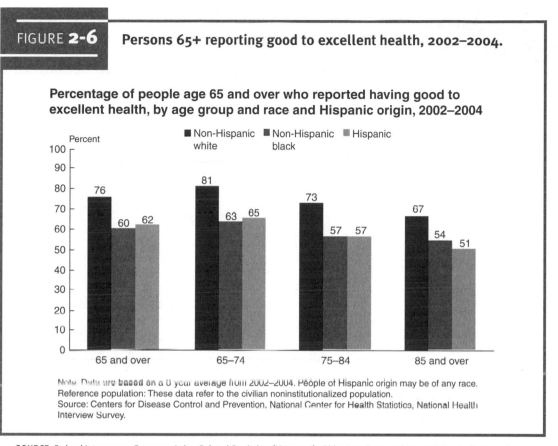

FIGURE 2-6 **Persons 65+ reporting good to excellent health, 2002–2004.**

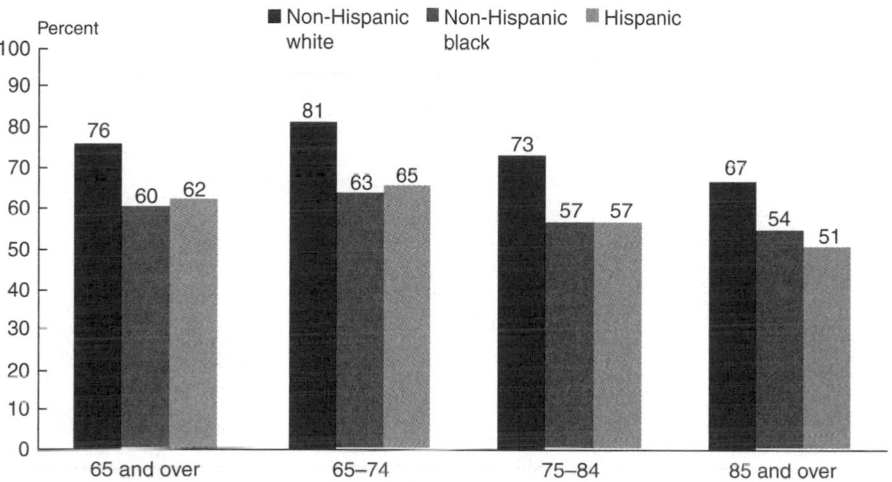

SOURCE: Federal Interagency Forum on Aging-Related Statistics. (May 2006). *Older Americans update 2006: Key indicators of well-being.* Washington, DC: U.S. Government Printing Office. Retrieved September 17, 2007, from http://www.agingstats.gov/Agingstatsdotnet/Main_Site/default.aspx

pens; it is just the same thing as turning out an old horse. (Fleming et al., 2003, p. 915)

Harriet Jacobs (1861, p. 27) noted:

Slaveholders have a method, peculiar to their institution, of getting rid of old slaves, whose lives have been worn out in their service. I knew an old woman, who for seventy years faithfully served her master. She had become almost helpless, from hard labor and disease. Her owners moved to Alabama, and the old black woman was left to be sold to any body who would give twenty dollars for her.

There were no national or state social supports for the poor in early America. Rather, the townships assisted the poor. In some communities, the rising taxes needed for relief of the poor led the communities to rid themselves of the poor by auctioning them off to farms for labor. Some communities even denied refuge to nonresidents, forcing the elderly to go from town to town in search of assistance. Citizens often divided the poor into two categories: the "worthy poor" who were unable to support themselves because of illness, disability, or old age, through no fault of their own, and the immoral, lazy, alcoholic poor. The elderly who had failed to save for their older years were also

TABLE 2-3 Persons 65+ Reporting Good to Excellent Health, 1994–1996

Percentage of Persons Age 65 or Older Who Reported Good to Excellent Health, by Age Group, Sex, and Race and Hispanic Origin, 1994 to 1996

	All Persons	Non-Hispanic White	Non-Hispanic Black	Hispanic
Total				
65 or Older	72.2	74.0	58.4	64.9
Men				
65 or Older	72.0	73.5	59.3	65.4
65 to 74	74.6	76.3	61.6	68.7
75 to 84	68.3	69.4	56.4	59.7
85 or Older	65.0	67.3	45.0	50.9
Women				
65 or Older	72.4	74.3	57.8	64.6
65 to 74	75.2	77.5	59.3	68.5
75 to 84	69.8	71.7	55.3	59.3
85 or Older	65.1	66.4	56.0	55.1

NOTE: Data are based on a 3-year average from 1994 to 1996. Hispanics may be of any race.

REFERENCE POPULATION: These data refer to the civilian noninstitutional population.

SOURCE: National Health Interview Survey, www.aoa.gov/prof/Statistics/minority_aging/facts_minority_aging.asp

deemed by some to be unworthy of assistance by the community (Fleming et al., 2003; The Poorhouse Story, 2005). The poor were often sent to poorhouses, which were warehouses for the old, insane, widowed, unmarried mothers, criminals, and drunks. They were often filthy and unsafe. Physical abuse, lack of waste facilities, rats, and poor food made poorhouses dangerous places for the elderly, yet the poor elderly often ended up supported by the community and placed in the poorhouse.

Military pensions were initiated by the U.S. government in 1861. In 1904, President Theodore Roosevelt established old age as a disability. By 1910, 25% of the elderly U.S. population (Northern white soldiers and their widows) was receiving military pensions. Military pensions accounted for 43% of federal expenditures. This first pension system did not last—it dissolved after supporting the last Union veterans and their families (Fleming et al., 2003).

After the Civil War, elderly blacks worked as sharecroppers or became dependent upon their extended families. Black, white, and Hispanic tenant farmers worked well into their old age, lacking the education and resources to do otherwise. Older blacks migrated to the cities as the mechanical cotton picker forced them from their land. Those who did not migrate to the cities suffered ever-worsening poverty (Fleming et al., 2003).

By 1900, poorhouses had changed into old-age homes. The costs of old-age homes became a burden for many counties, so in these counties elders were transferred to state-funded mental institutions. Charitable homes came into being, run by religious organizations, benevolent societies, and ethnic organizations. For-profit homes also developed, serving the chronically ill or disabled. Standards and oversight on all of these facilities were minimal (Fleming et al., 2003).

By the 1920s, the elderly population in the United States was increasingly seen as obsolete. The workplace denigrated older workers, seeing them as less productive and with too few attributes for working in the factories. Older workers were more likely to be injured on the job. Unions pushed for older workers to leave to make room for younger workers. Firms began to introduce mandatory retirement. Persons over 45 years of age began to have trouble finding work. Older workers suddenly found themselves without work, health insurance, unemployment insurance, or retirement savings (Fleming et al., 2003).

The 1920s also brought the fall of the stock market and inflation, and led to the Great Depression of the 1930s. In 1920, 25% of older adults were impoverished. This increased to 30% before the Depression, to 50% in 1935, and to 66% by 1940 (Fleming et al., 2003). There was mass unemployment, and poor families could no longer afford to support their elders. Old people became dependent upon local and state governments for support.

Franklin Roosevelt signed the Social Security Act in 1935. This act provided income assistance for the elderly. Roosevelt's purpose was to enact a law that would give some measure of protection to the average U.S. citizen and his or her family against a poverty-ridden old age. But then, medical costs began to rise, forcing the elderly to again rely on the government for assistance. Medicare and Medicaid were signed into law in 1965 by President Johnson. Medicare and Medicaid offered a form of health insurance to those who previously had been seen as uninsurable families (Fleming et al., 2003).

County "poor farms" continued to exist. The Social Security Act of 1935, however, denied funding to these facilities. Private care homes flourished in the 1940s, again with few standards or oversights. Social pressures begat the for-profit long-term care industry. In the 1950s, a federal relationship flourished with the providers. By 1960, however, there was still a shortage of 500,000 long-term care beds in the United States. By 1997, nearly 4% of the U.S. population was being cared for in nursing homes. Currently, about 55% of persons 85 or older are impaired and require long-term care (Carbonell, 2005).

In 1880, 75% of men 65 or older were employed, being too poor to retire. They left work due to poor health or the inability to find work. With the emphasis on youth and the passage of the Social Security and Medicare/Medicaid bills, the number of older men who are employed has steadily dropped throughout the years. In 2003, less than 20% of men 65 or older worked full- or part-time (Carbonell, 2005).

SUCCESSFUL AGING

Some may consider successful aging an oxymoron. The idea of aging successfully may not be considered a possibility in our youth-obsessed society. The later years of life are most often considered a time of decline, disability, dissatisfaction, and loneliness. There is no consensus on a definition of successful aging. One view is to consider success as reaching the extreme in health and function at an advanced age. An alternative view is successfully adapting to changes in the aging process, while another perspective might be accomplishing individual goals or experiencing an ultimate feeling of well-being (vonFaber et al., 2001). It might be best to consider a combination of psychosocial and biomedical paradigms. A psychosocial view includes acceptance of death, life satisfaction, and feelings of well-being. A biomedical model is seen more as an avoidance of disease and disability. One must not look at successful aging as merely an avoidance of disease and disability, however, but as an achievement of a sense of autonomy, dignity, and absence of suffering (Glass, 2003).

It may be argued that all or a combination of views may describe success in reaching old age. A study conducted in Leiden, Netherlands, explored the meaning of successful aging in those reaching 85 years of age. Data obtained from 599 elderly showed greater than 45% qualified as successful in the area of well-being whereas only 10% met criteria as successful in the area of functioning. In qualitative interviews, subjects identified successful aging as more of an adaptive process than reaching a state of being. Social function and feelings of well-being were valued more than physical and psychosocial well-being (vonFaber et al., 2001).

Numerous studies have been conducted on identifying characteristics of or predictors to old age. Two cohorts of adolescent boys (college students

Notable Quotes

The hard fact is that aging will bring unpleasant changes, among them, aches and pains; decreased vigor, healing ability, sensory acuity, muscle tone, bone density, and sexual energy; memory deficits; wrinkles, loss of beauty, friends, family, and independence; increased reliance on doctors and pills; and social isolation. We can mask the outward sign of the process and try to keep up old routines in spite of it, but cannot change the fact that we are all moving toward physical decline and death.

—Andrew Weil, MD, best-selling author, from his book *Healthy Aging*

and core-city youth) were followed for 60 years or until death. Physical and psychosocial data were gathered intermittently over this time. Predictor variables at age 50 included uncontrollable factors and personally controlled factors that distinguished "happy-well" and "sad-sick" elderly. Protective factors included personally controlled factors of smoking, driving, exercise, weight, and education. Two additional factors considered modifiable included a stable marriage and maturity of defenses. An absence of alcohol and cigarette use before age 50 was most protective (Valliant & Mukamal, 2001). This would point to the concept that poor health in late life is not inevitable and modifiable risk factors contribute to successful aging.

A group of over 6,000 elderly Japanese men in Hawaii were studied over 28 years noting survival rates, development of clinical illness, and physical and cognitive functioning over time. Predictors of healthy aging were identified as low blood pressure, low serum glucose, not smoking cigarettes, and not being obese. Risk factors present at young and middle life are considered possible markers for late life morbidity and disability. This study further noted that changes made to these factors at any time, even in late life, could provide a benefit (Reed et al., 1998).

Centenarians

Centenarians make up the fastest growing segment of our population in the United States, with the over-85-year-olds making up the second fastest growing segment. The U.S. Bureau of the Census estimates that there were 67,473 centenarians in the United States on November 1, 2005 (U.S. Census Bureau, 2006). The U.S. Census of 1990 found that four in five centenarians are women, and 78% of this age group is non-Hispanic white. African Americans make up the second largest group at 16%. This correlates with 76% and 12% of the total population, respectively. In the next 40 years, the number of centenarians may reach 850,000, depending upon changes in life expectancy over these years. Hispanics and Asian Americans will share a greater percentage of this age group, with non-Hispanic whites nearing 55%.

Centenarians were found to be a predominately lower educated, more impoverished, widowed, and more disabled population as compared to other elderly **cohorts** (U.S. Department of Health and Human Services, 1999). The lower education level of this cohort is not surprising considering the increase in levels of education noted over the span of the past century. The marital status of centenarians was overwhelmingly widowed, with 84% of 100-year-old women widowed as compared to 58% of men. Poverty status is more varied in this group and is dependent on race. Women generally were more likely to live in poverty in this age group. White centenarians were less likely than other races except Asian and Pacific Islanders to live in poverty. Disability, identified as having mobility and self-care limitations, was seen across all races. Not surprisingly, consistent with disability trends, all races of centenarians except American Indians, Eskimos, and Aleuts were noted to be not living alone. The increased likelihood of living in a nursing home at this age was noted in all race categories.

The New England Centenarian study was a population-based study conducted within the New England area. The researchers noted a surprising heterogeneity in this group including a wide range of economic status, educational attainment, racial background, and origin of birth. Physical status varied widely as well. Fifteen percent of centenarians in this study were still living independently at home while 50% lived in nursing homes and the remainder lived with family. Three-quarters of the study group suffered from some form of cognitive impairment. Health histories noted 95% of subjects enjoyed unimpaired health well into their ninth decade (Perls, Silver, & Lauerman, 1999). Most notable in this study is the observation that the older one gets, the healthier one has been. It is suspected the centenarians have not necessarily survived disease but have avoided chronic/acute diseases, successfully navigating through obstacles and the physical/psychosocial challenges of their lives (Griffith, 2004).

Secrets of Aging

Why do some people live longer than others? Why is there such a discrepancy in functionality at very old age? As noted previously, several factors may contribute to reaching old age. Lifestyle choices including diet, exercise, socialization, and coping with stress play a large part. Genetics also play a role, especially in those surviving over the age of 80. Lifestyle changes can maximize the genetic potential, but to attain the age of 100 requires a special genetic makeup. This is seen in a study comparing people with siblings who lived to 100 to people (the same age as the other group) whose siblings died at age 73 (average life expectancy of the late 1800s). The centenarian siblings were 3.5 times more likely to reach 80 and 4 times more likely to reach 90 years. These centenarian siblings were noted to weigh less, take fewer medications, and have fewer chronic diseases (e.g., heart disease, hypertension). The impact of genetic makeup vs. familial exposure to diet and exercise practices or longevity in general is not yet known.

A goal of the national health initiative, *Healthy People 2010*, is to increase the quality and extend the years of healthy life. A shift in attitudes by society, including health care professionals, is needed to ensure this is accomplished. Dispelling myths and correcting stereotypes of the aged are a starting point (**Figure 2-7**). A positive view of aging as a normal process not necessarily including illness and disease is needed. Improved insight by Americans into the benefits of successful aging may decrease the feelings of denial and foreboding when faced with this milestone (Gavan, 2003). Keys to successful aging supported by current research are further discussed in Chapters 10, 11, and 22.

BOX 2-1 Resource List

Aging Statistics

Administration on Aging:
http://www.hhs.gov/about/opdivs/aoa.html

American Association of Retired Persons:
http://www.aarp.org

American Geriatrics Society:
http://www.americangeriatrics.org

Centers for Disease Control and Prevention:
http://www.cdc.gov/nchs/agingact.htm

Federal Interagency Forum on Aging-Related Statistics:
http://www.agingstats.gov

Gray Panthers:
http://www.graypanthers.org

Merck Manual of Health and Aging:
http://www.merck.com/pubs/mmanual_ha/sec1/ch03/ch03a.html

Online Journals

BMC Geriatrics:
http://www.biomedcentral.com/bmcgeriatr

Geriatrics:
http://www.geri.com/geriatrics/

Geriatrics and Aging:
http://www.geriatricsandaging.com

Longevity
Estimate your longevity potential by accessing the Life Expectancy Calculator at:
http://www.livingto100.com

CDC/National Center for Health Statistics
http://www.cdc.gov/nchs/fastats/lifexpec.htm

FIGURE **2-7** **The majority of people are healthy, active, and continue to be engaged in society after retirement.**

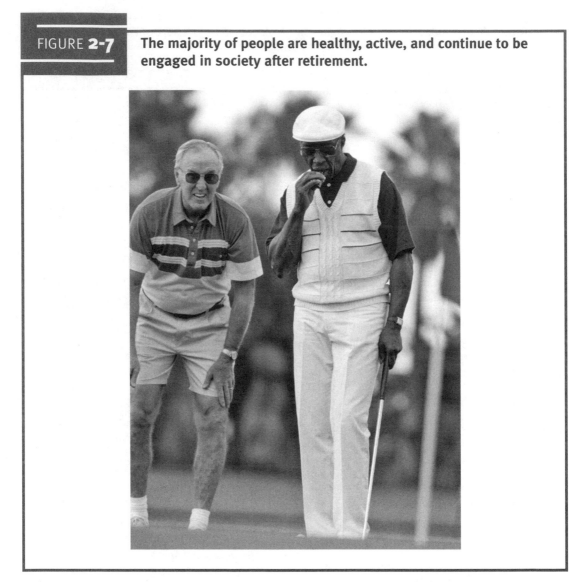

SOURCE: © Photodisc.

SUMMARY

This chapter has reviewed some of the important facts and statistics about the aging population. Aging in the United States may make new impact on society as the baby boomers enter the older age group. Health disparities already exist among minority elderly groups and are likely to continue. Other groups considered vulnerable older adults include U.S. veterans, those with disabilities, and prisoners. Last, successful aging is thought to be possible with wise lifestyle choices and avoidance of risk factors. These are further discussed throughout this text.

Critical Thinking Exercises

1. You will be one of the nurses caring for the baby boomers as they age. How will the prevalence of aged patients affect your nursing practice? What are the implications for your ongoing nursing education?
2. Healthful living becomes ever more important to prevent the chronic diseases of the aged. Fewer chronic diseases in the aged could mean that more health care services are available for those without chronic diseases. What is healthful living? What will your role be in promoting healthful living to your patients? Should nurses be responsible for promoting healthful living when they could be caring for sick patients?
3. The health care of the baby boomers will likely be affected by changes in Social Security, Medicare, and Medicaid. What implications does this have for your nursing practice? How might you address this issue as a nurse? How might you address this issue as a citizen?
4. The population of the United States is becoming ever more ethnically and culturally diverse. What health care issues can you foresee as this ethnically diverse population ages?
5. Think about older celebrities in the United States and abroad, and compare your thoughts about them to your thoughts about older people in general. Do you have different thoughts and feelings about Sean Connery than you do about a nursing home patient? How about those celebrities who are growing older—Cher, The Rolling Stones, Paul McCartney, Clint Eastwood, Chuck Norris? Compare and contrast a well-known senior celebrity with an aged patient you have recently met.

Personal Reflections

The aging of America will affect you both personally and professionally. Government resources will become more and more strained as the baby boomers become elders and begin to use these resources. Medicare, Medicaid, and Social Security may not continue to exist as we know them. There will be fewer beds available in both acute and chronic care facilities to care for the growing aged population. There may not be enough geriatric specialty physicians and nurses to care for the vast numbers of older adults. How could these circumstances affect you and your family? What are your personal plans for your own aging? Have you started to save money for retirement? Are you living a healthy lifestyle, eating "right," and exercising? Are you or your children overweight? Do you smoke or drink alcohol excessively? Are you ready to become involved in the political process so that your opinion is heard?

References

Administration on Aging. (2000). *Facts and figures: Statistics on minority aging in the U.S.* Retrieved May 31, 2005, from http://www.aoa.gov/prof/Statistics/minority_aging/facts_minority_aging.asp

Administration on Aging (2003). *Comparability index for tables in Older Americans: Key indicators*. Available at http://www.agingstats.gov/agingstatsdotnet/Main_Site/Data/compare/Population.pdf

Administration on Aging. (2006a). *A profile of older Americans: 2006*. Washington, DC: U.S. Department of Health and Human Services.

Administration on Aging. (2006b). *A statistical profile of black older Americans aged 65+*. Washington, DC: U.S. Department of Health and Human Services. Retrieved September 17, 2007, from http://www.aoa.gov/press/fact/pdf/attachment_1302.pdf

Administration on Aging. (2006c). *A statistical profile of Hispanic older Americans aged 65+*. Washington, DC: U.S. Department of Health and Human Services. Retrieved September 17, 2007, from http://www.aoa.gov/press/fact/pdf/attachment_1303.pdf

Administration on Aging, Department of Health and Human Services (2007). *A profile of older Americans: 2007*. Available at http://www.state.ia.us/elderaffairs/Documents/2007profile.pdf

Angel, R. J., & Angel, J. L. (1997). Health service use and long-term care among Hispanics. In K. S. Markides & M. R. Miranda (Eds.), *Minorities, aging and health* (pp. 343–366). Thousand Oaks, CA: Sage.

Aranda, M. P., & Miranda, R. M. (1997). Hispanic aging, social support, and mental health: Does acculturation make a difference? In K. S. Markides & M. R. Miranda (Eds.), *Minorities, aging and health* (pp. 271–294). Thousand Oaks, CA: Sage.

Carbonell, J. (May 17, 2005). *Testimony before the Subcommittee on Retirement Security and Aging, Committee on Health, Education, Labor and Pensions, United States Senate.* Retrieved May 27, 2005, from http://www.aoa.gov/press/speeches/2005/05_May/HHS%20Statement%20May%2017.pdf

Centers for Disease Control and Prevention (CDC). (2005). Health disparities experienced by Black or African Americans—United States. *Morbidity and Mortality Weekly Report, 54*(1), 1–3.

Chapleski, E. E. (1997). Long term care among American Indians: A broad lens perspective on service preference and use. In K. S. Markides & M. R. Miranda (Eds.), *Minorities, aging and health* (pp. 367–394). Thousand Oaks, CA: Sage.

Connolly, B. H. (1998). General effects of aging on persons with developmental disabilities. *Topics in Geriatric Rehabilitation, 13*(3), 1–18.

Egendorf, L. (Ed.). (2002). *An aging population*. San Diego: Greenhaven Press. Retrieved June 5, 2005, from http://www.enotes.com/aging-population/40151

Elo, I. (1997). Adult mortality among Asian Americans and Pacific Islanders: A review of the evidence. In K. S. Markides & M. R. Miranda (Eds.), *Minorities, aging and health* (pp. 41–78). Thousand Oaks, CA: Sage.

Experience Corps. (2005). *Fact sheet on aging in America*. Retrieved May 27, 2005, from http://www.experiencecorps.org/research/factsheet.html

Federal Interagency Forum on Aging-Related Statistics. (November 2004). *Older Americans 2004: Key indicators of well-being*. Washington, DC: U.S. Government Printing Office. Retrieved May 27, 2005, from http://www.agingstats.gov/chartbook2004/default.htm

Federal Interagency Forum on Aging-Related Statistics. (May 2006). *Older Americans update 2006: Key indicators of well-being*. Washington, DC: U.S. Government Printing Office. Retrieved September 17, 2007, from http://www.agingstats.gov/agingstatsdotnet/Main_Site/Default.aspx

Fleming, K., Evans, J. M., & Chutka, D. S. (2003). A cultural and economic history of old age in America. *Mayo Clinic Proceedings, 78*(7), 914–921.

Gavan, C. S. (2003). Successful aging families: A challenge for nurses. *Holistic Nursing Practice, 17*(1), 11–18.

Glass, T. (2003). Assessing the success of successful aging. *Annals of Internal Medicine, 139*(5, Part 1), 382–383.

Griffith, R. W. (2004). *The centenarian study*. Retrieved April 18, 2005, from http://www.healthandage.com

Hazuda, H. P., & Espino, D. V. (1997). Aging, chronic disease, and physical disability in Hispanic elderly. In K. S. Markides & M. R. Miranda (Eds.), *Minorities, aging and health* (pp. 127–148). Thousand Oaks, CA: Sage.

He, W. (2000). *The older foreign-born population of the United States: 2000*. Washington, DC: U.S. Census Bureau, U.S. Department of Health and Human Services, U.S. Department of Commerce.

Illinois Department on Aging. (2001). A look at health issues for older minorities. *Facts on Aging*, 29. Retrieved April 18, 2005, from http://www.state.il.us

Jacobs, H. (1861). *Incidents in the life of a slave girl: Written by herself.* Child, M. L. (Ed.). Boston: Published for the author. Retrieved June 5, 2005, from http://afroamhistory.about.com/library/bljacobs_chapter3.htm

Kitano, H. H., Tazuko, S., & Kitano, K. J. (1997). Asian American elderly mental health. In K. S. Markides & M. R. Miranda (Eds.), *Minorities, aging and health* (pp. 295–315). Thousand Oaks, CA: Sage.

Kramer, B. J. (1997). Chronic diseases in American Indian populations. In K. S. Markides & M. R. Miranda (Eds.), *Minorities, aging and health*. Thousand Oaks, CA: Sage.

Markides, K. S. & Miranda, M. R. (Eds.). (1997). *Minorities, aging and health*. Thousand Oaks, CA: Sage.

McMahon, P. (2003). Aging inmates present prison crisis. *USA Today*. Retrieved June 6, 2005, from http://www.usatoday.com/news/nation/2003-08-10-prison-inside-usat_x.htm

Merck Institute of Aging and Health (MIAH), Centers for Disease Control and Prevention (CDC), & Gerontological Society of America (GSA). (2004). *The state of aging and health in America 2004*. Retrieved May 20, 2005, from http://www.cdc.gov/aging/pdf/State_of_Aging_and_Health_in_America_2004.pdf

Mitka, M. (2004). Aging prisoners stressing the health care system. *Journal of the American Medical Association, 292*(4), 423–424.

Munnell, A. H. (2004). Population aging: It's not just the baby boom. *An Issue in Brief: Center for Retirement Research at Boston College, 16*, 1–7.

Perls, T. *The living to 100 life expectancy calculator*. Retrieved September 14, 2008, from http://calculator.livingto100.com/calculator

Perls, T., Silver, M., & Lauerman, J. (1999). *Living to 100: Lessons in living to your maximum*. New York: Basic Books.

The Poorhouse Story. (2005). Retrieved June 5, 2005, from http://www.poorhousestory.com/index.htm

Reed, D., Foley, D., White, L. R., Heimovitz, H., Burchfiel, C. M., Masaki, K., et al. (1998). Predictors of healthy aging in men with high life expectancies. *American Journal of Public Health, 88*(10), 1463–1468.

Ross, H. (2000). Growing older: Health issues for minorities: Closing the gap. *Newsletter of the Office of Minority Health*. Washington, DC: U.S. Department of Health and Human Services.

Sahyoun, N. R., Lentzner, H., Hoyert, D., & Robinson, K. N. (2001). Trends in causes of death among the elderly. *Aging Trends*, 1. Hyattsville, MD: National Center for Health Statistics.

Schreiber, C. (July 19, 1999). Behind bars: Aging prison population challenges correctional health system. *NurseWeek*. Retrieved June 6, 2005, from http://www.nurseweek.com/features/99-7/prison.html

U.S. Census Bureau. (2001). *The 65 years and over population: 2000. Census 2000 Brief.* Washington, DC: U.S. Department of Commerce, Economics and Statistics Administration.

U.S. Census Bureau. (2006). *Facts for features. Older Americans month: May 2006*. Retrieved September 17, 2007, from http://www.census.gov/Press-Release/www/releases/archives/facts_for features_special_editions/006537.html

U.S. Department of Health and Human Services. (1999). *Centenarians in the United States*. Available at http://www.census.gov/prod/99pubs/p23-199.pdf

Valliant, G. E., & Mukamal, K. (2001). Successful aging. *American Journal of Psychiatry, 158*(6), 839–847.

vonFaber, M., Bootsma-van der Wiel, A., van Exel, E., Gussekloo, J., Lagaay, A., van Dongen, E., et al. (2001). Successful aging in oldest old: Who can be characterized as successfully aged? *Archives of Internal Medicine, 161*(22), 2694–2700.

Winokur, J. (2005). *Aging in America*. Retrieved May 27, 2005, from http://www.msnbc.com/modules/ps/010524_AgingInAmerica/intro.asp?0sp=n9c1

CHAPTER 3

Theories of Aging

Jean Lange, PhD, RN, CNL

Sheila Grossman, PhD, FNP, APRN-BC

LEARNING OBJECTIVES

At the end of this chapter, the reader will be able to:

- Identify the major theories of aging.
- Compare the similarities and differences between biological and psychosocial theories.
- Describe the process of aging using a biological and a psychosocial perspective.
- Analyze the rationale for using multiple theories of aging to describe the complex phenomenon of aging.
- Describe a general theoretical framework, taken from all of the aging theories, that will assist nurses in making clinical decisions in gerontology.

KEY TERMS

- Apoptosis
- Free radicals
- Immunomodulation
- Lipofuscin
- Melatonin
- Mitochondria
- Nonstochastic theories of aging
- Reactive oxygen species (ROS)
- Senescence
- Stochastic theories of aging
- Telomerase
- Telomere

From the beginning of time, the elusive phenomenon of preserving youth has been a topic of discussion in science, health care, technology, and everyday life. Is there anyone who would not be interested in knowing how the human organism ages? Doesn't everyone want to live a long and healthy life? There are few who would not want to see what the future holds for our bodies and minds; even more curiosity surrounds what advances have been made or will possibly be made to alter and slow the aging process. Understanding what knowledge theories of aging have generated and reviewing the validity of these findings and how they impact evolution and scientific advances is a first step toward understanding the mystery of aging. Troen (2003) suggests: "The beneficial paradox may be that the maximum lifespan potential of humans may have been achieved, in part, due to our ability to grow old" (p. 5).

Complex physiological, social, economic, and psychological challenges present themselves as we age. Older adults may face declines in health and physical functioning that may necessitate moving to supportive care environments that drain financial resources. Death of friends or loved ones, grappling with questions about the meaning of life, maintaining a satisfactory quality of life in the face of increasing disability, adapting to retirement, and contemplating death are just a few of the psychological challenges that aging adults may face. Theories that can effectively guide nursing practice with older adults must be comprehensive yet consider individual differences. Cultural, spiritual, regional, socioeconomic, educational, and environmental factors as well as health status impact older adults' perceptions and choices about their health care needs. According to Haight and colleagues, "a good gerontological theory integrates knowledge, tells how and why phenomena are related, leads to prediction, and provides process and understanding. In addition, a good theory must be holistic and take into account all that impacts on a person throughout a lifetime of aging" (Haight, Barba, Tesh, & Courts, 2002, p. 14).

Since the early 1950s, sociologists, psychologists, and biologists have proposed varied theories about the aging process. Although there is increased emphasis in the nursing literature on issues regarding the growing elderly population, limited work has been done to develop nursing-specific aging theories. Increasingly, there is recognition that aging is a distinct discipline that requires aging theories having an interdisciplinary perspective. A recent model by Alkema and Alley (2006) attempts to address this need. The purpose of this chapter is to review the chronological development of biopsychosocial aging theories, the evidence supporting or refuting these theories, and their application to nursing practice. CINAHL, the National Library of Medicine, the Web of Science, PsycINFO, and Sociological Abstracts databases were reviewed to assess support for and clinical application of the theories of aging.

PSYCHOSOCIAL THEORIES OF AGING

The earliest theories on aging came from the psychosocial disciplines (**Table 3-1**). Psychosocial theories attempt to explain aging in terms of behavior, personality, and attitude change. Development is viewed as a lifelong process characterized by transitions. Psychological theories are concerned with personality or ego development and the accompanying challenges associated with various life stages. How mental processes, emotions, attitudes, motivation, and personality influence adaptation to physical and social demands are central issues.

Sociological theorists consider how changing roles, relationships, and status within a culture or society impact the older adult's ability to adapt. Societal norms can affect how individuals envision their role and function within that society, and thus impact role choices as well as how roles are enacted. The role of women in the United States has been redefined greatly since the 1960s. Such cohort or generational variables are a key component of sociological theories of aging.

Sociological Theories of Aging

Activity Theory

Sociological theorists have attempted to explain older adult behavior in relationship to society with such concepts as disengagement, activity, and continuity. One of the earliest theories addressing the aging process was begun by Havighurst and Albrecht in 1953 when they discussed the concept of activity engagement and positive adaptation to aging. From studying a sample of adults, they concluded that society expects retired older adults to remain active contributors. Activity theory was conceived as an actual theory in 1963 and purports that remaining occupied and involved is a necessary ingredient to satisfying late-life (Havighurst, Neugarten, & Tobin, 1963). The authors do not qualify the activity characteristics that are most directly linked to life satisfaction. Havighurst and Albrecht associate activity with psychosocial health and suggest activity as a means to prolong middle age and delay the negative effects of old age. An assumption of this theory is that inactivity negatively impacts one's self-concept and perceived quality of life and hastens aging.

Arguments against this point of view are that it fails to consider that activity choices are often constrained by physical, economic, and social resources. Furthermore, roles assumed by older adults are highly influenced by societal expectations (Birren & Schroots, 2001). Maddox (1963) suggests, however, that leisure time presents new opportunities for activities and roles such as community service that may be more consistent with these limitations. A second criticism of activity theory is the unproven assertion that continued activity delays onset of the negative effects of aging.

Despite these criticisms, the central theme of activity theory—that remaining active in old age is desirable—is supported by most research. Lemon and colleagues found a direct relationship between role and activity engagement and life satisfaction

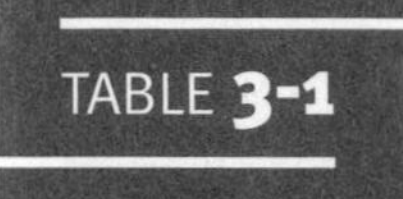

TABLE 3-1 Psychosocial Theories of Aging

Theory	Description
Sociological Theories	Changing roles, relationships, status, and generational cohort impact the older adult's ability to adapt.
Activity	Remaining occupied and involved is necessary to a satisfying late-life.
Disengagement	Gradual withdrawal from society and relationships serves to maintain social equilibrium and promote internal reflection.
Subculture	The elderly prefer to segregate from society in an aging subculture sharing loss of status and societal negativity regarding the aged. Health and mobility are key determinants of social status.
Continuity	Personality influences roles and life satisfaction and remains consistent throughout life. Past coping patterns recur as older adults adjust to physical, financial, and social decline and contemplate death. Identifying with one's age group, finding a residence compatible with one's limitations, and learning new roles postretirement are major tasks.
Age stratification	Society is stratified by age groups that are the basis for acquiring resources, roles, status, and deference from others. Age cohorts are influenced by their historical context and share similar experiences, beliefs, attitudes, and expectations of life course transitions.
Person-Environment-Fit	Function is affected by ego strength, mobility, health, cognition, sensory perception, and the environment. Competency changes one's ability to adapt to environmental demands.
Gerotranscendence	The elderly transform from a materialistic/rational perspective toward oneness with the universe. Successful transformation includes an outward focus, accepting impending death, substantive relationships, intergenerational connectedness, and unity with the universe.
Psychological Theories	Explain aging in terms of mental processes, emotions, attitudes, motivation, and personality development that is characterized by life stage transitions.
Human needs	Five basic needs motivate human behavior in a lifelong process toward need fulfillment.
Individualism	Personality consists of an ego and personal and collective unconsciousness that views life from a personal or external perspective. Older adults search for life meaning and adapt to functional and social losses.
Stages of personality development	Personality develops in eight sequential stages with corresponding life tasks. The eighth phase, integrity versus despair, is characterized by evaluating life accomplishments; struggles include letting go, accepting care, detachment, and physical and mental decline.
Life-course/life span development	Life stages are predictable and structured by roles, relationships, values, and goals. Persons adapt to changing roles and relationships. Age group norms and characteristics are an important part of the life course.
Selective optimization with compensation	Individuals cope with aging losses through activity/role selection, optimization, and compensation. Critical life points are morbidity, mortality, and quality of life. Selective optimization with compensation facilitates successful aging.

among older adults (Lemon, Bengston, & Peterson, 1972). The authors also observed that the quality of activities, as perceived by older adults, is more important than the quantity. Other investigators add that informal activities such as meeting friends for lunch or pursuing hobbies through group activities are more likely to improve life satisfaction than formal or solitary activities (Longino & Kart, 1982). In a more recent study of older Americans, participation in shared tasks was an important predictor of life satisfaction, particularly among retirees (Harlow & Cantor, 1996). According to Schroots (1996), successful aging means being capable of doing activities that are important to the older adult despite limitations. One recent study, however, found that in a convenience sample of 386 older women, engaging in the social activity of shopping was not predictive of life satisfaction (Hyun-Mee & Miller, 2007). This suggests that the type of activity may be an important consideration rather than merely the frequency of engagement.

> **Notable Quotes**
>
> *"Grow old along with me! The best is yet to be."*
>
> —Robert Browning

Disengagement Theory

In stark contrast to activity theorists, sociologists Cumming and Henry (1961) assert that aging is characterized by gradual disengagement from society and relationships. The authors contend that this separation is desired by society and older adults, and serves to maintain social equilibrium. Persons are freed from social responsibilities and gain time for internal reflection, while the transition of responsibility from old to young promotes societal functioning without interruption from lost members. Diminishing social contacts lead to further disengagement in a cyclical process that is systematic and inevitable. The outcome of disengagement, authors propose, is a new equilibrium that is ideally satisfying to both the individual and society. In support of this theory, a recent instrument measuring change in activity among older adults supports a tendency for less social contact among those over age 75 (Adams, 2004). The author reports, "In almost all instances, the group 75 years old and older reported a higher proportion of disengaged responses; they were particularly less invested than their younger counterparts in keeping up with hobbies, making plans for the future, making and creating things, and taking care of others" (p. 102).

The emphasis this theory places on social withdrawal has been challenged by other theorists who argue that a key element of life satisfaction among older adults appears to be engagement in meaningful relationships and activities (Baltes, 1987; Lemon et al., 1972; Neumann, 2000; Schroots, 1996). Others contend that the decision to withdraw varies across individuals and that disengagement theory fails to account for differences in sociocultural settings and environmental opportunities (Achenbaum & Bengtson, 1994; Marshall, 1996). Rapkin and Fischer (1992) found that demographic disadvantages and age-related transitions were related to a greater desire for disengagement, support, and stability. Elders who were married and healthy were more likely to report a desire for an energetic lifestyle. Cumming and Henry's notion of a necessary fit between society's needs and older adult activity is supported, however (Back, 1980; Birren & Schroots, 2001; Riley, Johnson, & Foner, 1972). Until recently, Social Security laws placed economic barriers against retirement before the mid-60s, but as years of healthy life expectancy increase, society is reframing its notions about the capability of older adults to make valuable contributions (Uhlenberg, 1992). Many adults are working past retirement age or begin part-time work in a new field. Others are actively engaged in a variety of volunteer projects that may substantially benefit their communities. The many examples of what is now termed "successful aging" are challenging the common association of aging with disease.

Subculture Theory

Unlike activity theorists, Rose (1965) views older adults as a unique subculture within society formed as a defensive response to society's negative attitudes and the loss of status that accompanies aging. As in disengagement theory, Rose proposes that although this subculture segregates the elderly from the rest of society, older adults prefer to interact among themselves. Rose contends that in the United States, one's degree of health and mobility is more critical in defining social status than occupation, education, or income. Older adults have a social disadvantage regarding status and associated respect because of the functional decline that accompanies aging.

Rose's theory argues for social reform. Growing numbers of older adults make it necessary to pay more attention to the needs of this age group and are challenging the prevailing view of aging as negative, undesirable, burdensome, and lacking status. Questions are beginning to be asked about whether society should be more supportive of older adults in terms of their environment, health care, work opportunities, and social resources. The emphasis on whether societal or older adults' needs take precedence is beginning to shift in favor of older adults. McMullen (2000) argues that sociological theories need to more clearly address the diversity among older adults as well as the disparity from other age groups. Research that supports or refutes Rose's theory is needed.

Continuity Theory

In the late 1960s, Havighurst and colleagues recognized that neither activity nor disengagement theories fully explain successful aging from a sociological point of view (Havighurst, Neugarten, & Tobin, 1968). Borrowing from psychology, they hypothesized that personality influences the roles one assumes, how roles are enacted, and one's satisfaction with living. They explained their new perspective in the continuity theory, also known as development theory. Continuity theory suggests that personality is well developed by the time one reaches old age and tends to remain consistent across the life span. Coping and personality patterns provide clues as to how an aging individual will adjust to changes in health, environment, or socioeconomic conditions, and what activities he or she will choose to engage in; thus, continuity theory acknowledges that individual differences produce varied responses to aging.

Havighurst and associates identified four personality types from their observations of older adults: integrated, armored-defended, passive-dependent, and unintegrated. Integrated personality types have adjusted well to aging, as evidenced by activity engagement that may be broad (reorganizers), more selective (focused), or disengaged. Armored-defended individuals tend to continue the activities and roles held during middle age, whereas passive-dependent persons are either highly dependent or exhibit disinterest in the external world. Least well-adjusted are unintegrated personality types who fail to cope with aging successfully. Havighurst (1972) later defined adjusting to physical, financial, and social decline; contemplating death; and developing a personal and meaningful perspective on the end of life as the tasks of older adulthood. Successful accomplishment of these tasks is evidenced by identifying with one's age group, finding a living environment that is compatible with physical functioning, and learning new societal roles postretirement.

Research suggests that self-perception of personality remains stable over time, and attitude and degree of adaptation to old age are related to life satisfaction. When older adults were asked how they thought they had changed over the years, almost all respondents thought they were still essentially the same person. Degree of continuity related to a more positive affect in these subjects (Troll & Skaff, 1997). In another study, Efklides and colleagues investigated effects of demographics, health status, attitude, and adaptation to old age on quality of life perceptions among older adults. The authors reported that positive attitude and adaptation to old age were associated with better perceptions about quality of life in this Greek sample (Efklides, Kalaitzidou, & Chankin, 2003). Recently, Agahi and colleagues used continuity theory to examine patterns of change in older adults' participation in leisure activities over time. Consistent with continuity as well as activity and disengagement theories, the authors found that active participation tends to decline over time, and that lifelong participation patterns predict involvement later in life (Agahi, Ahacic, & Parker, 2006). Critics of continuity theory, however, caution that the social context within which one ages may be more important than personality in determining what and how roles are played (Birren & Schroots, 2001).

Age Stratification Theory

In the 1970s, sociologists began to examine the interdependence between older adults and society, recognizing that aging and society are interrelated and cause reciprocal changes to individuals, age group cohorts, and society (Riley et al., 1972). Riley and colleagues observed that society is stratified into different age categories that are the basis for acquiring resources, roles, status, and deference from others in society. In addition, age cohorts are influenced by the historical context in which they live; thus, age cohorts and corresponding roles vary across generations. People born in the same cohort have similar experiences with shared meanings, ideologies, orientations, attitudes, and values as well as expectations regarding the timing of life course transitions. Individuals in different generations have different experiences that may cause them to age in different ways (Riley, 1994).

Age stratification transitioned aging theory from a focus on the individual to a broader context that alerted gerontologists to the influence of cohort groups and the socioeconomic and political impact on how individuals age (Marshall, 1996). Uhlenburg (1996) borrowed from age stratification theory in developing a framework for understanding what social changes are needed to reduce the burden that aging cohorts place on society in terms of their care needs at different stages of later life.

Newsom and Schulz (1996) demonstrated that physical impairment is associated with fewer social contacts, less social support, depression, and lower life satisfaction. This finding suggests that social networks are an important element in how individuals age. Yin and Lai (1983) used age stratification theory to explain the changing status of older adults due to differences among cohort groups. Investigators studying age segregation versus integration in residential settings learned that outcomes were less favorable among settings with single cohort groups (Hagestad & Dannefer, 2002; Uhlenberg, 2000).

Person-Environment-Fit Theory

In addition to the broadened view of aging that emerged in the 1970s, another shift in aging theory in the early 1980s blended existing theories from different disciplines. Lawton's (1982) person-environment-fit theory introduced functional competence in relationship to the environment as a central theme. Functional competence is affected by multiple intrapersonal conditions such as ego strength, motor skills, biologic health, cognitive capacity, and sensori-perceptual capacity as well as external conditions posed by the environment. The degree of competency may change as one ages, affecting functional ability in relationship to environmental demands. A person's ability to meet these demands is affected by his or her level of functioning and influences the ability to adapt to the environment. Those functioning at lower levels can tolerate fewer environmental demands.

Lawton's (1982) theory is useful for exploring optimal environments for older adults with functional limitations and identifying needed modifications in older adult residential settings. Building on Lawton's work, Wahl (2001) developed six models to explain relationships between aging and the environment, home, institution, and relocation decision making. O'Connor and Vallerand (1994) used Lawton's theory to examine the relationship between long-term care residents' adjustment and their motivational style and environment. Older adults with self-determined motivational styles were better adjusted when they lived in homes that provided opportunities for freedom and choice, whereas residents with less self-determined motivational styles were better adjusted when they lived in high constraint environments. The authors conclude that their findings support the person-environment-fit theory of adjustment in old age.

In a more recent study, Iwarsson's (2005) findings partially support a relationship between environmental fit and functioning. Dependence with activities of daily living (ADLs) was significantly related to activities of daily living among only the most frail older adults in his longitudinal study.

Gerotranscendence Theory

One of the most recent aging theories is Tornstam's (1994) theory of gerotranscendence. This theory proposes that aging individuals undergo a cognitive transformation from a materialistic, rational perspective toward oneness with the universe. Characteristics of successful transformation include a more outward or external focus, accepting impending death without fear, an emphasis on substantive relationships, a sense of connectedness with preceding and future generations, and spiritual unity with the universe. Gerotranscendence borrows from

BOX 3-1 Research Highlight

Aim: This longitudinal study investigated the patterns of leisure activities among Swedish men and women over a 34-year period.

Methods: Responses to questions about leisure activities were collected from a nationally representative data set of 495 Swedish men and women who participated in a series of three interviews between 1968 and 1992. Participants' ages ranged from 43–65 during the first interview and from 77–99 during the final interview. A regression analysis was used to determine whether mobility, vision, cognition, age, gender, or education would predict participation in leisure activities. Continuity theory was used as a theoretical framework for the study.

Findings: The typical participant was a cognitively intact, 83-year-old female with a grade-school level of education and some mobility impairment by the conclusion of the study. Declining participation over time in leisure activities (e.g., reading, hobbies, gardening, fishing, hunting, cultural activities, coursework, dance) was the predominant pattern ($p < .001$). Only eating out and attendance at religious services did not significantly decline. The tendency to participate in activities at a younger age predicted the likelihood of participation at later ages; gender, education, and age were not predictive. Impaired mobility, vision, and cognition were predictors for the degree of engagement in activities such as dancing, eating out, gardening, hobbies, and reading. Impaired mobility or cognition had a significantly predicted participation in four of these five activities; visual impairment affected only engagement in reading and hobbies.

Application to practice: These findings are consistent with continuity as well as activity and disengagement theories. The authors report that active participation tends to decline over time, and that lifelong participation patterns do predict involvement later in life. Encouraging elders to continue the activities they enjoyed earlier in life is suggested.

Source: Agahi, N., Ahacic, K., & Parker, M. G. (2006). Continuity of leisure participation from middle age to old age. *The Journals of Gerontology, 61B*(6), S340–S346.

disengagement theory but does not accept the idea that social disengagement is a necessary and natural development. Tornstam asserts that activity and participation must be the result of one's own choices, which differ from one person to another. Control over one's life in all situations is essential for the person's adaptation to aging as a whole.

Gerotranscendence has been tested in recent studies. In an ongoing longitudinal study based on the principles of gerodynamics, Schroots (2003) is investigating how people manage their lives, cope with transformations, and react to affective-positive and negative life events. In nursing, Wadensten (2002) used the theory of gerotranscendence to develop guidelines for care of older adults in a nursing home. The results indicate that these guidelines may be useful for facilitating the process of gerotranscendence in nursing home residents.

Psychological Theories of Aging

Human Needs Theory

At the same time as activity theory was being developed, Maslow (1954), a psychologist, published the human needs theory. In this theory, Maslow surmised that a hierarchy of five needs motivates human behavior: physiologic, safety and security, love and belonging, self-esteem, and self-actualization. These needs are prioritized such that more basic needs like physiological functioning or safety take precedence over personal growth needs (love and belonging, self-esteem, and self-actualization). Movement is multidirectional and dynamic in a lifelong process toward need fulfillment. Self-actualization requires the freedom to express and pursue personal goals and be creative in an environment that is stimulating and challenging.

Although Maslow does not specifically address old age, it is clear that physical, economic, social, and environmental constraints can impede need fulfillment of older adults. Maslow asserts that failure to grow leads to feelings of failure, depression, and the perception that life is meaningless. Since inception, Maslow's theory has been applied to varied age groups in many disciplines. Ebersole, Hess, and Luggen (2004) link the tasks of aging described by several theorists (Butler & Lewis, 1982; Havighurst, 1972; Peck, 1968) to the basic needs in Maslow's model. Jones and Miesen (1992) used Maslow's hierarchy to present a nursing care model for working with aged persons with specific needs in an attempt to relate all patient needs to universal, rather than exceptional, needs. The model is designed to be used by caregivers in residential settings.

Theory of Individualism

Like Maslow's theory, Jung's theory of individualism is not specific to aging. Jung (1960) proposes a lifespan view of personality development rather than attainment of basic needs. Jung defines personality as being composed of an ego or self-identity with a personal and collective unconsciousness. Personal unconsciousness is the private feelings and perceptions surrounding significant persons or life events. The collective unconscious is shared by all persons and contains latent memories of human origin. The collective unconscious is the foundation of personality on which the personal unconsciousness and ego are built. Individual personalities tend to view life primarily either through the self or through others; thus, extroverts are more concerned with the world around them, whereas introverts interpret experiences from the personal perspective. As individuals age, Jung proposes that elders engage in an "inner search" to critique their beliefs and accomplishments. According to Jung, successful aging means acceptance of the past and an ability to cope with functional decline and loss of significant others. Neugarten (1968) supports Jung's association of aging and introspection and asserts that "interiority" promotes positive inner growth. Subsequent theorists also describe introspection as a part of healthy aging (Erikson, 1963; Havighurst et al., 1968).

Stages of Personality Development Theory

Similar to other psychologists' theories at the time, Erikson's theory focuses on individual development. According to Erikson (1963), personality develops in eight sequential stages that have a corresponding life task that one may succeed at or fail to accomplish. Progression to a subsequent life stage requires that tasks at prior stages be completed successfully. Older adults experience the developmental stage known as "ego integrity versus despair." Erikson proposes that this final phase of development is characterized by evaluating one's life and accomplishments for meaning. In later years, Erikson and colleagues expanded upon his original description of integrity versus despair, noting that older adults struggle with letting go, accepting the care of others, detaching from life, and physical and mental decline (Erikson, Erikson, & Kivnick, 1986).

Several authors have expanded upon Erikson's work. Peck (1968) refined the task within Erikson's stage of ego integrity versus despair into three challenges: ego differentiation versus work role reoccupation, body transcendence versus body preoccupation, and ego transcendence versus ego preoccupation. Major issues such as meaningful life after retirement, the empty nest syndrome, dealing with the functional decline of aging, and contemplating one's mortality are consistent with Peck's conceptualization. Butler and Lewis (1982) later defined the challenges of late life as adjusting to infirmity, developing satisfaction with one's lived life, and preparing for death, mirroring those tasks described earlier by Peck.

Erikson's theory is widely employed in the behavioral sciences. In nursing, Erikson's model is often used as a framework for examining the challenges faced by different age groups. In a study of frail elderly men and women, Neumann (2000) used Erikson's theoretical framework when asking participants to discuss their perceptions about the meaning of their lives. She found that older adults who expressed higher levels of meaning and energy described a sense of connectedness, self-worth, love, and respect that was absent among participants who felt unfulfilled. This finding is consistent with the potential for positive or negative outcomes described by Erikson and colleagues (1986) in his stage of "integrity versus despair." In a qualitative study with six participants, five of whom were women, Holm and colleagues examined the value of storytelling among dementia patients. The investigators told stories linked to Erikson's developmental stages to stimulate sharing among the participants. The authors report that these stages were clearly evident among the experiences related by the participants (Holm, Lepp, & Ringsberg, 2005).

Life-Course (Life Span Development) Paradigm

In the late 1970s, the predominant theme of behavioral psychology moved toward the concept of "life course," in which life, although unique to each individual, is divided into stages with predictable patterns (Back, 1980). The significance of this shift was the inclusion of late as well as early life. Most theorists up to this point had focused primarily on childhood in their research. The substance of the life-course paradigm drew from the work of a European psychologist in the 1930s (Bühler, 1933). This new emphasis on adulthood occurred because of a demographic shift toward increasing numbers of older adults, the emergence of gerontology as a specialty, and the availability of subjects from longitudinal studies of childhood begun during the 1920s and 1930s (Baltes, 1987).

The central concepts of the life-course perspective blend key elements in psychological theories such as life stages, tasks, and personality development with sociological concepts such as role behavior and the interrelationship between individuals and society. The central tenet of life-course is that life occurs in stages that are structured according to one's roles, relationships, internal values, and goals. Individuals may choose their goals but are limited by external constraints. Goal achievement is associated with life satisfaction (Bühler, 1933). Individuals must adapt to changed roles and relationships that occur throughout life, such as getting married, finishing school, completing military service, getting a job, and retiring (Cunningham & Brookbank, 1988). Successful adaptation to life change may necessitate revising beliefs in order to be consistent with societal expectations. The life-course paradigm is concerned with understanding age group norms and their characteristics. Since the 1970s, the work of many behavioral psychologists such as Elder, Hareven, and Jackson has emerged from the life-course perspective, which remains a dominant theme in the psychology literature today. Selective optimization with compensation, discussed in the following section, is one example of a theory that emerged from the life-course perspective.

Selective Optimization with Compensation Theory

Baltes's (1987) theory of successful aging emerged from his study of psychological processes across the lifespan and, like earlier theories, focuses on the individual. He asserts that individuals learn to cope with the functional losses of aging through processes of selection, optimization, and compensation. Aging individuals become more selective in activities and roles as limitations present themselves; at the same time, they choose those activities and roles that are most satisfying (optimization). Finally, individuals adapt by seeking alternatives when functional limits prohibit sustaining former roles or activities. As people age, they pass through critical life points related to morbidity, mortality, and quality of life. The outcome of these critical junctures may result in lower or higher order functioning that is associated with higher or lower risk, respectively, for mortality. Selective optimization with compensation is a positive coping process that facilitates successful aging (Baltes & Baltes, 1990).

Much of the research testing psychosocial theories centers on life-course concepts (Baltes, 1987; Caspi, 1987; Caspi & Elder, 1986; Quick & Moen, 1998; Schroots, 2003). In an ongoing longitudinal study called "Life-Course Dynamics," Shroots examines the self-organization of behavior over the course of life. He has found that life structure tends to be consistent over time and is influenced by life events and experiences. The relationship of life events to structure does change, however, as we age. In an effort to outline the temporal and situational parameters of social life, Caspi (1987) developed a model for personality analysis using life-course concepts such as interactions among personality, age-based roles, and social transitions in a historical context. Life-course principles have also been used to examine gender differences in retirement satisfaction. Quick and Moen (1988) report that retirement quality for women is associated with good health, a continuous career, earlier retirement, and a good postretirement income. For men, good health, an enjoyable career, low work-role prominence, preretirement planning, and retiring voluntarily impacted satisfaction. The authors conclude that a gender-sensitive life-course approach to life transitions is essential.

Caspi and Elder (1986) criticized the life-course perspective of aging because it assumes that adaptation is governed by factors beyond the immediate situation. In a small sample of women, the authors examined how social and psychological factors experienced by women in the 1930s relate to life satisfaction in their older age. They report relationships among intellect, social activity, and life satisfaction in older, working-class women, but emotional health was a better predictor of life satisfaction among older women from higher class origins. Differences in how the Depression impacted adaptation to old age among women from distinct social classes are described. The authors conclude that the influence of social change on life course is intertwined with individual factors.

BIOLOGICAL THEORIES OF AGING

The biological theories explain the physiologic processes that change with aging. In other words, how is aging manifested on the molecular level in the cells, tissues, and body systems; how does the body-mind interaction affect aging; what biochemical processes impact aging; and how do one's chromosomes impact the overall aging process? Does each system age at the same rate? Does each cell in a system age at the same rate? How does chronological age influence an individual who is experiencing a pathophysiological disease process—how does the actual disease, as well as the treatment, which might include drugs, **immunomodulation**, surgery, or radiation, influence the organism? Several theories purport to explain aging at the molecular, cellular, organ, and system levels; however, no one predominant theory has evolved. Both genetics and environment influence the multifaceted phenomenon of aging.

Some aging theorists divide the biological theories into two categories:

1. A stochastic or statistical perspective, which identifies episodic events that happen throughout one's life that cause random cell damage and accumulate over time, thus causing aging
2. The nonstochastic theories, which view aging as a series of predetermined events happening to all organisms in a timed framework

Others believe aging is more likely the result of both programmed and stochastic concepts as well as allostasis, which is the process of achieving homeostasis via both behavioral and physiological change (Carlson & Chamberlain, 2005; Miquel, 1998). For example, there are specific programmed events in the life of a cell, but cells also accumulate genetic damage to the **mitochondria** due to **free radicals** and the loss of self-replication as they age. The following discussion presents descriptions of the different theories in the stochastic and nonstochastic theory categories, and also provides studies that support the various theoretical explanations.

Stochastic Theories

Studies of animals reflect that the effects of aging are primarily due to genetic defects, development, environment, and the inborn aging process (Harman, 2006). There is no set of statistics to validate that these same findings are true with human organisms. The following **stochastic theories of aging** are discussed in this section: free radical theory, Orgel/error theory, wear and tear theory, and connective tissue theory.

Free Radical Theory

Oxidative free radical theory postulates that aging is due to oxidative metabolism and the effects of free radicals, which are the end products of oxidative metabolism. Free radicals are produced when the body uses oxygen, such as with exercise. This theory emphasizes the significance of how cells use oxygen (Hayflick, 1985). Also known as superoxides, free radicals are thought to react with proteins, lipids, deoxyribonucleic acid (DNA), and ribonucleic acid (RNA), causing cellular damage. This damage accumulates over time and is thought to accelerate aging.

Free radicals are chemical species that arise from atoms as single unpaired electrons. Because a free radical molecule is unpaired it is able to enter reactions with other molecules, especially along membranes and with nucleic acids. Free radicals cause:

- Extensive cellular damage to DNA, which can cause malignancy and accelerated aging, due to oxidative modification of proteins that impact cell metabolism
- Lipid oxidation that damages phospholipids in cell membranes, thus affecting membrane permeability
- DNA strand breaks and base modifications that cause gene modulation

This cellular membrane damage causes other chemicals to be blocked from their regularly friendly receptor sites, thus mitigating other processes that may be crucial to cell metabolism. Mitochondrial deterioration due to oxidants causes a significant loss of cell energy and greatly decreases metabolism. Ames (2004) and Harman (1994) suggest some strategies to assist in delaying the mitochondrial decay, such as:

- Decrease calories in order to lower weight.
- Maintain a diet high in nutrients using antioxidants.
- Avoid inflammation.
- Minimize accumulation of metals in the body that can trigger free radical reactions.

Dufour and Larsson (2004) cite evidence of mitochondrial DNA damage accumulation and the aging process in mice. With the destruction of membrane integrity comes fluid and electrolyte loss or excess, depending on how the membrane was affected. Little by little there is more tissue deterioration. The older adult is more vulnerable to free radical damage because free radicals are attracted to cells that have transient or interrupted perfusion. Many older adults have decreased circulation because they have peripheral vascular as well as coronary artery disease. These diseases tend to cause heart failure that can be potentially worsened with fluid overload and electrolyte imbalance.

The majority of the evidence to support this theory is correlative in that oxidative damage increases with age. It is thought that people who limit calories, fat, and specific proteins in their diet may decrease the formation of free radicals. Roles of **reactive oxygen species (ROS)** are being researched in a variety of diseases such as atherosclerosis, vasospasms, cancers, trauma, stroke, asthma, arthritis, heart attack, dermatitis, retinal damage, hepatitis, and periodontitis (Lakatta, 2000). Lee, Koo, and Min (2004) report that antioxidant nutraceuticals are assisting in managing and, in some cases, delaying some of the manifestations of these diseases. Poon and colleagues (Poon, Calabrese, Scapagnini, & Butterfield, 2004) describe how two antioxidant systems (glutathione and heat shock proteins) are decreased in age-related degenerative neurological disorders. They also cite that free radical–mediated lipid peroxidation and protein oxidation affect central nervous system function. And now, for the first time, there is the possibility of investigating genetically altered animals to determine the impact of oxidative damage in aging (Bokov, Chaudhuri, & Richardson, 2004).

Examples of some sources of free radicals are listed in **Box 3-2**. In some instances, free radicals reacting with other molecules can form more free radicals, mutations, and malignancies. The free radical theory supports that as one ages, an accumulation of damage has been done to cells and, therefore, the organism ages. Grune and Davies

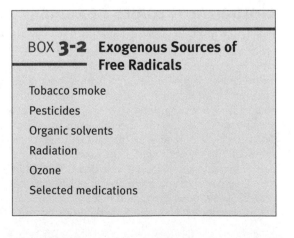

BOX 3-2 Exogenous Sources of Free Radicals

Tobacco smoke

Pesticides

Organic solvents

Radiation

Ozone

Selected medications

(2001) go so far as to describe the free radical theory of aging as "the only aging theory to have stood the test of time" (p. 41). They further describe how free radicals can generate cellular debris rich in lipids and proteins called **lipofuscin**, which older adults have more of when compared to younger adults. It is thought that lipofuscin, or age pigment, is a nondegradable material that decreases lysosomal function, which in turn impacts already disabled mitochondria (Brunk & Terman, 2002). Additionally lipofuscin is considered a threat to multiple cellular systems including the ubiquitin/proteasome pathway, which leads to cellular death (Gray & Woulfe, 2005).

Orgel/Error Theory

This theory suggests that, over time, cells accumulate errors in their DNA and RNA protein synthesis that cause the cells to die (Orgel, 1970). Environmental agents and randomly induced events can cause error, with ultimate cellular changes. It is well known that large amounts of x-ray radiation cause chromosomal abnormalities. Thus, this theory proposes that aging would not occur if destructive factors such as radiation did not exist and cause "errors" such as mutations and regulatory disorders.

Hayflick (1996) does not support this theory, and explains that all aged cells do not have errant proteins, nor are all cells found with errant proteins old.

Wear and Tear Theory

Over time, cumulative changes occurring in cells age and damage cellular metabolism. An example is the cell's inability to repair damaged DNA, as in the aging cell. It is known that cells in heart muscle, neurons, striated muscle, and the brain cannot replace themselves after they are destroyed by wear and tear. Researchers cite gender-specific effects of aging on adrenocorticotropic activity that are consistent with the wear and tear hypothesis of the ramifications of lifelong exposure to stress (Van Cauter, Leproult, & Kupfer, 1996). There is some speculation that excessive wear and tear due to exercising may accelerate aging by causing increased free radical production, which supports the idea that no one theory of aging incorporates all the causes of aging, but rather a combination of factors is responsible.

Studies of people with osteoarthritis suggest that cartilage cells age over time, and this degeneration is not due solely to strenuous exercise but also to general wear and tear. The studies point out that aged cells have lost the ability to counteract mechanical, inflammatory, and other injuries due to their senescence (Aigner, Rose, Martin, & Buckwalter, 2004).

Connective Tissue Theory

This theory is also referred to as cross-link theory, and it proposes that, over time, biochemical processes create connections between structures not normally connected. Several cross-linkages occur rapidly between 30 and 50 years of age. However, no research has identified anything that could stop these cross-links from occurring. Elastin dries up and cracks with age; hence, skin with less elastin (as with the older adult) tends to be dried and wrinkled. Over time, due to decreased extracellular fluid, numerous deposits of sodium, chloride, and calcium build up in the cardiovascular system. No clinical application studies were found to support this theory.

Nonstochastic Theories

The **nonstochastic theories of aging** are founded on a programmed perspective that is related to genetics or one's biological clock. Goldsmith (2004) suggests that aging is more likely to be an evolved beneficial characteristic and results from a complex structured process and not a series of random events. The following nonstochastic theories are discussed in this section: programmed theory, gene/biological clock theory, neuroendocrine theory, and immunologic/autoimmune theory.

Programmed Theory

As people age, more of their cells start to decide to commit suicide or stop dividing. The Hayflick phenomenon, or human fibroblast replicative **senescence** model, suggests that cells divide until they can no longer divide, whereupon the cell's infrastructure recognizes this inability to further divide and triggers the **apoptosis** sequence or death of the cell (Sozou & Kirkwood, 2001). Therefore, it is thought that cells have a finite doubling potential and become unable to replicate after they have done so a number of times. Human cells age each time they replicate due to the shortening of the telomere. **Telomeres** are the most distal appendages of the chromosome arms. This theory of programmed cell death is often alluded to when the aging process is discussed. The enzyme **telomerase**, also called a "cellular fountain of youth," allows human cells grown in the laboratory to continue to replicate long past the time they normally stop dividing. Normal human cells do not have telomerase.

It is hypothesized that some cancer, reproductive, and virus cells are not restricted, having a seemingly infinite doubling potential, and are thus immortal cell lines. This is because they have telomerase, which adds back DNA to the ends of the chromosomes. One reason for the Hayflick phenomenon may be that chromosome telomeres become reduced in length with every cell division and eventually become too short to allow further division. When telomeres are too short, the gene notes this and causes the cell to die or apoptosize. Shay and Wright (2001) suggest that telomerase-induced manipulations of telomere length are important to study to define the underlying genetic diseases and those genetic pathways that lead to cancer.

Although it is unknown what initial event triggers apoptosis, it is generally acknowledged that apoptosis is the mechanism of cell death (Thompson, 1995). Henderson (2006) reviewed how fibroblast senescence is connected to wound healing and discussed the implications of this theory for chronic wound healing. Increased cell apoptosis rates do cause organ dysfunction, and this is hypothesized to be the underlying basis of the pathophysiology of multiple organ dysfunction syndrome (MODS) (Papathanassoglou, Moynihan, & Ackerman, 2000).

Notable Quotes

"Positive aging means to love, to work, to learn something we did not know yesterday, and to enjoy the remaining precious moments with loved ones."

—George E. Vaillant, MD, from his book *Aging Well* (2002)

Gene/Biological Clock Theory

This theory explains that each cell, or perhaps the entire organism, has a genetically programmed aging code that is stored in the organism's DNA. Slagboom and associates (Slagboom, Bastian, Beekman, Wendendorf, & Meulenbelt, 2000) describe this theory as comprising genetic influences that predict physical condition, occurrence of disease, cause and age of death, and other factors that contribute to longevity.

A significant amount of research has been done on circadian rhythms and their influence on sleep, melatonin, and aging (Ahrendt, 2000; Moore, 1997; Richardson & Tate, 2000). These rhythms are defined as patterns of wakefulness and sleep that are integrated into the 24-hour solar day (Porth, 2005). The everyday rhythm of this cycle of sleep-wake intervals is part of a time-keeping framework created by an internal clock. Research has demonstrated that people who do not have exposure to time cues such as sunlight and clocks will automatically have sleep and wake cycles that include approximately 23.5 to 26.5 hours (Moore, Czeisler, & Richardson, 1983). This clock seems to be controlled by an area in the hypothalamus called the suprachiasmatic nucleus (SCN) that is located near the third ventricle and the optic chiasm. The SCN, given its anatomic location, does receive light and dark input from the retina, and demonstrates high neuronal firing during the day and low firing at night. The SCN is connected to the pituitary gland, explaining the diurnal regulation of growth hormone and cortisol. Also due to the linkage with the hypothalamus, autonomic nervous system, and brain stem reticular formation, diurnal changes in metabolism, body temperature, and heart rate and blood pressure are explained (Porth, 2005). It is thought that biological rhythms lose some rhythmicity with aging.

Melatonin is secreted by the pineal gland and is considered to be the hormone linked to sleep and wake cycles because there are large numbers of melatonin receptors in the SCN. Researchers have studied the administration of melatonin to humans and found a shift in humans' circadian rhythm similar to that caused by light (Ahrendt, 2000). The sleep-wake cycle changes with aging, producing more fragmented sleep, which is thought to be due to decreased levels of melatonin.

This theory indicates that there may be genes that trigger youth and general well-being as well as other genes that accelerate cell deterioration. Why do some people have gray hair in their late 20s and others live to be 60 or beyond before graying occurs? It is known that melanin is damaged with ultraviolet light and is the ingredient that keeps human skin resilient and unwrinkled. People who have extensive sun exposure have wrinkles earlier in life due to damage of collagen and elastin. But why, if we know that people have a programmed gene or genes that trigger aging, wouldn't we prevent the gene(s) from causing the problems they are intending to promote?

For example, hypertension, arthritis, hearing loss, and heart disease are among the most common chronic illnesses of older adults (Cobbs, Duthie, & Murphy, 1999). Each of these diseases has a genetic component to it. So if the health care profession can screen people when they are younger before they develop symptoms of target organ disease due to hypertension, loss of cartilage and hearing, and aspects of systolic and diastolic dysfunction, it is possible for people to live longer without experiencing the problems connected to these chronic illnesses.

The knowledge being acquired from the genome theory is greatly impacting the possibility of being able to ward off aging and disease. Studies of tumor suppressor gene replacement, prevention of angiogenesis with tumor growth, and regulation of programmed cell death are in process (Daniel & Smythe, 2003). Parr (1997) and Haq (2003) cite that caloric restriction extends mammalian life. By restricting calories there is a decreased need for insulin exposure, which consequently decreases growth factor exposure. Both insulin and growth factor are related to mammals' genetically determined clock controlling life span. So there is more evidence supportive of aging being influenced by key pathways such as the insulin-like growth factor path (Haq, 2003).

Neuroendocrine Theory

This theory describes a change in hormone secretion, such as with the releasing hormones of the hypothalamus and the stimulating hormones of the pituitary gland, which manage the thyroid, parathyroid, and adrenal glands, and how it influences the aging process. The following major hormones are involved with aging:

- Estrogen decreases thinning of bones, and when women age less estrogen is produced by the ovaries. As women grow older and experience menopause, adipose tissue becomes the major source of estrogen.
- Growth hormone is part of the process that increases bone and muscle strength. Growth hormone stimulates the release of insulin-like growth factor produced by the liver.
- Melatonin is produced by the pineal gland and is thought to be responsible for coordinating seasonal adaptations in the body.

There is a higher chance of excess or loss of glucocorticoids, aldosterone, androgens, triiodothyronine, thyroxine, and parathyroid hormone when the hypothalamus-pituitary-endocrine gland feedback system is altered. When the stimulating and releasing hormones of the pituitary and the hypothalamus are out of synch with the endocrine glands, an increase in disease is expected in multiple organs and systems. Of significance are the findings of Rodenbeck and Hajak (2001), who cite that with physiological aging and also with certain psychiatric disorders there is increased activation of the hypothalamus-pituitary-adrenal axis, which causes increased plasma cortisol levels. The increased cortisol levels can be linked with several diseases.

Holzenberger, Kappeler, and De Magalhaes Filho (2004) cite that by inactivating insulin receptors in the adipose tissue of mice, the life span of the mice increases because less insulin exposure occurs. This further supports that the neuroendocrine system is connected to life span regulation. Thyagarajan and Felten (2002) suggest that as one ages there is a loss of neuroendocrine transmitter function that is related to the cessation of reproductive cycles as well as the development of mammary and pituitary tumors.

Immunologic/Autoimmune Theory

This theory was proposed 40 years ago and describes the normal aging process of humans and animals as being related to faulty immunological function (Effros, 2004). There is a decreased immune function in the elderly. The thymus gland shrinks in size and ability to function. Thymus hormone levels are decreased at the age of 30 and are undetectable by the age of 60 (Williams, 1995). Involution of the thymus gland generally occurs at about 50 years. The elderly are more susceptible to infections as well as cancers. There is a loss of T-cell differentiation so that the body incorrectly perceives old, irregular cells as foreign bodies and attacks them.

There is also an increase in certain autoantibodies such as rheumatoid factor and a loss of interleukins. Some think that this change increases the chance of the older adult developing an autoimmune disease such as rheumatoid arthritis. Concurrently, resistance to tumor cells declines as one ages (Williams, 1995). Older adults are more prone to infection such as wound and respiratory infections, as well as to nosocomial infections if they are hospitalized.

Venjatraman and Fernandes (1997) cite that active and healthy older adults who participated in endurance exercises had a significantly increased natural killer cell function that, in turn, caused increased cytokine production and enhanced T-cell function, which improves general well-being. In contrast, those not exercising see a loss of immunological function as they age. The idea that increased exercise causes new growth of muscle fibers is not new, but that it also causes an increased immunological function, sense of well-being, and level of general health is significant. So it is supportive of the fact that there is a combination of factors that influence the prevention or, in some cases, the promotion of aging. Also important to note is that there should be a balance of exercising and resting because overdoing exercise can lead to injuries, and this would support the wear and tear theory of aging.

Table 3-2 summarizes the major theories of aging originating from a biological perspective. It seems that no one theory fully describes the etiology of aging. Kirkwood (2000) cites the impact that single gene mutations and various environmental interventions such as diet and stress have on aging.

TABLE **3-2** **Biological Theories of Aging**

Theory	Description
Stochastic Theories	Based on random events that cause cellular damage that accumulates as the organism ages.
Free radical theory	Membranes, nucleic acids, and proteins are damaged by free radicals, which causes cellular injury and aging.
Orgel/error theory	Errors in DNA and RNA synthesis occur with aging.
Wear and tear theory	Cells wear out and cannot function with aging.
Connective tissue/ cross-link theory	With aging, proteins impede metabolic processes and cause trouble with getting nutrients to cells and removing cellular waste products.
Nonstochastic Theories	Based on genetically programmed events that cause cellular damage that accelerates aging of the organism.
Programmed theory	Cells divide until they are no longer able to, and this triggers apoptosis or cell death.
Gene/biological clock theory	Cells have a genetically programmed aging code.
Neuroendocrine theory	Problems with the hypothalamus-pituitary-endocrine gland feedback system cause disease; increased insulin growth factor accelerates aging.
Immunological theory	Aging is due to faulty immunological function, which is linked to general well-being.

Of all the theories discussed in this section, it appears the gene theory and free radical theory seem to have the most support.

IMPLICATIONS FOR NURSING

For many years, nursing has incorporated psychosocial theories such as Erikson's personality development theory into its practice (Erikson, 1963). Psychological theories enlighten us about the developmental tasks and challenges faced by older adults and the importance of finding and accepting meaning in one's life. From sociologists, nursing has learned how support systems, functionality, activity and role engagement, cohorts, and societal expectations can influence adjustment to aging and life satisfaction. These broadly generalized theories, however, lack the specificity and holistic perspective needed to guide nursing care of older adults who have varied needs and come from different settings and sociocultural backgrounds (see **Case Study 3-1**).

In a quest for a theoretical framework to guide caregiving in nursing homes, Wadensten (2002) and Wadensten and Carlsson (2003) studied 17 nursing theories that were generated from the 1960s to the 1990s and found that none of the theorists discussed what aging is, nor did the theorists offer advice on how to apply their theory to caring for the older adult. Wadensten wrote that existing "nursing theories do not provide guidance on how to care for older people or on how to support them in the developmental process of aging. There is a need to develop a nursing care model that, more than contemporary theories, takes human aging into consideration" (2002, p. 119). Others concur that nursing needs to develop more situation-specific theories of aging to guide practice (Bergland & Kirkevold, 2001; Haight et al., 2002; Miller, 1990; Putnam, 2002). Two new theories, the functional consequences theory (Miller) and the theory of thriving (Haight et al.) are nurse authored and attempt to address this need.

Nursing Theories of Aging

FUNCTIONAL CONSEQUENCES THEORY

Functional consequences theory (**Table 3-3**) was developed to provide a guiding framework that would address older adults with physical impairment

Case Study 3-1

Mr. Ronald Dea, 64 years old, had been planning for many years to retire from his position as an accountant at a software company at his 65th birthday. Then his wife of 40 years died of lymphoma last year. He now finds that he only gets out of his house to work. He has let his racquetball membership, swimming club, and night out with his neighborhood friends slide. He finds he does not go out socially at all anymore except for visiting his two children and their families, who live out of town, when invited. He is no longer active in the Lions Club nor does he regularly attend his church where he and his wife used to be very involved.

Now he is deliberating whether to retire or not because he is aware that his work has become the only thing in his life. He is finding he does not have the energy he used to and that he is not excited about the weekend time he used to enjoy so much. He also has found he does not enjoy food shopping, so Mr. Dea generally buys his main meal at work and then snacks on crackers and cheese at night. He generally eats a donut or a bagel for breakfast. On the weekends, Mr. Dea stays in bed until noon and does not eat anything until night when he goes to the nearby fast food drive-in window to pick up fried chicken or has a pizza delivered.

He has not changed anything in his bedroom since his wife died nor removed any of his wife's belongings from the home. Mr. Dea has been delaying his regularly scheduled visits to his hematologist for management of his hemochromatosis. He has been gaining weight, approximately 14 pounds, since his wife was first diagnosed with cancer about 2½ years ago. He has also started smoking a cigar just about every evening. It was after his nightly smoke when he was walking up the hill in his backyard one evening that he fell and fractured his hip.

Mr. Dea has just been discharged home from the rehabilitation center, and you are the visiting nurse assigned to him. He has planned judiciously for his retirement but has been afraid to prepare the paperwork. Mr. Dea confides in you that he wants to remain independent as long as possible.

He shares his concerns with you and inquires what your opinion is of how he should proceed. One of his daughters is at his home for the next 2 weeks to assist him and is pushing him to retire and move in with her and her family.

Drawing from aging theory, what are some of the challenges you believe Mr. Dea is dealing with? What would you, given the knowledge you have learned regarding aging theories, recommend to Mr. Dea regarding retirement? Would you recommend he sell his house and move out of the town he has lived in for so many years? What other living arrangements might be conducive for Mr. Dea? Who would you suggest he and his daughter talk with regarding his everyday needs if he chooses to stay in his house during his convalescence? What are his priority needs for promoting his health? How would these be best managed? Use aging theory to support your responses.

and disability (Miller, 1990). Miller's theory borrows from several nursing and non-nursing theories including functional health patterns; systems theory; King's (1981) conceptualization of person, health, environment, and the nurse-client transaction; Lawton's (1982) person-environment fit; and Rose and Killien's (1983) conceptual work defining risk and vulnerability. Miller asserts that aging adults experience environmental and biopsychosocial consequences that impact their functioning. The nurse's role is to assess for age-related changes and accompanying risk factors, and to design interventions directed toward risk reduction and minimizing age-associated disability. Nursing's goal is to maximize functioning and minimize dependency to improve the safety and quality of living (Miller, 1990).

Functional consequences theory assumes that quality of life is integrated with functional capacity and dependency needs, and that positive consequences are possible despite age-related limitations. In addition to those experiencing negative functional consequences, Miller (1990) applies her theory to highly functioning older adults as well as to adult caregivers. She distinguishes the focus and goal of nursing interventions in varied settings (inpatient, outpatient, acute, or long-term care); thus, her theory can be used in many settings. Interventions are broadly interpreted as those of nurses, other health care providers, older adults, or significant others; therefore, this theory may be useful in other health care disciplines. This theory was used to create an assessment tool for the early detection of hospitalized elderly patients experiencing acute confusion and to prevent further complications (Kozak-Campbell & Hughes, 1996). Further testing is needed to determine the utility of the functional consequences theory in other settings.

Theory of Thriving

The theory of thriving (Haight et al., 2002) is based on the concept of failure to thrive and Bergland and Kirkevold's (2001) application of thriving to the experience of well-being among frail elders living in nursing homes. They discuss the concept in three

TABLE 3-3 Nursing Theories of Aging

Theory	Description
Functional consequences theory	Environmental and biopsychosocial consequences impact functioning. Nursing's role is risk reduction to minimize age-associated disability in order to enhance safety and quality of living.
Theory of thriving	Failure to thrive results from a discord between the individual and his or her environment or relationships. Nurses identify and modify factors that contribute to disharmony among these elements.

BOX 3-3 Web Exploration

End-of-Life Nursing Education Consortium (www.aacn.nche.edu/ELNEC/About.htm): The core curriculum in end of life consists of nine content modules with syllabus, objectives, student note-taking outlines, detailed faculty content outlines, slide copy, reference lists, and supplemental teaching materials available in hard copy and CD-ROM.

The Geriatric Nursing Education Project (www.aacn.nche.edu/Education/Hartford): Offers faculty development institutes, online interactive case studies, a guide for integrating gerontology into nursing curricula, and a complimentary catalog of geriatric nursing photos that may be used free of charge for print or Web-based media by schools of nursing.

Consult GeriRN (http://consultgerirn.org): An evidence-based online resource for nurses in clinical and educational settings. Includes many resources on a wide variety of topics related to aging including evidence-based geriatric protocols, hospital competencies for older adults, continuing education contact hours, the "Try This" series of assessment tools, information related to common geriatric problems, and links to additional age-related agencies and references.

The John A. Hartford Foundation Institute for Geriatric Nursing (www.hartfordign.org): A wealth of resources including core curriculum content for educators in academic and practice settings including detailed content outlines, case studies, activities, resources, PowerPoint slides, an online gerontological nursing certification review course, research support programs, best practice guidelines, consultation services, and geriatric nursing awards.

Mather LifeWays Institute on Aging (www.matherlifeways.com/re_researchandeducation.asp): Offers programs for faculty development (Web-based), long-term care staff, and family caregivers.

National Institute on Aging (www.niapublications.org): Free publications about older adults for health professionals and patients.

Toolkit for Nurturing Excellence at End-of-Life Transition (www.tneel.uic.edu/tneel.asp): A package for palliative care education on CD-ROM that includes audio, video, graphics, PowerPoint slides, photographs, and animations of individuals and families experiencing end-of-life transitions. An evidence-based self-study course on palliative care will soon be available for the national and international nursing community.

contexts: an outcome of growth and development, a psychological state, and an expression of physical health state. Failure to thrive first appeared in the aging literature as a diagnosis for older adults with vague symptoms such as fatigue, cachexia, and generalized weakness (Campia, Berkman, & Fulmer, 1986). Other disciplines later defined undernutrition, physical and cognitive dysfunction, and depression as its major attributes (Braun, Wykle, & Cowling, 1988). In their concept analysis of failure to thrive, Newbern and Krowchuk (1994) identified attributes under two categories: problems in social relatedness (disconnectedness and inability to find meaning in life, give of oneself, or attach to others) and physical/cognitive dysfunction (consistent unplanned weight loss, signs of depression, and cognitive decline).

Haight and colleagues (2002) view thriving in a holistic, life span perspective that considers the impact of environment as people age. They assert that thriving is achieved when there is harmony among a person and his or her physical environment and personal relationships. Failure to thrive is due to discord among these three elements. Nurses caring for patients can use this theory to identify factors that may impede thriving and plan interventions to address these concerns.

CONCLUSION

Both types of nursing theories contribute to our understanding of aging from the perspectives of thriving and functionality; however, neither encompasses all of the holistic elements (cultural, spiritual, geographic, psychosocioeconomic, educational, environmental, and physical) of concern to nursing. Until nursing has a comprehensive theoretical framework to guide its practice that is tested with diverse patients in varied settings, there remains much that can be useful from the theories of other disciplines. From the stochastic and programmed biological theories of aging, nurses can better manage nutrition, incontinence, sleep rhythms, immunological response, catecholamine surges, hormonal and electrolyte balance, and drug efficacy for older adults with chronic illnesses. Using psychosocial aging theories, nurses can assist both the older adult and his or her family in recognizing that the life they have lived has been one of integrity and meaning and facilitate peaceful death with dignity. Ego integrity contributes to older adults' well-being and reduces the negative psychological consequences that are often linked to chronic illness and older age. Finally, being cognizant of older adults' socioeconomic resources will assist the nurse and older adult in planning cost-effective best practices to improve symptom management and treatment outcomes.

Using knowledge gained from aging theories, nurses can:

- Help people to use their genetic makeup to prevent comorbidities
- Facilitate best practices for managing chronic illnesses
- Maximize individuals' strengths relative to maintaining independence
- Facilitate creative ways to overcome individuals' challenges
- Assist in cultivating and maintaining older adults' cognitive status and mental health

In conclusion, aging continues to be explained from multiple theoretical perspectives. Collectively, these theories reveal that aging is a complex phenomenon still much in need of research. How one ages is a result of biopsychosocial factors. Nurses can use this knowledge as they plan and implement ways of promoting health care to all age groups. As in other disciplines, the state of the science on aging is rapidly improving within the nursing profession. Nursing is developing a rich body of knowledge regarding the care of older adults. Programs and materials developed by the Hartford Institute for Geriatric Nursing, the End of Life Nursing Education Consortium, the American Association of Colleges of Nursing, and the Mather Institute provide a strong foundation for developing and disseminating our current knowledge. Nursing research must continue to span all facets of gerontology so that new information will be generated for improved patient outcomes.

BOX 3-4 Recommended Reading

Goldsmith, T. (2003). *The evolution of aging: How Darwin's dilemma is affecting your chance for a longer and healthier life*. Retrieved October 20, 2007, from http://www.azinet.com/aging

Kirkwood, T. (2002). Evolution of ageing. *Mechanisms of Ageing and Development, 123*, 737–745.

Taaffe, D., & Marcus, R. (2000). Musculoskeletal health and the older adult. *Journal of Rehabilitation Research and Development, 37*, 245–254.

Critical Thinking Exercises

1. Mrs. Smith, 72 years old and recently diagnosed with a myocardial infarction, asks why she should take an anticholesterol drug for her hyperlipidemia at her age. Why should she engage in the lifestyle changes her nurse is recommending?
2. Your 82-year-old patient, Rodney Whitishing, has been healthy most of his life and now is experiencing, for the second winter in a row, an extremely severe case of influenza. He has never taken a flu shot as a preventive measure because he felt he was very strong and healthy. Explain how you would discuss the older adult's immune system and why the elderly seem to be more vulnerable to influenza.
3. John, an 85-year-old man with emphysema, is brought to your clinic by his family because of increasing complaints about shortness of breath. John uses oxygen at home, but states that he is afraid to walk more than a few steps or show any emotion because he will become unable to get enough air. John tells you that he feels his life is not worth living. Using the theories of aging, how might you respond to this situation?

Personal **Reflections**

1. Develop a philosophy of how theories of aging can support or refute the idea of categorizing people in the young-old, middle-old, and old-old classifications according to chronological age. What other characteristics could be used to categorize people as they age? Give an example of how you would perceive a relative or friend of yours who is in the sixth or seventh decade of life.
2. Comparable to infant-child development stages, generate five or six stages of development for older adults to accomplish as they complete their work stage and begin their retirement era.
3. Using theories of aging with biological, psychological, and sociological perspectives, hypothesize how these frameworks influence the older adult's development.

References

Achenbaum, W. A., & Bengtson, B. L. (1994). Re-engaging the disengagement theory of aging: On the history and assessment of theory development in gerontology. *Gerontologist, 34*, 756–763.

Adams, K. B. (2004). Changing investment in activities and interests in elders' lives: Theory and measurement. *International Journal of Aging & Human Development, 58*(2), 87–108.

Agahi, N., Ahacic, K., & Parker, M. G. (2006). Continuity of leisure participation from middle age to old age. *The Journals of Gerontology, 61B*(6), S340–S346.

Ahrendt, J. (2000). Melatonin, circadian rhythms, and sleep. *New England Journal of Medicine, 343*, 1114–1115.

Aigner, T., Rose, J., Martin, J., & Buckwalter, J. (2004). Aging theories of primary osteoarthritis: From epidemiology to molecular biology. *Rejuvenation Research, 7*(2), 134–145.

Alkema, G. E., & Alley, D. E. (2006). Gerontology's future: An integrative model for disciplinary advancement. *The Gerontologist, 46*, 574–582.

Ameri, G., Govari, F., Nazari, T., Rashidinejad, M., & Afsharzadeh, P. (2002). The adult age theories and definitions.

Hayat Journal of Tehran Faculty Nurse Midwifery, 8(14).

Ames, B. (2004). Mitochondrial decay, a major cause of aging, can be delayed. *Journal of Alzheimer's Disease, 6*(2), 117–121.

Back, K. (1980). *Life course: Integrated theories and exemplary populations*. Boulder, CO: Westview Press.

Baltes, P. B. (1987). Theoretical propositions of life-span developmental psychology: On the dynamics between growth and decline. *Developmental Psychology, 23*, 611–626.

Baltes, P. B., & Baltes, M. M. (1990). Psychological perspectives on successful aging: The model of selective optimization with compensation. In P. B. Baltes & M. M. Baltes (Eds.), *Successful aging: Perspectives from the behavioral sciences* (pp. 1–34). New York: Cambridge University Press.

Bergland, A., & Kirkevold, M. (2001). Thriving: A useful theoretical perspective to capture the experience of well-being among frail elderly in nursing homes? *Journal of Advanced Nursing, 36*, 426.

Birren, J. E., & Schroots, J. J. F. (2001). History of geropsychology. In J. E. Birren (Ed.), *Handbook of the psychology of aging* (5th ed., pp. 3–28). San Diego: Academic Press.

Bokov, A., Chaudhuri, A., & Richardson, A. (2004). The role of oxidative damage and stress in aging. *Mechanisms of Ageing Development, 125*(10–11), 811–826.

Braun, J. V., Wykle, M. N., & Cowling, W. R. (1988). Failure to thrive in older persons: A concept derived. *Gerontologist, 28*, 809–812.

Brunk, U., & Terman, A. (2002). The mitochondrial-lysosomal axis theory of aging—Accumulation of damaged mitochondria as a result of imperfect autophagocytosis. *European Journal of Biochemistry, 269*(8), 1996–2002.

Bühler, C. (1933). *Der menschliche Lebenslauf als psychologisches Problem* [Human life as a psychological problem]. Oxford, England: Hirzel.

Butler, R. N., & Lewis, M. I. (1982). *Aging & mental health* (3rd ed.). St. Louis: Mosby.

Campia, E., Berkman, B., & Fulmer, T. (1986). Failure to thrive for older adults. *Gerontologist, 26*(2), 192–197.

Carlson, E., & Chamberlain, R. (2005). Allostatic load and health disparities: A theoretical orientation. *Research in Nursing & Health, 28*(4), 306–315.

Caspi, A. (1987). Personality in the life course. *Journal of Personality and Social Psychology, 53*, 1203–1213.

Caspi, A., & Elder, G. H. (1986). Life satisfaction in old age: Linking social psychology and history. *Psychology and Aging, 1*, 18–26.

Cobbs, E., Duthie, E., & Murphy, J. (Eds.). (1999). *Geriatric review syllabus: A core curriculum in geriatric medicine* (4th ed.). Dubuque, IA: Kendall/Hunt for the American Geriatric Society.

Cumming, E., & Henry, W. (1961). *Growing old*. New York: Basic Books.

Cunningham, W., & Brookbank, J. (1988). *Gerontology: The physiology, biology and sociology of aging*. New York: Harper & Row.

Daniel, J., & Smythe, W. (2003). Gene therapy of cancer. *Seminars of Surgical Oncology, 21*(3), 196–204.

Dufour, E., & Larsson, N. (2004). Understanding aging: Revealing order out of chaos. *Biochimica et Biophysica Acta-Bioenergetics, 1658*(1–2), 122–132.

Ebersole, P., Hess, P., & Luggen, A. S. (2004). *Toward healthy aging: Human needs and nursing response* (3rd ed.). St. Louis: Mosby.

Effros, R. (2004). From Hayflick to Walford: The role of T cell replicative senescence in human aging. *Experimental Gerontology, 39*(6), 885–890.

Efklides, A., Kalaitzidou, M., & Chankin, G. (2003). Subjective quality of life in old age in Greece: The effect of demographic factors, emotional state, and adaptation to aging. *European Psychologist, 8*, 178–191.

Erikson, E. (1963). *Childhood and society*. New York: W. W. Norton.

Erikson, E. H., Erikson, J. M., & Kivnick, H. Q. (1986). *Vital involvement in old age: The experience of old age in our time*. New York: W. W. Norton.

Goldsmith, T. (2004). Aging as an evolved characteristic—Weismann's theory reconsidered. *Medical Hypotheses, 62*(2), 304–308.

Gray, D., & Woulfe, J. (2005). Lipofuscin and aging: A matter of toxic waste. *Science of Aging Knowledge Environment, 5*, 1.

Grune, T., & Davies, K. (2001). Oxidative processes in aging. In E. Masoro & S. Austad (Eds.), *Handbook of the biology of aging* (5th ed., pp. 25–58). San Diego: Academic Press.

Hagestad, G. O., & Dannefer, D. (2002). Concepts and theories of aging: Beyond microfication in social sciences approaches. In R. H. Binstock & L. K. George (Eds.), *Handbook of aging and the social sciences* (5th ed., pp. 3–21). San Diego: Academic Press.

Haight, B. K., Barba, B. E., Tesh, A. S., & Courts, N. F. (2002). Thriving: A life span theory. *Journal of Gerontological Nursing, 28*(3), 14–22.

Haq, R. (2003). Age-old theories die hard. *Clinical Investigative Medicine, 26*(3), 116–120.

Harlow, R. E., & Cantor, N. (1996). Still participating after all these years: A study of life task participation in later life. *Journal of Personality and Social Psychology, 71*, 1235–1249.

Harman, D. (1994). Aging: Prospects for further increases in the functional life-span. *Age, 17*(4), 119–146.

Harman, D. (2006). Understanding and modulating aging: An update. *Annals of the New York Academy of Sciences, 1067*, 10–21.

Havighurst, R. (1972). *Developmental tasks and education*. New York: David McKay.

Havighurst, R. J., & Albrecht, R. (1953). *Older people*. Oxford, England: Longmans, Green.

Havighurst, R. J., Neugarten, B. L., & Tobin, S. S. (1963). Disengagement, personality and life satisfaction in the later years. In P. Hansen (Ed.), *Age with a future* (pp. 419–425). Copenhagen: Munksgoasrd.

Havighurst, R. J., Neugarten, B. L., & Tobin, S. S. (1968). Disengagement and patterns of aging. In B. L. Neugarten (Ed.), *Middle age and aging* (pp. 67–71). Chicago: University Press.

Hayflick, L. (1985). Theories of biologic aging. *Experimental Gerontology, 10*, 145–159.

Hayflick, L. (1996). *How and why we age*. New York: Ballantine Books.

Henderson, E. (2006). The potential effect of fibroblast senescence on wound healing and the chronic wound environment. *Journal of Wound Care, 15*(7), 315–318.

Holm, A. K., Lepp, M., & Ringsberg, K. C. (2005). Dementia: Involving patients in storytelling—a caring intervention. A pilot study. *Journal of Clinical Nursing, 14*(2), 256–263.

Holzenberger, M., Kappeler, L., & De Magalhaes Filho, C. (2004). IGF-1 signaling and aging. *Experimental Gerontology, 39*(11–12), 1761–1764.

Hyun-Mee, J., & Miller, N. J. (2007). Examining the effects of fashion activities on life satisfaction of older females: Activity theory revisited. *Family & Consumer Sciences Research Journal, 35*(4), 338–356.

Iwarsson, S. (2005). A long-term perspective on person-environment fit and ADL dependence among older Swedish adults. *Gerontologist, 45*(3), 327–336.

Jones, G. M., & Miesen, B. L. (Eds.). (1992). *Care-giving in dementia: Research and applications*. New York: Tavistock/Routledge.

Jung, C. G. (1960). *The structure and dynamics of the psyche. Collected works* (Vol. VIII). Oxford, England: Pantheon.

King, I. M. (1981). *A theory for nursing*. New York: John Wiley & Sons.

Kirkwood, T. (2000). Molecular gerontology: Bridging the simple and complex. *Annals of the New York Academy of Sciences, 908*, 14–20.

Kozak-Campbell, C., & Hughes, A. M. (1996). The use of functional consequences theory in acutely confused hospitalized elderly. *Journal of Gerontological Nursing, 22*(1), 27–36.

Lakatta, E. (2000). Cardiovascular aging in health. *Clinical Geriatric Medicine, 16*, 419–444.

Lawton, M. P. (1982). Competence, environmental press, and the adaptation of older people. In M. P. Lawton, P. G. Windley, & T. O. Byerts (Eds.), *Aging and the environment: Theoretical approaches* (pp. 33–59). New York: Springer.

Lee, J., Koo, N., & Min, D. (2004). Reactive oxygen species, aging, and antioxidative nutraceuticals. *Comprehensive Reviews in Food Science and Food Safety, 3*(1), 21–33.

Lemon, B. W., Bengston, V. L., & Peterson, J. A. (1972). An exploration of the activity theory of aging: Activity types and life satisfaction among in-movers to a retirement community. *Journal of Gerontology, 27*, 511–523.

Longino, C. F., & Kart, C. S. (1982). Explicating activity theory: A formal replication. *Journal of Gerontology, 35*, 713–722.

Maddox, G. L. (1963). Activity and morale: A longitudinal study of selected elderly subjects. *Social Forces, 42*, 195–204.

Marshall, V. W. (1996). The stage of theory in aging and the social sciences. In R. H. Binstock & L. K. George (Eds.), *Handbook of aging and the social sciences* (4th ed., pp. 12–26). San Diego: Academic Press.

Maslow, A. H. (1954). *Motivation and personality*. New York: Harper & Row.

McMullin, J. A. (2000). Diversity and the state of sociological aging theory. *Gerontologist, 40*, 517–530.

Miller, C. A. (1990). *Nursing care of older adults: Theory and practice*. Glenview, IL: Scott, Foresman/Little, Brown Higher Education.

Miquel, J. (1998). An update on the oxygen stress-mitochondrial mutation theory of aging: Genetic and evolutionary implications. *Experimental Gerontology, 33*(1–2), 113–126.

Moore, M., Czeisler, C., & Richardson, G. (1983). Circadian time-keeping in health and disease. *New England Journal of Medicine, 309*, 469–473.

Moore, R. (1997). Circadian rhythms: Basic neurobiology and clinical application. *Annual Review of Medicine, 48*, 253–266.

Neugarten, B. L. (1968). Adult personality: Toward a psychology of the life cycle. In B. L. Neugarten (Ed.), *Middle age and aging: A reader in social psychology* (pp. 137–147). Chicago: University Press.

Neumann, C. V. (2000). *Sources of meaning and energy in the chronically ill frail elder*. The University of Wisconsin-Milwaukee. Retrieved January 5, 2005, from http://www.uwm.edu/Dept/Grad_Sch/McNair/Summer00/cneumann.htm

Newbern, V. B., & Krowchuk, H. V. (1994). Failure to thrive in elderly people: A conceptual analysis. *Journal of Advanced Nursing, 19*, 840–849.

Newsom, J. T., & Schulz, R. (1996). Social support as a mediator in the relation between functional status and quality of life in older adults. *Psychology, 3*, 34–44.

O'Connor, B. P., & Vallerand, R. J. (1994). Motivation, self-determination, and person-environment fit as predictors of psychological adjustment among nursing home residents. *Psychology and Aging, 9*(2), 189–194.

Orgel, L. (1970). The maintenance of the accuracy of protein synthesis and its relevance to aging: A correction. *Proceedings of the National Academy of Sciences, 67*, 1476.

Papathanassoglou, E., Moynihan, J., & Ackerman, M. (2000). Does programmed cell death (apoptosis) play a role in the development of multiple organ dysfunction in critically ill patients? A review and a theoretical framework. *Critical Care Medicine, 28*(2), 537–549.

Parr, T. (1997). Insulin exposure and aging theory. *Gerontology, 43*(3), 182–200.

Peck, R. C. (1968). Psychological development in the second half of life. In B. L. Neugarten (Ed.), *Middle age and aging: A reader in social psychology* (pp. 88–92). Chicago: University Press.

Poon, H., Calabrese, V., Scapagnini, G., & Butterfield, D. (2004). Free radicals in brain aging. *Clinics in Geriatric Medicine, 20*(2), 329–359.

Porth, C. (2005). *Pathophysiology: Concepts of altered health states*. Philadelphia: Lippincott Williams & Wilkins.

Putnam, M. (2002). Linking aging theory and disability models: Increasing the potential to explore aging with physical impairment. *Gerontologist, 42*, 799–806.

Quick, H. E., & Moen, P. (1998). Gender, employment, and retirement quality: A life course approach to the differential experiences of men and women. *Journal of Occupational Health Psychology, 3*, 44–64.

Rapkin, B. D., & Fischer, K. (1992). Personal goals of older adults: Issues in assessment and prediction. *Psychology and Aging, 7*, 127–137.

Richardson, G., & Tate, B. (2000). Hormonal and pharmacological manipulation of the circadian clock: Recent developments and future strategies. *Sleep, 23*(Suppl. 3), S77–S88.

Riley, M. W. (1994). Age integration and the lives of older people. *Gerontologist, 34*, 110–115.

Riley, M. W., Johnson, M., & Foner, A. (1972). *Aging and society: A sociology of age stratification* (Vol. 3). New York: Russell Sage Foundation.

Rodenbeck, A., & Hajak, G. (2001). Neuroendocrine dysregulation in primary insomnia. *Reviews of Neurology, 157*(11 Pt 2), S57–S61.

Rose, A. M. (1965). The subculture of the aging: A framework for research in social gerontology. In A. M. Rose & W. Peterson (Eds.), *Older people and their social worlds* (pp. 3–16). Philadelphia: F. A. Davis.

Rose, M. H., & Killien, M. (1983). Risk and vulnerability: A case for differentiation. *Advances in Nursing Science, 5*, 60–73.

Schroots, J. J. F. (1996). Theoretical developments in the psychology of aging. *Gerontologist, 36*, 742–748.

Schroots, J. J. F. (2003). Life-course dynamics: A research program in progress from the Netherlands. *European Psychologist, 8*, 192–199.

Shay, J., & Wright, W. (2001). Telomeres and telomerase: Implications for cancer and aging. *Radiation Research, 155*(1), 188–193.

Slagboom, P., Bastian, T., Beekman, M., Wendendorf, R., & Meulenbelt, I. (2000). Genetics of human aging. *Annals of the New York Academy of Science, 908*, 50–61.

Sozou, P., & Kirkwood, T. (2001). A stochastic model of cell replicative senescence based on telomere shortening, oxidative stress, and somatic mutations in nuclear and mitochondrial DNA. *Journal of Theoretical Biology, 213*(4), 573–586.

Thompson, C. (1995). Apoptosis in the pathogenesis and treatment of disease. *Science, 267*, 1456–1462.

Thyagarajan, S., & Felten, D. (2002). Modulation of neuroendocrine-immune signaling by L-deprenyl and L-desmethyldeprenyl in aging and mammary cancer. *Mechanisms of Ageing Development, 123*(8), 1065–1079.

Tornstam, L. (1994). Gerotranscendence: A theoretical and empirical exploration. In L. E. Thomas & S. A. Eisenhandler (Eds.), *Aging and the religious dimension* (pp. 203–226). Westport, CT: Greenwood.

Troen, B. (2003). The biology of aging. *Mount Sinai Journal of Medicine, 70*(1), 3–22.

Troll, L. E., & Skaff, M. M. (1997). Perceived continuity of self in very old age. *Psychology and Aging, 12*, 162–169.

Uhlenberg, P. (1992). Population aging and social policy. *Annual Review of Sociology, 18*, 449–474.

Uhlenberg, P. (1996). The burden of aging: A theoretical framework for understanding the shifting balance of care giving and care receiving as cohorts age. *Gerontologist, 36*, 761–767.

Uhlenberg, P. (2000). Why study age integration? *Gerontologist, 40*, 261–266.

Van Cauter, E., Leproult, R., & Kupfer, D. (1996). Effects of gender and age on the levels and circadian rhythmicity of plasma cortisol. *Journal of Clinical Endocrinology Metabolism, 81*(7), 2468–2473.

Venjatraman, F., & Fernandes, G. (1997). Exercise, immunity and aging. *Aging, 9*(1–2), 42–56.

Wadensten, B. (2002). *Gerotranscendence from a nursing perspective: From theory to implementation*. Uppsala University. Retrieved January 7, 2005, from http://www.samfak.uu.se/Disputationer/Wadensten.htm

Wadensten, B., & Carlsson, M. (2003). Nursing theory views on how to support the process of ageing. *Journal of Advanced Nursing, 42*(2), 118–124.

Wahl, H. W. (2001). Environmental influences on aging and behavior. In J. E. Birren & K. W. Schaie (Eds.), *Handbook of the psychology of aging* (5th ed., pp. 215–237). San Diego: Academic Press.

Williams, M. (1995). *The American Geriatric Society's complete guide to aging and health*. New York: Harmony Books.

Yin, P., & Lai, K. H. (1983). A reconceptualization of age stratification in China. *Journal of Gerontology, 38*, 608–613.

SECTION

2

COMMUNICATION

(Competencies 3, 4)

CHAPTER 4

Aging Changes That Affect Communication

Liat Ayalon, PhD
Leilani Feliciano, PhD, MA
Patricia A. Areán, PhD

LEARNING OBJECTIVES

At the end of this chapter, the reader will be able to:

- Identify sensorimotor, cognitive, and psychological changes associated with aging.
- Understand the mechanisms behind changes in sensory-motor, cognitive, and psychological functioning of older adults.
- Distinguish between normal age-related changes and pathological ones.
- Understand the impact that sensory-motor, cognitive, and psychological changes associated with aging have on communication with older adults.
- Identify and refine communication skills and techniques with older adults.

KEY TERMS

- Activities of daily living (ADLs)
- Agnosia
- Agraphia
- Alzheimer's disease
- Anarthria
- Anhedonia
- Aphasia
- Apraxia
- Broca's area
- Cataracts
- Chronic obstructive pulmonary disease (COPD)
- Compensation
- Conductive problems
- Confabulation
- Cortex
- Crystallized intelligence
- Delirium
- Dementia
- Depression
- Diabetic retinopathy
- Disability
- Disturbed executive functioning
- Divided attention
- Dysarthria
- Electroconvulsive therapy
- Electrolarynx
- Expressive (nonfluent) aphasia
- Fine motor movement
- Fluid intelligence
- Forebrain
- Glaucoma
- Gross motor movement
- Gustation
- Hearing
- Hyperorality
- Hypothermia
- Information processing speed
- Instrumental activities of daily living (IADLs)
- Iris
- Irreversible dementia
- Language
- Laryngectomy
- Lens

- Long-term memory
- Macular degeneration
- Mixed hearing loss
- Movement
- Olfaction
- Ototoxic substances
- Parkinson's disease (PD)
- Pitch
- Presbycusis
- Presbyopia
- Pressure ulcers
- Primary aging
- Pseudodementias
- Pupil
- Receptive (fluent) aphasia
- Retinal detachment
- Reversible dementia
- Senile cataracts
- Senile miosis
- Sensorineural
- Short-term memory
- Somatosensory system
- Speech
- Sustained attention
- Thalamus
- Timber
- Tinnitus
- Touch
- Velocity
- Verbal apraxia
- Vision
- Visual acuity
- Visual illusions
- Wernicke's area

Communication is an important skill that allows us to survive in and interact with our world. Through our ability to communicate, we express our needs and wishes, understand the needs and wishes of others, negotiate adversity, and convey our feelings. Losing our ability to communicate effectively compromises our independence. As an example, imagine yourself at a hospital, trying to find your way to the nearest restroom. You are trying to ask for directions but no one understands what you say or, even worse than that, you move your lips and there is no sound. You would be forced to determine another way to reach your goal, but the method would be far more complicated than if you were simply able to say, "Where is the nearest restroom?" This example underscores the importance of communication and how changes in the ability to communicate may require special adaptation. This adaptation can be frustrating and anxiety provoking.

The ability to communicate depends on both physiological and psychological processes. Physical processes include listening, speaking, gesturing, reading, writing, touching, and moving. These processes, in turn, are dependent on adequate sensory abilities. The psychological aspects involve cognitive processes such as attention, memory, self-awareness, organization, and reasoning. The physiological/sensory and psychological/cognitive work together in a rather elegant and orchestrated manner. In this chapter, we will provide an overview of: 1) the sensory modalities involved in communication, 2) the role of the brain in communication, and 3) normal and pathological changes associated with aging and their impact on communication.

SENSORY MODALITIES INVOLVED IN COMMUNICATION

We receive information about the environment through our senses (seeing, hearing, smelling, touching, tasting, and vestibular). **Vision** has an important role in communication, with approximately 70% of all sensory information coming through the eyes (Springhouse, 2001). We use visual information to make sense of interactions and to add meaning to a verbal message. Gestures and other nonverbal behaviors, such as a smile, an eye blink, or tears, allow us to decipher the emotional tone of an interaction. Visual information provides us with important context with which to interpret communication. For example, being asked to take your shirt off would be experienced quite differently depending on whether the request was conveyed by a nurse or by a neighbor. In addition to the use of visual information in face-to-face interactions, we rely heavily on visual information in other modes of communication. Books, newspapers, television, computers, and traffic signs are all common modalities that rely on visual ability to convey information.

Hearing is another prominent sense involved in the reception of communication. A major source of communication is the content of auditory verbal information that is conveyed in conversations as well as via radio, television, or computers. Hearing not only allows us to determine the source of the information (e.g., who is speaking or where the sound is coming from), but also allows for interpretation of the meaning of spoken words. To accomplish this task, we rely heavily on nonverbal auditory information. The physical properties of the sound, such as **pitch** (how high or low a tone sounds) and **timber** (the quality of the sound) tell us whether a person is angry or whimsical, young or old, healthy or sick. Nonverbal auditory information also plays an important role, such as warning of impending danger or building a relaxing atmosphere.

On the surface, other sensory modalities may not seem as important for communication as vision and hearing; however, our other senses may communicate danger, serve as useful adjuncts, or substitute in the case of impairment or loss of either visual or auditory abilities. For example, **touch** may be used as a substitute for sight, allowing a visually impaired person to "read" his or her environment. Touch initiated by others can convey meaning such as anger or love. Touch also may serve as a communication of impending danger. For example, the sensation of cold air on your skin may convey a need to put on more clothing to stay warm, or heat may warn someone to move away from the heat source so as not to get burned.

The chemical senses of smell (**olfaction**) and taste (**gustation**) also seem to be unrelated to communication. However, olfaction can trigger feelings and memories. These memories may convey either comfort (e.g., the smell of fresh baked cookies may remind you of home, the scent of lavender may calm an agitated patient) or discomfort (e.g., the smell of certain medicines may make someone nauseous). Gustation also is used to convey meaning (e.g., we give chocolate on Valentine's day).

Similarly, **movement** provides us with important information about our environment. For some, movement combined with the sense of touch will allow the receipt of information from the environment. Orienting toward the source of communication is yet another way in which movement improves our ability to receive information from our environment. In addition to its role in the actual articulation of verbal information, movement allows us to convey meaning by the use of nonverbal gestures and facial expressions.

Speech is the primary form of communication with our environment. Speech is a very complex process that requires both visual and auditory input, motor output to both facial and vocal muscles, and central processing that takes place in multiple brain locations (Beers & Berkow, 2000). Speech involves both articulation and pronunciation, and is distinguished from **language**, which involves the actual selection of words and the integration of words into sentences. In contrast to speech, language can be either written or spoken, as well as either verbal or nonverbal (Finlayson & Heffer, 2000).

Disability (physical impairment) also plays a major role in affecting communication. Disability may affect our ability to convey or receive information. In addition, disability results in other people modifying their style of communication toward disabled older adults and, thus, is an important part of any discussion on communication.

THE ROLE OF THE BRAIN IN COMMUNICATION

The brain has a major role in attending to new information, making sense of and organizing information, and deciding on a response. The information we receive through our senses is not an exact representation of the real world. Our nervous system is limited in its ability to receive information from the physical world. For example, our hearing is limited to frequencies of 20 to 20,000 hertz and our vision is limited to wavelengths of 400 to 700 nanometers. Thus, we may be completely oblivious to stimuli that exceed these physical characteristics. Furthermore, our brain is set to respond to change rather than to continuity and, thus, tends to adapt by responding at a lower rate after a stimulus has been present for a while. This may result in perceiving certain stimuli as more intense just because of their novelty. Last, we tend to perceive incomplete information as complete and recognizable, because this is more efficient, less ambiguous, and makes better sense for us (Atrens & Curthoys, 1978; Howard Hughes Medical Institute, 2005).

Areas of the Brain Important for Communication

The **cortex** is a large, wrinkly sheet of neurons that covers the brain. The cortex contains all the brain's sensory and motor information as well as our thoughts. Information that is perceived through our sensory system goes to the **thalamus**, a relay station in the center of our brain. It is then transferred via the neurons into the sensory cortex. The sensory area of the cortex is located on a vertical strip near the center of the skull. Sensory information is represented on this strip in relation to the sensitivity of each body part, and not in relation to its actual size. For example, the tongue is very sensitive and, thus, captures a large area of the sensory cortex despite its relative small size. From the sensory cortex, information is sent to higher-order parts of the brain, such as the **forebrain**. These areas integrate the sensory information and interpret it based on past experiences, overall arousal level, and the array of sensory information already available to us (Atrens & Curthoys, 1978; Howard Hughes Medical Institute, 2005).

When one or more sensory systems do not function, our brain compensates by relying on other sensory modalities for information. For example, Helen Keller lost her vision and hearing at 19 months of age, but she was able to develop an extraordinary sense of touch that allowed her to communicate with the world (Howard Hughes Medical Institute, 2005). Although the brain is more flexible at such a young age, even older adults may use one modality to replace other modalities that function inadequately. For example, an older adult who has lost the ability to see might be able to learn how to use touch to "read" books written in Braille. Similarly, in the case of neurodegenerative diseases such as **dementia**, when the brain's ability to understand information and to communicate verbally deteriorates, older adults may resort to alternative forms of communication. For example, an older adult may put an item in his or her mouth in order to better recognize the item, or he or she may scream to communicate distress.

NORMAL AND PATHOLOGICAL AGE-RELATED CHANGES THAT AFFECT COMMUNICATION

Sensory changes are commonly seen with aging. The 2000 U.S. Census reported that of the 33 million noninstitutionalized elders over the age of 65 surveyed, approximately 14% had some type of sensory deficit (Waldrop & Stern, 2003). The number of individuals with sensory deficits increases with age, with 35% of people age 85 or older reporting a sensory disability. It is important for providers to learn about and distinguish normal aging changes from pathological ones, and to have an appreciation for how sensory changes interact with social, psychological, and communications abilities. The following sections will provide a discussion of age-related changes in the sensory systems, as well as aging changes in cognitive and psychological functioning. Because not all age-related changes are "normal" and expected, we will also discuss the pathological changes that are commonly seen in older adults. These will be followed by a discussion of the impact of these changes on communication. **Table 4-1** provides a concise summary of this section.

Vision

TYPICAL AGE-RELATED CHANGES IN THE EYE

The Lens. With age, the **lens** changes in color, becoming more yellowed or amber, and more opaque. This makes it difficult for the aging eye to distinguish colors on the blue-green hue range. The lens becomes flattened, denser, and less flexible (Gray, 1995). As a result, the lens's ability to accommodate (adjust focus) is compromised (Kline & Scialfa, 1996). These changes begin after the age of 40 and impact our ability to see certain colors, focus on objects, and so on.

The Iris and Pupil. Starting at the age of 50, the pupillary reflex responds more slowly, and the **pupil** does not dilate completely (the size of the pupil declines—**senile miosis**), making it more difficult to see in lower light and thus adapt to the dark quickly. Because less light enters the eye, older adults require more light than younger adults at a rate of approximately 10% more every 10 years (Stuen & Faye, 2003). The pupil also contracts less quickly, which makes it more difficult to deal with sudden illumination such as when walking from indoors into direct sunlight. By age 60, these changes in the **iris** (see Chapter 6), pupil, and lens result in a tremendous reduction (70%) in the amount of light that reaches the retina (Pirkl, 1995).

TABLE 4-1 **Normal and Pathological Changes and Their Impact on Communication**

Modality	Normal Changes	Pathological Changes	Impact on Communication
Vision	Changes in lens, pupil, and iris Results in poor visual acuity, presbyopia, increased sensitivity to light and glare	Macular degeneration Diabetic retinopathy Glaucoma Senile cataracts Retinal detachment	Isolation, insecurity, decrease in exchange of communication, embarrassment, depression
Hearing	Conductive problems Sensorineural problems Presbycusis Results in loss in sensitivity to pitch with high-frequency consonants, poor word recognition	Hearing loss due to exposure to: noise, ototoxic substances, medications, poisons, acute trauma, certain medical conditions	Inattention, repetitive questions, isolation, insecurity, decrease in social functioning, depression, loneliness, difficulties in following instructions
Speech and language	Decreased respiration Overproduction of mucus/reduced saliva Loss of teeth Decreased elasticity and muscle tone Results in shaky and breathy voice, voice may sound tremulous, frequent attempts at throat clearing, changes in articulation, semantic errors	Dysarthria Verbal apraxia Aphasia Chronic obstructive pulmonary disease Mechanical ventilation Laryngectomy	Deficits vary dramatically but may result in: difficulties producing language, difficulties in producing coherent and meaningful verbal communication, or difficulties in understanding verbal communication
Touch	Reduction in number of receptors Reduction in blood flow Results in a reduction in tactile and vibration sensations, decreased sensitivity to warm or cold stimuli	Many medical conditions such as dementia, Parkinson's, or diabetes can impact somatosensory functioning	Use of the mouth to explore the quality of the objects, safety might be compromised
Movement	Due to decline in many sensory organs, cognitive functioning, and bodily strength	Parkinson's disease Disability	Reduced ability to communicate nonverbal information, insecurity, and loss of independence

Modality	Normal Changes	Pathological Changes	Impact on Communication
	Results in reduced velocity and accuracy and greater variability across individuals		
Cognitive	Decline in information processing speed, divided attention, sustained attention, ability to perform visuospatial tasks, and short-term memory	Delirium Dementia: Alzheimer's disease	Depending on cognitive impairment, loss may result in complete disorientation and inappropriate response, difficulties finding words, depression, loss of insight, isolation, or impairment in ability to learn new information
Psychological	In general, older adults report levels of satisfaction that are similar to those of younger adults	Depression	Slowed response, lack of motivation, decrease in social activity

Typical Vision Problems

Visual problems are some of the most common sensory deficits in older adults. Most people experience testable visual losses that show up in a lab, but these losses are subtle and do not actually impair daily existence because of adaptation and **compensation** behaviors. Blindness or low vision affects 1 in 28 Americans over the age of 40 (Congdon et al., 2004). Prevalence rates are predicted to increase as the population of older adults increases. About 95% of adults over the age of 65 report needing glasses to assist with vision. Unfortunately, the effectiveness of glasses in correcting vision decreases with age. It is notable that in elders over the age of 85, less than half report that their glasses corrected all of their visual problems (AgeWorks, 2000; Ebersole & Hess, 2001).

Typical vision problems include the following:

- *Poor visual acuity or clarity:* Our ability to identify objects (stationary or moving) at a distance declines with age. **Visual acuity** is directly related to the amount of light that reaches the retina (the less light, the poorer the acuity) and is affected by age-related changes such as senile miosis and yellowing of the lens.
- *Presbyopia:* Latin for "old eyes"; the person cannot focus as clearly when objects are up close. These losses occur gradually from childhood, but do not typically become problematic until around 40–50 years old, as the lens begins to lose flexibility. Eyes become easily fatigued. **Presbyopia** is easily correctible with glasses, and by age 55 most people begin to wear glasses part time (e.g., for reading).
- Other problems include increased sensitivity to light and glare, senile miosis, and problems with color contrast. Increased sensitivity to light may lead to excessive watering of the eyes and blurred vision (National Institute on Aging, 2004). Sometimes the eyes produce too few tears, which can lead to itching and burning sensations, and sometimes reduce vision. Under conditions of glare, direct light narrows the visual field and limits peripheral vision. These individuals are typically blinded by direct beams of light, thus impairing their ability to drive at night. In addition, a decrease in the amount of light that hits the retina leads to a decrease in contrast sensitivity. An inability to detect shadows can impair an older adult's depth perception (e.g., an elder may not be able to detect a change in shadow that

indicates the edge of a step) and increase the risk of falls.

Behavioral Cues to Visual Deficits

One common symptom of vision problems is when people start to adjust the distance at which they hold a newspaper or book in front of them when they read. This is to compensate for loss of vision for items that are closer in distance. Also common is for people to begin to squint in an attempt to bring items farther in distance in focus. Squinting helps cut down some of the visual glare that may be impairing sight. These behavioral accommodations may be sufficient to counteract vision problems for several years, until vision deteriorates to the point where elders seek assessment and/or treatment.

Other behavioral cues include difficulties with **activities of daily living (ADLs)**. Visual deficits may lead to coordination difficulties in which the person has problems buttoning his or her shirt or finding food on a plate, leading the older person to eat less. They may have difficulty distinguishing an object from its background, leading to clumsy navigation of daily activities. Other cues include a decreased ability to "recognize familiar faces" and "locate 'small' objects, such as jewelry or keys" (Berry, Mascia, & Steinman, 2004, p. 37). This difficulty in distinguishing objects may also result in an older adult choosing brightly colored objects over more dull ones because the heightened color contrast assists the older adult in distinguishing them (Family Development and Resource Management, 2004); it also may lead to the older adult wearing stained or torn clothing (Berry et al., 2004).

Common Visual Diseases

The following are some of the common visual disorders associated with aging:

- *Macular degeneration:* **Macular degeneration** affects 10% or more of older adults and is a leading cause of blindness in the United States. The condition, which usually occurs bilaterally, is caused when neurons in the center of the retina (macula) are damaged and no longer function (due to hardening and blocking of the retinal arteries), resulting in blurred vision and loss of central vision.
- *Diabetic retinopathy:* **Diabetic retinopathy** is a long-term effect of diabetes. The blood vessels to the eyes grow weak and rupture, causing leakage into the eye and vision loss (creating blind spots), and may lead to blindness. New blood vessels form and "scar tissue may form along these new vessels, pulling on the retina causing macular distortion and possibly leading to retinal detachment" (Springhouse, 2001, p. 1158).
- *Glaucoma:* **Glaucoma** affects 2% of adults over the age of 40 (Springhouse, 2001). Glaucoma refers to a collection of eye disorders characterized by a buildup of viscous fluid (aqueous humor) in the intraocular cavity. The most common type of glaucoma (wide-angle glaucoma) occurs when the normal method of fluid drainage (out of the back of the eye through a small channel known as the trabecular meshwork) becomes blocked. This buildup of fluid creates pressure and damages the optic nerve. The cause of this blockage is as yet unknown, but the condition appears to be heritable. Glaucoma results in gradual loss of vision, and if left untreated, can lead to blindness.
- *Senile cataracts:* **Senile cataracts** are most commonly found in adults over the age of 70. **Cataracts** refer to a clouding of the lens, which blocks the path of light through the lens and can blur the image that is reflected onto the retina, resulting in hazy vision. Cataracts are most likely caused by changes in the proteins within the lens, which can cause blindness when severe. However, with surgical removal of the lens, cataracts can be corrected; 95% of surgery cases are effective (Eliopoulos, 2005; Springhouse, 2001).
- *Retinal detachment:* **Retinal detachment** is more common in men than in women; this condition occurs when the retina separates from the back of the eye and fills with vitreous fluid. Once separated, the retina is cut off from its blood supply, impairing its ability to function. This may result in severe visual impairment or blindness; however, this is usually correctable through surgical reattachment. In adults, this is typically caused by degenerative changes in the eye that lead to a torn retina,

but may also result from trauma, disease, or intraoccular pressure.

Students are encouraged to visit Lighthouse International's Web site at www.lighthouse.org/medical for simulations of common eye diseases. Chapter 13 provides additional information on the most common eye problems among older adults.

"The goal of low-vision care and other vision rehabilitation services is to maximize a person's usable sight and utilization of other sensory functions in combination with adaptive technologies and devices to perform usual, routine tasks" (Stuen & Faye, 2003, p. 9). Without rehabilitative care, elders are at risk for **depression**, anxiety, and communicative difficulties. Consider the following example:

Linda is a 79-year-old woman who has been completely independent up until 2 months ago. At that time, she had a car accident. Reportedly, Linda's vision became blurred and cloudy on that night and she just "missed" the car in front of her. An eye exam revealed 20/40 visual acuity. Further tests of contrast sensitivity and glare disability revealed severe impairment and suggested the presence of a cataract. Linda was instructed to refrain from driving and her physician discussed the pros and cons of cataract surgery with her.

In this case we see that Linda's impaired vision resulted in a car accident that could have seriously injured herself or others. This underscores the need for older adults to have regular eye examinations that can help detect the presence of problems before they interfere with the person's ability to perform daily routines.

The Impact of Visual Deficits on Communication

Declining visual skills may result in gradual isolation and a decrease in exchange of communication with the environment. As the person becomes less able to navigate outside of his or her home, he or she may become less socially active. Visual impairment may be a source of embarrassment to the older adult and serve to decrease the likelihood that he or she will engage in public activities (e.g., eating out in a restaurant, attending social gatherings) and further his or her isolation.

Communication Tips

When interacting with older adults with visual problems, it is important to position objects within their visual field. This includes positioning yourself within their visual field when speaking with the person. This helps the person to locate the object of conversation and to orient him or her to the topic of conversation.

When assisting elders with their care needs, it may be useful to give them a verbal indication of the actions you are about to impart, so as to avoid startling or scaring them needlessly (Family Development and Resource Management, 2004). It may be necessary to assist the person in labeling objects or to simplify what is in their visual field (e.g., reduce unnecessary clutter).

A more extreme situation is the case of **visual illusions** (distorted perceptions of vision). Due to the aging eye's decreased elasticity and accommodation abilities, an older adult may perceive objects or the difference between light and shadow at the edge of the field of vision as visual illusions. Other visual misperceptions include seeing little flecks or spots in the visual field when in bright light, or seeing shadows as people. The following excerpt is a real-life example:

It's mid-afternoon in an adult day care program, and the filtered afternoon sunlight is shining through the trees and bay window and onto one of the chairs at the table. Ethel, an 82-year-old female with some ambulation difficulties, is being escorted to the lunchroom when she stops suddenly and refuses to enter the kitchen. After persuasion and coaxing to enter the room were met with denial, Ethel was finally asked why she did not want to enter the room. Ethel proclaimed to the staff, "Look at all that water spilling from that chair onto the floor!"

Clearly Ethel did not want to enter the room for fear of slipping in the water. If staff were not aware of the possible interaction of her visual deficits and the environmental conditions (low lighting), it is possible that her behavior could have been misinterpreted as a behavioral problem, a symptom of dementia, or the presence of some other mental illness (e.g., psychosis—visual hallucinations).

Concomitant loss of other senses, particularly hearing, is common and can lead to further reductions in functional ability and independence (see **Box 4-1**). Among adults over the age of 70 with visual impairment, between 9% and 70% also have significant hearing loss (Brennan, 2003; Heine & Browning, 2002). This dual sensory loss (of both vision and hearing) can be particularly devastating given how much reliance we place on these senses to inform us about our environment.

BOX 4-1 Research Highlight

Aim: The study evaluated the relationship between auditory and visual sensory loss and depression.

Methods: A 2-year, population-based, prospective, observational study of 3,782 older adults age 65 or older was selected from the English Longitudinal Study of Ageing Waves 1 and 2. Sensory loss in vision and hearing, the eight-item Center for Epidemiologic Studies Depression Scale (CES-D), socioeconomic variables, health indicators, and social support were assessed.

Findings: Vision loss was a consistent predictor of the onset of and ongoing depression. On the other hand, the association between dual sensory loss and depression was no longer significant once health indicators (e.g., self-rated health and the presence of chronic conditions) were entered into the model.

Application to practice: Visual impairment is a specific risk for depression in older adults and has a more robust effect than hearing impairment. In any preventive or treatment efforts geared toward alleviating psychological disorders, clinicians need to take this information into consideration.

Chou, K. L. (2008). Combined effect of vision and hearing impairment on depression in older adults: Evidence from the English Longitudinal Study of Ageing. *Journal of Affective Disorders, 106*, 191–196.

Hearing

Mrs. Smith, the following fictional patient, typifies the difficulties experienced by many older adults and their discomfort in seeking help:

> *Margaret Smith, a 79-year-old widow and grandmother of four, used to look forward to the children's visits at holidays and other special occasions, but no longer enjoys the family gatherings. Margaret still attends them out of a sense of family duty and in order to make her children happy, but tends to sit apart from everyone, seemingly lost in thought. When her children attempt to get her involved in the conversation, she often keeps her statements short and noncommittal, and often appears to be off-topic. Her children worry about her cognitive status, but with the music and background noise, Margaret simply cannot hear what is being said. Margaret admits to her primary care physician that "I don't always hear so good, especially with the grandkids" but is afraid of telling her family, for fear that they will want to put her in "an old person's home."*

Typical Age-Related Changes in Hearing

Hearing loss is a commonly observed phenomenon in older adults and is one of the most common chronic disabilities in the United States. But hearing loss does not just affect older adults. In fact, hearing begins to decline on average in our 30s and continues more rapidly with age (Pirkl, 1995). Beginning at or around age 50–55, most adults start to lose sensitivity to pitch, with the very high frequency consonants (*t, p, k, f, s,* and *ch*) being lost first (Scheuerle, 2000). Background noise such as the hum of traffic or air conditioners (or in Margaret's case, music) may drown out voices, making conversation harder to hear. Higher pitched voices may not be understandable (Springhouse, 2001). Of course, there is variability in the extent of decline, with some people losing hearing in their 20s and some later on (Belsky, 1999). However, the general pattern is a decline with age, with 20–30% of Americans experiencing a hearing loss over the age of 65 years and 40–50% over the age of 75 (Jerger, Chmiel, Wilson, & Luchi, 1995; National Institute of Deafness and Communication Disorders [NIDCD], 2004); some researchers report even higher rates with over 89% of Americans over the age of 80 experiencing hearing loss (Cruickshanks et al., 1998).

Types of Hearing Loss

Conductive Problems. **Conductive problems** result in a reduction of sound transmission such that sound waves are blocked as they travel from the outer ear canal to the inner ear, resulting in a decrease in hearing sensitivity. Conductive loss can be caused by anything that blocks the external ear, but excessive wax (cerumen) buildup is the most common cause of conductive problems (Springhouse, 2001), with nearly one in three older adults having their hearing reduced by up to 35% (AgeWorks, 2000). Other causes of conduction problems include benign tumors (if left untreated), infections, and otosclerosis. Membranes in the middle ear become less flexible with age. The small bones (ossicles) become stiffer. Sometimes malformed or fused bones (otosclerosis) can lead to impaired movement of the stapes, thus preventing the transmission of sound waves. This is twice as likely to occur in women than in men, and usually occurs between adolescence and middle age (Springhouse, 2001).

Sensorineural Problems. Sound wave transmission can be interrupted from the inner ear to the auditory cortex of the brain, most likely due to damage to the cochlea and/or auditory nerve. **Sensorineural** loss is caused by both genetic and acquired factors (e.g., noise pollution, ototoxic substances). The most common form of age-related hearing loss is called **presbycusis** ("old man's hearing") (Bagai, Thavendiranathan, & Detsky, 2006). Presbycusis is the fourth-ranked chronic disability in older adults (age 65 or older) (Jerger et al., 1995). Presbycusis has a gradual onset and is typified by problems hearing high-pitched tones and a decrease in speech discrimination. Presbycusis occurs following loss of hair and supporting cells and nerve fibers in the cochlea. Loss of neurons in the cochlea can lead to poor word recognition (Springhouse, 2001) and thus difficulty understanding speech.

Mixed Hearing Loss. **Mixed hearing loss** is simply a mixture of both sensorineural and conductive hearing loss.

Pathological Changes to Hearing

Persistent Exposure to Noise Pollution

Not all hearing loss is due to **primary aging** factors. A weak tympanic membrane (the ear drum) may become damaged due to environmental noise or pressure changes. Employment-related damage in noisy environments—as with construction workers, racecar drivers or pit crews, and people who staff concerts—and combat/hunting-related damage are all common causes. This type of hearing loss is more likely to affect men because a larger proportion of men tend to work or engage in these activities. This form of hearing loss can be either temporary or permanent depending on the extent of the exposure. Long term exposure to environmental noise can also result in **tinnitus**, a condition in which the person experiences a persistent ringing, buzzing, humming, roaring, or other noise in the ears that only the person can hear. Tinnitus is often perceived as annoying or distracting, and has been associated with reduced quality of life in older adults (Nondahl et al., 2007).

Certain chemicals, substances, or conditions may damage an older adults' hearing. Such ototoxic conditions can lead to temporary changes in hearing or permanent hearing loss. These are discussed in the following section.

Exposure to Ototoxic Substances

Ototoxic substances

- Medications: Some medications, including aspirin, antibiotics, diuretics, and antidepressants, can cause symptoms of tinnitus. These losses are typically permanent and do not remit after removal of the medication.
- Poisons: Poisons such as arsenic, lead, or mercury are toxic to the inner ear and typically affect the eighth cranial nerve. Exposure to these substances may lead to either temporary or permanent hearing loss (Springhouse, 2001).

- Certain medical conditions may also predispose older adults to hearing problems.

Medical Conditions

- Acute trauma, or damage at the level of the central nervous system, can be due to head trauma (most likely caused by falls). If the damage is to the eighth cranial nerve, then sensorineural loss will be observed. If the damage is to the temporal lobe (the cortex), a loss of certain frequencies and pitches occurs.
- Cardiovascular disease—high blood pressure is a treatable cause of tinnitus.
- Cigarette smoking can aggravate tinnitus.
- Chronic viral or bacterial infections in the middle ear, if poorly treated, can result in hearing loss.
- Exposure to measles, mumps, or meningitis can lead to sensorineural deficits.

Difficulties Detecting Hearing Loss

Despite the fact that hearing loss is a common occurrence in older adults, it is not routinely assessed (Tsuruoka et al., 2001). It is estimated that only 20% of primary care physicians routinely assess older adults for hearing loss. Compounding this problem is that the patients themselves may not be aware of their deficit. This may be due to several factors including compensation, a failure to report due to its gradual onset (if presbycusis), ignorance of their condition, and/or embarrassment.

People often compensate for mild hearing loss by engaging in such behaviors as turning up the volume of the television, pretending to understand conversation, or attempting to fill in the gaps in conversation by using contextual cues. Missing sounds may not be detected by the person, and he or she may miss entire events and not know it. Thus, it is not surprising that in studies of hearing loss, some researchers have found that the affected person judges his or her impairment as less severe than the spouse does (Chmiel & Jerger, 1993). Conversely, because of social stigma and embarrassment, individuals may not report their hearing loss to others, and instead may withdraw socially to prevent others from detecting their hearing loss.

Older adults who do seek assistance with hearing problems have typically experienced some hearing loss for years before help is sought. One estimate of the time between the experienced loss and treatment seeking is as high as 10 years (Jerger et al., 1995). Think of the amount of suffering that may have needlessly been incurred.

Indications of Hearing Loss

Hearing impairment may lead to the following behaviors:

- Inattentiveness and/or inappropriate responses or no response to questions
- Asking repetitious questions, or asking for things to be repeated
- Complaints that other people are "mumbling" or have some other speech impediment
- An increased reaction to loud sounds (as in presbycusis)
- Increased or unusually loud speech in conversation, especially in areas with some type of background noise
- Tilting/cocking head toward a sound in an attempt to facilitate hearing
- Turning the volume up on the radio or television to higher than normal levels

Isolation and/or emotional upset often occur as a result of problems in communicating with others, either in group settings or individually.

The Impact of Hearing Deficits on Communication

Hearing loss has adverse effects on multiple domains including cognitive, emotional, behavioral, and social functioning. Hearing impairment can lead to negative results such as decreased quality of life, depression, isolation, impaired communication, and decreased social interactions (Jerger et al., 1995). Thus, it is imperative that individuals be assessed, treated, and routinely reassessed.

Hearing loss can be devastating to both individuals and their families. As with other age-related sensory changes, hearing loss can result in loss of functional independence and a reduction in quality of life (National Institutes of Health [NIH], 1999). In a large population-based longitudinal study of older adults with hearing impairment, Dalton and colleagues (2003) found that over 50% of participants had difficulties with communication. With increasing severity of impairment, participants were increasingly more likely to report communication problems (mild = 3 times more likely, moderate to severe = 8 times more likely) than nonimpaired controls. Severity of loss was also found to be associated with decreased "vitality, social functioning, role emotional, mental health, role physical, and physical functioning" domains as measured by a standardized measure, the Short-Form 36 Health Survey (SF-36) (Dalton et al., 2003, p. 667). Other researchers have found that older adults with hearing impairment commonly report experiencing isolation and loneliness (Chen, 1994). Clearly, hearing loss affects many areas beyond just the physical and sensory deficits.

Several studies have also examined the emotional impact of hearing loss. It has been well established that hearing impairment is significantly associated with generally lower mood and depression (e.g., Carabellese et al., 1993; Tsuruoka et al., 2001), isolation (e.g., Mulrow et al., 1990; Weinstein & Ventry, 1982), and increased risk of developing an anxiety disorder (Mehta et al., 2003).

Individuals with hearing loss also may have trouble functioning independently. They may find it difficult to understand (and therefore follow) their primary care doctor's advice and they may be prone to more accidents (difficulty responding to warnings or alarms) (National Institute on Aging, 2004). In addition, mild to moderate hearing loss is more likely to lead to social isolation. This may be related to the hearing-impaired individual becoming frustrated with having to constantly ask others to repeat themselves. This also may be related to feeling embarrassment over having failed at conversation (Tsuruoka et al., 2001). Conversely, the social isolation may sometimes be due to others, who may unconsciously stay away from those persons with whom having a conversation is difficult.

Communication Tips

When communicating with a person who presents with hearing impairment, do not shout. Shouting increases the intensity and pitch of the words, but does not aid in hearing what is being said (Family Development and Resource Management, 2004) because the high-frequency consonants are still not heard. A better suggestion is to attempt to project voice from the diaphragm (deepens tone). Make use of the person's other unimpaired senses. For example, alert the person that you are addressing him or her by touching him or her lightly or by using a visual cue, and wait for him or her to visually orient to you before speaking. Ensure that you are standing in front of the person in a well-lit room. This will help to assist him or her with lip-reading. If the person has better hearing in one of his or her ears, attempt to speak to that side if possible. If the person wears a hearing aid, ensure that it is turned on. Use gestures or objects to assist with communication (Family Development and Resource Management, 2004).

Other useful tips include limiting background noise. If conversing with a hearing-impaired elder, it is helpful to close the windows and turn off televisions, radios, and air conditioning units that may make it difficult for the person to distinguish voices from the background noise. In addition, make sure to allow adequate time for a response. Rewording the question may only serve to further confuse the person. It may be more helpful to use short sentences and speak clearly, taking care to enunciate words (Springhouse, 2001). At times, you may have to resort to writing or using a pictogram grid for communication. Again, consider the use of other modes of communication, such as gestures or touch, that might be helpful.

Speech and Language

Normal Aging Changes in Speech and Language

Normal age-related changes in speech and language occur as a result of physiological and cognitive changes. For example, decreased respiration strength may cause the voice to become deeper and speech may become more shaky and breathy. In addition, pitch may vary and voice may sound tremulous as a result of changes of the laryngeal structure. Some older adults may experience an overproduction of mucus, which may result in frequent attempts at throat clearing. Reduced saliva, loss of teeth, and decreased elasticity and muscle tone of the face also are common and may cause changes in articulation. Cognitive changes associated with aging also may be responsible for older adults using fewer words and making more semantic errors than younger adults (Beers & Berkow, 2000). As you will see in the following section, together, normal aging changes and pathological changes in the body systems result in impaired communication processes.

Pathological Changes in Speech and Language

Several conditions experienced by older adults may lead to changes in speech and language. For example, stroke is a common health problem in this age group and one which can leave significant deficits in the ability to speak and understand. Some pathological problems related to communication are discussed here.

- **Dysarthria** is disturbed articulation caused by disturbance in the control of the speech muscles. This disturbance is caused by brain lesions in motor areas in the central nervous system or the brain stem or disruption in the coordination of information from the basal ganglia, cerebellum, and motor neurons. Dysarthria-related lesions can be caused by stroke, brain tumor, degenerative diseases, metabolic diseases, or toxins. The location of the brain lesion determines the nature of the disturbance, which can manifest in many ways, with the most severe form being **anarthria** (complete inability to move the articulators for speech). People with dysarthria may present with slurred speech, breathiness, slow or rapid rate of speech, limited mouth or facial movement, monotonous voice, or weak articulation. A person who has dysarthria may be able to read, write, and gesture normally and comprehension may remain intact (Duffy, 1995; Finlayson & Heffer, 2000).
- **Verbal apraxia** is a disorder caused by damage primarily to the parietal lobe (the part of the brain involved with somatosensory processing). This is a neurological disorder characterized by impairment in initiation, coordination, and sequencing of muscle movement, which results in difficulties executing mouth and speech movements. People with verbal apraxia have the intention and the physical capacity to move the muscles that are involved in speech, but have difficulties producing speech, because of loss of volitional control over the muscles. This condition often accompanies aphasia (Beers & Berkow, 2000).
- **Aphasia** is the most common language disorder in the elderly and occurs in up to a third of the patients in an acute phase following stroke (Wade, Hewer, David, & Menderby, 1986). Aphasia is an inability to express or understand the meaning of words due to damage in the language areas. Damage is most frequently due to stroke in the left hemisphere, but can be due to brain tumor, trauma, infection, dementia, or surgery. In addition to spoken language, writing, reading, and the ability to gesture also may be impaired. **Receptive (fluent) aphasia** is characterized by an inability to comprehend spoken or written language but intact expressive ability. However, although the production of speech is intact, the meaning of spoken language is severely distorted and words do not hang together. This is a result of damage to **Wernicke's area** in the brain, which is in charge of the meaning of language. **Expressive (nonfluent) aphasia** is characterized by an inability to produce language in either an oral or a written form, but relatively intact language comprehension. The person produces very few effortful words, short sentences, and many pauses. This aphasia is due to damage to **Broca's area**, which is in charge of speech production. In most cases, however, a combination of deficits exists and aphasia is never purely expressive or receptive. Global aphasia is the most severe form of aphasia and is characterized by severe impairment in the production of recognizable words as well as in the understanding of spoken language (Duffy, 1995; Finlayson & Heffer, 2000).

Other medical conditions may also result in impairment in speech. For example:

- **Chronic obstructive pulmonary disease (COPD)** is a common condition in older adults that is characterized by blockage of airflow in the lungs. Speech is likely to be low in volume and the pitch restricted in range. Because of frequent coughing and dyspnea, people may also present with chronic hoarseness (Duffy, 1995).
- Some older adults may require support by mechanical ventilation because of respiratory failure. Those who require mechanical ventilation

often need to communicate by writing or by using an **electrolarynx**, which is a voice box that produces sounds based on air vibrations. Others may learn to communicate with a tracheostomy tube.

- Another medical procedure that affects communication is **laryngectomy**. This is an operation used to treat patients with laryngeal or hypopharyngeal cancers. After total laryngectomy, patients can no longer use their own voice. Instead, writing, mouthing words, gesturing, or an electrolarynx may be used. Surgical procedures to restore speech can also be performed, but this requires some additional practice and adaptation (Duffy, 1995).

The Impact of Speech and Language Deficits on Communication

Deficits in speech and/or language are not necessarily global and are likely to vary from person to person. For example, one elder may not be able to produce spoken language, but will have no difficulties in comprehending language, whereas another person may have deficits in both comprehension and production of language. Our interactions should, of course, be adapted according to the specific needs and deficits of the affected elderly person. Consider the following example:

> *John is a 78-year-old man who has been at the hospital for the past 3 weeks following a car accident. He is connected to a mechanical ventilator and is able to communicate only in writing. He also has a hearing problem; hence, staff members also need to communicate in writing. To improve his ability to communicate with others, the social worker suggested the use of a pocket talker. This allows individuals to communicate with persons who are hard of hearing by amplifying sounds and voices in the immediate environment. John also learned how to communicate using the talking tracheostomy tubes. A few days later, John reported a significant improvement in his mood.*

Communication Tips

Individuals with speech or language difficulties might be more anxious or self-aware when communicating and, thus, an environment that is low in distractions and that allows the elderly to feel relaxed might be helpful. Position yourself in close proximity to the elderly person and face him or her so that eye contact is maintained and facial expressions and body language are easily conveyed. In addition, being open and prepared to use multiple forms of communication, such as body language, or written or pictorial information, are important. Using short uncomplicated sentences that offer simple choices may also be helpful. Constantly rephrasing and using physical demonstrations can be helpful for those who have comprehension difficulties.

In cases when speech production is impaired, summarizing the message in order to check for accuracy may be helpful. It also is important not to correct every error and to respect the elder's limitations. Constant correction can be damaging to self-esteem and may result in punishing the affected person's efforts. Rather, being patient and accepting, even when communication takes time and effort, is of utmost importance and is likely to teach the elderly person and his or her family members to accept his or her challenges and limitations.

Touch

Touch, pressure, vibration, pain, and temperature are sensations that we receive through our skin and are part of the **somatosensory system**. The skin responds to external stimuli, which are then interpreted by the brain as softness, pain, or heat. Research has demonstrated that despite wide variability across individuals, there is a reduction in tactile and vibration sensations as well as decreased sensitivity to warm or cold stimuli as we age (Kenshalo, 1986; Stevens & Patterson, 1995; Thomson, Masson, & Boulton, 1993; Thornbury & Mistretta, 1981). Reduced touch sensitivity is more prevalent in the fingertips than in other locations, such as the forearm and lip (Stevens & Patterson, 1995).

Reduction in somatosensory sensitivity has been attributed to a reduction in the number of receptors and a reduction in the blood flow to the receptors that occur as we age (Gescheider, Beiles, Checkosky, Bolanowski, & Verrillo, 1994; Verrillo, Bolanowski, & Gescheider, 2002). However, not all older adults present with somatosensory deficits, and certain medical conditions associated with aging such as dementia, diabetes, arthritis, and

Parkinson's disease may exacerbate changes in the somatosensory system (McBride & Mistretta, 1982; Mold, Vesely, Keyl, Schenk, & Roberts, 2004; Muller, Richter, Weisbrod, & Klingberg, 1992).

Somatosensory information plays an important role in ensuring our safety. For example, the experiences of pain or heat alert us to change our position in the environment, to avoid certain situations, or to change the environment altogether. Reduced somatosensory sensitivity in the elderly has been associated with an increase in injuries, such as **hypothermia**, burns, or **pressure ulcers**. Reduced tactile perception also has been associated with postural instability and with the difficulties of older adults to position and orient their bodies in space (Corriveau, Hebert, Raiche, Dubois, & Prince, 2004; Toshiaki et al., 1995).

The Impact of Somatosensory Deficits on Communication

When older adults present with injuries, it is important not to blame or interpret the injuries as intentional, but instead try to identify alternative means to communicate the very essential somatosensory information. For example, teaching older adults to read the thermostat in order to detect the water temperature might help those with somatosensory deficits to notice excessive hot or cold temperatures. Encouraging older adults to move out of their chair frequently can prevent pressure ulcers.

Some older adults might grasp objects tightly or use their mouth to explore the quality of objects. It is important to recognize that these behaviors might be a result of sensory deficits, and the mouth becomes a tool for making sense of the world. It might be useful to describe the objects verbally or pictorially and to allow the person to explore them using all means (as long as they do not pose a danger to the individual).

Communication Tips

When engaging in physical activity with older adults, it is important to use verbal explanations to describe the physical activities as they take place. Some older adults may avoid tactile sensations altogether because of their deficits; however, in the presence of other sensory deficits, touch is often used as a substitute. Recall that we briefly discussed the important role of touch in other aspects of communication. For example, the receipt of touch initiated by others can convey meaning and add context that serves to facilitate communication. Touch can communicate comfort, strong emotions (e.g., anger), or danger. Therefore, sensory and somatosensory deficits may cause a person to have even further reductions in functional ability.

When older adults avoid activities that require touch, such as sewing or painting, you might want to encourage them to revert to enjoyable activities that capitalize on strengths and abilities they have maintained; for example, encouraging older adults to sing as a replacement for sewing to alleviate feelings of boredom, uselessness, or depression.

Movement

Movement is an important ability that fosters independence and promotes interaction and understanding of the environment (Wang, Badley, & Gignac, 2004). Movement is a function of many variables, such as posture, balance, flexibility, tone, strength, sensory integration, reflexes, and motor planning. Movement produced by the large muscle groups is called **gross motor movement**, while movement produced by the small muscle groups is called **fine motor movement**. Research has shown that both gross and fine motor movements are affected by the aging process, aging-related diseases, and a sedentary lifestyle associated with aging. In general, as we age, movement is characterized by reduced **velocity** (speed) and accuracy and greater variability across individuals (Fozard, Vercruyssen, Reynolds, Hancock, & Quilter, 1994; Mattay et al., 2002; Smith et al., 1999; Welford, 1982) (see **Box 4-2**).

Movement Disorders in Older Adults

Parkinson's disease (PD) is a chronic neurodegenerative condition characterized by impairment in the nerves that control movement. This is a progressive disease that affects the basal ganglia in the brain. People with PD have a shortage of dopamine. The etiology of Parkinson's disease is unclear. The major symptoms of PD include tremor, rigidity and stiffness, slowness of movement, postural instability, and/or impaired balance and coordination. Other symptoms may include memory problems, depression,

BOX 4-2 **Web Exploration**

The best way to understand physiological changes associated with aging and their impact on communication is to have a "first-hand" experience of some of these changes. Family Development and Resource Management offers a wonderful Web site with multiple exercises to stimulate some of the aging-related processes. Go to its Web site http://fcs.tamu.edu/families/aging/aging_simulation/index.php and try to gain "hands on" experiences by simulating at least two sensory-motor deficits. Write a short paragraph about your experiences and how these experiences affected your ability to communicate with others in your surroundings.

hallucination, and mild vision loss. The course and rate of progression vary. Currently, there is no cure for PD; however, medications that increase the presence of dopamine in the brain improve some of its symptoms (Ebersole & Hess, 1998).

Although the course of PD varies and deficits are not uniformly present, this condition is likely to impair communication in a variety of ways:

- Speech may become more slurred, soft, hoarse, or have an inappropriate rhythm.
- Writing may become smaller, shaky, and difficult to read.
- Facial expressions may be lost.

Thus, the presence of PD may impact the ability to communicate using written and spoken language as well as nonverbally.

Disability

With advanced age, older persons experience more chronic illnesses and disability. A decrease in the ability to perform ADLs and IADLs independently can have a negative impact on the older person's quality of life as discussed below.

Activities of Daily Living/ Instrumental Activities of Daily Living

Activities of daily living (ADLs) are basic tasks that one needs to perform in order to survive. These include eating, bathing, toileting, transferring, and grooming. **Instrumental activities of daily living (IADLs)** are more complex tasks that include handling finances, preparing meals, or managing one's medications. Because of their basic nature, impairments in ADLs are considered to be more severe than IADL impairments.

ADLs and IADLs are often used to assess functioning. Impairment in ADLs/IADLs is most prevalent among the elderly. It is estimated that about 26% of people between the ages of 65 and 74 report functional limitations, whereas almost 50% of people over the age of 75 report such limitations. Research has shown that 14% of older adults have ADL limitations and as many as 21% of older adults have impairment in IADLs (Administration on Aging, 2002). The rates of unmet needs associated with ADL impairments are very high. Unfortunately, research has shown that as many as 20% of those who had at least one ADL impairment did not receive adequate assistance to meet their needs (Allen & Mor, 1997; Desai, Lentzner, & Weeks, 2001).

Risk Factors for Impairment in ADLs/IADLs

In addition to age, other risk factors for ADL/IADL impairment include female gender (Collison, Cicuttini, Mead, & Savio, 1999; Oman, Reed, & Ferrara, 1999), cognitive impairment (Hebert, Brayne, & Spiegelhalter, 1993), the presence of a chronic disease (Collison et al., 1999), lack of exercise (Stessman, Hammerman-Rozenberg, Maaravi, & Cohen, 2002), depression (Han, 2002), subjective health problems (Collison et al., 1999), and low socioeconomic status (Kaplan, Strawbridge, Camacho, & Cohen, 1993). Research has shown that the trajectory of ADL changes across time is highly individualized. Often, people show a steep decline in their ADL functioning a few months prior to their death or hospitalization. Others, on the other hand, remain relatively unchanged in their ADL functioning (Li, 2005).

Measuring ADLs/IADLs

Measures of ADLs/IADLs have become increasingly popular because they are very sensitive indicators of hospital stay, nursing home placement, and mortality (Mast, Armin, MacNeill, & Lichtenberg, 2004). Most of the time, the presence or absence of a medical diagnosis would be less indicative of level of function than ADL/IADL functioning. Thus, information about ADL/IADL functioning can be used not only as a prognostic tool, but also to tell whether to treat a disease and to determine the person's level of need for care. Additionally, information about ADLs/IADLs can assist in setting realistic goals for treatment, developing an appropriate treatment plan, and monitoring change over time.

Notable Quotes

"To keep your brain young and protect yourself from age-related cognitive decline, learn to use a computer if you do not now use one, change your operating system frequently, and learn another language."

—Andrew Weill, MD
and best-selling author,
in *Healthy Aging* (p. 279)

Both ADLs and IADLs have their limitations as indicators of functional impairment. ADLs are very basic and, thus, may not be sensitive enough to capture less severe disability. IADLs, on the other hand, may not be relevant in long-term settings where one's opportunities to engage with the environment are limited. Additionally, some IADLs tend to be gender-specific (e.g., cooking a meal) and, thus, not applicable to the entire population, especially in the older cohort that is used to more traditional gender role standards.

Self-report measures of ADLs/IADLs are easy to use and require no prior training. However, research has shown that older adults often overestimate their abilities, whereas family members underestimate their loved one's abilities (Rubenstein et al., 1988). Furthermore, physicians were found to be poor judges of ADLs/IADLs (Elam et al., 1989). To complicate things, simple wording changes of questionnaire items resulted in major differences in prevalence estimates of functional disability (Picavet & van de Bos, 1996).

Direct observation of someone's performance is considered to be more objective and replicable than self-report measures; however, it is important to consider level of motivation when judging someone's functioning level. Additionally, performance-based measures may assess tasks that are irrelevant to the everyday life of the elderly. Thus, a combination of the two is warranted.

Compensating for ADL/IADL Impairments

Depending on the impairment in ADLs/IADLs, a person might use assistive devices such as a calendar or a pill organizer to overcome difficulties in managing medications. Others might use clothes with large buttons or with no buttons at all when faced with dressing difficulties. Changes in the environment, such as the addition of handrails to prevent falls, also can be implemented.

Cognitive Changes

There is a high variability in cognitive functioning both within individuals and across individuals. Some cognitive functions decline with age, some remain stable, and others improve. However, most studies suggest that people in their 30s and 40s have the highest cognitive abilities, which decline thereafter. Yet, it is estimated that cognitive changes become noticeable only when people are in their 70s.

A distinction between **fluid intelligence** (the acquisition of new information) and **crystallized intelligence** (the accumulation of knowledge over the life span) is often used. Fluid intelligence is believed to decline over time, whereas crystallized intelligence is believed to remain stable (Abeles et al., 1998). Some of the skills that decline with age include **information processing speed** (the time it takes to analyze data), **divided attention** (the ability to attend to and analyze two stimuli presented simultaneously), **sustained attention** (the ability to focus cognitive activity on a stimulus), performance on visuospatial tasks (e.g., drawing and block construction), word finding, rapid naming ability, abstraction, mental flexibility, and **long-term memory** (large storage capacity for information for long periods of time or even indefinitely). In contrast, **short-term memory** (modest capacity for storing information for a few seconds) shows a milder decline with age, while verbal comprehension and expression remain stable. Vocabulary may improve with age. It also is believed that wisdom and the accumulation of practical expertise continue to improve throughout the life span (Abeles et al., 1998).

Pathological Cognitive Changes

Delirium. **Delirium** is quite common in hospital settings, accounting for 10–15% of admissions in elders, while another 10–40% may be diagnosed during their hospital stay (American Psychiatric Association [APA], 1994). Delirium is prevalent in the terminally ill, with up to 80% developing this condition as they near death. The *Diagnostic and Statistical Manual of Mental Health Disorders*, 4th edition (APA, 1994), defines delirium as:

> 1. *Disturbance of consciousness with reduced ability to focus, sustain, or shift attention*
> 2. *A change in cognition (such as memory deficit, disorientation, language disturbance) or the development of a perceptual disturbance that is not better accounted for by a preexisting, established or evolving dementia*
> 3. *The disturbance develops over a short period of time (usually hours to days) and tends to fluctuate over the course of the day*
> 4. *There is evidence from the history, physical examination or laboratory findings that the disturbance is caused by several different possible events including general medical conditions (cancer, AIDS), metabolic disturbances (including electrolyte disturbances as occurs with dehydration, drug intoxication, drug withdrawal, drug side effects, and multiple etiologies).*

Without a good history and intake, delirium could easily be misinterpreted as any number of disorders including psychotic disorders, dementia, and mood disorders with psychotic features.

The prognosis for an individual with delirium is good to excellent if correctly identified, but full recovery is unlikely in the geriatric population, with estimates ranging from 4% to 40% (APA, 1994). Particularly in the medically ill, delirium is associated with increased risk of developing medical complications and functional decline. If misdiagnosed, delirium can be life threatening, leading to coma, seizures, and eventual death.

Given that a person with delirium commonly experiences hallucinations and tends to be disoriented and confused, communication is often fraught with misinterpretation (e.g., as when the person has delusions of persecution) and the person is likely to respond inappropriately (Springhouse, 2001).

The following are guidelines for communicating with the delirious elderly:

- Keep discussions simple and questions concise.
- Use large-print calendars and clocks to assist with orientation to time.
- Pictures of family members and loved ones might assist in reorienting the elder.
- Some older adults may experience an increased state of delirium in the darkness; thus, a well-lit place might be helpful.
- Offer frequent reassurance, because the person is likely to be anxious and fearful. Physical restraints are *not* recommended, because they may increase fear and agitation. Distraction and soothing conversation should be tried instead.

Dementia. There are over 35 million elderly people over age 65 in the United States (U.S. Bureau of the Census, 2000). This number is projected to increase to 70 million by the year 2030, which is a dramatic increase in those with the highest vulnerability to dementia. Dementia is not a disease, but rather a grouping of symptoms known as a syndrome, which may be caused by a number of different sources (Anthony & Aboraya, 1992). This is a progressive illness that impairs social and occupational functioning (APA, 1994). The APA (1994) defines the criteria for dementia as:

1. Development of cognitive deficits:
   - The person cannot recall new or previously learned information.
   - Memory problems must be present.
2. One or more of the following:
   a. **Apraxia**: Impaired motor activities due to damage to motor cortex (e.g., the person cannot use a key)
   b. *Aphasia:* Language disturbance (e.g., cannot find words or put sentences together)
   c. **Agnosia**: Failure to recognize or identity objects (e.g., the person may see something but cannot label it or tell what it is used for)

d. **Disturbed executive functioning**: Planning, organizing, sequencing, and abstracting problems due to frontal lobe damage

In addition to general loss of cognitive functioning, it is typical to see changes in personality, affect, and behavior over the course of the disease as a result of pathophysiological changes in the brain (Kasl-Godley & Gatz, 2000).

Dementia can have irreversible or reversible causes. **Irreversible dementia** refers to the inability to cure or reverse the symptoms with medical or psychological treatment. Examples of irreversible causes of dementia include head trauma (repeated blows to the head, as happens in professional boxing), infections such as those related to HIV and AIDS, brain tumors, and genetic diseases (Holland, 1999). Other irreversible causes include dementias due to other progressive diseases such as Alzheimer's disease (responsible for 50–60% of all dementias after the age of 60), Huntington's disease, and Parkinson's disease. Dementia can also be caused by vascular disease including multi-infarct dementia, which is caused by a series of small strokes (Kasl-Godley & Gatz, 2000).

Approximately 10–20% of dementias are **reversible** (Cooper, 1999). These are sometimes referred to as **pseudodementias**. The potential for reversibility depends on the etiology and treatment availability (Kaplan & Sadock, 1998). Typical causes include depression, hypothyroidism, drug toxicity, and hydrocephalus. Depression may mask itself as dementia (Teri, 1996). With treatment, dementia secondary to depression is reversible, although research has indicated that a large number of these individuals may go on to develop irreversible dementia later (Raskind & Peskind, 1992).

Alzheimer's Disease. As previously mentioned, dementia can be caused by a number of different sources. **Alzheimer's disease** is responsible for 50–60% of all dementias in adults over the age of 60. The progression of dementia of the Alzheimer's type is commonly detailed into three stages (Mayo Clinic, 2008):

1. *Stage 1* (duration 2–4 years, leading up to and including diagnosis)
    - Progressive memory loss (e.g., forgetfulness, misplaced objects) and confusion (e.g., easily overwhelmed by tasks, disorientation)
    - Mood and personality changes—may become more labile or depressed
    - Loss of spontaneity and initiative in verbal and nonverbal communication and activity engagement
    - Decreased concentration abilities
    - Impaired judgment and thinking
2. *Second stage* (duration 2–8 years)
    - Increasing memory loss and confusion
    - Difficulty recognizing loved ones
    - Poor impulse control with frequent outbursts, mood lability
    - May display aggressive behavior
    - Hallucinations or delusions
    - Aphasia and **confabulation** (filling in words or memory gaps with information that is made up in order to compensate for memory loss)
    - **Agraphia** (inability to write)
    - Agnosia
    - Repetitive behaviors are common; wandering and restlessness
    - **Hyperorality** (the need to taste and orally examine objects small enough to be placed in the mouth)
3. *Third stage* (duration 1–3 years)
    - Loss of weight or conversely binge eating and weight gain
    - Loss of most self-care skills
    - Incontinence of urine and bowel
    - Minimal to no communication, may scream
    - Multiple physical health problems and eventual death
    - Progressive decrease in ability to respond to environmental stimuli

Alzheimer's disease has been deemed a disease of "rule out." Although neuropsychological testing can be very useful in clinical diagnosis, currently no definitive diagnosis can be made until after death, when an autopsy can be performed and the hallmark pathophysiological features can be identified. However, excellent screening tools help to make a diagnosis so that treatment may be initiated early. See Chapter 15 for further information.

Delirium and dementia are not necessarily mutually exclusive. Delirium can occur in a person with dementia, making accurate diagnosis and treatment difficult. It is important, therefore, to develop an understanding of the similarities and differences between the two. A good history is important in helping with differentiation. However, given the person's symptom presentation (e.g., confusion and disorientation), the person is unlikely to be a good historian. Collateral information is important to gather, if possible. Refer to **Table 4-2** for a comparison of the two conditions.

TABLE 4-2 Diagnostic Comparison Between Delirium and Dementia

	Delirium	Dementia
Onset	Sudden	Depending on the type of dementia • Alzheimer's disease: onset is gradual and progressive. • Vascular dementia: onset can be sudden but progression is in a step-wise decline. • Pick's: onset is sudden and decline is progressive and rapid.
Prognosis and duration	If identified properly, the condition is temporary and reversible. Lasting from days to months	Depending on the type of dementia • If irreversible: process can be slowed by use of medications, but decline is inevitable. • If reversible type (pseudodementia): process is reversible with treatment of underlying cause; however, some researchers suggest that dementia secondary to depression is a prelude to later irreversible dementia. Lasting from months to years
Symptoms		
Orientation	Waxing and waning throughout the day with periods of lucidity	Progressive loss of orientation to time, place, and lastly person
Attention	Impairments in ability to attend	Relatively intact immediate attention skills
Memory	Impaired recent and remote memory	Progressive loss of memory with recent affected prior to remote
Learning and abstract thinking	Impaired	Impaired
Psychological	Hallucinations, delusion, and visual illusions common	Personality change, suspicion, paranoia, compulsive behavior, hallucinations/delusions possible

TABLE 4-2 (continued)

	Delirium	Dementia
Affect	Labile	Labile, prone to apathy and depression in early stages
Behavior	Impulsive, loss of typical social behaviors Loss of self-care skills due to inability to sequence steps for correct performance	Decreased inhibition, agitation, routine becomes important, withdrawal, loss of spontaneous engagement, wandering and hoarding common Loss of self-care abilities in later stage
Object naming	Intact to mild	Aphasia, agnosia
Treatment	• Maintain proper nutritional intake • Maintain fluid intake and balance • One-to-one observation • Repetitive orientation; do not reinforce hallucinations	• Behavior plans • Ensure medication compliance • Encourage group and social interaction as well as activity engagement • Clear simple instructions, memory prompts, reminiscence therapy

Dementia is also discussed in more depth in Chapter 15.

The Impact of Dementia on Communication. Communication with an individual with dementia is extremely important to successful interaction and completion of caregiving duties. In the early stages of dementia, individuals may have difficulty finding the words to express what they are trying to say (aphasia) and they may substitute one word for another. They may not be able to understand abstract concepts or more complicated language phrases. In either of these cases, elders and caregivers can become frustrated, embarrassed, and upset about their inability to communicate with each other effectively. This can lead to a reduction in social contact and reduced feelings of self-worth for the patient.

In individuals with more moderate to severe dementia, verbal abilities are likely to be severely limited. Many times individuals with cognitive impairment can become agitated because they do not understand what is expected of them. In addition, they can become easily frustrated if their attempts at communication are misunderstood. It may be important to use other means of communication to facilitate understanding. Sometimes touch can assist in conveying a message and comfort. The caregiver should be attentive to the person's responses, because some people may recoil from touch. In such cases, simple gestures or visual aids may be more effective (e.g., hold up the shirt if you are trying to get the person to dress). Other methods of communication can involve use of familiar songs/music or doing activities together (e.g., going for a walk) to convey care and concern.

Communication Tips. Robinson, Spenser, and White (1999) recommend that a nondemanding approach for communication is best. The caregiver's attitude or approach can often set the tone for the interaction. If you are calm, reassuring, and confident, the person is likely to respond in a relaxed and trusting manner. Elders with dementia generally are still attuned to nonverbal cues. If you are angry and tense, you are likely to find the person responding to you in a like fashion. Keep the pitch of your voice low, especially when interacting with a person with hearing impairments. Remember that shouting does not help with understanding and is likely to startle/upset the person with dementia.

When interacting with a person with dementia, make sure that the person is attending to you prior to beginning a conversation. Face the person and speak slowly and clearly. If you do not have the person's attention, wait a moment and try again. A gentle touch can be helpful, but be careful not to startle the person. Try to be eye level with the person so as not to create feelings of defensiveness or vulnerability. Begin by orienting the person to yourself (i.e., introduce yourself) and refer to the person by name (assists in preserving self-identity and relaxing the person). It is often helpful to reduce or eliminate background noise to improve the chances of maintaining the person's attention and having him or her hear you more clearly (e.g., turn down radios or television sets to eliminate distraction).

It might be helpful to break tasks into small manageable steps and provide very simple, clear directions. Taking a bath can be overwhelming or confusing to an individual when taken as a whole event and will need to be simplified. When helping someone to undress for bathing, the first step might be to begin with unbuttoning his or her shirt. The next step might be taking one arm out of the sleeve. Sometimes contextual cues may be helpful. Throughout the process, remember to keep telling the person what it is you are planning to do next and what it is you are currently doing. Leading a person slowly to the bathroom may assist in understanding what task is about to occur. Likewise, utilizing props may also assist with task recognition (e.g., handing the person a washcloth). Encourage the person to do as much as they can and praise efforts. If an instruction needs to be repeated, repeat it in the same way. This will facilitate comprehension. Assist with steps that may be more difficult for the person to accomplish on their own. This may be a little more time consuming than other approaches, but it is likely to be met with much less confusion and more pleasant interaction.

Use concrete terms and familiar words. Saying phrases such as "Here is your toast" may be more readily understood than "It's breakfast time" (Robinson et al., 1999). Try to offer choices whenever possible. When offering choices, simplicity is better. Use a paired choice procedure ("Would you like orange juice or water?") rather than using open-ended questions, which could generate confusion ("What would you like to drink this morning?"). Use of concrete terms is helpful here, as well. Allow the person adequate time to respond, because the processing of verbal material is slower in individuals with cognitive impairment. Refrain from arguing or attempting to reason with someone regarding delusions or hallucinations, because this can serve to further agitate the patient (Robinson et al., 1999). Instead, speak in soothing tones and attempt to distract the person, if possible.

Encourage discussion of significant life events, family traditions, remote memories, and other past events to encourage social contact and a sense of comfort and security. Utilize memory aids such as large-print calendars or organizers to enhance memory. Labeling items with large print helps in identification and recognition of objects. Encouraging individuals to refer to these aids can reduce the anxiety and paranoia associated with being in unfamiliar surroundings (e.g., a hospital room) and enhance self-dignity.

The physical environment can be important for stimulating cognitive functioning, managing behaviors, reducing depression and anxiety, and promoting and maintaining as high a level of independence as possible (National Institute on Aging, 2004). It may be helpful to establish a familiar environment, changing it as little as possible. When you do change the environment (e.g., moving from home to an assisted living facility), incorporate familiar items from the old environment. Include items that are *personally* familiar. You may wish to contact family members to have them bring cherished and familiar items from home to facilitate this (Robinson et al., 1999).

Psychological Changes

The prevalence of mental illness (with the exception of cognitive impairment) in older adults is lower than in the general population. However, some older adults may suffer from mental illness in late life (see **Case Study 4-1**). The reasons for developing mental illness in late life vary widely. Some older adults may have suffered from mental illness throughout their lives, whereas others may

Case Study 4-1

Mrs. Schmidt is a 64-year-old woman who has been staying at an acute care facility for over 3 months now. She has been suffering for several years from chronic obstructive pulmonary disease and was placed on mechanical ventilation last fall. She was initially admitted to your facility for a weaning trial from the mechanical ventilator. For the past 3 months, she has failed several trials of weaning. Last night, the physician informed her that she was to leave the acute facility, connected to the mechanical ventilation, and that no further trials will be initiated. This morning, you asked Mrs. Schmidt about her preparations for leaving the facility. In response, Mrs. Schmidt starts crying dramatically and asks to see the attending physician. She is extremely upset, stating that "no one had told her anything about this." She is adamantly asking for an extension of her stay and for another weaning trial. Two weeks later, Mrs. Schmidt is completely weaned from the mechanical ventilation. However, she still has a Foley catheter (a thin, sterile tube inserted into the bladder to drain urine) in place, which she refuses to let go, saying that, she "cannot be without it."

Questions:

1. What are some of the potential challenges for communicating with Mrs. Schmidt?
2. How would you assess for these challenges?
3. What are some of the potential explanations for the communication difficulties described in this vignette?
4. Is there anything that should have been done differently?
5. How would you explain Mrs. Schmidt's miraculous ability to wean?
6. How would you explain Mrs. Schmidt's refusal to "let go" of the Foley catheter?

experience mental illness for the first time in old age due to changes in their social, medical, or physical circumstances. However, in general, older adults tend to report satisfaction with life at similar rates as the general population (Abeles et al., 1998).

Pathological Psychological Changes

Depression. Depression is a very serious condition characterized by at least five of the following symptoms: sadness, **anhedonia** (lack of interest or pleasure in activities that one once used to enjoy), significant weight loss or gain, a marked decrease or increase in sleep, psychomotor agitation or retardation, fatigue or loss of interest, feelings of worthlessness or inappropriate guilt, impaired ability to concentrate or think, and recurrent thoughts of death including suicide ideation or attempts (APA, 1994). Although we all feel "depressed" or "blue" sometimes, clinical depression is more intense, broader, and lasts for at least 2 weeks.

Depression is a very serious condition that is associated with increased risk of death (either from medical conditions or from suicide), a greater number of medical conditions, higher health care costs, and longer hospital stays (Callahan, Hui, Nienaber, Musick, & Tierney, 1994; Frasure-Smith, Lesperance, & Talajic, 1993; Givens, Sanft, & Marcantonio, 2008; Jiang et al., 2001). Furthermore, the risk of suicide in older Caucasian men is the highest in the nation (Centers for Disease Control and Prevention, 2007). In addition to the negative consequences associated with depression for the elderly sufferer, depression affects the entire family. Research has shown that caregivers of depressed elderly have poorer mental health and perceived quality of life than others (Sewitch, McCusker, Dendukuri, & Yaffe, 2004). Caregiving for depressed elderly is associated with many hours of informal care and, as a result, is very costly to society as well as to the caregivers themselves (Langa, Valenstein, Fendrick, Kabeto, & Vijan, 2004).

Unique Characteristics of Depression in the Elderly. Depression in the elderly often is associated with multiple medical conditions that limit functioning and mobility. It also is associated with life transitions and with a change in status and role, as many older adults transition out of the workforce and have to find a new sense of purpose and meaning in their life. Loss of family members and friends also is common in older adults, who may experience a reduced support system. Many times, depressed older adults do not report depressed mood, but instead present with lack of interest and enjoyment as well as sleep and appetite problems that are mistaken for other medical conditions (Abeles et al., 1998).

What Causes Depression? Depression is a very common condition, with a 12-month prevalence of 6.6% (Mojtabai & Olfson, 2004). However, in long-term care, these rates are several times higher. Although depression is common in the elderly, it is *not* a normal part of aging. It is *not* normal to be depressed even when you are old or disabled. Depression also is *not* a sign of weakness or a punishment from God. There are many possible reasons for why one becomes depressed. Depression has been associated with chemical changes in the brain and with chemical imbalance (Leonard, 2000). Depression also has been associated with experiencing helplessness and with the sense of having no control over one's life (Seligman, Maier, & Geer, 1968). Others suggest that depression is associated with negative views of oneself, the world, and others and that these views color one's experiences in the world (Beck, 1964). Research also has shown that exposure to severe and prolonged stress results in depression (Horesh, Klomek, & Apter, 2008). Most likely, the cause of depression is some combination of all of these explanations.

Treatment for Depression. Research has shown that both medications and talk therapy are effective in treating depression in older adults (Lebowitz et al., 1997). **Electroconvulsive therapy** (ECT; the delivery of an electrical shock that causes electrical activity in the brain) also is an effective alternative, especially when antidepressant medications cannot be taken due to their side effects or due to interaction with other medications. Unfortunately, however, only a small fraction of depressed older adults receive treatment. This can be due to several reasons, including the stigma attached to mental illness, difficulties accessing care, or lack of awareness of available services. Difficulties recognizing and distinguishing depression from other medical conditions that present with similar symptoms is particularly common in the elderly (Charney et al., 2003). Nursing strategies for intervening with the older adult who experiences depression can be found in Chapter 14.

The Impact of Depression on Communication. Many times, depressed older adults lose the inclination to interact with others and become increasingly withdrawn. Furthermore, because of their depressed mood, multiple physical complaints, and lack of interest in pleasurable activities, others may prefer not to interact with depressed elderly. This results in depressed elderly being prone to isolation at times of greatest need for support. As a health care professional, you should become aware of your own feelings working with depressed elderly and of potential "urges" to avoid depressed elderly altogether. Realizing one's own biases is the first step toward providing better care for the elderly.

It also is important to remember that depression is not a willful condition and, therefore, encouraging the elderly to "just snap out of it" is not likely to help. Instead, gently and persistently encouraging older adults to engage in even minor activities is likely to eventually result in an improvement in their mood. It also is important to be aware of the potential stigma associated with mental illness. Many older adults may not express their depressed feelings openly and may not wish to share their depression with others. Being respectful and understanding of a person's concerns is essential. However, at the same time, try to engage and to communicate your availability to older adult patients.

Lack of concentration and indecisiveness are potential symptoms of depression. This is likely to make communication with the elderly slightly more challenging and may require repetition of information or the use of memory aids (e.g., sticky notes or a notebook) to improve the ability of the elderly to retain information.

SUMMARY

In this chapter, we discussed a variety of changes that can take place in older adults. These changes include sensory, somatosensory, cognitive, and psychological domains. Changes vary dramatically within and across individuals. Some are normal age related changes, whereas others are pathological. In addition, some have a profound effect on communication, whereas others have a negligible effect. Identifying the exact deficit and its etiology as well as the way it affects communication has the potential to improve the communication ability of older adults. Health care professionals need to be cautious and creative when working with older adults who present with deficits in communication. The next chapter will discuss more deeply some of the psychosocial interventions that improve communication with older adults who present with sensory-motor or cognitive deficits.

Critical Thinking Exercises

1. Mr. Robert Smith is a 79-year-old man who was recently diagnosed with severe hearing problems. Mr. Smith is very upset about his diagnosis and refuses to wear his hearing aids. What are some of the potential reasons for this emotional reaction? What are some potential alternatives to hearing aids? What would be your recommendations for Mr. Smith?
2. Mrs. Williams is an 81-year-old woman. She has been increasingly withdrawn and disengaged. Her appetite has declined and she has lost 15 pounds. Her primary care provider recommended a course of antidepressant treatment in order to boost up her energy and mood. Mrs. Williams took the medication for 2 weeks and stopped. What are some of the reasons for lack of adherence to depression treatment in older adults? What can be done to increase the use of depression treatment in older adults? What information could be most useful for Mrs. Williams?
3. Mr. Roberts was recently diagnosed with Alzheimer's disease. His wife and two daughters are extremely upset, calling you in order to learn more about Mr. Roberts's condition. How would you communicate about Alzheimer's disease with Mr. Roberts's family? What information would be most useful for family members of patients with Alzheimer's disease? What should they expect? Is there anything the family can do to help?
4. What information would be most useful for Mr. Roberts himself? Should he be present when you discuss his diagnosis with his family members? What are some of the pros and cons for doing so? How would you decide?
5. Mr. Brown is a 71-year-old man with a history of arthritis. During a recent fall at home, he fractured his hip. Mr. Brown has now been admitted to the nursing home where you work. What information would you seek out in order to assess Mr. Brown's risk for future falls? What would you be most concerned about?
6. John is an 85-year-old man who suffers from severe dementia. His caretaker reports that lately he has been extremely violent and sexual during dressing. How are these behaviors related to communication deficits?

Personal Reflections

1. What are some of the difficulties you might experience as a nurse who has to take care of older adults with sensory deficits? What skills would be most important for you to gain in order to overcome these difficulties?
2. What are your thoughts and feelings about treating older adults with depression? What are some of the advantages and disadvantages of treating depression?
3. What alternative modes of communication have you used in the past? Which ones were most effective and why? Which ones were most challenging and why?

References

Abeles, N., Cooley, S., Deitch, I. M., Harper, M. S., Hinrichsen, G., Lopez, M. A., et al. (1998). What practitioners should know about working with older adults. *Professional Psychology: Research and Practice, 29*(5), 413–427.

Administration on Aging. (2002). *Statistics: A profile of older Americans 2002: Health, health care, and disability.* Retrieved August 21, 2007, from http://www.aoa.dhhs.gov/prof/statistics/profile/12_pf.asp

AgeWorks. (2000). *Module 3: Normal change of aging.* Retrieved August 21, 2007, from http://www.ageworks.com/course_demo/513/module3/module3.htm

Allen, S. M., & Mor, V. (1997). The prevalence and consequences of unmet need: Contrasts between older and younger adults with disability. *Medical Care, 35*(11), 1132–1148.

American Psychiatric Association. (1994). *Diagnostic and statistical manual of mental disorders* (4th ed.). Washington, DC: Author.

Anthony, J. C., & Aboraya, A. (1992). Epidemiology of selected disorders. In J. E. Birren, R. B. Sloane, & G. D. Cohen (Eds.), *Handbook of mental health and aging* (pp. 27–73). San Diego, CA: Academic Press.

Atrens, D., & Curthoys, I. (1978). *The neurosciences and behavior: An introduction.* Sydney: Australia: Academic Press.

Bagai, A., Thavendiranathan, M.D., & Detsky, A. S. (2006). Does this patient have hearing impairment? *Journal of the American Medical Association, 295*(4), 416–428.

Beck, A. T. (1964). Thinking and depression: Theory and therapy. *Archives of General Psychiatry, 10,* 561–571.

Beers, M. H., & Berkow, R. (2000). *The Merck manual of geriatrics* (3rd ed.). West Point, PA: Merck & Co.

Belsky, J. (1999). *The psychology of aging: Theory, research, and interventions* (3rd ed.). Pacific Grove, CA: Brooks/Cole.

Berry, P., Mascia, J. L., & Steinman, B. A. (2004). Vision and hearing loss in older adults: "Double trouble." *Care Management Journals, 5*(1), 35–40.

Brennan, M. (2003). Impairment of both vision and hearing among older adults: Prevalence and impact on quality of life. *Generations, 28*(1), 52–56.

Callahan, C. M., Hui, S. L., Nienaber, N. A., Musick, B. S., & Tierney, W. M. (1994). Longitudinal study of depression and health services use among elderly primary care patients. *Journal of American Geriatric Society, 42*(8), 833–888.

Carabellese, C., Appollonio, I., Rozzini, R., Bianchetti, A., Frisoni, G. B., Frattola, L., et al. (1993). Sensory impairment and quality of life in a community elderly population. *Journal of the American Geriatric Society, 41*(4), 401–407.

Centers for Disease Control and Prevention. (2007). *Suicide: Facts at a glance.* Retrieved October 14, 2008, at http://www.cdc.gov/ncipc/dvp/Suicide/Suicide-DataSheet.pdf

Charney, D. S., Reynolds, C. F. 3rd, Lewis, L., Lebowitz, B. D., Sunderland, T., Alexopoulos, G. S., et al., for the Depression and Bipolar Support Alliance. (2003). Depression and Bipolar Support Alliance consensus statement on the unmet needs in diagnosis and treatment of mood disorders in late life. *Archives of General Psychiatry, 60*(7), 664–672.

Chen, H. L. (1994). Hearing in the elderly: Relation of hearing loss, loneliness, and self-esteem. *Journal of Gerontological Nursing*, 20, 22–28.

Chmiel, R., & Jerger, J. (1993). Some factors affecting assessment of hearing handicap in the elderly. *Journal of the American Academy of Audiology, 4*(4), 249–257.

Collison, S., Cicuttini, F., Mead, V., & Savio, F. (1999). Low level disability in activities of daily living in elderly people living independently: Risk factors and implications. *Australasian Journal on Ageing, 18*(1), 38–40.

Congdon, N., O'Clomain, B., Klaver, C. C., Klein, R., Munoz, B., Friedman, D. S., et al. (2004). Causes and prevalence of visual impairment among older adults in the United States. *Archives of Ophthalmology, 122,* 477–485.

Cooper, J. W. (1999). Nonpharmacologic and pharmacologic treatment of dementia-associated agitation, aggression and disruptive behavior. *Journal of Geriatric Drug Therapy, 12,* 5–28

Corriveau, H., Hebert, R., Raiche, M., Dubois, M .F., & Prince, F. (2004). Postural stability in the elderly: Empirical confirmation of a theoretical model. *Archives of Gerontology and Geriatrics, 39,* 163–177.

Cruickshanks, K. J., Wiley, T. L., Tweed, T. S., Klein, B. E. K., Klein, R., Mares-Perlman, J. E., et al. (1998). Prevalence of hearing loss in older adults in Beaver Dam, Wisconsin: The Epidemiology of Hearing Loss study. *American Journal of Epidemiology, 148*(9), 879–886.

Dalton, D. S., Cruickshanks, K. J., Klein, B. E. K., Klein, R., Wiley, T. L., & Nondahl, D. M. (2003). The impact of hearing loss on quality of life in older adults. *Gerontologist, 43*(5), 661–668.

Desai, M. M., Lentzner, H. R., & Weeks, J. D. (2001). Unmet need for personal assistance with activities of daily living among older adults. *Gerontologist, 41(1),* 82–88.

Duffy, J. R. (1995). *Motor speech disorders: Substrates, differential diagnosis, and management.* Elsevier Science, Health Science Division.

Ebersole, P., & Hess, P. (1998). Mobility. In: (ed.), *Toward healthy aging: Human needs and healthy response* (5th ed., pp. 389–436). Boston: Mosby.

Ebersole, P., & Hess, P. (2001). Sensory changes in aging. In: *Geriatric nursing and healthy aging* (pp. 140–159). St. Louis, MO: Mosby.

Elam, J. T., Beaver, T., El Derwi, D., Graney, M. J., Applegate, W. B., & Miller, S. T. (1989). Comparison of sources of functional report with observed functional ability of frail older persons. *Gerontologist, 29*(Suppl.), 308A.

Eliopoulos, C. (2005). Sensory deficits. In: (ed.). *Gerontological nursing* (pp. 385–402). Philadelphia: Lippincott Williams & Wilkins.

Family Development and Resource Management. (2004). Retrieved January 14, 2007, from http://fcs.tamu.edu/aging/sensory.htm

Finlayson, C., & Heffer, C. (2000). Impairment of speech and language. *Liverpool Handbook of Geriatric Medicine.* Retrieved February 4, 2008, from http://www.liv.ac.uk/GeriatricMedicine/TextbookFrame1.htm

Fozard, J. L., Vercruyssen, M., Reynolds, S. L., Hancock, P. A., & Quilter, R. E. (1994). Age differences and changes in reaction time: The Baltimore longitudinal study of aging. *Journal of Gerontology: Psychological Sciences, 49,* 179–189.

Frasure-Smith, N., Lesperance, F., & Talajic, M. (1993). Depression following myocardial infarction. Impact on 6-month survival. *Journal of the American Medical Association, 270,* 1819–1825.

Gescheider, G. A., Beiles, E. J., Checkosky, C. M., Bolanowski, S. J., & Verrillo, R. T. (1994). The effects of aging on information-processing channels in the sense of touch: II. Temporal summation in the P channel. *Somatosensory Motor Research, 11*(4), 359–365.

Givens, J. L., Sanft, T. B., & Marcantonio, E. R. (2008). Functional recovery after hip fracture: The combined effects of depressive symptoms, cognitive impairment, and delirium. *Journal of the American Geriatrics Society, 56,* 1075–1079.

Gray, H. (1995). *Gray's anatomy, descriptive and surgical* (15th ed.). New York: Barnes and Noble.

Han, B. (2002). Depressive symptoms and self-rated health in community-dwelling older adults: A longitudinal study. *Journal of the American Geriatrics Society, 50,* 1549–1556.

Hebert, R., Brayne, C., & Spiegelhalter, D. (1993). Factors associated with functional decline in physical functioning in the elderly: A six-year prospective study. *Journal of Aging Health, 5,* 140–153.

Heine, C., & Browning, C. J. (2002). Communication and psychosocial consequences of sensory loss in older adults: Overview and rehabilitations directions. *Disability and Rehabilitation, 24*(15), 763–773.

Holland, M. (1999). Pressing issues in the dementias and dementia services. *Hospital Medicine, 60*(7), 522.

Horesh, N., Klomek, A. B., & Apter, A. (2008). Stressful life events and major depressive disorder. *Psychiatry Research, 160,* 192–199.

Howard Hughes Medical Institute. (2005). *It's all in the brain: Illusions reveal the brain's assumptions.* Retrieved August 2, 2007, from http://www.hhmi.org/senses/a110.html

Jerger, J., Chmiel, R., Wilson, N., & Luchi, R. (1995). Progress in geriatrics. Hearing impairment in older adults: New concepts. *Journal of the American Geriatrics Society, 43*(8), 928–935.

Jiang, W., Alexander, J., Christopher, E., Kuchibhatla, M., Gaudlen, L. H., Cuffe, M. S., et al. (2001). Relationship of depression to increased risk of mortality and rehospitalization in patients with congestive heart failure. *Archives of Internal Medicine, 161,* 1849–1856.

Kaplan, G. A., Strawbridge, W. J., Camacho, T., Cohen, R. D. (1993). Factors associated with change in physical functioning in the elderly: A six year prospective study. *Journal of Aging and Health, 5,* 140–153.

Kaplan, H. I., & Sadock, B. J. (1998). *Kaplan & Sadock's synopsis of psychiatry* (7th ed.). Baltimore: Williams & Wilkins.

Kasl-Godley, J., & Gatz, M. (2000). Psychosocial interventions for individuals with dementia: An integration of theory, therapy, and a clinical understanding of dementia. *Clinical Psychology Review, 20,* 755–782.

Kenshalo, D. (1986). Somesthetic sensitivity in young and elderly humans. *Journal of Gerontology, 41*(6), 732–742.

Kline, D. W., & Scialfa, C. T. (1996). Visual and auditory aging. In J. E. Birren & K. W. Schaie (Eds.), *Handbook of the psychology of aging* (4th ed., pp. 181–203).

Langa, K. M., Valenstein, M. A., Fendrick, A. M., Kabeto, M. U., & Vijan, S. (2004). Extent and cost of informal caregiving for older Americans with symptoms of depression. *American Journal of Psychiatry, 161*(5), 857–863.

Lebowitz, B. D. (1997). Diagnosis and treatment of depression in late life. Consensus statement update. *Journal of the American Medical Association, 248*(14), 1186–1190.

Leonard, B. E. (2000). Evidence for a biochemical lesion in depression. *Journal of Clinical Psychiatry, 61*, 12–17.

Li, L. W. (2005). Trajectories of ADKL disability among community-dwelling frail older persons. *Research on Aging, 27*(1), 56 –79.

Lin, S. Y., Davey, R. C., & Cochrane, T. (2004). Community rehabilitation for older adults with osteoarthritis of the lower limb: A controlled clinical trial. *Clinical Rehabilitation, 18*(1), 92–101.

Maki, B. E. (1997). Gait changes in older adults: Predictors of falls or indicators of fear. *Journal of the American Geriatric Society, 45*(11), 313–320.

Mast, B. T., MacNeill, S. E., Lichtenberg, P. A. (2004). Post-stroke and clinically-defined vascular depression in geriatric rehabilitation patients. American Journal of Geriatric Psychiatry, *12*, 84–92.

Mattay, V. S., Fera, F., Tessitore, A., Hariri, A. R., Das, S., Callicott, J. H., et al. (2002). Neurophysiological correlates of age-related changes in human motor function. *Neurology, 58*, 630–635.

Mayo Clinic. (2008). *Alzheimer's stages: How the disease progresses*. Retrieved July 20, 2008, from http://www.mayoclinic.com/health/alzheimers-stages/AZ00041

McBride, M. R., & Mistretta, C. M. (1982). Light touch thresholds in diabetic patients. *Diabetes Care, 5*(3), 311–315.

McGibbon, C. A., & Krebs, D. E. (2004). Discriminating age and disability effects in locomotion: Neuromuscular adaptations in musculoskeletal pathology. *Journal of Applied Physiology, 96*(1), 149–160.

Mehta, K. M., Simonsick, E. M., Penninx, B. W. J. H., Schulz, R., Rubin, S. M., Satterfield, S., et al. (2003). Prevalence and correlates of anxiety symptoms in well-functioning older adults: Findings from the Health Aging and Body Composition Study. *Journal of the American Geriatrics Society, 51*(4), 499–504.

Mojtabai, R., & Olfson, M. (2004). Major depression in community dwelling middle aged and older adults: Prevalence and 2- and 4-year follow up symptoms. *Psychological Medicine, 34*, 623–634.

Mold, J. W., Vesely, S. K., Keyl, B. A., Schenk, J. B., & Roberts, M. (2004). The prevalence predictors and consequences of peripheral sensory neuropathy in older patients. *Journal of the American Board of Family Practice, 17*(5), 309–318.

Morely, J. E. (2001). Decreased food intake with aging. *The Journals of Gerontology Series A: Biological Sciences and Medical Sciences, 56*, 81–88.

Muller, G., Richter, R. A., Weisbrod, S., & Klingberg, F. (1992). Impaired tactile pattern recognition in the early stage of primary degenerative dementia compared with normal aging. *Archives of Gerontology and Geriatrics, 14*, 215–225.

Mulrow, C. D., Aguilar, C., Endicott, J. E., Velez, R., Tuley, M. R., Charlip, T. S., et al. (1990). Association between hearing impairment and quality of life of elderly individuals. *Journal of the American Geriatric Society, 38*(1), 45–50.

National Institute on Aging, NIH SeniorHealth. (2004). *Caring for someone with Alzheimer's. Frequently asked questions.* Retrieved January 31, 2005, from http://nihseniorhealth.gov/alzheimerscare/faq/faqlist.html

National Institute of Deafness and Communication Disorders (NIDCD). (2004). *Age-related changes in the prevalence of smell/taste problems among the United States adult population: Results of the 1994 Disability Supplement to the National Health Interview Survey (NHIS).*

National Institutes of Health (NIH). (1999). *The aging senses: Relationships among multiple sensory systems* (PA-99-123). Washington, DC: U.S. Government Printing Office.

Nondahl, D. M., Cruickshanks, K. J., Dalton, D. S., Klein, B. E., Klein, R., Schubert, C. R., et al. (2007). The impact of tinnitus on quality of life in older adults. *Journal of the American Academy of Audiology, 18*(3), 257–266.

Oman, D., Reed, D., & Ferrara, A. (1999). Do older women have more physical disability than men do? *American Journal of Epidemiology, 150*, 834–842.

Picavet, H. S. J., & van de Bos, G. A. M. (1996). Comparing survey data on functional disability: The impact of some methodological differences. *Journal of Epidemiology & Community Health, 50*(1), 86–93.

Pirkl, J. J. (1995). Transgenerational design: Prolonging the American dream. *Generations, 19*, 32–36.

Popelka, M. M., Cruickshanks, K. J., Wiley, T. L., Tweed, T. S., Klein, B. E. K., & Klein, R. (1998). Low prevalence of hearing aid use among older adults with hearing loss: The Epidemiology of Hearing Loss study. *Journal of the American Geriatrics Society, 46*(9), 1075–1078.

Raskind, M. A., & Peskind, E. R. (1992). Alzheimer's disease and other dementing disorders. In J. E. Birren, R. B. Sloane, & G. D. Cohen (Eds.), *Handbook of mental health and aging* (pp. 477–513). San Diego, CA: Academic Press.

Robinson, A., Spenser, B., & White, L. (1999). *Understanding difficult behaviors: Some practical suggestions for coping with Alzheimer's disease and related illnesses.* Ypsilanti, MI: Eastern Michigan University.

Rubenstein, L. V., Calkins, D. R., Greenfield, S., Jette, A. M., Meenan, R. F., Nevins, M. A., et al. (1988). Health status assessment for elderly patients: Effects of different data sources. *Journal of Gerontology,* 39, 686–691.

Scheuerle, J. (2000). Hearing and aging. *Educational Gerontology, 26*(3), 237–247.

Seligman, M. E. P., Maier, S. F., & Geer, J. (1968). The alleviation of learned helplessness in dogs. *Journal of Abnormal Psychology,* 73, 256–262.

Sewitch, M .J., McCusker, J., Dendukuri, N., & Yaffe, M. J. (2004). Depression in frail elders: Impact on family caregivers. *International Journal of Geriatric Psychiatry, 19,* 655–665.

Smith, C. D., Umberger, G. H., Manning, E. L., Slevin, J. T., Wekstein, D. R., Schmitt, F. A., et al. (1999). Critical decline in fine motor hand movement in human aging. *Neurology, 53*(7), 1458–1461.

Sorri, M., Luotonen, M., & Laitakari, K. (1984). Use and nonuse of hearing aids. *British Journal of Audiology, 18*(3), 169–172.

Springhouse. (2001). *Diseases* (3rd ed.). Springhouse, PA: Springhouse Corporation.

Stessman, J., Hammerman-Rozenberg, R., Maaravi, Y., & Cohen, A. (2002). Effect of exercise on ease in performing activities of daily living and instrumental activities of daily living from age 70 to 77: The Jerusalem Longitudinal Study. *Journal of the American Geriatrics Society, 50*(12), 1934–1938.

Stevens, J. C., & Patterson, M. Q. (1995). Dimensions of spatial acuity in the touch sense: Changes over the life span. *Somatosensory Motor Research, 12*(1), 29–47.

Stuen, C., & Faye, E. E. (2003). Vision loss: Normal and not normal changes among older adults. *Generations, 27*(1), 8–14.

Teri, L. (1996). Depression in Alzheimer's disease. In M. Hersen & V. V. Van Hasselt (Eds.), *Psychological treatment of older adults: An introductory text* (pp. 209–222). New York: Plenum Press.

Thomson, F. J., Masson, E. A., & Boulton, A. J. (1993). The clinical diagnosis of sensory neuropathy in elderly people. *Diabetes Medicine, 10*(9), 843–846.

Thornbury, J. M., & Mistretta, C. M. (1981). Tactile sensitivity as a function of age. *Journal of Gerontology, 36*(1), 34–39.

Toshiaki, T., Nobuya, H., Seiji, N., Shuichi, I., et al. (1995). Aging and postural stability: Change in sensorimotor function. *Physical and Occupational Therapy in Geriatrics, 13*(3), 1–16.

Tsuruoka, H., Masuda, S., Ukai, K., Sakakura, Y., Harada, T., & Majima, Y. (2001). Hearing impairment and quality of life for the elderly in nursing homes. *Auris Nasus Larynx, 28,* 45–54.

U.S. Bureau of the Census. (2000). *United States Census 2000.* Available at http://www.census.gov/main/www/cen2000.html.

Verrillo, R. T., Bolanowski, S. J., & Gescheider, G. A. (2002). Effect of aging on the subjective magnitude of vibration. *Somatosensory Motor Research, 19*(3), 238–244.

Wade, D. T., Hewer, R. L., David, R. M., & Menderby, P. M. (1986) Aphasia after stroke: Natural history and associated deficits. *Journals of Neurology, Neurosurgery, and Psychiatry, 49,* 11–16.

Waldrop, J., & Stern, S. M. (2003). *Disability status: 2000, Census 2000 brief.* Washington, DC: U.S. Government Printing Office.

Wang, P. P., Badley, E. M., & Gignac, M. (2004). Activity limitation, coping efficacy and self-perceived physical independence in people with disability. *Disability Rehabilitation, 26*(13), 785–793.

Weinstein, B. E., & Ventry, I. M. (1982). Hearing impairment and social isolation in the elderly. *Journal of Speech and Hearing Research, 25,* 593–599.

Welford, A. T. (1982). Motor skills and aging. In J. A. Mortimer, F. J. Pirozzolo, & G. J. Maletta (Eds.), *The aging motor system* (pp. 152–187). New York: Praeger.

CHAPTER 5

Therapeutic Communication with Older Adults

Kathleen Stevens, PhD, RN, CRRN

LEARNING OBJECTIVES

At the end of this chapter, the reader will be able to:

- Communicate effectively, respectfully, and compassionately with older adults and their families.
- Identify physiological and psychosocial barriers to communication among older adults.
- Recognize and use common augmentative and alternative communication devices.
- Acknowledge the nurse's role and responsibility in the process of communication.
- Utilize basic principles when communicating with older adults.
- Discuss strategies to overcome communication barriers.
- Facilitate the communication of older adults with a particular focus on the use of assistive technology.
- Describe potential safety issues when communicating health care information and strategies to enhance clear, effective communication.

KEY TERMS

- Affective communication
- Aphasia
- Assistive technology
- Augmentative and alternative communication (AAC)
- Communication
- Dysarthria
- Health literacy
- Instrumental or task-focused communication
- Language

"There may be no single thing more important in our efforts to achieve meaningful work and fulfilling relationships than to learn to practice the art of communication."

—*Max DePree*

Communication is a core skill in the health care professions. We rely on our ability to communicate effectively to gather and share information as well as to build relationships with patients and families. Learning and practicing the art of communication is one key to success as clinicians.

For many clinicians, communicating with older adults can be anxiety producing and fraught with challenges. The challenges may be associated with our memories of past difficulties communicating with older adults, be they family members, clergy, teachers, or neighbors, or they may be related to the physiological or psychosocial characteristics associated with aging. The purpose of this chapter is to review basic principles of communication and present strategies for communicating with older adults. This information should promote development of the skills needed to communicate effectively and promote optimal health for older adults.

ANATOMY AND PHYSIOLOGY OF COMMUNICATION

The term **communication** is used frequently in our language and in our work. The term originates from the Latin word "commune," which means "to hold in common." By virtue of its origins, the word implies that communication is a process that involves more than one person. Communication is the process or means by which an individual relates experiences, ideas, knowledge, and feelings to another. Communication is a reciprocal process involving minimally two people, a sender and a receiver. Effective communication depends on the ability of both to engage in the process of sharing not merely words, but also concepts, emotions, and thoughts.

Physiologically, communication occurs as a result of a complex interaction of cognition, hearing, speech, and language centers. Cognition is essential to sending, receiving, and interpreting information in our communications. Cognitive centers in the brain are the basis for storing memory, developing emotion, forming judgments, and creating knowledge. From the time of birth, as we process new sensory information, cognitive centers in the brain are storing memories that will, over time, allow us to recognize patterns, forming complex thoughts and judgments. The cortex of the brain is the primary repository for cognition. Within the cortex are a multitude of interlinked storage areas that help store, retrieve, and make sense of messages coming from the world. The ability to store and use this knowledge is dependent upon many factors, including age, nutrition, activity, chemical balance, and the presence of any cerebrovascular disorders that could interfere with function.

The second cortical function that is important for communication is language production and the ability to speak. **Language** is the use of symbols or gestures that are common to groups and serve as a means of sharing thoughts, ideas, and emotions. Infants learn to assign specific sounds, known as words, to objects, activities, and ultimately emotions. This is often referred to as our primary language. As we age we learn not only to speak, but also to read and write the symbols associated with our primary language. Throughout our lifetime we may learn a number of different languages. The ability to speak and understand multiple languages depends on frequency of use and environment. There may be many different dialects or meanings assigned to words within a language based on geography or age. No matter how many languages we learn over the course of a lifetime, however, initial memories of our primary language serve as the foundation for all future learning.

Cortical centers located in the parietal lobe of the dominant hemisphere, often referred to as the speech center, are the primary area of language development and speech production. Broca's area at the junction of the parietal and frontal lobes in the dominant hemisphere is responsible for speech production, whereas Wernicke's center at the intersection of the parietal and temporal lobes is the area of speech recognition. Damage to these areas will result in **aphasia**, an acquired loss or impairment of language. The most common cause of aphasia is the brain damage that occurs with a stroke.

Speech refers to oral communication of the sounds or words associated with language. In addition to the speech centers in the brain, speech production is dependent upon muscles and structures responsible for ventilation, phonation, and articulation. Important structures of speech are the diaphragm, intercostal muscles, larynx, vocal cords, tongue, and muscles of the mouth and face. When damage occurs to the oral muscles the individual may have difficulty producing sounds or words that can be understood by others; this is called **dysarthria**. Dysarthria refers to a group of neuromuscular disorders that affect the speed, strength, range, timing, or accuracy of speech movements, which often result in reduced intelligibility of speech. Dysarthria can be present from birth as a result of cerebral palsy or other birth injuries, or may develop later in life as a result of facial injury, tumors, or paralysis associated with a stroke. Individuals with dysarthria may use **assistive technology** to augment or replace vocal communication.

Individuals may also be nonvocal due to illness, injury, or secondary to treatment interventions such as radiation, surgery to the neck, or mechanical ventilation. If hand function is not significantly impaired, these individuals may using writing, typing, or a communication board to communicate with others. Neurological diseases such as amyotrophic lateral sclerosis (ALS) or a pontine stroke may result in quadriparesis and a total paralysis of the muscles required for phonation and vocalization. These individuals cannot produce speech or use their hands to express their thoughts. They are aware of the environment and conversations around them; however, with no motor function below the level of the eyes it is difficult to effectively communicate to others. Participants in a phenomenological study described the experience of being nonvocal as "being trapped in a silent world" (Carroll, 2007, p. 1168). Without the ability to speak, these individuals reported feelings of frustration and being incomplete (Carroll, 2007). The ability to communicate with others is an essential part of our being. It is important for nurses to assess and establish a viable means of communication with each patient.

VERBAL AND NONVERBAL COMMUNICATION

Communication can be verbal or nonverbal. Nonverbal communication refers to behaviors or gestures that convey a message without the use of verbal language. Nonverbal communication can either enhance the delivery of a message or create a barrier to understanding. For example, when a school crossing guard says "STOP" loudly and raises her hand with all five fingers extended, the individual is using a common nonverbal gesture to enhance the message delivered verbally. When we use eye contact in addition to a verbal greeting, we are using a nonverbal gesture along with words to welcome the individual. When similar verbal

BOX 5-1 Research Highlight

Aim: The purpose of this secondary analysis was to interpret narratives from a previous study to gain a better understanding of the common meanings and experiences of persons using augmentative and alternative communication (AAC) devices.

Methods: The researchers analyzed original data obtained from a Web-based focus group. Data came from online responses to questions at a conference Web site with free expression of dialogue by 16 participants, though responses were monitored. A research team used Heideggerian hermeneutics for the secondary analysis.

Findings: Six themes and one pattern emerged: "1) maintaining effective communication, 2) interacting in various situations, 3) AAC device-imposing limitations, 4) wading through prepackaged technology, 5) AAC device giving more than a voice, and 6) accepting the AAC device" (p. 215). Researchers summarized that "communication technology enables humanness" (p. 215).

Application to practice: AAC devices were more than technology to the users. They provided a means of remaining human and connected with the world through communicating with others. In addition, nurses should realize that users of such devices may require more time in use, but that these devices have personal meaning to users and allow them to participate in society, certainly a goal of rehabilitation for those of any age.

Source: Dickerson, S. S., Stone, V. I., Pnachura, C., & Usiak, D. (2002). The meaning of communication: Experiences with augmentative communication devices. *Rehabilitation Nursing, 27*(6), 215–220.

communication and nonverbal gestures are together, they can help us to deliver our message and improve communications.

Vocal nonverbal communication refers to the tone, pitch, speech rate, or fluency of verbal communication. In the preceeding example, the school crossing guard used pitch and tone to say "STOP" loudly, thereby catching our attention. What if the guard said the same word but in a normal voice—would it convey the same meaning? A nurse, directing a patient to a clinic exam room, who says in a loud, harsh tone, "Come here to this room," may be perceived by the patient to be stern and uninterested in him or her as a person. To communicate effectively we should be aware of our verbal and nonverbal vocal communications. What we say and how we say it are essential to therapeutic communication.

Nonvocal nonverbal communication refers to the use of facial gestures, body posture, eye contact, and touch as a means of communication. This chapter already mentioned how the use of eye contact along with a verbal word of welcome can enhance communication. Let's now picture a staff member looking intently at a chart, avoiding any eye contact or facial expression while greeting a new patient. In this example, the staff member's nonverbal communication speaks louder than his words. In this case, the patient may report the service was poor and staff was uninterested.

Nonverbal communication on the part of the patient is also an important factor in therapeutic communication in a health care setting. Look at **Case Study 5-1**. The staff nurse used a simple verbal comment to clarify the meaning of the patient's nonverbal behavior and determine her next action. A patient's nonverbal communication can provide nurses insight into the person's feelings and emotions. Learning to read the patient's nonverbal gestures is important for nurses.

Communication involves more than one person, so both the sender and the receiver must be attentive and demonstrate good communication skills. The goal of effective communication "is interpreting the messages and responding in an appropriate manner" (Caris-Verhallen, Kerkstra, & Bensing, 1997, p. 916). Through our communications we are not merely sending a message, but creating a shared meaning and understanding of an event, experience, or memory. Understanding and respecting the message of the sender are essential to effective communications. The receiver must be open to the ideas of the sender and provide respect during the conversation. Being silent, showing attentiveness, and listening to the sender are critical. Good listening starts with allowing time for conversation to occur; when we are rushed it is difficult to give the time and attention needed to truly understand the meaning associated with the words spoken. Understanding is enhanced when we share our interpretation with the sender, asking him or her to validate our interpretation or clarify misinterpretations. Try to approach each conversation with an open mind and a willingness to listen. Effective communication does not require agreement, but it does necessitate listening and taking into account the meaning of an idea, event, or experience described by the other person. By using communication and conversation we learn together and build

Case Study 5-1

A student nurse on rounds enters a patient's room and finds an older woman sitting comfortably in a wheelchair in no apparent distress staring out the window with her back to the nurse. Is this patient inviting communication from the nurse? Based on the patient's position and posture, the nurse may elect to not speak or say anything, fearing she might disturb the patient. Shortly, the staff nurse enters the room and comments, "Mrs. Hale, are you waiting for someone? Can I do anything to help you get ready for a visit?" Mrs. Hale responds, "I am waiting for my son. He is generally on time. I hope nothing bad has happened. I would like to go to the bathroom before he arrives so I don't have to worry about that during his visit."

- What is the nurse's most appropriate response in this situation?
- Should the student nurse have done anything differently during her visit to the room on rounds? If so, what?
- What nonverbal communication would the nurse expect to see from Mrs. Hale?
- What nonverbals should the nurse include in her care of this woman?

a common bond through our understanding and respect for others.

ALTERNATIVE COMMUNICATION AND ASSISTIVE TECHNOLOGY

Assistive technology can help individuals improve their mobility, communication, self-care, or vocational skills. Assistive technology is "any item, piece of equipment, or product system, whether acquired commercially off the shelf, modified, or customized, that is used to increase, maintain, or improve functional capabilities of individuals with disabilities" (Olson & DeRuyter, 2002, p. 4). It is important to remember that assistive technology is a tool, not a solution, and individuals vary in their willingness to use assistive devices. The type of impairment, degree of impairment, and illness severity are important factors in the rate of use of assistive technology among older adults (Mann, Hurren, & Tomita, 1993). Pape, Kim, and Weiner (2002) reported in a review of the personal factors influencing assistive technology use that approximately 25% of persons over 65 years of age own an assistive device and many have multiple devices. Two types of assistive technology can enhance communication, those that improve hearing and those that improve the ability to communicate.

> **Notable Quotes**
>
> *"Hearing impairment of any type and degree is a barrier to incidental learning."*
>
> —Carol Flexer, PhD, audiologist, author, and distinguished professor

In an evidence-based review of nursing management of hearing impairment in nursing facility residents, Adams-Wendling and Pimple (2007) reported a high prevalence of hearing loss in nursing facility residents. Risk factors associated with hearing impairment among older adults include physiological changes associated with aging; nursing facility residence; cognitive decline; history of chronic otitis media; exposure to excessive noise; use of ototoxic medications, especially early antibiotics; visual impairments; and gender. Hearing loss is also now a common impairment in middle-age individuals, and the incidence is expected to increase secondary to lifestyle and exposure to excessive noise among this group (AARP, 2007). Advances in technology and improved access to assistive devices mandated by the Americans with Disabilities Act have contributed to the development of assistive devices to improve hearing. There are two major types of assistive devices used to improve hearing: assistive listening devices and hearing aids.

According to the American Speech-Language-Hearing Association (ASHA, 1998), an assistive listening device (ALD) is any type of device that can help an individual function better in day-to-day living. An assistive listening device may be used with or without a hearing aid. There are four major types of assistive listening devices: personal frequency modulation systems, infrared systems, induction loop systems, and one-to-one communicators. An assistive listening device typically transmits sound waves to a microphone worn by the individual, which increases sound volume and reduces interference from environmental noise, thus improving the listening experience for the individual without impacting the sounds heard by others. These devices are often available in theaters, concert halls, or schools to allow individuals to hear the performance or speaker.

A hearing aid is an ear-level or body-worn electronic device that uses a tiny microphone to pick up sound waves, change weaker sounds, and modify sound signals so they then can be conveyed to the ear via a tiny speaker. There are different types of aids based on style and technology. Style differences are based on where the hearing aid is worn. The common styles are listed in **Table 5-1**.

For many years, hearing aids used analog technology to amplify sound. Newer models of hearing aids use digital programming to convert sound waves to digital signals that are converted by a computer chip within the device to sound. Digital devices are typically more expensive models.

Given the prevalence of hearing loss, a hearing screening should be included in health assessments in community and institutional settings. Demers (2007) recommends health care providers use a simple self-report screening instrument, such as the Brief Hearing Loss Screener, in health assessments of

TABLE 5-1 Types of Hearing Aids

BTE (behind the ear)	BTEs are about 1 inch long and worn behind the outer ear. A small tube connects with the amplification device behind the ear and delivers amplified sound into the ear canal. The device has an adjustable volume control and is battery powered. It is the most common style of hearing aid. These devices are suitable for the entire range of hearing loss.
OTE (over the ear)	This is a new style that is very small and sits on top of the outer ear.
ITE (in the ear)	ITEs are custom-fitted devices molded to the contour of the outer ear. The device has an adjustable volume control and a battery; however, both are much smaller than ones used in a BTE device. Some users have difficulty seeing or manipulating the control and battery. These devices are used for mild to moderate hearing loss.
ITC (in the canal)	ITCs are tiny devices that fit into the ear canal and are barely visible. They are customized to fit the size and shape of the ear canal. Although cosmetically appealing, their small size is a drawback for some individuals.
CIC (completely in the canal)	CICs are the smallest type of device in the in the ear class. The entire device fits within the canal. Although cosmetically flattering, the small size is a true disadvantage because of difficulty handling and positioning the device. This device is the most expensive model of hearing aid.

SOURCE: Adapted from AARP. (2007). *Consumer guide to hearing aids.* Washington, DC: Author.

non-institutionalized older adults. Due to the prevalence of hearing loss among residents in nursing facilities, all residents should be screened and evaluated for hearing impairment on admission and on an ongoing basis (Adams-Wendling & Pimple, 2007). These tools are designed to assist nurses with making timely and accurate referrals to a speech language pathologist or certified audiologist. Before a hearing aid is fitted, the individual should have an audiologic assessment by a certified audiologist (ASHA, 1998) to determine which model will best improve hearing and be most functional for the individual.

An **augmentative and alternative communication (AAC)** system is "an integrated group of components, including symbols, aids, strategies and techniques used by individuals to enhance communication" (Henderson & Doyle, 2002, p. 127). A speech language pathologist and an occupational therapist must conduct a thorough evaluation to assess the individual's abilities, limitations, and ability to effectively use a prescribed communication system. Augmentative communication systems range from simple low tech devices such as an alphabet or icon communication board to high tech computer devices that record and translate the spoken word into print.

If a patient who uses an AAC system to communicate is admitted to your unit, it is important to learn from the patient or his or her caregiver how to use the device. Out of courtesy, ask permission from the individual with a disability prior to using or handling any assistive technology, and always be respectful by storing it in a place that is accessible to the patient and that provides the greatest degree of safety for the device. All nursing staff and health care professionals who work with the patient should learn to use the device and allow time for the patient to use the device to communicate. Staff should be aware of basic operations (e.g., battery charging) necessary to keep the unit in functional order and provide the patient with the opportunity to safely store and charge the device as needed.

Communication in Health Care

Communication is the essence of nursing. Communication is a two-way process, so it is important to look at communication in health care from the consumer or patient perspective. Caris-Verhallen, Kerkstra, and Bensing (1997), in a review of the literature on the role of communication in nursing care of the older adult, discuss the distinction between instrumental or task-focused communication and affective communication from the perspective of the consumer. **Instrumental or task-focused communication** refers to behavior necessary for assessing and solving problems. Think about the conversations you have with patients that are focused on "caring for" the person. In these conversations, the primary interest of the health care provider is to gather information that will help them provide care for the person. These conversations may be formal and structured, such as the admission interview, a health assessment, discussion of advance directives, or patient-family education. In these conversations, the health care provider is initiating the conversation with a specific intent of gathering information from the patient that will be of assistance in diagnosing or treating patient problems. Instrumental communication can include informal conversations as well, such as when the nurse asks the patient, "What time do you want to eat?" or "What would you like me to order for your meal today?" Once again, the conversation is focused on the health care provider requesting information necessary for caring for the patient. In all these cases the conversation is generally initiated by the health care provider and the focus is a question about how best to care for the patient. Patients want to be cared for, but they often also want more—to be "cared about" as a person.

The second type of communication from the patient perspective is **affective communication**, which focuses on how the health care provider is caring about the patient and his or her feelings and emotions. Affective communications tend to be more informal and more difficult for health care providers. There is a greater degree of vulnerability for the health care provider in affective or psychosocial communications to develop an emotional or personal relationship with the patient. Look at the example in **Case Study 5-2**. By electing to spend time with the patient and allowing him time to talk about his life and emotions, the nurse conveyed her interest in knowing him as a person. During the conversation the nurse gained information that would be of assistance in care planning for the patient; however, this was not the primary intent of the conversation. From the patient's perspective, the nurse showed interest in caring about him rather than caring for him.

Affective communication is important in long-term health care relationships, be it a nurse practitioner treating a patient with chronic illness in the clinic or a nurse working with a patient in long-term care or in the home. Think about ways a nurse can demonstrate caring about the person rather than merely caring for the person.

Case Study 5-2

A nurse walks into the day room of an assisted living unit and sees an older male resident playing cards alone. The nurse approaches the man and asks if he would like to play with a partner. The nurse proceeds to play a hand of cards with him. During the card game, the two converse about how the resident enjoyed playing cards with his wife while she was alive. The resident talks about how he misses his wife and the impact her death has had on him.

- How did the nurse facilitate therapeutic communication in this case?
- What types of nonverbals would you expect to see on the part of the nurse? On the part of the older man? What does this situation remind us about with regards to communication?
- How might the nurse have handled this situation differently?
- What might have happened if the nurse had taken a different approach to conversation?

Communicating with the Older Adult

Communication with older adults can be quite rewarding, though at times it is fraught with challenges for both the sender and the receiver. Physiological changes associated with aging or secondary to chronic illness and disease can pose a barrier to communication. Common physiological changes associated with aging that interfere with communication include high-frequency hearing loss, loss of dentition, reduced vital capacity, and reduced oral motor function. Chapter 6 provides more detailed information about these changes.

Communicating with others can be facilitated by paying attention to the basic principles of conversation. In her book *Making Contact* (1976), renowned family therapist and author Virginia Satir describes the basic principles for making contact and communicating with others. The basic principles are invite, arrange environment, maximize communication, maximize understanding, and follow through.

Inviting

An invitation says to the other person that you are interested in them and sharing time with them. Health care providers can make a number of gestures that show respect and interest in the patient as a person. It can be as simple as arranging time for a conversation rather than doing an assessment on the run. As the new patient arrives on the unit, the nurse extends a greeting and conducts a triage assessment of the individual's health status while saying to the patient, "I will be coming to your room in about 15 minutes to meet with you and get some information to help us care for you here." Meanwhile, the nurse makes arrangements to minimize distractions during the admission interview.

Another inviting strategy is to greet the person by name and ask a nonthreatening open-ended question, thereby engaging the person in conversation. Think about the difference between an interrogation and a conversation—which is more pleasant? "Tell me about yourself and what brought you here today" invites the person to share information about themselves in a nonthreatening manner. See **Table 5-2** for other types of open-ended questions.

Arranging the Environment

The second basic principle is to arrange an environment conducive to communication. The environment should be comfortable, provide privacy, and minimize distractions that could be barriers to communication, such as noise or poor lighting. At times, nurses invite patients to come into our space; for example, when we bring the patient to a treatment room in the clinic, the exam room often includes two chairs, which the health care provider can use to position themselves face to face with the interviewee in order to facilitate communication. Other times health care providers enter a patient's home or room in a long-term care setting, in which case we are entering the patient's territory and space. It is important to respect personal space and territory when arranging an environment conducive to conversation. When entering an older patient's space, simple gestures such as asking permission to sit or move the furniture conveys a sense of respect for the person. If the individual uses assistive equipment such as a wheelchair, cane, or communication device, ask permission before touching the equipment. It is equally important to ask where items should be placed prior to leaving the room to facilitate independence and provide safety. Organizations such as the United Spinal Association (2008) and the Rehabilitation Institute of Chicago (2006) publish materials on disability etiquette and tips to enhance communications with individuals with disability.

The ideal position when communicating with a patient is one whereby the sender and receiver are seated 3–6 feet apart with chairs positioned to allow for eye-to-eye contact. When having a conversation with a person in a wheelchair, remember to pull up a chair and position yourself at equal height to the person. For patients with impaired vision, reposition the chair so you can be seen within their field of vision.

Maximizing Communication

The third principle is to use communication strategies that maximize the individual's ability to understand the message. Communication is critical in health care, yet many consumers have difficulty understanding the language of health care due to language barriers, illiteracy, or limited literacy. In the Healthy People 2010 report (2000), health literacy was identified as an important component of health communication. **Health literacy** is defined in this report as "the degree to which individuals have the capacity to obtain, process, and understand basic health information and services needed to make appropriate health decisions" (Healthy People, 2000). In order to obtain essential health

TABLE 5-2 Open-Ended Questions for Starting a Conversation

Ask questions about the past.	"Out of all the places you have lived, what made some better than others?" "Tell me about the places you have visited in your lifetime." "Tell me what kind of work you did and how you got into that field of employment." "I see you have been coming to this hospital for a number of years. Can you tell me about these visits and how I can make your stay more comfortable?" "According to your records you have seen a number of our home health staff. Can you tell me about services you have received?"
Ask personal questions.	"Tell me about your family." "I see you have grandchildren. Can you tell me about them and where they are located?" "How did you meet your husband? Tell me about your courtship and wedding."
Inquire about what is new and different.	"You have been coming to the clinic more often this year. Can you tell me why and what changes have occurred?" "Tell me about your session with the physical therapist yesterday." "I see you have a new roommate. Can you tell me how things are working out between the two of you?" "Tell me about the meals you are receiving."
Ask about their hopes and dreams.	"When you were younger what did you wish for?" "What do you wish for your family?"
Talk about facts or mutually shared events.	"Your physician just left; tell me about your conversation." "I saw you were watching the news at breakfast; tell me what's going on in the world today." "What's the headline in today's newspaper?"
Ask how and why questions.	"I see you had quite a few children. How did you manage raising them?" "You are on a number of medications. Tell me how you keep track of what to take and when." "What do you do to stay so active?"
Reference current events that are meaningful to most people.	"This summer is so hot. What's your favorite summer experience?" "Today is Valentine's Day. Tell me about a special valentine in your life."

SOURCE: Adapted from Cox, B. J., & Waller, L. L. (1991). *Bridging the communication gap with the elderly.* Chicago, IL: American Hospital Association.

care services, consumers need to understand instructions on how and when to call a physician's office or seek medical assistance. For many individuals with literacy problems, the hospital can be intimidating due to the unfamiliar environment, maze of departments, number of questions asked, and diversity of health care providers encountered during a visit. It has been estimated that nearly half of all American adults, approximately 90 million, have some degree of difficulty understanding health care information (Nielsen-Bohlman, Panzer, & Kindig, 2004). Due to lack of educational opportunities, cognitive decline, and sensory impairments associated with aging and/or chronic illness, older adults are an at-risk population for problems associated with health literacy.

Advocacy groups such as the Joint Commission (2007), the Partnership for Clear Health Care Communication, and AARP have initiated campaigns encouraging patients to speak up and ask questions of health care providers to improve understanding essential for decision making. These same groups have published guidelines for health care providers to improve communication with individuals with limitations in health literacy. Providers should assess literacy and comprehension whenever providing diagnostic or treatment information.

When communicating with patients, the Partnership for Clear Health Communication (2008) recommends health care providers follow these simple tips:

- Create a safe environment for patients.
- Sit down and face the individual when speaking, and talk slowly.
- Use simple language. Avoid technical terms; if they must be used, provide a simple and clear definition of their meaning.
- Encourage patients to ask questions.
- Organize information so important points stand out.
- Limit the amount of information provided at each visit.
- Use pictures or visual models to explain important concepts.
- Ask patients to "teach back"; that is, to repeat back to you what they have heard (Joint Commission, 2007).
- Ask patients what they will do when they return home, or ask the patient to tell you when it is important to seek medical care in order to validate their understanding.

Good communication in health care is the foundation for optimal outcomes.

It is our responsibility as the sender to use language appropriate for the receiver. When an individual has difficulty understanding English, it may be necessary to use an interpreter to present the information to the individual in his or her primary language. Many hospitals provide phone access to interpreters to improve communication between health care providers and consumers.

It is equally important to use age-appropriate language in communication. This is particularly important when communicating with older adults. Show respect by addressing the patient by his or her surname. Avoid familiar terms such as "honey," "bud," or "sweetie," which can be demeaning to the individual. During the initial interview, ask the patient how he or she prefers to be addressed and make note of this in the care plan or medical record. Our language should demonstrate respect for the individual as an adult.

Periodically ask the receiver to clarify what he or she is hearing as a means of ensuring accurate interpretation of your message. Mistakes occur when we make assumptions and fail to validate understanding. Take the case of the nurse who told her patient to take a medication prescribed TID—"take after each meal." Based on her physician's recommendation, the patient eats 5–6 small meals per day. Several days postdischarge the patient called for a prescription refill, and the nurse learned the patient was taking the medication after each meal, thus taking a minimum of five pills per day. To maximize understanding, ask the individual to repeat or "teach back" what was said or told to them and what this means for them in their life. This simple step can be a life saver and helps you avoid communication errors.

Maximizing Understanding

The next principle is to maximize understanding. The most important skill to help maximize understanding is to learn to listen. Learning to listen is essential to good communications. It is much easier to hear than it is to listen. Listening requires not only hearing the words spoken, but also understanding their meaning and the context in which they are spoken. We must be open-minded and provide opportunities for the individual to share their thoughts with us. It means allowing time to communicate and focusing attention on the person at the time of the conversation. Minimizing environmental distractions not only helps the individual with whom we are communicating, but also helps us maintain our focus.

Following Through

The final principle is to follow up and follow through. Words backed by actions help develop trust. A relationship built on trust and concern for the welfare of others is critical to optimal health outcomes. These simple techniques can be applied to all of our communications.

CHALLENGES IN COMMUNICATING WITH OLDER ADULTS

Memory or Cognitive Deficits

Physiological changes associated with chronic illness have various presentations. Although the basic principles of communication still apply, they need to be modified to overcome barriers associated with the individual's disability. Cognitive damage may occur secondary to metabolic damage, stroke, or hormonal or degenerative disease. Chapters 7 and 11 provide information about screening and treatment for those with memory or cognitive problems. The Mini Mental State Examination (MMSE) is a reliable screening tool to assess cognitive function. Individuals with cognitive deficits secondary to diffuse cortical damage present with signs of dementia, including decreased attention span, memory loss, word finding problems, and perseveration. These individuals often have difficulty with conversation and are dependent upon others to initiate conversation. All too often the individual's posture and nonverbal communication convey a sense of disinterest; thus, staff members are reluctant to initiate conversations. Early on in the disease process, conversation and the opportunity to share memories with others can be rewarding and energizing for the person. Regular conversation helps orient the individual to daily activities and creates a structure that promotes independence. Conversation that encourages thought and reflection can help keep the mind active. Just as exercise is important to the maintenance of physical function and mobility, mental exercise is equally important. **Table 5-3** outlines the basic principles of communication and strategies that benefit individuals with memory or cognitive deficits.

> **Notable Quotes**
>
> *"Tell me and I'll forget. Show me and I'll remember. Involve me and I'll understand."*
>
> —Confucius

One of the most common problems affecting cognition and memory among the elderly is Alzheimer's disease. The *Rush Manual for Caregivers* (Rush Alzheimer's Disease Center, 2002) offers several suggestions for making communication easier with those who have dementia. Frazier-Rios and Zembrzuski (2007), in an issue of the *Try This* series published by the Harford Foundation, provide a guide to assessing and tailoring communications for hospitalized older adults with dementia. Minimize use of the bedside intercom, which can be confusing. Use face-to-face communication as much as possible. Dialogue should be encouraged for as long as possible. Use simple instructions and ask yes or no questions. Use cues from the person's behavior and reactions to decide whether to modify your approach. Be aware of your own body language and tone of voice as well. Nurses may need to experiment with various types of communication, and approaches may need to be modified as the person's dementia progresses.

Speech Deficits or Impairments (Aphasia)

Aphasia is an acquired loss or impairment of language that occurs as a result of damage to the speech centers in the dominant hemisphere of the brain. There are many types of aphasia. Individuals with aphasia should be evaluated by a speech language pathologist who can provide instruction on the best strategies to use with each person. The

TABLE 5-3 Communicating with Individuals with Memory or Cognitive Deficits

Invite, respect	Approach persons in a nonthreatening manner within their visual field. Sit quietly with the person and gently touch her or his hand. Be respectful of the patient's belongings. At times patients can get overly upset when an outsider touches their belongings, even basic items such as the tissue box or washcloth. Ask permission before moving objects. Show concern; stop and have a conversation—don't limit communication to times when you need information.
Environment	Post a few pictures, a calendar, or a daily schedule in the patient's room and use it to enhance conversation or promote recall. Sit so you are facing the person when speaking. Avoid a setting with a lot of sensory stimulation—it can be distracting to the person. Maintain eye contact; it will help keep the patient focused on you and the topic. Be respectful of space. If the individual chooses to get up and start walking mid-conversation, ask if you may follow.
Understanding	Speak in normal tones. Use age-appropriate language. Start with a familiar topic. Sometimes this means talking about the past, then through conversation bringing the person back to current circumstances. Talk about people or events known to the person. This may mean referring to a deceased family member—the individual will let you know if this reference is comforting—or distressing. For many individuals, pleasant memories from the past are a source of comfort. Orientation questions can be confusing and frustrating for the person, so rather than asking, "What's today's date?" consider "Where's the calendar? Let's find today's date and mark it so we can find it later." Ask one question at a time. If the individual becomes upset or agitated, ease up and use distraction to change the topic or provide a period of quiet to allow a cool-down period.
Communication	Show interest in the person. If it is difficult to hear the person, gently ask him or her to speak louder. Provide time for conversation. Sometimes it will take a while to get the message out. Sometimes it is easier for the person to tell a story than respond to a direct question. Don't laugh at responses, no matter how bizarre. Acknowledge your inability to understand and your frustration. It's probably a mutual feeling that both parties share.

SOURCE: Adapted from ElderCare Online. (1998). *Communicating with impaired elderly persons.* Retrieved February 1, 2008, from http://www.ec-online.net/Knowledge/Articles/communication.html

most common types of aphasia are global aphasia, Broca's aphasia, and Wernicke's aphasia. Patients with a global aphasia typically have problems understanding language as well as producing speech. Language is typically nonfunctional in all modalities—speaking, reading, and writing. At times the individual may repeat a sound or word over and over. Although the individual may have difficulty speaking he or she may understand nonverbal gestures. Nonverbal gestures, such as nodding toward the individual as you address them, make the individual feel included. It is important to include all patients with aphasia in social groups.

Broca's aphasia is a nonfluent, agrammatic expressive aphasia. Individuals with Broca's aphasia typically have good auditory comprehension. They are able to understand what is said to them; however, they have difficulty producing intelligible speech. This is often quite frustrating for these individuals, because they know what they want to say but just can't get it out in words that have meaning to the receiver. Communication requires great patience. It is important to give the patient an opportunity to speak, because with time and therapy these individuals may make important gains in learning to communicate with others.

Wernicke's aphasia is a fluent aphasia. The individual is able to speak and produce language, although the speech may contain many odd words and sounds. Wernicke's aphasia is characterized by impaired auditory comprehension, so in this case the individual has great difficulty understanding what is said. Often he or she must rely on our nonverbal gestures to understand directions or questions.

It takes time and patience to communicate with individuals with aphasia. Nurses should structure activities and provide opportunities for these individuals to be engaged in some form of communication. Without opportunities to communicate with others, individuals may withdraw and become socially isolated. The expertise of the speech therapist can be invaluable in helping patients to regain maximal communication patterns. See **Table 5-4** for tips regarding communicating with individuals with aphasia.

TABLE 5-4 Communicating with Individuals with Aphasia

Invite, respect	Include the individual in conversations. Look at the person as well as others during conversation. Treat the person as an adult. Provide time for the individual to speak. Getting the message across is more important than perfection. If you don't understand the person, politely say so: "I'm sorry, I can't understand what you are saying to me." Remember, frustration works both ways—it's always better to end the conversation with a smile rather than a frown.
Environment	Position yourself across from the person so they can see your face and you can see theirs.
Understanding	Speak naturally. Don't raise your voice—it won't help. Speak slowly using simple words and sentences. Use simple gestures to supplement your message. (This isn't a game of Charades or Pictionary—don't get carried away with your gestures.) Tell the patient one thing at a time. Announce topic changes and allow a few minutes before proceeding.

Communication	Provide time for the individual to speak. Look at the person and listen as they speak. If you don't understand, ask them to describe the word, use another word, say or write the first letter, point to the item, or describe the context for use. If the individual is able to write, ask them to write the word or use a word board. Follow instructions from the speech language pathologist to improve the consistency of communication.

SOURCE: Adapted from ElderCare Online. (1998). *Communicating with impaired elderly persons*. Retrieved February 1, 2008, from http://www.ec-online.net/Knowledge/Articles/communication.html

Speech Impairments (Dysarthria)

Dysarthria can occur secondary to a number of diseases. Even the loss of dentition that occurs with aging may predispose the individual to dysarthria. Individuals with dysarthria may be difficult to understand when they are speaking. Patience and practice are key to understanding individuals with dysarthria. As one gets accustomed to the language sounds it becomes easier to understand what the individual is trying to say. As the receiver, it is important not to fake or pretend you understand. If the message is not clear, ask the individual to repeat, write, or communicate key words by using gestures. **Table 5-5** outlines the basic principles of communication and specific strategies that can be used to enhance communication with individuals with dysarthria.

Visual Impairments

Individuals with visual impairments have no difficulty hearing or speaking; however, they will miss nonverbal communications. These individuals will have difficulty reading signs or relying on visual

TABLE 5-5 Communicating with Individuals with Dysarthria

Invite, respect	Remember, speech impairment is not related to intelligence. Use age-appropriate language. Make a note in the medical record if the individual uses an AAC device. If you know the individual uses an AAC device, store it in an accessible location so it is readily available for use.
Environment	A quiet environment with minimal distractions can help facilitate understanding. Face the person as they are speaking for facial cues and gestures that can enhance understanding.
Understanding	Remember, the individual has no problem hearing you. Speak in a normal tone.
Communication	Encourage the person to speak slowly and use simple sentences or single words. Allow time for the patient to respond. Don't try to complete their words or sentences. If there is no speech (aphasia, presence of an artificial airway, postoperatively after oral surgery): • Assess the individual's yes/no reliability.

(continues)

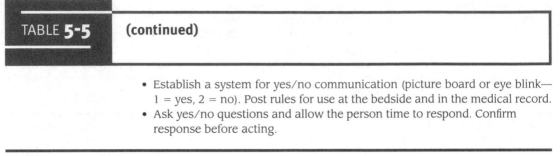

TABLE 5-5 (continued)

- Establish a system for yes/no communication (picture board or eye blink—1 = yes, 2 = no). Post rules for use at the bedside and in the medical record.
- Ask yes/no questions and allow the person time to respond. Confirm response before acting.

SOURCE: Adapted from ElderCare Online. (1998). *Communicating with impaired elderly persons.* Retrieved February 1, 2008, from http://www.ec-online.net/Knowledge/Articles/communication.html

cues for orientation or education purposes. Printed materials may need to be large or translated into Braille to maximize understanding. **Table 5-6** outlines the basic principles of communication and techniques that can enhance communications with individuals with visual impairments.

Hearing Impairments

Individuals with hearing loss fall into one of two groups, the hearing impaired and those who are deaf. Individuals with a hearing impairment have a reduced ability to hear across the spectrum of sound. Typically, with age it becomes more difficult to hear soft, high-pitched sounds. Based on the severity of the damage, the individual may or may not elect to use a hearing aid. Unless the hearing loss poses a significant disability, the individual may elect to just get by without the hearing aid, at times much to the dismay of other family members. Many hearing-impaired elders have learned language and

TABLE 5-6 Communicating with Individuals with Visual Impairments

Invite, respect	Gently call out to the individual when entering the room and identify yourself and anyone with you in the room. If the individual can see shapes or outlines, stand where he or she can see you. The best location will vary—make a note on the medical record alerting other staff to the patient's needs.
Environment	Minimize distractions. Describe the environment and where you are located in relation to the person. Explain what you are doing, especially when you are moving and creating sounds in the room (e.g., storing dressing supplies in the closet, preparing equipment to draw blood). Make certain not to move frequently used objects.
Understanding	Alert the person when you will be touching them.
Communication	Oral communication with touch is more important than nonverbal gestures that they cannot see; use an appropriate tone of voice.

SOURCE: Adapted from ElderCare Online. (1998). *Communicating with impaired elderly persons.* Retrieved February 1, 2008, from http://www.ec-online.net/Knowledge/Articles/communication.html

lived in an aural world, so they tend to rely on lip reading, which matches oral movements with sounds that are familiar to them. **Table 5-7** outlines the basic principles to use when communicating with individuals with hearing impairments. **Figure 5-1** displays different types of hearing aids that may be used.

Older adults who participate in an audiologic rehabilitation program and have positive social support have been shown to perceive less of a self-handicap than other hearing-impaired elderly (Taylor, 2003). This study by Taylor suggests that adults with hearing impairments would benefit from more formal training, of both them and their spouse or supportive family members, related to facilitating long-term communication at home.

In contrast, individuals who are deaf cannot hear. They rely on one of several forms of sign language as their primary language. Sign language is a different language, much like German is different from the English language. Therefore, with few exceptions, qualified sign language interpreters should be used to ensure effective communication with deaf persons in emergency and other health care situations where the rapid exchange of

TABLE 5-7 Communicating with Individuals with Hearing Impairment

Invite, respect	To get the attention of the person, touch the person gently, wave, or use another physical sign. Store assistive devices—hearing aid, notepad, and pen—within reach of the individual. Make certain any emergency alarms essential for safety have a light or visual alert to get the individual's attention in case of emergency. Allow time for the conversation.
Environment	If the individual uses a hearing aid, check to see whether he or she is wearing it and that it is turned on. Minimize background noise (turn off the radio or TV and close the door to minimize distractions from the hall). When speaking, face the person directly so he or she can see your lips and facial expressions. The preferred distance is 3-6 feet from the person.
Understanding	Speak clearly in a low-pitched voice; avoid yelling or exaggerating speaking movements—it won't help. Use short sentences. Don't hesitate to use written notes to maximize understanding and involve the person in the conversation. Avoid chewing, eating, or smoking as you speak; they will make reading your speech more difficult. Keep objects (e.g., scarf, hands) away from your face when speaking. Allow the individual to be involved in making decisions—don't assume it takes too much time to ask.
Communication	Provide time for the individual to speak. Ask questions to clarify the message; if needed, have the individual write a response.

SOURCE: Adapted from ElderCare Online. (1998). *Communicating with impaired elderly persons.* Retrieved February 1, 2008, from http.//www.ec-online.net/Knowledge/Articles/communication.html

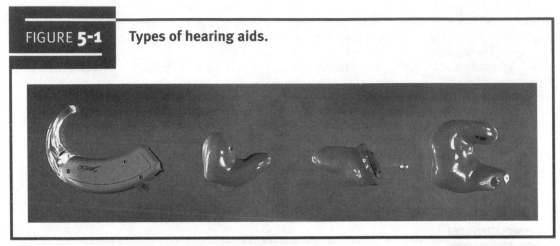

FIGURE 5-1 **Types of hearing aids.**

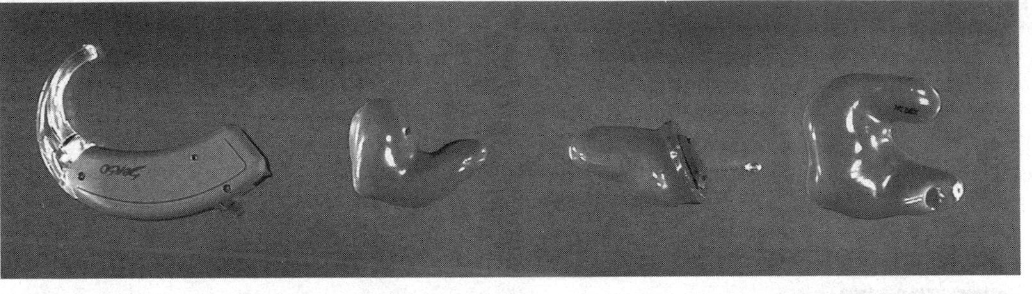

SOURCE: © Jones and Bartlett Publishers. Courtesy of MIEMSS.

BOX 5-2 **Resource List**

American Speech-Language-Hearing Association: www.asha.org

Ask Me 3: www.askme3.org

Canadian National Institute for the Blind: www.cnib.ca

Deaf Empowerment: www.deafe.org

Deaf Resource Library: www.deaflibrary.org

ElderCare Online, Communicating with Impaired Elderly Persons: www.ec-online.net/knowledge/articles/communication.html

Gallaudet University: www.gallaudet.edu

Institute for Disabilities Research and Training: www.idrt.com

National Association of the Deaf: www.nad.org

National Patient Safety Foundation, Partnership for Clear Health Communication: www.npsf.org/pchc2/

Paralyzed Veterans of America: www.pva.org

Rehabilitation Institute of Chicago: www.ric.org

United Spinal Association: www.united-spinal.org

accurate information is critical. The use of qualified sign language interpreters communicates respect and ensures that deaf individuals and hearing health care professionals will be able to communicate with each other at a rate and level of complexity equal to, or as effective as, the communication rate of persons who speak directly to each other in the same language. **Table 5-8** lists strategies that can be used to enhance communications with individuals who are deaf.

SUMMARY

In conclusion, communication with older adults may present some unique challenges, including physical changes from normal aging as well as those associated with common disease processes. By using the basic techniques discussed in this chapter, nurses can facilitate effective communication with older adults within a variety of situations and settings.

TABLE 5-8 Communicating with Individuals Who Are Deaf

Invite, respect	Note on the patient's record that the individual is deaf and may need an interpreter. Document whether the individual uses American Sign Language or other assistive communication. Use a TDD phone or relay service to communicate with the person. Use an interpreter for conversations regarding health care decision making. To get the attention of the person, touch the person gently, wave, or use another physical sign. Store assistive devices—notepad and pen—within reach of the individual. Make certain any emergency alarms essential for safety have a light or visual alert to get the individual's attention in case of emergency. Allow time for the conversation—functional as well as social.
Environment	When speaking, face the person directly so that he or she can see your lips and facial expressions. The preferred distance is 3–6 feet from the person.
Understanding	Don't hesitate to use written notes to maximize understanding and involve the person in the conversation. Avoid chewing, eating, or smoking as you speak—they will make reading your speech more difficult. When using an interpreter, face the individual not the interpreter—when asking as well as listening to a response. Be mindful of your nonverbal expressions during conversations—remember you are conversing with the person, not the interpreter.
Communication	Allow the individual to be involved in making decisions—don't assume it takes too much time to ask. Provide time for the individual to return communication and keep your focus on the person. Ask questions to clarify the message; if needed, have the individual write his or her response.

SOURCE: Adapted from ElderCare Online. (1998). *Communicating with impaired elderly persons.* Retrieved February 1, 2008, from http://www.ec-online.net/Knowledge/Articles/communication.html

Critical Thinking *Exercises*

1. Mrs. Rodgers is a 68-year-old retired sales clerk. For many years she worked in the sewing and fabrics department at the local store. She is admitted to the hospital after a fall. Her daughter reports her mother has been withdrawn and it is difficult to get her attention when she is watching television.

continues

Critical Thinking Exercises

According to the CT scan, it appears Mrs. Rodgers has an acoustic neuroma that may have contributed to her fall. Describe factors that may impact your communications with Mrs. Rodgers.

2. Dr. Knowles is an 85-year-old man who has had cerebral palsy since birth. He has dysarthria, which has gotten noticeably worse since he has lost his teeth. He is admitted to your unit with complaints of chest pain. The nursing assistant tells you, "I just can't understand him, so I always say yes to his questions." What advice would you give to the nursing assistant to communicate better with Dr. Knowles?
3. Mr. Riley lives at home with his son and two high school–age grandchildren. According to the son, Mr. Riley has transient episodes of confusion and disorientation. He tends to get his son and grandson confused. On a home visit with Mr. Riley he acknowledges his confusion and comments, "No one talks to me so I guess I just drift off and get lost in time." What recommendations would you make to Mr. Riley's son?
4. Ms. Zorica is an elderly Russian woman who is being seen in the clinic for multiple chronic conditions including diabetes, high blood pressure, and venous ulcers. On this visit the physician changed her Lasix dose from 40 mg daily to 40 mg and 60 mg on alternating days. You are assigned to do the discharge medication reconciliation. What can you do to explain the change in medication and new dosing schedule?

Personal **Reflections**

1. Language and the meaning of words may change over time so that as we age terms that were meaningful and relevant to our life at an early age are either no longer in use or have a different meaning to others not of our generation. (Example: "to mimeograph": A method of printing multiple documents that has since been replaced by Xerox or digital printing methods.)
   a. List terms used by older adults that are no longer used in daily language (e.g., phonograph).
   b. List terms that are part of your world but may be unfamiliar to older adults (e.g., MP3, iPod, TiVo).
   c. Discuss how age differences between sender and receiver can have an impact on communications.
2. Think about a time you visited the dentist and your mouth was anesthetized for a dental procedure. Describe how you felt communicating with others. To what degree were they able to understand what you were trying to say? If you needed emergency care, could you communicate this need to others?

   In this example you experienced a temporary or transient episode of dysarthria. You may have been frustrated communicating with others or relied on alternative means, such as writing, to communicate. Imagine if the anesthesia never wore off and your speech never improved. Describe how you would feel in this circumstance.

Personal **Reflections**

3. You are a nurse admitting an 87-year-old man accompanied by his wife who is in a wheelchair. List 10 nonverbal behaviors you may use during the admission interview to enhance communication.
    1. ______
    2. ______
    3. ______
    4. ______
    5. ______
    6. ______
    7. ______
    8. ______
    9. ______
    10. ______
4. Reflect back on your last day at clinical. What types of conversations did you have with your assigned patient? Were there opportunities for you to engage in an affective conversation with your assigned patient? Did you observe other staff members engaging patients in affective communications? List barriers in health care that limit staff engaging in affective conversations with patients.
5. Call local hospitals and ask for information on language translation services. Ask for information on the policy for use of interpreter services at the facility.

References

AARP. (2007). *Consumer guide to hearing aids.* Washington, DC: Author.

Adams-Wendling, L., & Pimple, C. (2007). Nursing management of hearing impairment in nursing facility residents. Iowa City: University of Iowa Gerontological Nursing Interventions Research Center, Research Dissemination Core.

American Speech-Language-Hearing Association. (1998). *Guidelines for hearing aid fitting for adults.* [Guidelines]. Retreived December 4, 2008, from http://www.asha.org/policy

Caris Verhallen, W. M., Kerkstra, A., & Bensing, T. (1997). The role of communication in nursing care for elderly people: A review of the literature. *Journal of Advanced Nursing, 25,* 915–933.

Carroll, S. M. (2007). Silent, slow lifeworld: The communication experience of nonvocal ventilated patients. *Qualitative Health Research, 17*(9), 1165-1177.

Demers, K. (2007, November 12). Hearing screening in older adults: A brief hearing loss screener. In: *Try this: Best practices in nursing care of older adults.* Retrieved on October 23, 2008, from http://consultgerirn.org/uploads/File/trythis/issue_12.pdf

Dickerson, S. S., Stone, V. I., Pnachura, C., & Usiak, D. (2002). The meaning of communication: Experiences with augmentative communication devices. *Rehabilitation Nursing, 27*(6), 215–220.

ElderCare Online. (1998). *Communicating with impaired elderly persons.* Retrieved February 1, 2008, from http://www.ec-online.net/Knowledge/Articles/communication.html

Frazier-Rios, D., & Zembrzuski, A. (2007). Communication difficulties: Assessment and interventions in hospitalized older adults with dementia. In: *Try this: Best practices in nursing care for hospitalized older adults.* New York: The Hartford Institute for Geriatric Nursing.

Healthy People 2010. (2000). *11. Health communication.* Retrieved February 1, 2008, from http://www.healthypeople.gov/document/HTML/Volume1/11HealthCom.htm

Henderson, J., & Doyle, M. (2002). Augmentative and alternative communication. In D. A. Olson & F. DeRuyter (Eds.), *Clinician's guide to assistive technology* (pp. 127–151). St. Louis: Mosby.

Holland, L., & Halper, A. S. (1996). Talking to individuals with aphasia: A challenge for the rehabilitation team. *Topics in Stroke Rehabilitation, 2*, 27–37.

Joint Commission on Accreditation of Healthcare Organizations. (2007). *"What did the doctor say?": Improving health literacy to protect patient safety.* Oakbrook Terrace, IL: Joint Commission.

Mann, W., Hurren, D., & Tomita, M. (1993). Comparison of assistive technology use and needs of home-based older persons with different impairments. *American Journal of Occupational Therapy, 47*, 980–987.

Nielsen-Bohlman, L., Panzer, A. M., & Kindig, D. (Eds.). (2004). *Health literacy: A prescription to end confusion.* Washington, DC: National Academies Press.

Olson, D. A., & DeRuyter, F. (Eds.). (2002). *Clinician's guide to assistive technology*. St. Louis: Mosby.

Pape, T. L., Kim, J., & Weiner, B. (2002). The shaping of individual meanings assigned to assistive technology: A review of personal factors. *Disability and Rehabilitation, 24*(1/2/3), 5–20.

Partnership for Clear Health Communication. (2008). *What providers can do.* Retrieved February 1, 2008, from http://www.askme3.org/PFCHC/what_can_provid.asp

Rehabilitation Institute of Chicago LIFE Center. (2006). *Straight talk about disability*. Retrieved February 1, 2008, from http://lifecenter.ric.org/content/384/index.html?topic=&subtopic=

Rush Alzheimer's Disease Center. (2002). *The Rush manual for caregivers*. Chicago, IL: Author.

Satir, V. (1976). *Making contact*. Berkeley, CA: Celestial Arts.

Taylor, K. S. (2003). Effects of group composition in audiologic rehabilitation programs for hearing impaired elderly. *Audiology Online.* Retrieved October 2, 2005, from http://www.audiologyonline.com/articles/article_detail.asp?article_id=498

United Spinal Association. (2008). *Disability etiquette, tips on interacting with people with disabilities.* Jackson Heights, NY: Author.

SECTION

3

ASSESSMENT
(Competencies 5–8)

TECHNICAL SKILLS
(Competencies 9–10)

CHAPTER 6

REVIEW OF THE AGING OF PHYSIOLOGICAL SYSTEMS

JANICE M. HEINEMAN, PHD
JENNIFER HAMRICK-KING, PHDC
BETH SCAGLIONE SEWELL, PHD

LEARNING OBJECTIVES

At the end of this chapter, the reader will be able to:

- Describe the aging process of each physiological system.
- Distinguish between intrinsic aging and age-related disease.
- Describe how the aging process of each physiological system correlates with the functional ability of the older adult.
- Explain how the aging process of one system interacts with and/or affects other physiological systems.
- Acknowledge that not every aspect of every physiological system changes with age.
- Recognize that aging changes are partially dependent upon an individual's health behaviors and preventive health measures.

KEY TERMS

- α-adrenoceptors
- Acquired immunity
- Actin
- Adrenal cortex
- Adrenal glands
- Adrenal medulla
- Adrenocorticotropic hormone (ACTH)
- Aldosterone
- Alveoli
- Amino acid neurotransmitters
- Andropause
- Anemia
- Anorexia of aging
- Antibodies
- Antigen
- Apoptosis
- Arteries
- Atria
- Autoimmunity
- Autonomic nervous system
- B cells
- β-adrenoceptors
- Baroreceptor
- Baroreflex
- Basic multicellular unit (BMU)
- Calcitonin
- Cardiac output
- Cartilaginous joints
- Catecholamines
- $CD34^+$ cells
- Cell-mediated immunity
- Chemoreceptors
- Cholinergic neurons
- Chronological aging
- Clonal expansion
- Colon
- Complement system
- Cortical bone
- Corticotropin-releasing hormone (CRH)
- Cortisol

- Cytokines
- Dehydroepiandrosterone (DHEA)
- Dermis
- Detrusor
- Diaphragm
- Diastole
- Dopaminergic system
- Elastic recoil
- Epidermis
- Epinephrine
- Erythrocytes
- Esophagus
- Extrinsic aging
- Fast-twitch fibers
- Follicle-stimulating hormone (FSH)
- Forced expiratory volume (FEV)
- Free radicals
- Gallbladder
- Gastrointestinal immunity
- Glomerular filtration rate
- Glomeruli
- Glucagon
- Glucocorticoids
- Glucose tolerance
- GLUT4
- Gonadotropin-releasing hormone (GnRH)
- Growth hormone (GH)
- Hematopoiesis
- Homeostasis
- Hormones
- Humoral immunity
- Hypogeusia
- Hypophysiotropic
- Hypothalamic-pituitary-adrenal (HPA) axis
- Immovable joints
- Immunosenescence
- Inflammatory response
- Inhibin B
- Innate immunity
- Insulin
- Insulin resistance
- Islets of Langerhans
- Keratinocytes
- Killer T cells
- Langerhans cells
- Leukocytes
- Lipofuscin
- Liver
- Luteinizing hormone (LH)
- Macrophage
- Mechanoreceptors
- Melanin
- Melanocytes
- Melatonin
- Menopause
- Mineralocorticoids
- Monoaminergic system
- Motor unit
- Muscle quality
- Muscle strength
- Myocardial cells
- Myofibril
- Myosin
- Natural killer (NK) cells
- Nephrons
- Nerve cells
- Neurogenesis
- Neurotransmitter
- Nocturia
- Norepinephrine
- Olfaction
- Osteoblast
- Osteoclast
- Osteocyte
- Pancreas
- Parathyroid gland
- Parathyroid hormone (PTH)
- Pharynx
- Photoaging
- Pineal gland
- Plaques
- Plasma cell
- Plasticity
- Pluripotent stem cells
- Presbycusis
- Presbyopia
- Replicative senescence
- Reproductive axis
- Sarcomere
- Sarcopenia
- Sarcoplasmic reticulum
- Skeletal muscle
- Slow-twitch fibers
- Stem cell progenitors
- Subcutaneous layer
- Suppressor T cells
- Synapses
- Synaptogenesis

- Synovial fluid
- Synovial joint
- Synovium
- Systole
- T cells
- Tangles
- T-helper cells
- Thrombocytes
- Thyroid
- Thyroid-stimulating hormone (TSH)
- Thyroxine (T4)
- Total lung capacity
- Trabecular bone
- Triiodothyronine (T3)
- Ureters
- Urethra
- Vasopressin
- Ventilatory rate
- Ventricles
- Vital capacity

Without the physiological changes of aging we might never say that a person ages. The general population's concept of aging is generally, and almost instinctively, characterized by changes in physical appearance, functional decline, and chronic disease. All of these characteristics are the result of physiological change. Even the psychological and social changes associated with aging, such as depression and social withdrawal, are often rooted in changes in the structure and function of the body's physiological systems. Thus, it could be argued that the physiology of aging is true aging.

Aging processes that occur in one physiological system can directly or indirectly influence other physiological systems. Thus, although it is relatively easy to focus on changes in only one physiological system, a broader scope is necessary to truly understand the influences and consequences of aging on physiological structure and function. This is especially true given that people are now living longer and for longer periods of time in that stage of life that is currently considered to be old age. Although each cohort ages differently, general aging changes tend to remain stable. In this chapter we will review the aging process of each of the body's major physiological systems. We ask, however, that the reader remain mindful that physiological aging is an extremely individual process and that how the body ages is greatly affected by a person's genetic makeup, health behaviors, and availability of resources.

THE CARDIOVASCULAR SYSTEM

The cardiovascular system consists of the heart, associated vasculature, and blood. The heart and vasculature deliver the blood to every organ system in the body, maintaining oxygen levels, supplying nutrients, and carrying toxins away to be filtered by the spleen and liver. The structural and functional abilities of the cardiovascular system are crucial to sustaining the human body. Age-related changes to the cardiovascular structure and function will be evaluated in this section.

Overview of the Cardiovascular Structure and Function

The heart contains four chambers, consisting of the two upper **atria** and the two lower **ventricles** (Digiovanna, 2000). Blood from the venous system enters the two atria. Oxygen-rich blood from the lungs enters the left atrium, proceeds to the left ventricle, and is expelled into the aorta for delivery to the entire body, excluding the lungs. Oxygen-poor blood returns from the body's venous system to the right atrium. The right ventricle expels oxygen-poor blood into pulmonary **arteries** that carry the blood to the lungs for reoxygenation (Digiovanna, 2000; Moore, Mangoni, Lyons, & Jackson, 2003). When ventricles contract during **systole** or peak blood pressure, blood fills the arteries. Once the ventricles relax during **diastole**, or low pressure, blood is propelled into the capillaries (Digiovanna, 2000; Moore et al., 2003; Pugh & Wei, 2001).

Larger arteries are associated with the structure and function of the heart, whereas smaller arteries and arterioles are associated with systemic structure and function. The arterial system as a whole is responsible for the qualities of pressure and resistance that are characteristic of the cardiovascular system (Moore et al., 2003). The veins carry over half of the total blood in the cardiovascular system and are associated with the qualities of volume and conformity (Moore et al., 2003). **Figure 6-1** illustrates the arterial and venous systems

FIGURE 6-1 **The cardiovascular system.**

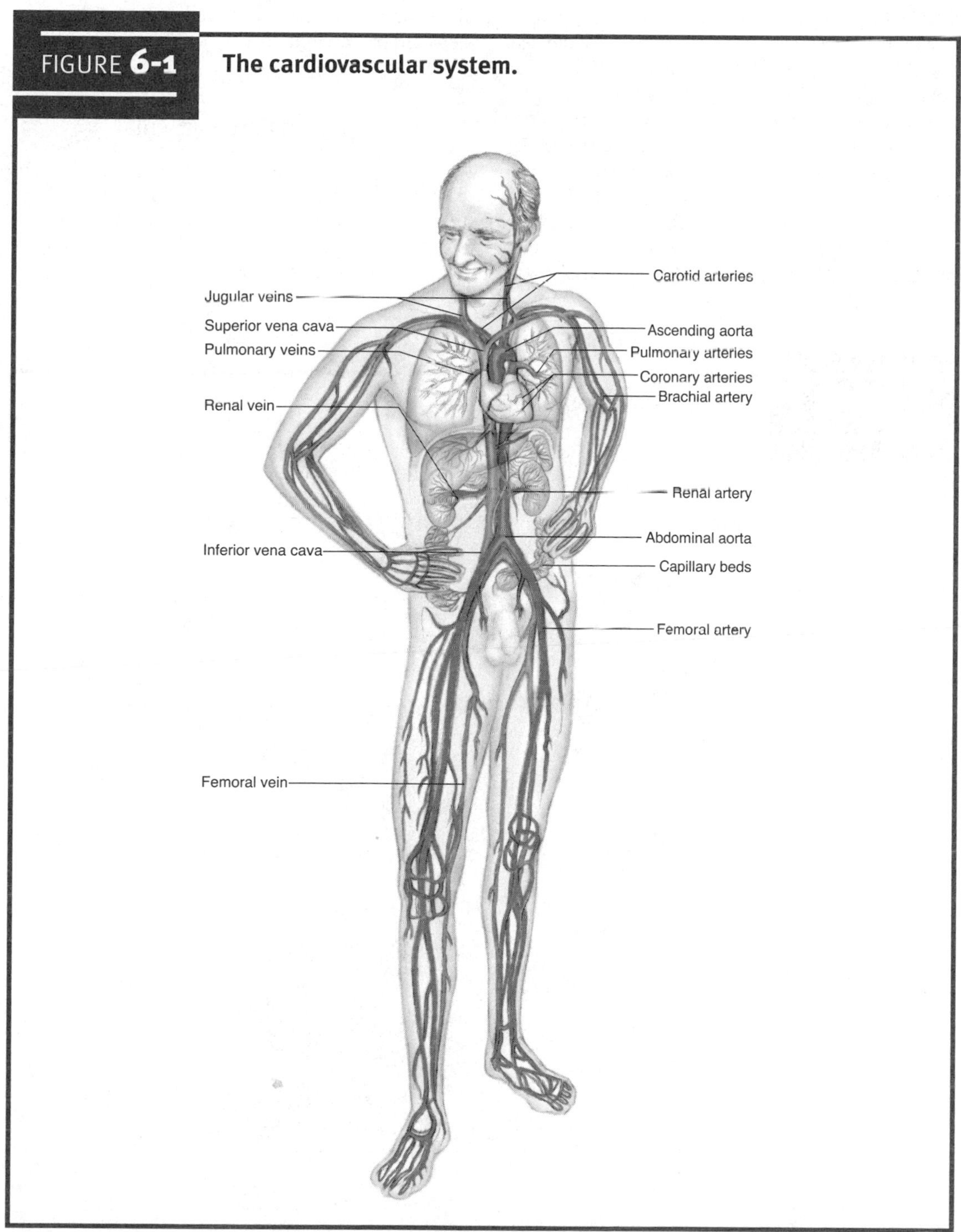

SOURCE: Anatomy and Physiology: Understanding the Human Body, Robert E. Clark, Jones and Bartlett Publishers 2005.

within the body and organ systems, and **Figure 6-2** demonstrates the structural overview of the heart and the path of blood flow into and out of the heart.

The main function of the cardiovascular system is to maintain **homeostasis** by transferring oxygen, nutrients, and hormones to other organ systems. The cardiovascular system also provides defense mechanisms through white blood cells. In addition, this physiological system regulates body temperature and contributes to acid-base balance within the range of pH 7.35 to 7.45 (Digiovanna, 2000). **Figure 6-3** illustrates the pathway of oxygen-rich and oxygen-depleted blood circulation to corresponding organs and body areas.

Aging Changes in Cardiovascular Structure

Cardiac Aging

Enlargement of heart chambers and coronary cells occurs with age, as does increased thickening of heart walls, especially in the left ventricle (Priebe,

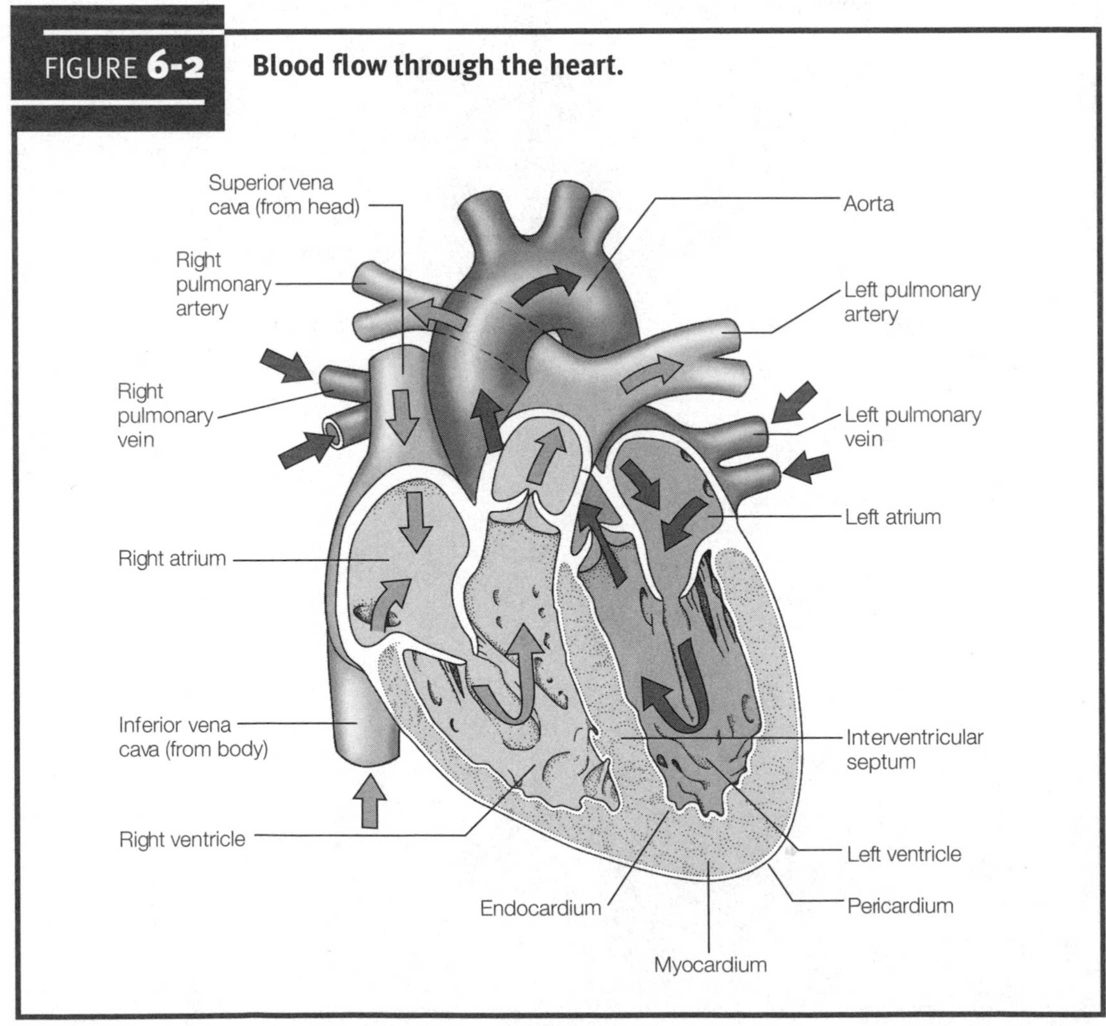

FIGURE **6-2** **Blood flow through the heart.**

SOURCE: Human Biology, 5e. Daniel D. Chiras, Jones and Bartlett Publishers 2005.

FIGURE 6-3 **The circulatory system.**

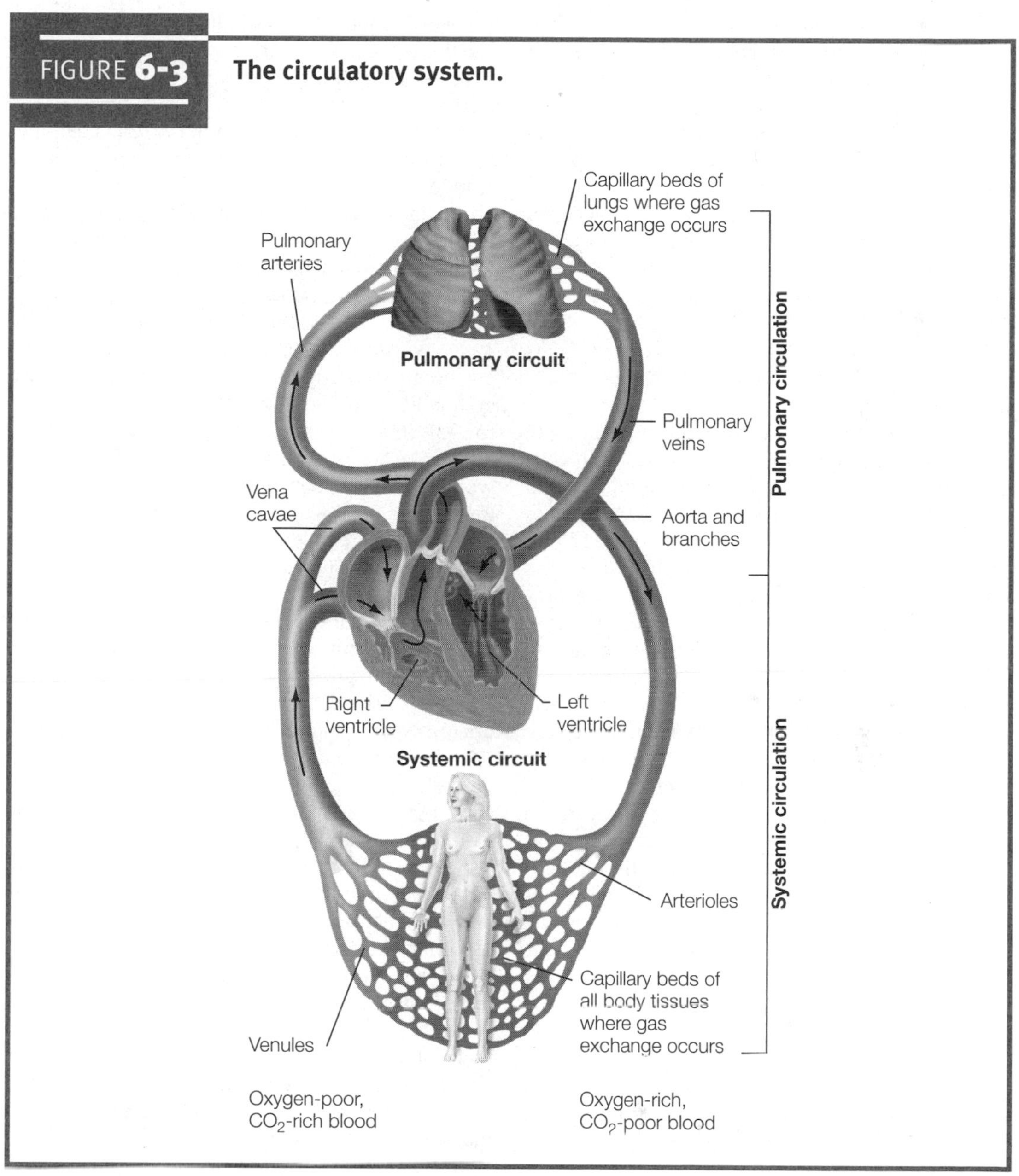

SOURCE: Human Biology, 5e. Daniel D. Chiras, Jones and Bartlett Publishers 2005.

2000; Pugh & Wei, 2001; Weisfeldt, 1998). This enlargement and thickening cause a decline in ventricle flexibility (Pugh & Wei, 2001) and an overall increase in heart weight of about 1.5 grams/year in women and 1.0 gram/year in men, measured from age 30 to age 90 years (Ferrari, Radaelli, & Centola, 2003; Lakatta, 1996). Ventricles in the heart also begin to thicken and stiffen in correlation with continued steady production of collagen. In addition, there is a decline in the number of **myocardial cells** and subsequent enlargement of the remaining cells (Ferrari et al., 2003; Olivetti, Melessari, Capasso, & Anversa, 1991; Pugh & Wei, 2001). Early studies found that the total number of myocardial cells declines by approximately 40% to 50% between the ages of 20 and 90 (Olivetti et al., 1991). However, recent investigations have concluded that women maintain myocardial cell numbers with age (Olivetti et al., 1991).

Vascular Aging

Aged arteries become extended and twisted. Alterations also occur in endothelial cells, and arterial walls thicken due to increased levels of collagen and decreased levels of elastin (Ferrari et al., 2003; Lakatta, 1999b; Virmani et al., 1991). With age, large arteries begin to dilate and stiffen, leading to hypertension pathophysiology characterized by increased blood velocity from the aorta to the systemic arterial system (Moore et al., 2003; O'Rourke & Hashimoto, 2007; Weisfeldt, 1998). Variable levels of arterial stiffness occur depending on differential changes in elastin and collagen levels. Arterial walls of the aging human, particularly in the aorta, are characterized by loss of muscle attachments due to disorganization of elastic tissue and accumulation of collagen (O'Rourke & Hashimoto, 2007). The level of arterial stiffness also depends on whether the affected arteries are central elastic arteries or peripheral muscular arteries (Pugh & Wei, 2001; Robert, 1999). Peripheral arteries can show increased stiffness due to accumulating mineral (calcium), lipid, and collagen residues (Lakatta, 1993a; Richardson, 1994; Robert, 1999). Although arteries stiffen due to alterations in elastin and collagen, arterioles undergo atrophy, affecting their ability to expand with pressure alterations (Richardson, 1994).

> **Notable Quotes**
>
> *"In the central place of every heart there is a recording chamber. So long as it receives a message of beauty, hope, cheer, and courage—so long are you young. When the wires are all down and our heart is covered with the snow of pessimism and the ice of cynicism, then, and only then, are you grown old."*
>
> —Douglas MacArthur

Although the aorta and other arteries begin to stiffen with age, the left ventricle pumps the same amount of blood. This combination of arterial stiffening and stable blood flow results in increased wave velocity of blood traveling toward the arterial system and increased pressure in late systole (Carroll, Shroff, Wirth, Halsted, & Rajfer, 1991; Lakatta, 1993a; O'Rourke & Hashimoto, 2007; Schulman, 1999; Weisfeldt, 1998). The aorta and proximal elastic arteries are able to stretch by 10% during systole in youth; however, this dilation is reduced to 2–3% in aged subjects (O'Rourke & Hashimoto, 2007). The flexibility of the aorta remains greater in women than in men until menopause, at which time aortic flexibility declines. However, estrogen replacement recovers some of the lost aortic expandability (Hayward, Kelly, & Collins, 2000; Rajkumar et al., 1997).

Overall vascular tone tends to decline with age due to deterioration in endothelium regulation of vascular relaxation (Pugh & Wei, 2001; Quyyumi, 1998). All four cardiac valves increase in circumference in older adults, with the greatest increase occurring in the aortic valve. In addition, calcium deposits accrue in the valves and may lead to stenosis (Pugh & Wei, 2001; Roffe, 1998; Tresch & Jamali, 1998).

In the cardiac conduction system, the sinoatrial (SA) node demonstrates some fibrosis as well as loss of pacemaker cells, down to approximately 10% of those observed at age 20 (Lakatta, 1993a; Wei, 1992). Also with age, the atroventricular (AV) node may be affected by nearby calcification of cardiac muscle (Pugh & Wei, 2001). In contrast to those of the arterial system, age-related changes to the venous system have not been well described in the literature (Moore et al., 2003). **Table 6-1** summarizes cardiovascular age-related structural changes.

Cardiovascular Aging Mechanisms

Finding the mechanism responsible for the aging of the cardiovascular system could lead to interventions and therapies aimed at reducing the

TABLE 6-1 Summarization of Cardiovascular Structural and Functional Changes That Occur with Age

Structural changes with age	Decreased myocardial cells, decreased aortic distensibility, decreased vascular tone
	Increased heart weight, increased myocardial cell size, increased left ventricle wall thickness, increased artery stiffness, increased elastin levels, increased collagen levels, increased left atrium size
Functional changes with age	Decreased diastolic pressure (during initial filling), decreased diastolic filling, decreased reaction to β-adrenergic stimulus
	Increased systolic pressure, increased arterial pressure, increased wave velocity, increased left ventricular end-diastolic pressure, elongation of muscle contraction phase, elongation of muscle relaxation phase, elongation of ventricle relaxation
No change with age	Ejection fraction, stroke volume, overall systolic function

age-associated physiological factors that alter cardiovascular structure and functioning. Some potential mechanisms include **free radicals**, apoptosis, inflammatory processes, advanced glycation end products, and gene expression (Pugh & Wei, 2001). Free radicals have been implicated in the overall aging process of the body, as described in Chapter 3 and also mentioned later in this chapter under "The Aging Brain." The presence of **lipofuscin**, a brown pigment found in aging cells, relates to oxidative mechanisms. In combination with mitochondrial dysfunction, lipofuscin may result in the increased production of free radicals (Roffe, 1998; Wei, 1992).

Increased levels of free radicals can foster **apoptosis**, or cell death. Due to the very limited regenerative properties of cardiomyocytes, or heart cells, apoptosis can have detrimental effects on cardiovascular structure and functioning (Pugh & Wei, 2001). The proposed triggers for induction of apoptosis include elevated levels of noradrenaline and initiation of the renin-angiotensin system with age (Sabbah, 2000). Another possible trigger for apoptosis is gene expression, which causes changes in the messenger RNA (mRNA) associated with the **sarcoplasmic reticulum** and the related enzyme ATPase (Lakatta, 1993a). These mRNA changes lead to both qualitative and quantitative alterations in the sarcoplasmic reticulum and ATPase. These alterations, in turn, lead to functional changes in relaxation of the heart and diastolic filling (Lakatta, 1993a; Lompre, 1998; Pugh & Wei, 2001). Aging mechanisms associated with the heart continue to be researched in depth, hopefully leading to new insights in the near future.

Aging Changes in Cardiovascular Function

Cardiac Aging

According to several studies, the ability of the heart to exert force or to contract does not change with age (Gerstenblith et al., 1997; Rodeheffer et al., 1984; Weisfeldt, 1998; Colcombe, et al. 2004). At rest, the aging heart adapts and maintains necessary functioning quite efficiently (Pugh & Wei, 2001). Although the ability of the cardiac muscle to exert force does not change with age, the actual muscle contraction as well as the relaxation phase does elongate with age (Lakatta, 1993a; Lakatta, Gerstenblith, Angell, Shock, & Weisfeldt, 1975; Roffe, 1998; Schulman, 1999). The prolonged contraction and relaxation phases with age correlate with extended release of calcium as well as decline in calcium reuptake (Roffe, 1998).

Ventricles also experience prolonged relaxation due to age-related declines in the sarcoplasmic reticulum pump and the associated enzyme ATPase, which produces energy for the cardiovascular system (Lompre, 1998; Pugh & Wei, 2001). The left atrium in the heart enlarges, contributing to functional changes in the filling. Furthermore, research has demonstrated that increased arterial stiffness along with the extended relaxation period leads to increased left ventricular end-diastolic pressure. This is demonstrated by a decline in pressure at the beginning of diastolic filling and an increase in pressure during late diastolic filling (Kane, Ouslander, & Abrass, 1999; Lakatta, 1993a; Miller et al., 1986; Pugh & Wei, 2001; Roffe, 1998). With age, diastolic filling declines at a rate of approximately 6% to 7% each decade both during exercise and at rest, but diastolic heart failure rarely occurs (Schulman, 1999). Increased pressure during ventricular systole due to increased aortic stiffening has been correlated with left ventricle hypertrophy (O'Rourke & Hashimoto, 2007). In turn, increased left ventricle mass has been correlated with age-related declines in initial diastolic filling (Salmasi, Alimo, Jepson, & Dancy, 2003). The increase in left ventricular mass correlates with increased total blood flow and elevated systolic blood pressure (Weisfeldt, 1998). Although no age-related change occurs in ejection fracture or stroke volume (Ferrari et al., 2003; Gerstenblith et al., 1997; Rodeheffer et al., 1984), the increase in left ventricular mass and concomitant increase in left ventricle oxygen requirements predisposes the development of left ventricular failure (Levy, Larsen, Vasan, Kannel, & Ho, 1996).

Vascular Aging

Aging does not appear to change the overall maximum capacity, the maximum vasodilation, or the perfusion of coronary vessels (Weisfeldt, 1998). However, resistance increases with age in the aorta, arterial wall, and vascular periphery. In addition, blood viscosity increases between the ages of 20 and 70 years (Lakatta & Levy, 2003; Morley & Reese, 1989). Cardiovascular symptoms of hypertension parallel the usual aging changes seen in older adults. Such symptoms, however, are exhibited at younger ages as well and are sometimes exaggerated. These differences have led to use of the term *muted hypertension* to describe cardiovascular aging changes (Lakatta, 1999b). Other changes such as moderate accumulation of cardiac amyloid and lipofuscin do not appear to alter functional abilities, but they are present in approximately half of individuals over age 70, and elevated levels could produce degenerative changes (Pugh & Wei, 2001). Small arteries (<400 μm), arterioles (<100 μm), and the capillaries comprise the microcirculation. Specific structural changes of the microcirculation are generally unnotable with aging (O'Rourke & Hashimoto, 2007). No age-related changes occur in blood-tissue exchange via the capillaries, suggesting a possible compensatory mechanism such as capillary thickening (Richardson, 1994).

Autonomic Nervous System Aging Effects

A few of the age-related changes in the cardiovascular system occur due to the **autonomic nervous system**. Orthostatic hypotension has a prevalence as high as 30% in individuals over 75 years of age (Gupta & Lipsitz, 2007). Changes related to orthostatic hypotension include decreased reaction of the entire system, both myocardial and vascular, to β-adrenergic stimulus as well as reduced **baroreflex** activity relating to an imbalance in neuroendocrine control (Lakatta, 1999b; Phillips, Hodsman, & Johnston, 1991; Pugh & Wei, 2001; Weisfeldt, 1998). **Norepinephrine** concentrations increase with age, causing overactivation of the sympathetic nervous system. This overactivation subsequently leads to overstimulation of **β-adrenoceptors**, even to the point of desensitization (Esler, Kaye, et al., 1995; Lakatta, 1993b, 1999a; Moore et al., 2003). With usual functional abilities, however, stimulation of the β-adrenoceptors triggers vessel dilation. In contrast, **α-adrenoceptors** that control vessel constriction remain stable with age (Priebe, 2000; Weisfeldt, 1998). Reduced arterial baroreflex activity, which controls peripheral vessels, has been correlated with several changes including arterial stiffening, neural modifications, and decreased stimulation of **baroreceptors** (Hunt, Farquar, & Taylor, 2001). These changes in baroreflex activity can lead to impaired sympathetic nerve response and resistance in peripheral vessels. As a result, blood pressure becomes unstable and hypotension may result (Ferrari et al., 2003). Table 6-1 summarizes age-associated changes in the functional abilities of the cardiovascular system.

Exercise and Aging

When older adults exercise, the cardiovascular response is different from the response of younger individuals. Cardiovascular condition during exercise is usually measured using maximum oxygen consumption (VO_{2max}), which equals the sum of **cardiac output** and systemic oxygen reserve. VO_{2max} shows age-related declines of around 10% per decade beginning in the second decade of life and reductions of around 50% by age 80 (Aronow, 1998; Maharam, Bauman, Kalman, Skolnick, & Perle, 1999). Furthermore, declines are accelerated as aging progresses, from 3–6% per decade in the 20s and 30s to more than 20% per decade in the 70s and beyond (Bearden, 2006; Fleg et al., 2005). Cardiovascular reserve is best measured using maximum cardiac output, which is equal to heart rate multiplied by stroke volume during exercise (Fleg, 1986). With age, the increased heart rate and contractility usually associated with exercise become less pronounced; however, opposition to blood flow increases (Weisfeldt, 1998). With these changes an overall decline in cardiac function and cardiac output is observed with initiation of exercise (Pugh & Wei, 2001; Weisfeldt, 1998).

A number of individuals from the Baltimore Longitudinal Study, ages 20 to 80 years and without heart disease, participated in an exercise program so that their cardiovascular functioning could be assessed (Rodeheffer et al., 1984). The researchers conducting this study observed and concluded that when older adults began to exercise their heart rate did not respond as well, a greater end-systolic volume existed, and heart contractility declined. However, as these older adults continued to exercise, the end-diastolic volume increased, producing greater stroke volume and ending with an unchanged cardiac output. Other research has shown similar conclusions with exercise including decreased heart rate and contractility, decreased peak heart rate and ejection fraction, decreased end-systolic volume, increased end-diastolic volume, and preserved stroke volume, further supporting the findings of increased left ventricle end-diastolic volume and maintained cardiac output during exercise (Fleg et al., 1995; Kane et al., 1999; Lakatta, 1993a, 1999a; Roffe, 1998; Wei, 1992). Exercise also increases vascular resistance and elevates both systolic and diastolic pressure (Lind & McNicol, 1986). Salmasi and colleagues (2003) conducted a research study involving 55 patients less than 50 years of age and 45 patients greater than 50 years of age, and evaluated them for left ventricle diastolic function at rest and during isometric exercise. These researchers concluded that degeneration in left ventricle diastolic functioning occurred in the 50-year and older group, both at rest and during isometric exercise, due to ventricle stiffening leading to decreased diastolic filling initially (Salmasi et al., 2003). Conclusions on cardiovascular change with exercise must be evaluated carefully in order to discern age-associated alterations across time and across individuals (**Table 6-2**).

Although structural and functional changes occur in the cardiovascular system with age, some changes remain variable across time and across individuals. Some research studies comparing cardiovascular function across different age cohorts do not take into account nutrition practices, exercise regimens or lack thereof, and other effects such as the lifestyle of older adults across time and space compared to younger individuals (Lakatta, 1999b). For example, older adults today often will say they grew up on a farm with large meals and a lack of concern for fat content; however, younger individuals today are very health conscious with tremendous focus on fat and calories. Nutrition and exercise habits as well as other health-related practices continually change over time, which brings up the question of how comparable younger individuals are to older individuals in terms of cardiovascular functioning (McReynolds & Rossen, 2004).

THE RESPIRATORY SYSTEM

The respiratory system refers to the parts of the body involved in breathing. This system works in close collaboration with the cardiovascular system

TABLE 6-2 Lifestyle Interventions to Maintain or Improve Physiological Functioning in Aging

Physical activity	1. Do some type of exercise at least 30 minutes a day and more involved exercise 3–5 days per week. 2. Include cardio training, weight-bearing exercise, resistance, balance training, and flexibility exercise.
Nutrition	1. Low calorie diet 2. Low fat diet 3. Low cholesterol diet 4. Low sodium diet 5. At least five fruits and vegetables per day 6. Plenty of whole grains 7. Eight glasses of water a day
Vitamins and minerals	1. Vitamins: B_6, B_{12}, D, K, A, C, E, beta carotene, and folic acid 2. Minerals: selenium, calcium, and iron
Examples of self-report assessment measures of physical activity and nutrition status	1. The Physical Activity Scale for the Elderly (PASE) (Washburn et al., 1993) 2. Nutritional Risk Index (Wolinsky et al., 1990) 3. The DETERMINE Screen (Nutrition Screening Initiative, 1992)
Prevalence rates of weight, dietary intake, and physical activity in individuals age 65 and over	1. Obese: Men—27%, Women—32% Age 65–74: Men—32%, Women—39% Age 75 and over: Men—18%, Women—24% Overweight: Men—73%, Women—66% Underweight: Men—1%, Women—3% 2. Diet (Healthy Eating Index): 19% good diet, 67% needed improvement, 14% poor diet *low score on daily fruit and dairy servings *high score on variety of food and cholesterol intake 3. Nonstrenuous physical activity: 21% total for 65 and over; Regular strenuous physical activity: Age 65–74: 26% Age 75–84: 18% Age 85 and over: 9%

SOURCE: Drewnowski & Evans, 2001; Federal Interagency Forum on Aging-Related Statistics, 2004; McReynolds & Rossen, 2004; Topp et al., 2004.

to provide the body with a continuous supply of oxygen necessary to produce energy and to eliminate unwanted carbon dioxide. This gaseous exchange is vital to life and, hence, proper functioning of the respiratory system and its constituent parts is critical to human survival.

Structure and Function of the Respiratory System

The respiratory system is composed of the mouth, nose, pharynx, trachea (or windpipe), and lungs, as well as the diaphragm and rib muscles. During respiration (**Figure 6-4a**), oxygen first passes through the mouth and nasal passages, where it is filtered of any large contaminants. It then enters the **pharynx**, where it absorbs water vapor and is warmed. The oxygen then flows through the trachea, a tube extending into the chest cavity, and into two smaller tubes called the bronchi, each of which splits into tubes called the bronchioles. Oxygen flows through the bronchi into the bronchioles and then into the lungs through many smaller tubes called alveolar ducts. From the alveolar ducts, oxygen travels into tiny, spongy air sacs called **alveoli** (**Figure 6-4b**), of which there are approximately 600 million in the average, healthy adult lung (Krauss Whitbourne, 2002). The alveoli are the functional units of the lungs and the site of gas exchange. Once in the alveoli, oxygen is diffused through the capillaries into the blood. The blood then carries the oxygen to the cells of the body. Carbon dioxide exits the body through the same, albeit reverse, pathway through which oxygen entered.

FIGURE **6-4a** **The respiratory system.**

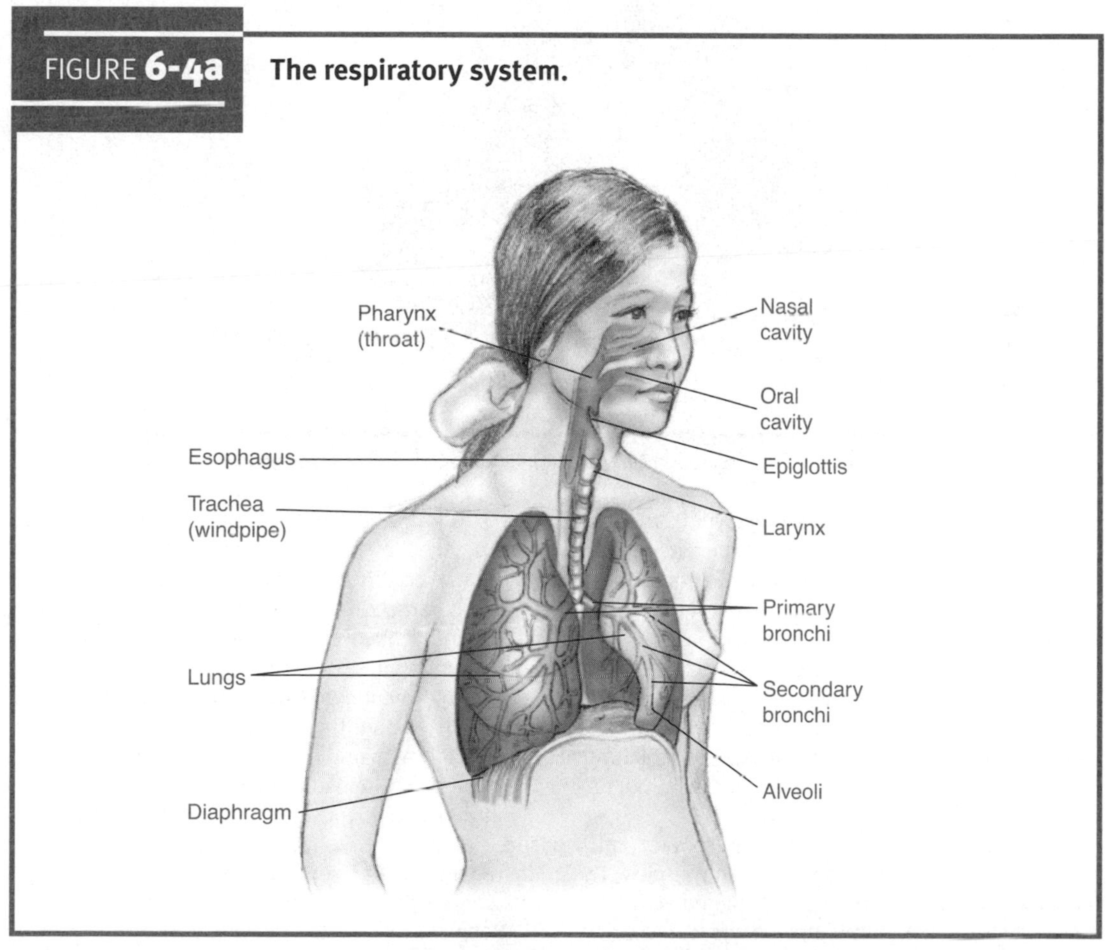

SOURCE: Anatomy and Physiology: Understanding the Human Body, Robert E. Clark, Jones and Bartlett Publishers 2005.

FIGURE 6-4b Alveolar structure.

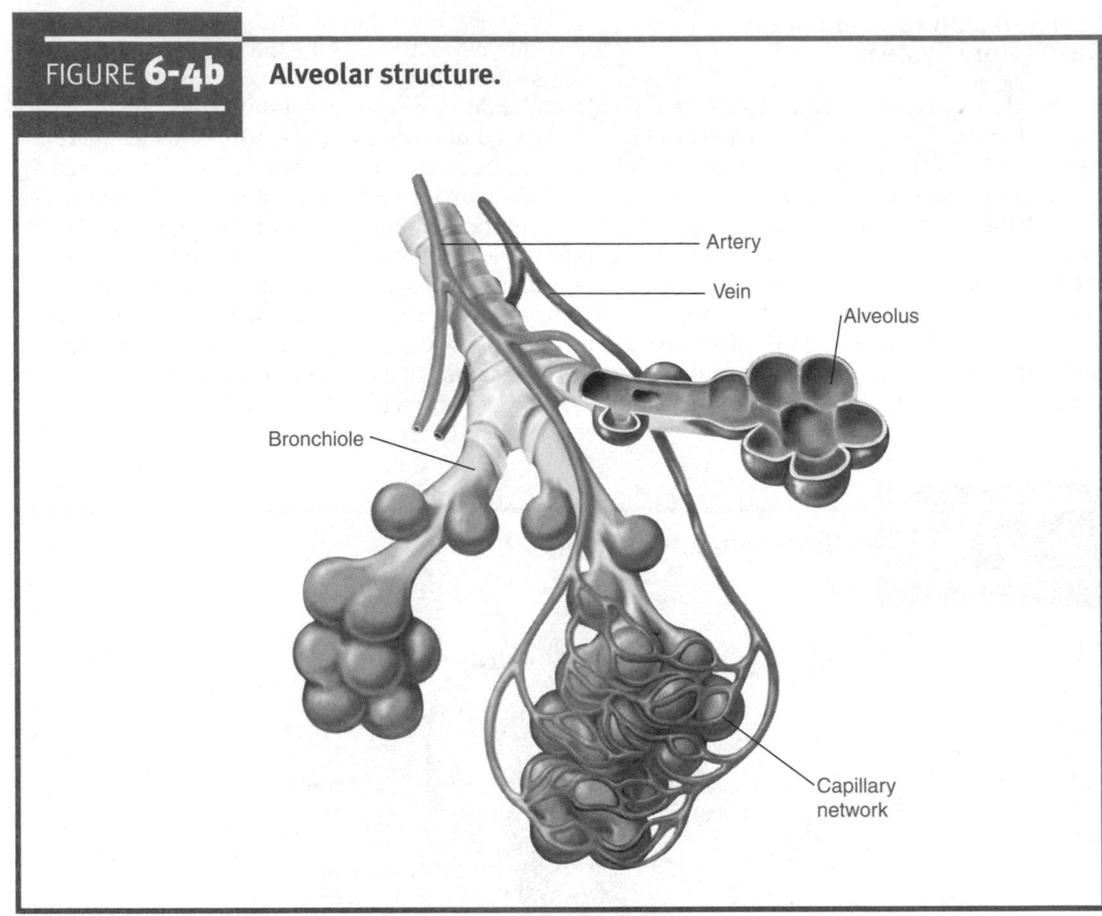

SOURCE: Anatomy and Physiology: Understanding the Human Body, Robert E. Clark, Jones and Bartlett Publishers 2005.

The lungs, more specifically the alveoli, are composed of elastic tissue that allows them to expand and recoil during inhalation and exhalation, respectively. The more the alveoli can expand and recoil, the more oxygen they can bring in and the more carbon dioxide they can expel. The alveoli also secrete a substance known as surfactant, which reduces the surface tension within the lungs. This reduction in surface tension helps to keep the lungs from collapsing after each breath. Hence, surfactant aids in maintaining lung stability.

Respiration is highly controlled by respiratory muscles, including the diaphragm and rib muscles. The **diaphragm** is a sheet of muscles located across the bottom of the chest. Respiration occurs with contraction and relaxation of the diaphragm and the rib muscles. To allow for the intake of oxygen, the rib muscles contract and push the ribs up and out while the diaphragm contracts and is pulled downward. These muscle contractions increase the volume of the chest cavity and reduce pressure within the cavity. The change in volume and pressure allows oxygen to be sucked into the lungs. Expansion of the lung during inhalation expands the elastic tissue. Upon relaxation of the diaphragm and rib muscles, the lung tissue and the ribs relax. Supplementing the relaxation of the diaphragm and rib muscles is the recoil of the lung tissue. Consequently, the volume of the chest cavity decreases while its pressure increases and carbon dioxide is forced out of the lungs.

Respiratory function is measured in terms of both lung volumes and lung capacities. The names

TABLE **6-3** **Respiratory Volumes and Capacities**

Volumes	Definition	Age-Related
Tidal volume (TV)	Amount of air inspired and expired during a normal breath	Decrease
Inspiratory reserve volume (IRV)	Amount of air that can be inspired after maximum inspiration	Decrease
Expiratory reserve volume (ERV)	Amount of air that can be expired after maximum expiration	Decrease
Residual volume (RV)	Amount of air remaining in the lungs following maximum expiration	Increase
Forced expiratory volume (FEV)	Amount of air that can be forcefully expelled in 1 second	Decrease
Capacity	**Definition**	**Age-Related**
Total lung capacity (TLC)	Maximum capacity to which the lungs can expand during maximum inspiratory effort	No change
Vital capacity (VC)	Amount of air that can be expelled following maximum inspiration	Decrease
Inspiratory capacity (IC) (IC 5 TV1 IRV)	Maximum amount of air that can be inspired after reaching the end of a normal expiration	Decrease
Functional residual capacity (FRC)	Amount of air remaining in the lungs following a normal expiration	Increase

SOURCE: Author.

and definitions of these various measurements are presented in **Table 6-3** and **Figure 6-5**. This table and this figure should be referred to throughout the following discussion of age-related changes in the respiratory system.

Aging of the Respiratory System

Alveoli

As a person ages, the alveoli of the lungs become flatter and shallower, and there is a decrease in the amount of tissue dividing individual alveoli. In addition, there is a decrease in the alveolar surface area. A person 30 years of age has an alveolar surface area of approximately 75 square meters. This surface area decreases by 4% per decade thereafter to around 60 square meters by age 70 years (Carpo & Campbell, 1998). The volume of blood distributed to pulmonary circulation declines with age due to a decreasing number of capillaries per alveolus (Meyer, 2005; Nitzan et al., 1994). Because gas exchange occurs over the surface of the alveoli, the age-related reduction in alveolar surface area as well as the reduced number of capillaries per alveolus impairs efficient passage of oxygen from the alveoli to the blood (De Martinis & Timiras, 2003; Meyer, 2005).

Lung Elasticity

With age there is a decrease in the lungs' elasticity, which in turn causes a change in the **elastic recoil** properties of the lungs. During expiration, elastic recoil helps to keep the lungs open until all

FIGURE **6-5** **Measuring lung capacity.**

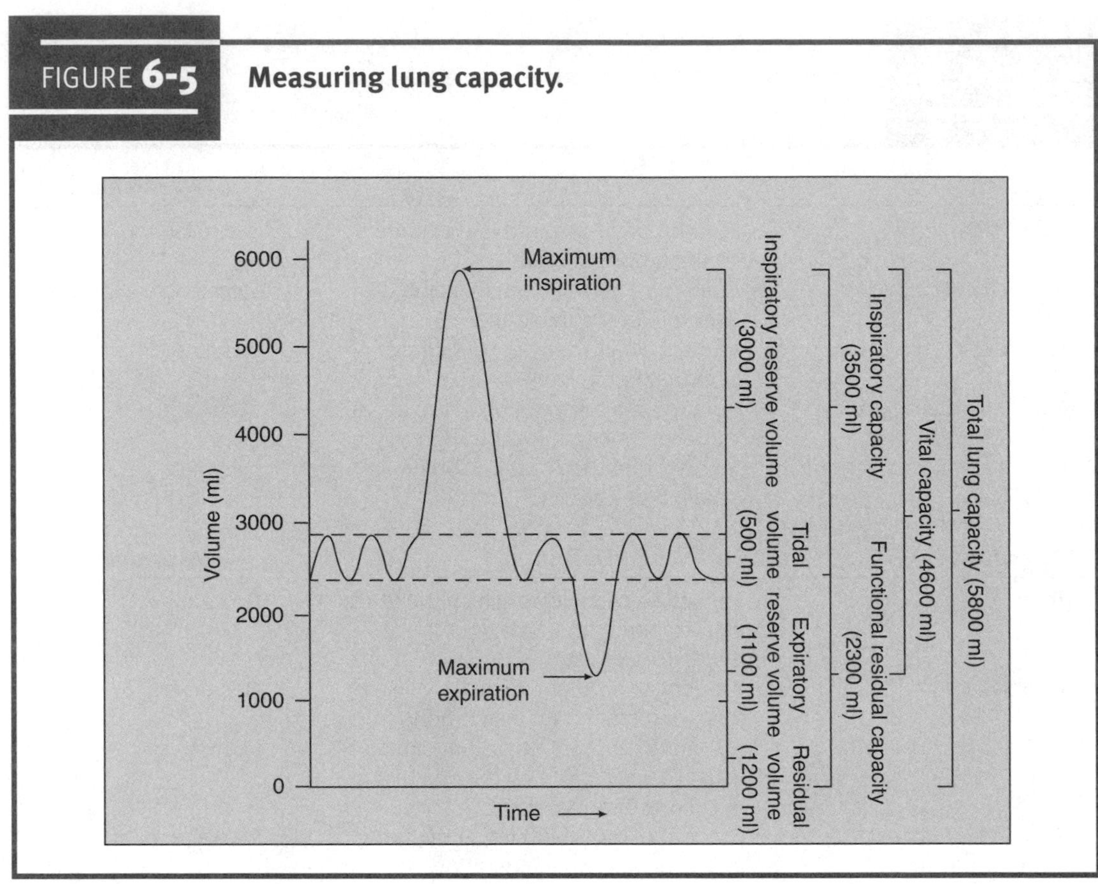

SOURCE: Reprinted from Human physiology: Foundations & frontiers (2nd ed.), D. Moffett, S. Moffett, & C. L. Schauff, pg. 458, 1993, with permission from Elsevier.

air is expelled and the lungs are forced to collapse due to the action of the respiratory muscles. Loss of elastic recoil causes the lungs to close prematurely, trapping air inside and preventing the lungs from emptying completely. As a result, unexpired air remains in the lungs and, consequently, during the next inhalation less air can be inspired (Krauss Whitbourne, 2002). Despite the reduced inspiratory capacity, **total lung capacity**—the maximum volume to which the lungs can expand during greatest inspiratory effort—remains virtually unchanged with age. After adjustment for age-related decreases in height, total lung capacity of both men and women decreases by less than 10% between the ages of 20 and 60 years (De Martinis & Timiras, 2003).

Changes in lung elasticity can decrease the efficiency of oxygen delivery. Due to the effects of gravity, more blood flows through the lower than the upper portion of the lungs. However, because of the reduced ability of the aging lungs to expand during inhalation, less air reaches the lower portion of the lungs. Air is more likely to flow through the upper portion of the lungs; yet, it is the lower lung that has a greater capillary network and blood supply for oxygen delivery. Thus, the decrease of air flow through the lower lung results in less efficient delivery of oxygen to the body. Consequently, as individuals age they must breathe in more air in order to achieve the same amount of gas exchange, a task that is difficult to accomplish with a loss of lung elasticity. This same upper–lower lung disparity is seen in young people. However, because of their greater lung elasticity, younger individuals are better able to compensate for the disparity by bringing more air into the lungs (Krauss Whitbourne, 2002).

The Chest Wall

The chest wall becomes stiffer with advancing age, decreasing the ease with which the thoracic cavity can expand. The increase in stiffness is largely due to a loss of rib elasticity as well as age-related calcification of the cartilage that attaches the ribs to the breastbone. The stiffness of the chest reduces its ability to expand during inhalation and contract during exhalation. Age related vertebral kyphosis, arthritis of the costavertebral joints, as well as the increased rigidity of the thoracic cavity lead to increased anteroposterior diameter, which results in flattening of the diaphragm (El Solh & Ramadan, 2006). Older persons rely heavily on the diaphragm for expansion and contraction of the chest cavity when they breathe (Digiovanna, 1994). However, the diaphragm may weaken by up to 25% (Beers & Berkow, 2000) with age. This weakening, combined with an age-associated loss of overall muscle mass, reduces the contractual abilities of the diaphragm, limiting respiration.

Changes in Respiratory Measures

As a result of the age-related changes in lung tissue and the chest wall, the respiratory system of older adults is less able to provide sufficient gas exchange to meet the body's demand for oxygen, particularly at times of maximum physical exertion (Arking, 1998). This insufficiency is demonstrated by age-related changes in respiratory measures (Table 6-3).

Research has shown that **vital capacity**—the maximum amount of air that can be expelled following a maximum inspiration—decreases with advancing age. Between the ages of 20 and 70 years, vital capacity is reduced by approximately 40% (Krauss Whitbourne, 2002), and in some cases vital capacity in the seventh decade may decrease to almost 75% of its value at 17 years of age (De Martinis & Timiras, 2003). Residual volume, however, increases nearly 50% with age (De Martinis & Timiras, 2003). This increase, in combination with reduced vital capacity, leads to a reduction in the amount of air that can be inspired. In addition, any fresh air that is inhaled is mixed with stale, residual air. This mixing, together with diminished inhalation, contributes to the lungs' reduced ability to deliver sufficient oxygen to the body (Krauss Whitbourne, 2002).

Residual volume is inversely related to **forced expiratory volume (FEV)**, the amount of air that can be forcefully expelled in 1 second. As residual volume increases, FEV decreases. Thus, evidence supporting a marked decrease in FEV with age is congruent with the age-related increase in residual volume (Arking, 1998, Hollenberg, Yang, Haight, & Tager, 2006).

Another respiratory measure known to change with age is the **ventilatory rate**, or the minute respiratory rate. Ventilatory rate is defined as the volume of air inspired in a normal breath (i.e., tidal volume) multiplied by the frequency of breaths per minute. At low levels of exertion, age does not appear to have any effect on ventilatory rate. However, at maximal exertion levels the ventilatory rate shows an age-related decline. Young adult males have a maximum capacity for inspiration of about 125 to 170 liters of air per minute, but this rate can be sustained for only approximately 15 seconds. A ventilatory rate of 100 to 120 liters of air per minute can be maintained for prolonged periods of time. However, by the age of 85 years, the ventilatory rate has decreased to approximately 75 liters per minute (Arking, 1998).

Age-Related Pathologies of the Respiratory System

The proportion of deaths due to respiratory disease is at its highest, approximately 30%, in the first year of life. By late adolescence and early adulthood only about 5% of deaths are attributed to respiratory disease. However, from the fifth decade of life on, there is a steady increase in the incidence of respiratory disease, and among persons over 85 years of age, respiratory disease accounts for 25% of all deaths (De Martinis & Timiras, 2003). Two of the most prevalent respiratory diseases among older adults are chronic obstructive pulmonary disease (COPD) and pneumonia.

Chronic Obstructive Pulmonary Disease (COPD)

COPD is characterized by limited airflow and impaired gas exchange. COPD encompasses chronic bronchitis, chronic obstructive bronchitis, and emphysema, or a combination of these disorders (Barnes, 2000). The pathology of COPD is characterized by a decreased ability of the lungs to respire properly. Environmental irritants such as cigarette smoke promote the production of excessive amounts of mucus within the airways. As this mucus builds up, the airways become restricted. The result is inefficient respiration in which excessive air accumulates in the alveoli, causing them to remain perpetually inflated. This constant inflation damages the alveolar walls, and the body repairs this damage by replacing the normally elastic tissue with fibrous tissues that are much less permeable to gas exchange. In addition, the fibrous tissue decreases elastic recoil, further contributing to inefficient and difficult respiration (Arking, 1998). Individuals with COPD often experience excessive cardiac workload as the heart tries to compensate for impaired airflow by pumping more blood to the lungs (Arking, 1998).

Pneumonia

Pneumonia is characterized by lung inflammation generally brought on by infection. The impaired immune response with age (see "The Immune System" later in this chapter) is thought to play a significant role in the high prevalence of pneumonia seen among elderly persons. Older individuals are more susceptible to severe pneumonia and complications of pneumonia than are younger persons. In addition, mortality from pneumonia is known to be significantly higher in those age 60 years or older (Naughton, Mylotte, & Tayara, 2000).

THE GASTROINTESTINAL SYSTEM

Aging in Key Components of the Gastrointestinal Tract

Overall, the gastrointestinal system (**Figure 6-6**) appears to be relatively preserved in aging with only minor changes. The two gastrointestinal areas most affected by age are the upper tract (the pharynx and **esophagus**) and the **colon**, also referred to as the large intestine (Hall, 2002). Changes in the gastrointestinal system can have multiple and varied effects, including effects upon consumption and absorption of nutrients and waste secretion. In this section, age-related changes of the gastrointestinal system, from the mouth to the large intestine and the accompanying glands and organs, will be evaluated.

The Mouth

The gastrointestinal system begins at the mouth, which shows some signs of age-related changes that affect the ability to chew. Changes in taste also occur, as described in this chapter's "The Nervous System" section. The mouth is utilized for mastication, or chewing. It is responsible for moistening food with saliva. The chewing and moistening of food allows for easier passage of the processed content to the pharynx and esophagus (Arking, 1998; Hall & Wiley, 1999).

Dental decay and tooth loss affect many older individuals today, making it more difficult to chew and prepare food to be swallowed (Hall & Wiley, 1999). Age-related changes in teeth cause them to be less sensitive and more brittle (Devlin & Ferguson, 1998). However, in the near future tooth decay and loss may decline due to increased health awareness, improved dentistry practices, and higher availability of fluoride toothpaste and floss that were not available when today's generation of older adults was maturing.

With age, there is atrophy of those muscles and bones of the jaw and mouth that control mastication. Consequently, it is more difficult for older adults to chew their food (Devlin & Ferguson, 1998; Digiovanna, 2000; Karlsson, Persson, & Carlsson, 1991; Newton, Yemm, Abel, & Menhinick, 1993). Along with changes in the skeletal muscle, changes occur in the nerves that innervate the oral region. As a result, there is some change in the ability of the nerves and muscles to coordinate functioning (Digiovanna, 2000). Refer to "The Muscle" later in this chapter for additional information regarding aging changes in skeletal muscle.

Saliva produced and secreted by salivary glands and the oral mucosa assists in removing food from teeth, neutralizing acid, replacing minerals in enamel, inhibiting bacteria and fungi growth, and breaking down starch molecules (Devlin & Ferguson, 1998; Digiovanna, 2000). Salivary flow is controlled by the autonomic nervous system and is influenced by food touching the mouth, by jaw

FIGURE 6-6 **The gastrointestinal system.**

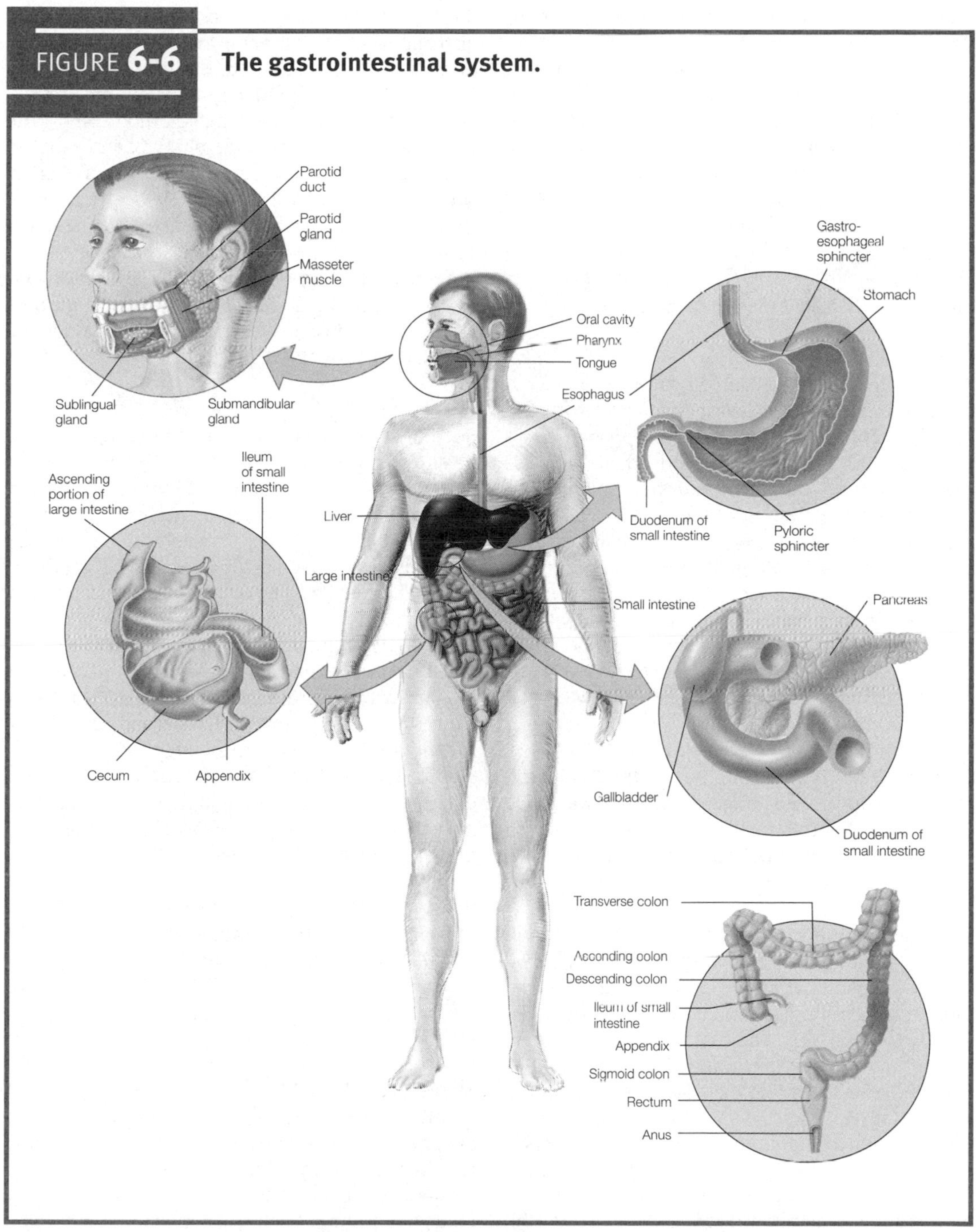

SOURCE: Human Biology, 5e. Daniel D. Chiras, Jones and Bartlett Publishers 2005.

movement, and by olfaction and gustation input (Bourdiol, Mioche, & Monier, 2004; Digiovanna, 2000). Although almost 40% of older adults complain of dry mouth, salivary gland function remains stable with age due to the large secretory reserve in the main salivary glands (Bourdiol et al., 2004; Devlin & Ferguson, 1998; Ghezzi & Ship, 2003; Tepper & Katz, 1998). Dry mouth can be attributed to prescription and over-the-counter medications, nutritional deficiencies, disease, and treatment therapies such as chemotherapy (Devlin & Ferguson, 1998; Ghezzi & Ship; Ship, 2003; Pillemer, & Baum, 2002).

The Esophagus

A study in 1964 showing impaired esophageal motility function in older individuals led to the development of the term *presbyesophagus*; however, the study included many individuals with diseases such as diabetes and neuropathy that confounded the findings (Soergel, Zboralske, & Amber, 1964). Studies have since demonstrated preservation of esophageal functioning in aging until around age 80, when some changes occur. These changes include decline in upper esophageal sphincter pressure, increased time for the upper esophageal sphincter to relax, and decreased intensity of esophageal contractions, potentially caused by loss of muscle abilities and nerve innervations (Fulp, Dalton, Castell, & Castell, 1990; Hall & Wiley, 1999; Orr & Chen, 2002; Schroeder & Richter, 1994). The lower esophageal sphincter was once thought to demonstrate age-related declines in contractions and impaired relaxation; however, recent work has shown that no real changes occur to the lower sphincter (Hall & Wiley, 1999).

Swallowing is controlled by the brain through cortical input to the medulla oblongata swallowing centers, which have nerve endings in the skeletal muscle controlling the pharynx and esophagus (Hall & Wiley, 1999). The esophagus also contains smooth muscle that is controlled by nerve endings from the intestines and by the vagus nerve in the brain (Hall & Wiley, 1999). Rao and colleagues (2003) conducted a study evaluating sensory and mechanical changes in both skeletal and smooth muscle located in the esophagus, and found that older adults demonstrated stiffening of the esophageal wall and less sensitivity to discomfort and pain in the esophagus. These changes affect the older patient's ability to swallow. The gag reflex also appears to be absent in around 40% of healthy older adults (Davies, Kidd, Stone, & MacMahon, 1995). Dysphagia (difficulty swallowing), reflux, heartburn, and chest pain are common complaints that relate to changes in the pharynx and esophagus. Approximately 35% of older individuals report such complaints (Hall & Wiley, 1999; Orr & Chen, 2002; Reinus & Brandt, 1998; Shaker, Dua, & Koch, 1998). Although frequency of reflux episodes does not appear to vary with age, the duration of gastroesophageal episodes appears to be more prolonged in older adults (Ferriolli, Oliveira, Matsuda, Braga, & Dantos, 1998).

The Stomach

Several studies have determined that age-related declines in peristaltic contractions and stomach emptying do not appear to be clinically significant (Brogna, Ferrara, Bucceri, Lanteri, & Catalano, 1999; O'Mahony, O'Leary, & Quigley, 2002). A study by Madsen and Graff (2004) assessing gastrointestinal motility in aging concluded that no changes in gastric emptying occurred with age. Furthermore, enteric nerves or nerves innervating the intestinal system that control gastric motility do not change with age (Madsen & Graff, 2004). Other studies have shown that peristalsis and gastric contractile force are mildly reduced in the elderly and that the reduction reaches significance in less active elderly subjects rather than in those who maintain an active lifestyle (O'Donovan et al., 2005; Shimamoto, Hirata, & Hiraike, 2002). Gastric acid secretions do not appear to change with age, but pepsin, bicarbonate, and sodium ion secretions and prostaglandin content do show age-related decline (Hall & Wiley, 1999). These secretion changes cause a decline in gastric defense mechanisms and create an increased potential for mucosal injury in the stomach (Hall & Wiley, 1999).

The Small Intestine

Small intestine motility needed for digestion and absorption of nutrients has been reported to show no change or only minor changes in contraction intensity with age (Brogna et al., 1999; O'Mahony et al., 2002; Orr & Chen, 2002; Shaker et al., 1998). Madsen and Graff (2004) also discovered no age-related change in small intestine transit rate (the time needed for digested material to move through the length of the small intestine). This finding supports results from other studies. The endocrine and nervous system aid in motility functioning in the intestines, and any changes in these specific systems could potentially cause changes in intestinal abilities (Shaker et al., 1998). However, no clinically significant motility changes appear to occur in the small intestine with age.

A common consequence of prolonged gastric emptying is a decrease in gastric acid secretion in approximately 32% of elderly people (Saffrey, 2004). This decreased acid production along with motility disturbances in the small intestine can lead to bacterial overgrowth in the small intestine, a common clinical finding in the older population, causing malabsorption and malnutrition (Madsen & Graff, 2004; O'Mahony et al., 2002; Orr & Chen, 2002; Salles, 2007). Absorption of nutrients does not change with age. Changes in vitamin absorption are seen with particular vitamins but not others (Hall & Wiley, 1999). For instance, vitamin A absorption increases in older adults whereas vitamin D, zinc, and calcium absorption decreases. Absorption of vitamins B_1, B_{12}, C, and iron does not change with age (Baik & Russell, 1999; Hall & Wiley, 1999; Simon, Leboff, Wright, & Glowacki, 2002; Tepper & Katz, 1998).

The Large Intestine

The large intestine, also referred to as the colon, measures approximately 5 feet long when stretched out and covers the area from the small intestine to the anus (Digiovanna, 2000). In aging, a loss of enteric, or intestinal, neurons and nerve connections to the smooth muscle in the colon occurs (Gomes, deSouza, & Liberti, 1997; Shaker et al., 1998). Madsen and Graff (2004) concluded that older adults experience longer colonic transit time (the amount of time needed for fluid and excrement to travel the length of the colon). This change again relates to age-related loss of neurons and receptors in the enteric nervous system. Increased colonic transit time also correlates with increased fibrosis in the colon (Hall, 2002). Colonic pressure in the intra-lumen also increases with age, but can be lowered with fiber supplementation (Hall, 2002).

The rectum, a colonic structure that is located before the anus, shows an age-related increase in fibrous tissue. This increase reduces the rectum's ability to stretch as feces pass through (Digiovanna, 2000). In the anus, the external anal sphincter shows an age-related decrease in motor neurons responsible for sphincter control. This sphincter also thins with age. However, the internal anal sphincter thickens with age, possibly as a compensatory mechanism. Nonetheless, it shows a decline in contractile abilities (Digiovanna, 2000; Nielson & Pedersen, 1996; O'Mahony et al., 2002; Rociu, Stoker, Eijkemans, & Lameris, 2000). Aging women experience a greater risk of anal sphincter changes due to laxity of the pelvic floor, decreased pressure in the rectum, and even menopause (Hall, 2002).

Aging in Accessory Glands and Organs

As people age, relatively no changes occur in the secretions of the liver, pancreas, and gallbladder (Hall, 2002). However, these accessory glands and organs, which work in close association with the gastrointestinal system, remain crucial for intestinal stability.

The Liver

The **liver** is the largest gland in the body and contributes to the conversion of food by secreting bile into the small intestine and by screening blood from the stomach and small intestine for toxic substances, excess nutrients, and ammonia (Digiovanna, 2000). With age, the liver's size as well as its blood flow and perfusion can decrease by 30% to 40%. In addition, hepatocytes, or liver cells, can undergo structural alterations. However, due to the liver's large reserve capacity and the hepatocytes' ability to regenerate after damage, no functional changes result from the changes in structure (Digiovanna, 2000; Hall & Wiley, 1999; James, 1998; Marchesini et al., 1988; Schmucker, 1998; Wynne et al., 1989). Decreased drug clearance in the older population can occur due to the declines in liver size and blood flow as well as age-related changes in the kidneys, but this is highly variable among individuals (James, 1998; Le Couteur & McLean, 1998; McLean & Le Couteur, 2004).

The Gallbladder

The **gallbladder** is a small sac located below the liver that stores the bile sent from the liver. Bile is stored until the gallbladder receives intestinal and pancreatic signaling via the hormone cholecystokinin. This signaling indicates a readiness for digestion and, in response, bile is released into the ducts of the small intestine (Digiovanna, 2000; MacIntosh et al., 2001). Refer to Figure 6-6 for the location and anatomical structure of the gallbladder. With age, no overall structural changes occur in the gallbladder with the exception of the bile ducts (Digiovanna, 2000). However, in older adults the gallbladder appears to demonstrate declines in emptying rates so that less bile is secreted when food is digested (Hall & Wiley, 1999). Increased bile volume in the gallbladder has been correlated with gallstones in older adults. This increase in bile volume is more common in older women than men (Bates, Harrison, Lowe, Lawson, & Padley, 1992; Hall & Wiley, 1999). The bile ducts tend to widen with age, allowing potential gallstones to pass through more easily; however, the duct near the opening of the small intestine becomes narrower, trapping the gallstones and leading to abnormal changes (Digiovanna, 2000).

The Pancreas

The **pancreas** is a gland located below the stomach and above the small intestine. Refer to Figure 6-6 for pancreatic location and structure. The pancreas secretes pancreatic fluid that neutralizes stomach acid and accelerates the transport of large nutrients into ducts that eventually converge with the bile duct leading into the small intestine (Digiovanna, 2000; Hall & Wiley, 1999). The pancreas decreases in weight with age and shows some histological changes such as fibrosis and cell atrophy (Hall & Wiley, 1999). However, due to the large reserve capacity of the pancreas, the small changes that occur, including changes in the enzymes that aid in stomach acid neutralization and nutrient breakdown, do not affect overall pancreatic function as a person ages (Digiovanna, 2000; Hall & Wiley, 1999).

Gastrointestinal Immunity

The gastrointestinal tract, with a mucosal lining containing immunological properties, is the largest organ (Hall & Wiley, 1999). The immune response in the gastrointestinal system depends on the congruent work of lymphoid and epithelial cells (Schmucker, Thoreux, & Owen, 2001). Secretion of antibodies into the intestinal mucosa works to neutralize toxins, block bacteria from adhering to surfaces, and block antigens from crossing the mucosa (Holt, 1992; Schmucker et al., 2001). Research has suggested a decline in immunological function in the aging gastrointestinal system. This decline can increase rates of infections that occur via the gastrointestinal system. Infection may, in turn, lead to mortality and morbidity (Arranz, O'Mahony, Barton, & Ferguson, 1992; Schmucker, Heyworth, Owen, & Daniels, 1996; Schmucker, Owen, Outenreath, & Thoreux, 2003; Schmucker et al., 2001). A decline in **gastrointestinal immunity** can be attributed to a change in lymphoid cells or epithelial cells, or possibly both cell types (Schmucker et al., 2001).

Although relatively few changes occur in the aging gastrointestinal system, changes that do occur increase the risk for diseases and disorders. Age-related changes, compounded by other influential factors such as comorbidity and medication use, place older individuals at increased risk for gallstones, constipation, fecal incontinence, and infection.

THE GENITOURINARY SYSTEM

Overview of the Genitourinary System

The genitourinary system (**Figure 6-7**) in both males and females contains the kidneys and associated renal arteries and veins, the **ureters**, the bladder, and the **urethra** running through the genitalia (Digiovanna, 2000; Lindeman, 1995). The urinary system provides many functions that help the body to maintain homeostasis, or balance of the organ systems. For instance, the urinary system: 1) removes wastes and toxins such as ammonia, uric acid, and some medications from the blood; 2) regulates osmotic pressure in the blood and interstitial fluid; 3) regulates concentration levels of calcium, sodium, potassium, magnesium, and phosphorus; 4) controls the acid–base balance by making necessary adjustments; 5) regulates blood pressure; 6) activates vitamin D in order to maintain calcium levels; and 7) regulates oxygen level through stimulation of erythropoietin, the hormone responsible for increased red blood cell production in the bone marrow (Digiovanna, 2000; Lye, 1998). The kidneys form urine through a process of filtration, reabsorption, and secretion with constant homeostasis maintained throughout the process (Digiovanna, 2000). Under usual living conditions the kidneys can be maintained

FIGURE 6-7 The genitourinary system.

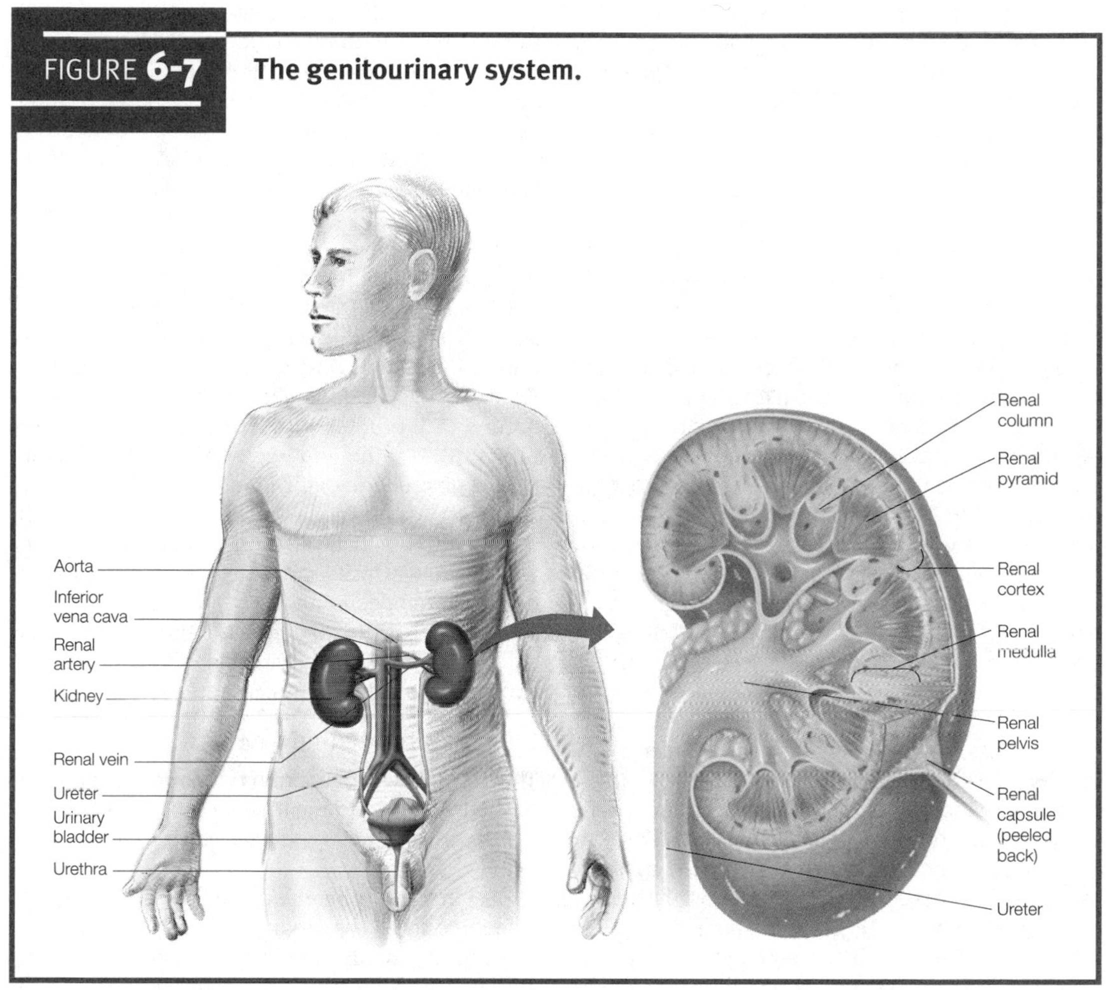

SOURCE: Human Biology, 5e. Daniel D. Chiras, Jones and Bartlett Publishers 2005.

on as little as 30% capacity, but under stressful conditions such as high temperatures kidney reserves are needed to maintain proper functioning (Digiovanna, 2000). In this section, aging structural and functional changes in the urinary system will be evaluated. For age-related changes in genitalia, refer to the section "The Reproductive System."

Urinary Structural Changes with Age

The Kidneys

With age, the kidneys shrink in length and weight. At 30 years of age, the average kidney weighs 150 to 200 g. By age 90, weight has declined to between 110 and 150 g (Beck, 1998, 1999a; Jassal, Fillit, & Oreopoulos, 1998; Lindeman, 1995; Minaker, 2004). The number of **glomeruli** decreases by as much as 30% to 40% by age 90 due to glomerulosclerosis. Remaining glomeruli decrease in size but increase in basement membrane thickness (Beck, 1999a; Lindeman; Musso, Ghezzi, & Ferraris, 2004). The size and number of **nephrons**, the combination of the Bowman's capsule and renal tubule with the glomerulus, also decrease with age (Jassal & Oreopoulos, 1998; Jassal et al., 1998; Minaker, 2004). On average, renal blood flow declines 10% per decade beginning as early as

20 years of age. Young adults (20 years) average a renal blood flow of 600 ml/min whereas average blood flow in older adults (80 years) averages only 300 ml/min (Beck, 1999a; Digiovanna, 2000; Jassal et al., 1998; Lindeman, 1995; Minaker, 2004). Furthermore, blood flow declines with age due to changes in the arteries and capillaries in the kidneys (Digiovanna, 2000; Jassal et al., 1998; McLean & Le Couteur, 2004). Renal blood flow in the cortical section of the kidneys declines at a much quicker rate compared to the average renal blood flow rate. This indicates that cortical nephrons are severely affected by age (Lindeman, 1995). Changes in blood flow and **glomerular filtration rate (GFR)** account for a majority of functional disability in the kidneys with age. With disease and some medications, blood flow and GFR can be further compromised (Beck, 1999a; Digiovanna, 2000; Lindeman, 1995). The GFR variably declines with age. This decline is measured by creatinine or **insulin** clearance and usually begins in the third decade as a result of changes in glomeruli, clustering of capillaries, and renal blood flow rate (Digiovanna, 2000; Jassal et al., 1998; McLean & Le Couteur, 2004; Rowe, Andres, Tobin, Norris, & Shock, 1976). A decline in GFR becomes significant as people age because elimination of waste and toxins declines, causing an accumulation of harmful substances such as uric acid and medications in the body (Digiovanna, 2000; McLean & Le Couteur, 2004). Renal tubules also show age-related changes, including decreased number and length. There is also evidence of age-related interstitial fibrosis and thickening of renal tubule basement membranes. This can affect reabsorption and excretion (Beck, 1999a; Jassal & Oreopoulos, 1998; Jassal et al., 1998). Despite age-related structural changes, the kidneys contain a large reserve capacity, and functional abilities remain relatively stable unless stressed (Beck, 1999a; Jassal et al., 1998; Minaker, 2004).

The Bladder

The bladder is a hollow organ lined with a mucous membrane, contains smooth muscle including the **detrusor** muscle, and consists of two components, the bladder body and the base (Andersson & Arner, 2004; Kevorkian, 2004). With age, the bladder decreases in size and develops fibrous matter in the bladder wall, changing its overall stretching capacity and contractibility (Digiovanna, 2000). The filling capacity of the bladder also declines along with the ability to withhold voiding (Diokno, Brown, Brock, Herzog, & Normolle, 1988; Elbadawi, Diokno, & Millard, 1998; Resnick, Elbadawi, & Yalla, 1995). The ability of the detrusor to contract declines in both aging men and women, and there is an increase in incidence of detrusor overactivation (Diokno et al., 1988; Minaker, 2004; Resnick et al., 1995). However, other research has not shown any age-related changes in detrusor contractility, but has demonstrated that the detrusor in usual aging remains stable with unchanged contractility and no observable obstructions (Elbadawi, Yalla, & Resnick, 1993; Madersbacher et al., 1998). In around 50% of men with benign prostatic hyperplasia (BPH), the enlargement of the prostate causes obstruction of the bladder outlet and results in urinary dysfunction (Resnick et al., 1995). In response to bladder outlet obstruction, the bladder walls become thicker and stronger in order to recompense for declining function (Elbadawi et al., 1998). Overall, the bladder goes through few variable structural changes with age, but these changes can impact a person physically.

Ureters and the Urethra

The urinary system contains two ureters that connect each kidney to the bladder, but ureters do not demonstrate any age-specific changes (Digiovanna, 2000).

The urethra forms the canal that leads from the bladder out of the body, and also functions in response to excitatory or inhibitory stimuli (Andersson & Arner, 2004; Brading, Teramoto, Dass, & McCoy, 2001; Digiovanna, 2000). In the male, the sphincter elevates from the prostate encompassing the urethra (Strasser et al., 1996). In the female, the urethra extends about 3 to 4 cm. Males have longer urethras; this is due to the urethra's anatomical location in the penis (Digiovanna, 2000; Kevorkian, 2004). With age, the length of the urethra and the pressure needed to close off the urethra both decline in women (Elbadawi et al., 1998; Madersbacher et al., 1998; Resnick et al., 1995). Also, the urethra thins with age, and striated muscle that controls sphincters also thins and weakens (Digiovanna, 2000; Kevorkian, 2004). In men, the prostate gland surrounds the urethra directly below the bladder (see Figure 6-7), and prostate enlargement around the bladder and urethra can cause urinary dysfunction (Digiovanna, 2000; Hollander & Diokno, 1998; Resnick et al., 1995).

Urinary Functional Changes with Age

Urination

Urination involves both the central and peripheral nervous systems and requires that bladder contraction and urethral relaxation occur simultaneously (Andersson & Arner, 2004; Kevorkian, 2004). The amount of urine expelled from the body decreases with age correlating with increases of around 50–100 ml in postvoid residual (PVR) with age (Madersbacher et al., 1998; Minaker, 2004). Renal changes affect the ability to concentrate and dilute the urine, causing electrolyte imbalance (Jassal & Oreopoulos, 1998). Urine osmolality in the older adult only reaches about half of that in a younger adult, leading to increased water loss in the aged (Beck, 1999b). Older individuals also experience an increase in **nocturia** or an increased number of fluid voids occurring at night, which can disturb sleep patterns (Asplund, 2004; Kirkland, Lye, Levy, & Banerjee, 1983; Lubran, 1995; Muhlberg & Platt, 1999).

Prostate volume increases in aging males, and it is possible that, with longevity, every male will experience benign prostatic hyperplasia (BPH) (Madersbacher et al., 1998). BPH can lead to prostatic changes that influence lower urinary tract function as well as erectile and ejaculatory disorders (Hafez & Hafez, 2004; Hollander & Diokno, 1998, 1998; Paick, Meehan, Lee, Penson, & Wessells, 2005; Rosen et al., 2003). More specifically, in BPH the prostate enlarges enough to encroach on the urethra and bladder causing urinary retention, difficulty voiding, urinary tract infections, and, in advanced stages, renal failure (Hollander & Diokno, 1998; Resnick et al., 1995). Nerve stimulations to the smooth muscle of the prostate, bladder, and urethra occur in BPH, causing voiding difficulty. However, blocking the stimulus allows the muscle to relax, improving voiding abilities in BPH (Hollander & Diokno, 1998).

Glomerular Filtration Rate

The glomerular filtration rate (GFR), usually measured by creatinine clearance, declines in older individuals, but there is no resultant increase in blood creatinine concentration (Beck, 1999a; Minaker, 2004). Creatinine clearance is measured by the Cockcroft-Gault equation (1976):

$$\frac{140 - \text{age (years)} \times \text{IBW (ideal body weight) (kg)}}{72 \times \text{serum creatinine (mg/dl)}}$$

*Note: Multiply by 0.85 for females.

Measuring creatinine does not yield an accurate concentration rate because 1) the creatinine production rate is variable, 2) the tubules also secrete creatinine, and 3) elders have decreased muscle mass. Inaccuracy in measurement generally results in an overestimation of creatinine level of about 20% to 30% (Fliser et al., 1997; Lindeman, 1995; McLean & Le Couteur, 2004). The Cockcroft-Gault equation can be used to predict renal disease but may not reflect the usual aging process. As a result, use of the equation can lead to medication underdosing in healthy older adults and overdosing in compromised older adults (Fliser et al., 1997; Lubran, 1995; McLean & Le Couteur, 2004; Rule et al., 2004). A closer estimation of actual GFR comes from inulin clearance or non-radio-labeled iothalamate (Lubran, 1995; Muhlberg & Platt, 1999; Rule et al., 2004).

Adverse drug reactions occur approximately 3 to 10 times more often in the older population as compared to younger cohorts (Muhlberg & Platt, 1999). Adverse drug reactions in the older population occur as a result of changes in the kidneys, more specifically changes in GFR and renal clearance. Adverse drug reactions can also occur due to changes in tubular filtration (Abernathy, 1999; Muhlberg & Platt, 1999). Estimates of GFR among older adults correlate with aging tubular filtration and are often used to determine the amount of drug to use in the older population (Lindeman, 1990). The key phrase in geriatric pharmacy remains "start low and go slow" because of renal changes that affect pharmacokinetics and pharmacodynamics with age (Abernathy, 1999; Muhlberg & Platt, 1999). Furthermore, polypharmacy and medication compliance are also associated with increased adverse events in the older population (Abernathy, 1999).

Homeostasis Changes

Overall, the aging kidneys function relatively well in maintaining fluid levels and electrolyte concentration balance; however, age-related changes are more readily observed under conditions of stress such as dehydration and high temperatures (Arking, 1998; Minaker, 2004). Age-related structural changes in the kidneys lead to some functional declines such as deterioration in the ability to regulate sodium concentrations under usual conditions. In addition, there is a decline in the ability to maintain sodium and potassium homeostasis and to conserve water during times of stress (e.g., dehydration; Jassal & Oreopoulos, 1998; Minaker, 2004). The inability to properly regulate sodium can be attributed to malfunctioning of the ascending loop of Henle in addition to increases in prostaglandin levels and tubular unresponsiveness to aldosterone (Musso et al., 2004). A decline in overall potassium level in the body also occurs with age due to low potassium secretion resulting from the decline in tubular reaction to aldosterone (Jassal & Oreopoulos, 1998; Muhlberg & Platt, 1999; Musso et al, 2004). Older adults also experience changes in the ability to reabsorb water and, in conjunction with decreased thirst in older adults, the body can become dehydrated more quickly (Lye, 1998; Musso et al., 2004). Acid–base homeostasis appears to be relatively stable (pH 6.9 to 7.7) in older adults under usual conditions; however, under conditions of acid overload older adults cannot excrete acid as quickly as younger adults (Lindeman, 1998; Muhlberg & Platt, 1999; Sorribas et al., 1995). The nephron functionally serves the kidneys by balancing sodium and water and eliminating waste from the bloodstream (Arking, 1998). With age, nephrons shrink in size and decrease in number. This is partly due to decreased blood flow in the glomeruli, which causes an increase in solute levels and eventually renders the nephron nonfunctional (Arking, 1998; Jassal et al., 1998; Minaker, 2004). Changes in homeostasis can negatively impact both the structural and functional capacity of the renal system.

Hormone Changes

Plasma renin and **aldosterone** concentration levels gradually decline with age, beginning around 40 years of age (Muhlberg & Platt, 1999). With age, the renin-angiotensin system undergoes a decline in its ability to maintain salt levels following salt deprivation (Corman et al., 1995; Mimran, Ribstein, & Jover, 1992). In addition, the renin-angiotensin-aldosterone axis fails to adequately respond to hormone volume changes in healthy older adults without deprivation; therefore, maximum sodium levels cannot be attained (Beck, 1999a; Muhlberg & Platt, 1999). During normal renal functioning, antidiuretic hormone release is responsible for reabsorption of fluid in the tubules and production of a concentrated urine to maintain blood osmolarity. Studies concerning changes in the basal levels of antidiuretic hormone in the elderly have been inconclusive. Several studies, however, have indicated that changes in reabsorption are related to loss of responsiveness of antidiuretic hormone receptors in the tubules, leading to nocturnal polyuria with frequent nighttime voiding (Jassal & Oreopoulos, 1998; Johnson, Miller, Pillin, & Auslander, 2003; Musso, Liakopoulos, Ioannidis, Eleftheriadias, & Stefandis, 2006). Aging changes also occur in the calcium-parathormone-vitamin D_3 axis, as exhibited by decreased serum calcium levels, increased parathyroid hormone levels resulting from GFR decline, and declines in vitamin D metabolism by the aging kidneys (Chapuy, Durr, & Chapuy, 1983; Marcus, Masdirg, & Young, 1984; Massry et al., 1991; Muhlberg & Platt, 1999; Vieth, Ladak, & Walfish, 2003). Due to the decline in vitamin D metabolism by the kidneys, vitamin D supplementation is usually recommended in the older population (Vieth et al., 2003).

Age-related changes in the genitourinary system lead to alterations in genital structures, voiding behaviors, toxin and medication clearance, hormone levels, and overall physiological homeostasis of the body. Overall structural and functional changes can vary with age, but these changes can impact a person physically, emotionally, psychologically, and socially, especially when urinary function declines and becomes abnormal, as seen with incontinence. Although aging changes in the kidneys can vary among older adults, as seen with GFR, as a whole these changes are quite common and should be considered when evaluating and treating an older population.

THE REPRODUCTIVE SYSTEM

Female changes in the reproductive system are most notably associated with the onset of

menopause and subsequent declines in estrogen. Menopause and symptoms associated with menopause serve as the physical reminder of reproductive aging, but underlying neuroendocrine and ovarian changes occur years earlier (Randolph et al., 2004). Male changes in the reproductive system are mostly associated with androgen deficiency and physical syndromes such as impotency. However, changes in reproductive hormones affect not only the reproductive system, but also other physiological systems. This section will provide an overview of all of the changes associated with reproductive aging in both women and men. The reader should refer to **Figures 6-8** and **6-9** for illustrations of the female and male reproductive systems.

Female Reproductive Aging

Neuroendocrine Function

The **reproductive axis** refers to the integration of the hypothalamus, pituitary, and gonads (ovaries for women). The axis controls reproductive hormones and ovulatory cycles (Chakraborty & Gore, 2004; Hall, 2004). The hypothalamus releases **gonadotropin-releasing hormone (GnRH)**, which binds to corresponding gonadotrope receptors in the pituitary, stimulating the synthesis and release of **follicle-stimulating hormone (FSH)** and **luteinizing hormone (LH)** (Hall, 2004, 2007). FSH regulates ovarian follicle development and the conversion of androstenedione to estrogen. LH regulates ovulation, supports the corpus luteum, and helps synthesize androgens (Hall, 2004, 2007; Yialamas & Hayes, 2003). Reproductive function relies heavily on hormone signaling from the ovaries to the hypothalamus and pituitary, as demonstrated by FSH secretion in the development of mature oocytes (Hall, 2004, 2007). The menstrual cycle functions on a negative feedback system, but also relies on positive feedback with estrogen in order to produce the LH surge for ovulation (Hall, 2004, 2007). **Figure 6-10** demonstrates the menstruation cycle along with corresponding changes in ovarian hormone levels throughout the cycle.

Age-related changes in neuroendocrine function include a change in gonadotropin levels. This change occurs before ovarian age-related changes, implicating involvement of the hypothalamus. With age, FSH levels begin increasing before menopause occurs and continue to increase throughout and after menopause. Estradiol levels tend to increase right before and while transitioning into menopause and then drastically decrease during menopause (Joffe, Soares, & Cohen, 2003). **Inhibin B**, a glycoprotein synthesized in the ovaries that usually suppresses FSH, also decreases in older women, explaining the observed increase in FSH (Hansen et al., 2005; Klein et al., 1996; Santoro, Adel, & Skurnick, 1999). Age-related changes in circulating hormones (estrogen and progesterone) strongly affect hypothalamic and pituitary responses to positive and negative hormone feedback systems. Finally, age-related changes occur in estrogen and progestin receptors located in the brain. These changes occur independently of changes in circulating hormone levels in the body (Chakraborty & Gore, 2004; Gill, Sharpless, Rado, & Hall, 2002; Hall, Lavoie, Marsh, & Martin, 2000; Rossmanith, Handke-Vesel, Wirth, & Scherbaum, 1994).

Age-related decline in estrogen affects the brain, resulting in some cognitive changes, insomnia, or even depression. Estrogen decline also affects other areas of the body that contain estrogen receptors and estrogen-dependent tissue (Smith, 1998; Wise, Dubal, Wilson, Rau, & Bottner, 2001; Wise, Krajnak, & Kashon, 1996). For example, with decreased estrogen levels the skin contains less collagen and becomes thin, sweat and sebaceous glands become dry, hair follicles begin to dry, bones lose calcium and undergo increased bone resorption, breasts lose connective tissue but gain adipose tissue, lipoproteins increase, bladder function decreases, cardiovascular function and blood pressure change, and the absorption and metabolism of nutrients become less efficient (Smith, 1998; Wise et al., 1996). A majority of the emphasis concerning estrogen has been on neuroprotective effects, including delay of onset in Alzheimer's disease and Parkinson's disease as well as protection against nerve cell death and brain injury (Roof & Hall, 2000; Wise, Dubal, Wilson, Rau, & Bottner, 2001; Wise, Dubal, Wilson, Rau, & Liu, 2001).

Female System Changes

The Ovaries. With age, the ovaries atrophy to such a small size that they can become impalpable during an exam (Smith, 1998). The number of ovarian

FIGURE **6-8** **The female reproductive system.**

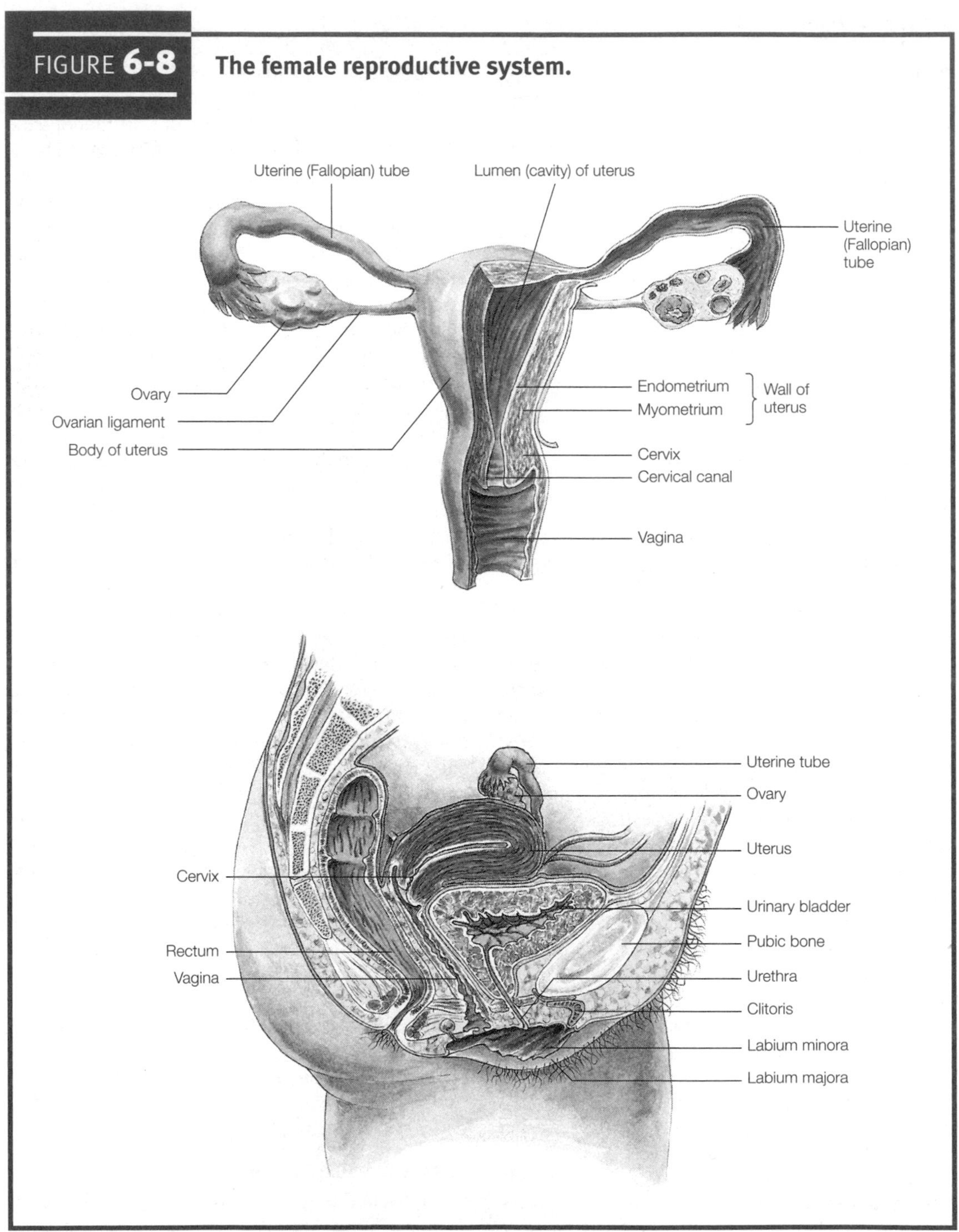

SOURCE: Human Biology, 5e. Daniel D. Chiras, Jones and Bartlett Publishers 2005.

FIGURE 6-9 **The male reproductive system.**

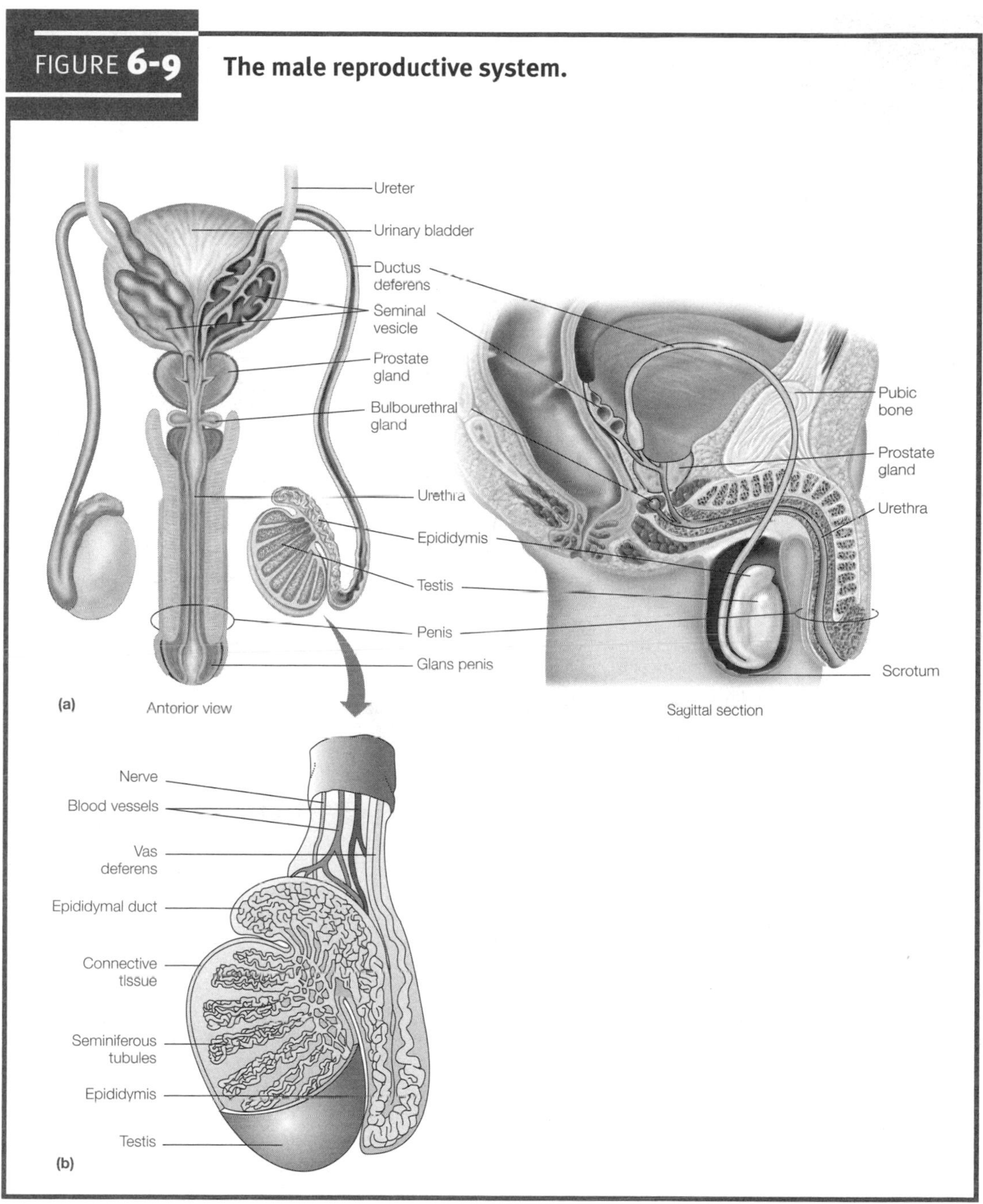

SOURCE: Human Biology, 5e. Daniel D. Chiras, Jones and Bartlett Publishers 2005.

FIGURE 6-10 The menstrual cycle.

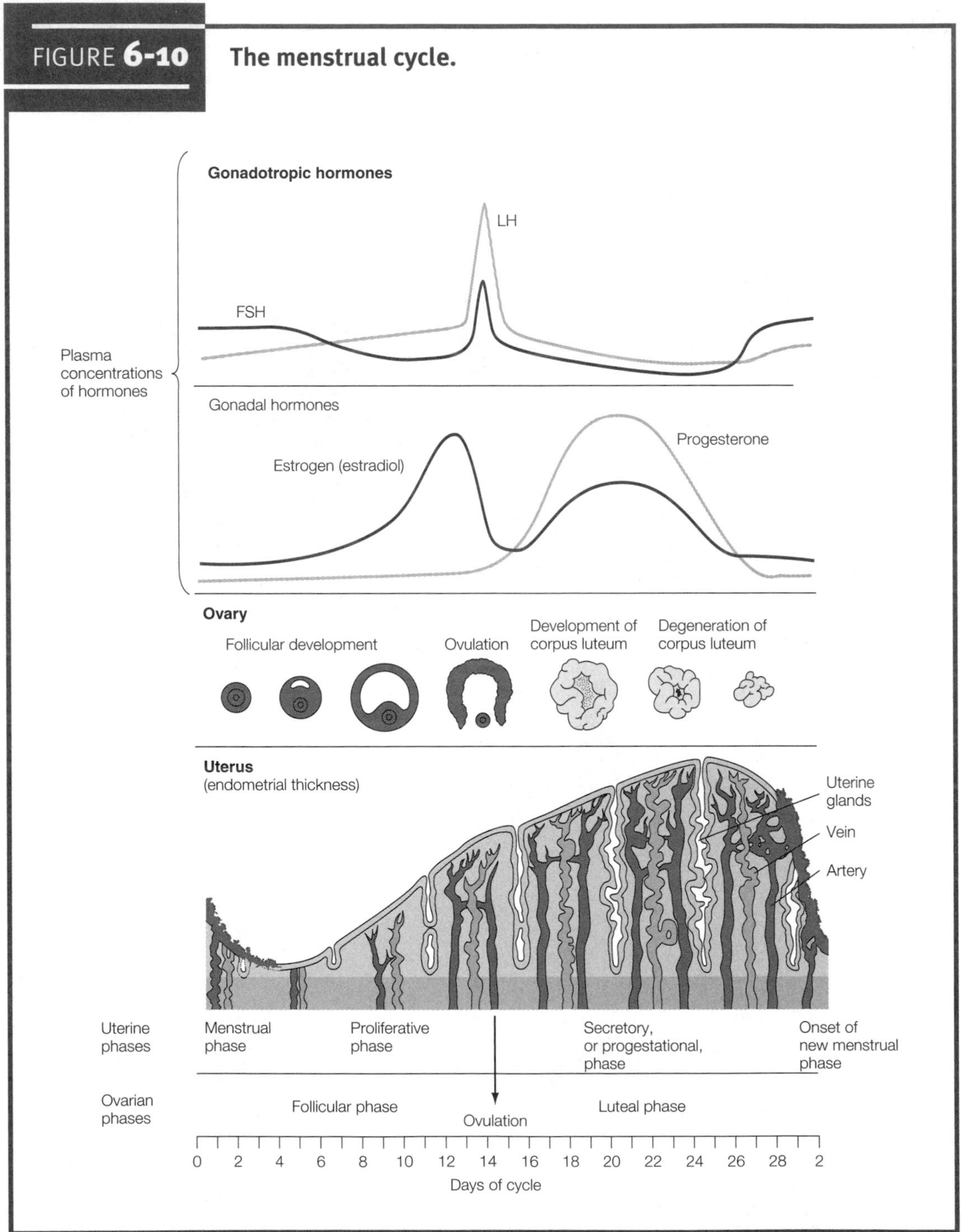

SOURCE: Human Biology, 5e. Daniel D. Chiras, Jones and Bartlett Publishers 2005.

follicles decreases with age leading to a decline in fertility. This decline usually begins in the 30s or 40s, and more rapid declines occur after age 35 (Digiovanna, 2000; Hall, 2004; Smith, 1998). The ovarian follicles that remain through these declining years tend to be underdeveloped and only a few follicles ovulate and form a corpus luteum. Eventually, by the age of 50 to 65 years, a woman will have no remaining viable follicles (Digiovanna, 2000; Smith; Wise et al., 1996).

In the late reproductive years, around age 45, when fertility declines, FSH levels tend to increase earlier in the follicular phase due to age-related decline in inhibin B. The earlier decline in FSH occurs even before increases in levels of LH or decreases in levels of estradiol (Hall, 2004; Wise et al., 1996). The increase in FSH levels is attributed to the drastic age-related decline in inhibin B, a glycoprotein synthesized in the ovaries that suppresses FSH secretion in younger individuals (Hall, 2004; Wise et al., 1996). Decline in inhibin B along with the increase in FSH establishes the earliest age-related changes in the ovaries (Hall, 2004). In the clinical setting, FSH values are determined at day 3 of the menstrual cycle in order to indicate the stage of reproductive age (Hall, 2004). Reproductive aging causes a decline in estrogen due to a decrease in ovarian follicles. A decline in progesterone also occurs (Chakraborty & Gore, 2004; Smith, 1998). The ovaries also produce about 25% of the testosterone in women. The rest is supplied by the adrenal glands and conversion of androstenedione, a testosterone precursor (Horton & Tait, 1966; Yialamas & Hayes, 2003). However, testosterone in women is only about one-tenth of that found in men (Judd & Yen, 1973; Yialamas & Hayes, 2003). These changes in the ovaries, including ovarian failure and oocyte depletion, are causally linked to the triggering of menopause (Hall, 2004; Wise et al., 1996).

The Uterus. Age-related decreases in uterine endometrial thickening during menstrual cycles occur as the result of decreased estrogen and progesterone levels (Digiovanna, 2000). This thickening leads to a decline in menstrual flow, eventually causing missed menstrual cycles and permanent cessation of ovulation and menstruation (Digiovanna, 2000). The supporting ligaments attached to the uterus are weakened with age, causing the uterus to tilt backward (Digiovanna, 2000). Over the postmenopausal period the uterus decreases in size by as much as 50% and may become so small as to be impalpable in women over the age of 75 (Digiovanna, 2000; Smith, 1998). As a result of stenosis and possible retraction, the cervix, the structure at the opening of the uterus, may also be unidentifiable upon physical exam in postmenopausal women (Smith, 1998).

The Vagina. With age, the vagina becomes shorter and narrower and the vaginal walls tend to thin and weaken (Smith, 1998). These structural changes, especially thinning of the vaginal walls and loss of elasticity, increase the chances for vaginal injury in the older female (Digiovanna, 2000). A loss of mucosal layers in the vagina as well as a large decrease in discharge causes a loss of lubrication. As a result, the vagina can become very dry, causing sexual intercourse to be painful (Digiovanna, 2000; Smith, 1998). With age, vaginal pH levels also shift from an acidic environment (3.8–4.2) toward an alkaline environment (6.5–7.5). The shift occurs due to decreased glycogen levels in vaginal tissue, which results in an environment where microbes flourish (Digiovanna, 2000; Smith, 1998). With all of these changes, vaginal infections tend to increase with age (Digiovanna, 2000). The increased rate of infection may also be due in part to shrinkage of the labia majora, part of the external genitalia. As a result of this shrinkage, the labia become separated. This separation in turn exposes a greater surface area upon which microbes and infectious agents can nest (Digiovanna, 2000).

Menopause

On average, menopause occurs around 51 years of age, but the reproductive changes described in this section begin years earlier (Digiovanna, 2000; Hall, 2004; Joffe et al., 2003). The late reproductive stage begins around 35 years of age with a decrease in fertility marked by a decrease in inhibin B, a decrease in progesterone, a slight increase in estradiol, and an increase in FSH (Hall, 2004, 2007; Joffe et al., 2003; Soules et al., 2001). The menopausal transition is defined by declines in estradiol along with the onset of variable menstrual cycles in both early and late stages. Periods of amenorrhea trigger the move into the late stage (Hall, 2004; Soules et al., 2001). Menopause is said to have occurred 1 year after the final menstrual period (Digiovanna,

2000; Hall, 2004, 2007; Soules et al., 2001). The postmenopausal period is characterized by drastic decreases in ovarian hormone functioning and changes in corresponding hormone-related systems such as bone formation and resorption (Hall, 2004, 2007; Soules et al., 2001). **Table 6-4** classifies the stages of menopause along with corresponding changes that occur within each stage.

Menopause is usually causally linked with ovarian failure and complete oocyte depletion, but recent research also implicates the hypothalamus and pituitary via a decline in estrogen negative feedback on LH release (Soules et al., 2001; Weiss, Skurnick, Goldsmith, Santoro, & Park, 2004). Estrogen and progesterone are still present in small amounts during early postmenopausal years, but ovarian production of these hormones eventually declines and ceases completely during late postmenopausal years (Chakraborty & Gore, 2004; Digiovanna, 2000). Estrogen levels decrease by 80% by postmenopausal years and progesterone decreases by 60% (Smith, 1998). During menopause, ovaries decrease production of androstenedione by 50%. This decline could help explain loss of libido and energy in the older female (Yialamas & Hayes, 2003). Although some studies have shown that there are slight declines in testosterone levels during and after menopause, others have shown no change in testosterone levels (see **Case Study 6-1**). Thus, the question of whether androgen deficiency occurs in older women remains unanswered (Laughlin, Barrett-Connor, Kritz-Silverstein, & von Muhlen, 2000; Yialamas & Hayes, 2003; Zumoff, Strain, Miller, & Rosner, 1995).

Physical symptoms that are often described by menopausal women include hot flashes, mood disturbance, weight gain, vaginal dryness, bladder infections, loss of sex drive, fatigue, insomnia,

TABLE 6-4 Classification of the Stages of Menopause and the Characteristics Associated with Each Stage as Defined by STRAW

Reproductive	Menopausal Transition	Menopause	Postmenopause
Late	Early/Late		Early/Late
Variable symptoms: vasomotor (hot flashes), breast tenderness, insomnia, migraines, premenstrual anxiety, and/or depression	Early: Menstrual cycle lengths vary Late: Two or more skipped cycles and some amenorrhea	Begins 12 months after the final menstrual period	Early: 5 years since the final menstrual period; ovarian hormone function decreases; increased bone loss Late: 5 years after the final menstrual period until death
Begin FSH elevation, decreased inhibin B, slight increase in estradiol, decreased progesterone	FSH elevation, LH elevation, decreased inhibin B, decreased estradiol	FSH elevation, LH elevation, decreased inhibin B, decreased estradiol	FSH elevation, LH elevation, decreased inhibin B, decreased estradiol, increased GnRH

SOURCE: Soules et al., 2001 and Hall, 2004.

Case Study 6-1

H.M. is a 72-year-old Caucasian female with a history of osteopenia for the past 4 years and shortness of breath related to 42 years of smoking. She presents today with complaints of painful sexual intercourse and a constant feeling of being cold. Upon questioning, she reports sometimes experiencing dizziness and light-headedness upon standing from a chair; however, she never loses consciousness when standing. She also reports a few episodes of forgetting her two grandchildren's names in the past several months. On evaluation of mental status using the Mini Mental State Exam (MMSE) she scores a 26. On physical exam, she has a blood pressure of 140/89, a weight loss of 6 pounds, and a loss of a 1/2 inch from her height from the previous visit 8 months ago. She reports no discomfort in her back or neck regions. She has no history of stroke, seizure, heart disease, or thyroid disease. H.M. did not begin hormone therapy at any point during or after menopause by her own choosing. She did begin taking calcium supplements during menopause and within the past 5 years began taking over-the-counter herbal estrogen to self-treat some of her noted symptoms.

Questions:

1. What steps would you take to address H.M.'s chief complaints for today's visit?
2. List possible labs, tests, therapeutic options, and recommendations for the patient during this visit.
3. Would you address other existing issues or would you reevaluate at the next visit?
4. List potential areas that will be noted for continuing evaluation and possible future treatment.

cognitive decline, hair loss, backaches, and joint pain (Hafez & Hafez, 2004; Joffe et al., 2003). Aging effects on the entire reproductive axis contribute to reproductive aging and eventual menopause in women.

Male Reproductive Aging

Neuroendocrine Changes

The male reproductive axis also involves the integration of the hypothalamus and pituitary, but for males the gonad involved is the testes (Sampson, Untegassan, Plas, & Berger, 2007; Schlegel & Hardy, 2002; Yialamas & Hayes, 2003). Similar to the female reproductive axis, the hypothalamus secretes GnRH into the blood. GnRH then travels to the pituitary where it stimulates the secretion of the gonadotropins FSH and LH (Schlegel & Hardy, 2002; Seidman, 2003). The gonadotropins travel to the testes where LH stimulates the Leydig cells to produce testosterone while FSH stimulates the Sertoli cells to initiate and maintain sperm production (Schlegel & Hardy, 2002; Seidman, 2003; Yialamas & Hayes, 2003). Sertoli cells, however, have the ability to suppress FSH secretion via inhibin B (Schlegel & Hardy, 2002). In males, a negative feedback system among the testes, the hypothalamus, and the pituitary controls the rate of sperm production and testosterone release. This is demonstrated by the relationship between FSH and Sertoli cells as well as by the effect of testosterone on GnRH and gonadotropin secretion (Schlegel & Hardy, 2002; Seidman, 2003; Yialamas & Hayes, 2003). Testosterone is the most available androgen in the male reproductive system, with secretory bursts occurring around six times per day (Partin & Rodriguez, 2002; Seidman, 2003). Testosterone binds to androgen receptors located in the brain and spinal cord, activating cellular mechanisms that influence androgen-dependent tissues (Seidman, 2003).

Age-related changes to the male reproductive axis include increases in FSH and LH levels, decreases in both serum and bioavailable testosterone levels, and a decline in Leydig cell function (Kandeel, Koussa, & Swerdloff, 2001; Morley et al., 1997; Sampson et al., 2007; Schlegel & Hardy, 2002). Testosterone levels in men decline with age, but can show variability from small decreases to major decreases depending on health status (Seidman, 2003). As testosterone levels decline in older males the amount of estrogen remains stable, leading to a decline in the testosterone-to-estrogen ratio (Kandeel et al., 2001). A decline in testosterone is often associated with decreases in libido, spontaneous erections, sexual desire, and sexual thoughts (Seidman, 2003).

Male System Changes

The Testes. In aging, the testes decrease in both size and weight, but with high variability among men (Digiovanna, 2000). The Leydig cells decrease in number but not in structure. In addition, these cells decrease their production of testosterone (Digiovanna, 2000; Yialamas & Hayes, 2003). In contrast, the small amount of estrogen secreted by the testes does not decline with age, nor does the estrogen that is aromatized from androstenedione. As a result, the ratio of estrogen to testosterone increases in older males (Partin & Rodriguez, 2002). In stages over time, the seminiferous tubules show thinning of the walls and narrowing of lumen. The lumen can become so narrow that the seminiferous tubules become blocked (Digiovanna, 2000). Other dynamics that may contribute to or enhance the aging of the structure and function of the seminiferous tubules include decreased blood flow and changes in testosterone production (Digiovanna, 2000). Although a decline in sperm production occurs in aging males, the production never ceases. As a result, the older male remains fertile (Digiovanna, 2000).

Glands. The seminal vesicles and the bulbourethral glands demonstrate no age-related changes (Digiovanna, 2000). However, the biggest concern in older males is changes in the prostate gland. The lining and muscle layer of the prostate gland become thinner with age, probably due to the reduced blood flow to the area (Digiovanna, 2000). Benign prostatic hyperplasia (BPH), which is dependent on age and androgen production, remains very common in aging males with approximately 50% of men experiencing nodules by age 60 and around 90% by age 85 (Hollander & Diokno, 1998; Letran & Brawer, 1999). By age 60, approximately 13% of males will be diagnosed with clinical BPH that requires medical attention. By age 85, this percentage has increased to 23% (Letran & Brawer, 1999). BPH causes the prostate to grow very large, which may result in urethral blockages (Hafez & Hafez, 2004; Hollander & Diokno, 1998). Common complaints with BPH include increased frequency and discomfort with urination, bladder and kidney infections, and erectile and ejaculatory dysfunction (Hafez & Hafez, 2004; Hollander & Diokno, 1998; Paick et al., 2005; Rosen et al., 2003).

The Penis. The penis begins to show fibrous changes in erectile tissue around the urethra starting in the 30s and 40s. By ages 55 to 60 years, increased fibrosis occurs in all erectile tissues (Digiovanna, 2000). This fibrosis in erectile tissue causes an increase in the amount of time it takes to achieve an erection in the older male; however, the ability to have an erection is maintained with age and is usually most affected by medication or disease (Digiovanna, 2000; Kandeel et al., 2001). In addition to the increase in time to obtain an erection, older males also require more stimulation in order to maintain the erection. In addition, older males generally experience less intense orgasms and ejaculation, decreases in ejaculatory volume, and an increase in the refractory period following ejaculation (Kandeel et al., 2001; Schlegel & Hardy, 2002).

Andropause

Andropause is classified as a decline in testosterone levels and eventual deficiency significant enough to cause clinical symptoms (American Society for Reproductive Medicine [ASRM] Practice Committee, 2004; Hafez & Hafez, 2004; Yialamas & Hayes, 2003). Unlike menopause, andropause occurs gradually over time and does not occur in all aging males (Hafez & Hafez, 2004). A decline in the functional ability of the entire reproductive axis causes decreased production of testosterone in aging males (Yialamas & Hayes, 2003). When testosterone is produced in the adult male it stimulates negative feedback of GnRH, FSH, and LH secretion. In the older adult male this negative feedback is enhanced (Yialamas & Hayes, 2003). During andropause, when testosterone becomes extremely low, a recovery mechanism triggers increases in FSH and LH in an attempt to elevate testosterone levels (Hafez & Hafez, 2004). Androgen deficiency in the aging male (ADAM) includes symptoms of low libido; decreased energy, strength, and stamina; increased irritability; and cognitive changes (ASRM Practice Committee, 2004; Janowsky, Oviatt, & Orwoll, 1994; Korenman et al., 1990; Sternbach, 1998; van den Beld, de Jong, Grobbee, Pols, & Lamberts, 2000; Yialamas & Hayes, 2003). Physiological symptoms of ADAM include erectile dysfunction, osteopenia, osteoporosis, breast enlargement, decreased muscle mass, shrinkage of the testes, and increased fat deposition (ASRM Practice Committee, 2004; Greendale, Edelstein, & Barrett-Connor, 1997; Hafez & Hafez, 2004; Turner & Wass, 1997; Vermeulen, Goemaere, & Kaufman, 1999; Yialamas & Hayes, 2003). Diagnosis of andropause generally occurs via measurement of total serum testosterone levels; however, measures of the true testosterone level should be based on total testosterone and testosterone metabolites as well as androgen receptor activity (Yialamas & Hayes, 2003).

Although the hypothalamus-pituitary-gonadal axis controls both male and female reproductive systems, the age-related changes in the axis and the physiological effects are very diverse. All males and females experience age-related changes in the reproductive system; however, these changes occur with tremendous variability among individuals.

THE NERVOUS SYSTEM

Introduction to the Nervous System

The two components of the nervous system, central and peripheral, have the potential to affect the entire body through continual communication via nerve innervations and signals. As a person ages, natural changes occur in the nervous systems that can have direct or indirect effects on the rest of the body. The central nervous system consists of the brain and the spinal cord whereas the peripheral nervous system encompasses the motor and sensory neurons located in the sensory-somatic system and the autonomic system (**Figure 6-11**). The autonomic nervous system consists of the motor and sensory neurons that maintain homeostasis within the body. It can be further divided into the parasympathetic and sympathetic systems. Communication among the brain, spinal cord, and peripheral nerves is responsible for maintenance of homeostasis. This communication process within the nervous system and between organ systems and the nervous system is demonstrated in **Figure 6-12**.

The process of aging in the nervous system could lead to profound effects on other organ systems, considering the constant communication that occurs. Any change in the nervous system has the potential to influence the stability of the entire body, even if minimally. In this section, the age-related changes that occur in the brain, spinal cord, and peripheral nerves will be discussed.

The Aging Brain

The human brain goes through many developmental changes throughout a person's life span.

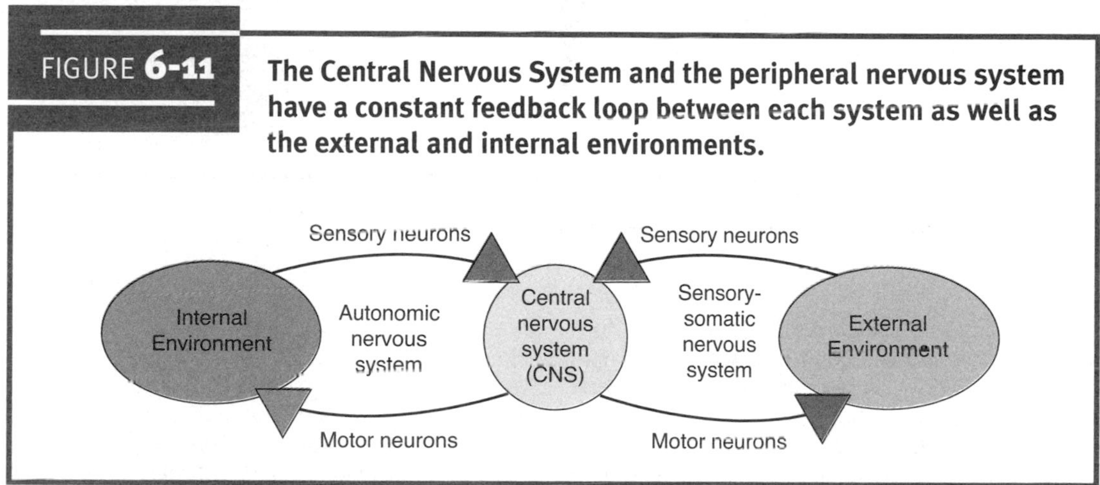

FIGURE **6-11** **The Central Nervous System and the peripheral nervous system have a constant feedback loop between each system as well as the external and internal environments.**

SOURCE: Adapted from John Kimball, PhD; Organizations of the Nervous System; Kimball's Biology page http://users.rcn.com/jkimball.ma.ultranet/BiologyPages/P.PNS.htm.

FIGURE 6-12 The autonomic nervous system.

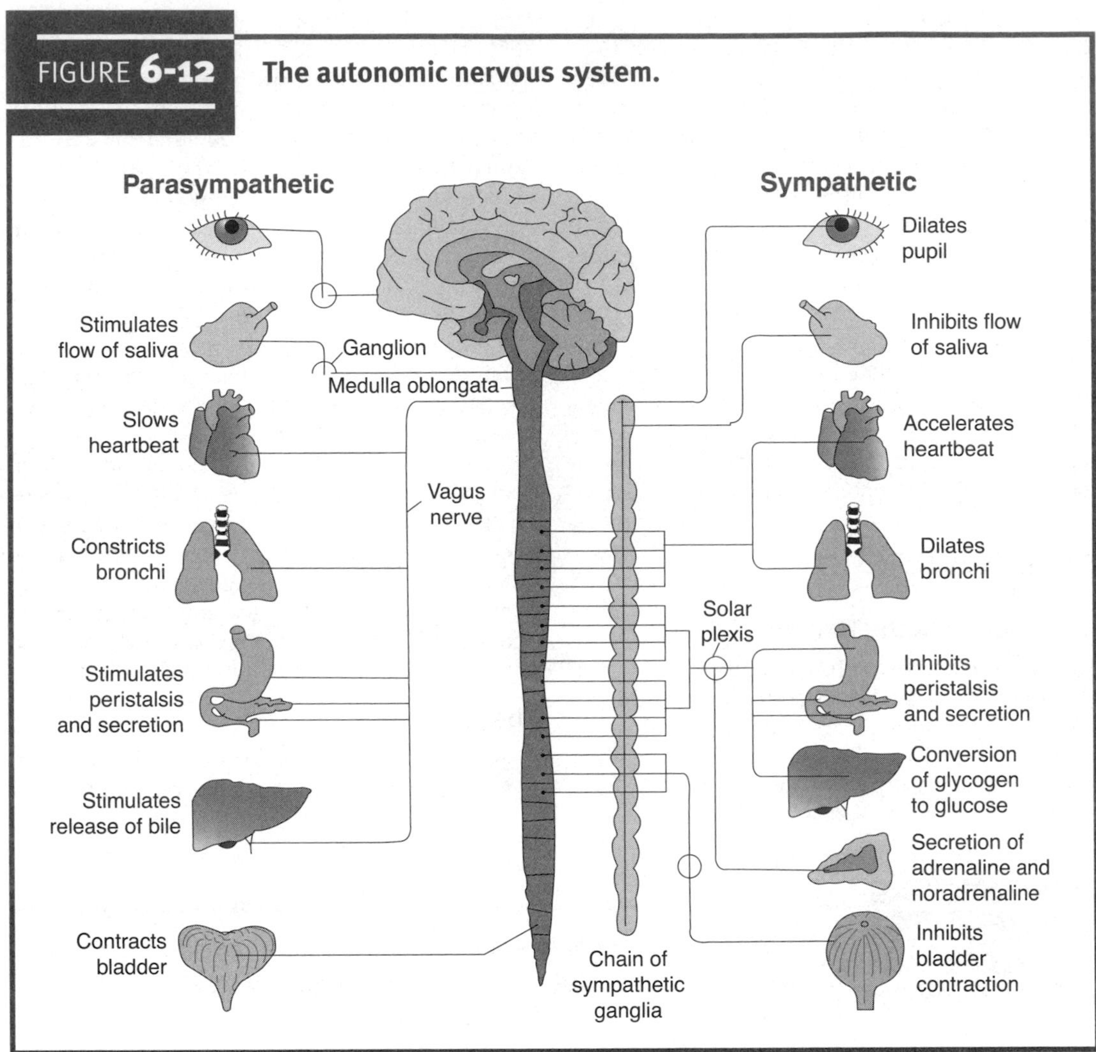

SOURCE: Adapted from John Kimball, PhD; Organization of the Nervous System, Kimball's Biology Page http://users.rcn.com/jkimball.ma.ultranet/BiologyPages/P/PNS.html.

Aging should still be considered on a developmental scale, not a decrement scale. Although brain changes do occur as humans grow older, one should not assume that cognitive function will automatically decline. Memory changes can be observed by the fifth decade, but changes remain variable among individuals. There is also great variation in the type of memory affected (Erickson & Barnes, 2003).

Overall Structural Changes

The brain decreases in size and weight as men and women age (Arking, 1998; Digiovanna, 1994; Minaker, 2004). At birth, the brain weighs approximately 357 grams. Brain weight peaks at about 1,300 grams around the age of 20 years. This weight is maintained until 55 years of age (Arking, 1998). After age 55 there is a decline in brain weight. This decline can result in a brain weight that is 11%

BOX 6-1 Research Highlight

Aim: The authors conducted two studies for the purpose of examining the hypothesis that cardiovascular fitness can offset declines in cognitive function.

Method: In study 1, a cross-sectional assessment of 41 community dwelling older adults was used to test physical fitness. In study 2, a randomized clinical trial with a separate sample of 29 highly fit older adults was examined. Participants were asked to complete various physical tasks including using a treadmill, and then specific cortical measures were noted on MRIs and compared.

Findings: Study findings showed that increases in cardiovascular fitness resulted in increased functioning of the brain's attentional network during a cognitive challenge. Highly fit individuals exhibited greater brain activity than did either low- or unfit individuals.

Application to practice: The study results suggest that improvements in cardiovascular fitness can have a positive influence on the plasticity of the aging brain. Nurses can encourage older adults about engaging in regular exercise to improve cardiovascular fitness can have a positive effect on brain activity.

Source: Colcombe, S. J., Kramer, A. F., Erickson, K. I., Scalf, P., McAuley, E., Cohen, J. J., Webb, A., Jerome, G. J., Marquez, D. X., & Elavsky, S. (2004). Cardiovascular fitness, cortical plasticity and aging. *Proceedings of the National Academy of Sciences USA, 101*(9), 3316–3321.

smaller than that observed in the young adult brain (Arking, 1998); however, measurements of brain weight may show bias due to individual differences in head size and body weight. Measuring changes in individual brain volume helps to diffuse this inherent bias. Brain volume appears to be stable from age 20 to 60 followed by a significant decline of between 5% and 10% (Arking, 1998; Minaker, 2004). Magnetic resonance imaging (MRI) studies have demonstrated that, compared to women, men demonstrate greater age-related volume loss in the brain as a whole as well as in the temporal and frontal lobes (Leon Carrion, Salgado, Sierra, Marquez-Rivas, & Dominguez-Morales, 2001; Murphy, DeCarli, Schapiro, Rapoport, & Horwitz, 1992). In the same MRI study, researchers showed that women had a greater loss of volume in the hippocampus and parietal lobes than that observed in men. From ages 30 to 90 years both men and women experience a volume loss of 14% in the cerebral cortex, 35% in the hippocampus, and 26% in the cerebral white matter (Anderton, 2002). Ventricles within the brain enlarge throughout the aging process. Ventricle size at age 90 may be as much as three to four times ventricle size at age 20. Ventricle enlargement may help to explain some loss of brain volume (Arking, 1998; Beers & Berkow, n.d.; Digiovanna, 1994). Although the ventricles on the inside of the brain enlarge, the gyri—raised ridges on the surface of the brain—shrink, and the sulci—grooves between the gyri—become wider (Digiovanna, 1994).

Neuron Changes

The brain is composed of gray matter and white matter. The gray matter is located on the surface of the brain, known as the cerebral cortex, and contains the nerve cell bodies. The white matter contains no cell bodies or dendrites, but is strictly myelinated nerve fibers (Arking, 1998). **Figure 6-13** demonstrates the composition of a nerve cell and fibers. The average number of neocortical neurons is 19 billion in female brains and 23 billion in male brains, a 16% difference. A study by Pakkenberg and Gundersen (1997) that focused on neuron numbers in 20- to 90-year-old individuals showed that approximately 10% of all neocortical neurons are lost over the life span in both sexes. Cell loss remains minimal in some parts of the brain whereas other areas show tremendous neuron decrease (Katzman, 1995). According to Beers and Berkow (n.d.), neuronal cell loss remains minimal in the brain stem nuclei, paraventricular nuclei, and supraoptic nuclei. Losses in other areas can be great: 10% to 60% in the hippocampus, 55% in the superior temporal gyrus, and 10% to 35% in the temporal lobe. However, recent anatomical studies have not shown any statistically significant age-related change in neuron numbers in the hippocampus, the primary center for learning and memory (Erickson & Barnes, 2003). Unlike previous studies, these recent anatomical studies have taken into account age-related tissue shrinkage and have utilized better-controlled stereological methods in making the determination that no neuronal decreases occur (Anderton, 2002; Peters, 2002). Other sources describe a significant decline of neurons in the cerebrum, which controls voluntary movement, vision, hearing, and other senses. Only a minimal neuronal loss is seen in the cerebellar cortex and the basal ganglia, which are responsible for muscle movement and control (Digiovanna, 1994, 2000). The brainstem demonstrates some loss of neurons in the nucleus of Meynert (acetylcholine production) and the locus coeruleus (norepinephrine production), which aids in sleep regulation (Digiovanna, 1994, 2000).

Early reports of neuron loss should be considered carefully because more recent studies have used more carefully controlled human tissue samples, study design, and neuron counting techniques (Peters, 2002). A loss of neurons in the aging brain is present, but not to the extent that researchers have reported in the past (Morrison & Hof, 1997; Peters, 2002; Peters, Morrison, Rosene, & Hyman, 1998). The myelin sheath, which surrounds the axon on every neuron and promotes faster electrical signaling along each neuron, breaks down in aging (Bartzokis et al., 2004; Dickson, 1997; Peters, 2002). Myelination of the axon appears to continue until middle age, followed by a breakdown in the structural integrity of the myelin (Bartzokis et al., 2004; Dickson, 1997). This degradation of myelin may cause neuronal disruption by slowing the nerve impulses as they travel through the nervous system. This may help to explain mild age-related declines in cognition and motor control (Dickson, 1997).

The loss of a neuron or a decrease in neuron participation causes disruption of neural circuits and hence neural signaling. Dendrites serve as the system through which nerve impulses are relayed to the neuron. The **synapse** serves as the messenger system between dendrites. **Figure 6-14**

FIGURE 6-13 **A neuron.**

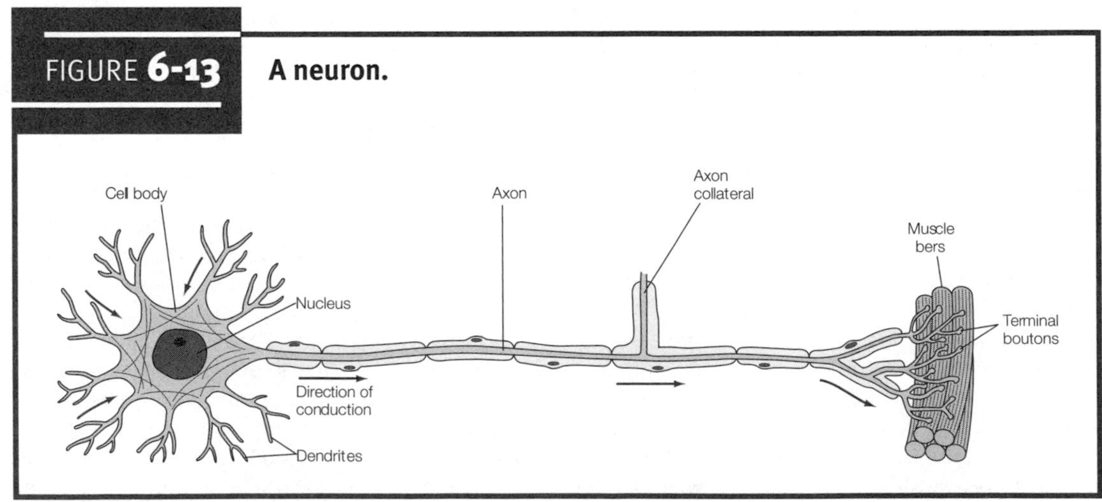

SOURCE: Human Biology, 5e. Daniel D. Chiras, Jones and Bartlett Publishers 2005.

FIGURE 6-14 **A synapse and synaptic transmission.**

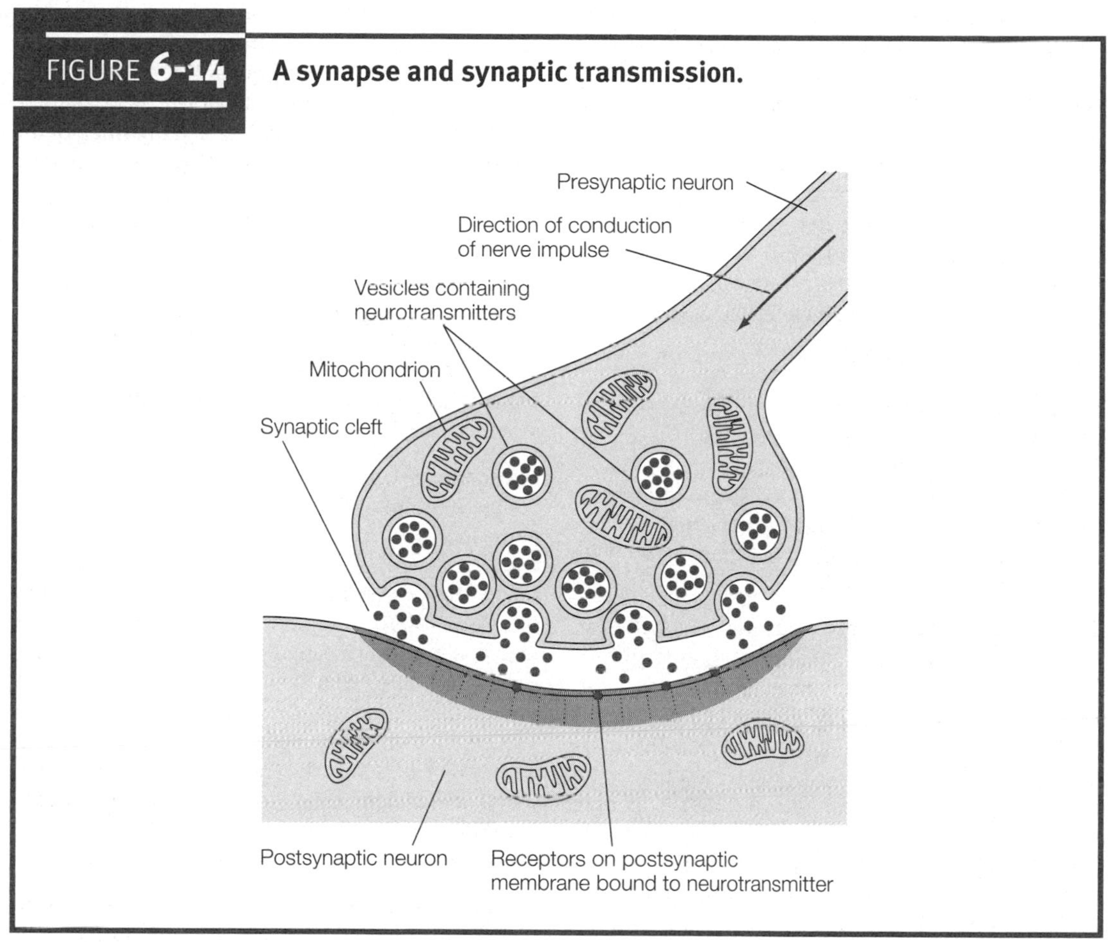

SOURCE: Human Biology, 5e. Daniel D. Chiras, Jones and Bartlett Publishers 2005.

demonstrates how a synapse works to relay chemical messages between neurons. The number of dendrites and dendritic spines decreases with age, but not uniformly in the brain (Arking, 1998). Several human studies focusing on synapse change in different areas of the brain throughout the life span have shown no significant change (Scheff, Price, & Sparks, 2001). However, significant synapse loss has been shown in multiple brain areas in postmortem Alzheimer's disease tissue when compared to control tissue (Lippa, Hamos, Pulaski, Degennaro, & Drachman, 1992; Scheff & Price, 1998, 2001; Scheff, Sparks, & Price, 1996).

The brain demonstrates remarkable compensatory mechanisms to recover from loss, even in old age. **Plasticity**, or the ability to lengthen and/or form new neuronal connections onto available existing neurons, is one of these compensatory mechanisms (Beers & Berkow, n.d.; Digiovanna, 1994, 2000). Plasticity can occur through many avenues including **neurogenesis**, **synaptogenesis**, synaptic alteration, synaptic efficacy, long-term potentiation, axon sprouting, and dendrite transformation (Teter & Ashford, 2002). An example of synaptic alteration is synapses' ability to broaden and cover more surface area, possibly compensating for synapse loss in some brain areas (Digiovanna, 1994, 2000; Terry, DeTeresa, & Hansen, 1987). In aging or injury, new neuronal connections specifically compensate for the loss of neurons in certain brain areas in order to aid in preservation of function (Beers & Berkow, n.d.). Plasticity does diminish with age, but is not completely lost. Aging effects include a decrease in long-term potentiation and synaptogenesis in addition to delays in axon sprouting that in turn affect the formation of new connections (Teter & Ashford, 2002).

Neurotransmitter Changes

A **neurotransmitter** is a chemical messenger encapsulated in synaptic vesicles that is released from the axon into the synaptic space and onto corresponding receptors on the postsynaptic neuron. Neurotransmitter changes during the aging process can influence memory and cognition as well as behavior and motor function.

Cholinergic. Cholinergic neurons, which release the neurotransmitter acetylcholine, play a significant role in learning and memory in humans and animals (Arking, 1998; Mattson, 1999). Acetylcholine induces learning and memory via cholinergic input to the hippocampus and neocortex in the brain (Kelly & Roth, 1997; Mattson, 1999). With age, acetylcholine synthesis and release from synaptic vesicles begin to decline. The postsynaptic acetylcholine receptors, known as nicotinic and muscarinic receptors, and transport of choline also demonstrate age-related deficits (Beers & Berkow, n.d.; Kelly & Roth, 1997; Mattson, 1999). In Alzheimer's disease these cholinergic deficits are more pronounced, which led to the development of acetylcholinesterase inhibitor medications now on the market to treat the disease. The objective of the medication is to decrease the degradation of acetylcholine in the synaptic space, thereby increasing the amount of acetylcholine available to bind with postsynaptic receptors.

Dopaminergic. The **dopaminergic system** involves the neurotransmitter dopamine, mainly in the substantia nigra and striatum (Arking, 1998). In aging, dopamine levels decrease by around 10% per decade, and dopamine transport in the neuron also diminishes (Katzman, 1995; Mattson, 1999; Peters, 2006). Age-related changes are also found in dopamine receptors. In addition, the ability of dopamine to bind to postsynaptic receptors also decreases (Katzman, 1995; Mattson, 1999). Positron emission tomography (PET) studies have shown a decline in dopamine receptors located in the caudate and putamen of the aging brain (Mozaz & Monguio, 2001). In Parkinson's disease, dopamine levels are greatly decreased, leading to the hallmark symptom of diminished motor control and compromised cognitive performance (Peters, 2006). Decreases in dopamine with age may explain some age-related motor deficits as well as motor dysfunction resulting from the use of medications targeting the dopaminergic neurotransmitter system (Kelly & Roth, 1997; Mattson, 1999; Mozaz & Monguio, 2001; Volkow et al., 1998).

Monoaminergic. The **monoaminergic system** consists mainly of the neurotransmitters norepinephrine and serotonin located in the locus coeruleus and the raphe nucleus (brainstem), respectively (Arking, 1998; Kelly & Roth, 1997; Mattson, 1999). Norepinephrine tends to increase with age in certain brain regions, but corresponding receptors have been shown to decrease in both humans and animals (Gruenewald & Matsumoto, 1999; Mattson, 1999). Serotonin levels and receptor binding sites both decrease with age, which may play a role in depression and sleep changes later in life (Mattson, 1999; Mattson, Maudsley, & Martin, 2004; Ramos-Platon & Beneto-Pascual, 2001).

Amino Acid Transmitters. The **amino acid neurotransmitters** consist mainly of glutamate, the major excitatory neurotransmitter, and gamma-aminobutyric acid (GABA), the major inhibitory neurotransmitter (Kelly & Roth, 1997; Mattson, 1999). The hippocampus, a central location for learning and memory, contains high levels of glutamate. This relationship between glutamate and memory leads to a questioning of the idea that memory decline is strongly tied solely to acetylcholine depletion (Kelly & Roth, 1997). Glutamate receptors decline with age, but the change in glutamate with age is unknown (Mattson, 1999). The overstimulation and release of glutamate may be significant in Alzheimer's disease, Parkinson's disease, and Huntington's disease as well as stroke (Mattson, 1999). GABA concentrates in the brain areas of the substantia nigra and the globus pallidus (Kelly & Roth, 1997). Age-related changes in the GABA neurotransmitter are unknown; however, decreases in GABA have been correlated with aggressive behavior (Jimenez, Cuartero, & Moreno, 2001; Mattson, 1999). GABA can synthesize glutamate, which can convert to GABA via the enzyme glutamic acid decarboxylase (Gluck, Thomas, Davis, & Haroutunian, 2002). So, changes in glutamate could have a direct or indirect effect on GABA in the aging brain and vice versa.

Neuroendocrine Changes

Age-related changes to neuroendocrine functioning affect many other systems in the body. **Figure 6-15** demonstrates body systems that are controlled and/or affected by changes in neuroendocrine functioning with an emphasis on the pituitary gland. Aging changes in secretion of hypothalamic-releasing hormone are studied indirectly by observing changes in pituitary secretion response to hypothalamic-releasing hormone, to chemicals that block feedback mechanisms, and to chemicals that stimulate the release of hypothalamic-pituitary hormone (Gruenewald & Matsumoto, 1999). One example of a neuroendocrine age-related change is the reproductive axis or the hypothalamic-pituitary-gonadal axis that controls the regulation of male and female hormones (Chakraborty & Gore, 2004; Hall, 2004). (Refer to "The Reproductive System" earlier in this chapter for further discussion of age-related neuroendocrine function of gonadal hormones.) Another example is the **hypothalamic-pituitary-adrenal (HPA) axis** that integrates the endocrine, immune, and nervous systems. This integration allows for great adaptability (Ferrari et al., 2001). The HPA axis regulates glucocorticoid levels in the body and allows the body to respond to stressful conditions (Ferrari et al., 2001; Gruenewald & Matsumoto, 1999). Age changes in the negative feedback system of glucocorticoids on the HPA axis may cause glucocorticoids to circulate for longer periods of time. Consequently, damage may occur to hippocampal neurons needed for cognitive function (Gruenewald & Matsumoto, 1999).

In the central nervous system, the neurotransmitters dopamine and norepinephrine affect hypothalamic and pituitary hormone release, and with age these neurotransmitters cause changes in hormone secretions (Gruenewald & Matsumoto, 1999). Hypothalamic neurons release dopamine that inhibits prolactin release from the pituitary. Prolactin stimulates dopaminergic neurons in the hypothalamus, but with age dopaminergic changes can lead to deregulation of prolaction secretion (Gruenewald & Matsumoto, 1999). Norepinephrine levels have been shown to increase in certain brain areas even with a decrease in noradrenergic neurons and receptors (Mattson, 1999). An age-related increase in norepinephrine could affect the release of **growth hormone (GH)**, **thyroid-stimulating hormone (TSH)**, and leutinizing hormone (LH) from the pituitary gland (Gruenewald & Matsumoto, 1999). Neuroendocrine changes with age have the potential to affect many systems in the body via hormone alterations. These changes are an example of how the nervous system plays an integral role in every aspect of the human body.

Vascular Changes

Cerebral blood flow decreases with age, reportedly by an average of 20%. Decreased blood flow is accompanied by decreased glucose utilization and metabolic rate of oxygen in the brain (Arking, 1998; Beers & Berkow, n.d.; Dickson, 1997; Mattson, 1999). According to Katzman (1995), the National Institute of Mental Health longitudinal study revealed that individuals with an average age of 70 years were comparable in cerebral blood flow to individuals with an average age of 20.8 years. However, an 11-year follow-up showed that the older cognitively intact participants had a significant reduction in cerebral blood flow, leading to the conclusion that the eighth decade of life was a turning point. The rate of blood flow in women decreases slightly more rapidly than in men; however, blood flow is usually greater in women than in men until age 60 (Beers & Berkow, n.d.). Potential explanations for decreased cerebral blood flow include cerebrovascular disease, structural changes in cerebral blood vessels, and neuron loss accompanied by a reduction in blood flow need (de la Torre, 1997). Cerebral blood vessels display less elasticity and increased fibrosis, which may lead to increased vascular resistance (Mattson, 1999).

The blood–brain barrier shows age-related degradation of capillary walls. This degradation affects the ability of nutrients such as glucose and oxygen to nourish the brain (Arking, 1998; de la Torre, 1997; Mattson, 1999). In conjunction with the inability to effectively nourish the brain, changes in

FIGURE 6-15 The pituitary gland.

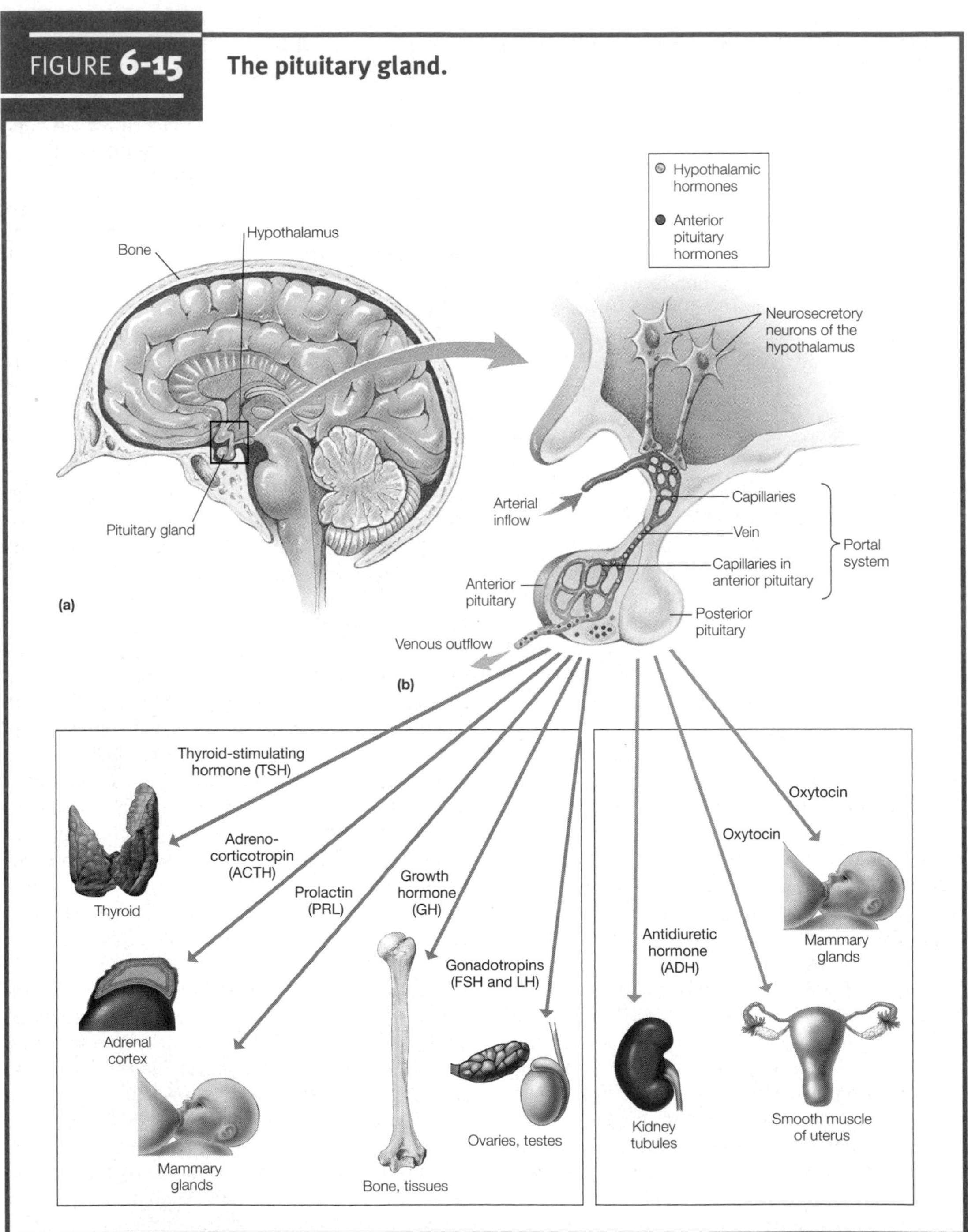

SOURCE: Human Biology, 5e. Daniel D. Chiras, Jones and Bartlett Publishers 2005.

capillaries could also prevent waste by-products from effectively exiting the blood–brain barrier, in turn causing a build-up of potentially neurotoxic substances (de la Torre, 1997).

A number of studies have associated increased lesions in myelinated areas, known as white matter lesions, with increased cerebral vascular risk, a reduced cerebral blood flow, and loss of vascular density (Artero, Tiemeier, & Prins, 2004; Atwood et al., 2004; Moody et al., 2004). It remains unclear, however, whether these lesions are a causative step or a result of the vascular compromise.

Plaques and Tangles

β-amyloid **plaques** and neurofibrillary **tangles** are considered hallmarks of Alzheimer's disease (**Figure 6-16**), but both also can be found in older individuals without evidence of dementia (Anderton, 2002; Beers & Berkow, n.d.; Dickson, 1997; Schmitt et al., 2000). Plaques occur outside of the neuronal

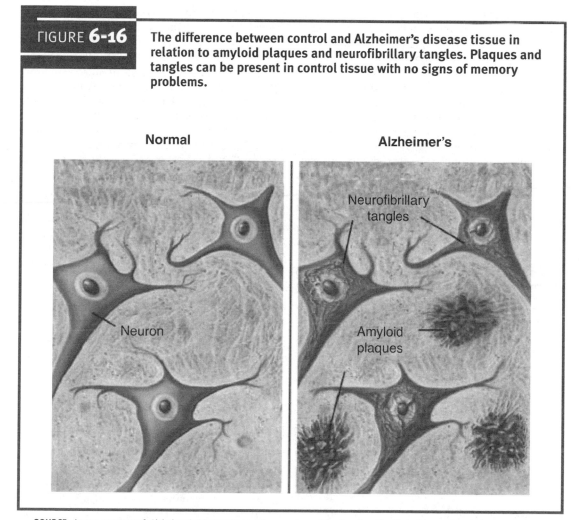

FIGURE 6-16 **The difference between control and Alzheimer's disease tissue in relation to amyloid plaques and neurofibrillary tangles. Plaques and tangles can be present in control tissue with no signs of memory problems.**

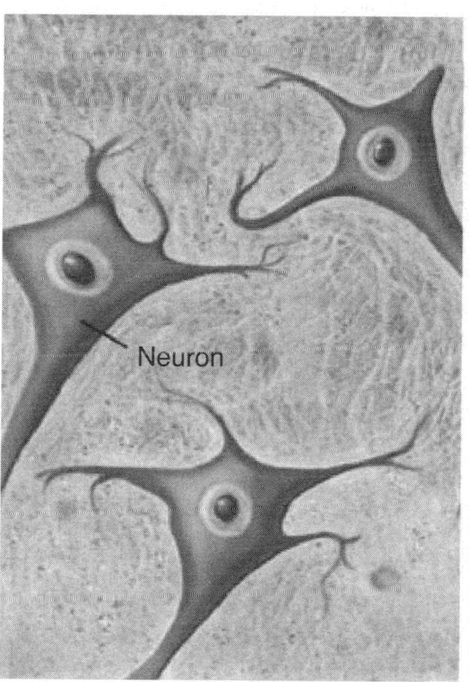

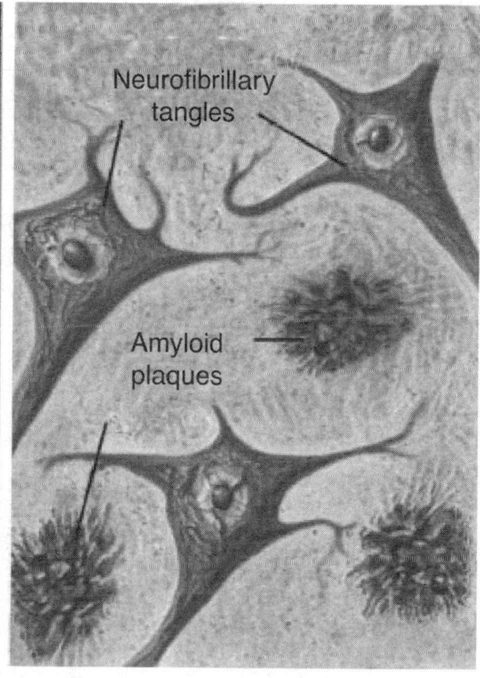

SOURCE: Image courtesy of: Alzheimer's Disease Research, a program of the American Health Assistance Foundation http://www.ahaf.org/alzdis/about/plaques_tanglesBorder.jpg.

cell and consist of gray matter with a protein core surrounded by abnormal neurites (Anderton, 2002). Each plaque consists of a core of protein, with the dominant protein being amyloid β-peptide, which is formulated from a larger protein known as amyloid precursor protein (Anderton, 2002; Dickson, 1997). This amyloid β-peptide has been shown to be neurotoxic, inducing oxidative stress and stimulating inflammatory processes (Mattson, 1999). However, in the aging brain plaques are disseminated, unlike in the Alzheimer's disease brain where plaques are very numerous and dense (Dickson, 1997).

Neurofibrillary tangles occur in the neuronal cell body and consist of paired helical filaments and a few straight filaments (Anderton, 2002; Dickson, 1997). The main protein associated with neurofibrillary tangles is known as tau, a phosphoprotein that supports microtubule stability (Binder, Guillozet-Bongaarts, Garcia-Sierra, & Berry, 2005; Dickson, 1997). In neurofibrillary tangles, tau protein undergoes abnormal phosphorylation and increases in density (Dickson, 1997). In aging, tangles are found in very low numbers and usually concentrate in areas of the entorhinal cortex, hippocampus, and amygdala (Anderton, 2002; Dickson, 1997; Mattson, 1999). In the aged brain, the greatest density of tangles appears in the entorhinal cortex, whereas in the Alzheimer's disease brain plaques spread throughout the entire cortex (Dickson, 1997).

Free Radicals

A free radical is a molecule with an unpaired electron in the outer shell of electrons. A free radical remains unstable until paired with another molecule (Mattson, 1999). In humans, oxygen is the major molecule in the generation of free radicals. Although the brain makes up only 2% of total body weight, it consumes around 20% of the total oxygen uptake (Benzi & Moretti, 1997; Tortora & Derrickson, 2006). In the cell, mitochondria continuously emit oxygen free radicals during the electron transport process, which manifests oxidative stress and can cause oxidative damage (Benzi & Moretti, 1997; Mattson, 1999; Sohal, Mockett, & Orr, 2002). Antioxidants and repair mechanisms for oxidative stress in biological systems are covered under the oxidative stress hypothesis (see Chapter 2). Oxygen free radicals, or oxyradicals, continually increase and accumulate with age, causing oxidative damage to lipids, proteins, and DNA in human tissue including the brain (Mattson, 1999; Sohal et al., 2002). Oxidative damage to proteins, such as cell membrane proteins, could be highly significant in brain aging. Such damage can result in loss of structural integrity and subsequent cell dysfunction and neuron degeneration (Mattson, 1999; Sohal et al., 2002). Nuclear DNA in the nervous system does not incur much oxidative damage in aging; however, oxidative damage is tremendous in mitochondrial DNA because mitochondria are the main source of free radical production (Mattson, 1999). A decrease in available cell energy and impairment in cell metabolism could be mechanisms in promoting free radical production with age (Mattson, 1999; Sohal et al., 2002).

BOX 6-2 Web Exploration

Explore the findings from the Nun Study, which provide some unique insight into the development and manifestations of Alzheimer's disease. Go to http://www.mc.uky.edu/nunnet/ and follow the links, or visit http://www.mc.uky.edu/nunnet/AWGExcerpt.htm to read an excerpt from *Aging with Grace*, a book about the Nun Study by David Snowdon (2001).

Source: Author.

The Aging Spinal Cord

Cells

Overall, the number of spinal cord cells remains stable until around age 60, and then declines thereafter (Beers & Berkow, n.d.; Digiovanna, 1994). Interneuron loss in the lower spinal cord has been reported. Neuron decrements of up to 25% to 45% are observed in those neurons of the spinal layer that correlate to the cerebral cortex (Arking, 1998).

Nerve Conduction

According to Abrams and colleagues (1995), the aging spine may narrow due to pressure on the spinal cord resulting from bone overgrowth. Due to this narrowing, spinal cord axons decrease and can eventually cause changes in sensation. However, these effects may be correlated not only with age, but also with degenerative disease processes or compression of spinal disks that clamp nerves (Beers & Berkow, n.d.). An MRI study by Ishikawa and colleagues (2003) focused on age-associated changes of the cervical spinal cord and spinal canal. These researchers concluded that the transverse area of the cervical spinal cord decreased with age and the spinal canal narrowed with age. These aging changes may directly or indirectly affect motor control and/or sensory systems in the body.

The Aging Peripheral Nervous System

The peripheral nervous system contains approximately 100 billion **nerve cells**. These cells form nerve fibers that cascade throughout the body, connecting the central nervous system to the rest of the body. Hence, these cells work as a relay messenger system (Abrams, Beers, & Berkow, 1995). The somatic nervous system connects the brain and spinal cord to skeletal muscles and sensory receptors. The autonomic nervous system regulates organ function through activation of nervous system response and through inhibition of parasympathetic response (Abrams et al., 1995). See Figure 6-12 for a diagram of the autonomic pathway of the peripheral nervous system. Nerve conduction speed slows with age as a result of the degradation of the myelin sheaths that coat axons (Bartzokis et al., 2004; Beers & Berkow, n.d.; Mozaz & Monguio, 2001; Peters, 2002). In addition, calcium modulation appears to be functionally compromised with advancing age. Calcium is a key regulator of nervous signaling, from excitability to neurotransmitter release. Calcium's disregulation has also been implicated in loss of cell viability in nervous tissue (Buchholz, Behringer, Pottorf, Pearce, & Vanterpool, 2007). Changes in motor speed, such as reaction times to stimuli, and changes in sensory abilities, such as changes in taste or smell, may be explained by these age-related changes in the peripheral nervous system.

Sensory Neurons

Sensory neuron function declines with age, leading to alterations in reflexes and voluntary actions and influencing certain quality of life areas such as memories, thoughts, and emotion (Digiovanna, 1994, 2000). The sense of touch changes with age due to changes in the touch receptors, or Meissner's corpuscles, and the pressure receptors, or Pacinian corpuscles. However, only small changes in sensory neurons related to touch are observed (Digiovanna, 1994, 2000). Sensory neurons for smell, or olfactory neurons, decrease with age, causing a lessened ability to detect and identify certain smells. This dampened ability could affect eating habits and, due to the inability to detect toxic fumes, may also place older adults in potentially dangerous situations (Digiovanna, 1994, 2000). The sense of taste involves the flavors of salty, sweet, sour, bitter, and umami. Aging changes occur on an individual basis, usually affecting salty and bitter flavors, with salty flavors declining the most (Digiovanna, 1994, 2000). However, the sense of smell may also play a significant role in the age-related changes in taste. This may occur because of the strong link between certain food aromas and taste expectations. The sense of taste has a rapid compensatory response to injury, such as burning the tongue with hot food, and even aging. This compensatory response is characterized by replacement of taste receptors and sensory neurons (Digiovanna, 1994, 2000). Other sensory neurons that decline with age affect the monitoring of blood pressure, thirst, urine in the bladder, and fecal matter in the intestine and rectum. Bone, joint, and muscle position and function are also affected by age-related changes in sensory neurons (Digiovanna, 1994, 2000).

Somatic Motor Neurons

With age, there is a decrease in the number of motor neurons. As a result, there is a reduction in the number of muscle cells and consequent muscle degeneration and weakness (Digiovanna, 1994, 2000). Age changes in the remaining motor neurons include myelin breakdown and cell membrane damage. These changes lead to slower relay of messages that in turn alters the ability of the muscle to contract and relax (Bartzokis et al., 2004; Digiovanna, 1994, 2000). Changes in both sensory and motor peripheral nerve pathways cause voluntary movements to become slower, less accurate, and less coordinated with age (Digiovanna, 1994). These aging changes that affect muscle strength and movement abilities can be lessened with daily exercise aimed at increasing and retaining the performance of remaining muscle.

Autonomic Motor Neurons

Aging causes changes to both the sympathetic and parasympathetic pathways to organ systems. One example of these changes is seen in the body's response to change in blood pressure. When blood pressure drops too low, sympathetic neurons usually help to increase blood pressure by stimulating the heart and constricting blood vessels. However, with age the sympathetic response is delayed, causing low blood pressure and subsequent orthostatic hypotension. When blood pressure rises, the parasympathetic pathway helps to slow the heart rate. But with age this function declines, resulting in elevated blood pressure as well as a decrease in the time required to return to homeostasis (Digiovanna, 1994, 2000). Autonomic neuron age-related changes can also affect thermoregulation. The sympathetic pathway normally acts to constrict blood vessels, thereby preventing heat loss in cold conditions. However, with age there is a decline in this action and this decline, together with age-related changes in blood vessels, results in increased risk of hypothermia (Digiovanna, 1994, 2000). Other age-related changes in the autonomic pathway that affect vision, swallowing, and sexual arousal will be covered in other sections of this chapter.

Injury Responsiveness

Throughout life, peripheral nerve injury is usually repaired through new axon growth and nerve reinnervation of the damaged area, but age decreases these reparative properties (Beers & Berkow, n.d.). These changes in the peripheral nervous system cause older individuals to become slower in detecting and recognizing stimuli, thereby making actions and reactions more difficult (Digiovanna, 1994).

The nervous system remains the most integral organ system in the body due to its influence on every other organ system. Age-related changes that occur at the central and peripheral nerve levels can directly and indirectly influence the homeostasis of the entire body. When observing an age-related change in the older adult, professionals need to broaden their scope of observation to integrate other body systems so that they may better understand the aging changes in the person as a whole.

The Endocrine System

The endocrine system consists of various glands, groups of cells that produce and secrete chemical messengers known as **hormones**. Hormones transfer information from one set of cells to another as they work to maintain overall homeostasis and regulate the body's growth, metabolism, and sexual development and function. The major glands comprising the endocrine system are the hypothalamus, pituitary gland, thyroid, parathyroids, pineal gland, adrenal glands, and the reproductive glands (ovaries and testes). The pancreas together with its hormones is also considered part of the endocrine system. Age-related changes to the endocrine system as a whole are best presented through individual discussion of the glands, their hormones, and the functions they perform.

The Hypothalamus and Pituitary Gland

The hypothalamus is a collection of cells located in the lower, central portion of the brain, and it provides a link between the nervous system and endocrine system. Nerves within the hypothalamus produce **hypophysiotropic** hormones that either stimulate or suppress the secretion of hormones from the pituitary gland. Thus, the hypothalamus acts primarily as a mechanism of control for pituitary hormone secretion. The hypothalamus provides hormonal messages to the pituitary, which in turn produces and secretes its own hormones.

The pituitary gland, only the size of a pea, is located just below the hypothalamus at the base of the brain. It is often termed the "master gland" because it produces hormones that regulate numerous other endocrine glands. These regulatory hormones include growth hormone, vasopressin, thyrotropin, and corticotropin. Growth hormone and vasopressin will be discussed here, and thyrotropin and corticotropin will be discussed with the thyroid and adrenal glands, respectively.

Growth Hormone. Growth hormone (GH) is released from the pituitary gland in response to growth hormone–releasing hormone (GRH) secreted by the hypothalamus. GH stimulates the uptake of amino acids into cells and the synthesis of proteins from these amino acids. In so doing, GH promotes the growth of bone, muscle, and other body tissues. Growth hormone also plays a role in the body's handling of nutrients because it causes increased breakdown of fat for energy. In addition, GH is known to act antagonistically to insulin and increase blood sugar levels. (See the discussion of the pancreas and its function later in this chapter.)

Evidence suggests that with advancing age there is a decline in the level of GH. The reason for this observed decline has not been well defined, but may involve changes in the diurnal rhythm of GH secretion or decreases in GRH output from the hypothalamus (Russell-Aulet, Jaffe, Mott-Friberg, & Barkans, 1999). In young adults, GH secretion and blood levels of GH rise during the night, reaching a nocturnal peak during the first 4 hours of sleep (P. S. Timiras, 2003a), and taper off toward morning, with GH levels reaching a minimum during the day. Results from studies examining age-related changes in GH show an overall decrease in nightly GH secretion as well as a dampening of the hormone's nocturnal peak (Prinz, Weitzman, Cunningham, & Karacan, 1983). It is thought that over time the nightly increase in GH secretion may cease completely and become constant at all times (Digiovanna, 1994). Whatever the mechanisms behind it, the age-related decline in GH is of great importance because it contributes to age-associated loss of muscle mass, decreased bone formation, reduced protein synthesis, reduced tissue repair, and decline in immune function (Chahal & Drake, 2007; P. S. Timiras, 2003a).

Vasopressin. Vasopressin, also known as antidiuretic hormone (ADH), is secreted by neurons that originate in the hypothalamus and extend into the pituitary gland. Vasopressin works to regulate homeostatic levels of osmotic pressure and blood pressure. The release of vasopressin is stimulated by either a decrease in blood pressure or an increase in osmotic pressure. Once secreted, vasopressin promotes water reabsorption by the kidneys. This reabsorption of water prevents increases in the body's osmotic pressure and helps to maintain a substantial blood volume, thereby preventing blood pressure from becoming too low. Vasopressin secretion also helps to maintain blood pressure by stimulating the constriction of blood vessels. The release of vasopressin is inhibited by increased blood pressure or decreased osmotic pressure as well as by alcohol. Decreased levels of vasopressin result in the loss of water through the urine. This fluid loss leads to increases in osmotic pressure as well as decreases in blood volume and blood pressure.

With age there is an average increase in levels of circulating vasopressin. However, this age-related increase does not produce a subsequent rise in water reabsorption as would be expected, possibly due to the loss of vasopressin receptor responsiveness noted in the genitourinary section (Johnson et al., 2003; P. S. Timiras, 2003a). The reason for this is unclear, but most research suggests that the failure to respond to increased vasopressin levels with increased water reabsorption occurs primarily in individuals with kidney infections or hypertension and, thus, should not be viewed as a usual characteristic of the aging process (P. S. Timiras, 2003a). In general, age-related changes in vasopressin levels are not known to have significant effects on body homeostasis. Furthermore, the ability of vasopressin to respond appropriately to low blood pressure remains unchanged with age.

The Thyroid Gland

T4 and T3

The **thyroid** is a small, butterfly-shaped gland located in the lower front portion of the neck. The secretion of the thyroid hormones, **thyroxine (T4)** and **triiodothyronine (T3)**, occurs through collaboration with the hypothalamus and pituitary glands. The hypothalamus produces and secretes thyrotropin-releasing hormone (TRH), which in turn stimulates the secretion of thyroid-stimulating hormone (TSH) from the pituitary gland. Finally, TSH stimulates the synthesis and secretion of T4 and T3. Utilizing a negative feedback loop, T4 and T3 inhibit TSH secretion. Thus, with higher levels of T4 and T3, levels of TSH are lower and vice versa. In addition to its role of regulating the T4 and T3 levels, TSH acts to maintain the growth and structural integrity of the thyroid gland. An absence or deficit of TSH results in atrophy of the thyroid (P. S. Timiras, 2003c).

During the early years of life, the thyroid gland is essential for growth of the whole body and its organs as well as development and maturation of the central nervous system. In adulthood, however, the thyroid functions mainly to regulate the body's metabolic rate. T4 and T3 both promote an increase in metabolic rate. Heat is a by-product of the metabolic process and, hence, increased metabolic rate leads to an increase in heat production. Thus, the thyroid hormones also act to regulate body temperature. The thyroid gland is not essential for life (P. S. Timiras, 2003c); however, without this gland there is a slowing of the metabolic rate, general lethargy, and a poor resistance to cold. In contrast, abnormally high levels of the thyroid hormones result in a potentially dangerous elevation of metabolic rate.

As the body ages, thyroid hormone levels decrease slightly yet remain in the lower range of normal. Because there is less negative feedback, due to lower T3 and T4 levels, the level of TSH increases with age (Tortora & Derrickson, 2006). Borderline abnormal values of T4, T3, and TSH are more common in women than men (P. S. Timiras, 2003c). However, there is a large degree of variability in these hormone levels among older adults, and hormone levels may depend on age and general health as well as gender. Yet, in general, the ability of the thyroid and its hormones to provide metabolic and thermal regulation is not impaired with age.

CALCITONIN

Most thyroid cells produce T4 and T3, but some cells—known as c cells—produce a hormone called **calcitonin**. Calcitonin promotes a decrease in blood calcium by stimulating increased uptake of calcium by bone-forming cells. Conversely, calcitonin inhibits the action of cells involved in the breakdown of bone. Unlike secretion of T4 and T3, calcitonin secretion does not involve the hypothalamus or pituitary. Instead, calcitonin release is regulated by blood calcium levels. High levels of calcium trigger the secretion of calcitonin. Calcitonin then causes calcium to be removed from the blood, thereby lowering blood calcium levels. The lower calcium levels then feed back and inhibit calcitonin secretion.

Little is known about age-related changes in calcitonin; however, there have been some reports of decreased calcitonin levels with age. Such a decrease would have profound effects on older persons' risk of osteoporosis given the effects of calcitonin on bone formation and breakdown.

The Parathyroid Gland

The **parathyroid gland** consists of groups of cells located on the back of the thyroid gland. The parathyroid gland secretes a hormone known as **parathyroid hormone (PTH)**. PTH acts antagonistically to calcitonin, and homeostasis of blood calcium depends heavily on a proper balance between PTH and calcitonin. PTH release is stimulated by low blood calcium levels whereas elevated calcium levels inhibit PTH secretion. Thus, PTH works to raise blood calcium levels. It does this through a variety of mechanisms including the removal of calcium from bone, the decline of calcium release into the urine by the kidneys, and the activation of vitamin D by the kidneys, which in turn stimulates calcium absorption by the small intestine. Blood levels of PTH increase with aging, possibly due to decreases in calcium intake (Tortora & Derrickson, 2006).

In children and young adults, calcium levels are maintained through the consumption and subsequent intestinal absorption of dietary calcium. At these ages maintenance of blood calcium levels has no effect on bone (P. S. Timiras, 2003c). However, in older persons calcium levels are maintained primarily through calcium reabsorption from bone. The reason for this shift in mechanisms of calcium level regulation is not fully understood. However, it is thought that with age, PTH may have a decreased ability to stimulate production of active vitamin D by the kidneys and/or that active vitamin D may be impaired in its ability to stimulate intestinal absorption of calcium.

The Pineal Gland

The **pineal gland**, a tiny gland located deep within the brain, secretes the hormone **melatonin**. Secretion of melatonin is highly influenced by light properties, including light intensity, length of light exposure, and light wavelength (i.e., color; Digiovanna, 1994). Detection of increased light exposure (day) inhibits melatonin secretion whereas detection of decreased light exposure (night) stimulates hormone secretion. Hence, blood levels of melatonin follow a diurnal rhythm with hormone levels highest at night and lowest during the day. It is melatonin that synchronizes internal body functions with a day–night cycle that shifts in response to seasonal changes in the length of the day–night cycle (P. S. Timiras, 2003c; Tortora & Derrickson, 2006).

Age is accompanied by a decline in melatonin levels. This decline can have a negative impact on other diurnal rhythms such as sleep patterns. Melatonin is known to reach peak concentrations during sleep, and administration of doses of melatonin equivalent to nighttime levels have been shown to promote and sustain sleep (P. S. Timiras, 2003c). Thus, age-related declines in melatonin may be linked to the poor sleep quality and insomnia of some elderly persons.

The Adrenal Glands

The **adrenal glands** are paired glands located above the kidneys. Each gland is composed of an outer region known as the adrenal cortex and an inner region known as the adrenal medulla.

The Adrenal Cortex

The **adrenal cortex** secretes three types of hormones: **glucocorticoids**, **mineralocorticoids**, and sex hormones. Secretion of both glucocorticoids and sex hormones from the adrenal cortex is stimulated by pituitary **adrenocorticotropic hormone (ACTH)**. The secretion of ACTH follows a diurnal rhythm and is itself stimulated by **corticotropin-releasing hormone (CRH)** from the hypothalamus. Thus, release of glucocorticoids and sex hormones from the adrenal cortex relies on a hypothalamic-pituitary-adrenal pathway or axis.

Glucocorticoids. Glucocorticoids have several metabolic functions. These include increased amino acid uptake and glucose production by the liver, decreased amino acid uptake and protein synthesis in muscle, inhibition of somatic (nonreproductive) cell growth, suppression of growth hormone secretion from the pituitary gland, and mobilization of lipids and cholesterol. Glucocorticoids also have anti-inflammatory actions including the inhibition of inflammatory and allergic reactions.

The primary glucocorticoid in humans is **cortisol**. Cortisol is synthesized from cholesterol, and its synthesis follows the diurnal rhythm of ACTH release. Cortisol levels are highest in the early morning hours and lowest in the evening. However, both ACTH and cortisol can be secreted independent of this diurnal rhythm under periods of physical or psychological stress (Aeron Biotechnology, 2005). Cortisol is, in fact, often referred to as the stress hormone because it promotes the production of increased energy necessary for dealing with stress.

When cortisol is secreted it stimulates a breakdown of muscle protein, releasing amino acids that can in turn be used by the liver to produce glucose for energy. Cortisol also makes fatty acids, an energy source from fat cells, available for use. The net effect is an increase in energy supply that allows the brain to more effectively coordinate the body's response to a stressor. The increased energy supply also helps the muscles to respond quickly and efficiently to a stressor or threat that requires a physical response.

Early research suggested that cortisol secretion decreases slightly with advancing age, but that this decreased secretion is compensated for by a simultaneous decrease in cortisol excretion from the body. As a result, normal cortisol levels would be maintained as a person ages. More recent studies, however, suggest that as long as individuals are healthy, cortisol secretion remains unchanged with age (P. S. Timiras, 2003a, 2003c).

Studies conducted in animals have provided evidence that under stressful conditions corticosterone (equivalent to the human cortisol) is more elevated among old than young animals. In addition, this elevated level persists for a longer period of time in some older animals. It has been hypothesized that the high levels of corticosterone following a stressor represent a loss of resiliency of the HPA axis such that the axis fails to decrease ACTH in response to elevated corticosterone levels and, consequently, fails to stop corticosterone release once the stress has passed. In rats, there is evidence that the elevated levels of corticosterone may be toxic to the brain, particularly the hippocampus. To date there is little evidence to support an age-related decline in the competence of the HPA axis among humans. However, given the age-associated changes found in animal models, further study of the changes in the HPA axis among older humans is warranted (P. S. Timiras, 2003a).

Clearly, glucocorticoids stimulate a beneficial response during times of stress. However, glucocorticoids also have some undesirable effects including suppression of cartilage and bone formation, stimulation of bone demineralization, inhibition of portions of the immune response, and promotion of gastrointestinal tract bleeding and ulcer formation (Digiovanna, 1994). When glucocorticoids are administered therapeutically for their anti-inflammatory effects, their concentration in the blood can rise to extremely high levels. Excessively high levels of glucocorticoids exacerbate their aforementioned negative physiological effects. Given that older persons are generally at greater risk for osteoporosis and infection as well as high blood pressure, therapeutic administration of glucocorticoids in this population should be carefully monitored.

Mineralocorticoids. The mineralocorticoids derive their name from their critical role in regulating extracellular concentrations of minerals, principally sodium and potassium. The primary mineralocorticoid is aldosterone, which targets the kidneys. Aldosterone has three major physiological effects: increased renal reabsorption of sodium or decreased urinary secretion of sodium, increased renal reabsorption of water and consequent expansion of extracellular fluid volume, and increased renal excretion of potassium. These physiological effects of aldosterone aid in the maintenance of fluid–electrolyte balance within the body. In addition, aldosterone helps to maintain blood pressure through its effects on sodium and water retention and increased fluid (i.e., blood) volume (P. S. Timiras, 2003a).

Secretion of aldosterone is stimulated primarily through the release of the enzyme renin from the kidneys and activation of the renin-angiotensin-aldosterone system. Renin is released in response to low blood pressure, increased osmotic pressure, and adverse changes in sodium concentrations. Once released, renin promotes the production of angiotensin, a peptide that then stimulates secretion of aldosterone (P. S. Timiras, 2003a). Conversely, high blood pressure, decreased osmotic pressure, and favorable changes in sodium concentrations will inhibit the release of renin and activation of the renin-angiotensin system. As a result, the production and release of aldosterone is suppressed (Digiovanna, 1994).

The stimulation and suppression of aldosterone also have secondary regulatory mechanisms. The release of aldosterone is secondarily stimulated by pituitary ACTH. Suppression of aldosterone release is secondarily controlled by high sodium concentrations, potassium deficiency, and the release of atrial natriuretic factor, a hormone released by the heart in response to increased blood volume (Digiovanna, 1994).

Aldosterone levels decrease with age. The primary reason for this decrease is thought to be a decline in renin activity and subsequent decline in the activity of the renin-angiotensin-aldosterone system. The release of aldosterone in response to ACTH does not appear to undergo age-related changes (University of California Academic Geriatric Resource Program, 2004). Because aldosterone stimulates sodium retention, decreased levels of aldosterone predispose older persons to sodium loss and possible hyponatremia, a condition characterized by water–mineral imbalance.

In addition to the overall decrease in aldosterone levels, older persons have an impaired ability to increase aldosterone secretion and aldosterone blood levels when necessary. Thus, there is a decline in aldosterone reserve capacity. This decline is not due to age-related changes in the adrenal cortex; rather, it is thought to be the result of decreased ability of the kidneys to secrete renin when needed (Digiovanna, 1994).

Adrenal Sex Hormones. The primary adrenal sex hormone of interest among aging persons is **dehydroepiandrosterone (DHEA)**. DHEA is, in fact, the most abundant hormone in the human body (Chahal & Drake, 2007; Shealy, 1995, Yen & Laughlin, 1998). As a neurosteroid, it is thought that DHEA may have antidiabetic, anti-obesity, cardioprotective, and immune-enhancing properties (Chahal & Drake, 2007; Yen & Laughlin, 1998). The exact physiological function of DHEA is not well understood; however, it is known to convert to a multitude of other hormones, mainly the sex hormones testosterone and estrogen. The major effects of DHEA are largely the result of the actions of those hormones to which it is converted (Dhatariya & Nair, 2003).

DHEA levels are high at birth but then undergo a precipitous drop until between the 6th and 10th year of life, at which time DHEA levels begin to steadily increase, achieving maximal concentrations during the third decade (Arlt, 2004). By age 70–80 years DHEA levels are only 5–10% of peak values achieved in early adulthood (Hinson & Raven, 1999). Very low levels of DHEA are also observed in a variety of often age-related disease states including diabetes, cardiovascular disease, Alzheimer's disease, and various cancers. Thus, DHEA appears to be one of the most critical hormones in predicting disease. It has been hypothesized that low DHEA levels may be a marker of poor health status and, as a result, are associated with not only increased risk of disease, but also increased mortality (Arlt, 2004). As a result of DHEA's association with aging and disease, DHEA replacement has been touted as a means of slowing, if not reversing, the aging process as well as the chronic disease and disability with which it is often accompanied.

DHEA replacement studies in humans have produced equivocal results. For example, research has shown positive effects of DHEA replacement on muscle strength and body composition including increased muscle strength and decreased fat mass. Positive effects on bone, including increased bone mineral density, have also been demonstrated. However, numerous other studies have found no change in muscle strength, body composition, or bone density with DHEA replacement (Dhatariya & Nair, 2003). Overall, there is no consensus regarding the benefits of DHEA replacement. Although low levels of DHEA may predispose an individual to disease, there is no evidence that these low levels of DHEA cause disease. In addition, most studies of DHEA replacement have been short term and, thus, there is a paucity of information regarding the benefits (or risks) of DHEA use over long periods of time (Hinson & Raven, 1999). DHEA is currently available without a prescription, but given the relative lack of information regarding the risks and benefits of its use, especially in the long term, caution should be taken in self-administration of the hormone without medical supervision.

Adrenal Medulla

The **adrenal medulla** is part of the sympathetic division of the autonomic nervous system. Hormones called **catecholamines**, mainly **epinephrine** (adrenaline) and norepinephrine (noradrenaline), are produced in the adrenal medulla and released in response to sympathetic nervous system activity. Much like cortisol, epinephrine and norepinephrine play a critical role in the body's stress response, and their release is greatly increased under stressful conditions. Major physiological effects mediated by epinephrine and norepinephrine hormones include increased heart rate and blood pressure, increased metabolic rate, and increased blood glucose levels and hence increased energy. There is also an inhibition of nonessential activities such as gastrointestinal secretion. This preparing of the body to respond to stress or threat is often termed the "fight or flight" response. Activation of adrenal medullary hormones is stimulated through a variety of means including low blood sugar, hemorrhage, threat of bodily harm, emotional distress, and even exercise.

With aging there is a decrease in epinephrine secretion from the adrenal medulla. One study has reported that, under resting conditions, epinephrine secretion is 40% less in older men as compared to younger men; however, there is a 20% simultaneous age-related decrease in epinephrine clearance from the circulation (Esler, Kaye et al., 1995). As a result, levels of epinephrine concentration do not change significantly with age (Seals & Esler, 2000). Mechanisms for the age-related decline in epinephrine secretion have not been well investigated. Hypothesized mechanisms include 1) age-related attenuation in the adrenal medulla's response to nervous system activity, and 2) an overall age-associated decrease in nervous system activity to the adrenal medulla. It also has been hypothesized that reduced epinephrine secretion with age may be the result of decreased synthesis and storage of epinephrine in the adrenal medulla (Seals & Esler, 2000).

Under stressful conditions there is a characteristic increase in epinephrine secretion. This increase is markedly attenuated in older persons. Research has found that the increase in epinephrine secretion in response to a stressor is reduced by 33–44% in older men as compared to their younger counterparts (Seals & Esler, 2000). Thus, the ability of the adrenal medulla to effectively respond to stressful situations is greatly impaired, even in healthy older adults.

Reproductive Hormones

Please refer to the previous discussion of the reproductive system for a review of age-related changes in the reproductive axis and female and male reproductive hormones.

The Pancreas

The hormone-secreting cells of the pancreas occur in tiny clusters known as the **islets of Langerhans**. Four islet cell types have been identified: the alpha (A), beta (B), delta (D), and pancreatic polypeptide (PP) cells. These cells secrete, respectively, **glucagon**, insulin, somatostatin, and pancreatic polypeptide. Of these hormones, only insulin is secreted exclusively by its cell type (B cells). The other hormones are also secreted by the gastrointestinal mucosa, and somatostatin can be found in the brain. The function of PP cells has not been well identified, and therefore will not be discussed here.

Both insulin and glucagon are integral parts of metabolism regulation, and their secretion is regulated principally by blood glucose levels. High blood glucose levels stimulate the release of insulin and inhibit glucagon secretion. The released insulin then stimulates the cells of the body to absorb an amount of glucose from the blood that is sufficient to meet the body's energy needs. It also acts to promote storage of excess glucose in the liver, muscle, and fat cells and to suppress the release of this stored glucose. The result is a lowering of blood glucose levels. Conversely, low blood glucose levels stimulate glucagon release and inhibit insulin secretion. Secreted glucagon then promotes the release of stored glucose, and the result is a rise in blood glucose level. Somatostatin can inhibit the release of both insulin and glucagon, but the overall role of this hormone in regulation of blood glucose levels has not been firmly established.

Blood Glucose Levels

Blood glucose level is generally expressed as the amount (in milligrams) of glucose per deciliter (100 ml) of blood. According to the guidelines of the American Diabetes Association (ADA), normal fasting plasma glucose (FPG) level is below 100 mg/dl. When the FPG level lies between 100 and 125 mg/dl, an individual is said to have impaired fasting glucose, or impaired glucose tolerance, meaning that he or she is unable to reverse a dramatic rise in blood glucose levels and restore glucose homeostasis. An FPG of >126 mg/dl indicates a diagnosis of diabetes (American Diabetes Association, 2005).

In addition to the FPG, a person's ability to respond to increased blood glucose levels can also be measured by the oral glucose tolerance test (OGTT). The OGTT involves drinking a solution of concentrated glucose after having fasted for at least 10 hours. Blood glucose levels are measured at the beginning of the test and then periodically thereafter for 3 hours. Individuals with normal glucose tolerance will exhibit a rise in glucose levels following consumption of the glucose solution, but glucose levels will return to normal within 2 hours. In persons with impaired glucose tolerance, blood glucose levels will remain high for longer than 2 hours. According to ADA guidelines, a person whose blood glucose level is 140 mg/dl or less after 2 hours is considered to have a normal glucose response. A person whose blood glucose level falls to between 140 and 199 mg/dl after 2 hours is said to be glucose intolerant. When, after 2 hours, blood glucose levels are elevated to 200 mg/dl or above, a person has diabetes (American Diabetes Association, 2005).

Age-Related Glucose Intolerance

First documented by Spence (1921) and since confirmed by numerous others, biological aging is associated with a decline in **glucose tolerance**. This decline is generally associated with impaired response to a glucose challenge such as the OGTT rather than with fasting glucose levels. Although a small rise in fasting glucose of 1–2 mg/dl per decade has been observed by some, it is postprandial (following a meal) glucose levels that show the greatest increase, up to 15 mg/dl per decade (Morrow & Halter, 1994). Thus, the glucose intolerance of aging is associated primarily with response to glucose challenge or oral glucose load (Jackson, 1990). Approximately 40% of individuals ages 65 to 74 years have some degree of impairment in glucose homeostasis. This percentage rises to 50% in those over the age of 80 years (Harris, 1990; Minaker, 1990). The altered glucose metabolism that comes with increased age has potentially important pathophysiological consequences, because these age-related changes have been associated with an accumulation of advanced glycosylation end products (AGEs) that are believed to contribute to varying age-related pathologies as well as long-term complications in those who have diabetes (Halter, 2000). Mechanisms proposed as contributing to age-related glucose intolerance include impaired insulin secretion, insulin resistance, and alterations in glucose counterregulation.

Insulin Secretion. Studies of the effects of aging on insulin secretion provide some evidence that aging may be associated with subtle impairment in insulin release (Chen, Halter, & Porte, 1987). Other research, however, has found no alteration in insulin secretion with age (Peters & Davidson, 1997), and overall, results from various studies have provided equivocal results regarding the role of insulin secretion in the impaired glucose tolerance of aging. Although the inability to secrete sufficient amounts of insulin to overcome the heightened blood glucose levels and insulin resistance associated with aging may contribute to the phenomenon, impaired insulin secretion is generally not regarded as the primary cause of age-related glucose intolerance.

Insulin Resistance. A defect in insulin action is generally presented as the greatest contributing factor in impaired glucose tolerance among elderly persons. Evidence suggests that the primary effect of the aging process on glucose homeostasis is the development of a resistance to the actions of insulin, that is, **insulin resistance** (Peters & Davidson, 1997). This resistance leads to an impaired ability to suppress glucose release from the liver as well as an impaired glucose uptake, with the latter defect predominating. Skeletal muscle is considered the primary site of the impaired glucose uptake (Jackson, 1990). The mechanism(s) through which this impairment develops is still poorly understood. However, because insulin receptors on cell membranes appear to be unchanged with age (Fink, Kolterman, Griffin, & Olefsky, 1983; Rowe, Minaker, Pallotta, & Flier, 1983), the principal cause of resistance to insulin uptake is assumed to be a postreceptor defect. It is hypothesized this defect may involve the transportation of glucose from the membrane receptor into the cell. Glucose uptake in virtually all cells is mediated by transporter proteins. **GLUT4** is an insulin-mediated transporter located within vesicles in the cells' cytoplasm. Upon stimulation by insulin, these vesicles travel to the cell membrane and release the GLUT4 transporters, which in turn serve as a port of cell entry for glucose. In the absence of insulin stimulation, GLUT4 is transferred back to vesicles and the entry of glucose is slowed (Czech, Erwin, & Sleeman, 1996). Thus, GLUT4 plays a central role in the maintenance of glucose homeostasis, and it is hypothesized that impaired GLUT4 synthesis, transfer, and activity may lead to insulin resistance (Halter, 2000).

Glucose Counterregulation. Research has reported that glucose counterregulation by glucagon, as well as other hormones—such as epinephrine, cortisol, and growth hormone—that tend to raise blood glucose levels, is impaired in healthy elderly individuals (Marker, Cryer, & Clutter, 1992; Meneilly, Cheung, & Tuokko, 1994b). Rather than contributing to an elevation of plasma glucose levels, such a defect in glucose counterregulation results in delayed recovery from the hypoglycemic (low blood sugar) state. Thus, the impaired glucose homeostasis characterizing aging is marked not only by elevated fasting plasma glucose but also by periods of prolonged hypoglycemia. The latter gains even greater importance when it is recognized that in comparison to younger subjects, elders demonstrate reduced awareness of the autonomic warning signs of hypoglycemia (Meneilly, Cheung, & Tuokko, 1994a). Furthermore, they exhibit impaired psychomotor performance during hypoglycemic episodes and thus are less likely to take the action necessary to return glucose levels to normal even if they are aware of the existing hypoglycemia (Meneilly, 2001).

Confounding Factors of the Glucose Intolerance of Aging

A general consensus exists that the processes of biological and physiological aging are themselves the most important contributors to impaired glucose homeostasis among elders (Meneilly, 2001). However, other factors exist that may contribute to the severity of the impairment. These include genetic predisposition (Halter, 2000) as well as various lifestyle and environmental factors.

Adiposity. Aging is associated with a decrease in lean body mass (Peters & Davidson, 1997) and an overall increase in adiposity as well as a redistribution of adipose tissue to the intra-abdominal region (Kotz, Billington, & Levine, 1999). This tissue redistribution places the elderly population at increased risk for development of insulin resistance and glucose intolerance because clinical studies have shown that persons with this adipose distribution pattern exhibit greater insulin resistance as well as increased risk of diabetes (Despres & Marette, 1999; Garg, 1999). Research shows that adipose tissue in the abdominal region is metabolically more active than that in other regions of the body due to elevated fatty acid concentrations in this area (Bjorntorp, 1997; Garg, 1999). It is hypothesized that this increased metabolic activity may be the cause of the increased insulin resistance associated with overweight and obesity (Despres & Marette, 1999). Indeed, it has been shown that older people who are classified as having normal glucose tolerance have less adiposity, particularly less intra-abdominal or central adiposity, and they do not experience a detectable difference in sensitivity to insulin (Halter, 2000).

Physical Activity. Physical activity is known to increase insulin action through heightened insulin sensitivity (Dela, Mikines, & Galbo, 1999; Jackson, 1990). Thus, decreased levels of physical activity may contribute to the development of insulin resistance. Aging is generally associated with declines in functional mobility and a decrease in physical activity, thereby placing elders at greater risk for impaired glucose tolerance. Older individuals with greater degrees of physical activity exhibit better glucose tolerance and less evidence of insulin resistance than do less active older people (Halter, 2000). It has been shown that glucose uptake is high in elderly athletes and low in bed-ridden elders compared with elderly controls (Dela et al., 1999). Furthermore, among elders endurance training has been shown to produce improvements in insulin-mediated glucose uptake similar to those observed in young subjects (Dela et al., 1999). It must be noted, however, that elders who are more physically active are also more likely to have less body fat and less central adiposity (Halter, 2000). Thus, it is most likely the combined effects of reduced abdominal adiposity and increased levels of physical activity that give rise to greater insulin sensitivity and glucose tolerance.

Diet. There is some evidence that impaired glucose tolerance in aging may be due at least in part to the diminished dietary carbohydrate intake often observed in elderly persons (Peters & Davidson, 1997). It has been shown that increased carbohydrate intake improves glucose tolerance in both young and old subjects. However, the older subjects exhibit decreased glucose tolerance at each level of matched carbohydrate intake when compared to the younger population (Chen et al., 1987). This idea is supported by studies showing that when old and young subjects are fed diets comparable in carbohydrate levels, age differences in glucose tolerance, insulin secretion, and insulin action are diminished but still persistent (Halter, 2000). Thus, age itself appears to be correlated with decreased glucose tolerance. However, poor levels of dietary carbohydrate intake are likely to exacerbate the age-related impairments in glucose metabolism.

Polypharmacy. Several pharmacologic agents are known to affect glucose metabolism, and older adults are frequent users of such agents. Therefore, when evaluating alterations in blood glucose levels among elders, their medication regimens must be considered and attention must be paid to potential drug interactions (Minaker, 1990; Morley & Perry, 1991). Drugs known to affect glucose metabolism include, but are not limited to, β-blockers, calcium channel blockers, glucocorticoids, and other nonpharmacologic agents such as alcohol, caffeine, and nicotine (Bressler & DeFronzo, 1997). Furthermore, in treating the elderly diabetic patient, sulphonylureas should be used with caution. These pharmacologic agents stimulate insulin secretion and can contribute to the development of hypoglycemia (Graal & Wolffenbuttel, 1999). In addition, the interaction of sulphonylureas with some drugs can increase the hypoglycemic effect of the sulphonylureas (Peters & Davidson, 1997). Thus, elderly persons are at increased risk for the development of prolonged hypoglycemia when treated with sulphonylureas.

THE MUSCLE

The body's muscular system is composed of three types of muscle—skeletal muscle, smooth muscle, and cardiac muscle. **Skeletal muscles**, examples of which include the bicep, tricep, quadricep, hamstring, and gastrocnemius (calf) muscle, make up the majority of the body's overall muscle mass. Skeletal muscle is also the muscle type in which most age-related changes occur. Thus, skeletal muscle and its changes with age will be the focus of our discussion about the aging muscle.

Skeletal Muscle: Structure and Function

Skeletal muscles are composed of several thin muscle bundles (**Figure 6-17**). These bundles are held together with connective tissue but are able to move independently of one another (Arking, 1998). The muscle bundles are composed of several muscle fibers, each of which is formed from the fusion of numerous individual **myofibrils**.

Myofibrils contain two types of protein molecules—**actins** and **myosins**. Actin and myosin molecules are arranged in a parallel, overlapping manner within compartments called **sarcomeres**. The overlap of actin and myosin within the sarcomere results in a pattern of alternating light and dark bands, which accounts for the striated, or striped, appearance of skeletal muscle. In a state of rest, actin molecules overlap both ends of the myosin molecules, which are centered within the sarcomere. Muscle contraction results when actin molecules are pulled toward the center of the sarcomere in a ratcheting motion (**Figure 6-18**). This contraction of skeletal muscle is controlled by an individual's own volition; hence, skeletal muscle has also been termed voluntary muscle.

Although muscle fibers have a common basic structure, they can be divided into two distinct physiological types, **fast-twitch fibers** and **slow-twitch fibers**. These two fiber types produce the same amount of force per contraction; however, they produce this force at different rates. White fast-twitch fibers contract quickly and provide short bursts of energy, but they fatigue quickly. As a result of these contractile properties, fast-twitch fibers are generally used for high-intensity, low-endurance, generally anaerobic activities such as sprinting and weight lifting. Red slow-twitch fibers contract slowly but steadily and are not easily fatigued. Therefore, these fibers are best suited for use in aerobic activities of low intensity but high endurance, such as long-distance running. Slow-twitch fibers are also used for postural activities, such as the supporting of the head by the neck.

Every person is born with a fixed ratio of fast-twitch to slow-twitch muscle fibers. However, the ratio may vary from one body location to another, and one person may have a greater ratio of fast-twitch to slow-twitch fibers in a particular location than does another person. This phenomenon is part of what can result in one individual being, for example, a better sprinter or better long-distance runner than another.

Notable Quotes

"Men do not quit playing because they grow old; they grow old because they quit playing."

—Oliver Wendell Holmes

Aging of the Skeletal Muscle

Sarcopenia

A reduction in muscle mass occurs to at least some degree in all elderly persons as compared to young, healthy, physically active young adults (Roubenoff, 2001; Tortora & Derrickson, 2006). This reduction in muscle mass is known as **sarcopenia** (from the Greek meaning poverty of flesh) and is distinct from muscle loss due to disease or starvation. One population-based study estimated that the prevalence of sarcopenia rises from 13–24% in individuals under the age of 70 years to greater than 50% in persons over the age of 80 years (Baumgartner et al., 1998). Sarcopenia is of great consequence to older persons because it is associated with tremendous increases in functional disability and frailty. Older sarcopenic men are reported to have 4.1 times higher rates and women 3.6 times higher rates of disability than their gender specific counterparts with normal muscle mass (Baumgartner et al., 1998).

FIGURE 6-17 **Structure of the skeletal muscle fiber, myofibril and sarcomere.**

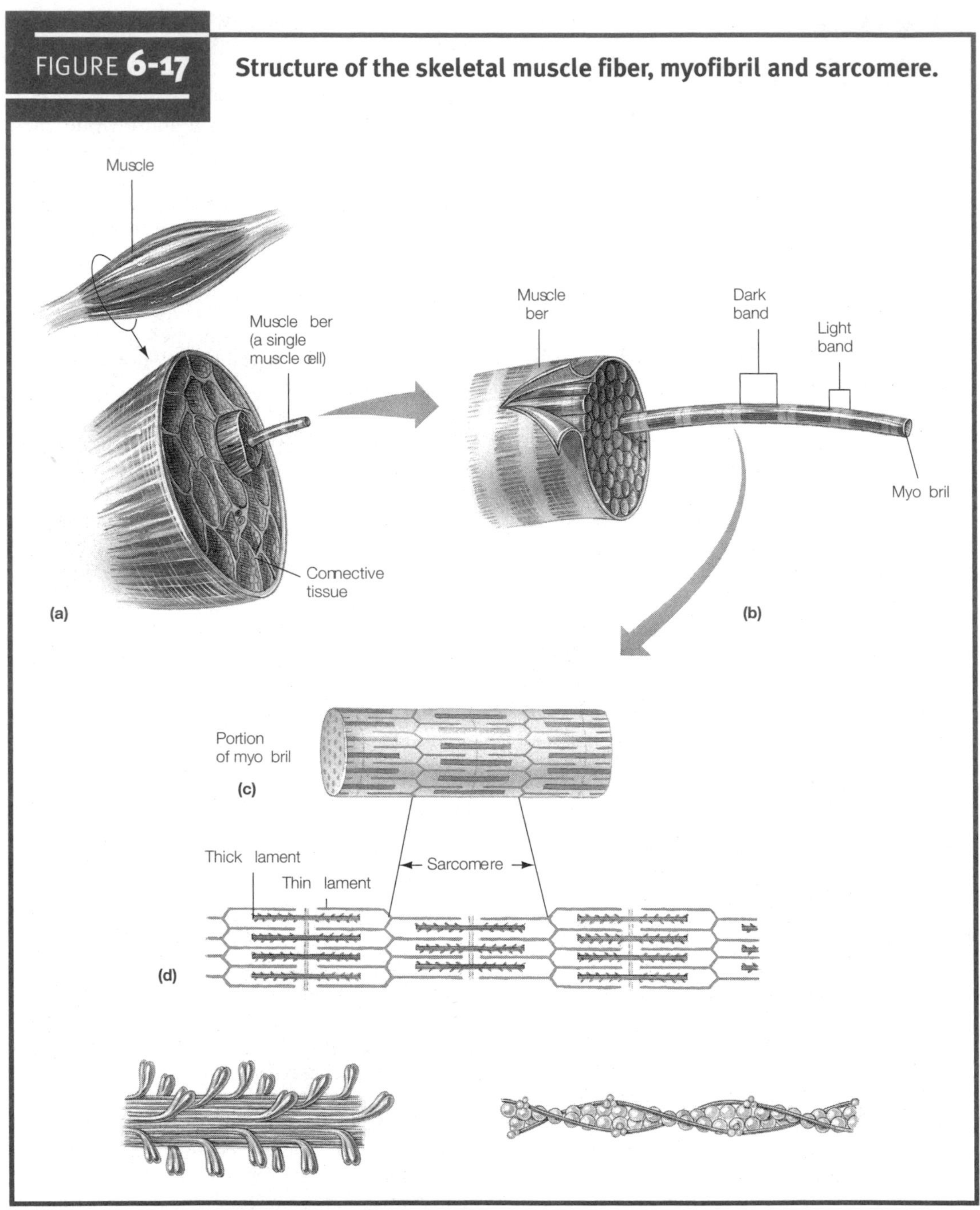

SOURCE: Human Biology, 5e. Daniel D. Chiras, Jones and Bartlett Publishers 2005.

FIGURE 6-18 The interaction of actin and myosin to produce skeletal muscle contraction. Inorganic phosphate (P_i) and ADP may be released during the contraction.

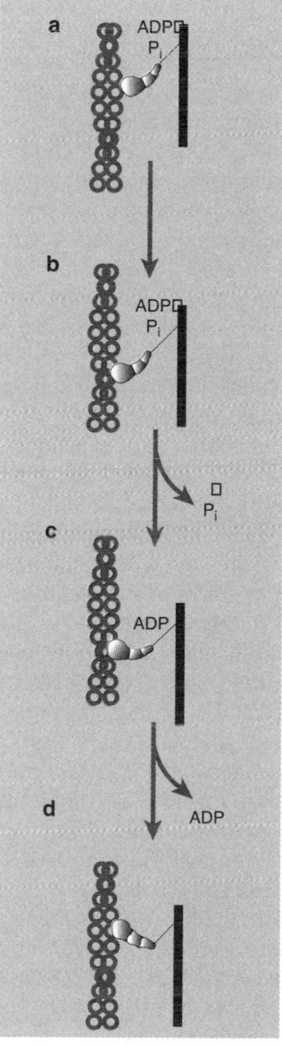

SOURCE: Reprinted with permission from Nature Publishing Group.

The total cross-sectional area of skeletal muscle is reported to decrease by as much as 40% between the ages of 20 and 60 years (Doherty, 2003), with the greatest loss occurring in the lower limbs (Doherty, 2003; Vandervoot & Symons, 2001). Men are known to have greater total muscle mass than women; however, men experience greater relative muscle loss with age than do their female counterparts (Janssen, Heymsfield, Wang, & Ross, 2000). The reason for this gender difference has not been clearly defined, but it is postulated to relate to hormonal factors (Janssen et al., 2000). Although men experience greater relative muscle loss, it has been noted that sarcopenia may be of greater concern for older women given their longer life expectancy and higher rates of disability in old age (Roubenoff & Hughes, 2000).

Gender is not the only factor contributing to differences in the rate of sarcopenia. The loss of muscle mass is highly individualized and greatly dependent upon genetic, lifestyle, and other factors that influence the varied mechanisms proposed to underlie sarcopenia. The most commonly proposed mechanisms include a decline in the number and size of muscle fibers, loss of **motor units**, hormonal influences, altered protein synthesis, nutritional factors, and lack of physical activity, all of which are discussed below.

Changes in Muscle Fibers. With age, there is an overall loss in the number of both fast- and slow-twitch muscle fibers. By the ninth decade, approximately 50% fewer muscle fibers are present in the vastus lateralis muscle (the lateral portion of the quadriceps) than are observed in the same muscle of a 20-year-old (Lexell, Taylor, & Sjostrom, 1988). In addition, a reduction in the size of muscle fibers has been observed, with the greatest reduction seen in fast-twitch muscle fibers. Reduction in the size of fast-twitch fibers ranges from 20% to 50% with age, whereas slow-twitch fibers have been shown to reduce in size by only 1% to 25% as a person ages (Doherty, 2003).

Loss of Motor Units. Muscle fibers are innervated by motor nerves, which extend from the spinal cord. Each nerve innervates several muscle fibers. The combination of a single nerve and all the fibers it innervates is known as a motor unit, and it is this motor unit that allows muscles to contract. Beginning about the seventh decade of an individual's life, the number of functional motor units begins to decline precipitously (Vandervoot & Symons, 2001). One group of researchers found that the estimated number of motor units in the bicep-brachialis muscle declined by nearly half, from an average of 911 motor units in subjects less than 60 years of age to 479 in subjects older than 60 years of age (Brown, Strong, & Snow, 1988). A similar degree of motor unit loss was shown in a group of subjects ages 60 to 80 years compared with a group of subjects ages 20 to 40 years (Doherty & Brown, 1993).

The loss of motor units with age is due to an age-related loss of muscle innervation (Deschenes, 2004). As motor units are lost, surviving motor nerves adopt muscle fibers that have been abandoned due to their loss of innervation (Roubenoff, 2001). This results in an increase in the size of the adopting motor unit. Thus, older persons generally have larger, yet less efficient, motor units than do younger persons (Roubenoff, 2001). Because these enlarged motor units are now responsible for the contraction of a greater number of muscles, they are generally less efficient. This inefficiency can lead to tremors and weakness (Enoka, 1997) and, together with the atrophy of fast-twitch muscle fibers, can result in a decline in coordinated muscle action (Morley, Baumgartner, Roubenoff, Mayer, & Nair, 2001). Furthermore, abandoned muscle fibers that are not adopted by surviving motor units begin to atrophy as a result of disuse secondary to their loss of innervation. This atrophy contributes to an overall loss of muscle mass. Muscle atrophy secondary to nerve cell death is clearly demonstrated through the loss of muscle mass observed in persons who have suffered a stroke (Roubenoff, 2001).

Hormonal Influences. Estrogen and testosterone are anabolic hormones—hormones that promote the build-up of muscle. With age, levels of these hormones decline, thereby contributing to muscle atrophy and sarcopenia. Accelerated loss of muscle around the time of menopause lends support to the idea that estrogen may play a role in the maintenance of muscle mass (Poehlman, Toth, & Gardner, 1995). There is evidence supporting estrogen replacement therapy as a means of attenuating the loss of muscle mass among older women (Dionne, Kinaman, & Poehlman, 2000; Phillips, Rook, Siddle, Bruce, & Woledge, 1993). However, some research suggests that the beneficial effects of estrogen replacement are most pronounced in the perimenopausal period and may have little to no effect on the loss of muscle mass among postmenopausal women (Doherty, 2003). Among older men, testosterone supplementation has been shown to increase muscle mass; however, studies performed to date have been conducted among healthy older men. It is not known whether testosterone supplementation would have the same beneficial effects on muscle mass in older men with physical impairments, chronic disease, or frailty (Bhasin, 2003). Testosterone supplementation has also been shown to increase muscle strength among elderly women (Davis, McCloud, Strauss, & Burger, 1995).

Growth hormone (GH) (see "The Endocrine System" earlier in this chapter) is another anabolic hormone that declines with age. The decline in GH begins during the fourth decade of life and parallels the decline in muscle mass (Roubenoff, 2001). Because of the strong association between GH and muscle mass, administration of GH has been suggested as a potential method by which age-related loss of muscle mass might be attenuated. However, research investigating the effects of GH on muscle mass has produced equivocal results, and there is no evidence that GH administration results in any increase in muscle strength (Borst, 2004). In addition, the use of GH is accompanied by numerous side effects including fluid retention, hypotension, and carpal tunnel syndrome, and these side effects are reported to be more severe among older persons (Borst, 2004). Given the equivocal results regarding its efficacy as well as the side effects associated with its use, GH is not recommended as an intervention for sarcopenia (Doherty, 2003).

Protein Synthesis. Excluding water, protein is the primary component of skeletal muscle and accounts for approximately 20% of its weight (Proctor, Balagopal, & Nair, 1998). Furthermore, muscle is the body's largest repository for protein (Balagopal, Rooyackers, Adey, Ades, & Nair, 1997; Proctor et al., 1998). When protein breakdown within the body exceeds protein synthesis, muscle atrophy occurs. Some research findings suggest that aging is associated with a reduced capacity of skeletal muscle to synthesize protein. Such a reduction is likely to lead to a decrease in muscle mass among elderly persons. However, other research (Volpi, Sheffield-Moore, Rasmussen, & Wolfe, 2001) has found no difference in the synthesis rate of muscle protein with age. Thus, further studies are needed to elucidate the role that protein synthesis plays in sarcopenia.

Nutritional Factors. Food intake declines with age, with greater decline occurring among men than women (Morley et al., 2001). This decline is often referred to as the **anorexia of aging**, and it is hypothesized to be associated with a decrease in the senses of smell and taste as well as an earlier rate of satiation with age (Morley et al., 2001). It is thought that the anorexia of aging may result in protein intake below the level necessary to maintain muscle mass and consequently contribute to sarcopenia (Morley et al., 2001; Drewnowski & Evans, 2001); however, the degree to which alterations in protein intake with age may play a role in age-related loss of muscle mass is unknown and requires further study.

Muscle Strength

Loss of **muscle strength**, the muscle's capacity to generate force, is thought to be secondary to declines in muscle mass (Ivey et al., 2000), and decreases in muscle strength are seen with advancing age. Data from one study demonstrated that 71% of men between the ages of 40 and 59 and 85% of men age 60 or older had declines in muscle strength over a 9-year period (Kallman, Plato, & Tobin, 1990). Age-related decreases in strength are reported to range from 20–40%, with even greater decreases of 50% or more occurring in persons in their ninth decade or beyond (Doherty, 2003). Older men experience greater absolute declines in muscle strength than women; however, because men have greater total muscle mass than women, relative losses in strength are similar between males and females (Doherty, 2003). The rate at which the decline in muscle strength occurs has not been well defined, but longitudinal studies have shown rates of strength loss of about 1–3% per year (Doherty, 2003).

Muscle Quality

In addition to declines in muscle mass and strength, advancing age is also associated with a loss of **muscle quality**, strength generated per unit of muscle mass. However, research shows that age-related declines in muscle quality differ by both gender and muscle group. Studies (Lynch et al., 1999; Ostchega, Dillon, Lindle, Carroll, & Hurley, 2004) of arm and leg muscle quality in men and women found that age-related differences in arm muscle quality declined more among males than females, yet leg muscle quality declined at similar rates among both genders. In addition, among men the rates of decline of leg and arm muscle quality were similar. However, among women there was a greater rate of decline of leg muscle quality than arm muscle quality. Lower limb weakness is of particular concern because it results in an inability to perform most daily tasks, such as standing up from a chair, walking, or stair climbing (Olivetti et al., 2007; Ostchega et al., 2004).

Resistance Training and Aging Muscle

Older persons who are less physically active have less muscle mass and greater rates of disability and debilitating falls than persons who remain physically active as they age (Evans, 2002; Moreland, Richardson, Goldsmith, & Clase, 2006). There is a large body of evidence demonstrating that exercise can not only slow or prevent muscle loss with age, but also increase muscle mass as well as muscle strength among older persons. Resistance exercise, exercise aimed at increasing the force generated by muscle, has been shown to have the most beneficial effects on aging muscle. One study of 66-year-old men found that a 12-week program of resistance training resulted in significant increases in the cross-sectional area of both fast-twitch and slow-twitch muscle fibers (Frontera, Meredith, O'Reilly, Knuttgen, & Evans, 1988). In addition, muscle strength improved significantly. Even among very elderly persons, resistance exercise has shown benefits for age-related changes in muscle. An 8-week resistance training program conducted among men and women in their 90s resulted in a

15% increase in muscle cross-sectional area and a nearly 175% increase in the amount of weight subjects were capable of lifting (Fiatarone et al., 1990). Numerous other studies have shown that resistance training programs of 10 to 12 weeks' duration, with training 2–3 days per week, result in significant increases in muscle strength among older persons (Doherty, 2003). It has been reported that resistance training may restore approximately 75% of lost muscle mass and 40% of lost muscle strength (Roubenoff, 2003). Significant increases in muscle strength are also achieved using weight-bearing exercise regimes (Olivetti et al., 2007).

Resistance training has also been shown to improve muscle quality. Following a 9-week training program, older men and women showed statistically significant increases in muscle quality. Furthermore, subsequent to the initial 9-week program there was a 31-week detraining period after which levels of muscle quality remained significantly greater than levels measured before the start of the 9-week program (Ivey et al., 2000).

Finally, there is also evidence to support an increase in protein synthesis with resistance exercise. One study reported an approximately 50% increase in protein synthesis among 65- to 75-year-old men following a 16-week progressive resistance training program (Yarasheski, Zackwieja, Campbell, & Bier, 1995). Improvements in protein synthesis have also been demonstrated among frail elderly men and women ages 76–92 years (Yarasheski et al., 1999). Other research has reported increases in protein synthesis of over 100% following resistance training (Hasten, Pak-Loduca, Obert, & Yarasheski, 2000).

The plethora of benefits to muscle that result from resistance training demonstrate the extreme importance of regular physical activity, especially of the resistance type, among aging men and women. It is no wonder that many have cited resistance training as the most important factor in preventing and even reversing the losses in muscle mass, strength, and power that come with advancing age.

THE SKELETAL SYSTEM

The skeletal system is composed of the 206 bones of the body as well as the joints that connect them. The skeleton, extremely strong yet relatively light in weight, gives shape and support to the human body. It also acts to protect the body; for example, the skull protects the brain and eyes while the ribs protect the heart and the vertebrae protect the spinal cord. The skeleton also provides a structure to which muscles can attach by tendons, enabling the body to move. Furthermore, it acts as a set of levers to modify movement provided by the muscles, increasing or decreasing the distance, speed, and force obtained from muscle contraction (Digiovanna, 1994; Marieb & Hoehn, 2007; Tortora & Derrickson, 2006). When one considers the importance of the functions performed by the skeletal system, it becomes apparent that any alteration or destruction of the skeletal system would have potentially serious consequences for the overall health and physical functioning of the human body.

Bone

In addition to the aforementioned functions of the skeletal system, each component of bone has its own unique function(s). A principal function of bone is mineral storage and the maintenance of free mineral homeostasis. The predominant mineral stored within bone is calcium. Calcium is necessary for, among other things, muscle contraction and nerve impulse conduction. If it is to aid in these functions, calcium must be readily and continuously available in a free form. Yet too much free calcium may be toxic and too little calcium may impair or prevent cell functioning. Thus, there must be a means of maintaining mineral homeostasis. Bone cells assist in this maintenance.

Bone cells are of four types: osteogenic cells, **osteoblasts**, **osteocytes**, and **osteoclasts** (**Figure 6-19**). Osteogenic cells are unspecialized stem cells capable of cell division. The resulting cells develop into osteoblasts. Osteoblasts secrete collagen and minerals to produce a bone matrix; hence, it is these cells that are responsible for the construction of new bone and the repair of damaged or broken bone. They mature into osteocytes, the main cells in bone tissue that maintain daily activities of the bone such as exchange of nutrients and wastes with the blood (Tortora & Derrickson, 2006). The fourth bone cell type is the osteoclasts, which break down or resorb existing bone, dissolving minerals of the bone matrix so that these minerals can be used by the body.

FIGURE 6-19 **Cross section through a bony trabecula.**

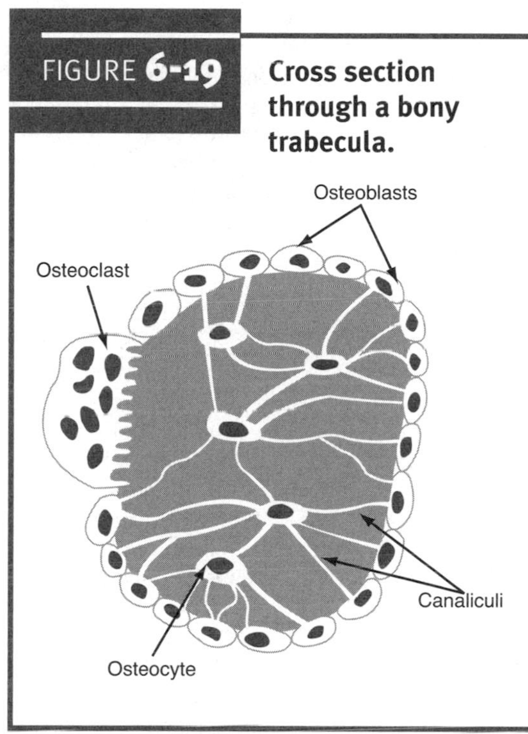

SOURCE: Reprinted from Basic Medical Endocrinology (3rd ed.). H. M. Goodman, p. 261 (2003) with permission from Elsevier.

The formation and resorption of bone are not separately regulated processes. Osteoblasts and osteoclasts occur together in temporary anatomic structures known as **basic multicellular units (BMUs)**. A mature BMU is composed of both cell types, a vascular supply, a nerve supply, and connective tissue (Manolagas, 2000). A BMU has a life span of approximately 6–9 months, longer than the life span of osteoblasts and osteoclasts. Thus, the BMU must be continually supplied with new cells.

During development and growth, BMUs mold bone to achieve proper size and shape by osteoclastic removal of bone from one site and osteoblastic deposition at a different one. This process is known as modeling. By adulthood, the skeleton has reached maturity and modeling no longer occurs. However, in adulthood there is periodic replacement of old bone with new bone, and this process is known as bone remodeling. Through bone remodeling, the human skeleton is completely regenerated every 10 years (Manolagas, 2000). The purpose of bone remodeling is not well understood; however, it is hypothesized that remodeling occurs to repair fatigue and damage and to prevent excessive aging. Thus, the primary purpose of bone remodeling may be to attenuate if not prevent the accumulation of old bone (Manolagas, 2000).

Bone remodeling by the osteoblasts and osteoclasts is principally controlled through hormonal regulation. As previously noted in the discussion of the endocrine system, thyroid calcitonin inhibits bone resorption, lowering blood calcium levels. Parathyroid hormone from the parathyroid gland has the opposite effect—it increases bone resorption and mobilizes calcium, thereby increasing blood calcium levels. Other hormones are also involved in bone remodeling, yet often indirectly. Glucocorticoids promote bone resorption, and growth hormone and insulin work to increase bone formation.

Bone Types

There are two types of bone—cortical or compact bone and trabecular or spongy bone. **Cortical bone** comprises the outer layer of bone and is composed of numerous osteons—long, narrow cylinders of bone matrix. The osteons are tightly fused to one another and possess a complex system of blood vessels and nerves. Osteons are continually dissolved and replaced anew. Cortical bone surrounds and protects trabecular bone and provides the majority of skeletal strength.

Trabecular bone makes up the inner portion of bone and is composed of small pieces of bone matrix known as trabeculae. The trabeculae are arranged in very irregular patterns. Compared to cortical bone, trabecular bone provides only minimal skeletal strength. The ratio of cortical bone to trabecular bone varies throughout the body. Cortical bone is predominant in the limbs whereas trabecular bone is predominant in bones of the axial skeleton, such as the ribs, vertebrae, and skull.

Aging of the Bone

Bone Loss

In order to ensure that there is no net loss of bone, the amount of bone resorbed by the BMU must not exceed the amount formed. As the body ages, it loses the ability to maintain this balance between bone resorption and formation (Tortora & Derrickson, 2006). The BMU is said to be in a negative balance and bone loss occurs. Negative BMU balance begins as early as the third decade, long before menopause in women (Seeman, 2003a). After several decades have passed, skeletal mass may be reduced to half of what it was at 30 years of age (P. S. Timiras, 2003b).

Estrogen promotes apoptosis or programmed cell death of osteoclasts. Thus, the osteoclast life span is increased by estrogen deficiency whereas the life span of osteoblasts declines with such a deficiency (Tortora & Derrickson, 2006). Consequently, BMU balance becomes more negative. Thus, estrogen deficiency is a key contributor to bone loss, and bone loss accelerates in women after menopause due to a decline in estrogen levels (Seeman, 2003a). Simultaneously, as osteoclast activity increases and more bone is resorbed, the remaining bone becomes more porous. The result of this increased porosity is a decline in bone mineral density. Unfortunately, bone loss continues from the lower density bone and at a higher rate than before menopause. The increased rapidity of bone loss is explained by 1) the increasingly negative BMU, 2) a higher remodeling rate, and 3) reduction in the mineral content of bone due to the replacement of older, more densely mineralized bone with younger, less densely mineralized bone (Seeman, 2003b).

Estrogen deficiency also plays a role in bone loss among men. Although men do not undergo the midlife acceleration in bone resorption characteristically seen in women, decreased bone mineral density among men is due to a decline in levels of estrogen, not testosterone (Seeman, 2003a). It has been suggested that estrogen may regulate bone resorption whereas both estrogen and testosterone may regulate bone formation (Falahati-Nini et al., 2000). At any given age bone mass is greater in men than in women, but the rate of bone loss is generally accelerated among women (Arking, 1998). However, the overall loss of bone is quantitatively similar in persons of both genders, suggesting that bone loss may occur over a longer period of time in men than in women (Seeman, 2003b).

Bone Type

The majority of bone resorption occurs within trabecular bone, and in both men and women bone loss occurs at least a decade earlier in trabecular bone than in cortical bone (Arking, 1998). As the body ages, trabeculae become thinner and weaker. In addition, some may disappear entirely and cannot be replaced. As a result of these changes the bone becomes permanently weaker at the site of trabeculae thinning or loss. Furthermore, some trabeculae may become disconnected from the others, resulting in a decline in bone strength (Digiovanna, 1994).

Corticol bone loss is not detected until about 40 years of age, at which time the rate of loss begins to increase. However, the loss of cortical bone still occurs at only half the rate of trabecular bone loss (Digiovanna, 1994). Loss of trabecular bone occurs from the inside of the bone outward. Normally, old osteons shrink and are dissolved while new osteons form next to them and eventually fill the space left by the old ones. With age, however, new osteons are unable to fill this space completely, leaving larger and larger gaps between existing osteons. The result is a weakening of the bone.

Bone Strength

With age there is not only a loss of bone, but also a loss of bone strength. This loss of strength has been attributed to at least two different processes. The first is the increased porosity of bone that occurs due to continuous bone remodeling. Greater porosity reduces the structural strength of bone. The second is an age-related loss of collagen due to decreased protein synthesis, which increases the ratio of bone minerals to collagen, leading to increased brittleness of bone (Arking, 1998; Tortora & Derrickson, 2006). Reduction in collagen fiber strength may be related to decreases in growth hormone production, which was noted earlier in the endocrine section. In childhood approximately two-thirds of bone is composed of collagen and connective tissues whereas in aged individuals minerals comprise two-thirds of bone structure (P. S. Timiras, 2003b).

Bone tensile strength is a property that allows bone to withstand forces applied to the skeleton during movements such as bending and stretching. Strong, young bones will respond to force with flexibility and resilience, bending as needed. But aged bones are more likely to snap when subjected to force. Consequently, the age-associated decline in bone strength increases older persons' risk of bone fracture (Arking, 1998). See the following section for further discussion of bone fractures among older persons.

Age-Related Disease and Injury of the Bone

Osteoporosis

Osteoporosis is a disease that results from reductions in bone quantity and strength that are greater than the usual age-related reductions. Bones of those with osteoporosis are generally very porous, containing numerous holes or empty pockets. In addition, they are thin and fragile and, consequently, extremely prone to fracture (discussed in the following section). An estimated 10 million Americans suffer from osteoporosis and another 34 million have low bone mass that puts them at increased risk for the disease. The majority of osteoporosis cases, 8 million (80%), occur in women whereas only 2 million (20%) occur in men (National Osteoporosis Foundation, 2007).

Bone Fracture

Osteoporosis and the general progressive loss of bone mass with age leads to increased risk of fracture among older persons. Fifty percent of women and 25% of men over the age of 50 years will experience an osteoporosis-related fracture in their lifetime. Fractures in elderly persons often occur as the result of only minimal or moderate trauma whereas in younger persons considerable force is required to fracture a bone. In addition, the fractures that occur in old age generally occur at different sites than those that occur at younger ages. Among younger persons the most common site of fracture is the bone shaft, whereas in older persons fractures generally occur next to a joint (P. S. Timiras, 2003b). Regardless of the site of fracture, fractures among older adults are generally more difficult to prevent or repair, and recovery from fracture occurs much more slowly in older persons than in young individuals.

In young adults, fractures occur more frequently among males than females. This is hypothesized to be the result of males' generally more frequent engagement in physical activity and exposure to accidental falls (P. S. Timiras, 2003b). In older adults, however, women generally experience greater fracture rates than men. This gender difference may be due, at least in part, to the fact that women begin life with a smaller skeleton that adapts less well to aging than that of men (Seeman, 2002). This gender difference in fracture incidence with age is most evident in fractures of the vertebrae, forearm, and hip (P. S. Timiras, 2003b).

There are also racial differences in the rate of fracture. The rates of fracture associated with old age are significantly lower among African Americans than Caucasians, specifically three times lower among African American women and five times lower among African American men. These racial differences may be explained by the 10% to 20% greater bone mass and density of adult bone among African Americans. In addition, bone remodeling occurs more slowly among African Americans than Caucasians (P. S. Timiras, 2003b).

Joints

Joints or articulations are junctions between two or more bones. Three types of joints comprise the body's articular system. **Immovable joints** or fibrous joints consist of collagen fibers that bind bones tightly together. The toughness of collagen allows minimal, if any, shifting of bones, and as such the joints are immovable. Skull bones are examples of immovable joints. These joints keep the skull in place, allowing support and protection of the brain.

Cartilaginous joints have a layer of cartilage that separates the two connected bones. These joints may also have ligaments to aid in holding bones together. Cartilaginous joints allow for slight movement. Examples of this type of joint include the joints between vertebrae. These cartilaginous joints are known as intervertebral disks, and together with strong ligaments they hold the vertebrae together and aid the vertebrae in supporting the weight of the body. They also allow the vertebral column to bend and twist slightly.

The third and most common type of joint is the **synovial joint**. The bones that this type of joint connects contain smooth cartilage on their opposing ends. This cartilage minimizes friction when the joint moves. A sleeve of connective tissue encapsulates the ends of the two bones that have been joined. The joint capsule is lined with the **synovium**, a membrane that secretes **synovial fluid**. The fluid is thick and slippery, allowing easy movements of the bones. In addition, it absorbs part of the shock sustained by the joint. Although synovial joints, together with reinforcing ligaments, bind two bones tightly together, they are characterized by free range of motion. Nearly all the joints in the arms, legs, shoulders, and hips are synovial joints.

Aging of the Joints

Immovable Joints. With increasing age the collagen between the bones of immovable joints becomes coated with bone matrix. As a result, the space between bones gets even narrower and the bones may eventually fuse together completely. Consequently, the joints become stronger. Therefore, with age immovable joints actually improve.

Cartilaginous Joints. The aging process is associated with a stiffening of the cartilage comprising cartilaginous joints. Ligaments also become stiffer and less elastic. The result of these changes is a reduction in the amount of movement allowed by the cartilaginous joints. Vertebral movement is decreased and there is a decline in the ability of intervertebral disks to support the body and cushion the spinal cord. With age the vertebrae weaken and, as a result, the weight of the body forces the intervertebral disk to expand into the vertebrae, forming a concave region. This change appears to force more of the weight of the body onto the outer edge of the intervertebral disk, compressing the disk (Digiovanna, 1994). The result is a shortening of the spinal column and a decrease in body height.

Synovial Joints. The functional ability of synovial joints begins to decline around 20 years of age (Digiovanna, 1994). As a person ages both the joint capsule and the ligaments become shorter, stiffer, and less able to stretch. In addition, the cartilage lining the bones becomes calcified, thinner, and less resilient (Arking, 1998; Tortora & Derrickson, 2006). Consequently, it becomes more difficult to move, and range of motion and efficiency of the joint are reduced. As a result, both the initiation and speed of movement begin to slow with age. This leads to a lessened ability to maintain balance and makes it difficult to act quickly to minimize the force of impact resulting from a fall or other physically harmful event.

With age the synovial membrane also becomes stiffer and less elastic. In addition, it loses some of its vasculature, which in turn reduces its ability to produce synovial fluid. The fluid that is produced is thinner and less viscous (Arking, 1998). As a result of these changes in the synovial membrane and fluid, there is a decline in the ease and comfort with which the joints move within the joint capsule as a person ages.

The net result of the aging of synovial joints is often increased injury and decreased activity performance. However, there is evidence to demonstrate that this net result can be slowed or minimized through continual physical activity. Exercise can increase flexibility of the joint components and also appears to increase circulation to the joints (Digiovanna, 1994; Tortora & Derrickson, 2006).

It should be noted here that at least some, if not many, of the changes in joints with age may be due not to the aging process but to repeated injuries the joints experience over time due to the performance of regular daily activities. It is often difficult to distinguish these latter effects from true biological aging (Digiovanna, 1994).

Diseases of the Joints

Osteoarthritis. Age-related changes in the joints often result in or are compounded by arthritis, a disease characterized by inflammation of the joints and accompanied by joint pain and injury. There are more than 100 different types of arthritis, but the two most common forms are osteoarthritis and rheumatoid arthritis.

Osteoarthritis is by far the most common form of arthritis, accounting for more than half of all arthritis cases (Digiovanna, 1994). More than 20 million people in the United States have osteoarthritis, and the disease is much more common among older persons. More than half of people 65 years of age or older would show x-ray evidence of osteoarthritis in at least one joint. Before age 45, osteoarthritis is more common among men, but after age 45 it becomes more common in women (National Institute of Arthritis and Musculoskeletal and Skin Diseases, 2006).

Osteoarthritis frequently affects the weight-bearing joints, such as the hips, knees, and lower spine. Finger joints also are common sites of osteoarthritis. This form of arthritis causes a breakdown and weakening of cartilage, which results in a decreased ability to cushion the ends of the bones. If enough cartilage is lost, the bones will begin to rub against each other. The bones then respond by producing more bone matrix, which builds up and can lead to an enlargement of the joints and difficulty in joint movement. In addition, the bone matrix produced may be rough and jagged and, when it rubs against soft tissues, can cause pain. Furthermore, with age there is a decrease in synovial fluid concentration and viscosity. This decrease may lower the lubricating and cushioning properties of the joints, making movement of the joint difficult and painful (Moskowitz, Kelly, & Lewallen, 2004).

THE SENSORY SYSTEM

The sensory system provides constant stimulation to the body and relays important messages to the mind and body. The sensory system can evoke emotion and memories, and when disrupted can influence quality of life (Arking, 1998; Digiovanna, 1994; Weiffenbach, 1991). Age-related changes to touch, smell, taste, vision, and hearing lead older individuals to interact with the environment differently than they did at a younger age.

Touch

The ability to touch and distinguish texture and sensation tends to decline with age due to a decrease in the number and alteration in the structural integrity of touch receptors, or Meissner's corpuscles, and pressure receptors, or Pacinian corpuscles (Arking, 1998; Digiovanna, 1994, 2000). Receptors that are related to the sense of touch are also known as **mechanoreceptors**. See **Figure 6-20** for an illustration and location of mechanoreceptors in the integumentary system. Changes to these touch and pressure receptors lead to a decrease in the ability to acknowledge that an object is touching or applying pressure to the skin, a decrease in the ability to identify where the touch or pressure is occurring, an inability to distinguish how many objects are touching the skin, and a decreased ability to identify objects just by touch (Digiovanna, 1994, 2000). Aging changes to the skin as well as changes in surface hair may also play a role in diminished touch. (See the following section, "The Integumentary System.") Arking (1998) suggests that the skin on the hands, the most sensitive to touch, undergoes the most age-related change in touch. In addition to the hands, Stevens and Choo (1996) found that the feet undergo major declines in touch sensitivity with age. This conclusion may be explained by a higher concentration of receptors in the hands and feet whereas the rest of the body has a larger surface area over which receptors are dispersed.

Stevens and Patterson (1995) conducted a spatial acuity study of touch that involved changes in stimuli related to discontinuity, skin location, and area on the skin as well as changes in the orientation of stimuli in older versus younger adults. Conclusions from this study showed that all four acuity measures declined with age at a rate of 1% per year between the ages of 20 and 80. Furthermore, these researchers demonstrated that acuity at sites such as the forearm and lip declined less quickly than acuity in the fingertips. These changes to touch can be related to a decline in the number of sensory neurons and a decreased ability of the remaining sensory neurons to efficiently relay signals critical to the detection, location, and identification of touch or pressure on the skin (Digiovanna, 1994, 2000).

Of particular concern for the elderly is loss of sensation and proprioception, or reception of information regarding body movements and position (Shaffer & Harrison, 2007). Recent data suggest that aging results in loss of lower limb sensory fibers and receptors for vibration and discriminative touch as well as impaired lower extremity proprioception. These compromises along with declines in ability to initiate corrective movements leave elderly adults more prone to imbalances and falls (Maki & McIlroy, 2006; Shaffer & Harrison, 2007).

Smell

Olfactory System Anatomy

The chemical senses of smell and taste work together and influence each other as a functional entity (Weiffenbach, 1991). The olfactory system contains supporting cells for mucus production, olfactory receptors, and basal cells that replenish every 2 months and eventually transform into new olfactory receptors (Sherwood, 2007). When basal cells transform into receptors, the entire neuron, including the axon that projects into the brain, is completely replaced (Sherwood, 2007). The olfactory axons connect to the olfactory bulb and the olfactory nerve layer. The nerve layer synapses into the glomerulus, sending messages to the primary olfactory cortex of

FIGURE **6-20** **General sense receptors.**

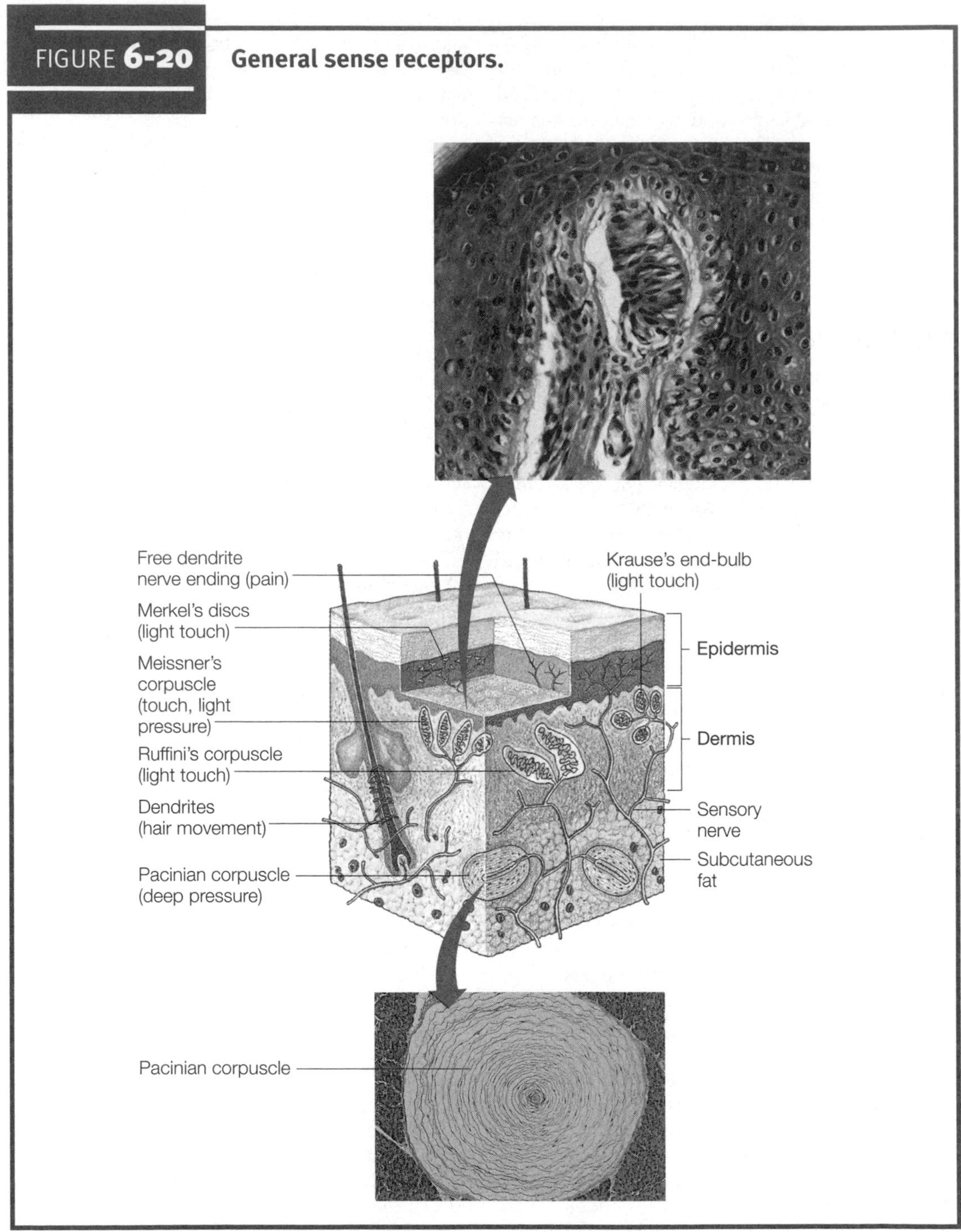

SOURCE: Human Biology, 5e. Daniel D. Chiras, Jones and Bartlett Publishers 2005.

the brain (Kovacs, 2004). Approximately 5 million olfactory receptors of about 1,000 different types are located in the nose. Each receptor type detects one miniscule component of an odor instead of the odor as a whole (Sherwood, 2007).

Age-Related Olfactory Changes

Olfaction, or the sense of smell, appears to be reduced with age, as demonstrated by threshold studies of stimulus strength. A decrease in smell is also referred to as hyposmia (Seiberling & Conley, 2004). Evidence shows peaks in the senses of smell and taste during the 20s and 40s, but by the 60s and 70s there is a decline in olfaction. This decline includes reduced ability for both odor detection and identification, especially among males. Over 50% of people age 65 years or older have significant olfactory dysfunction (Arking, 1998; Kovacs, 2004; Marieb & Hoehn, 2007; Seiberling & Conley, 2004). A decrease in the number of olfactory neurons and weakening of olfactory neural pathways to the brain lead to a reduction in the ability to identify and distinguish aromas (Digiovanna, 1994, 2000; Seiberling & Conley, 2004). At the age of 25 years, the olfactory bulb contains approximately 60,000 mitral cells. By the age of 95 years, there are only 14,500 mitral cells. This decline in cell numbers decreases the functional ability of the olfactory neural system (Bhatnagar, Kennedy, Baron, & Greenberg, 1987). As discussed in "The Nervous System" section, neurofibrillary tangles and amyloid plaques can be observed in the aging brain and have been documented in the olfactory bulb (Kovacs, 1999, 2004). See **Figure 6-21** to identify olfaction pathways and neural correlates. Age-related gender differences include that males show greater declines in

FIGURE **6-21** **The olfactory system.**

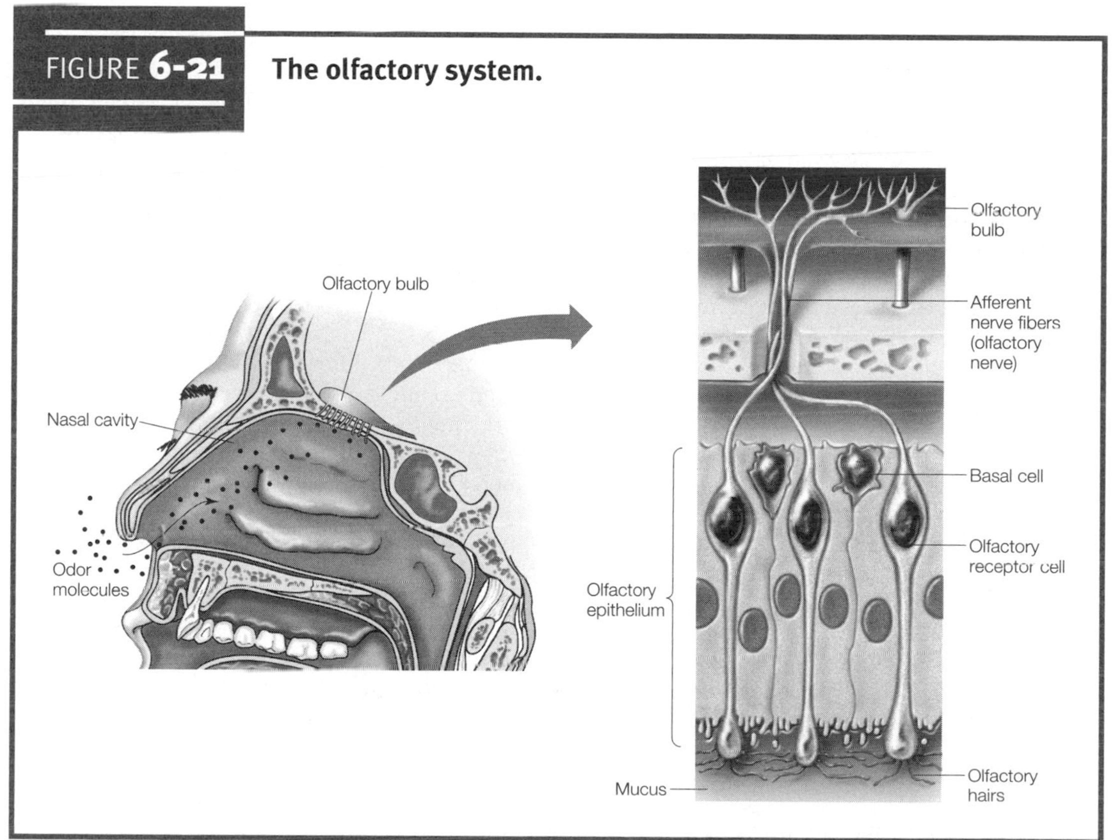

SOURCE: Human Biology, 5e. Daniel D. Chlras, Jones and Bartlett Publishers 2005.

detection and identification of odors than do females (Arking, 1998; Kovacs, 2004).

Concerns associated with the declining sense of smell in older populations include the inability to smell harmful odors such as gas or smoke in the home and the inability to smell pleasurable memory-invoking aromas such as flowers (Digiovanna, 1994, 2000; Kovacs, 2004; Stevens, Cain, & Weinstein, 1987). A decline in the ability to smell can also influence the sense of taste, often causing older individuals to change their eating habits and to receive less enjoyment from food (Cowart, 1989; Marieb & Hoehn, 2007; White & Ham, 1997). The decline in smell is much more predominant than the decline in taste, but individuals often say that the sense of taste has changed when actually it is the sense of smell that is impaired (Seiberling & Conley, 2004).

Taste

Anatomy of Gustation

Taste, or gustation, and the **chemoreceptors** for taste are located in approximately 10,000 taste buds found mostly on the tongue, but also in the rest of the oral cavity and throat (Sherwood, 2007). Taste receptors constantly renew about every 10 days through generation of new receptor cells (Sherwood, 2007). The four primary tastes are sweet, salty, bitter, and sour; a fifth primary taste known as umami, a sensation related to the presence of the amino acid glutamate, has also been discovered (Digiovanna, 1994, 2000; Lindemann, 2000; Sherwood, 2007).

Age-Related Gustation Changes

Aging causes a decrease in taste, also known as **hypogeusia**, usually more noticeable around the age of 60 with more severe declines occurring after the age of 70 (Seiberling & Conley, 2004). However, the sense of taste seems to decrease only slightly with age and can be variable among individuals (Digiovanna, 1994, 2000). Threshold studies, or studies that evaluate the lowest level of stimulus needed to reach threshold to invoke a response, are often used to measure taste (Digiovanna, 1994, 2000). Threshold studies have demonstrated some age-related, quality-specific changes in taste. The ability to detect salt changes the most with age whereas detection of sugar does not appear to change (Bartoshuk & Duffy, 1995; Cowart, 1989; Digiovanna, 1994, 2000; Weiffenbach, 1991; Weiffenbach, Baum, & Burghauser, 1982). Taste changes with age are not as well understood as changes in smell, but it has been hypothesized that there is a decrease in the number of taste buds as well as a change in taste receptors and cell membrane ion channels with age (Mistretta, 1984; Seiberling & Conley, 2004). Because taste buds have the ability to regenerate every 10 days, any changes in taste are most likely correlated with disruptions in taste receptors and cell membranes. Of course, taste sensation can be disrupted for other reasons including medication use, smoking, disease, infections, and poor oral health (Schiffman, 1997; Seiberling & Conley, 2004; Wilson et al., 2005). The most common concerns related to changes in taste, which are strongly tied to changes in smell, are food poisoning and malnutrition (Marieb & Hoehn, 2007; Schiffman, 1997; Wilson et al., 2005).

Vision

The eyes monitor objects and conditions around the body, continually sending sensory messages to the brain such that the body can elicit appropriate responses to the outside environment (Digiovanna, 2000).

Anatomy and Age-Related Changes in Eye Structure

Many older adults experience dry eyes and/or a feeling of irritation, as if an object is in the eye. This condition is known as dry eye syndrome (Kollarits, 1998). Dry eye syndrome may be explained by age-related decline in the amount of tears produced by the lacrimal glands. The conjunctiva, which also normally helps to lubricate the eye and eyelid with a mucous secretion, may have functional declines (Digiovanna, 1994, 2000; Kalina, 1999). The cornea, a transparent structure behind the conjunctiva, refracts or bends light rays traveling through the eye; with age the cornea tends to decrease in transparency. This decrease can cause a reduction in the amount of light entering the eye as well as an increase in light scattering (Digiovanna, 1994, 2000). The scattered light still reaches the retina, albeit in incorrect areas causing bright areas in the field of view. This phenomenon is known as glare (Digiovanna, 1994, 2000). See **Figure 6-22** for an overview of the physiology of the eye. Behind the cornea lies the iris, which contains a hole called the

FIGURE **6-22** **Anatomy of the human eye.**

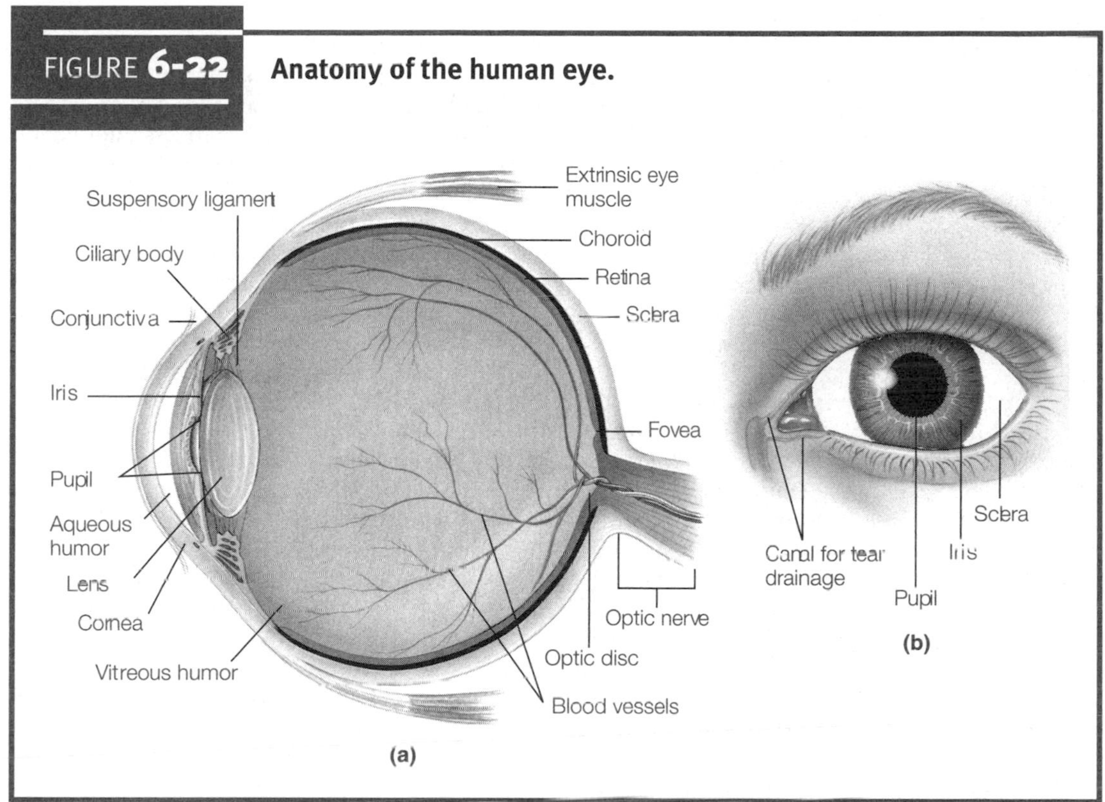

SOURCE: Human Biology, 5e. Daniel D. Chiras, Jones and Bartlett Publishers 2005.

pupil. The pupil allows light to pass into the eye (Digiovanna, 1994, 2000).

Collagen fibers in the eye begin to thicken and muscle cell numbers decrease with age. These changes reduce the ability of the pupil and iris to work together to constrict and dilate. As a result, the eye is unable to appropriately adapt to changing light intensities (Digiovanna, 1994, 2000; Kalina, 1999). The lens of the eye demonstrates an age-related loss of elasticity that has also been attributed to changes in collagen fibers. With age, the lens of the eye becomes less curved and more flat. In addition, there is a decreased transparency to colors of light, especially blue, and formation of opaque spots that block and scatter light (Digiovanna, 1994, 2000; Marieb & Hoehn, 2007). Retinal rods of the eye that are responsible for low-light vision demonstrate age-related changes, whereas retinal cones remain relatively stable (Kalina, 1999). The center of the eye contains vitreous humor, a gel containing collagen fibrils. With age, the vitreous humor loses transparency and there is an increase in the scattering of light, which may potentially cause floaters (Digiovanna, 2000; Kalina, 1999; Kollarits, 1998). The amount of aqueous humor, or fluid between the cornea and lens, produced declines with age, resulting in structural corneal changes such as flattening (Digiovanna, 2000; Kalina, 1999). All of these age-related structural changes in the eye explain many of the age-associated changes in vision.

Age-Related Changes in Visual Function

One of the most common visual concerns in aging that occurs over time, but which becomes most notable around 40 years of age and older, is **presbyopia** or the inability to focus on nearby objects, such as newsprint. This inability is also known as farsightedness (Digiovanna, 1994; Jackson & Owsley, 2003). Presbyopia is generally corrected using bifocals and trifocals in lenses (Jackson & Owsley, 2003). Several studies have shown a decline in visual acuity, or the smallest object or detail that can be seen, even in individuals wearing corrective lenses. This decline may be correlated with a decrease in the neurons along the visual pathway as well as changes in the actual lens of the eye (Jackson & Owsley, 2003). Sensitivity to contrast, or the ability to observe a pattern in different light and intensity, also declines with age as a result of changes in the optics of the eye. Contrast sensitivity further declines under conditions of low light. Such a decline is likely due to changes in the neural pathways (Jackson & Owsley, 2003; Owsley, Sekular, & Siemsen, 1983; Sloane, Owsley, & Alzarez, 1988). Decline in contrast sensitivity is demonstrated by older individuals' complaints that driving and seeing road signs at night is very difficult, prompting them to drive only in daylight. All of these changes can be associated with aging of the cornea. Corneal aging is characterized by decreased transparency, greater scattering of light, and a flattening effect that results in reduced refraction, as previously described (Digiovanna, 1994). Another common complaint among older individuals pertains to changes in the visual field. Studies have demonstrated a narrowing of both the central and peripheral visual fields in older adults as compared to those of young adults. Narrowing is greater in peripheral fields as a result of disruption in the visual neural pathway (Haas, Flammer, & Schneider, 1986; Jackson & Owsley, 2003; Johnson, Adams, & Lewis, 1989). This decrease in the visual field area causes a lessened ability to visually search environmental surroundings, making it difficult to identify and discriminate objects and moving targets (Jackson & Owsley, 2003). Other consequences of aging changes in the visual neural pathway are demonstrated by decreased detection and awareness of moving objects as well as a diminished ability to distinguish one motion from another very similar motion (Ball & Sekuler, 1986; Gilmore, Wenk, Naylor, & Stuve, 1992; Jackson & Owsley, 2003). For instance, a police officer directs traffic around an accident scene on a two-lane highway by motioning one lane to slow and stop while motioning a car in the opposite lane to proceed slowly around. From a distance the older driver may not be able to clearly distinguish the hand movements of the officer until he or she is much closer to the scene. The speed with which individuals can visually process information also tends to slow in the older adult. As a result, older adults need to focus on an object for a longer period of time in order to identify and describe it (Jackson & Owsley, 2003; Salthouse, 1993).

Visual attention, divided attention, and selective attention also decrease with aging, with more pronounced deficits occurring when objects or information are shown very quickly (Jackson & Owsley, 2003). Impaired divided attention can be observed when an older adult is given two simultaneous tasks to complete, such as viewing a series of two pictures side by side on a computer screen for 5 seconds. If the older adult is instructed to learn the name on a building in one picture and to count how many animals are in the other picture, he or she will eventually begin to focus on only one picture.

Age-related changes in color vision lead to impaired color discrimination, especially along the blue–yellow color continuum. This indicates increased absorption of short wavelengths and a deficiency in those cones associated specifically with short wavelengths (Jackson & Owsley, 2003). The photoreceptors—rods and cones—also demonstrate age-related changes. The rod photoreceptors aid vision in the dark and in other low-light situations and demonstrate a greater age-related decline in density than do cone photoreceptors. Cone photoreceptors aid vision in regular and bright light situations and are involved in color vision. These photoreceptors maintain relative stability in density with age (Curcio, Millican, Allen, & Kalina, 1993; Jackson & Owsley, 2003). The decline in rod photoreceptors also provides evidence to support the common complaint of older individuals that they do not see as well at night, especially when driving.

Age-Related Eye Diseases

The most common causes of vision loss in the older adult population are cataracts, glaucoma, macular degeneration, and diabetic retinopathy (Heine & Browning, 2002; Jackson & Owsley, 2003; Kollarits, 1998; Marieb & Hoehn, 2007). These are all eye diseases or conditions that present more frequently in the aging population, but should not be considered a part of usual aging (National Eye Institute, 2002). The presence of cataracts, or a decrease in the transparency of the lens in the eye, is fairly common in the older population and everyone who lives long enough will experience some degree of cataracts (Digiovanna, 1994; Kollarits, 1998). By the age of 75 approximately 50% of older adults will show signs of cataracts and about 25% of these cases will be advanced cataracts, with more instances occurring in women than men (Klein, Klein, & Linton, 1992a). Risk of glaucoma, increased intraocular pressure, is partly genetic but is also subject to environmental influences. Glaucoma causes loss in the peripheral visual field (Duggal et al., 2005; Kollarits, 1998). In general, intraocular pressure increases with age (Kalina, 1999). Around 2% of individuals in the United States over the age of 40 experience glaucoma, with a higher prevalence in African Americans (Kollarits, 1998). Adults age 75 or older also demonstrate a high incidence of macular degeneration (Klein et al., 1992b), which is a major cause of irreversible vision impairment and blindness. It accounts for 22% of cases of blindness in one eye and 75% of cases of legal blindness in adults 50 years of age or older (Klein, Wang, Klein, Moss, & Meuer, 1995). Diabetic retinopathy relates directly to the presence of diabetes. Diabetes is a disease state and not a part of usual aging; therefore, this topic will not be covered in this section (National Eye Institute, 2002).

Hearing

The External Canal

The external canal of the ear consists of the visible external ear opening, known as the pinna or auricle, and the canal that extends to the eardrum or tympanic membrane (Digiovanna, 2000; Patt, 1998; Tortora & Derrickson, 2006). Small vellus hairs cover the entire ear canal, and larger tragus hairs concentrate only in the most external portion of the canal (Patt, 1998). Cerumen glands situated in the ear canal open into hair follicles and onto skin, producing the odor associated with cerumen, or ear wax (Patt, 1998). Age-related shrinkage of cerumen glands causes cerumen to become dryer. In turn, there is often blockage of the external canal and a decreased ability to hear (Digiovanna, 2000; Patt, 1998; Rees, Duckert, & Carey, 1999). In aging, the outer ear loses elasticity, the external ear canal narrows, and the tympanic membrane stiffens (Heine & Browning, 2002; Schuknecht, 1974). The skin on the ear becomes thinner and more susceptible to tears and infection (Rees et al., 1999). Hair on the external ear becomes longer and denser (Digiovanna, 2000; Patt, 1998).

The Middle Ear

The middle ear consists of three small bones called the auditory ossicles. These bones are the malleus, incus, and stapes (Digiovanna, 2000; Tortora & Derrickson, 2006). The ossicles amplify the vibrations sent from the external ear so as to maintain intensity of the sound wave traveling to the cochlea of the inner ear (Digiovanna, 2000; Tortora & Derrickson, 2006). The middle ear also loses elasticity and the ossicles tend to shrink with age (Heine & Browning, 2002; Patt, 1998; Schuknecht, 1974). Narrowing of the joint space between ossicles occurs as a result of age-related calcification of the joint capsule and deterioration of the cartilage; however, this narrowing does not seem to cause loss of sound waves in the middle ear (Jerger, Chmiel, Wilson, & Luchi, 1995; Patt, 1998; Rees et al., 1999).

The Inner Ear

The cochlea of the inner ear, also called the hearing organ, is spiral in shape and is filled with perilymph liquid (Digiovanna, 2000; Patt, 1998; Tortora & Derrickson, 2006). Within the cochlea, vibrations pass from the perilymph through the vestibular membrane into endolymph, another cochlear liquid, and finally to the basilar membrane (Digiovanna, 2000). See **Figure 6-23** for a representation of ear anatomy as well as changes to the ear and hearing processes.

Age-related hearing loss occurs as a result of changes in the inner ear (Digiovanna, 2000; Rees et al., 1999; Tortora & Derrickson, 2006).The inner ear shows a loss of elasticity in the basilar membrane as well as degeneration of the organ of Corti, manifested as increased shrinkage and loss of hair cells (Heine & Browning, 2002; Schuknecht, 1974). Degeneration of small blood vessels in the cochlea leads to a reduction in endolymph production and a diminished ability of vibrations to travel through the ear (Digiovanna,

FIGURE 6-23 The anatomy of the ear and the parts of the ear that show changes with age.

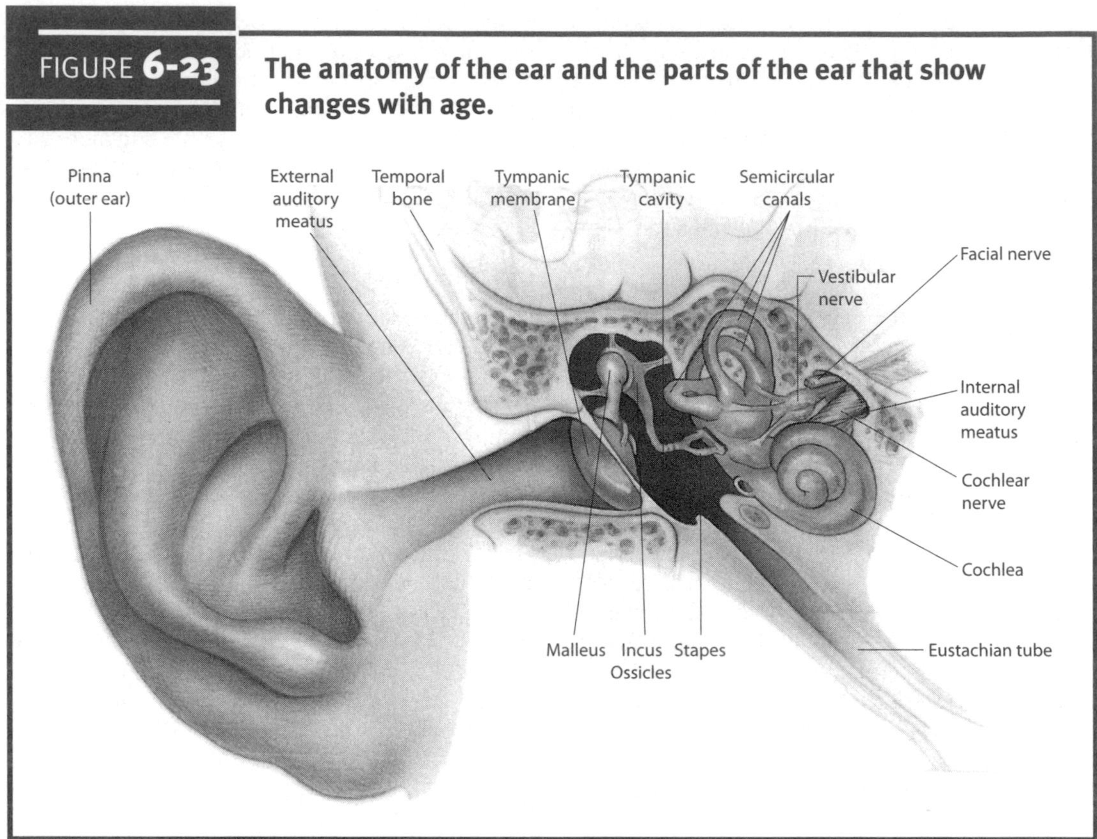

SOURCE: Beth Hartwell, MD http://medic.med.uth.tmc.edu/Lecture/Mainear3.gif.

2000; Tortora & Derrickson, 2006). In the auditory portion of the brain, the cortex displays shrinkage, loss of neurons, and decreased blood flow (Heine & Browning, 2002; Schuknecht, 1974).

The Vestibular System

The inner ear encompasses the cochlea as well as the vestibule and balance organs (Patt, 1998). In the vestibular system, age-related decline occurs in hair cells, ganglion cells, and sensory nerve fibers (Patt, 1998; Rees et al., 1999). The vestibular system together with the eye and proprioceptors helps to maintain the body's physical balance or equilibrium (Rees et al., 1999). Compromises in vestibular balance occur with more frequency in the elderly and may lead to one of the most common complaints among older adults—dizziness. Among those age 65 or older, 90% of reports of vertigo or other imbalance result in physician office visits (Patt, 1998; Rees et al., 1999).

Hearing Mechanism

Hearing is the result of sound waves entering the external ear and canal, traveling to the tympanic membrane, and sending vibrations according to sound wave intensity. These vibrations are relayed to the ossicles and on toward the cochlea, which is considered the hearing organ (Jerger et al., 1995). The vibrations initiate a wave motion in the cochlea, causing changes in the basilar membrane and, in turn, stimulating the hair cells in the cochlea. Eventually signals are sent through nerve fibers to the central auditory system (Jerger et al., 1995).

Hearing Loss

Aging changes that cause hearing loss include the alteration and decline in threshold sensitivity, the ability to hear high frequency sounds, and the ability to discern speech (Rees et al., 1999). Age-related hearing loss, also known as **presbycusis**, remains the most common sensory deficit in the older population. Approximately 35% of men and women age 60 to 70 years and 39% of those over the age of 75 report difficulty with conversation when they are in areas with background noise (Fransen, Lemkens, Van Laer, & Van Camp, 2003; Rees et al., 1999). Ringing in the ears, or tinnitus, is also a frequent occurrence in the elderly (Tortora & Derrickson, 2006). Typically, hearing loss, observed more often among males than females, occurs in both ears. The ability to hear higher frequency sounds is generally affected the most. Hearing loss is most closely correlated with sensorineural disruption (Fransen et al., 2003; Rees et al., 1999).

A constant decline in hearing is observed in aging. Higher frequencies are affected first and then, with decreased hearing ability, the frequencies become more variable. Hearing acuteness varies with age at the onset of hearing loss as well as with progressive states and hearing severity (Fransen et al., 2003; Rees et al., 1999). Hearing loss has been physiologically correlated to loss of hair cells and cochlear neurons as well as degeneration of the stria vascularis in the ear (Fransen et al., 2003). Four categories of presbycusis correlate the deterioration in hearing function with the changes in ear physiology, particularly changes in the cochlea. High-frequency hearing loss, or sensory presbycusis, results from the loss of hair cells in the cochlea of the ear. Strial presbycusis results from shrinkage of the stria vascularis. Neural presbycusis develops as a result of cochlear neuron deterioration and can cause a loss of the ability to discriminate words. Finally, cochlear conductive presbycusis causes gradual threshold loss correlated with potential changes in the cochlear duct in the ear (Rees et al., 1999; Schuknecht & Gacek, 1993). Along with usual aging processes, intrinsic and extrinsic factors such as occupation, loud noise, nutrition, cholesterol, and arteriosclerosis also affect the auditory system (Digiovanna, 2000; Rees et al., 1999).

Changes in the sensory system include changes in the anatomy of sensory organs and corresponding neural circuits and brain areas. Age-related changes occur variably for every individual, meaning that one person may not experience noticeable changes while another experiences severe decrements or even complete loss of a sensory system. These changes impact the older adult's quality of life on a variety of levels.

THE INTEGUMENTARY SYSTEM

The integumentary system consists of the skin and its accessory structures including hair, nails, and the sweat and sebaceous (oil) glands. The integumentary system protects the body's tissues and internal organs, serves as a barrier against injury and infection, helps regulate body temperature, and acts as a receptor for stimuli of touch, pressure, and pain. It is also the physiological system most visible to the human eye, and thus the system that most readily displays the signs of aging.

Skin: Structure and Function

The skin, the largest of all human organs, is composed of three primary layers—the **epidermis**, the **dermis**, and the **subcutaneous layer** (see Figure 6-20 earlier in the chapter). Each layer has a unique structure and function.

The Epidermis

The epidermis is the thin, outermost layer of the skin. It is composed of three primary cell types—keratinocytes, melanocytes, and Langherans cells. **Keratinocytes** produce the protein keratin. As keratin accumulates in the cells, the cells die. Eventually these dead cells are pushed outward by the production of new cells beneath them The keritinized cells begin to form a superficial layer of the epidermis known as the stratum corneum that serves to protect the surface of the human body. These cells are exfoliated, or shed, and replaced by new cells. This process of cell exfoliation and replacement is cyclical, with one cycle normally lasting 14 to 28 days, depending on the region of the body (Marieb & Hoehn, 2007; M. L. Timiras, 2003).

The **melanocytes** produce melanin, a pigment essential to protecting the body from ultraviolet (UV) rays. Exposure to UV radiation leads to DNA and other damage in cells of both the epidermis and dermis. **Melanin** blocks and absorbs UV radiation and, in so doing, protects against cellular dysfunction and lowers the risk of tumor formation. Because of their role in protection against UV radiation, melanocytes are found in increased numbers in sun-exposed skin.

The **Langerhans cells**, although they comprise only 1–2% of epidermal cells (Fossel, 2004), play a critical role in the body's immune defense system, particularly cutaneous immune reactions. These cells recognize foreign antigens and, in response, activate immune defenses. The main functions of Langerhans cells include antigen binding, processing, and presentation to naïve T cells (see "The Immune System" later in this chapter; Schmitt, 1999). Langerhans cells, in addition to responding to antigens, launch immune responses to tumor cells. Thus, Langerhans cells help to protect the body against both infection and skin cancer.

In addition to these cellular functions, the epidermis plays a critical role in the production of vitamin D_3, which is produced when its epidermal precursor form is activated through the skin's exposure to UV radiation, that is, sunlight (Yaar & Gilchrest, 2001). Ninety percent of the body's supply of vitamin D is produced in this manner (Holick, 2003). Vitamin D_3 plays a significant role in calcium homeostasis and bone metabolism, and deficiencies in vitamin D_3 have been associated with osteoporosis and osteomalacia as well as numerous other diseases, including cardiovascular disease, multiple sclerosis, diabetes, and a variety of cancers (Holick, 2003).

The Dermis

The dermis is composed primarily of the connective tissue fibers of collagen and elastin. Collagen provides structure to the skin. Due to its flexibility and extreme strength, collagen offers resistance against pulling forces (Arking, 1998), and thus helps protect the skin from being torn when stretched. Elastin, woven throughout collagen, adds resilience and flexibility to skin. Elastin is responsible for maintaining skin tension while simultaneously allowing skin to stretch to permit necessary movement of muscles and joints.

In addition to its connective tissue structure, the dermis is rich in vasculature. This dense vasculature allows for the provision of nutrients to the epidermis and assists in the control of body temperature through regulation of blood flow. The dermis also contains an abundance of nerves that relay information to the brain in response to a variety of sensory stimuli. Pressure and touch stimuli are detected and responded to by nerve endings known, respectively, as Pacini's and Meissner's corpuscles (see "The Sensory System" earlier in this chapter).

The Subcutaneous Layer

The subcutaneous layer is made up of loose collagen and subcutaneous fat. Collagen provides structure to the skin, much as it does in the dermis. Subcutaneous fat, with its rich vasculature, acts as an insulator against extensive heat loss. Thus, this layer of the skin plays an extremely important role in thermoregulation. Fat also serves as a shock absorber to prevent injury and trauma to bone, muscle, and internal organs. In addition, subcutaneous fat acts as a storage area for caloric reserves.

The Aging Skin

Changes in skin structure and function can be classified as either chronological (intrinsic) aging or extrinsic aging. **Chronological aging** refers to those changes considered to be due only to the passage of time (**Table 6-5**). **Extrinsic aging** is the result of chronic exposure of the skin to external factors such as smoking, poor nutrition, and especially UV light, which induces **photoaging** (Baumann, 2007). Chronologically aged skin is characterized by thinness and a reduction in elasticity. The wrinkles caused by chronological aging are usually very fine and thus the skin appears relatively smooth. In contrast, photoaged skin is characterized by deep wrinkles, sagging, and a leathery appearance (Scharffetter-Kochanek et al., 2000). Generally, chronological aging and photoaging become superimposed upon one another and compound each other's effects. However, as can be seen in **Figure 6-24**, most of the visible changes in aged skin are the result of photoaging. Chronological aging primarily affects skin's function rather than its appearance.

With age, there is an overall decrease in the turnover rate of epidermal keratinocytes. By the

TABLE 6-5 Chronological or Intrinsic Aging Changes of the Integumentary System

	Structure	Function	Consequence
Skin			
Epidermis	Decreased turnover rate of keratinocytes	Prolonged exposure of the epidermal cells to the environment	Increased risk of skin cancer
			Slower wound repair
	Decreased number of active melanocytes	Weakening of the protective barrier against UV radiation	Increased risk of tumor formation and skin cancer
	Reduction in pigment granules in melanocytes		Reduced ability to tan
	Grouping and increased size of melanocytes		Age spots
	Reduction in number of Langerhans cells	Dampened cell-mediated immune response	Increased susceptibility to infection and tumor development
	Decline in vitamin D_3 production		Increased risk of osteoporosis, osteomalacia, and other diseases
Dermis	Loss of thickness	Reduced ability to maintain skin suppleness	Increased likelihood of sagging and wrinkling
	Loss of collagen elasticity and overall loss of collagen	Reduced ability to return skin to normal tension	Sagging
	Elastin loses resiliency and becomes more brittle		
	Loss of vascularity	Decline in blood flow; impaired thermoregulation	Decrease in skin temperature; dampened ability to adapt to temperature change; reduction in sweat and oil production
	Decline in number of Pacini's and Meissner's corpuscles	Reduced response to pressure and touch	Increased risk of injury; impaired ability to perform fine maneuvers with hands
Subcutaneous layer	Loss of thickness	Impaired ability to insulate and protect	Increased risk of heat loss and hypothermia; increased risk of injury and bruising

continues

TABLE 6-5 Chronological or Intrinsic Aging Changes of the Integumentary System (continued)

	Structure	Function	Consequence
Skin Derivatives			
Hair	Thinning and loss; changes in length, appearance, and site of growth; graying		
Nails	Decline in linear growth rate; change in color, texture, and shape		
Eccrine glands	Decreased number of glands	Reduced efficiency of sweat production	Impaired thermoregulation; increased risk of heat exhaustion and heat stroke
Sebaceous glands		Reduction of oil and wax production	Increased roughness, dryness, and itchiness of skin

SOURCE: Author.

eighth decade (Fossel, 2004), turnover rate has decreased by as much as 50%. The reduced turnover rate slows the exfoliation-replacement rate of dead keratinocytes. As a result, exposure of epidermal cells to harmful carcinogens is prolonged and the risk of skin cancer increases (M. L. Timiras, 2003). Risk of infection also increases. In addition, decreased epidermal turnover rate contributes to the slower wound repair seen in elderly persons.

The number of active melanocytes also declines with age, at a rate of 10% to 20% per decade (Fossel, 2004). This decline weakens the body's protective barrier against UV radiation, resulting in an increased risk of UV-induced DNA damage. Such damage greatly increases the risk of tumor formation and the development of skin cancer, especially among the elderly population in which the DNA repair rate is slowed (Yaar & Gilchrest, 2001). With age, the remaining melanocytes generally have fewer pigment granules, making aged skin less likely to tan (Krauss Whitbourne, 2002). In addition, the melanocytes tend to increase in size and group together. This results in the so-called age spots that appear on elderly skin.

Langerhans cells show an age-associated numerical decline of 20% to 50% from early adulthood to late adulthood (Yaar & Gilchrest, 2001). As a result, cell-mediated immune response is dampened with age. In fact, both animal and human studies have found immune system abnormalities to be associated with defects in the structure and function of skin cells (Arking, 1998). A depressed immune response can increase susceptibility to skin infection as well as skin allergens. In addition, when coupled with the reduction in melanocytes' protective action, the weakened immune response only further increases older persons' risk of tumor development.

Finally, vitamin D_3 production by the epidermis declines with age. This is the result of both a

FIGURE 6-24 **Photoaging (a) vs chronological aging (b).**

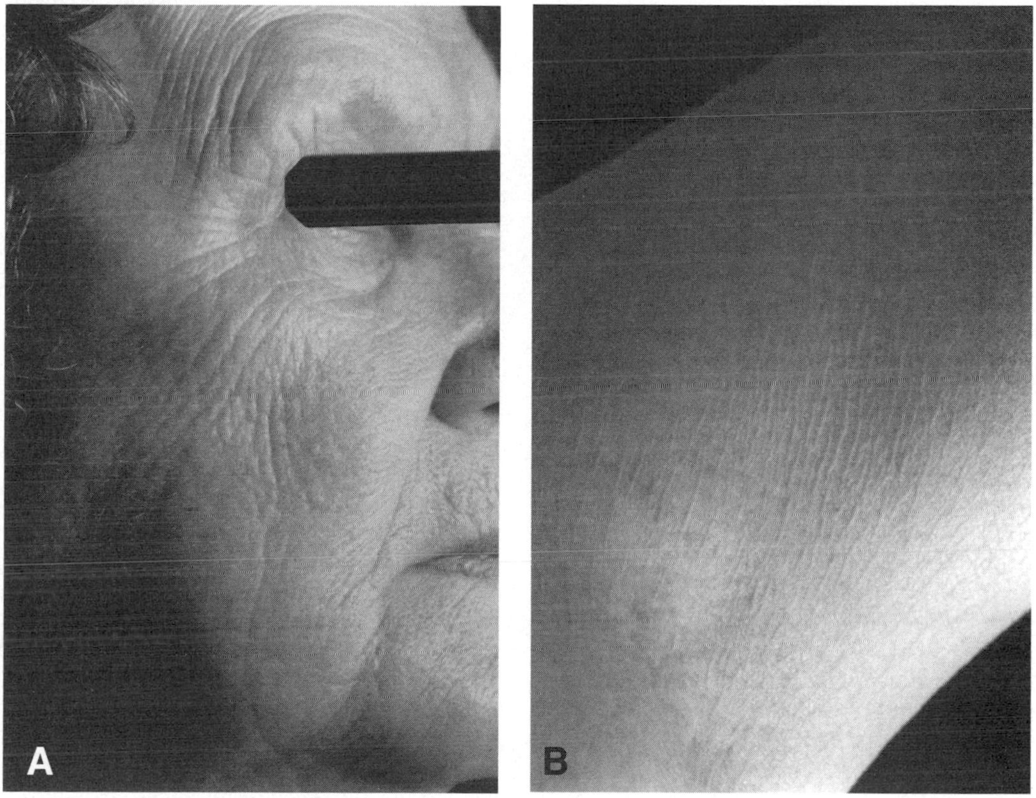

SOURCE: Reprinted from Experimental Gerontology, Vol. 35, Scharffetter-Kochanek, K., Brenneisen, P., Wenk, J., Herrmann, G., Ma, W., Kuhr, L., Meewes, C., & Wlaschek, M. Photoaging of the skin from phenotype to mechanisms, pg 307-316, Copyright (2000) with permission from Elsevier.

decrease in epidermal vitamin D_3 precursor and a reduction in sun exposure among older adults. The lower levels of vitamin D_3 put older adults at greater risk for poor overall bone health, osteoporosis, and numerous other diseases, as mentioned earlier.

In young skin, the epidermal and dermal layers are held tightly together through a series of interdigitations called dermal papillae, and it is nearly impossible to separate this epidermal-dermal junction. With age, however, there is a flattening of the epidermal-dermal junction as its interdigitated structure is lost. This flattening of the junction allows the epidermis to more easily separate from the underlying dermis. In turn, this separation renders older persons more susceptible to bruising and tearing of the skin as well as to blister formation. Furthermore, the decreased area of surface contact between the epidermis and dermis may compromise communication and nutrient transfer between these two layers of the skin (Baumann, 2007; Yaar & Gilchrest, 2001). The rate of change in the epidermal-dermal junction differs among women and men. In women, changes occur rather sharply between 40 and 60 years of age, most likely as a result of hormonal changes with menopause. Among men, the rate of change is much more constant throughout adulthood (Yaar & Gilchrest, 2001).

The greatest changes in aging skin are seen in the dermis. There is a general thinning of the dermal layer, with loss of thickness averaging 20% in older persons (Baumann, 2007; Beers & Berkow; 2000). This thinning of the dermis is due in large part to a general loss of collagen—approximately a 1% loss per year in adulthood (M. L. Timiras, 2003)—as well as a decrease in its flexibility. In addition, elastin becomes increasingly brittle and less resilient. This change in elastin results in a loss of its ability to return to its original tension after it is stretched by the movement of underlying muscles and joints. Consequently, skin is more likely to sag. The overall effect of these changes in the connective tissues of the dermis is the looseness, loss of suppleness, and increased fine wrinkling that is characteristic of old, chronologically aged skin. It is of interest to note that the dermal layer is generally thicker in males than females, and this may account for the apparently greater rate of deterioration of female skin, especially following menopause (Arking, 1998).

With age the dermis also undergoes a decline in vascularity, and blood flow is reduced by approximately 60% (Beers & Berkow, 2000). This reduction results in a decrease in skin temperature, making the skin of older adults generally cool to the touch. Diminished vascularity also contributes to impaired thermoregulation. The avascularity characterizing older skin can give a paler appearance to the skin, and generally the bones and remaining blood vessels beneath the skin become more visually prominent.

Nerve endings in the dermis also undergo changes as a person ages. In particular, the number of Pacini's and Meissner's corpuscles decreases, leading to a decline in the sensations of pressure and touch. Consequently, older persons are more prone to injuries resulting from poor detection of sensory stimuli. In addition, sensory loss leads to a decline in the ability to perform fine maneuvers with the hands.

The skin's subcutaneous layer thins dramatically with age. This loss of thickness occurs primarily in the skin of the face and hands (Arking, 1998). There is a general redistribution of body fat to the intra-abdominal region with age. Thus, subcutaneous thickness of the skin around the hips and abdomen may, in fact, increase (Fenske & Lober, 1986). The subcutaneous layer ordinarily acts as an insulator against excessive loss of body heat. Thus, as it thins, the ability to conserve heat declines, making the older person more prone to low body temperature and possible hypothermia when exposed to the cold (Krauss Whitbourne, 2002). The thinning of the subcutaneous layer also limits its ability to act as a protective cushioning. Consequently, bones, major organs, arteries, and nerves receive more concentrated impacts (Fossel, 2004), in turn increasing the risk of injury and bruising.

Estrogen and Aging Skin

Sex hormones greatly influence the aging process, and the skin is a target organ for these hormones. Therefore, a change in sex hormone levels with age will affect any skin functions that are under hormonal control (Sator, Schmidt, Rabe, & Zouboulis, 2004). Estrogen is a sex hormone and has been extensively studied for its influence on skin aging. Research has shown that the reduction in estrogen associated with menopause is associated with impaired structure and function of the skin (Phillips, Demircay, & Sahu, 2001; Shah & Maibach, 2001). Postmenopausal women receiving hormone replacement therapy (HRT) have been shown to have thicker, healthier skin. Women on HRT show statistically greater collagen content than those not receiving HRT (Phillips et al., 2001). In addition, the skin of those receiving hormonal treatment exhibits less loss of elasticity, in turn exerting a positive effect on skin sagging (Pierard, Letawe, Dowlati, & Pierard-Franchimont, 1995). One national study found that estrogen use may prevent both skin drying and skin wrinkling (Dunn, Damesyn, Moore, Reuben, & Greendale, 1997).

Aging of Skin Accessory Structures

Hair

Hair is produced by hair follicles underneath the surface of the skin. With age, the germination centers that produce hair follicles undergo changes and may, in fact, be destroyed (Baumann, 2007; Krauss

Whitbourne, 2002). As a result, thinning and loss of scalp hair occurs with age, in both men and women. There may also be a thinning of facial hair in men. Simultaneously, however, the hair on older men's eyebrows and inside their ears may become longer and coarser. Similarly, women may develop unwanted facial hair, especially following the hormonal changes associated with menopause.

Hair also tends to gray over time. Graying is due primarily to gradual loss of functional melanocytes from hair bulbs and a general decline in melanin production. The age of onset of graying varies somewhat based on heredity and racial background. For Caucasians, the average age of graying onset is the mid-30s, for Asians, late-30s, and for African Americans, mid-40s. Despite these variations, however, it can generally be said that by 50 years of age 50% of people have 50% gray hair (Tobin & Paus, 2001).

Nails

The linear growth rate of nails decreases with age (M. L. Timiras, 2003). In addition, nails tend to become thinner, drier, and more brittle as a person ages. Nails also undergo a change in shape, generally become flat or concave instead of convex (Beers & Berkow, 2000). Longitudinal grooves or ridges may also form on the nails.

Glands

Both sweat glands and sebaceous glands undergo changes with age. The number of sweat glands decreases by approximately 15% during adulthood (Beers & Berkow, 2000; Tortora & Derrickson, 2006). In addition, the glands' efficiency declines and less sweat is produced. The result is impaired thermoregulation and difficulty in staying cool. This leaves older adults at greater risk for heat exhaustion and heat stroke.

Sebaceous glands do not decrease in number with age; however, the size of the glands decreases with age as does glandular activity. Soon after puberty, oil production declines at a rate of 23% per decade in men and 32% per decade in women (Jacobsen et al., 1985). Clinical manifestations associated with age-related changes of the sebaceous glands include increased dryness, roughness, and itchiness of the skin as well as, in rare cases, sebaceous gland carcinoma (Zouboulis & Boschnakow, 2001).

THE IMMUNE SYSTEM

The immune system is a network of cells and biochemicals responsible for defending the body against foreign microorganisms such as bacteria, viruses, fungi, and parasites. Whenever the immune system is compromised, the body is left vulnerable to a variety of infections and infectious diseases, from the flu and common cold to tuberculosis and AIDS. The numerous and, at times, life-threatening consequences of a weakened immune system illustrate the tremendous importance of the system in maintaining good health.

The crucial feature of the immune system that makes it such a remarkable system of defense is its ability to distinguish the body's own cells ("self") from any foreign cells or microorganisms ("nonself"). A foreign substance invading the body is known as an **antigen**. Antigens carry marker molecules on their surface that identify them as foreign. It is these marker molecules that allow for the discernment of self and nonself. In cases where this discernment process fails, the immune system will attack its own cells. This attack of self is termed **autoimmunity** and can lead to a variety of autoimmune diseases, such as rheumatoid arthritis and multiple sclerosis. Once again, these consequences of a disrupted immune system demonstrate its critical role in protecting the health of an organism.

The defense mechanisms of the immune system are divided into two primary types, innate (or nonspecific) immunity and acquired (also called specific or adaptive) immunity. Each type of immunity is characterized by its own components and method of function. However, the two must work in close collaboration, often through the use of cytokines, to fulfill their common responsibility—the protection of the body against infection and disease.

Innate Immunity

The innate immune system is the one with which a person is born. It is always present and is activated almost immediately upon exposure to an antigen. It is the body's initial attempt at ridding the body of foreign substances. Although **innate immunity** allows for the general discernment of self vs. nonself, it does not have the ability to recognize a specific antigen. Thus, even if the body is repeatedly exposed to the same antigen, the body will react each time to that particular antigen as if it had never before been encountered. Innate immunity does not adapt to or remember a specific antigen. Consequently, it is unable to improve the effectiveness of its defense against that antigen. Innate immunity, therefore, is antigen-independent and results in no immunologic memory of prior encounters with an antigen.

Innate immunity operates through a variety of mechanisms. One of these mechanisms involves the use of physical barriers, in particular the skin and mucosal membranes. The skin may be the most basic and yet one of the most important mechanisms of immunity, because it is the first site most antigens encounter and the site at which many are stopped. Mucosal membranes, such as those lining the eyes, airways, and gastrointestinal and genitourinary tracts, also provide physical barriers of protection. So too do mucosal secretions, such as saliva and tears, which contain enzymes that destroy potential infectious agents.

If an antigen manages to breach physical barriers such as skin and mucosa, the innate immune system continues its attack on the antigen by launching additional defense mechanisms. These include the actions of **macrophages**, **natural killer (NK) cells**, and the **complement system** as well as the inflammatory response.

Macrophages act through a process called phagocytosis. During phagocytosis an antigen is completely engulfed and, through the use of destructive enzymes, literally consumed by the macrophage. Macrophages also secrete cytokines that stimulate the actions of NK cells. When NK cells are activated, they work to kill cells that have been altered through infection by an antigen. Destruction of these cells occurs through two mechanisms. First, NK cells literally punch holes in the membranes of the altered cells and release enzymes that promote self-induced death (or apoptosis) of the altered cells. Second, NK cells release cytokines that target macrophages and enhance their destructive action. Thus, macrophages and NK cells work synergistically to augment each other's actions and thereby provide a stronger defense against invading antigens.

The complement system is a collection of proteins that can kill antigens directly or help to destroy antigens by attaching to and marking them for destruction by macrophages and other cells of the immune system. The complement system also initiates the **inflammatory response**, which results in the release of several chemical messengers that signal macrophages and other phagocytic cells to destroy the antigen. These chemical messengers also increase blood flow and cause blood vessels to release fluid, resulting in redness and swelling, respectively, at the site of invasion. The swelling helps to isolate an antigen and prevent if from coming in further contact with body tissues. The inflammatory response also generates heat, and thus fever, in an attempt to overheat and kill antigens.

Innate immunity provides an early and strong line of defense against foreign antigens. In addition, the very occurrence of the innate immune response serves as a signal for initiation of the acquired immune response, effectively stimulating further mechanisms of defense. When they act in concert, innate and acquired immunity provide the body with its most powerful protection against infection and disease.

Acquired Immunity

Acquired immunity consists of two branches (**Table 6-6**). The first, **humoral immunity**, is mediated by antigen-attacking proteins called **antibodies** and is responsible for defending the body against extracellular antigens found in the blood and other body fluids or "humors." The second branch, **cell-mediated immunity**, is responsible for destroying intracellular antigens. Acquired immunity involves the actions of two primary types of leukocytes—**B cells** and **T cells**. Both cell types are produced in the bone marrow; however, only B cells continue to mature in the marrow. T cells are transported to the thymus, a small organ behind the breast bone, for maturation. Once both cell types have reached maturity they reside mainly in the lymph nodes and spleen. B cells are involved primarily in humoral immunity and T cells principally in cell-mediated immunity. However, there is strong communication between the two cell types, reflecting the collaborative action of the two branches of acquired immunity.

Humoral Immunity

B cells are activated through encounters with antigens; however, not just any antigen will activate any B cell. Each B cell is programmed to respond to only one specific antigen. Once activated by this antigen, the B cell undergoes a process known as **clonal expansion** in which it multiplies to produce a multitude of B cell clones. These clones then differentiate into antibody-producing B cells, or **plasma cells**. Plasma cells are capable of producing and secreting antibodies against only the specific antigen that initiated the humoral immune response. The antibodies are released into the bloodstream where they bind with the targeted antigen. This binding action neutralizes the antigen and prompts other immune cells, such as macrophages, into action.

Following clonal expansion, not all B cell clones will differentiate into antibody-producing cells. Some will become memory B cells. Upon formation, these memory cells do not produce antibodies; however, they effectively remember the antigen against which they were produced and retain the ability to produce antibodies in the future should the antigen be reintroduced. The memory cells survive, perhaps for years, and circulate in the bloodstream, primed to launch a rapid response if and when they again encounter their antigen. Thus, humoral immunity is characterized by immunologic memory.

Cell-Mediated Immunity

T cells are of three types—**T-helper cells**, **killer T cells**, and **suppressor T cells** (**Table 6-7**).

T-helper cells are the primary regulatory agents of the immune system. They identify foreign antigens and, in response, proliferate through clonal expansion and release chemical messengers that stimulate action of the killer T cells. T-helper cells also have an indirect role in humoral immunity. Only nonprotein antigens have the ability to cause direct activation of B cells. Protein antigens require that B cells first interact with and receive chemical signals from T-helper cells before the B cells can be activated and an antibody-mediated humoral response launched. This T-helper cell activation of the B cells provides an excellent example of the interaction between humoral and cell-mediated immunity.

Killer T cells, also known as cytotoxic T cells, directly attack and destroy infected cells within the body. Most commonly killer T cells operate against virally infected cells; however, they are also responsible for ridding the body of cells that have been transformed by cancer. In addition, killer T cells are the cells responsible for the rejection of organ and tissue grafts.

Suppressor T cells are the final players in an immune response. These cells counteract the actions of T-helper and killer T cells as well as B cells, bringing an end to the immune response once

TABLE 6-6 Comparison of Humoral and Cell-Mediated Immunity

Humoral	Cell-Mediated
Principal cellular agent is the B cell.	Principal cellular agent is the T cell.
B cells respond to bacteria, bacterial toxins, and some viruses.	T cells respond to cancer cells, virus-infected cells, single-cell fungi, parasites, and foreign cells in an organ transplant.
When activated, B cells form memory cells and plasma cells, which produce antibodies to these antigens.	When activated, T cells differentiate into memory cells, cytotoxic cells, suppressor cells, and helper cells; cytotoxic T cells attack the antigen directly.

SOURCE: Human Biology, 5e. Daniel D. Chiras, Jones and Bartlett Publishers 2005.

TABLE 6-7 Summary of T- Cells

Cell Type	Action
Cytotoxic T cells	Destroy body cells infected by viruses, and attack and kill bacteria, fungi, parasites, and cancer cells
Helper cells	Produce a growth factor that stimulates T cells, B-cell proliferation and differentiation, and antibody production by plasma cells; enhance activity of cytotoxic T cells
Suppressor cells	May inhibit immune reaction by T cells, decreasing B- and T-cell activity and B- and T-cell division
Memory cells	Remain in the body awaiting contact with the antigen they remember, at which time they proliferate and differentiate into cytotoxic T cells, helper T cells, suppressor T cells, and additional memory cells

SOURCE: Human Biology, 5e. Daniel D. Chiras, Jones and Bartlett Publishers 2005.

an infection has passed. In addition, suppressor T cells act to dampen the immune response when it becomes overactive. This dampening action is crucial given that overaction of the immune response can lead to both allergic reactions and autoimmune disease. Thus, the action of suppressor T cells is critical to ensuring that the overall immune response remains properly balanced.

Like humoral immunity, cell-mediated immunity is characterized by immunologic memory. During proliferation T cells produce a pool of memory cells. These cells remain dormant until they again come in contact with the antigen they remember; they then unleash a faster and more powerful immune response than the first. Some memory cells are able to survive for the lifetime of an individual. This ability is what provides us with lifelong immunity to diseases such as chicken pox and measles.

Immunosenescence

The term **immunosenescence** refers to the aging of the immune system. To date the aging process is thought to involve primarily innate immunity and the T cells of acquired immunity. B cells are less highly affected by immunosenescence; however, the majority of investigations have been performed only in animal models (Aw, Silva, & Palmer, 2007).

Innate Immunity

Clinical evidence suggests a dysfunction in the innate immune system. With aging, elevated levels of proinflammatory cytokines released from fibroblasts and macrophages are believed to be linked to age-associated diseases such as diabetes, osteoporosis, and atherosclerosis that appear to have an inflammatory pathway involved (Aw et al., 2007; Gomez, Boehmer, & Kovacs, 2005; Licastro et al., 2005). A number of studies have also indicated that phagocytosis is reduced in the aging immune system and that the destructive capacity of neutrophils and macrophages is inhibited by decreased levels of production of the superoxide anion, which is responsible for the destruction of ingested material (Aw et al., 2007, Plackett, Boehmer, Faunce, & Kovacs, 2004). Some studies have also implicated depressed NK function in some of the decline in innate immunity (Aw et al., 2007; Gruver, Hudson, & Sempowski, 2007; Mocchegiani & Malavolta, 2004; Solana & Mariani, 2000).

Thymus Involution

The most prominent morphological change characterizing immunosenescence is the involution, or atrophy, of the thymus (Aw et al., 2007). The thymus begins to atrophy around puberty and continues as an individual ages. Extrapolating from known rates of thymic involution, it has been postulated that if an individual were to live to 120 years of age, the thymus would atrophy completely (Aspinall & Andrew, 2000). Given that the thymus is responsible for T cell maturation and differentiation, it is not surprising that the involution of this organ results in changes in the T cell population.

Naïve/Memory T Cell Ratio

At any given time, both naïve and memory T cells are present in the body. Naïve T cells are those that have not yet been exposed to an antigen; these are the cells that respond to any new antigen that might attack the body. Memory T cells, as discussed earlier, are T cells that are programmed to respond to specific and previously encountered antigens. With age there is a shift in the ratio of naïve T cells to memory T cells. In young persons, this ratio is quite high, with more naïve T cells than memory T cells. Over time, however, many more naïve cells become exposed to antigens and converted to memory T cells. In addition, as a result of thymic involution, fewer naïve T cells are produced with age. As a result of these changes, the population of naïve T cells is depleted over time. Therefore, the ratio of naïve T cells to memory T cells is very low in older persons. Consequently, elderly persons respond much less efficiently to new antigens that may threaten the body (Gruver et al., 2007; Linton & Dorshkind, 2004; Whitman, 1999), leaving them more vulnerable to infection and disease.

Replicative Senescence

The greater the number of B or T cells available to fight off infection and disease, the more likely it is that the immune response will be effective. Thus, the replication or proliferation of immune cells subsequent to stimulation by an antigen is crucial to efficient immune function. However, cells can undergo only a finite number of divisions, after which there can be no further proliferation of cells. This phenomenon is known as **replicative senescence**. Replicative senescence is the result not of the passage of time per se, but of repeated cell division (Effros & Pawelec, 1997). Nonetheless, over time older cells will have experienced more demands for cell division than younger cells. Consequently, older cells are more likely to have exhausted their ability to divide and to have reached a state of replicative senescence. This is particularly true of immune cells that repeatedly encounter their antigens (Effros, Dagarag, & Valenzuela, 2003) (e.g., antigens giving rise to the common cold). In addition to the increased number of cells that reach replicative senescence as a person ages, research has also shown that replicative senescence occurs earlier (i.e., after fewer divisions) in T cells from old individuals. This suggests that T cells may have a reduced ability to proliferate in old age (Wick & Grubeck-Loebenstein, 1997)

The primary result of replicative senescence is a decline in the overall number of immune cells available to ward off invading antigens. In addition, if immune cells reach replicative senescence during an active immune response, they will be unable to continue cell division, thereby leading to premature termination of the immune response (Effros & Pawelec, 1997). Thus, with age the immune response is greatly weakened due to the inability of immune cells to divide indefinitely. Replicative senescence appears to be of particular concern for T cells and cell-mediated immunity.

Cell Signaling

Effective cell-mediated immunity requires that when a T cell binds to its antigen, the presence of that antigen must be communicated or signaled to the interior of the cell. One of the key molecules involved in this signaling process is CD28, located on the surface of T cells. Without the presence of CD28, the cell is unable to respond to an invading antigen and thus remains inactive. With age, there is a progressive increase in the number of T cells lacking CD28. Consequently, there is increased likelihood of disruption to the signaling pathway and, ultimately, T cell function is impaired (Hirokawa, 1999).

Calcium, essential for numerous biochemical reactions, is also crucial for effective cell signaling. In general, calcium deficiency becomes more likely as a person ages. In addition, calcium mobilization from intracellular stores is inhibited in older subjects compared to younger subjects (Aw et al., 2007). This deficiency contributes to impaired cell signaling within the immune system of older persons. Calcium is also a central player in the production of cytokines. Thus, calcium deficiency can inhibit production of these chemical messengers, thereby hindering immune system communication and the overall coordination of the immune response (Whitman, 1999).

Autoimmunity

Despite the age-related decrease in immune response to foreign antigens, there is an increase in autoimmunity. There is an overall increase in the percentage of T cells and B cell–generated antibodies that are directed against many of the body's own cells. The reason for the increase in autoimmunity is not well understood; however, it has been hypothesized that although T cells directed against the body's own cells are normally destroyed in the thymus before they are fully matured, involution of the thymus with age allows these cells to persist. In turn these T cells could also prompt B cells to produce autoantibodies—antibodies against the body's own cells. Ultimately, there is an increase in autoimmunity.

Clinical Implications of Immunosenescence

Vaccinations. Due to changes characterizing immunosenescence, older individuals are more susceptible to infection and disease than are younger individuals. One method of strengthening the immune defenses is to administer vaccines such as those against influenza and pneumonia. By introducing the body to a foreign antigen, vaccines stimulate the production of antibody-producing B cells as well as memory T cells against the antigen. However, older individuals' antibody response to vaccines is slower and weaker than that seen in younger individuals (Whitman, 1999). In addition, due to the decrease in naïve T cells with age, the T cell response of older persons to a new antigen, such as that introduced by vaccine, may be particularly impaired (Wick & Grubeck-Loebenstein, 1997). T cells of older adults have, in fact, been shown to respond less quickly to vaccines. Overall, the age-related changes in response to vaccines generally render them less effective in older patients.

Infection and Disease. Immunosenescence is associated with increased incidence of infectious disease such as bronchitis and influenza. It is also implicated in the increased incidence of tumors and cancer that occurs with age. In addition, immunosenescence has been associated with a number of age-related autoimmune diseases and inflammatory reactions, including diabetes, arthritis, osteoporosis, cardiovascular disease, and dementia. Inarguably, the aging of the immune system has widespread implications for disease incidence and overall health within the elderly population.

THE HEMATOPOIETIC SYSTEM

The hematopoietic system is responsible for the production, differentiation, and proliferation of mature blood cells from stem cells. The site of blood cell production, or **hematopoiesis**, changes with the developmental stage of an organism. In the fetus, blood cells are produced in the liver, spleen, and yolk sac. In children and adults, blood cells are produced in the bone marrow. At birth, the cavities of nearly all bones are filled with active bone marrow; however, by adulthood active bone marrow is found only in the femur, humerus, sternum, vertebrae, and ribs as well as the pelvic bones and some skull bones.

Hematopoiesis

Hematopoiesis begins with **pluripotent stem cells**. Pluripotent describes the cells' ability to differentiate into any of several different types of progeny cells, or **stem cell progenitors**. Each type of progenitor is committed to the production of only one particular type of mature blood cell (e.g., red blood cells, white blood cells, platelets, as discussed below). (See **Table 6-8**.) Pluripotent stem cells and stem cell progenitors comprise the body's stem cell pool. The stem cells are capable of self-renewal and, thus, the stem cell pool is maintained throughout an individual's life. The self-renewal capacity of stem cells together with the unlimited differentiation potential of pluripotent stem cells allow for regeneration of all hematopoietic cells as needed.

Hematopoiesis is regulated by a network of several biochemical messengers known as **cytokines**. Any imbalance in cytokine production or decreased sensitivity to cytokines by pluripotent stem cells and/or stem cell progenitors can result in disruption of hematopoiesis. Likewise, disruption may result

TABLE 6-8 Summary of Blood Cells

Name	Light Micrograph	Description	Concentration (Number of Cells/mm^3)	Life Span	Function
Red blood cells (RBCs)		Biconcave disk; no nucleus	4 to 6 million	120 days	Transports oxygen and carbon dioxide
White blood cells Neutrophil		Approximately twice the size of RBCs; multi-lobed nucleus; clear-staining cytoplasm	3,000 to 7,000	6 hours to a few days	Phagocytizes bacteria
Eosinophil		Approximately same size as neutrophil; large pink-staining granules; bilobed nucleus	100 to 400	8–12 days	Phagocytizes antigen-antibody complex; attacks parasites
Basophil		Slightly smaller than neutrophil; contains large, purple cytoplasmic granules; bilobed nucleus	20 to 50	Few hours to a few days	Releases histamine during inflammation
Monocyte		Larger than neutrophil; cytoplasm grayish-blue; no cytoplasmic granules; U- or kidney-shaped nucleus	100 to 700	Lasts many months	Phagocytizes bacteria, dead cells, and cellular debris
Lymphocyte		Slightly smaller than neutrophil; large, relatively round nucleus that fills the cell	1,500 to 3,000	Can persist many years	Involved in immune protection, either attacking cells directly or producing antibodies
Platelets		Fragments of megakaryocytes; appear as small dark-staining granules	250,000	5–10 days	Play several key roles in blood clotting

SOURCE: Human Biology, 5e. Daniel D. Chiras, Jones and Bartlett Publishers 2005.

from a reduction in the number of pluripotent stem cells available for differentiation into mature blood cells. The hematopoietic system is responsible for a variety of functions, including oxygen delivery to cells, the immune response, and hemostasis, or the control of blood loss. Given the importance of these functions, any interruption to hematopoiesis will have potentially serious consequences for efficient and proper functioning of the body.

The Blood Cells

Erythrocytes

Erythrocytes (Table 6-8), or red blood cells, are biconcave in shape and have no nuclei. They are red due to the presence of hemoglobin, an iron-containing protein pigment. Erythrocytes are responsible for the transport of oxygen, which binds to hemoglobin molecules and is then carried from the lungs to the cells where it is needed for metabolism. The efficient delivery of oxygen is a key function of erythrocytes, and the production and functional activity of erythrocytes increases in response to hypoxia, or oxygen deprivation.

Once produced in the bone marrow, erythrocytes mature in 24 to 48 hours. They have a life span of approximately 120 days, after which they die and are removed from circulation. Erythrocytes, however, have the capacity for continual self-renewal, allowing for the replenishment of the red blood cell supply. This replenishment balances the routine destruction of erythrocytes and, thus, a relatively constant number of red blood cells is maintained in the circulation.

Leukocytes

Leukocytes (Table 6-8), or white blood cells, are classified on the basis of their nuclear shape as well as the presence or absence of cytoplasmic granules. Leukocytes are of two primary types, granular and agranular, and function principally within the immune system. Granular leukocytes, or granulocytes, include the neutrophils, basophils, and eosinophils. Neutrophils are phagocytic cells that ingest and kill bacteria. Basophils and eosinophils are involved in inflammatory reactions. Agranular leukocytes, also termed mononuclear leukocytes, consist of lymphocytes and monocytes. The lymphocytes include B-lymphocytes and T-lymphocytes, which are involved in humoral and cell-mediated immunity, respectively. (See "The Immune System" earlier in this chapter.) Monocytes are also involved in the immune response. These cells leave the blood and enter tissues where they mature into macrophages, cells necessary for the destruction of infectious agents.

Thrombocytes

Thrombocytes (Table 6-8), or platelets, are responsible for hemostasis, the prevention of blood loss. Hemostasis involves the aggregation of thrombocytes to form a clot. The clot then acts to seal off and impede blood loss from wounds.

Aging of the Hematopoietic System

Changes that are most often discussed in regard to the aging hematopoietic system include the reduced proliferative and self-replicative capacity of stem cells and changes in the cytokine network. However, the degree to which these changes are the result of aging per se remains controversial. There is a great deal of evidence to suggest that functioning of the hematopoietic system, when under basal or steady-state conditions, undergoes no significant changes with aging. Many of the changes in the hematopoietic system of older individuals are evidenced only under circumstances, such as hemorrhaging or anemia, in which the system is under stress and experiencing an increase in functional demand.

Stem Cells and Aging

The Proliferative Capacity of Stem Cells. Some research suggests that stem cells' proliferative capacity is limited and may decrease with age, reaching a state of exhaustion (Globerson, 1999). As discussed in Chapter 3, reduction in proliferative capacity is thought to result from continual shortening of telomeres, the terminal sections of chromosomes. Once telomeres become too short to allow for further cell replication, cell proliferation ceases. If and when stem cell proliferation is stopped, the body becomes limited in its ability to renew the supply of mature hematopoietic cells. A reduction in mature hematopoietic cells would in turn affect the efficiency with which these cells perform their respective functions, such as oxygen delivery and the immune response.

Telomerase is the enzyme that stimulates the addition of telomeric portions to the end of chromosomes, thereby maintaining the self-renewal capacity of cells. Telomerase activity is up-regulated in response to chemical messages from cytokines and down-regulated in response to cell proliferation. Although the action of telomerase may act to limit telomere shortening and subsequent reductions in proliferative capacity, it has not been shown to entirely prevent reduction in telomere length (Engelhardt et al., 1997; Kamminga & DeHaan, 2006). Thus, potential methods by which telomerase activity is increased will not lead to a cessation of the loss of proliferative capacity. Furthermore, research has suggested that indeed other factors besides the action of telomerase are involved in regulation of telomere shortening (Lansdorp et al., 1997). Thus, certainly the mechanisms influencing loss of proliferative capacity with age have yet to be clarified and will require further research.

As mentioned earlier, many of the age-related changes in the hematopoietic system are most evident not when the body is in the basal state but when the body is under hematopoietic stress. Hematopoietic stress requires a fairly rapid increase in the number of functional blood cells, thereby necessitating an efficient process of stem cell proliferation. Hence, the reduction of stem cell proliferative capacity illustrates well how age-related changes would be most clearly evident under conditions of stress.

CD34$^+$ Progenitor Stem Cells. CD34$^+$ cells, the primary circulating progenitor stem cells, are believed to decrease in number with age. This decrease is evidenced by one study, which found that among normal human volunteers (ages 20–90 years) CD34$^+$ cells exhibited an inverse correlation with age (Egusa, Fujiwara, Syahruddin, Isobe, & Yamakido, 1998). The decline in CD34$^+$ cells witnessed among older adults ages 66–73 years was similar to that witnessed in centenarians. This research suggests that reduction in CD34$^+$ cell counts is primarily an early age-related phenomenon. Centenarians and those with great longevity are unlikely to exhibit decreases in CD34$^+$ progenitor cells beyond that which they experienced in the early stages of aging (Bagnara et al., 2000).

Age-Related Changes in the Cytokine Network

Cytokines involved in the regulation of hematopoiesis include interleukin 3 (IL-3), granulocyte-macrophage colony-stimulating factor (GM-CSF), interleukin 6 (IL-6), and tumor necrosis factor alpha (TNF-α). IL-3 and GM-CSF stimulate proliferation of hematopoietic cells. Conversely, IL-6 and TNF-α act to inhibit hematopoiesis (Balducci, Hardy, & Lyman, 2000; Baraldi-Junkins, Beck, & Rothstein, 2000). These cytokines show changes in older populations, which may implicate them in many of the age-related changes in the hematopoietic system.

The peripheral blood of older individuals is reported to have a reduced capacity to produce IL-3 and GM-CSF (Bagnara et al., 2000), thereby limiting their efficiency in stimulating the production of hematopoietic cells. IL-6 and TNF-α, in contrast, show an increased concentration with age in both animals and humans (Balducci et al., 2000). This increase has the potential to disrupt homeostatic regulation of hematopoiesis and may be partially responsible for poor response to hematopoietic stress with age. Furthermore, increased IL-6 concentrations show an association with increased risk of death, anemia, and functional decline in older persons (Balducci et al., 2003).

Anemia and Aging

Anemia is a condition in which a deficiency in the number of erythrocytes or the amount of hemoglobin they contain limits the exchange of oxygen and carbon dioxide between the blood and tissues. Anemia is a common condition among older persons. Eight percent to 44% of the elderly population suffers from anemia, with a higher prevalence among older men (Nilsson-Ehle, Jagenburg, Landahl, & Svanborg, 2000). These prevalence statistics are based on the World Health Organization's (WHO) criteria for a diagnosis of anemia—hemoglobin less than 12 g/dl blood in women and less than 13 g/dl blood in men (De Martinis & Timiras, 2003).

Despite the relatively ubiquitous nature of anemia among elderly persons, it is important to note that most forms of anemia in this population are due to causes other than aging. This is demonstrated by the fact that hemoglobin and hematocrit remain essentially unchanged among healthy older persons. In addition, when anemia is diagnosed in older adults there is almost always another comorbid medical condition present and underlying the anemia (De Martinis & Timiras, 2003). Thus, anemia should not be considered an age-related disease; it is not a universal or even usual condition that develops as the body ages.

SUMMARY

As the content in this chapter has discussed, there are many biological and physiological changes that occur with normal aging. Even in the absence of pathology, normal changes to the human body may necessitate older persons making adjustments in their activities and lifestyle to safely accommodate some of these changes. Recognizing normal changes in the various systems of the aging body will assist the nurse in identifying subtle changes that could indicate the beginning of a health problem. Readers are encouraged to refer to this chapter as needed while learning from the following chapters, and to use this material for comparison in recognizing common abnormalities of aging.

Critical Thinking Exercises

1. Choose an age-related disease in which you have a particular interest and discuss how this disease might impact the functional ability, independence, and psychosocial well-being of an older adult.
2. Many people within and outside the field of geriatrics and gerontology use the term *normal aging* to refer to physiological changes that occur over the passage of time. Do you believe there is such a thing as "normal aging"? Why or why not? How do you believe the use of the term *normal aging* might impact the clinical care received by older adults?
3. Read "No Truth to the Fountain of Youth" by S. Jay Olshansky, Leonard Hayflick, and Bruce A. Carnes in *Scientific American*, Vol. 286, No. 6, pp. 92–95 (June 2002). This article can also be found online at http://www.midwestscc.org/archives/Olshansky3.pdf. Do you agree with the arguments made by the authors of this article? Discuss your reactions to and thoughts on the article with your classmates. You may also want to consider reviewing the two articles on anti-aging medicine listed in this chapter's Recommended Readings list (**Box 6-3**).

BOX 6-3 Recommended Readings

de Haan, G. (2002). Hematopoietic stem cells: Self-renewing or aging? *Cells Tissues Organs, 171*(1), 27–37.

DeVault, K. (2002). Presbyesophagus: A reappraisal. *Current Gastroenterology Reports, 4*(3), 193–199.

Enoch, J., Werner, J., Haegerstrom-Portnoy, G., Lakshminarayanan, V., & Rynders, M. (1999). Forever young: Visual functions not affected or minimally affected by aging: A review. *Journal of Gerontology Series A: Biological Sciences and Medical Sciences, 54*(8), B336–B351.

Federal Interagency Forum on Aging-Related Statistics. (2004). *Older Americans 2004: Key indicators of well-being.* Washington, DC: U.S. Government Printing Office.

Finch, C. (2005). Developmental origins of aging in brain and blood vessels: An overview. *Neurobiology of Aging, 26*(3), 303–307.

Fukunaga, A., Uematsu, H., & Sugimoto, K. (2005). Influences of aging on taste perception and oral somatic sensation. *Journal of Gerontology Series A: Biological Sciences and Medical Sciences, 60A*(1), 109–113.

Greenwald, D. (2004). Aging, the gastrointestinal tract, and risk of acid-related disease. *American Journal of Medicine, 117*(Suppl. 5A), 8S–13S.

Harman, S., & Blackman, M. (2004). Use of growth hormone for prevention and treatment of effects of aging. *Journals of Gerontology Series A: Biological Sciences and Medical Sciences, 59*(7), 652–658.

Hazzard, W. R., Blass, J. P., Halter, J. B., Ouslander, J. G., & Tinetti, M. E. (Eds.). (2003). *Principles of geriatric medicine and gerontology* (5th ed.). New York: McGraw-Hill Professional.

Henderson, V., Paganini-Hill, A., Miller, B., Elble, R., Reyes, P., Shoupe, D., et al. (2000). Estrogen for Alzheimer's disease in women: Randomized, double-blind, placebo-controlled trial. *Neurology, 54*, 295–301.

Hurwitz, J., & Santaro, N. (2004). Inhibins, activins, and follistatin in the aging female and male. *Seminars in Reproductive Medicine, 22*(3), 209–217.

Jackson, R. (2001). Elderly and sun-affected skin. Distinguishing between changes caused by aging and changes caused by habitual exposure to sun. *Canadian Family Physician, 47*, 1236–1243.

Linton, P., & Thoman, M. (2001). T cell senescence. *Frontiers in Bioscience, 1*(6), D248–D261.

Marder, K., & Sano, M. (2000). Estrogen to treat Alzheimer's disease: Too little, too late? So what's a woman to do? *Neurology, 54*, 2035–2037.

Nikolaou, D., & Templeton, A. (2004). Early ovarian ageing. *European Journal of Obstetrics and Gynecology and Reproductive Biology, 113*(2), 126–133.

O'Dononvan, D., Hausken, T., Lei, Y., Russo, A., Keough, J., Horowitz, M., & Jone, K. (2005). Effects of aging on transpyloric flow, gastric emptying and intragastric distribution in healthy humans—impact on glycemia. *Digestive Diseases and Sciences, 50*(4), 671-676.

continues

BOX 6-3 Recommended Readings

Olshansky, J., Hayflick, L., & Perls, T. T. (2004). Anti-aging medicine: The hype and the reality—Part I. *Journals of Gerontology Series A: Biological Sciences and Medical Sciences, 59A*(6), B513–B514.

Olshansky, J., Hayflick, L., & Perls, T. T. (2004). Anti-aging medicine: The hype and the reality—Part II. *Journals of Gerontology Series A: Biological Sciences and Medical Sciences, 59A*(7), B649–B651.

Rosenzweig, E., & Barnes, C. (2003). Impact of aging on hippocampal function: Plasticity, network dynamics, and cognition. *Progress in Neurobiology, 69*, 143–179.

Salvador, J., Adams, E., Ershler, R., & Ershler, W. (2003). Future challenges in analysis and treatment of human immune senescence. *Immunology and Allergy Clinics of North America, 23*(1), 133–148.

Scharffetter-Kochanek, K., Brenneisen, P., Wenk, J., Herrmann, G., Ma, W., Kuhr, L., et al. (2000). Photoaging of the skin from phenotype to mechanisms. *Experimental Gerontology, 35*(3), 307–316.

Sullivan, M., & Yalla, S. (2002). Physiology of female micturition. *Urology Clinics of North America, 29*, 499–514.

Timiras, P. S. (Ed.). (2003). *Physiological basis of aging and geriatrics* (3rd ed.). Boca Raton, FL: CRC Press.

Topp, R., Fahlman, M., & Boardley, D. (2004). Healthy aging: Health promotion and disease prevention. *Nursing Clinics of North America, 39*(2), 411–422.

Troncale, J. (1996). The aging process. Physiologic changes and pharmacologic implications. *Postgraduate Medicine, 99*(5), 111–114, 120–122.

Uylings, H., & De Brabander, J. (2002). Neuronal changes in normal human aging and Alzheimer's disease. *Brain and Cognition, 49*, 268–276.

Van Zant, G., & Liang, Y. (2003). The role of stem cells in aging. *Experimental Hematology, 31*(8), 659–672.

Vijg, J., & Suh, Y. (2005). Genetics of longevity and aging. *Annual Review of Medicine, 56*, 193–212.

Wade, P., & Cowen, T. (2004). Neurodegeneration: A key factor in the ageing gut. *Neurogastroenterology and Motility, 16*(Suppl. 1), 19–23.

Wakamatsu, M. (2003). What affects bladder function more: Menopause or age? *Menopause, 10*(3), 191–192.

Personal Reflections

1. Discuss with an older adult (such as a grandparent or great-grandparent) the significant physical changes that occurred as a consequence of the aging process without disease over his or her life course. Focus on changes that led to lifestyle alterations and changes that most affected him or her personally. What specific alterations stand out the most in your mind? Which ones most affect quality of life?
2. Review several Web sites about aging and discuss what healthy aging means from a media perspective versus a research or personal perspective. Compare your own experiences of aging processes with those found in other arenas. How could you use these resources in your nursing practice?
3. Identify preventive techniques that may enhance the aging experience or delay aging processes throughout the life course. Discuss how these techniques work on the body for every organ system and how they might help delay aging or maintain a healthy aging status. Correlate your discussion with older individuals you know. How could you use this knowledge to make you more sensitive toward caring for the aged?

BOX 6-4 Resource List

American Federation for Aging Research: http://www.afar.org

American Society on Aging: http://www.asaging.org

Baltimore Longitudinal Study of Aging: http://www.grc.nia.nih.gov/branches/blsa/blsa.htm

Centers for Disease Control and Prevention, Healthy Aging: http://www.cdc.gov/aging/

Geriatrics & Aging: http://www.geriatricsandaging.com

National Council on Aging: http://www.ncoa.org/index.cfm

National Institute on Aging (NIA): http://www.nia.nih.gov

National Institute on Aging Age Pages: http://www.healthandage.com/html/min/nih/content/booklets/research_new_age/page3.htm

The Nun Study: http://www.mc.uky.edu/nunnet/

University of California at San Francisco Academic Geriatric Resource Center Online Curriculum: http://www.ucsfagrc.org

U.S. Administration on Aging (AOA): http://www.aoa.gov

References

Abernathy, D. (1999). Aging effects on drug disposition and effect. *Geriatric Nephrology and Urology, 9*, 15–19.

Abrams, W., Beers, M., & Berkow, R. (Eds.). (1995). *The Merck manual of geriatrics* (2nd ed.). Whitehouse Station, NJ: Merck & Company.

Aeron Biotechnology. (2005). *Salivary hormone monitoring: Cortisol.* Retrieved March 10, 2005, from http://www.aeron.com/new_page_27.htm

American Diabetes Association. (2005). *Frequently asked questions about pre-diabetes.* Retrieved March 10, 2005, from http://www.diabetes.org/pre-diabetes/faq.jsp

Andersson, K., & Arner, A. (2004). Urinary bladder contraction and relaxation: Physiology and pathophysiology. *Physiological Reviews, 84*(3), 935–986.

Anderton, B. (2002). Ageing of the brain. *Mechanisms of Ageing and Development, 123*, 811–817.

Arking, R. (1998). *Biology of aging: Observations and principles* (2nd ed.). Sunderland, MA: Sinauer Associates.

Arlt, W. (2004). *Adrenal androgens.* Retrieved March 10, 2005, from http://www.endotext.org/aging/aging12/aging12.htm

Aronow, W. (1998). Effects of aging on the heart. In R. Tallis, H. Fillit, & J. Brocklehurst (Eds.), *Brocklehurst's textbook of geriatric medicine and gerontology* (5th ed., pp. 255–262). London: Churchill Livingstone.

Arranz, E., O'Mahony, S., Barton, J., & Ferguson, A. (1992). Immunosenescence and mucosal immunity: Significant effects of old age on secretrory IgA concentrations and intraepithelial lymphocyte counts. *Gut, 33*(7), 882–886.

Artero, S., Tiemeier, H., & Prins, N. (2004). Neuroanatomical localization and clinical correlates of white matter lesions in the elderly. *Journal of Neurology and Neurosurgery Psychiatry, 75*, 1304–1308.

Aspinall, R., & Andrew, D. (2000). Thymic involution in aging. *Journal of Clinical Immunology, 20*(4), 250–256.

Asplund, R. (2004). Nocturia, nocturnal polyuria, and sleep quality in the elderly. *Journal of Psychosomatic Research, 56*(5), 511–525.

American Society for Reproductive Medicine Practice Committee. (2004). Treatment of androgen deficiency in the aging male. *Fertility and Sterility, 82*(Suppl. 1), S46–S50.

Atwood, L., Wolf, P., Heard-Costa, N., Massaro, J., Beiser, A., D'Agostino, R., et al. (2004). Genetic variation in white matter hyperintensity volume in the Framingham study. *Stroke, 35*, 1609–1613.

Aw, D., Silva, A., & Palmer, D. (2007). Immunosenescence: Emerging challenges for an ageing populatation. *Immunology, 120*, 435–446.

Bagnara, G. P., Bonsi, L., Strippoli, P., Bonifazi, F., Tonelli, R., D'Addato, S., et al. (2000). Hemopoiesis in healthy old people and centenarians: Well-maintained responsiveness of CD34+ cells to hemopoietic growth factors and remodeling of cytokine network. *Journals of Gerontology: Biological Sciences, 55A*(2), B61–B66.

Baik, H., & Russell, R. (1999). Vitamin B12 deficiency in the elderly. *Annual Review of Nutrition, 19*, 357–377.

Balagopal, P., Rooyackers, O. E., Adey, D. B., Ades, P. A., & Nair, K. S. (1997). Effects of aging on in vivo synthesis of skeletal muscle myosin heavy-chain and sarcoplasmic protein in humans. *American Journal of Physiology, 273*(4 Pt 1), E790–E800.

Balducci, L. (2003). Anemia, cancer, and aging. *Cancer Control, 10*(6), 478–486.

Balducci, L., Hardy, C. L., & Lyman, G. H. (2000). Hemopoietic reserve in the older cancer patient: Clinical and economic considerations. *Cancer Control, 7*(6), 539–547.

Ball, K., & Sekuler, R. (1986). Improving visual perception in older observers. *Journal of Gerontology, 41*, 176–182.

Baraldi-Junkins, C., Beck, A., & Rothstein, G. (2000). Hematopoiesis and cytokines. Relevance to cancer and aging. *Hematology and Oncology Clinics of North America, 14*(1), 45–61.

Barnes, P. J. (2000). Chronic obstructive pulmonary disease. *New England Journal of Medicine, 343*(4), 269–280.

Bartoshuk, L., & Duffy, V. (1995). Taste and smell. In E. Masoro (Ed.), *Handbook of physiology: Section 11, Aging* (pp. 363–376). New York: Oxford Press.

Bartzokis, G., Sultzer, D., Lu, P., Nuechterlein, K., Mintz, J., & Cummings, J. (2004). Heterogeneous age-related breakdown of white matter structural integrity: Implications for cortical "disconnection" in aging and Alzheimer's disease. *Neurobiology of Aging, 25*(7), 843–851.

Bates, T., Harrison, M., Lowe, D., Lawson, C., & Padley, N. (1992). Longitudinal study of gallstone prevalence at necropsy. *Gut, 33*(1), 103–107.

Baumann, L. (2007). Skin aging and its treatment. *Journal of Pathology, 211*, 241–251.

Baumgartner, R., Koehler, K., Gallagher, D., Romero, L., Heymsfield, S., Ross, R., et al. (1998). Epidemiology of sarcopenia among the elderly in New Mexico. *American Journal of Epidemiology, 147*(8), 755–763.

Bearden, S. (2006). Effect of aging on the structure and function of skeletal muscle microvascular networks. *Microcirculation, 13*, 305–314.

Beck, L. (1998). Changes in renal function with aging. *Clinical Geriatric Medicine, 14*, 199–209.

Beck, L. (1999a). Aging changes in renal function. In W. Hazzard, J. Blass, W. Ettinger Jr., J. Halter, & J. Ouslander (Eds.), *Principles of geriatric medicine and gerontology* (4th ed., pp. 767–776). New York: McGraw-Hill.

Beck, L. (1999b). Fluid and electrolyte balance in the elderly. *Geriatric Nephrology and Urology, 9*, 11–14.

Beers, M. H., & Berkow, R. (Eds.). (2000). *The Merck manual of geriatrics* (3rd ed.). New York: John Wiley & Sons.

Beers, M., & Berkow, R. (Eds.). (n.d.). *The Merck manual of geriatrics* (Internet 3rd ed.). Merck & Company, Inc. Retrieved January 20, 2005, from http://www.merck.com/mrkshared/mm_geriatrics/home.jsp

Benzi, G., & Moretti, P. (1997). Contribution of mitocondrial alterations to brain aging. *Advances in Cell Aging & Gerontology, 2*, 129–160.

Bhasin, S. (2003). Testosterone supplementation for aging-associated sarcopenia. *Journals of Gerontology: Medical Sciences, 58A*(11), 1002–1008.

Bhatnagar, K., Kennedy, R., Baron, G., & Greenberg, R. (1987). Number of mitral cells and the bulb volume in the aging human olfactory bulb: A quantitative morphological study. *Anatomical Record Part A, 218*, 73–87.

Binder, L., Guillozet-Bongaarts, A., Garcia-Sierra, F., & Berry, R. (2005). Tau, tangles, and Alzheimer's disease. *Biochimic et Biophysica Acta (BBA)—Molecular Basis of Disease, 1739*(2–3), 216–223.

Bjorntorp, P. (1997). The relationship between obesity and diabetes. In K. Alberti, P. Zimmet, R. DeFronzo, & H. Keen (Eds.), *International textbook of diabetes mellitus* (Vol. 1, pp. 611–627). New York: John Wiley & Sons.

Borst, S. E. (2004). Interventions for sarcopenia and muscle weakness in older people. *Age and Ageing, 33*(6), 548–555.

Bourdiol, P., Mioche, L., & Monier, S. (2004). Effect of age on salivary flow obtained under feeding and non-feeding conditions. *Journal of Oral Rehabilitation, 31*, 445–452.

Brading, A., Teramoto, N., Dass, N., & McCoy, R. (2001). Morphological and physiological characteristics of urethral circular and longitudinal smooth muscle. *Scandinavian Journal of Urology and Nephrology: Supplementum, 207*, 12–18.

Bressler, P., & DeFronzo, R. (1997). Drug effects on glucose homeostasis. In K. Alberti, P. Zimmet, R. DeFronzo, & H. Keen (Eds.), *International textbook of diabetes mellitus* (2nd ed., Vol. 1, pp. 231–254). New York: John Wiley & Sons.

Brogna, A., Ferrara, R., Bucceri, A., Lanteri, E., & Catalano, F. (1999). Influence of aging on gastrointestinal transit time. An ultrasonographic and radiologic study. *Investigative Radiology, 34*(5), 357–359.

Brown, W., Strong, M., & Snow, R. (1988). Methods of estimating numbers of motor units in biceps-brachialis muscles and losses of motor units with aging. *Muscle and Nerve, 11*(5), 423–432.

Buchholz, J., Behringer, E., Pottorf, W., Pearce, W., & Vanterpool, C. (2007). Age-dependent changes in $Ca2^{+}$ homeostatis in peripheral neurones: Implications for changes in function. *Aging Cell, 6*, 285–296.

Carpo, R., & Campbell, E. (1998). Aging of the respiratory system. In A. P. Fishmen (Ed.), *Pulmonary diseases and disorders* (pp. 251–264). New York: McGraw-Hill.

Carroll, J., Shroff, S., Wirth, P., Halsted, M., & Rajfer, S. (1991). Arterial mechanical properties in dilated cardiomyopathy: Aging and the response to nitroprusside. *Journal of Clinical Investigation, 87*, 1002–1009.

Chahal, H., & Drake, W. (2007). The endocrine system and ageing. *Journal of Pathology, 211*, 173–180.

Chakraborty, T., & Gore, A. (2004). Aging-related changes in ovarian hormones, their receptors, and neuroendocrine function. *Experimental Biology and Medicine, 229*, 977–987.

Chapuy, M., Durr, F., & Chapuy, P. (1983). Age-related changes in parathyroid hormone and 25-hydroxycholecalciferol levels. *Journal of Gerontology, 38*, 19–22.

Chen, M., Halter, J., & Porte, D. (1987). The role of dietary carbohydrate in the decreased glucose tolerance of the elderly. *Journal of the American Geriatrics Society, 35*(5), 417–424.

Cockcroft, D., & Gault, M. (1976). Prediction of creatinine clearance from serum creatinine. *Nephron, 16*, 31–41.

Colcombe, S. J., Kramer, A. F., Erickson, K. I., Scalf, P., McAuley, E., Cohen, N. J., et al. (2004). Cardiovascular fitness, cortical plasticity, and aging. *Proceedings of the National Academy of Sciences of the United States of America, 101*(9), 3316–3321.

Corman, B., Barrault, M., Klingler, C., Houot, A., Michel, J., Della Bruna, R., et al. (1995). Renin gene expression in the aging kidney: Effect of sodium restriction. *Mechanisms of Ageing and Development, 84*(1), 1–13.

Cowart, B. (1989). Relationships between taste and smell across the adult life span. *Annals of the New York Academy of Science, 561*, 39–55.

Curcio, C., Millican, C., Allen, K., & Kalina, R. (1993). Aging of the human photoreceptor mosaic: Evidence for selective vulnerability of rods in central retina. *Investigative Ophthalmology & Visual Science, 34*(12), 3278–3296.

Czech, M., Erwin, J., & Sleeman, M. (1996). Insulin action on glucose transport. In D. LeRoith, S. Taylor, & J. Olefsky (Eds.), *Diabetes mellitus: A fundamental and clinical text* (pp. 205–213). Philadelphia: Lippincott-Raven.

Davies, A., Kidd, D., Stone, S., & MacMahon, J. (1995). Pharyngeal sensation and gag reflex in healthy subjects. *Lancet, 345*, 487–488.

Davis, S., McCloud, P., Strauss, B., & Burger, H. (1995). Testosterone enhances estradiol's effects on postmenopausal bone density and sexuality. *Maturitas, 21*(3), 227–236.

Dela, F., Mikines, K., & Galbo, H. (1999). Physical activity and insulin resistance in man. In G. Reaven & A. Laws (Eds.), *Insulin resistance: The metabolic syndrome X* (pp. 97–120). Totowa, NJ: Humana Press.

de la Torre, J. (1997). Cerebrovascular changes in the aging brain. In P. Timiras & E. Bittar (Eds.), *Advances in cell aging and gerontology: The aging brain* (Vol. 2, pp. 707–717). Greenwich, CT: Jai Press.

De Martinis, M., & Timiras, P. S. (2003). The pulmonary respiration, hematopoiesis, and erythrocytes. In P. S. Timiras (Ed.), *Physiological basis of aging and geriatrics* (pp. 319–336). Boca Raton, FL: CRC Press.

Deschenes, M. (2004). Effects of aging on muscle fiber type and size. *Sports Medicine, 34*(12), 809–824.

Despres, J.-P., & Marette, A. (1999). Obesity and insulin resistance: Epidemiologic, metabolic, and molecular aspects. In G. Reaven & A. Laws (Eds.), *Insulin resistance: The metabolic syndrome X* (pp. 51–81). Totowa, NJ: Humana Press.

Devlin, H., & Ferguson, M. (1998). Aging and the orofacial tissues. In R. Tallis, H. Fillit, & J. Brocklehurst (Eds.), *Brocklehurst's textbook of geriatric medicine and gerontology* (5th ed., pp. 789–802). London: Churchill Livingstone.

Dhatariya, K. K., & Nair, K. S. (2003). Dehydro-epiandrosterone: Is there a role for replacement? *Mayo Clinic Proceedings, 78*, 1257–1273.

Dickson, D. (1997). Structural changes in the aging brain. In P. Timiras & E. Bittar (Eds.), *Advances in cell aging and gerontology: The aging brain* (Vol. 2, pp. 51–76). Greenwich, CT: Jai Press.

Digiovanna, A. G. (1994). *Human aging: Biological perspectives.* New York: McGraw-Hill.

Digiovanna, A. G. (2000). *Human aging: Biological perspectives* (2nd ed.). Boston: McGraw-Hill.

Diokno, A., Brown, M., Brock, B., Herzog, A., & Normolle, D. (1988). Clinical and cystometric characteristics of continent and incontinent noninstitutionalized elderly. *Journal of Urology, 140*, 567–571.

Dionne, I., Kinaman, K., & Poehlman, E. (2000). Sarcopenia and muscle function during menopause and hormone-replacement therapy. *Journal of Nutrition, Health, and Aging, 4*(3), 156–161.

Doherty, T., & Brown, W. (1993). The estimated numbers and relative sizes of thenar motor units selected by multiple point stimulation in young and older animals. *Muscle and Nerve, 16*(4), 355–366.

Doherty, T. J. (2003). Invited review: Aging and sarcopenia. *Journal of Applied Physiology, 95*, 1717–1727.

Drewnowski, A., & Evans, W. (2001). Nutrition, physical activity, and quality of life in older adults: Summary. *Journals of Gerontology Series A: Biological Sciences and Medical Sciences, 56A*(Special Issue II), 89–94.

Duggal, P., Klein, A., Lee, K., Iyengar, S., Klein R., Bailey-Wilson, J., et al. (2005). A genetic contribution to intraocular pressure: The Beaver Dam Eye Study. *Investigative Ophthalmology and Visual Science, 46*(2), 555–560.

Dunn, L. B., Damesyn, M., Moore, A. A., Reuben, D. B., & Greendale, G. A. (1997). Does estrogen prevent skin aging? Results from the First National Health and Nutrition Examination Survey (NHANES I). *Archives of Dermatology, 133*(3), 339–342.

Effros, R. B., Dagarag, M., & Valenzuela, H. F. (2003). In vitro senescence of immune cells. *Experimental Gerontology, 38*(11–12), 1243–1249.

Effros, R. B., & Pawelec, G. (1997). Replicative senescence of T cells: Does the Hayflick limit lead to immune exhaustion? *Immunology Today, 18*(9), 450–454.

Egusa, Y., Fujiwara, Y., Syahruddin, E., Isobe, T., & Yamakido, M. (1998). Effect of age on human peripheral blood stem cells. *Oncology Reports, 5*(2), 397–400.

Elbadawi, A., Diokno, A., & Millard, R. (1998). The aging bladder: Morphology and urodynamics. *World Journal of Urology, 16*(Suppl. 1), S10–S34.

Elbadawi, A., Yalla, S., & Resnick, N. (1993). Structural basis of geriatric voiding dysfunction. II. Aging detrusor: Normal vs. impaired contractility. *Journal of Urology, 150*, 1657–1667.

ElSolh, A., & Ramadan, F. (2006). Overview of respiratory failure in older adults. *Journal of Intensive Care Medicine, 21*, 345–351.

Engelhardt, M., Kumar, R., Albanell, J., Pettengell, R., Han, W., & Moore, M. (1997). Telomerase regulation, cell cycle, and telomere stability in primitive hematopoietic cells. *Blood, 90*(1), 182–193.

Enoka, R. (1997). Neural strategies in the control of muscle force. *Muscle and Nerve, 5*(Suppl.), S66–S69.

Erickson, C., & Barnes, C. (2003). The neurobiology of memory changes in normal aging. *Experimental Gerontology, 38*, 61–69.

Esler, M., Kaye, D., Thompson, J., Jennings, G., Cox, H., Turner, A., et al. (1995). Effects of aging on epinephrine secretion and regional release of epinephrine from the human heart. *Journal of Clinical Endocrinology and Metabolism, 80*(2), 435–442.

Esler, M., Turner, A., Kaye, D., Thompson, J., Kingwell, B., Morris, M., et al. (1995). Aging effects on human sympathetic neuronal function. *American Journal of Physiology, 268*, R278–R285.

Evans, W. J. (2002). Effects of exercise on senescent muscle. *Clinical Orthopaedics and Related Research, 403S*, S211–S220.

Falahati-Nini, A., Riggs, B. L., Atkinson, E. J., O'Fallon, W. M., Eastell, R., & Khosla, S. (2000). Relative contributions of testosterone and estrogen in regulating bone resorption and formation in normal elderly men. *Journal of Clinical Investigation, 106*(12), 1553–1560.

Fenske, N., & Lober, C. (1986). Structural and functional changes of normal aging skin. *Journal of the American Academy of Dermatology, 15*(4 Pt 1), 571–585.

Ferrari, A., Radaelli, A., & Centola, M. (2003). Invited review: Aging and the cardiovascular system. *Journal of Applied Physiology, 95*(6), 2591–2597.

Ferrari, E., Cravello, L., Muzzoni, B., Casarotti, D., Paltro, M., Solerte, S., et al. (2001). Age-related changes of the hypothalamic-pituitary-adrenal axis: Pathophysiological correlates. *European Journal of Endocrinology, 144*, 319–329.

Ferriolli, E., Oliveira, R., Matsuda, N., Braga, F., & Dantos, R. (1998). Aging, esophageal motility and gastroesophageal reflux disease. *Journal of the American Geriatric Association, 46*, 1534–1537.

Fiatarone, M., Marks, E., Ryan, N., Meredith, C., Lipsitz, L., & Evans, W. (1990). High-intensity strength training in nonagenarians: Effects on skeletal muscle. *Journal of the American Medical Association, 263*(22), 3029–3034.

Fink, R., Kolterman, O., Griffin, J., & Olefsky, J. (1983). Mechanisms of insulin resistance in aging. *Journal of Clinical Investigation, 71*, 1523–1535.

Fleg, J. (1986). Alterations in cardiovascular structure and function with advancing age. *American Journal of Cardiology, 57*, 33C–44C.

Fleg, J., Morrell, C., Bos, A., Brant, L., Talbot, L., Wright, J., et al. (2005). Accelerated longitudinal decline of aerobic capacity in healthy older adults. *Circulation, 112*, 674–682.

Fleg, J., O'Connor, F., Gerstenblith, G., Becker, L., Clulow, J., Schulman, S., et al. (1995). Impact of age on the cardiovascular response to dynamic upright exercise in healthy men and women. *Journal of Applied Physiology, 78*, 890–900.

Fliser, D., Franek, E., Joest, M., Block, S., Mutschler, E., & Ritz, E. (1997). Renal function in the elderly: Impact of hypertension and cardiac function. *Kidney International, 51*, 1196–1204.

Fossel, M. B. (2004). *Cells, aging, and human disease.* New York: Oxford University Press.

Fransen, E., Lemkens, N., Van Laer, L., & Van Camp, G. (2003). Age-related hearing impairment (ARHI): Environmental risk factors and genetic prospects. *Experimental Gerontology, 38*, 353–359.

Frontera, W., Meredith, C., O'Reilly, K., Knuttgen, H., & Evans, W. (1988). Strength conditioning in older men: Skeletal muscle hypertrophy and improved function. *Journal of Applied Physiology, 64*, 1038–1044.

Fulp, S., Dalton, C., Castell, J., & Castell, D. (1990). Aging-related alterations in human upper esophageal sphincter functions. *American Journal of Gastroenterology, 85*, 1569–1572.

Garg, A. (1999). The role of body fat distribution in insulin resistance. In G. Reaven & A. Laws (Eds.), *Insulin resistance: The metabolic syndrome X* (pp. 83–96). Totowa, NJ: Humana Press.

Gerstenblith, G., Frederiksen, J., Yin, F., Fortuin, N., Lakatta, E., & Weisfeldt, M. (1977). Echocardiographic assessment of a normal adult aging population. *Circulation, 56*(2), 273–278.

Ghezzi, E., & Ship, J. (2003). Aging and secretory reserve capacity of major salivary glands. *Journal of Dentistry Research, 82*(10), 844–848.

Gill, S., Sharpless, J., Rado, K., & Hall, J. (2002). Evidence that GnRH decreases with gonadal steroid feedback but increases with age in postmenopausal women. *Journal of Clinical Endocrinology and Metabolism, 87*, 2290–2296.

Gilmore, G., Wenk, H., Naylor, L., & Stuve, T. (1992). Motion perception and aging. *Psychology and Aging, 7*(4), 654–660.

Globerson, A. (1999). Hematopoietic stem cells and aging. *Experimental Gerontology, 34*(2), 137–146.

Gluck, M., Thomas, R., Davis, K., & Haroutunian, V. (2002). Implications for altered glutamate and GABA metabolism in the dorsolateral prefrontal cortex of aged schizophrenic patients. *American Journal of Psychiatry, 159*, 1165–1173.

Gomes, O., deSouza, R., & Liberti, E. (1997). A preliminary investigation of the effects of ageing on the nerve cell number in the myenteric ganglia of the human colon. *Gerontology, 43*, 210–217.

Gomez, C., Boehmer, E. D., & Kovacs, E. (2005). The aging innate immune system. *Current Opinion in Immunology, 17*, 457–462.

Graal, M., & Wolffenbuttel, B. (1999). The use of sulphonylureas in the elderly. *Drugs and Aging, 15*(6), 471–481.

Greendale, G., Edelstein, S., & Barrett-Connor, E. (1997). Endogenous sex steroid and bone mineral density in older women and men. The Rancho Bernardo Study. *Journal of Bone Mineral Research, 12*, 1833–1843.

Gruenewald, D., & Matsumoto, A. (1999). Aging of the endocrine system. In W. Hazzard, J. Blass, W. Ettinger Jr., J. Halter, & J. Ouslander (Eds.), *Principles of geriatric medicine and gerontology* (4th ed., pp. 949–966). New York: McGraw-Hill.

Gruver, A., Hudson, L., & Sempowski, G. (2007). Immunosenescence of ageing. *Journal of Pathology, 211*, 144–156.

Gupta, V., & Lipsitz, L. (2007). Orthostatic hypotension in the elderly: Diagnosis and treatment. *American Journal of Medicine, 120*, 841–847.

Haas, A., Flammer, J., & Schneider, U. (1986). Influence of age on the visual fields of normal subjects. *American Journal of Ophthalmology, 101*, 199–203.

Hafez, B., & Hafez, E. (2004). Andropause: Endocrinology, erectile dysfunction, and prostate pathophysiology. *Archives of Andrology, 50*, 45–68.

Hall, J. (2004). Neuroendocrine physiology of the early and late menopause. *Endocrinology and Metabolism Clinics of North America, 33*(4), 637–659.

Hall, J. (2007). Neuroendocrine changes with reproductive aging in women. *Seminars in Reproductive Medicine, 25*, 344–355.

Hall, J., Lavoie, H., Marsh, E., & Martin, K. (2000). Decrease in gonadotropin-releasing hormone (GnRH) pulse frequency with aging in postmenopausal women. *Journal of Clinical Endocrinology and Metabolism, 85*, 1794–1800.

Hall, K. (2002). Aging and neural control of the GI tract. II. Neural control of the aging gut: Can an old dog learn new tricks? *American Journal of Physiology: Gastrointestinal and Liver Physiology, 283*, G827–G832.

Hall, K., & Wiley, J. (1999). Age-associated changes in gastrointestinal function. In W. Hazzard, J. Blass, W. Ettinger Jr., J. Halter, & J. Ouslander (Eds.), *Principles of geriatric medicine and gerontology* (4th ed., pp. 835–842). New York: McGraw-Hill.

Halter, J. (2000). Effects of aging on glucose homeostasis. In D. LeRoith, S. Taylor, & J. Olefsky (Eds.), *Diabetes mellitus, a fundamental and clinical text* (2nd ed., pp. 576–582). Philadelphia: Lippincott Williams & Wilkins.

Hansen, K., Thyer, A., Sluss, P., Bremner, W., Soules, M., & Klein, N. (2005). Reproductive ageing and ovarian function: Is the earlier follicular phase FSH rise necessary to maintain adequate secretory function in older ovulatory women? *Human Reproduction, 20*(1), 89–95.

Harris, M. (1990). Epidemiology of diabetes mellitus among the elderly in the United States. *Clinics in Geriatric Medicine, 6*(4), 703–719.

Hasten, D., Pak-Loduca, J., Obert, K., & Yarasheski, K. (2000). Resistance exercise acutely increases MHC and mixed muscle protein synthesis rate in 78–84 and 23–32 yr olds. *American Journal of Physiology, 278*(4), E620–E626.

Hayward, C., Kelly, R., & Collins, P. (2000). The role of gender, the menopause and hormone replacement on cardiovascular function. *Cardiovascular Research, 46*, 28–49.

Heine, C., & Browning, C. (2002). Communication and psychosocial consequences of sensory loss in older adults: Overview and rehabilitation directions. *Disability and Rehabilitation, 24*(15), 763–773.

Hinson, J., & Raven, P. (1999). DHEA deficiency syndrome: A new term for old age? *Journal of Endocrinology, 163*, 1–5.

Hirokawa, K. (1999). Age-related changes of signal transduction in T cells. *Experimental Gerontology, 34*(1), 7–18.

Holick, M. F. (2003). Vitamin D: A millennium perspective. *Journal of Cellular Biochemistry, 88*(2), 296–307.

Hollander, J., & Diokno, A. (1998). Prostate gland disease. In E. Duthie & P. Katz (Eds.), *Practice of geriatrics* (3rd ed., pp. 535–545). Philadelphia: W. B. Saunders.

Hollenberg, M., Yang, J., Haight, T., & Tager, I. (2006). Longitudinal changes in aerobic capacity: Implications for concepts of aging. *Journals of Gerontology, 61A*(8), 851–858.

Holt, P. (1992). Clinical significance of bacterial overgrowth in elderly people. *Age and Ageing, 21*, 1–4.

Horton, R., & Tait, J. (1966). Androstenedione production and interconversion rates measured in peripheral blood and studies on the possible site of its conversion to testosterone. *Journal of Clinical Investigation, 45*, 301–313.

Hunt, B., Farquar, W., & Taylor, J. (2001). Does reduced vascular stiffening fully explain preserved cardiovagal baroreflex function in older, physically active men? *Circulation, 103*, 2424–2427.

Ishikawa, M., Matsumoto, M., Fujimura, Y., Chiba, K., & Toyama, Y. (2003). Changes of cervical spinal cord and cervical spinal canal with age in asymptomatic subjects. *Spinal Cord, 41*, 159–163.

Ivey, F., Tracy, B., Lemmer, J., NessAiver, M., Metter, E., Fozard, J., et al. (2000). Effects of strength training and detraining on muscle quality: Age and gender comparisons. *Journals of Gerontology: Biological Sciences, 55A*(3), B152–B157.

Jackson, G., & Owsley, C. (2003). Visual dysfunction, neurodegenerative diseases, and aging. *Neurology Clinics of North America, 21*, 709–728.

Jackson, R. (1990). Mechanisms of age-related glucose intolerance. *Diabetes Care, 13*(Suppl. 2), 9–19.

Jacobsen, E., Billings, J., Frantz, R., Kinney, C., Stewart, M., & Downing, D. (1985). Age-related changes in sebaceous wax ester secretion rates in men and women. *Journal of Investigative Dermatology, 85*(5), 483–485.

James, O. (1998). The liver. In R. Tallis, H. Fillit, & J. Brocklehurst (Eds.), *Brocklehurst's textbook of geriatric medicine and gerontology* (5th ed., pp. 841–862). London: Churchill Livingstone.

Janowsky, J., Oviatt, S., & Orwoll, E. (1994). Testosterone influences spatial cognition in older men. *Behavioral Neuroscience, 108*, 325–332.

Janssen, I., Heymsfield, S., Wang, Z., & Ross, R. (2000). Skeletal muscle mass and distribution in 468 men and women aged 18–88 yr. *Journal of Applied Physiology, 89*, 81–88.

Jassal, S., & Oreopoulos, D. (1998). The aging kidney. *Geriatric Nephrology and Urology, 8*, 141–147.

Jassal, V., Fillit, H., & Oreopoulos, D. (1998). Aging of the urinary tract. In R. Tallis, H. Fillit, & J. Brocklehurst (Eds.), *Brocklehurst's textbook of geriatric medicine and gerontology* (5th ed., pp. 919–924). London: Churchill Livingstone.

Jerger, J., Chmiel, R., Wilson, N., & Luchi, R. (1995). Hearing impairment in older adults: New concepts. *Journal of the American Geriatrics Society, 43*(8), 928–935.

Jimenez, M., Cuartero, E., & Moreno, J. (2001). Neurobehavioral syndromes in patients with cerebrovascular pathology. In J. Leon-Carrion & M. Giannini (Eds.), *Behavioral neurology in the elderly* (pp. 337–362). Boca Raton, FL: CRC Press.

Joffe, H., Soares, C., & Cohen, L. (2003). Assessment and treatment of hot flashes and menopausal mood disturbance. *Psychiatric Clinics of North America, 26*, 563–580.

Johnson, C., Adams, A., & Lewis, R. (1989). Evidence for a neural basis of age-related visual field loss in normal observers. *Investigative Ophthalmology and Visual Science, 30*, 2056–2064.

Johnson, T., Miller, M., Pillin, D., & Auslander, J. (2003). Arginine vasopressin and nocturnal polyuria in older adults with frequent nighttime voiding. *Journal of Urology, 170*(2), 480–484.

Judd, H., & Yen, S. (1973). Serum androstenedione and testosterone levels during the menstrual cycle. *Journal of Clinical Endocrinology and Metabolism, 36*, 475–481.

Kalina, R. (1999). Aging and visual function. In W. Hazzard, J. Blass, W. Ettinger Jr., J. Halter, & J. Ouslander (Eds.), *Principles of geriatric medicine and gerontology* (4th ed., pp. 603–616). New York: McGraw-Hill.

Kallman, D., Plato, C., & Tobin, J. (1990). The role of muscle loss in the age-related decline of grip strength: Cross-sectional and longitudinal perspectives. *Journals of Gerontology, 45*, M82–M88.

Kamminga, L., & DeHaan, G. (2006). Cellular memory and hematopoietic stem cell aging. *Stem Cells, 24*, 1143–1149.

Kandeel, F., Koussa, V., & Swerdloff, R. (2001). Male sexual function and its disorders: Physiology, pathophysiology, clinical investigation, and treatment. *Endocrine Reviews, 22*(3), 342–388.

Kane, R., Ouslander, J., & Abrass, I. (1999). Cardiovascular disorders. In S. Zollo & M. Navrozov (Eds.), *Essentials of clinical geriatrics* (4th ed., pp. 292–317). New York: McGraw-Hill.

Karlsson, S., Persson, M., & Carlsson, G. (1991). Mandibular movement and velocity in relation to state of dentition and age. *Journal of Oral Rehabilitation, 18*, 1–8.

Katzman, R. (1995). Human nervous system. In E. Masoro (Ed.), *Handbook of physiology: Section 11, aging* (pp. 325–344). New York: Oxford University Press.

Kelly, J., & Roth, G. (1997). Changes in neurotransmitter signal transduction pathways in the aging brain. In

P. Timiras & E. Bittar (Eds.), *Advances in cell aging and gerontology: The aging brain* (Vol. 2, pp. 243–278). Greenwich, CT: Jai Press.

Kevorkian, R. (2004). Physiology of incontinence. *Clinics in Geriatric Medicine, 20*, 409–425.

Kirkland, J., Lye, M., Levy, D., & Banerjee, A. (1983). Patterns of urine flow and electrolyte excretion in healthy elderly people. *British Medical Journal, 287*, 1665–1667.

Klein, B., Klein, R., & Linton, K. (1992a). Prevalence of age-related lens opacities in a population: The Beaver Dam Eye Study. *Ophthalmology, 99*(4), 546–552.

Klein, B., Klein, R., & Linton, K. (1992b). Prevalence of age-related maculopathy: The Beaver Dam Eye Study. *Ophthalmology, 99*(6), 933–943.

Klein, N., Illingworth, P., Groome, N., McNeilly, A., Battaglia, D., & Soules, M. (1996). Decreased inhibin B secretion is associated with the monotropic FSH rise in older, ovulatory women: A study of serum and follicular fluid levels of dimeric inhibin A and B in spontaneous menstrual cycles. *Journal of Clinical Endocrinology and Metabolism, 81*, 2742–2745.

Klein, R., Wang, Q., Klein, B., Moss, S., & Meuer, S. (1995). The relationship of age-related maculopathy cataract, and glaucoma to visual acuity. *Investigative Ophthalmology and Visual Science, 36*(1), 182–191.

Kollarits, C. (1998). Ophthalmologic disorders. In E. Duthie & P. Katz (Eds.), *Practice of geriatrics* (3rd ed., pp. 457–466). Philadelphia: W. B. Saunders.

Korenman, S., Morley, J., Mooradian, A., Davis, S., Kaiser, F., Silver, A., et al. (1990). Secondary hypogonadism in older men: Its relation to impotence. *Journal of Clinical Endocrinology and Metabolism, 71*, 963–969.

Kotz, C., Billington, C., & Levine, A. (1999). Obesity and aging. *Clinics in Geriatric Medicine, 15*(2), 391–412.

Kovacs, T. (1999). β-amyloid deposition and neurofibrillary tangle formation in the olfactory bulb in ageing and Alzheimer's disease. *Neuropathology and Applied Neurobiology, 25*, 481–491.

Kovacs, T. (2004). Mechanisms of olfactory dysfunction in aging and neurodegenerative disorders. *Ageing Research Review, 3*, 215–232.

Krauss Whitbourne, S. (2002). *The aging individual: Physical and psychological perspectives* (2nd ed.). New York: Springer.

Lakatta, E. (1993a). Cardiovascular regulatory mechanisms in advanced age. *Physiological Reviews, 73*, 413–467.

Lakatta, E. (1993b). Deficient neuroendocrine regulation of the cardiovascular system with advancing age in healthy humans. *Circulation, 87*, 631–636.

Lakatta, E. (1996). Cardiovascular aging in health. In M. Chizner (Ed.), *Classic teachings in clinical cardiology* (Vol. 2, pp. 1369–1390). Cedar Grove, NJ: Laennec.

Lakatta, E. (1999a). Cardiovascular aging research: The next horizons. *Journal of the American Geriatrics Society, 47*, 613–625.

Lakatta, E. (1999b). Circulatory function in younger and older humans in health. In W. Hazzard, J. Blass, W. Ettinger Jr., J. Halter, & J. Ouslander (Eds.), *Principles of geriatric medicine and gerontology* (4th ed., pp. 645–660). New York: McGraw-Hill.

Lakatta, E., Gerstenblith, G., Angell, S., Shock, N., & Weisfeldt, M. (1975). Prolonged contraction duration in aged myocardium. *Journal of Clinical Investigation, 55*(1), 61–68.

Lakatta, E., & Levy, D. (2003). Arterial and cardiac aging: Major shareholders in cardiovascular disease enterprises: Part II aging arteries: A setup for vascular disease. *Circulation, 107*, 139–146.

Lansdorp, P., Poon, S., Chavez, E., Dragowska, V., Zijlmans, M., Bryan, T., et al. (1997). Telomeres in the hematopoietic system. *CIBA Foundation Symposium, 211*, 209–222.

Laughlin, G., Barrett-Connor, E., Kritz-Silverstein, D., & von Muhlen, D. (2000). Hysterectomy, oophorectomy, and endogenous sex hormone levels in older women: The Rancho Bernardo Study. *Journal of Clinical Endocrinology and Metabolism, 85*, 645–651.

Le Couteur, D., & McLean, A. (1998). The aging liver: Drug clearance and an oxygen diffusion barrier hypothesis. *Clinical Pharmacokinetics, 34*, 359–373.

Leon-Carrion, J., Salgado, H., Sierra, M., Marquez-Rivas, J., & Dominguez-Morales, M. (2001). Neuroanatomy of the functional aging brain. In J. Leon-Carrion & M. Giannini (Eds.), *Behavioral neurology in the elderly* (pp. 67–84). Boca Raton, FL: CRC Press.

Letran, J., & Brawer, M. (1999). Disorders of the prostate. In W. Hazzard, J. Blass, W. Ettinger Jr., J. Halter, & J. Ouslander (Eds.), *Principles of geriatric medicine and gerontology* (4th ed., pp. 809–822). New York: McGraw-Hill.

Levy, D., Larsen, M. G., Vasan, R. S., Kannel, W. B., & Ho, K. K. (1996). The progression from hypertension to congestive heart failure. *Journal of the American Medical Association, 275*(20), 1557–1562.

Lexell, J., Taylor, C., & Sjostrom, M. (1988). What is the cause of aging atrophy? Total number, size and proportion of different fiber types studied in whole vastus lateralis muscle from 15- to 83-year-old men. *Journal of the Neurological Sciences, 84*, 275–294.

Licastro, F., Candore, G., Lio, D., Porcellini, E., Colonna-Romano, G., Franceschi, C., et al. (2005). Innate immunity and inflammation in ageing: A key for understanding age-related diseases. *Immunity and Ageing, 2*, 8.

Lind, A., & McNicol, G. (1986). Cardiovascular response to holding and carrying weights by hand and shoulder harness. *Journal of Applied Physiology, 25*, 261–267.

Lindeman, R. (1990). Overview: Renal physiology and pathophysiology of aging. *American Journal of Kidney Diseases, 16*(4), 275–282.

Lindeman, R. (1995). Renal and urinary tract function. In E. Masoro (Ed.), *Handbook of physiology: Section 11, aging* (pp. 485–502). New York: Oxford University Press.

Lindeman, R. (1998). Renal and electrolyte disorders. In E. Duthie & P. Katz (Eds.), *Practice of geriatrics* (3rd ed., pp. 546–562). Philadelphia: W. B. Saunders.

Lindemann, B. (2000). A taste for umami. *Nature Neuroscience, 3*(2), 99–100.

Linton, P. J., & Dorshkind, K. (2004). Age-related changes in lymphocyte development and function. *Nature Immunology, 5*(2), 133–139.

Lippa, C., Hamos, J., Pulaski, S., Degennaro, L., & Drachman, D. (1992). Alzheimer's disease and aging: Effects on perforant pathway perikarya and synapses. *Neurobiology of Aging, 13*, 405–411.

Lompre, A. (1998). The sarco(endo)plasmic reticulum Ca2+-ATPases in the cardiovascular system during growth and proliferation. *Trends in Cardiovascular Medicine, 8*(2), 75–82.

Lubran, M. (1995). Renal function in the elderly. *Annals of Clinical and Laboratory Science, 25*, 122–133.

Lye, M. (1998). Disturbances of homeostasis. In R. Tallis, H. Fillit, & J. Brocklehurst (Eds.), *Brocklehurst's textbook of geriatric medicine and gerontology* (5th ed., pp. 925–948). London: Churchill Livingstone.

Lynch, N., Metter, E., Lindle, R., Fozard, J., Tobin, J., Roy, T., et al. (1999). Muscle quality. I. Age-associated differences between arm and leg muscle groups. *Journal of Applied Physiology, 86*(1), 188–194.

MacIntosh, C., Horowitz, M., Verhagen, M., Smout, A., Wishart, J., Morris, H., et al. (2001). Effect of small intestinal nutrient infusion on appetite, gastrointestinal hormone release, and gastric myoelectrical activity in young and older men. *American Journal of Gastroenterology, 96*(4), 997–1007.

Madersbacher, S., Pycha, A., Schatzl, G., Mian, C., Klingler, C., & Marberger, M. (1998). The aging lower urinary tract: A comparative urodynamic study of men and women. *Urology, 51*(2), 206–212.

Madsen, J. L., & Graff, J. (2004). Effects of aging on gastrointestinal motor function. *Age and Ageing, 33*(2), 154–159.

Maharam, L., Bauman, P., Kalman, D., Skolnik, H., & Perle, S. (1999). Masters athletes: Factors affecting performance. *Sports Medicine, 28*(4), 273–285.

Maki, B., & McIlroy, W. (2006). Control of rapid limb movements for balance recovery: Age-related change and implications for fall prevention. *Age and Aging, 35*(S2), ii12–ii18.

Manolagas, S. C. (2000). Birth and death of bone cells: Basic regulatory mechanisms and implications for the pathogenesis and treatment of osteoporosis. *Endocrine Reviews, 21*(2), 115–137.

Marchesini, G., Bua, V., Brunori, A., Bianchi, G., Pisi, P., Fabbri, A., et al. (1988). Galactose elimination capacity and liver volume in aging man. *Hepatology, 8*(5), 1079–1083.

Marcus, R., Masdirg, P., & Young, G. (1984). Age-related changes in parathyroid hormone and parathyroid hormone action in normal humans. *Journal of Clinical Endocrinology and Metabolism, 58*, 223–230.

Marieb, E., & Hoehn, K. (2007). *Human anatomy and physiology* (7th ed.). San Francisco, CA: Pearson/Benjamin Cummings.

Marker, J., Cryer, P., & Clutter, W. (1992). Attenuated glucose recovery from hypoglycemia in elderly. *Diabetes, 41*, 671–678.

Massry, S., Faddy, G., Zhou, X., Chandrasoma, P., Cheng, L., & Filburn, C. (1991). Impaired insulin secretion of aging: Role of renal failure and hyperparathyroidism. *Kidney International, 40*, 662–667.

Mattson, M. (1999). Cellular and neurochemical aspects of the aging human brain. In W. Hazzard, J. Blass, W. Ettinger Jr., J. Halter, & J. Ouslander (Eds.), *Principles of geriatric medicine and gerontology* (4th ed., pp. 1193–1208). New York: McGraw-Hill.

Mattson, M., Maudsley, S., & Martin, B. (2004). BDNF and 5-HT: A dynamic duo in age-related neuronal plasticity and neurodegeneration disorders. *Trends in Neuroscience*, 27(10), 589–594.

McLean, A., & Le Couteur, D. (2004). Aging biology and geriatric clinical pharmacology. *Pharmacological Reviews, 56*(2), 163–184.

McReynolds, J., & Rossen, E. (2004). Importance of physical activity, nutrition, and social support for optimal aging. *Clinical Nurse Specialist, 18*(4), 200–206.

Meneilly, G. (2001). Pathophysiology of diabetes in the elderly. In A. Sinclair & P. Finucane (Eds.), *Diabetes in old age* (2nd ed., pp. 17–23). New York: John Wiley & Sons.

Meneilly, G., Cheung, E., & Tuokko, H. (1994a). Altered responses to hypoglycemia of healthy elderly people. *Journal of Clinical Endocrinology and Metabolism, 78*(6), 1341–1348.

Meneilly, G., Cheung, E., & Tuokko, H. (1994b). Counterregulatory hormone responses to hypoglycemia in the elderly patient with diabetes. *Diabetes, 43*, 403–410.

Meyer, K. (2005). Aging. *Proceedings of the American Thoracic Society, 2*, 433–439.

Miller, T., Grossman, S., Schechtman, K., Biello, D., Ludbrook, P., & Ehsani, A. (1986). Left ventricular diastolic filling and its association with age. *American Journal of Cardiology, 58*, 531–535.

Mimran, A., Ribstein, J., & Jover, B. (1992). Aging and sodium homeostasis. *Kidney International Supplement, 37*, S107–S113.

Minaker, K. (1990). What diabetologists should know about elderly patients. *Diabetes Care, 13*(Suppl. 2), 34–46.

Minaker, K. (2004). Common clinical sequelae of aging. In L. Goldman & D. Ausiello (Eds.), *Cecil textbook of medicine* (22nd ed.). Philadelphia: W. B. Saunders. Retrieved January 10, 2005, from http://home.mdconsult.com/das/book/45511299-2/view/1231

Mistretta, C. (1984). Aging effects on anatomy and neurophysiology of taste and smell. *Gerodontology, 3*, 131–136.

Mocchegiani, E., & Malavolta, M. (2004). NK and NKT cell functions in immunosenescence. *Aging Cell, 3*, 177–184.

Moody, D., Thore, C., Anstrom, J., Challa, C., Langefield, C., & Brown, W. (2004). Quantification of afferent vessels shows reduced brain vascular density in subjects with leukoaraiosis. *Radiology, 233*, 883–890.

Moore, A., Mangoni, A., Lyons, D., & Jackson, S. (2003). The cardiovascular system in the ageing patient. *British Journal of Clinical Pharmacology, 56*, 254–260.

Moreland, J., Richardson, J., Goldsmith, C., & Clase, C. (2004). Muscle weakness and falls in older adults: A systemic review and meta-analysis. *Journal of the American Geriatrics Society, 52*, 1121–1129.

Morley, J., Kaiser, F., Perry, H., Patrick, P., Morley, P., Stauber, P., et al. (1997). Longitudinal changes in testosterone, leutinizing hormone, and follicle-stimulating hormone in healthy older men. *Metabolism, 46*(4), 410–413.

Morley, J., & Perry, H. (1991). The management of diabetes mellitus in older individuals. *Drugs, 41*(4), 548–565.

Morley, J., & Reese, S. (1989). Clinical implications of the aging heart. *American Journal of Medicine, 86*, 77–86.

Morley, J. E., Baumgartner, R., Roubenoff, R., Mayer, J., & Nair, K. S. (2001). Sarcopenia. *Journal of Laboratory and Clinical Medicine, 137*, 231–243.

Morrison, J., & Hof, P. (1997). Life and death of neurons in the aging brain. *Nature, 279*, 112–119.

Morrow, L., & Halter, J. (1994). Treatment of the elderly with diabetes. In C. Kahn & G. Weir (Eds.), *Joslin's diabetes mellitus* (13th ed., pp. 552–559). Philadelphia: Lea & Febiger.

Moskowitz, R., Kelly, M., & Lewallen, D. (2004). Understanding osteoarthritis of the knee—causes and effects. *American Journal of Orthopaedics, 33*(Suppl. 2), 5–9.

Mozaz, M., & Monguio, I. (2001). Motor functions and praxis in the elderly. In J. Leon-Carrion & M. Giannini (Eds.), *Behavioral neurology in the elderly* (pp. 125–150). Boca Raton, FL: CRC Press.

Murphy, D., DeCarli, C., Schapiro, M., Rapoport, S., & Horwitz, B. (1996). Age-related differences in volumes of subcortical nuclei, brain matter, and cerebrospinal fluid in healthy men as measured with magnetic resonance imaging (MRI). *Archives of Neurology, 49*(8), 839–845.

Musso, C., Ghezzi, L., & Ferraris, J. (2004). Renal physiology in newborns and old people: Similar characteristics but different mechanisms. *International Urology and Nephrology, 36*, 273–276.

Musso, C., Liakopoulos, V., Ioannidis, I., Eleftheriadias, T., & Stefandis, I. (2006). Acute renal failure in the elderly: Particular charactaristics. *International Journal of Urology and Nephrology, 38*, 787–793.

National Eye Institute. (2002). *Prevalence of blindness data*. Retrieved October 31, 2008, from http://www.nei.nih.gov/eyedata/pbd_tables.asp

National Institute of Arthritis and Musculoskeletal and Skin Diseases. (2006). *Handout on health: Osteoarthritis*. Retrieved November 2, 2007, from http://www.niams.nih.gov/hi/topics/arthritis/oahandout.htm

National Osteoporosis Foundation. (2007). *Fast facts on osteoporosis*. Retrieved November 5, 2007, from http://www.nof.org/osteoporosis/diseasefacts.htm

Naughton, B., Mylotte, J., & Tayara, A. (2000). Outcome of nursing home-acquired pneumonia: Derivation and application of a practical model to predict 30 day mortality. *Journal of the American Geriatrics Society, 48*(10), 1292–1299.

Newton, J., Yemm, R., Abel, R., & Menhinick, S. (1993). Changes in human jaw muscles with age and dental state. *Gerodontology, 10*(1), 16–22.

Nielson, M., & Pedersen, J. (1996). Changes in the anal sphincter with age. An endosonographic study. *Acta Radiologica, 37*, 357–361.

Nilsson-Ehle, H., Jagenburg, R., Landahl, S., & Svanborg, A. (2000). Blood haemoglobin declines in the elderly: Implications for reference intervals from age

70 to 88. *European Journal of Haematology, 65*(5), 297–305.

Nitzan, M., Mahler Y., Schechter, D., Yaffe, S., Bocher, M., & Chisn, R. (1994). A measurement of pulmonary blood volume increase during systole in humans. *Physiological Measures, 15*, 489–498.

Noblett, K., & Ostergard, D. (1999). Gynecologic disorders. In W. Hazzard, J. Blass, W. Ettinger Jr., J. Halter, & J. Ouslander (Eds.), *Principles of geriatric medicine and gerontology* (4th ed., pp. 797–808). New York: McGraw-Hill.

O'Donovan, D., Hausken, T., Lei, Y., Russo, A., Keough, J., Horowitz, M., et al. (2005). Effects of aging on transpyloric flow, gastric emptying and intragastric distribution in healthy humans—impact on glycemia. *Digestive Diseases and Sciences, 50*(4), 671–676.

Olivetti, G., Cigola, E., Maestri, R., Lagrasta, C., Conadi, D., & Quaini, F. (2000). Recent advances in cardiac hypertrophy. *Cardiovascular Research, 45*(1), 68–75.

Olivetti, G., Melessari, M., Capasso, J., & Anversa, P. (1991). Cardiomyopathy of the aging human heart: Myocyte loss and reactive cellular hypertrophy. *Circulation Research, 68*, 1560–1568.

Olivetti, L., Schurr, K., Sherrington, C., Wallbank, G., Pamphlett, P., Mun-San Kwan, M., et al. (2007). A novel weight-bearing strengthening program during rehabilitation of older people is feasible and improves standing up more than a non weight-bearing strengthening program: A randomised trial. *Austrian Journal of Physiotherapy, 53*, 147–153.

O'Mahony, D., O'Leary, P., & Quigley, E. (2002). Aging and intestinal motility: A review of factors that affect intestinal motility in the aged. *Drugs Aging, 19*(7), 515–527.

O'Rourke, M., & Hashimoto, J. (2007). Mechanical factors in arterial aging: A clinical perspective. *Journal of the American College of Cardiology, 50*, 1–13.

Orr, W., & Chen, C. (2002). Aging and neural control of the GI tract. IV. Clinical and physiological aspects of gastrointestinal motility and aging. *American Journal of Physiology: Gastrointestinal and Liver Physiology, 283*, G1226–G1231.

Ostchega, Y., Dillon, C., Lindle, R., Carroll, M., & Hurley, B. (2004). Isokinetic leg muscle strength in older Americans and its relationship to a standardized walk test: Data from the National Health and Nutrition Examination Survey 1999–2000. *Journal of the American Geriatric Society, 52*, 977–982.

Owsley, C., Sekular, R., & Siemsen, D. (1983). Contrast sensitivity throughout adulthood. *Vision Research, 23*, 689–699.

Paick, S., Meehan, A., Lee, M., Penson, D., & Wessells, H. (2005). The relationship among lower urinary tract symptoms, prostate specific antigen and erectile dysfunction in men with benign prostatic hyperplasia: Results from the Proscar Long-Term Efficacy and Safety Study. *Journal of Urology, 173*, 903–907.

Pakkenberg, B., & Gundersen, J. (1997). Neocortical neuron number in humans: Effect of sex and age. *Journal of Comparative Neurology, 384*, 312–320.

Partin, A., & Rodriguez, R. (2002). The molecular biology, endocrinology, and physiology of the prostate and seminal vesicles. In P. Walsh (Ed.), *Campbell's urology* (8th ed.). Philadelphia: W. B. Saunders. Retrieved January 10, 2005, from http://home.mdconsult.com/das/book/45511299-2/view/1049

Patt, B. (1998). Otologic fisorders. In E. Duthie & P. Katz (Eds.), *Practice of geriatrics* (3rd ed., pp. 449–456). Philadelphia: W. B. Saunders.

Peters, A. (2002). The effects of normal aging on myelin and nerve fibers: A review. *Journal of Neurocytology, 31*, 581–593.

Peters, A., & Davidson, M. (1997). Aging and diabetes. In K. Alberti, P. Zimmet, & R. Defronzo (Eds.), *International textbook of diabetes mellitus* (2nd ed., Vol. 2, pp. 1151–1176). Chichester: John Wiley & Sons.

Peters, A., Morrison, J., Rosene, D., & Hyman, B. (1998). Are neurons lost from the primate cerebral cortex during aging? *Cerebral Cortex, 8*, 295–300.

Peters, R. (2006) Ageing and the brain. *Postgrad Medical Journal, 82*, 84–85.

Phillips, P., Hodsman, G., & Johnston, C. (1991). Neuroendocrine mechanisms and cardiovascular homeostasis in the elderly. *Cardiovascular Drugs and Therapy, 4*(Suppl. 6), 1209–1213.

Phillips, S., Rook, K., Siddle, N., Bruce, S., & Woledge, R. (1993). Muscle weakness in women occurs at an earlier age than in men, but strength is preserved by hormone replacement therapy. *Clinical Science, 84*(1), 95–98.

Phillips, T. J., Demircay, Z., & Sahu, M. (2001). Hormonal effects on skin aging. *Clinics in Geriatric Medicine, 17*(4), 661–672.

Pierard, G. E., Letawe, C., Dowlati, A., & Pierard-Franchimont, C. (1995). Effect of hormone replacement therapy for menopause on the mechanical properties of skin. *Journal of the American Geriatrics Society, 43*(6), 662–665.

Plackett, T., Boehmer, E., Faunce, D., & Kovacs, E. (2004). Aging and innate immune cells. *Journal of Leukocyte Biology, 76*, 291–299.

Poehlman, E., Toth, M., & Gardner, A. (1995). Changes in energy balance and body composition at menopause. *Annals of Internal Medicine, 123*(9), 673–675.

Priebe, H. (2000). The aged cardiovascular risk patient. *British Journal of Anaesthesia, 85*(5), 763–778.

Prinz, P., Weitzman, E., Cunningham, G., & Karacan, I. (1983). Plasma growth hormone during sleep in young and aged men. *Journals of Gerontology, 38*(5), 519–524.

Proctor, D., Balagopal, P., & Nair, K. (1998). Age-related sarcopenia in humans is associated with reduced synthetic rates of specific muscle proteins. *Journal of Nutrition, 128*(Suppl. 2), 351S–355S.

Pugh, K., & Wei, J. (2001). Clinical implications of physiological changes in the aging heart. *Drugs & Aging, 18*(4), 263–276.

Quyyumi, A. A. (1998). Endothelial function in health and disease: New insights into the genesis of cardiovascular disease. *American Journal of Medicine, 105*, 325–395.

Rajkumar, C., Kingwell, B., Cameron, J., Waddell, T., Mehra, R., Christophidis, N., et al. (1997). Hormonal therapy increases arterial compliance in postmenopausal women. *Journal of the American College of Cardiology, 30*(2), 350–356.

Ramos-Platon, M., & Beneto-Pascual, A. (2001). Aging, sleep, and neuropsychological functioning outcomes. In J. Leon-Carrion & M. Giannini (Eds.), *Behavioral neurology in the elderly* (pp. 203–242). Boca Raton, FL: CRC Press.

Randolph, J., Sowers, M., Bondarenko, I., Harlow, S., Luborsky, J., & Little, R. (2004). Change in estradiol and follicle-stimulation hormone across the early menopausal transition: Effects of ethnicity and age. *Journal of Clinical Endocrinology and Metabolism, 89*(4), 1555–1561.

Rao, S., Mudipalli, R., Mujica, V., Patel, R., & Zimmerman, B. (2003). Effects of gender and age on esophageal biomechanical properties and sensation. *American Journal of Gastroenterology, 98*(8), 1688–1695.

Rees, T., Duckert, L., & Carey, J. (1999). Auditory and vestibular dysfunction. In W. Hazzard, J. Blass, W. Ettinger Jr., J. Halter, & J. Ouslander (Eds.), *Principles of geriatric medicine and gerontology* (4th ed., pp. 617–632). New York: McGraw-Hill.

Reinus, J., & Brandt, L. (1998). The upper gastrointestinal tract. In R. Tallis, H. Fillit, & J. Brocklehurst (Eds.), *Brocklehurst's textbook of geriatric medicine and gerontology* (5th ed., pp. 803–826). London: Churchill Livingstone.

Resnick, N., Elbadawi, A., & Yalla, S. (1995). Age and the lower urinary tract: What is normal? *Neurourology and Urodynamics, 14*, 577–579.

Richardson, D. (1994). Adjustments associated with the aging process. In N. Mortillaro & A. Taylor (Eds.), *The pathophysiology of the microcirculation* (pp. 200–204). Boca Raton, FL: CRC Press.

Robert, L. (1999). Aging of the vascular wall and atherosclerosis. *Experimental Gerontology, 34*, 491–501.

Rociu, E., Stoker, J., Eijkemans, M., & Lameris, J. (2000). Normal anal sphincter anatomy and age- and sex-related variations at high-spatial-resolution endoanal MR imaging. *Radiology, 217*(2), 395–401.

Rodeheffer, R., Gerstenblith, G., Becker, L., Fleg, J., Weisfeldt, M., & Lakatta, E. (1984). Exercise cardiac output is maintained with advancing age in healthy human subjects: Cardiac dilatation and increased stroke volume compensate for a diminished heart rate. *Circulation, 69*(2), 203–213.

Roffe, C. (1998). Ageing of the heart. *British Journal of Biomedical Science, 55*(2), 136–148.

Roof, R., & Hall, E. (2000). Gender differences in acute CNS trauma and stroke: Neuroprotective effects of estrogen and progesterone. *Journal of Neurotrauma, 17*, 367–388.

Rosen, R., Altwein, J., Boyle, P., Kirby, R., Lukacs, B., Meuleman, E., et al. (2003). Lower urinary tract symptoms and male sexual dysfunction: The multinational survey of the aging male (MSAM-7). *European Urology, 44*(6), 637–649.

Rossmanith, W., Handke-Vesel, A., Wirth, U., & Scherbaum, W. (1994). Does the gonadotropin pulsatility of postmenopausal women represent the unrestrained hypothalamic-pituitary activity? *European Journal of Endocrinology, 130*, 485–493.

Roubenoff, R. (2001). Origins and clinical relevance of sarcopenia. *Canadian Journal of Applied Physiology, 26*(1), 78–89.

Roubenoff, R. (2003). Sarcopenia: Effects on body composition and function. *Journals of Gerontology: Medical Sciences, 58A*(11), 1012–1017.

Roubenoff, R., & Hughes, V. A. (2000). Sarcopenia: Current concepts. *Journals of Gerontology: Medical Sciences, 55A*(12), M716–M724.

Rowe, J., Andres, A., Tobin, J., Norris, A., & Shock, N. (1976). The effect of age on creatinine clearance in men: A cross-sectional and longitudinal study. *Journal of Gerontology, 32*, 155–163.

Rowe, J., Minaker, K., Pallotta, J., & Flier, J. (1983). Characterization of the insulin resistance of aging. *Journal of Clinical Investigation, 71*, 1581–1587.

Rule, A., Gussak, H., Pond, G., Bergstralh, E., Stegall, M., Cosio, F., et al. (2004). Measured and estimated GFR in healthy potential kidney donors. *American Journal of Kidney Diseases, 43*(1), 112–119.

Russell-Aulet, M., Jaffe, C., Mott-Friberg, R., & Barkans, A. (1999). In vivo semiquantification of hypothalamus growth hormone releasing hormone (GHRH) output in humans:Evidence for relative GHRH deficiency in aging. *Journal of Clinical Endocrinology Metabolism, 84*(10), 3490–3497.

Sabbah, H. (2000). Apoptotic cell death in heart failure. *Cardiovascular Research, 45*, 704–712.

Saffrey, M. (2004), Aging of the enteric nervous system. *Mechanism of Ageing and Development, 125*, 899–906.

Salles, N. (2007). Basic mechanisms of the aging gastrointestinal tract. *Digestive Diseases, 25*, 112–117.

Salmasi, A., Alimo, A., Jepson, E., & Dancy, M. (2003). Age-associated changes in left ventricular diastolic function are related to increasing left ventricular mass. *American Journal of Hypertension, 16*, 473–477.

Salthouse, T. (1993). Speed mediation of adult age differences in cognition. *Developmental Psychology, 29*, 722–738.

Sampson, N., Untegassan, G., Plas, E., & Berger, P. (2007). The ageing male reproductive tract. *Journal of Pathology, 211*, 206–218.

Santoro, N., Adel, T., & Skurnick, J. (1999). Decreased inhibin tone and increased activin A secretion characterize reproductive aging in women. *Fertility and Sterility, 71*, 658–662.

Sator, P. G., Schmidt, J. B., Rabe, T., & Zouboulis, C. C. (2004). Skin aging and sex hormones in women—clinical perspectives for intervention by hormone replacement therapy. *Experimental Dermatology, 13*(Suppl. 4), 36–40.

Scharffetter-Kochanek, K., Brenneisen, P., Wenk, J., Herrmann, G., Ma, W., Kuhr, L., et al. (2000). Photoaging of the skin from phenotype to mechanisms. *Experimental Gerontology, 35*(3), 307–316.

Scheff, S., & Price, D. (1998). Synaptic density in the inner molecular layer of the hippocampal dentate gyrus in Alzheimer disease. *Journal of Neuropathology and Experimental Neurology, 57*(12), 1146–1153.

Scheff, S., & Price, D. (2001). Alzheimer's disease-related synapse loss in the cingulate cortex. *Journal of Alzheimer's Disease, 3*(5), 495–505.

Scheff, S., Price, D., & Sparks, D. (2001). Quantitative assessment of possible age-related change in synaptic numbers in the human frontal cortex. *Neurobiology of Aging, 22*, 355–365.

Scheff, S., Sparks, D., & Price, D. (1996). Quantitative assessment of synaptic density in the outer molecular layer of the hippocampal dentate gyrus in Alzheimer's disease. *Dementia, 7*(4), 226–232.

Schiffman, S. (1997). Taste and smell losses in normal aging and disease. *Journal of the American Medical Association, 278*(16), 1357–1362.

Schlegel, P., & Hardy, M. (2002). Male reproductive physiology. In P. Walsh (Ed.), *Campbell's urology* (8th ed., pp. 1358–1377). Philadelphia: W. B. Saunders.

Schmitt, D. (1999). Immune functions of the human skin. Models of in vivo studies using Langerhans cells. *Cell Biology and Toxicology, 15*, 41–45.

Schmitt, F., Davis, D., Wekstein, D., Smith, C., Ashford, J., & Markesbery, W. (2000). Preclinical AD revisited: Neuropathology of cognitively normal older adults. *Neurology, 55*, 370–376.

Schmucker, D. (1998). Aging and the liver: An update. *Journal of Gerontology Section A: Biological Sciences & Medical Sciences, 53*(5), B315–B320.

Schmucker, D., Heyworth, M., Owen, R., & Daniels, C. (1996). Impact of aging on gastrointestinal mucosal immunity. *Digestive Diseases and Sciences, 41*(6), 1183–1193.

Schmucker, D., Owen, R., Outenreath, R., & Thoreux, K. (2003). Basis for the age-related decline in intestinal mucosal immunity. *Clinical and Developmental Immunology, 10*, 167–172.

Schmucker, D., Thoreux, K., & Owen, R. (2001). Aging impairs intestinal immunity. *Mechanisms of Ageing and Development, 122*(13), 1397–1411.

Schroeder, P., & Richter, J. (1994). Swallowing disorders in the elderly. *Practical Gastroenterology, 18*, 19–41.

Schuknecht, H. (1974). *Pathology of the ear*. Cambridge, MA: Harvard University Press.

Schuknecht, H., & Gacek, M. (1993). Cochlear pathology in presbycusis. *Annals of Otology, Rhinology and Laryngology, 102*, 1–16.

Schulman, S. (1999). Cardiovascular consequences of the aging process. *Cardiology Clinics, 17*(1), 35–49.

Seals, D. R., & Esler, M. D. (2000). Human ageing and the sympathoadrenal system. *Journal of Physiology, 528*(3), 407–417.

Seeman, E. (2002). Pathogenesis of bone fragility in women and men. *Lancet, 359*, 1841–1850.

Seeman, E. (2003a). Invited review: Pathogenesis of osteoporosis. *Journal of Applied Physiology, 95*, 2142–2151.

Seeman, E. (2003b). Reduced bone formation and increased bone resorption: Rational targets for the treatment of osteoporosis. *Osteoporosis International, 14*(Suppl. 3), S2–S8.

Seiberling, K., & Conley, D. (2004). Aging and olfactory and taste function. *Otolaryngologic Clinics of North America, 37*(6), 1209–1228.

Seidman, S. (2003). The aging male: Androgens, erectile dysfunction, and depression. *Journal of Clinical Psychiatry, 64*(Suppl. 10), 31–37.

Shaffer, S., & Harrison, A. (2007). Aging of the somatosensory system: A translational perspective. *Physical Therapy, 87*(2), 193–207.

Shah, M. G., & Maibach, H. I. (2001). Estrogen and skin. An overview. *American Journal of Clinical Dermatology, 2*(3), 143–150.

Shaker, R., Dua, K., & Koch, T. (1998). Gastroenterologic disorders. In E. Duthie & P. Katz (Eds.), *Practice of geriatrics* (3rd ed., pp. 505–523). Philadelphia: W. B. Saunders.

Shealy, C. N. (1995). A review of dehydroepiandrosterone (DHEA). *Integrative Physiological and Behavioral Science, 30*(4), 308–313.

Sherwood, L. (Ed.). (2007). *Human physiology: From cells to systems* (6th ed). Belmont, CA: Thompson, Brooks/Cole.

Shimamoto, C., Hirata, I., & Hiraike, Y. (2002). Evaluation of gastric motor activity in the elderly by electro gastrography and the 13C-acetate breath test. *Gerontology, 48*, 381–386.

Ship, J., Pillemer, S., & Baum, B. (2002). Xerostomia and the geriatric patient. *Journal of the American Geriatrics Society, 50*, 535–543.

Simon, J., Leboff, M., Wright, J., & Glowacki, J. (2002). Fractures in the elderly and vitamin D. *Journal of Nutrition, Health, and Aging, 6*(6), 406–412.

Sloane, M., Owsley, C., & Alzarez, S. (1988). Aging, senile miosis and spatial contrast sensitivity at low luminance. *Vision Research, 28*, 1235–1246.

Smith, M. (1998). Gynecologic disorders. In E. Duthie & P. Katz (Eds.), *Practice of geriatrics* (3rd ed., pp. 524–534). Philadelphia: W. B. Saunders.

Soergel, K., Zboralske, F., & Amberg, J. (1964). Presbyesophagus: Esophageal motility in nonagenarians. *Journal of Clinical Investigation, 43*, 1972–1979.

Sohal, R., Mockett, R., & Orr, W. (2002). Mechanisms of aging: An appraisal of the oxidative stress hypothesis. *Free Radical Biology & Medicine, 33*(5), 575–586.

Solana, R., & Mariani, E. (2000). NK and NK/T cells in human senescence. *Vaccine, 18*, 1613–1620.

Sorribas, V., Lotscher, M., Loffing, J., Biber, J., Kaissling, B., Murer, H., et al. (1995). Cellular mechanisms of the age-related decrease in renal phosphate reabsorption. *Kidney International, 50*, 855–863.

Soules, M., Sherman, S., Parrott, E., Rebar, R., Santoro, N., Utian, W., et al. (2001). Executive summary: Stages of reproductive aging workshop (STRAW). *Fertility and Sterility, 76*(5), 874–878.

Spence, J. (1921, July). Some observations on sugar tolerance with special reference to variations found at different ages. *Quarterly Journal of Medicine*, 314–326.

Sternbach, H. (1998). Age-associated testosterone decline in men: Clinical issues for psychiatry. *American Journal of Psychiatry, 155*, 1310–1318.

Stevens, J., Cain, W., & Weinstein, D. (1987). Aging impairs the ability to detect gas odor. *Fire Technology, 23*(3), 198–204.

Stevens, J., & Choo, K. (1996). Spatial acuity of the body surface over the life span. *Somatosensory and Motor Research, 13*(2), 153–166.

Stevens, J., & Patterson, M. (1995). Dimensions of spatial acuity in the touch sense: Changes over the life span. *Somatosensory and Motor Research, 12*(1), 29–47.

Strasser, H., Tiefenthaler, M., Steinlechner, M., Bartsch, G., & Konwalinka, G. (1996). Urinary incontinence in the elderly. *Age and Ageing, 25*, 285–291.

Tepper, R., & Katz, S. (1998). Overview: Geriatric gastroenterology. In R. Tallis, H. Fillit, & J. Brocklehurst (Eds.), *Brocklehurst's textbook of geriatric medicine and gerontology* (5th ed., pp. 783–788). London: Churchill Livingstone.

Terry, R., DeTeresa, R., & Hansen, L. (1987). Neocortical cell counts in normal human adult aging. *Annals of Neurology, 21*(6), 530–539.

Teter, B., & Ashford, J. (2002). Neuroplasticity in Alzheimer's disease. *Journal of Neuroscience Research, 70*, 402–437.

Timiras, M. L. (2003). The skin. In P. S. Timiras (Ed.), *Physiological basis of aging and geriatrics* (3rd ed., pp. 397–404). Boca Raton, FL: CRC Press.

Timiras, P. S. (2003a). The adrenals and pituitary. In P. S. Timiras (Ed.), *Physiological basis of aging and geriatrics* (3rd ed., pp. 167–188). Boca Raton, FL: CRC Press.

Timiras, P. S. (2003b). The skeleton, joints, and skeletal and cardiac muscles. In P. S. Timiras (Ed.), *Physiological basis of aging and geriatrics* (3rd ed., pp. 375–395). Boca Raton, FL: CRC Press.

Timiras, P. S. (2003c). The thyroid, parathyroid, and pineal glands. In P. S. Timiras (Ed.), *Physiological basis of aging and geriatrics* (3rd ed., pp. 233–249). Boca Raton, FL: CRC Press.

Tobin, D., & Paus, R. (2001). Graying: Gerontobiology of the hair follicle pigmentary unit. *Experimental Gerontology, 36*, 29–54.

Tortora, G., & Derrickson, B. (2006). *Principles of anatomy and physiology* (11th ed.). Hoboken, NJ: John Wiley and Sons.

Tresch, D., & Jamali, I. (1998). Cardiac disorders. In E. Duthie & P. Katz (Eds.), *Practice of geriatrics* (3rd ed., pp. 353–374). Philadelphia: W. B. Saunders.

Turner, H., & Wass, J. (1997). Gonadal function in men with chronic illness. *Clinical Endocrinology, 47*, 379–403.

University of California Academic Geriatric Resource Program. (2004, December 22). *Module supplement: Endocrine system: Aldosterone.* Retrieved March 10, 2005, from http://ucsfagrc.org/supplements/endocrine/12_aldosterone.html

van den Beld, A., de Jong, F., Grobbee, D., Pols, H., & Lamberts, S. (2000). Measures of bioavailable serum testosterone and estradiol and their relationship with muscle strength, bone density, and body composition in elderly men. *Journal of Clinical Endocrinology and Metabolism, 85*, 3276–3282.

Vandervoot, A. A., & Symons, T. B. (2001). Functional and metabolic consequences of sarcopenia. *Canadian Journal of Applied Physiology, 26*(1), 90–101.

Vermeulen, A., Goemaere, S., & Kaufman, J. (1999). Sex hormones, body composition, and aging. *Aging Male, 2*, 8–15.

Vieth, R., Ladak, Y., & Walfish, P. (2003). Age-related changes in the 25-hydroxyvitamin D versus parathyroid hormone relationship suggest a different reason why older adults require more vitamin D. *Journal of Clinical Endocrinology and Metabolism, 88*(1), 185–191.

Virmani, R., Avolio, A., Margner, W., Robinowitz, M., Herderick, E., Cornhill, J., et al. (1991). Effect of aging on aortic morphology in populations with high and low prevalence of hypertension and atherosclerosis: Comparison between Occidental and Chinese communities. *American Journal of Pathology, 139*, 1119–1129.

Volkow, N., Gur, R., Wang, G., Fowler, J., Moberg, P., Ding, Y., et al. (1998). Association between decline in brain dopamine activity with age and cognitive and motor impairment in healthy individuals. *American Journal of Psychiatry, 155*(3), 344–349.

Volpi, E., Sheffield-Moore, M., Rasmussen, B. B., & Wolfe, R. R. (2001). Basal muscle amino acid kinetics and protein synthesis in healthy young and older men. *Journal of the American Medical Association, 286*(10), 1206–1212.

Wei, J. (1992). Age and the cardiovascular system. *New England Journal of Medicine, 327*, 1735–1739.

Weiffenbach, J. (1991). Chemical senses in aging. In T. Getchell, R. Doty, L. Bartoshuk, & J. Snow (Eds.), *Smell and taste in health and disease* (pp. 369–380). New York: Raven Press.

Weiffenbach, J., Baum, B., & Burghauser, R. (1982). Taste threshold: Quality specific variation with aging. *Journal of Gerontology, 37*, 372–377.

Weisfeldt, M. (1998). Aging, changes in the cardiovascular system, and responses to stress. *American Journal of Hypertension, 11*(3), 41S–45S.

Weiss, G., Skurnick, J., Goldsmith, L., Santoro, N., & Park, S. (2004). Menopause and hypothalamic-pituitary sensitivity to estrogen. *Journal of the American Medical Association, 292*(24), 2991–2996.

White, J., & Ham, R. (1997). Nutrition. In R. Ham & P. Sloane (Eds.), *Primary care geriatrics: A case-based approach* (3rd ed., pp. 108–127). New York: Mosby-Year Book.

Whitman, D. B. (1999, March). *The immunology of aging*. Retrieved January 31, 2005, from http://www.csa.com/hottopics/immune-aging/oview.html

Wick, G., & Grubeck-Loebenstein, B. (1997). Primary and secondary alterations of immune reactivity in the elderly: Impact of dietary factors and disease. *Immunological Reviews, 160*, 171–184.

Wilson, M., Thomas, D., Rubenstein, L., Chibnall, J., Anderson, S., Baxi, A., et al. (2005). Appetite assessment: Simple appetite questionnaire predicts weight loss in community-dwelling adults and nursing home residents. *American Journal of Clinical Nutrition, 82*(5), 1074–1081.

Wise, P., Dubal, D., Wilson, M., Rau, S., & Bottner, M. (2001). Minireview: Neuroprotective effects of estrogen—New insights into mechanisms of action. *Endocrinology, 142*(3), 969–973.

Wise, P., Dubal, D., Wilson, M., Rau, S., & Liu, Y. (2001). Estrogens: Trophic and protective factors in the adult brain. *Frontiers in Neuroendocrinology, 22*(1), 33–66.

Wise, P., Krajnak, K., & Kashon, M. (1996). Menopause: The aging of multiple pacemakers. *Science, 273*, 67–70.

Wynne, H., Cope, E., Mutch, E., Rawlins, M., Woodhouse, K., & James, O. (1989). The effect of age upon liver volume and apparent liver blood flow in healthy man. *Hepatology, 9*(2), 297–301.

Yaar, M., & Gilchrest, B. A. (2001). Skin aging: Postulated mechanisms and consequent changes in structure and function. *Clinics in Geriatric Medicine, 17*(4), 617–630.

Yarasheski, K., Pak-Loduca, J., Hasten, D., Obert, K., Brown, M., & Sinacore, D. (1999). Resistance exercise training increases mixed muscle protein synthesis rate in frail women and men. *American Journal of Physiology, 40*(1, Pt 1), E118–E125.

Yarasheski, K., Zackwieja, F., Campbell, J., & Bier, D. (1995). Effect of growth hormone and resistance exercise on muscle growth and strength in older men. *American Journal of Physiology, 268*(2, Pt 1), E268–E276.

Yen, S., & Laughlin, G. (1998). Aging and the adrenal cortex. *Experimental Gerontology, 33*(7–8), 897–910.

Yialamas, M., & Hayes, F. (2003). Androgens and the ageing male and female. *Best Practice and Research Clinical Endocrinology and Metabolism, 17*(2), 223–236.

Zouboulis, C. C., & Boschnakow, A. (2001). Chronological ageing and photoageing of the human sebaceous gland. *Clinical Dermatology, 26*, 600–607.

Zumoff, B., Strain, G., Miller, L., & Rosner, W. (1995). Twenty-four hour mean plasma testosterone concentration declines with age in normal premenopausal women. *Journal of Clinical Endocrinology and Metabolism, 80*, 1429–1430.

CHAPTER 7

Assessment of the Older Adult

Lorna W. Guse, PhD, RN

LEARNING OBJECTIVES

At the end of this chapter, the reader will be able to:

- Identify the major components of comprehensive assessment of older adults including functional, physical, cognitive, psychological, social, and spiritual assessments.
- Name tools that are frequently used in the assessment of older adults.
- Recognize the challenges of conducting comprehensive assessments of older adults.
- Discuss the role of other health professionals in the assessment of older adults.
- Describe some of the issues in relation to comprehensive assessment of older adults.

KEY TERMS

- Agnosia
- Aphasia
- Apraxia
- Cataracts
- Cerumen
- Dysphagia
- Functional incontinence
- Glaucoma
- Ketones
- Longevity
- Macular degeneration
- Osteoarthritis
- Osteoporosis
- Otosclerosis
- Overflow incontinence
- Polydipsia
- Polyphagia
- Polyuria
- Presbycusis
- Presbyopia
- Stress incontinence
- Urge incontinence

The basis of an individualized plan of care for an older adult is a comprehensive assessment. Enhanced skills in comprehensive geriatric assessment can improve health outcomes, increase nursing assessment confidence, and provide a role model for health care teams (Stolee et al., 2003). Assessment has been described as the cornerstone of gerontological nursing, and the goal is to conduct a systematic and integrated assessment (Olenek, Skowronski, & Schmaltz, 2003). The health and health care needs of older adults are complex, deriving from a combination of age-related changes, age-associated and other diseases, heredity, and lifestyle. Assessment requires knowledge and an understanding of these complex factors. In assessing and providing care to older adults, nurses are members of a health care team that includes physicians, therapists, social workers, spiritual care workers, pharmacists, nutritionists, and others. Each member of the team has a contribution to make, and nurses should draw upon the knowledge of other team members to enhance the assessment process.

Comprehensive assessments can be lengthy, and this presents a challenge to nurses because depending on health status and energy level, the older adult may not be well or strong enough for an extensive physical or verbal-based assessment. If the older adult is experiencing memory problems, the reliability of question-based assessment may be suspect. The role of the family and particularly family caregivers (often spouses and adult children) adds another dimension. The literature suggests that when family members act as proxies for health information, there can be underestimates and overestimates of functional ability, cognition, and social functioning (Ostbye, Tyas, McDowell, & Koval, 1997). Assessment tools do not always identify the source of information, and even experienced nurses sometimes rely too much on secondary sources such as family members and caregivers rather than focusing on the older adult as the primary source of information (Luborsky, 1997).

Since the early 1960s when major tools to measure function were introduced, the number of assessment tools from which nurses can choose has increased exponentially. Part of this increase has been due to the refinement of existing tools and the testing and tailoring of tools across client populations, as well as the creation of new tools. The current growth in the development of clinical practice guidelines has not yet reached the stage where nurses have identified a complete roster of the "best" tools to use with older adults across all settings for specific areas of assessment (see www.ConsultGeriRN.org for examples). However, certain tools are used by nurses because they have been used traditionally to provide a foundation for decision making and intervention strategies. In this chapter, we will identify these common tools and provide guidelines for assessment. In addition, several of the chapters in this text give examples of assessment tools related to specific content.

A cautionary note is needed. Comprehensive assessment is not a neutral process; the sources of information and tools used as well as the nurse's skill level have consequences for the older adult's individualized plan of care. The physical and social environment can support or suppress an older adult's abilities. Comprehensive assessment consists of objective and subjective elements, and how the assessment data are interpreted is of major importance. As Kane (1993) has suggested, interpretation is an art, and it is an art that nurses must aspire to master both as students and as practitioners.

FUNCTIONAL ASSESSMENT

Nurses typically conduct a functional assessment in order to identify an older adult's ability to perform self-care, self-maintenance, and physical activities, and plan appropriate nursing interventions. There are two approaches. One approach is to ask questions about ability, and the other approach is to observe ability through evaluating task completion. However, although we tend to speak of "ability," our verbal and observational tools tend to screen for "disability." Disability refers to the impact that health problems have on an individual's ability to perform tasks, roles, and activities, and it is often measured by asking questions about the performance of activities of daily living (such as eating and dressing) and instrumental activities of daily living (such as meal preparation and hobbies) (Verbrugge & Jette, 1994). The basis of our understanding of ability, disability, physical function, activities of daily living, and any contextual factors comes from work initiated by the World Health Organization (WHO) almost 30 years ago.

The *International Classification of Impairment, Disability and Handicap* (ICIDH) was first published by the WHO in 1980. It suggested relationships among impairment, disability, and handicap. In attempting to move away from a disease perspective and toward a health perspective, the WHO discontinued using the term *handicap* and made definitional changes, creating a new *International Classification of Functioning, Disability, and Health* (ICIDH-2) in 2001. The ICIDH-2 uses the term *disability* to reflect limitations in activities based on an interaction between the individual's health (including impairment, or problems in body function or structure) and the physical, social, and attitudinal environment. This broader perspective on health, activity, and environment is illustrated in the WHO definitions provided in **Box 7-1**. Kearney and Pryor (2004) have suggested that nursing has not yet integrated the ICIDH-2 framework into research, practice, and education. Specifically, they suggest that the ICIDH-2 framework provides nurses with a broad structure "to address more fully, activity limitations and participation restrictions associated with impairment" (2004, p. 166). Moreover, they argue that in nursing education, students should be encouraged to develop "a health care plan that outlines strategies to promote maximum health, function, well-being, independence and participation in life for the individual" (2004, p. 167). Kearney and Pryor are, in fact, promoting an "ability" perspective rather than emphasizing deficits.

Taking an ability perspective on comprehensive assessment of older adults builds upon the ICIDH-2 framework and is informed by the work of Kearney and Pryor (2004) and others. Functional assessment should first emphasize an older adult's ability and the appropriate nursing interventions to support, maintain, and maximize ability; second, it should focus on an older adult's disability and the appropriate nursing interventions to compensate for and prevent further disability. Nursing interventions that create excess disability are not appropriate. Excess disability is defined as "functional disability greater than that warranted by actual physical and physiological impairment of the individual" (Kahn, 1964, p. 112). For example, assisting an older adult in a nursing home to get dressed in the morning when that individual is mentally and physically able to do this task creates excess disability.

Tools to assess functional ability tend to address self-care (basic activities of daily living or ADLs), higher level activities necessary to live independently in the community (instrumental activities of daily living or IADLs), or highest level activities (advanced activities of daily living or AADLs) (Adnan, Chang, Arseven, & Emanuel, 2005). Advanced activities of daily living include societal, family, and community roles, as well as participation in occupational and recreational activities.

In selecting or using tools to measure functional ability, the nurse must be clear on two questions. First, is performance or capacity being assessed? Some tools ask, "Do you dress without help?" (performance) whereas others ask, "Can you dress without help?" (capacity). Asking about capacity places the emphasis on ability. The second question is, "Who is the source of information on functional ability?" Is information gained verbally from the

BOX 7-1 WHO (2001) ICIDH-2 Definitions

In the context of health:

Body functions are the physiological functions of body systems (including psychological functions).

Body structures are anatomical parts of the body such as organs, limbs, and their components.

Impairments are problems in body function or structure such as significant deviation or loss.

Activity is the execution of a task or action by an individual.

Participation is involvement in a life situation.

Activity limitations are difficulties an individual may have in executing activities.

Participation restrictions are problems an individual may experience in involvement in life situations.

Environmental factors make up the physical, social, and attitudinal environment in which people live and conduct their lives.

family or from the older adult? Does the nurse assess functional ability by direct observation or by relying on the observations of others?

In 1987, the Omnibus Budget Reconciliation Act (OBRA) mandated the use of the Minimum Data Set (MDS) in all Medicaid- and Medicare-funded nursing homes. This assessment tool attempted to identify a resident's strengths, preferences, and functional abilities in a systematic way in order to better address his or her needs. The MDS was revised in 1995 and a home-based version was also later developed. In this chapter, we will not be looking at this particular assessment tool. Instead, examples of tools to assess functional ability will be presented in relation to ADL, IADL, and AADL. In addition, the use of physical performance measures will be discussed in relation to functional assessment.

Activities of Daily Living (ADLs)

The original ADL tool was developed by Katz and his colleagues during an 8-year period at the Benjamin Rose Hospital, a geriatric hospital in Cleveland, Ohio, using observations of patients with hip fractures and their performance of activities during recovery (Katz, Ford, Moskowitz, Jackson, & Jaffee, 1963). The Katz Index of ADL (Katz et al., 1970) distinguished between independence and dependence in activities and created an ordered relationship among ADLs. It addressed the need for assistance in bathing, eating, dressing, transfer, toileting, and continence.

Other similar tools followed the Katz Index of ADL and are still being developed and refined. These tools can be divided into those that are generic and those that are disease- or illness-specific. Some tools are designed to provide a more sensitive assessment of ability for older adults with cognitive limitations. Such tools attempt to separate disability stemming from cognitive limitations from those caused by physical limitations. Generally speaking, since the early work of Katz and his colleagues, there has been an emphasis on more detailed assessments of ADL. Unfortunately, the development of different tools with different foci (for example, performance versus capacity) has tended to create confusion because these differences can lead to varying outcomes (Parker & Thorslund, 2007).

One widely used ADL tool is the Barthel Index (Mahoney & Barthel, 1965). This index was designed to measure functional levels of self-care and mobility, and it rates the ability to feed and groom oneself, bathe, go to the toilet, walk (or propel a wheelchair), climb stairs, and control bowel and bladder. Tasks typically assessed with ADL tools are listed in **Box 7-2**. In using the Barthel Index or any ADL assessment tool, it is critical that the assessment be detailed and individualized. For example, the Barthel item for "personal toilet" includes several tasks (wash face, comb hair, shave, clean teeth), and the older adult may be independent in some but not all of them and may require an assistive device for some but not all of them. A detailed assessment will provide information for appropriate nursing interventions, that is, those designed to promote ability and compensate for and prevent further disability for that individual.

Some older adults, specifically those with cognitive limitations but with good physical abilities, can manage their ADLs with direction and support (cueing and supervising). As pointed out by Tappen (1994), most ADL assessment tools were developed for physically impaired individuals and "are not sensitive to the functional difficulties experienced by the persons with Alzheimer's disease and related dementia" (1994, p. 38). The Refined ADL Assessment Scale is composed of 14 separate tasks within 5 selected ADL areas (toileting, washing, grooming, dressing, and eating) (Tappen, 1994). This scale represents an approach to ADL assessment known

BOX 7-2 Tasks Typically Assessed with ADL Assessment Tools

Eating
Dressing
Bathing/washing
Grooming
Walking/ambulation
Ascending/descending stairs
Communication
Transferring (e.g., from bed to chair)
Toileting (bowel and bladder)

as "task segmentation," which means breaking down the ADL activity into smaller steps (Morris & Morris, 1997). For example, the steps of washing one's hands or getting dressed in the morning are fairly complex for someone with cognitive limitations. However, by cueing as needed, the nurse can assess which of the steps are challenging and which are not. In getting dressed in the morning, some older adults with cognitive limitations will require help in selecting clothing, but once these clothing pieces are selected and laid out, the older adult may require limited cueing to progress through the complex task of dressing. Beck (1988) has developed a dressing assessment tool for persons with cognitive limitations that is particularly detailed. Another consideration for assessment is the use of assistive devices to support older adults and their activities of daily living. The development and use of assistive devices has increased among all segments of the older adult population from those in nursing homes to those living in the community. It is important to ask about such devices and how they are used to perform activities of daily living. More detailed content on the use of assistive technology is presented in Chapter 16.

The most common ADL scale used in rehabilitation of older adults is the Uniform Data System for Medical Rehabilitation (UDSMR) Functional Independence Measure (FIM). The FIM instrument scores a person from 1 (needing total assistance or not testable) to 7 (complete independence) and is considered an exceptionally reliable and valid tool. Categories measured include self-care, bowel and bladder, transfer, locomotion, communication, and social cognition (UDSMR, 1996). This measure is done at admission and discharge and several times in between to assess progress in rehabilitation.

Instrumental Activities of Daily Living (IADLs)

Instrumental activities of daily living include a range of activities that are considered to be more complex compared with ADLs and address the older adult's ability to interact with his or her environment and community. It is readily apparent that items in IADL assessment tools are geared more for older adults living in the community; for example, items often ask about doing the laundry or shopping for groceries. It has also been suggested that IADL tools emphasize tasks traditionally associated with women's work in the home (Lawton, 1972). IADLs include the ability to use the telephone, cook, shop, do laundry and housekeeping, manage finances, take medications, and prepare meals. Missing from most IADL tools are activities that may be more associated with men, such as fixing things around the house or lawn care. One of the earliest IADL measures was developed by Lawton and Brody (1969). Tasks typically assessed with IADL tools are listed in **Box 7-3**.

Advanced Activities of Daily Living (AADLs)

Advanced activities of daily living include societal, family, and community roles, as well as participation in occupational and recreational activities. AADL assessment tools tend to be used less often by nurses and more often by occupational therapists and recreation workers to address specific areas of social tasks. One tool that seems to combine elements of ADLs, IADLs, and AADLs is the Canadian Occupational Performance Measure (COPM) (Chan & Lee, 1997). Developed by Law and colleagues (1994), this tool is designed to detect changes in self-perception of occupational performance over time.

The COPM asks older adults to identify daily activities that are difficult for them to do but, at the same time, are self-perceived as being important

BOX 7-3 Tasks Typically Assessed with IADL Assessment Tools

Using the telephone
Taking medications
Shopping
Handling finances
Preparing meals
Laundry
Light or heavy housekeeping
Light or heavy yardwork
Home maintenance
Using transportation
Leisure/recreation

to do. The tool asks about self-care activities (personal care, functional mobility, and community management), productivity (paid/unpaid work, household management, and play/school), and leisure (quiet recreation, active recreation, and socialization). Consequently, interventions to enhance and support ability are planned to address those activities of importance to the older adult. The strength of the COPM is that it focuses on the older adult's functional priorities by asking about importance so that interventions can be tailored to enhance those priority activities and increase satisfaction.

Physical Performance Measures

One of the criticisms directed toward ADL and IADL assessment tools is that they are highly subjective, relying on the perspectives of older adults (and sometimes their family members) or on health care professionals who may tend to be more conservative in estimating ability (Guralnik, Branch, Cummings, & Curb, 1989). In contrast, physical performance measures involve direct observation of activities, such as observing the older adult prepare and eat a meal, but also include tasks related to balance, gait, and the ability to reach and bend. The Physical Performance Test (PPT) is one example of a physical performance assessment tool (Reuben & Sui, 1990). The seven-item version asks the individual to write a sentence, transfer five kidney beans from an emesis basin to a can (one at a time), put on and remove a jacket, pick up a penny from the floor, turn 360 degrees, and walk 50 feet (Reuben, Valle, Hays, & Sui, 1995).

The benefit of using physical performance measures is related to a potential relationship between physical ability and functional ability. The question is, does assessment of physical performance relate meaningfully to the ADL and IADL abilities of older adults? Does difficulty with walking and climbing stairs, for example, go hand-in-hand with ADL and IADL abilities such as toileting or grocery shopping? Findings have been inconsistent due at least in part to the several ways of measuring physical performance and functional ability. Some studies have suggested that physical performance measures provide good information to identify older adults who may be at risk for losing functional ability in ADL and becoming prone to falls (Gill, Williams, & Tinetti, 1995; Tinetti, Speechley, & Ginter, 1988).

PHYSICAL ASSESSMENT

Conducting a physical assessment of an older adult is based on technical competence in physical assessment, knowledge of the normal changes (Chapter 6) and diseases associated with aging, as well as good communication skills (Chapter 5). In this chapter, a basis in technical competence is taken for granted and the emphasis is on presenting physical assessment information that is particularly relevant to the older adult (see **Case Study 7-1**). Physical assessment with a "systems" approach reviews each body

Case Study 7-1

You are visiting an older couple in the community in order to assess the couple's functional ability and the potential for their needing assistance with ADLs or IADLs. Mr. and Mrs. Boyd are 72 and 67 years old, respectively, and have been married for 45 years. They have lived in the same neighborhood since Mr. Boyd retired from his bank manager job 12 years ago. Mrs. Boyd has been a housewife since her marriage. Mr. and Mrs. Boyd have one child, a son who lives in another city about 500 miles away. There are no other family members in their community.

As you sit with both of them at the kitchen table, Mrs. Boyd tells you to direct all your questions to her because Mr. Boyd has trouble understanding questions. She goes on to explain that Mr. Boyd used to garden and maintain the yard but no longer seems interested in doing anything. He sleeps a great deal, seems to be eating less, and is often uncommunicative when she speaks to him. She says that her husband is getting quite forgetful and that this worries her because he was always socially engaging and a man who could speak on several subjects.

Mrs. Boyd tells you that she makes all the decisions and spends most of her time planning meals, doing housework, and attending her ladies' church group. She says that she could really use some help with outdoor tasks because these tasks had been handled by Mr. Boyd until just recently. When you ask what she means by

(continued)

"recently," Mrs. Boyd replies that a change seems to have occurred within the last 6 months.

You thank Mrs. Boyd for sharing this information with you, and you indicate that most of the questions can be directed to her but that you will be asking Mr. Boyd some questions as part of the assessment. Mrs. Boyd seems concerned by this but agrees to give you an opportunity to try and ask some questions of Mr. Boyd. You begin your assessment by asking Mrs. Boyd about her functional abilities, including ADLs and IADLs, indicating that you will be asking the same questions of Mr. Boyd.

Questions:

1. Drawing from the 10 principles of comprehensive assessment and your knowledge of functional, physical, cognitive, psychological, social, and spiritual assessment of older adults, what are the areas of assessment that you think should be explored first with Mr. and Mrs. Boyd?
2. Will you be relying on self-report, proxy report, performance measures, or all of these for the assessment?
3. Mrs. Boyd seems to want to dominate the interview. How will this affect the assessment process?
4. Which other health professionals do you think should be involved directly or in consultation in relation to your assessment?

system by first taking a history and then conducting a physical examination. It is important to ask questions that produce an accurate description of the older adult's physical health status and furthermore to explore the meaning and implications of physical health status on an individual basis. The same changes in visual acuity for two older adults may have quite different meanings and implications. For one older adult, the changes may not affect their everyday activities whereas for the other, they may mean the loss of a driver's license and accompanying distress and hardship in relation to unmet transportation needs and decreased social contact.

Physical assessment by body systems usually involves a health care team approach. Physicians, including specialists such as a cardiologist, and nurses are key members of the team. Nurses often do an initial assessment or act as case finders in the community and in clinics. Other members of the health care team include a nutritionist, respiratory therapist, social worker, physical therapist, and psychologist.

Circulatory Function

Several factors play a role in older adults and their circulatory status. Age-related changes in the heart muscle and blood vessels result in overall decreased cardiac function. These changes plus lifestyle, including limited exercise and physical activity, increase the likelihood that older adults will experience diminished circulatory function. Other lifestyle factors that have an impact on circulatory function are smoking behaviors and the consumption of alcohol. When the current cohort of older adults was young, the benefits of exercise and physical activity and the detrimental effects of smoking were not common knowledge. The social context was different compared with our current one. The cumulative effects of age-related changes, heredity, and lifestyle mean that there can be great variation among older adults in relation to their circulatory function. In addition, through the use of medications and assistive devices, diminished circulatory function may have a greater or lesser impact on their day-to-day life. Although diseases of the circulatory system can occur at all ages, these diseases are associated with people in their older years, and comprehensive assessment will include taking a cardiac history and performing a physical examination.

The circulatory health assessment should address family history; current problems with chest pain or discomfort, especially if associated with exertion; current diagnoses and associated medications as well as over-the-counter and herbal medicines; sources of stress; and adherence to current medical regimens. The assessment should also include a physical examination, assessing blood pressure, listening to chest sounds, and taking a pulse rate. Other assessment protocols may include an exercise stress test, blood and serum tests, electrocardiograms, and other tests for imaging and assessing the condition of the heart and blood vessels. These advanced laboratory assessment protocols are usually ordered by physicians and the results are shared by the health care team as detailed assessment information.

Respiratory Function

Age-related changes to bones, muscles, lung tissue, and respiratory fluids all contribute to the respiratory difficulties experienced by some older adults. Older adults are particularly susceptible to respiratory diseases, and the signs of infection may not be as obvious as they are in younger adults. Therefore, assessment of respiratory function should occur more often, particularly with older adults who may have compromised respiratory function because of disease or injury. Older adults who have restricted mobility and have extended bed rest are especially at risk for respiratory infections and serious sequential complications.

The respiratory assessment should ask about current medications (including prescribed, over-the counter, and herbal) and take a history of smoking behavior and exposure to environmental pollutants during the life span. Other areas for assessment include current difficulties and anxieties associated with breathing, decreased energy to complete everyday tasks, frequent coughing, and production of excessive sputum. Physical examination includes observation of posture and breathlessness, and listening to chest sounds. Other assessment protocols include blood and pulmonary function tests, chest x-ray, and sputum analysis. Information from these tests assists the nurse in a total assessment of respiratory function.

Gastrointestinal Function

Age-related changes in the gastrointestinal system are not dramatic and therefore may not be noticed by many older adults. Smooth muscle changes mean decreased peristaltic action and reduced gastric acid secretion, which may affect gastric comfort and appetite. A concern of many older adults is constipation, which is usually defined as the lack of a bowel movement for 3 or more days. A lack of dietary fiber, low levels of physical activity, and lack of fluid are associated with constipation among healthy older adults (Annells & Koch, 2003). Although the problem of constipation does not always receive serious attention, a recent review reported that chronic constipation was associated with serious consequences including fecal impaction, incontinence, and delirium, leading to severe curtailment in ADLs and, in some cases, necessitating hospitalization (Tariq, 2007).

Assessment of gastrointestinal function begins with asking about the older adult's usual diet; appetite and changes in appetite; occurrence of nausea, vomiting, indigestion, or other stomach discomforts; and problems with bowel function, including constipation and diarrhea. In relation to constipation, the nurse should ask about exercise, diet, and fluid intake, and whether the older adult is using prescribed, over-the-counter, or herbal remedies to deal with constipation. A 3- to 7-day meal diary can illustrate eating habits that might have an impact on constipation. Limited ingestion of fresh fruits and vegetables and fluids contributes to constipation, as does limited exercise and mobility. Older adults have a diminished sense of thirst, and fluid intake may be inadequate to maintain normal bowel function. Diagnostic testing can include barium enemas and x-rays, stool analysis, and examination of the colon.

Special attention should be directed to changes in appetite and specifically to loss of appetite. Poor appetite with related declines in body weight and energy is often seen as a warning sign that signals future health problems (Morley, 2003). Decreased body weight is associated with negative changes to the skin, making it prone to injury, and reduced caloric intake affects energy levels needed for mobility and other activities of daily living. Poor appetite is not solely embedded in gastrointestinal function and instead includes aspects of social and psychological function. Mealtime is also a social experience and often involves interaction with others. One study of community-dwelling older adults reported that impaired appetite was associated with depression, poor self-rated health, smoking, chewing problems, visual impairment, and weight loss (Lee et al., 2006).

Oral health assessment is an area often overlooked with older adults, and nurses should routinely ask about oral health practices including brushing, flossing, and regular contact with a dentist. Poor oral care leads to dental caries, dry mouth, and mouth infections as well as systematic infections that can affect cardiac and respiratory function. Examination of the mouth should include observing the condition of the tongue, teeth, and gums for dehydration, infection, and poor oral hygiene. Check dentures to be sure they are well-fitting, particularly if a weight change has occurred. Especially at risk for oral health problems are older adults with limited incomes who cannot manage regular contact with a dentist and older adults in long-term care facilities who lack the physical or cognitive ability to maintain self-care in oral health (Bawden, 2006).

Genitourinary Function

Age-related changes in the genitourinary system along with age-related diseases such as diabetes and hypertension can have a major impact on everyday life. Bladder muscles weaken and bladder capacity is lessened. Difficulties in sensing that the bladder has not emptied may mean that residual urine stays within the bladder, creating a medium for potential infection. Older women are more likely to experience incontinence, which is often related to a history of childbirth or gynecologic surgeries. Gynecologic assessment of older women is an area of assessment that is sometimes neglected. Older women and their caregivers may mistakenly believe that because the childbearing years have passed or because of sexual inactivity, a gynecologic exam is no longer needed (Richman & Drickamer, 2007). The nurse should be asking questions about abnormal bleeding, vaginal discharge, and any urinary symptoms. Pelvic examinations and Pap smears are usually carried out by physicians, but nurses have an important role in identifying the need for this further assessment.

Older men may develop problems with an enlarged prostate that impedes the flow of urine through the urethra. Incontinence is not a normal part of aging; when incidents of incontinence occur regularly, this can lead to embarrassment, restricted social activity, and skin problems. Urinary incontinence can be managed and improved by nursing interventions that involve behavioral treatment options (McGuire, 2006). More detailed content on urinary incontinence, assessment, and nursing interventions are presented in Chapter 14. Unmanaged incontinence can have significant consequences to daily life, and unmanaged incontinence in the home environment is a major factor in the decision for nursing home placement.

A serious medical problem, chronic renal failure can arise as a complication of age-related diseases such as diabetes and hypertension. This is a potentially life-threatening illness that requires specialized care and may ultimately mean support through kidney dialysis.

Health history questions should attend to any previous or current difficulties related to the frequency and voluntary flow of urine during either the day or night. If incontinence is a problem, then questions should focus on the type of incontinence: **stress**, **urge**, **functional**, or **overflow** (see Chapter 14). Older adults who have problems with continence may restrict their fluid intake, which will have implications for other body systems including skin condition and the gastrointestinal system. The nurse should ask about fluid intake, especially caffeine and alcohol (because these substances affect bladder tone) and observe the skin for dehydration. The nurse also should ask about medication use (prescribed, over-the-counter, and herbal remedies). Diagnostic tests include urine analysis tests for blood, bacteria, and other components such as **ketones**. Other diagnostic tests may be ordered by the physician to assess bladder muscle tone and function and prostate size and potential obstructions.

Sexual Function

Two of the prevailing myths in our society are that older adults are neither sexually active nor interested in sexual relationships. This is not the case; however, several factors associated with aging do have an impact on sexual activity, including lack of partner (often through widowhood), chronic illnesses, and medication use that may negatively affect performance and sexual satisfaction. In conducting a comprehensive assessment with an older adult, asking about sexual function is appropriate. However, it is important to be knowledgeable about age-related and disease-associated changes in relation to sexual function and to be sensitive and respectful of privacy because this is clearly a very personal area of human function.

Age-related changes for men include a decrease in the speed and duration of erection; in women there is a decrease in vaginal lubrication. Health and social factors may have a great impact on sexual activity among older adults; chronic illness such as osteoarthritis and diminished positive self-image because of a societal emphasis on youthful beauty are two such factors. Lack of privacy inhibits the expression of sexuality; this in particular can be a deterrent in residential long-term care facilities (Richman & Drickamer, 2007).

Assessment questions should focus on sexual function and whether there have been any changes or concerns. Do not assume that older adults are sexually inactive. Instead ask about sexual activity and whether there have been changes or concerns in relation to sexuality and sexual activity. Asking these questions can open the door to further dialogue. In the past few years, there has been a great deal of advertising by pharmaceutical companies for erectile dysfunction drugs. The advertising is aimed at middle-aged and older adults, and there may be some natural curiosity about these new drugs. An older adult's questions about enhancement medications might be best answered in consultation with a pharmacist because of potential side effects and interactions with other medications.

Neurological Function

The neurological system affects all other body systems. Age-related changes involve declines in reaction time, kinetic and body balance problems, and sleep disturbances. Age-related diseases such as Alzheimer's disease and Parkinson's disease and other health problems such as stroke can lead to cognitive changes including memory loss, lack of spatial orientation, **agnosia**, **apraxia**, **dysphagia**, **aphasia**, and delirium. Dementia is a collection of diseases where the changes in brain cells and activity lead to progressive loss of mental capacity. Alzheimer's disease is the most common disease of dementia. Cognitive assessment for dementia will be discussed in a later section of this chapter.

Neurological assessment of older adults includes several components. The nurse should ask about medications (prescribed, over-the-counter, and herbal remedies) and any medical diagnosis related to the neurological system, such as history or family history of stroke. The nurse should observe and ask about previous and current impairments in speech, expression, swallowing, memory, orientation, energy level, balance, sensation, and motor function. Other areas of assessment relate to the occurrence of sleep disturbance, tremors, and seizures.

Musculoskeletal Function

Several age-related changes occur in the musculoskeletal system and lead to decreased muscle tone, strength, and endurance. The stiffening of connective tissue (ligaments and tendons) and erosion of articular surfaces of joints create restrictions in joint mobility. Declines in hormone production contribute to bone loss, and the ability to heal is reduced. Common musculoskeletal health problems include **osteoarthritis** and **osteoporosis**. Of particular concern are the risk of falls and the potential for fractures with associated morbidity and mortality. One commonly used assessment tool for the risk of falls is the Morse Fall Scale; a description of this scale is provided in Chapter 14.

The most commonly reported illness among older adults is osteoarthritis, and it is more likely to occur in the weight-bearing joints, especially the hips and knees. Because sore and stiff joints are universally associated with aging, older adults and health care professionals often take an accepting attitude about these complaints. The nurse should be asking about the history of sore joints: Which joints are affected? How long has there been pain? What kind of pain is it? Does it interfere with everyday activities? Is the pain managed? If so, how is it managed? Is there a history of bone and muscle injuries? Has there been surgery? Have alternative and complementary therapies such as acupuncture or herbal remedies been explored? What are the pertinent lifestyle factors for this older adult, including participating in exercise and physical activity?

Observation of posture, stance, and walking can assist in asking the appropriate questions: Does the older adult favor one side of the body while walking? Are assistive devices such as canes and walkers being used? Canes and walkers should be at the appropriate height in relation to body height. Ask whether an assessment was done by a therapist in selecting the height, weight, and type of cane or walker. In observing walking and rising from a chair, attend to body language and facial expressions that indicate discomfort. Observe and examine the kind of footwear being worn. Does the footwear offer adequate support while promoting good circulation?

The Up and Go Test provides a quick assessment of an older person's mobility and overall function.

The nurse should measure a distance of 10 feet from the person's chair and ask him or her to rise, walk to the line, turn, walk back, and sit down. An average time to do this is 10 seconds. Greater than 10 seconds may indicate functional problems with ambulation (Reuben et al., 2008).

Osteoporosis is a major health problem and has an increasingly large impact on disability and the need for supportive and rehabilitative health services (Stone & Lyles, 2006). Osteoporosis causes a gradual loss of bone mass, and bones become porous and vulnerable to fracture. It is associated with aging, heredity, poor calcium intake, hormonal changes, and a sedentary lifestyle. Older adults with osteoporosis experience symptoms of chronic back pain, muscle weakness, joint pain, loss of height, and decrease in mobility. Bone density tests can compare bone mass with individuals of comparable or younger ages as a marker. If needed, calcium intake can be increased through diet or supplements. The nurse should ask about symptoms and whether a bone density test has been carried out; if so, what were the subsequent recommendations?

Sensory Function

Age-related and disease-related changes in sensory function can have profound effects on older adults and their day-to-day functioning. Of the five senses—hearing, vision, smell, taste, and touch—it is the occurrence of diminished vision and hearing that seems to have the greatest impact on older adults. Problems with vision or hearing can have negative effects on social interaction and hence on social and psychological health. A recent study sited in complex continuing care facilities demonstrated that hearing impairment and mood were associated, and that improved hearing was directly related to improved mood and quality of life (Brink & Stones, 2007).

Presbyopia refers to an age-related change in vision. The lens of the eye becomes less elastic and this creates less efficient accommodation of near and distant vision. **Presbycusis** refers to age-related progressive hearing loss. Decrements in vision and hearing can affect communication ability with potential consequences to older adults' health, safety, everyday activities, socialization, and quality of life. Screening tools for vision and hearing are of two types: self-report and performance-based.

Specifically for vision, difficulty in reading has implications for safety in relation to reading instructions on prescription bottles and following other written directions for health care. Age-related **macular degeneration**, the deterioration of central vision, is the leading cause of severe vision loss in older adults in the United States. Older adults should undergo regular eye examinations for changes in vision (including the formation of **cataracts**) and screening for ocular pressure (for **glaucoma**). The American Academy of Ophthalmology recommends periodic eye examinations at 1- to 2-year intervals for older adults who do not experience symptoms or high risk factors (Jung, Coleman, & Weintraub, 2007). These performance-based tests are conducted by other health professionals—optometrists and ophthalmologists—but nurses are often in a key position to screen for vision problems and to encourage older adults to initiate and maintain regular visits with other health professionals to assess vision changes.

The following two screening procedures are simple tests for functional vision:

1. Ask the older adult to read a newspaper headline and story and observe for difficulty and accuracy.
2. Ask the older adult to read the prescription bottle and, again, observe for difficulty and accuracy.

It is important to follow up with specific questions that explore the vision problem from the perspective of the individual: Is vision a problem? Does it interfere with everyday activities or with hobbies and social life? Are magnification aids or enlarged printed material useful strategies? Is home lighting contributing to the problem? Is it more difficult to see in the evening compared with other times of the day?

Hearing loss is a major concern for many older adults. According to the U.S. Census Bureau (Bureau of the Census, 1997), about 30% of older adults between 65 and 74 years of age and 50% of those between 75 and 79 years of age experience some hearing loss. Most hearing loss in older adults is both symmetric and bilateral, and hearing problems are exacerbated in a noisy environment. Non-aging-related hearing loss can be attributed to **cerumen** impaction, infection, occurrence of a foreign body, or **otosclerosis**. Assessment questions

BOX 7-4 Research Highlight

Aim: To explore the nurses' knowledge of, understanding of, and implications for care of older adults with dementia in acute care hospital wards

Methods: The theoretical framework was Kitwood and Bredin's (1992) person-centered approach. The research used a vignette describing a patient with dementia in an acute care ward and asked closed- and open-ended questions to explore nurses' assessment knowledge and proclivity to provide person-centered care. Forty-nine registered nurses from one acute care hospital in England participated in the project. Data were analyzed using qualitative and quantitative methods.

Findings: Nurses demonstrated a lack of consistency in choosing the care alternative from the closed-ended questions that reflected a person-centered care approach with older adults with dementia. From the open-ended question on knowledge and understanding, 85% of nurses indicated that they only partly possessed the skills and knowledge to work with older adults with dementia.

Application to practice: Dementia is a complex condition and provides a challenge for nurses in acute care settings in relation to assessment and the provision of person-centered care. To improve care for older adults with dementia in hospitals, education is needed on the nature and progress of dementia, and on skills to enhance person-centered care, particularly in relation to social interaction and communication.

Source: Fessey, V. (2007). Patients who present with dementia: Exploring the knowledge of hospital nurses. *Nursing Older People, 19*(10), 29–33.

should ask about any hearing problems and how these problems affect the older adult's everyday life. The following question is useful in assessing ear and hearing problems: Are you experiencing a hearing problem or any ear pain, ringing in the ears, or ear discharge? One study reported that asking, "Do you have a hearing problem now?" was effective in screening for hearing loss among older adults (Gates, Murphy, Rees, & Fraher, 2003). An initial assessment question might be, "Tell me when your hearing loss is the biggest problem for you?" The nurse who assesses hearing function is in a good position to recommend further diagnostic testing with an audiologist.

For older adults who wear hearing aids, the condition and working order of these aids is often overestimated and should be regularly assessed and monitored. One study conducted in a retirement community reported that for most of those wearing hearing aids, a visual check indicated problems with either broken or missing components, inappropriate volume setting, or weak or dead batteries, and this was especially true for those older adults who were relatively dependent on nursing care (Culbertson, Griggs, & Hudson, 2004).

The other senses are taste, smell, and touch. Taste and smell are interrelated; the sense of smell influences the sense of taste for food as well as appetite. Although there are some age-related changes (for example, fewer taste receptors), older adults who are experiencing a noticeable loss of taste and smell generally have other medical conditions (Ferrini & Ferrini, 2000). Medical conditions, especially those affecting the nose; medication side effects; nutritional deficiencies; poor oral hygiene; and smoking can all detrimentally affect the senses of smell and taste. Assessments should ask generally about satisfaction with taste and smell, the duration and extent of the problem, and the impact of the problem on everyday life.

Integumentary Function

Age-related changes to the skin include loss of elasticity, slower regeneration of cells, diminished gland secretion, reduced blood supply, and structural changes including loss of fat. This means that the skin of older adults is more susceptible to injury and infection and less resilient in terms of repair. Older adults with decreased mobility and extended bed rest are at high risk for skin damage and breakdown. For many older adults, skin dryness and itching are two common complaints. Emollients and powders can bring relief for most minor skin conditions.

Asking questions about skin problems and concerns and inspecting the skin are basic elements of assessment and should be done on a regular basis. If skin injury has already occurred, close monitoring and treatment are essential. The nurse should ask about rashes, itching, dryness, frequent bruising, and any open sores. Skin conditions can be linked with nutritional status and body weight, and the nurse can work with a nutritionist to promote a healthy diet and appropriate weight. Any loss of sensation, particularly in extremities, is a cause of concern. Impeded circulation with lack of sensation can lead to untreated skin breakdown, and prevention is preferable to the more serious consequences of infection and disability. In the event of wounds, there are assessment tools to gauge the extent and level, such as the Braden Wound Index, which is described in more detail in Chapter 14. Nurses with expertise in wound care are usually available in acute and long-term care for consultation and advice. This is often a specialized area of nursing practice.

The older adult's skin should be observed for color, hydration, circulation, and intactness. Fluid intake may be less than optimal and result in severe dryness. The nurse should be asking questions about skin changes, signs and symptoms of infection, usual skin care, and problems with healing. The nurse should also observe the fingernails and toenails for splitting and tears.

Endocrine and Metabolic Function

Age-related changes in endocrine function include decreased hormone secretion and breakdown of metabolites. Of special concern for older adults is the onset of diabetes mellitus or thyroid disease because these diseases can be insidious and silent. Much damage to the body can occur even before these conditions are diagnosed. Diabetes mellitus becomes more prevalent with age, but the symptoms of **polydipsia**, **polyphagia**, and **polyuria** may go unnoticed for several years. Because the thirst sensation diminishes with age, older adults may not be aware of their polydipsia. By the time the disease is diagnosed, more serious complications such as impaired circulation, foot ulcers, and vision disturbances may have ensued.

The more common form of diabetes mellitus among older adults is type 2 or non-insulin-dependent diabetes mellitus. With age, there is an increased resistance to the action of insulin within the body, and this change in combination with lifestyle choices places some older adults at inordinate risk for developing this disease. Age-related changes, heredity, obesity, poor nutrition, inadequate physical activity, and other illnesses increase the likelihood of type 2 diabetes among older adults. Given that the disease may be silent for many years, it is critical that nurses be attuned to assessing for the risk for developing diabetes among older adults and monitor changes and symptoms at every opportunity. As part of the health history, the following areas should be addressed:

- Family history of diabetes
- Changes in weight and appetite
- Fatigue
- Increased thirst and fluid intake
- Vision problems
- Slow wound healing
- Headache
- Gastrointestinal problems

More specific symptoms should be further assessed including occurrence of polyphagia, polydipsia, and polyuria. Diagnostic tests such as fasting blood sugar can provide a definitive diagnosis. The oral glucose tolerance test is of little value by itself because the older adult may have impaired glucose tolerance but not diabetes (Armetta & Molony, 1999).

In terms of thyroid disease, the formation of nodules that interfere with normal thyroid functioning becomes more common with age. Unfortunately, hypothyroidism and associated symptoms of fatigue, forgetfulness, and cold sensitivity may be seen as normal "slowing down" with age and go undetected. Hyperthyroidism is much more likely in the older years, but among older adults, the typical symptom of restlessness and hyperactivity may be lacking.

For older adults, hyperthyroidism or an overproduction of thyroid hormone does not usually mean major changes to everyday life. Nursing observation and assessment questions should address the occurrence of nervousness, heat intolerance, weight loss, tremor, and palpitations. Hypothyroidism or below normal levels of thyroid hormone causes several changes that can be uncomfortable and distressing. In the health history, the nurse should be assessing for skin changes (dry, flaky), fluid retention (edema and weight gain), fatigue, forgetfulness, constipation, and unusual sensitivity to the cold. Diagnostic tests (TSH test, TRH test, and radioimmunoassay) provide definitive diagnosis.

Hematologic and Immune Function

Several factors affect older adults' hematologic and immune systems. In relation to hematologic function, anemia is a common disorder among older adults, especially among those in nursing homes. Although a slight decrease in hemoglobin occurs with aging, more often the anemia is attributable to an iron deficiency or another illness. About 40% of adults age 60 or older have iron-deficiency anemia. Assessment should focus on observation of the color and quality of the skin and nail beds, and address food choices and food habits. Of a more serious nature, iron deficiency can occur because of blood loss, and the nurse should ask questions about occurrence of blood in stools. Diagnostic tests include hemoglobin, hematocrit, complete blood count (CBC), and red blood cell (RBC) count.

The immune system functions to protect the body from bacteria, viruses, and other microorganisms. Age-related changes to the immune system include diminished lymphocyte function and antibody immune responses. These changes put older adults at risk for infections. Vaccines for influenza and pneumonia are given in the fall and are available in physicians' offices, public health agencies, and other sites. As part of the assessment, the nurse should ask about recent and current infections and access to and use of vaccines to prevent infections. In terms of the symptoms of infection, it is important to remember that in evaluating vital signs, older adults tend to have a diminished febrile response to infection.

Some nurses are uncomfortable talking with older adults about sexual activity, prophylaxis, and sexually transmitted disease (STD), but these questions are an essential part of the health assessment process. Sexually active older adults, particularly those with more than one partner, are at risk for STDs. Of particular concern is the lack of STD education ("safe sex") programs focused on older adults, specifically HIV education. Human immunodeficiency virus (HIV) is a human retrovirus that causes acquired immune deficiency syndrome (AIDS). The disease is spread through parenteral and body fluids. It can be sexually transmitted through anal, oral, and vaginal intercourse.

AIDS is epidemic in the United States, and the Centers for Disease Control and Prevention reports that 11% of those infected are 50 years of age or older. Older adults may not be tested for HIV because they do not believe that they are at high risk or they may be unwilling to discuss their risky sexual behaviors. In terms of assessment, it is important to address the topic of sexual activity and ask the same questions that would be asked of a younger person. Open-ended questions are preferable, and it will be more productive to say, "Tell me about your sex life" rather than simply asking, "Do you have sex?" (Anderson, 2003). Depending on the status of sexual activity, other questions related to sexual preference and number of partners should be pursued. Signs and symptoms associated with HIV such as weight loss, dehydration, ataxic gait, or fatigue may go unnoticed or be attributed to age-related changes. However, once risk factors are identified, diagnostic testing will confirm a diagnosis.

COGNITIVE ASSESSMENT

Changes in cognitive function with age vary among older adults and are difficult to separate from other comorbidities (physical and psychological conditions), other age-related changes (for example, hearing), the side effects of medications, and changes in intellectual activity. Generally speaking, older adults manifest a gradual and modest decline in short-term memory and experience a reduction in the speed with which new information is processed.

Cognitive function is usually understood in relation to the qualities of attention, memory, language, visuospatial skills, and executive capacity. The most extensively used cognitive assessment tool is the Mini Mental State Examination (MMSE) (Folstein, Folstein, & McHugh, 1975). The MMSE was originally developed to differentiate organic from functional disorders and to measure change in cognitive impairment, but it was not intended to be used as a diagnostic tool. It measures orientation, registration, attention and calculation, short-term recall, language, and visuospatial function. It does not measure executive function, and the results of the MMSE can vary by age and education, with older individuals and those with fewer years of formal education having lower scores (Crum, Anthony, Bassett, & Folstein, 1993). In addition, some of the MMSE items may be less relevant for older adults who are hospital inpatients or who are living in long-term care facilities. For example, orientation-based questions regarding dates and day or time may be less relevant for long-term care residents compared with questions that ask about location of their room in the facility. A sample of items from the MMSE is given in **Box 7-5**. The entire MMSE is purchased by agencies and facilities as part of the assessment process. It is also available in the document "Screening for Delirium, Dementia and Depression in Older Adults" (Registered Nurses' Association of Ontario, 2003) on the following Web site: www.rnao.org.

Notable Quotes

"Health care providers' lack of awareness of current geriatrics practice and persistence in holding the outdated belief that confusion is a normal part of aging contribute to significant underrecognition of dementia in all settings. Early recognition and diagnosis are critical to carrying out best practices in the care of older patients."

—Deirdre Mary Carolan Doerflinger, PhD, CRNP (2007), in *American Journal of Nursing*, p. 62.

The Mini-Cog is another screening tool that can be administered in 5 minutes or less and requires minimal training (Doerflinger, 2007). The screening consists of a three-item recall and a clock-drawing test. This reliable tool can assist nurses with early detection of cognitive problems. A full-text article about the Mini-Cog can be accessed through www.consultgerirn.org, and a video link demonstrating use of the tool can be viewed at http://links.lww.com/A204.

Dementia is a permanent progressive decline in cognitive function, and Alzheimer's disease is the most common form of dementia. The *Diagnostic and Statistical Manual of Mental Disorders*, 4th edition (DSM-IV), used by both the psychiatric and psychological communities, states that dementia of the Alzheimer's type typically is manifested by both impaired memory (long- or short-term) and inabil-

BOX 7-5 Sample Items from the MMSE

Orientation to Time:

"What day is it?"

Registration:

"Listen carefully. I am going to say three words. You say them back after I stop.

"Ready? Here they are . . .

"APPLE (pause), PENNY (pause), TABLE (pause). Now repeat those words back to me." [Repeat up to five times, but score only the first trial.]

Naming:

"What is this?" [Point to a pencil or pen.]

Reading:

"Please read this and do as it says." [Show examinee the words on the stimulus form.]

CLOSE YOUR EYES

ity to learn new information, or to recall recent information, and is distinguished by one (or more) of the following cognitive disturbances: aphasia, apraxia, agnosia, or disturbance in executive functioning (i.e., planning, organizing, sequencing, abstracting). These cognitive limitations have broad and major implications for occupational and social interaction, as well as safety. The declines associated with Alzheimer's disease are progressive and irreversible. Definitive diagnosis is possible only on autopsy, but diagnosis is made in the absence of alternatives (for example, brain tumor and other neurological conditions or diseases). Several tools are available to assess cognitive function, and the common element of most is the assessment of memory function.

For nurses, assessing cognitive function is a challenging task because of the combination of factors that may be interacting: physical and psychological comorbidities, age-related changes, the side effects of medications, and changes in environment, as some examples. Added to this is the concern that for older adults and their families, even the suspicion of Alzheimer's disease can be a frightening and discouraging experience. Concerns arise related to the loss of memory but even more so to the potential loss of the "person" as the disease progresses. An influential individual in our understanding of the course and nature of cognitive decline in dementia was Tom Kitwood, who pioneered the theory and practice of "person-centered care." Kitwood and Bredin (1992) argued that older persons with dementia should be recognized for their uniqueness, their experiential being, and their relatedness with others. Taking this perspective, nursing assessment emphasizes individualization, asking about and taking into account previous preferences for care directly expressed by the older adult with dementia, or from family members as proxies, when necessary.

A relatively new area of assessment of older adults with dementia is that of "social ability." Social abilities include giving and receiving attention, participating in conversation, recognizing social stimuli, appreciating humor, and being helpful to others (Baum, Edwards, & Morrow-Howell, 1993; Dawson, Wells, & Kline, 1993; Sabat & Collins, 1999). Dawson and her colleagues have developed and validated a social abilities assessment subscale that can be used as a basis for supporting and maintaining ability in social life as much as possible. The entire tool (Abilities Assessment for the Nursing Care of Persons with Alzheimer's Disease and Related Disorders) is available in the document "Caregiving Strategies for Older Adults with Delirium, Dementia and Depression" (Registered Nurses' Association of Ontario, 2004) on the following Web site: www.rnao.org.

PSYCHOLOGICAL ASSESSMENT

Psychological assessment of older adults presents a wide continuum from positive mental health to mental health problems, and the tendency seems to be weighted toward assessment of mental health disorders. In this chapter we will be looking at two areas of psychological assessment: quality of life,

BOX 7-6 Recommended Readings

American Geriatrics Society, AGS Panel. (Updated annually). *Geriatrics at your fingertips*. New York: Blackwell Publishing.

Baldwin, S., & Capstick, A. (2007). *Tom Kitwood on dementia: A reader and critical commentary.* McGraw-Hill Open University Press.

Kane, R. L., Ouslander, J. G., Abrass, I. B., & Resnick, B. (2008). *Essentials of clinical geriatrics* (6th ed.). New York: McGraw-Hill.

which may include several positive mental health constructs, and depression, a common mental health problem.

Quality of Life

Quality of life and successful aging are two central concepts in assessment and care of older adults. Broadly speaking, quality of life encompasses all areas of everyday life: environmental and material components, and physical, mental, and social well-being (Fletcher, Dickinson, & Philp, 1992). Quality of life among older adults is highly individualistic, subjective, and multidimensional in scope. With respect to what constitutes quality of life, what is important to one person may be quite unimportant to another. Related to quality of life is the concept of successful aging. Long associated with community living, successful aging has traditionally been linked with physical health, independence, functional ability, and **longevity**. However, other elements such as engagement in social life, self-mastery, optimism, personal meaning in life, and attainment of goals have been suggested as vital to the idea of successful aging (Reker, Peacock, & Wong, 1987; Rowe & Kahn, 1997). Elements of successful aging can include self-acceptance, positive relationships with others, and personal growth. A broad conceptualization of successful aging means broad applicability to older adults with varying abilities and disabilities. If we can go beyond the idea of physical health as the primary criterion for successful aging, then we can remove the labeling of frail older adults as being "unsuccessful" in their aging (Guse & Masesar, 1999).

Assessment of quality of life and successful aging can assist in better understanding the psychological health of older adults. Simply put, the following assessment questions will open dialogue on attitude, beliefs, and feelings about aging and mental health (**Figure 7-1**). For example, the nurse

FIGURE 7-1 **Quality care begins with comprehensive assessment.**

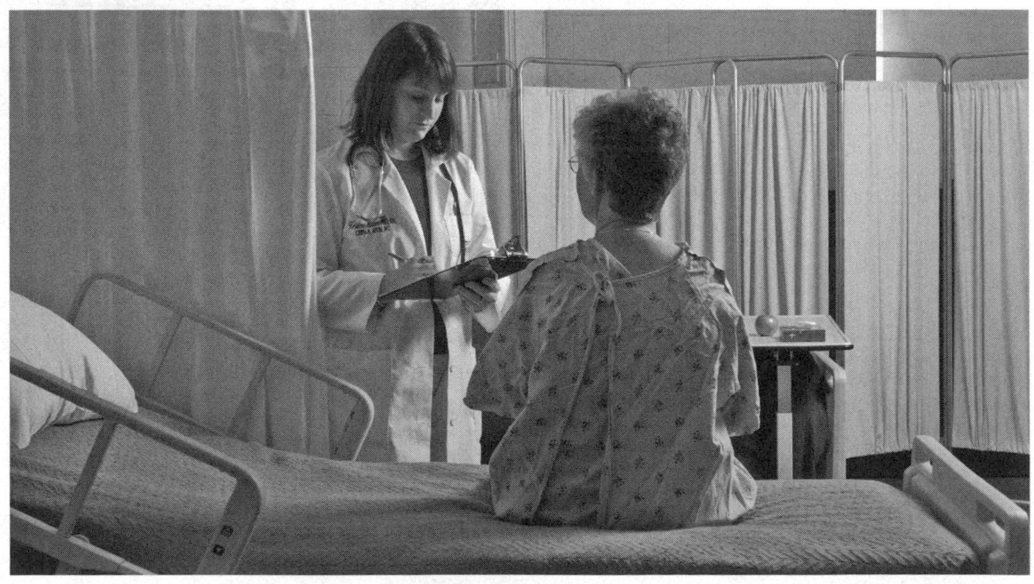

SOURCE: Photo courtesy of Don Battershall (Hartford Foundation)

can ask, "How would you describe your quality of life?" and "What would add to your quality of life?" Questions on successful aging are also informative. For example, "Would you describe yourself as someone who is aging successfully?" and "What would help you to age successfully?"

Depression

Clinical depression is the most common mental health problem among older adults, and it often goes undetected because clinicians attribute depressive symptoms to age-associated changes, chronic physical illness, medication side effects, or pain. The consequences of clinical depression can be serious and include suicidal ideation and suicide attempts. The prevalence of clinical depression in older Americans is estimated to be 14–20% among community-dwelling individuals, 30–40% among recently hospitalized individuals, and 15–30% among older persons residing in long-term care facilities (Anstey, von Sanden, & Sargent-Cox, 2007; Lebowitz et al., 1997; Wilson, Mottram, & Sexsmith, 2007). Minor depression can precede clinical or major depression and can be a response to stressors such as widowhood, loss of independence, or other losses. Older Americans may experience minor depression on a chronic basis but not meet the established criteria for clinical or major depression as outlined in the DSM-IV. To meet the DSM-IV criteria, an older adult must experience five or more of the following symptoms during a 2-week period (American Psychiatric Association, 2000):

- Sadness
- Lack of enjoyment of previously enjoyed activities
- Significant weight loss
- Sleep disturbance
- Restlessness
- Fatigue
- Feelings of worthlessness
- Impaired ability to think clearly or concentrate
- Suicide ideation or attempt

Depressed older adults may experience difficulty with sleeping, loss of appetite, physical discomfort, anxiety, hopelessness, bouts of crying, and thoughts of suicide. They may feel uncomfortable in social situations and curtail their usual social contacts and events, creating a downward spiral of depression and isolation. A recent study conducted among rural older adults in public housing facilities reported an association among symptoms of depression, poverty, and social isolation (Fisher & Copenhaver, 2006).

Depression is associated with cognitive limitations, and depressed older adults can experience disorientation, shortened attention span, emotional outbursts, and difficulty in intellectual functioning. Differentiating between dementia and depression when several of the same symptoms are present is a challenge for nurses. Chapter 13 provides more information on the relationship among dementia, depression, and delirium; another excellent source is the document "Screening for Delirium, Dementia and Depression in Older Adults" (Registered Nurses' Association of Ontario, 2003), found on the Web site www.rnao.org.

The Geriatric Depression Scale (GDS) is widely used by nurses to assess symptoms of depression. The interviewer asks the older person a set of 30 questions with possible answers of yes or no. A "negative" response, which depending on the question may be a yes or no answer, is scored as one point; a higher score indicates more symptoms of depression. A score of 0–30 is possible, with 0–9 being normal, 10–19 indicating mild depression, and 20–30 indicating severe depressive symptoms. The 30-item GDS is provided in **Box 7-7**, and the capitalized responses are to be used in the scoring of responses. A shortened version of the GDS is presented in Chapter 12, and this 15-item scale may be more appropriate for older adults who are fatigued or have a limited attention span.

Clinical depression may be chronic or have a shorter duration, and it is not the same as experiencing temporary feelings of unhappiness, confused thinking, and somatic complaints. Nurses are in a good position, whether it be in community, acute care, or long-term care practice, to screen for potential depression (Bruno & Ahrens, 2003). One study found that questions asking about functional ability decline, visual impairment, memory impairment, and using three or more medications provided a reasonably good screen for depressive symptoms and consequential health service

BOX 7-7 Geriatric Depression Scale (1983)

1. Are you basically satisfied with your life? Yes/NO
2. Have you dropped many of your activities or interests? YES/No
3. Do you feel that your life is empty? YES/No
4. Do you often get bored? YES/No
5. Are you hopeful about the future? Yes/NO
6. Are you bothered by thoughts you can't get out of your head? YES/No
7. Are you in good spirits most of the time? Yes/NO
8. Are you afraid that something bad is going to happen to you? YES/No
9. Do you feel happy most of the time? Yes/NO
10. Do you often feel helpless? YES/No
11. Do you often get restless and fidgety? YES/No
12. Do you prefer to stay at home, rather than going out and doing new things? YES/No
13. Do you frequently worry about the future? YES/No
14. Do you feel that you have more problems with memory than most? YES/No
15. Do you think that it is wonderful to be alive now? Yes/NO
16. Do you often feel downhearted and blue? YES/No
17. Do you feel pretty worthless the way you are now? YES/No
18. Do you worry a lot about the past? YES/No
19. Do you find life very exciting? Yes/NO
20. Is it hard to you to get started on new projects? YES/No
21. Do you feel full of energy? Yes/NO
22. Do you feel that your situation is hopeless? YES/No
23. Do you think that most people are better off than you are? YES/No
24. Do you frequently get upset over little things? YES/No
25. Do you frequently feel like crying? YES/No
26. Do you have trouble concentrating? YES/No
27. Do you enjoy getting up in the morning? Yes/NO
28. Do you prefer to avoid social gatherings? YES/No
29. Is it easy for you to make decisions? Yes/NO
30. Is your mind as clear as it used to be? Yes/NO

Source: Yesavage, J. A., Brink, T. L., Rose, T. L. Lum, O., Huang, V., Adey., M. M., & Leirer, V. O. (1983). Development and validation of a geriatric depression scale: A preliminary report. *Journal of Psychiatric Research, 17*, 37–49. (Reprinted with permission.)

utilization (Dendukuri, McCusker, & Belzile, 2004). Even asking the question, "Do you often feel sad or depressed?" is likely to open discussion and lead to further assessment of feelings of depression (Mahoney et al., 1994).

SOCIAL ASSESSMENT

Social functioning affects health and disease outcomes, and health status affects the ability to socialize and interact with others (Tomaka,

BOX 7-8 Resource List

Hospital Elder Life Program (http://elderlife.med.yale.edu): The Hospital Elder Life Program (HELP) is a patient-care program, developed by doctors and nurses at the Yale School of Medicine, that is designed to prevent delirium among hospitalized older patients.

The John A. Hartford Foundation Institute for Geriatric Nursing (http://www.hartfordign.org and http://www.ConsultGeriRN.org): These Web sites offer links to several assessment tools including SPICES (an overall assessment tool), Fall Risk Assessment, and the Geriatric Depression Scale.

National Institute for Health and Clinical Excellence (NICE) (http://www.nice.org.uk): This agency is an excellence-in-practice organization responsible for providing national guidance on the promotion of good health and the prevention and treatment of ill health in the United Kingdom. The Web site offers assessment and prevention tools in relation to falls and older adults.

Registered Nurses' Association of Ontario (http://www.rnao.org/bestpractices): This is the professional association of registered nurses in Ontario, Canada. It provides several best practices including assessment guidelines, for example, in the areas of pain, stage I to IV pressure ulcers, foot ulcers for people with diabetes, and screening for delirium, dementia, and depression in older adults.

Thompson, & Palacios, 2006). As people age, they may find that their social networks become smaller, and this may place them at risk in several ways. Decades of research have told us that individuals with low quantity and quality of social relationships have a higher morbidity and mortality risk compared with those who have a good quantity and quality of social contacts. A supportive social network and in particular the presence of a spouse can act to maintain an older adult in the community; the lack of a partner is a predictor of nursing home placement.

Social assessment of older adults includes collecting information on the presence of a social network and on the interaction between the older adult and family, friends, neighbors, and community. Kane, Ouslander, and Abrass (1989) developed a broad-based social assessment that includes asking questions about recent life events (such as death of a spouse), living arrangements, everyday activities requiring help (and who usually provides help), potential isolation (frequency of leaving the house and having visitors), adequacy of income, and sources of health care coverage. Posed by the nurse, these general questions can identify areas of limitation in social contact and social support.

Having a social network of friends and family does not necessarily mean that there are social supports. However, the Lubben Social Network Scale contains 10 items, 3 of which have been found to differentiate those who are isolated from those who are not (Kane, 1995). These questions are:

- Is there any one special person you could call or contact if you needed help?
- In general, other than your children, how many relatives do you feel close to and have contact with at least once a month?
- In general, how many friends do you feel close to and have contact with at least once a month?

The more important aspects of social support may be the number of supportive persons and the various types of support (emotional, instrumental, and informational) that are available. Seeman and Berkman (1988) have identified four questions that assess the adequacy of social support. These questions are:

- When you need help, can you count on anyone for house cleaning, groceries, or a ride?
- Could you use more help with daily tasks?
- Can you count on anyone for emotional support (talking over problems or helping you make a decision)?
- Could you use more emotional help (receiving sufficient support)?

Using these kinds of questions will help assess the adequacy and range of support available to an older adult. Nurses should be asking questions about social support and social function as part of the comprehensive assessment. The questions developed by Lubben can be used with older adults generally across settings (community and acute and long-term care settings), whereas some of the questions posed by Seeman and Berk clearly relate to older adults living in the community.

SPIRITUAL ASSESSMENT

Spiritual assessment is an integral part of comprehensive assessment and provides a basis for an individualized plan of care (Forbes, 1994). Although there is a link between religiosity and spirituality, the two concepts are not synonymous. Religiosity refers to believing in God, organized rituals, and specific dogma; spirituality refers more broadly to ideas of belief that encompass personal philosophy and an understanding of meaning and purpose in life. Having religious beliefs may foster spirituality, but those without formal religious beliefs still can experience spirituality. Most health service intake forms have a place for collecting information on formal religious affiliation, but this does not necessary mean that the older adult is practicing his or her faith, or is active in a place of worship.

One of the earliest guidelines for spiritual assessment was developed by Stoll (1979), and it contains questions that address both religiosity and spirituality. The guidelines are divided into four areas:

1. The concept of God or deity (for example, "Is religion or God significant to you?")
2. Personal source of strength and hope (for example, "What is your source of strength and hope?")
3. Significance of religious practices and rituals (for example, "Are there any religious practices that are important to you?")
4. Perceived relationship between spiritual belief and health (for example, "Has being sick made any difference in your feelings about God or the practice of your faith?")

Nurses may not be comfortable conducting a spiritual assessment because it may seem inappropriately invasive or because it is an area that some nurses do not feel adequately prepared to address as an unmet need. If the intake record indicates a formal religious affiliation, then it is fairly straightforward to ask, "Do you have any religious needs?" or "Would you like to speak with a pastoral care worker?" Questions that address spirituality can begin by asking, "Are you having a spiritual need? Is there some way that I might help with your spiritual needs?" Another spiritual assessment question asks, "Have your health problems affected your feelings of meaning or purpose?" Spiritual assessment is an area that would benefit greatly from more research.

OTHER ASSESSMENT: OBESITY

Obesity has become a major health problem among Americans, including older Americans, and it is associated with chronic disease and disability (Jenson, 2005). Given the obesity prevalence in middle-aged adults, the proportions and numbers of obese older adults are expected to increase substantially over the next decade (Arterburn, Crane, & Sullivan, 2004). Providing care to obese persons places caregivers, both family and staff members, at risk for injury. In 1998, the National Institutes of Health released the first federal overweight and obesity guidelines, which are based on the body mass index (BMI), a ratio of weight (in pounds) to height (in inches squared), as an assessment tool. The BMI is a number usually between 16 and 40. A BMI between 25 and 29 is considered "overweight" and more than 30 is considered "obese." For instructions on how to calculate a BMI, go to the Centers for Disease Control Web site: www.cdc.gov/nccdphp/dnpa/healthyweight/assessing/bmi/adult_BMI/english_bmi_calculator/bmi_calculator.htm.

The adverse effects of obesity in relation to cardiovascular disease, diabetes, osteoarthritis, and gallbladder disease are well documented (Fields & Strano 2005). Obese older adults are likely to experience balance and mobility problems that place them at risk for falls. One study reported obesity as being a risk factor for decline in functional ability (as assessed by needing assistance with ADLs and IADLs) (Jensen & Friedmann, 2002). Unfortunately, there has been little research conducted on obese older adults, and this remains an area for further research and tool refinement. It is not clear whether the markers for overweight and obesity are relevant to older adults who may experience illness-related weight gain or loss. It has been suggested that for many older adults, an emphasis on weight maintenance might be the best approach until more evidence is accumulated through research (Jensen & Friedmann, 2002).

Nurses can assess for overweight and obesity using the BMI and by asking about a history of weight change. If food intake is a concern, a common approach is to begin with a 3- to 7-day meal diary. This information can assist in determining a person's food habits. This is an area of assessment where nurses could benefit from working with the nutritionist and the dietician, who have a specialized knowledge base.

DEVELOPING AN INDIVIDUALIZED PLAN OF CARE

At the beginning of this chapter, we indicated that the basis of an individualized plan of care for an older adult is a comprehensive assessment, and we have reviewed functional, physical, cognitive, psychological, social, and spiritual assessment. **Box 7-9** provides 10 guidelines for comprehensive

BOX 7-9 Ten Principles of Comprehensive Assessment

1. The cornerstone of an individualized plan of care for an older adult is a comprehensive assessment.
2. Comprehensive assessment takes into account age-related changes, age-associated and other diseases, heredity, and lifestyle.
3. Nurses are members of the health care team, contributing to and drawing from the team to enhance the assessment process.
4. Comprehensive assessment is not a neutral process.
5. Ideally, the older adult is the best source of information to assess his or her health. When this is not possible, family members or caregivers are acceptable as secondary sources of information. When the older adult cannot self-report, physical performance measures may provide additional information.
6. Comprehensive assessment should first emphasize ability and then address disability. Appropriate interventions to maintain and enhance ability and to improve or compensate for disability should follow from a comprehensive assessment.
7. Task performance and task capacity are two difference perspectives. Some assessment tools ask, "Do you dress without help?' (performance) whereas others ask, "Can you dress without help?" (capacity). Asking about capacity will result in answers that emphasize ability.
8. Assessment of older adults who have cognitive limitations may require task segmentation, or the breaking down of tasks into smaller steps.
9. Some assessment tools or parts of assessment tools may be more or less applicable depending on the setting, that is, community, acute care, or long-term care settings.
10. In comprehensive assessment, it is important to explore the meaning and implications of health status from the older adult's perspective. For example, the same changes in visual acuity for two older adults may have quite different meanings and implications for everyday life.

assessment that form a basis with which to develop an individualized plan of care. Additionally, **Box 7-10** provides a summary of the quality assessment tools recommended as best practices by the John A. Hartford Foundation and the Nurse Competence in Aging initiative (see www.ConsultGeriRN.org) (**Box 7-11**).

SUMMARY

Comprehensive assessment of the older adult is an essential component of geriatric nursing care that involves both objective and subjective data collection. Nurses may obtain information about the older adult patient from a variety of sources including the

BOX 7-10 Assessment Tools Available Through the Try This Series

The following are available via http://www.hartfordign.org/resources/education/tryThis.html:

- SPICES: An Overall Assessment Tool of Older Adults
- Katz Index of Independence in Activities of Daily Living (ADL)
- The Mini Mental State Examination (MMSE)
- The Geriatric Depression Scale (GDS)
- Predicting Pressure Ulcer Risk
- The Pittsburgh Sleep Quality Index (PSQI)
- The Epworth Sleepiness Scale
- Assessing Pain in Older Adults
- Fall Risk Assessment
- Assessing Nutrition in Older Adults
- Sexuality Assessment
- Urinary Incontinence Assessment
- Hearing Screening
- Confusion Assessment Method (CAM)
- Caregiver Strain Index (CSI)
- Elder Mistreatment Assessment
- Beers' Criteria for Potentially Inappropriate Medication Use in the Elderly
- Alcohol Use Screening and Assessment
- The Kayser Jones Brief Oral Health Status Examination (BOHSE)
- Horowitz's Impact of Event Scale: An Assessment of Post-Traumatic Stress in Older Adults

Preventing Aspiration in Older Adults with Dysphagia
Immunizations for the Older Adult
Assessing Family Preferences for Participation in Care in Hospitalized Older Adults
The Lawton Instrumental Activities of Daily Living (IADL) Scale
The Hospital Admission Risk Profile (HARP)
Confusion Assessment Method for the Intensive Care Unit (CAM-ICU)
Avoiding Restraints in Patients with Dementia
Brief Evaluation of Executive Dysfunction: An Essential Refinement in the Assessment of Cognitive Impairment
Assessing Pain in Persons with Dementia
Therapeutic Activity Kits

BOX 7-10 (continued)

Recognition of Dementia in Hospitalized Older Adults
Wandering in the Hospitalized Older Adult
Communication Difficulties: Assessment and Interventions
Assessing and Managing Delirium in Persons with Dementia
Decision Making and Dementia
Working with Families of Hospitalized Older Adults with Dementia
Eating and Feeding Issues in Older Adults with Dementia: Part I: Assessment
Eating and Feeding Issues in Older Adults with Dementia: Part II: Interventions

patient, family, friends, caregivers, nursing staff, other team members, charts, and other written documentation. All aspects of the older adult person should be considered, including physical, psychological, socioeconomic, and spiritual. Particular challenges may be encountered when assessing older adults with cognitive impairments. This chapter presented many tools and web sites that can assist the nurse in assessing older adults as the initial step in individualizing a plan of care.

BOX 7-11 Web Exploration

Visit the Hartford Institute's Web site and browse the tools, videos, and articles available at http://www.hartfordign.org/resources/education/tryThis.html.

Critical Thinking Exercises

1. In this chapter, we have said that comprehensive assessment is not a neutral process. Reflect on what that really means and what kinds of things might constitute an unwanted bias to the assessment process.
2. In this chapter, we have emphasized that comprehensive assessment makes use of nursing knowledge and understanding of the combined factors of age-related changes, age-associated and other diseases, heredity, and lifestyle choices. Think of an older adult for whom you have provided care and describe that person. Try to outline the factors (age-related changes, age-associated and other diseases, heredity, and lifestyle choices) that are relevant for his or her health assessment.

Personal Reflections

1. In this chapter, we have underlined the importance of the health care team and consultation with team members. Reflect on your understanding of the contributions of team members in relation to the assessment of older adults. What are some of your personal qualities in terms of working as a member of the health care team?
2. How would you define "successful aging" in relation to your own aging? What are the implications of your definition in relation to decisions you might make during your lifetime? How might this definition affect the way you view the aging process of others?

References

Adnan, A., Chang, A., Arseven, O. K., & Emanuel, L. L. (2005). Assessment instruments. In L. L. Emanuel (Ed.), *Clinical geriatric medicine* (pp. 121–146). Philadelphia: Saunders.

American Psychiatric Association. (2000). *Diagnostic and statistical manual of mental disorders* (4th ed., text rev.). Washington, DC: Author.

Anderson, M. A. (2003). *Caring for older adults holistically* (3rd ed.). Philadelphia: F. A. Davis.

Annells, M., & Koch, T. (2003). Constipation and the breached trio: Diet, fluid intake, exercise. *International Journal of Nursing Studies, 40*, 843–852.

Anstey, K. J., von Sanden, C., & Sargent-Cox, C. (2007). Prevalence and risk factors for depression in a longitudinal, population-based study including individuals in the community and residential care. *American Journal of Geriatric Psychiatry, 15*(6), 497–505.

Armetta, M., & Molony, C. M. (1999). Topics in endocrine and hematologic care. In S. L. Molony, C. M. Waszynski, & C. H. Lyder (Eds.), *Gerontological nursing: An advanced practice approach* (pp. 359–387). Stamford, CT: Appleton & Lange.

Arterburn, D. E., Crane, P. K., & Sullivan, S. D. (2004). The coming epidemic of obesity in elderly Americans. *Journal of the American Geriatrics Society, 52*, 1007–1012.

Baum, C., Edwards, D. F., & Morrow-Howell, N. (1993). Identification and measurement of productive behaviours in senile dementia of the Alzheimer's type. *The Gerontologist, 33*, 403–408.

Bawden, M. E. (2006). Clean those teeth. *Perspectives, 30*(4), 15.

Beck, C. (1988). Measurement of dressing performance in persons with dementia. *American Journal of Alzheimer's Care and Related Disorders and Research, 3*, 21–25.

Brink, P., & Stones, M. (2007). Examination of the relationship among hearing impairment, linguistic communication, mood and social engagement of residents in complex continuing care facilities. *The Gerontologist, 47*(5), 633–641.

Bruno, L., & Ahrens, J. (2003, November). The importance of screening for depression in home care patients. *Caring*, 54–58.

Bureau of the Census. (1997). *Statistical abstract of the United States 1997* (117th ed.). Washington, DC: U.S. Department of Commerce.

Chan, C. C., & Lee, T. M. (1997). Validity of the Canadian Occupational Performance Measure. *Occupational Therapy International, 4*(3), 229–247.

Crum, R., Anthony, J., Bassett, S., & Folstein, M. (1993). Population-based norms for the Mini-Mental State Examination by age and educational level. *Journal of the American Medical Association, 269*(18), 2386–2391.

Culbertson, D. S., Griggs, M., & Hudson, S. (2004). Ear and hearing status in a multilevel retirement facility. *Geriatric Nursing, 25*, 93–98.

Dawson, P., Wells, D. L., & Kline, K. (1993). *Enhancing the abilities of persons with Alzheimer's disease and related dementias.* New York: Springer.

Dendukuri, N., McCusker, J., & Belzile, E. (2004). The Identification of Seniors at Risk screening tool: Further evidence of concurrent and predictive validity. *Journal of the American Geriatrics Society, 52*, 290–296.

Doerflinger, D. M. C. (2007). The Mini-Cog. *American Journal of Nursing, 107*(12), 62–71.

Ferrini, A., & Ferrini, R. (2000). *Health in the later years.* New York: McGraw-Hill Higher Education.

Fessey, V. (2007). Patients who present with dementia: Exploring the knowledge of hospital nurses. *Nursing Older People, 19*(10), 29–33.

Fields, S. D., & Stano-Paul, L. (2005). Preface: Obesity. *Clinics in Geriatric Medicine, 21*(4), xi–xiii.

Fisher, K. M., & Copenhaver, V. (2006). Assessing the mental health of rural older adults in public housing facilities. *Journal of Gerontological Nursing, 22*(9), 26–33.

Fletcher, A. E., Dickinson, E. J., & Philp, I. (1992). Review: Quality of life instruments for everyday use with elderly patients. *Age and Aging, 21*, 142–150.

Folstein, M. F., Folstein, S. E., & McHugh, P. R. (1975). A practical method for grading the cognitive state of patients for the clinician. *Journal of Psychiatric Research, 12*(3), 189–198.

Forbes, E. J. (1994). Spirituality, aging, and the community-dwelling caregiver and care recipient. *Geriatric Nursing, 15*(6), 297–302.

Gates, G. A., Murphy, M., Rees, T. S., & Fraher, M. A. (2003). Screening for handicapping hearing loss in the elderly. *Journal of Family Practice, 52*(1), 56–62.

Gill, T. M., Williams, C. S., & Tinetti, M. E. (1995). Assessing risk for the onset of functional dependence among older adults: The role of physical performance. *Journal of the American Geriatrics Society, 43*, 604–609.

Guralnik, J. M., Branch, L. G., Cummings, S. R., & Curb, J. D. (1989). Physical performance measures in aging research. *Journal of Gerontology: Medical Sciences, 44*(5), M141–M146.

Guse, L. W., & Masesar, M. (1999). Quality of life and successful aging in long-term care: Perceptions of residents. *Mental Health Nursing, 20*(6), 527–539.

Jensen, G. L. (2005). Obesity and functional decline: Epidemiology and geriatric consequence. *Clinics in Geriatric Medicine, 21*(4), 677–687.

Jensen, G. L., & Friedmann, J. M. (2002). Obesity is associated with functional decline in community-dwelling rural older adults. *Journal of the American Geriatrics Society, 50*, 918–923.

Jung, S., Coleman, A., & Weintraub, N. T. (2007). Vision screening in the elderly. *Journal of the American Medical Directors Association, 8*(6), 355–362.

Kahn, R. S. (1964). Comments. In M. P. Lawton & F. G. Lawton (Eds.), *Mental impairment in the aged* (pp. 109–114). Philadelphia: Philadelphia Geriatric Center.

Kane, R., Ouslander, J., & Abrass, J. (1989). *Social assessment: Essentials of geriatrics.* New York: McGraw-Hill.

Kane, R. A. (1995). Comment. In L. Z. Rubenstein, D. Wieland, & R. Bernabei (Eds.), *Geriatric assessment technology: The state of the art* (pp. 99–100). New York: Springer.

Kane, R. L. (1993). The implications of assessment. *Journals of Gerontology, 48*(special issue), 27–31.

Katz, S., Down, T. D., Cash, H. R., & Grotz, R. C. (1970). Progress in the development of the index of ADL. *The Gerontologist, 10*, 20–30.

Katz, S., Ford, A., Moskowitz, R., Jackson, B., & Jaffee, M. (1963). Studies of illness in the aged: The index of ADL, a standardized measure of biological and psychosocial functioning. *Journal of the American Medical Association, 185*, 94–101.

Kearney, P. M., & Pryer, J. (2004). The international classification of functioning, disability, and health (ICF) and nursing. *Journal of Advanced Nursing, 46*(2), 142–170.

Kitwood, T., & Bredin, K. (1992). Towards a theory of dementia care: Personhood and well-being. *Ageing and Society, 12*(3), 269–287.

Law, M., Polatajko, H., Pollock, N., McColl, M. A., Carswell, A., & Baptiste, S. (1994). Pilot testing of the Canadian Occupational Performance Measure: Clinical and measurement issues. *Canadian Journal of Occupational Therapy, 61*(4), 191–197.

Lawton, M. P. (1972). Assessing the competence of older people. In D. Kent & R. Kastenbaum (Eds.), *Research, planning and action for the elderly.* Sherwood, NY: Behavioral Publications.

Lawton, M. P., & Brody, E. M. (1969). Assessment of older people: Self-maintaining and instrumental activities of daily living. *The Gerontologist, 9*(3), 179–186.

Lebowitz, B. D., Pearson, J. L., Schneider, L. S., Reynolds, C. F., Aleropoulos, G. S., Bruce, M. F., et al. (1997). Diagnosis and treatment of depression in late life: Consensus statement update. *Journal of the American Medical Association, 278*, 1186–1190.

Lee, J. S., Kritchevsky, S. B., Tylavsky, F., Harrie, T. B., Ayonayon, H. N., & Newman, A. B. (2006). Factors associated with well-functioning community-dwelling older adults. *Journal of Nutrition for the Elderly, 26*(1), 27–43.

Luborsky, M. (1997). Attuning assessment to the client: Recent advances in theory and methodology. *Generations, 21*(1), 10–15.

Mahoney, F. I., & Barthel, D. W. (1965). Functional evaluation: The Barthel index. *Maryland State Medical Journal, 14*(2), 61–65.

Mahoney, J., Drinka, T., Abler, R., Gunter-Hunt, G., Matthews, C., Grenstein, S., et al. (1994). Screening for depression: Single question versus GDS. *Journal of the American Geriatrics Society, 42*, 1006–1008.

McGuire, K. (2006). Promotion of urinary continence: Management of urinary incontinence in the geriatric setting. *Perspective, 30*(2), 22–23.

Morley, J. E. (2003). Anorexia and weight loss among older persons. *Journal of Gerontology Biological Sciences, 58*(2), 131–137.

Morris, J. N., & Morris, S. A. (1997). ADL assessment measures for use with frail elders. In J. A. Teresi, M. P. Lawton, D. Holmes, & M. Ory (Eds.), *Measurement in elderly chronic care populations* (pp. 130–156). New York: Springer.

Olenek, K., Skowronski, T., & Schmaltz, D. (2003, August). Geriatric nursing assessment. *Journal of Gerontological Nursing*, 5–10.

Ostbye, T., Tyas, S., McDowell, I., & Koval, J. J. (1997). Reported activities of daily living: Agreement between elderly subjects with and without dementia and their caregivers. *Age and Ageing, 26*, 99–106.

Parker, M. G., & Thorslund, M. (2007). Health trends in the elderly population: Getting better and getting worse. *The Gerontologist, 47*(2), 150–158.

Registered Nurses' Association of Ontario. (2003). *Screening for delirium, dementia and depression in older adults*. Toronto, Canada: Author.

Registered Nurses' Association of Ontario. (2004). *Caregiving strategies for older adults with delirium, dementia and depression*. Toronto, Canada: Author.

Reker, G. T., Peacock, E. J., & Wong, P. T. P. (1987). Meaning and purpose in life and well-being: A life span perspective. *Journal of Gerontology, 42*, 44–49.

Reuben, D. B., Herr, K. A., Pacala, J. T., Pollock, B. G., Potter, J. F., & Semla, T. P. (2008). *Geriatrics at your fingertips*. Malden, MA: American Geriatrics Society.

Reuben, D. B., & Sui, A. L. (1990). An objective measure of physical function of elderly outpatients: The physical performance test. *Journal of the American Geriatrics Society, 38*, 1190–1193.

Reuben, D. B., Valle, L. A., Hays, R. D., & Siu, A. L. (1995). Measuring physical function in community-dwelling older persons: A comparison of self-administered, interviewer-administered and performance-based measures. *Journal of the American Geriatrics Society, 43*, 17–23.

Richman, S. M., & Drickamer, M. A. (2007). Gynecologic care of elderly women. *Journal of the American Medical Directors Association, 8*(4), 219–223.

Rowe, J. W., & Kahn, R. L. (1997). Successful aging. *The Gerontologist, 37*, 433–440.

Sabat, S. R., & Collins, M. (1999, January/February). Intact social, cognitive ability and selfhood: A case study of Alzheimer's disease. *American Journal of Alzheimer's Disease*, 112–119.

Seeman, T. E., & Berkman, L. F. (1988). Structural characteristics of social networks and their relationship with social support in the elderly: Who provides support? *Social Science and Medicine, 26*(7),737–749.

Stolee, P., Patterson, M. L., Wiancko, D. C., Esbaugh, J., Arcese, Z. A., Vinke, A. M., et al. (2003). An enhanced role in comprehensive geriatric assessment for community nurse case managers. *Canadian Journal on Aging, 22*(2), 177–184.

Stoll, R. L. (1979, September). Guidelines for spiritual assessment. *American Journal of Nursing*, 1574–1577.

Stone, L. M., & Lyles, K. W. (2006). Osteoporosis in later life. *Generations, 30*(3), 65–70.

Tappen, R. M. (1994). Development of the refined ADL assessment scale. *Journal of Gerontological Nursing, 20*(6), 36–41.

Tariq, S. H. (2007). Constipation in long-term care. *Journal of the American Medical Directors Association, 8*(4), 209–218.

Tinetti, M. E., Speechley, M., & Ginter, S. F. (1988). Risk factors for falls among elderly persons living in the community. *New England Journal of Medicine, 319*, 1701–1707.

Tomaka, J., Thompson, S., & Palacios, R. (2006). The relation of social isolation, loneliness and social support to disease outcomes among the elderly. *Journal of Aging and Health, 18*(3), 359–384.

Uniform Data System for Medical Rehabilitation. (1996). *Guide for the Uniform Data Set for Medical Rehabilitation (including the FIM instrument)*. Buffalo, NY: Author.

Verbrugge, L. M., & Jette, A. M. (1994). The disablement process. *Social Science and Medicine, 38*, 1–14.

Wilson, K., Mottram, P., & Sexsmith, A. (2007). Depressive symptoms in the very old living alone: Prevalence, incidence and risk factors. *International Journal of Geriatric Psychiatry, 22*, 361–366.

World Health Organization. (2001). *International classification of function, disability, and health (ICF)*. Geneva: Author.

Yesavage, J. A., Brink, T. L., Rose, T. L., Lum, O., Huang, V., Aday, M., et al. (1983). Development and validation of a geriatric depression screening scale. *Journal of Psychiatric Research, 17*, 37–49.

CHAPTER 8

Medications and Laboratory Values

Creaque V. Charles, PharmD, CGP
Cheryl A. Lehman, PhD, RN, CRRN-A

Learning Objectives

At the end of this chapter, the reader will be able to:

- Discuss demographics related to aging and medication use.
- Identify the effect of aging on drug metabolism.
- Describe common drug-related problems in the elderly.
- List medications that may be inappropriate for older adults.
- Distinguish the relationship between laboratory values and medication administration.
- Review the nurse's role in the older adult's adherence to a medication regimen.
- Critically evaluate selected case studies related to older adults and medication.
- Describe medications used for three common conditions in the elderly population.

Key Terms

- Absorption
- Activities of daily living
- Adherence
- Adverse drug reaction (ADR)
- Compliance
- Distribution
- Drug–disease interaction
- Drug–drug interaction
- Excretion
- Food–drug interaction
- Function
- Instrumental activities of daily living
- Metabolism
- Peak blood level
- Pharmacodynamics
- Pharmacokinetics
- Polypharmacy
- Random blood level
- Trough blood level

The older adult with medications requires much more than pouring and administering the drugs. The nurse must have basic knowledge about the indications for the medication, correct dosages, correct administration, anticipated side effects, potential adverse drug reactions, and contraindications for each medication. The nurse must also, however, have knowledge of the unique biopsychosocial aspects of medication administration in the elderly. These include knowing how aging affects the metabolism of medications ("bio"), being aware of psychological influences on adherence to medication regimens, and the social aspects that are integral to a successful outcome. This chapter will review the biopsychosocial aspects of medication administration, while stressing the influence of the nurse on successful medication outcomes.

DEMOGRAPHICS

Today, the geriatric population (persons older than 65 years of age) makes up about 13% of the general population. That number is expected to increase to greater than 20% by the year 2030. Elderly patients, however, consume about 33% of all prescription medications and over-the-counter drugs (Delafuente & Stewart, 2001). Overall, the elderly have more disease states than other age groups and therefore require the use of more medications. Thus, effective and safe drug therapy is one of the greatest challenges within the elderly population. One national survey of noninstitutionalized persons, published in 2002, found that 40% of adults older than 65 years used 5 or more different medications per week, and 12% used 10 or more different medications. Also, these persons randomly filled additional prescriptions when acute medical conditions arose, such as infections or pain. Elderly persons who reside in nursing homes and assisted living facilities typically use even more medications (Beers & Berkow, 2000).

THE EFFECTS OF AGING ON DRUGS

Normal aging is associated with certain physiological changes that can significantly influence drug response. Both pharmacokinetics and pharmacodynamics play a role in how a person will respond to a drug.

Pharmacokinetics

Pharmacokinetics is the time course by which the body absorbs, distributes, metabolizes, and excretes drugs (Beers & Berkow, 2000). In other words, pharmacokinetics speaks to how drugs move through the body and how quickly this occurs.

Absorption is defined as the movement of a drug from the site of administration, across biological barriers, into the plasma. Although the rate of drug movement through the body may decrease with age, the extent of drug absorption is least affected by age. Certain disease states, however, and the simultaneous use of several medications have been shown to decrease absorption of some medications (California Registry, 2004).

Distribution is the movement of a drug from the plasma into the cells. As patients age, total body water declines and fat stores increase. This physiological change affects the distribution phase of highly water-soluble and fat-soluble drugs. Therefore, the volume of distribution may be decreased for drugs that are highly water soluble and increased for drugs that are highly lipid soluble. For example, diazepam (Valium) is a highly lipid-soluble medication. Diazepam has a documented long half-life in a young adult (the time it takes for half of the drug taken to be metabolized), but in an elderly person the half-life is even longer due to the increase in the fat stores. For the elderly patient who may be more sensitive to the side effects of diazepam, the longer half-life may cause prolonged adverse effects.

With age, hepatic mass and hepatic blood flow decrease (Beers & Berkow, 2000). Therefore, the hepatic **metabolism** of medications is reduced. Also with age, the renal mass and renal blood flow are reduced. This physiological change will decrease the amount of drug that goes through renal **excretion**. This can result in higher, and potentially toxic, levels of drug in the body of the older adult, compared to the same dosage administered to a younger person. Because renal function tends to decline with age, drug doses should be reviewed and adjusted periodically in all elderly patients.

Pharmacodynamics

Pharmacodynamics is the time course and effect of drugs on cellular and organ function. In other words, pharmacodynamics is what drugs do once they're in the body.

The effects of similar drug concentrations at the site of action may be greater or less than those in younger patients. Therefore, the potential for increased sensitivity to medications at the cellular level must be considered when administering them to an elderly patient. For instance, in the elderly person, an increased receptor response is seen for benzodiazepines, opiates, and warfarin (Coumadin). This results in benzodiazepines producing increased sedation, opiates increasing analgesia and respiratory suppression, and warfarin producing an increased anticoagulant effect (California Registry, 2004).

DRUG-RELATED PROBLEMS IN THE ELDERLY

About one-third of drug-related hospitalizations occur in persons over 65 years old (Beers &

Berkow, 2000). Even though medications provide benefit by preventing and treating disease, older people are more susceptible to drug-related problems, including adverse drug reactions (ADRs), food–drug interactions, polypharmacy, inappropriate prescribing, and noncompliance.

Adverse Drug Reactions

The World Health Organization defines **adverse drug reactions (ADRs)** as "any noxious, unintended, and undesired effect of a drug, which occurs at doses used in humans for prophylaxis, diagnosis, or therapy" (Delafuente & Stewart, 2001, p. 289). Two different types of ADRs are **drug–drug interactions** and **drug–disease interactions**. Drug–drug interactions can be defined as the alteration of the pharmacokinetics or pharmacodynamics of drug A when taken at the same time as drug B. Drug–disease interactions are defined as the worsening of a disease by a medication (see **Table 8-1**).

Older patients, with multiple disease states, often consume many different medications to treat both acute and chronic medical conditions. As a result, ADRs occur often in older patients. Age-related alterations in drug distribution, hepatic metabolism, and renal clearance all play a significant role in the chances of an elderly patient developing an ADR. ADRs in elderly patients may decrease functional status, increase health services use, and in some rare cases have resulted in death. Overall, ADRs represent a major problem for elderly patients. In addition to better prescribing patterns from physicians, there's a need for nurses and pharmacists to increase medication monitoring.

Notable Quotes

"Medication toxic effects and drug-related problems can have profound medical and safety consequences for older adults and economically affect the health care system."

—Fick et al., 2003

Food–Drug Interactions

Undetected **food–drug interactions** may lead to serious morbidity and mortality in the older adult. The effect of certain foods on drugs metabolized by the CYP450 families and on drugs susceptible to chelation and absorption has recently been recognized. Foods may contain compounds that lead to failure of an intended drug effect; alternately, malnutrition can lead to poor metabolism of drugs (McCabe, 2004).

The presence or absence of food may reduce or increase the bioavailability of a medication, leading to unanticipated effects. The first "lethal" food–drug interaction recognized was that of cheese and monoamine oxidase inhibitors (MAOIs). The interaction of food and drug in this instance could lead to extremely high blood pressure and stroke. Grapefruit juice is known to interact with antihistamines, and greens with warfarin. Herbal and dietary supplements may interact with medications, affecting metabolism of the drug. Natural licorice may induce hypertension and interfere with certain drugs. Antibiotics may be susceptible to chelation and absorption by fortified cereals, calcium-fortified orange juice, or protein beverages. These interactions reduce the efficacy of the antibiotic and may lead to antibiotic-resistant bacteria (McCabe, 2004).

Malnutrition can also affect the metabolism of medications. Gut integrity is necessary for drug metabolism; a patient who goes without food for several days may change the integrity of the gut and thus negatively impact drug metabolism and absorption. Patients receiving nutritional supplementation are at increased risk for drug-induced nutritional problems. Medications can also cause malnutrition. Chemotherapeutic agents may change appetite, cause nausea and vomiting, and affect the intestinal mucosa. Anticonvulsants can create marginal nutrient states in older adults. Diuretics affect the fluid and electrolyte balance. And excessive, chronic alcohol intake can lead to poor nutritional intake and changes in drug metabolism (McCabe, 2004).

Polypharmacy

Many older patients are prescribed multiple drugs, take over-the-counter medications, and are often prescribed additional drugs to treat the side effects of the medications that they are already taking. The increase in the number of medications often leads to **polypharmacy**, which is defined as the prescription, administration, or use of more medications than are clinically indicated in a given patient.

TABLE 8-1 Drug–Disease Interactions in the Elderly

Disease	Drugs	Adverse Reactions
Benign prostatic hyperplasia	Anticholinergics	Urinary retention
Chronic obstructive pulmonary disease	β-blockers, opioids	Bronchoconstriction, respiratory depression
Dementia	Anticholinergics, opioids	Increased confusion, delirium
Depression	Alcohol, β-blockers, centrally acting antihypertensives, corticosteroids	Precipitation or exacerbation of depression
Diabetes	Corticosteroids	Hyperglycemia
Glaucoma	Anticholinergics	Exacerbation of glaucoma
Hypertension	NSAIDs	Increased blood pressure
Hypokalemia	Digoxin	Cardiac arrhythmias
Hyponatremia	Oral hypoglycemics, diuretics, carbamazepine, SSRIs	Decreased sodium concentration
Orthostatic	Diuretics, tricyclic antidepressants, vasodilators	Dizziness, falls, syncope, hip fracture
Osteopenia	Corticosteroids	Fracture
Parkinson's disease	Antipsychotics	Worsening movement disorder
Peptic ulcer disease	Anticoagulants, NSAIDs	Upper gastrointestinal bleeding
Peripheral vascular disease	β-blockers	Intermittent claudication
Renal impairment	Aminoglycosides, NSAIDs	Acute renal failure

Aminoglycosides (e.g., gentamicin)
Anticoagulants (e.g., warfarin)
β-blockers (e.g., metoprolol)
Centrally acting antihypertensives (e.g., clonidine)
Corticosteroids (e.g., prednisone)
NSAIDs = nonsteroidal anti-inflammatory drugs (e.g., ibuprofen)
Opioids = narcotic medications (e.g., morphine)
SSRIs = selective serotonin reuptake inhibitors (e.g., paroxetine)
Tricyclic antidepressants (e.g., amitriptyline)

SOURCE: Beers, M. H., & Berkow, R. (Eds.). (2000). Clinical pharmacology. In *Merck manual of geriatrics* (3rd ed., pp. 54–74). Whitestation, NJ: Merck Research Laboratories.

Potential adverse outcomes of polypharmacy include ADRs, increased cost, and noncompliance. See **Case Study 8-1**.

Several interventions that may help the prescriber to prevent polypharmacy include knowing all medications, by both brand and generic name, being used by the patient; identifying indications for each medication; knowing the side effect profiles of the medications; eliminating drugs with no benefit or indication; and avoiding the urge to treat a drug reaction with another drug. Patient education on the risks of polypharmacy may help the patient as well.

Case Study 8-1

Ms. Espinoza is a 90-year-old Hispanic woman admitted to the hospital from her assisted living facility. She has a history of hypertension and dementia, and had a stroke and a myocardial infarction 3 years ago. She has also had insomnia for the past month. Ms. Espinoza is admitted due to an alteration in her mental status. She has had a cold and a cough for a week, for which she took Coricidin (acetaminophen and chlorpheniramine) and Tylenol PM (acetaminophen and diphenhydramine). Her home medications include monthly Nascobal (vitamin B_{12}) injections; Toprol-XL (metoprolol succinate), 100 mg daily; Plendil (felodipine), 10 mg daily; Allegra (fexofenadine), 180 mg daily; Ecotrin (aspirin EC), 325 mg daily; and Colace (docusate sodium), 100 mg daily. She also has a very unsteady gait.

Ms. Espinoza's admitting diagnosis is pneumonia. The physicians order the following medications: Lasix (furosemide), 20 mg IV push, × 1; Pepcid (famotidine), 20 mg bid; Ecotrin (aspirin EC), 325 mg daily; Toprol-XL (metoprolol succinate), 100 mg daily; Colace (docusate sodium), 100 mg daily; Allegra (fexofenadine), 180 mg daily; Levoquin (levofloxacin), 250 mg daily IVPB; Plendil (felodipine), 10 mg po daily; and Ambien (zolpidem), 5 mg at bedtime as needed.

Questions

1. Which medication(s) may have contributed to Ms. Espinoza's altered mental status?
2. In addition to the drug regimen, does Ms. Espinoza have any other risk factors for altered mental status?
3. Would you alter her drug regimen in any way? If so, how?

The nurse plays a key role in screening for polypharmacy. When determining whether a medication is appropriate for a patient, the nurse should ask the following questions (Beers & Berkow, 2005):

- Is the medication necessary? For example, does the patient have a medical problem for every medication ordered?
- Do the risks outweigh the benefits? If there's a potential for an ADR, will the benefit of administering the medication outweigh the risk of the ADR? One example might be examining the benefit of administering vancomycin (Vancocin) to a renally impaired elderly patient who has methacillin-resistant staphylococcus aureus (MRSA) and who is resistant to all other antibiotics. In this case, the benefits of the medication probably outweigh the risks to the kidney, as long as renal function is carefully monitored and dosage is adjusted according to renal function as well as peak and trough levels.
- Is the frequency of the medication prescribed appropriately? For instance, sustained-release morphine (MS Contin) can be ordered every 12–24 hours whereas immediate-release morphine (MSIR) is ordered more frequently.
- Is the medication prescribed in the most appropriate dose, route, and/or form? Some elderly patients have difficulty swallowing; therefore, other dosage forms such as suppositories or topical patches may be more appropriate.

See **Table 8-2** for a quick summary of this topic.

Inappropriate Prescribing

Overall there is no generalized rule for prescribing drugs to the geriatric population. Numerous studies indicate that some prescribing patterns in the el-

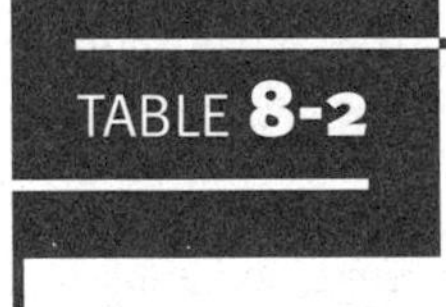

TABLE 8-2 Questions to Ask to Avoid Inappropriate Prescribing for Elderly Patients

- Is the treatment necessary?
- Is this the safest drug available?
- Is this the most appropriate dose, route of administration, and dosage form?
- Is the frequency appropriate?
- Do the benefits outweigh this risk?

SOURCE: *The Merck Manual of Geriatrics* (3rd ed., pp. 54–74), edited by Mark H. Beers and Robert Berkow. Copyright 2000 by Merck & Co., Inc., Whitehouse Station, NJ.

derly population are inappropriate, such as no indications for use of a drug, inappropriate frequency of medications, inadequate dosages, and the possibility of drug interactions or ADRs. Goulding (2004) found that, between 1995 and 2000, at least one inappropriate drug was administered to 7.8% of the elderly patients in her study. Also, at least one drug classified as "never or rarely appropriate" was prescribed to between 3.7% and 3.8% of patients. A large share of the inappropriate drugs in this study was pain medications and central nervous system drugs. The odds that female patients were being prescribed inappropriate medications were double that of males.

One example of the potential effects of inappropriate prescribing was described by Wagner et al. (2002). This research team analyzed the Medicaid claims data for a 42-month period in New Jersey. After statistical adjustment for age, sex, race, nursing home residence, exposure to "other" medications, diagnosis of epilepsy and dementia, and hospitalization in the last 6 months, the incidence of hip fracture was significantly higher in persons who took benzodiazepines. Not only were hip fractures associated with benzodiazepine use, short half-life benzodiazepines were not safer than long half-life benzodiazepines. Hip fracture risk was highest in the first 2 weeks after starting a benzodiazepine. Kudoh and colleagues (2004) found that long-term elderly users of benzodiazepines increased their risk of postoperative confusion, as well.

Compliance

Although age alone does not affect **compliance**, about 40% of elderly persons do not adhere to their medication regimen (Beers & Berkow, 2000, p. 69). The more complex the medication regimen, the less likely the patient will comply. For elderly patients, nonadherence may result from the patient trying to avoid side effects and therefore reducing the amount of drug consumed, lack of money, or forgetfulness (early dementia). Seniors may simply not be taking the medications they need because they cannot afford them. Compliance can be encouraged by establishing a good relationship with the patient, providing education about possible side effects, providing clear instructions for how the medication should be taken, encouraging questions from the patient, and providing home nursing support as needed.

POTENTIALLY INAPPROPRIATE MEDICATIONS FOR GERIATRIC PATIENTS

There is a benefit/risk relationship with the consumption of any medication. The benefit of medication use is to provide positive outcomes; the risk may include unwarranted side effects. There are several medications available on the market that provide excellent results but are not ideal for use in elderly patients. Although some medications cannot be avoided entirely due to the disease state, one should be aware of the possible side effects, especially when administering medications to an elderly patient who often has multiple comorbidities.

The Beers Criteria for Potentially Inappropriate Medication Use in the Elderly (Beers, 1997; Fick et al., 2003) is widely recognized as the standard of care for medication prescription. A panel of experts identified medications that have potential risks that would outweigh the benefits of the medication in the older adult population (Hartford Institute, n.d.). See **Case Study 8-2**.

If any of these medications are administered, the lowest and most effective dose should be started first, then titrated slowly upward until the desired effect is obtained. Remember the saying "Start low and go slow." This strategy will help to prevent ADRs that may prolong a hospital stay, lead to a hospitalization, and even cause harm to the patient and others.

Table 8-3 gives a partial list of commonly prescribed medications that should be avoided in the elderly. Readers are encouraged to review the entire list at http://archinte.ama-assn.org/cgi/reprint/163/22/2716.

LABORATORY VALUES

Due to physiologic changes, laboratory results for older adults may differ from those of younger adults; that is, the reference ranges or "normals" may be different. There has been, however, little study on this topic, and the "normal" values of most laboratory tests are not known for older adults. As persons age, they become less like each other. The rate of organ decline and aging will vary from person to person, making it more likely that each individual will have different individual "normals" for their laboratory

Case Study 8-2

Mrs. Tyler is an 84-year-old white woman with a past medical history of breast cancer, mastectomy, dementia, osteoporosis, depression, and a right hip fracture and repair 1 month ago. She also has a history of anxiety. Her home medications include Prozac (fluoxetine hydrochloride), 20 mg qd; Os-Cal (calcium carbonate), 500 mg tid; Aricept (donepezil hydrochloride), 10 mg qd; Zantac (ranitidine), 150 mg qd; Ecotrin (aspirin EC), 81 mg qd; Mellaril (thioridazine HCl), 10 mg qd; and Valium (diazepam), 10 mg at bedtime daily. She has no known drug allergies.

Mrs. Tyler was admitted to the emergency room after a fall at her assisted living facility. She suffered a fractured left hip. She was admitted to your nursing unit with the new fracture and constipation. Medications ordered on admission included: normal saline IV at 75 cc hour; Hep-Lock (heparin), 5,000 mg sq q 12 hours; MSIR (morphine), 2 mg IV push q 3–4 hrs prn pain; MS SR, 15 mg po bid; Oscal (calcium carbonate), 500 mg po tid; Mellaril (thioridazine HCl), 10 mg qd; Protonix (pantoprazole), 40 mg qd; Aricept (donepazil HCl), 5 mg qd; and Prozac (fluoxetine), 20 mg po qd. Fleet (sodium phosphate) enema × 2 and Citro-Mag (magnesium citrate) 150 ml × 1 were ordered to treat the constipation. Protonix (pantoprazole sodium), 40 mg qd, was also ordered for GI prophylaxis.

Postoperatively, Mrs. Tyler was put on Demerol (meperidine) per PCA pump, with promethazine as needed. Three days later, she presented with altered mental status and hallucinations. Her urine and blood cultures were negative for infection. The daughter states that Mrs. Tyler has never acted like this before and that she is very concerned about her mother's condition.

Questions

1. What home medications may have contributed to Mrs. Tyler's fall?
2. What symptoms does Mrs. Tyler display that may be drug related?
3. Would you alter Mrs. Tyler's hospital drug regimen in any way?

values (Merck, 2007). Age-related declines in cardiac, pulmonary, renal, and metabolic function can, however, be correlated with changes in laboratory values with aging (Merck, 2007).

Many variables can affect laboratory results for the older adult. For instance, leaving a tourniquet in place too long can cause an elevation in the results of a cholesterol test, as may exercise or position changes immediately before the blood is drawn. Or, the amount of anticoagulant in a vacutainer tube may vary, influencing the results. Results from venous and capillary sites can vary within the same individual. The same person may also vary in results over time, simply due to normal biologic events. And the normal aging process can cause variations in normals for the older population. For example, normal changes with aging occur in serum chemistry (alkaline phosphatase, serum albumin, serum magnesium, and uric acid), lipids (total and HDL cholesterol, triglycerides), blood glucose (fasting, 1- and 2-hour postprandial), renal function (creatinine clearance), thyroid (T4 and TSH), and hematology (leukocyte count, erythrocyte sedimentation rate, and vitamin B_{12}) (Brigden & Heathcote, 2000).

There is no general rule of thumb for interpreting laboratory tests for older adults. The results of some tests may increase in value, others may decrease, while still others do not change in older adults. It can be difficult to differentiate whether changes from the usually referenced "normal" values are due to normal aging, chronic disease, or medications. Laboratory values outside the normal ranges may indicate either a benign or a pathologic condition; however, values within the norms may indicate exactly the same thing. Nurses must be aware of this fact and consider the total assessment rather than relying on a single laboratory test for diagnosis (Edwards & Baird, 2005).

Drugs commonly used by the elderly may alter laboratory results. Isoniazid, levodopa, morphine, vitamin C, and penicillin G may lead to false-positive urine glucose results. Levodopa may produce an increase in serum bilirubin and uric acid (Merck, 2007).

Table 8-4 outlines which laboratory values can be expected to increase normally with age and which values can be expected to decrease normally with age. Remember, the absolute "normals" for the older adult are not known.

TABLE 8-3 Medications to Avoid in the Elderly

Medication	Effect
Propoxyphene (Darvon) and combination products (Darvon with ASA, Darvon-N, and Darvocet-N)	Offers few advantages over acetaminophen, yet has the same adverse effects as other narcotic medications
Amitriptyline (Elavil), chlordiazepoxide-amitriptyline (Limbitrol), and perphenazine-amytriptyline (Triavil)	Strong anticholinergic and sedation effects
Diphenhydramine (Benadryl)	May cause confusion and sedation; use in smallest possible dose for emergency allergic reactions
All barbiturates, except when used to control seizures	Highly addictive, more adverse effects in the older adult
Meperidine (Demerol)	May cause confusion
Short-acting nifedipine (Procardia and Adalat)	Potential hypotension and constipation
Clonidine (Catapres)	Potential for orthostatic hypotension and CNS adverse effects
Mineral oil	Potential for aspiration and adverse effects; other options readily available
Estrogens only	Lack of cardioprotective effect in older women; evidence of carcinogenic potential
Nitrofurantoin (Macrodantin)	Potential for renal impairment; other alternatives available
Cimetadine (Tagamet)	CNS effects including confusion
Indomethacin (Indocin and Indocin SR)	CNS adverse effects; other NSAIDs available with fewer adverse effects
Methocarbamol (Robaxin), carisoprodol (Soma), chlorzoxaxone (Paraflex), cyclobenzaprine (Flexeril), oxybutynin (Ditropan)	Anticholinergic effects, sedation, weakness
Short-acting dipyridamole (Persantine)	Orthostatic hypotension
Methyldopa (Aldomet) and methyldopa-hydrochlorothiazide (Aldoril)	May cause bradycardia and exacerbate depression in older adults

SOURCE: Fick, D. M., Cooper, J. W., Wade, W. E., Waller J. L., Maclean, J. R., & Beers, M. H. (2003). Updating the Beers criteria for potentially inappropriate medication use in older adults: Results of a U.S. consensus panel of experts. *Archives of Internal Medicine*, *163*(22), 2716–2724.

TABLE 8-4 Changes in Lab Values with Age

Increases with Age	Decreases with Age	Unchanged with Age
Alkaline phosphatase	Albumin	Hepatic function tests (serum bilirubin, AST, ALT, GGTP)
ANA	Aldosterone	Coagulation tests
C-reactive protein	Serum calcium	Biochemical tests (serum electrolytes, total protein*, serum folate)
Cholesterol, total	HDL cholesterol (women)	Arterial blood tests (pH, $PaCO_2$)
Clotting factors VII and VIII	Creatine kinase	Renal function tests (serum creatinine)
Copper	Creatinine clearance	Thyroid function tests (T4)
D-dimers	Dihydroepiandrosterone	Complete blood count (hematocrit, hemoglobin, erythrocyte indices)
Ferritin	1,25-dihydroxyvitamin D	
Fibrinogen	Estradiol	
Gastrin	Growth hormone	
2 h pp glucose	IGF-1	
Interleukin 6	Interleukin 1	
PSA	Magnesium	
PTH	PaO_2	
Rheumatoid factor	Phosphorus	
Sedimentation rate	Platelets	
Triglycerides	Free testosterone	
Uric acid	Total protein*	
	Zinc, serum	

* indicates conflicting information in literature
ALT: serum alanine aminotransferase
ANA: antinuclear antibody
AST: serum glutamine aminotransferase (also called SGOT)
GGTP: *gamma-glutamyl transpeptidase*
HDL: high density lipoprotein

SOURCE: ClinLab Navigator. (2007). *Aging effect on laboratory values*. Retrieved October 15, 2007, from http://www.clinlabnavigator.com; Geriatric Medicine in Clinical Practice. (2002). *Laboratory values.* Retrieved October 15, 2005, from http://geriatricsyllabus.com/syllabus/main.jsp?cid=AGE-LAB; Gliatto, M. F. (2000). Generalized anxiety disorder. *American Family Physician*. Retrieved June 14, 2005, from http://www.aafp.org/afp/20001001/1591. html; *Merck Manual of Geriatrics*. (2000). *Appendix 1: Laboratory values.* Retrieved October 15, 2007, from http://www.merck.com/mkgr/mmg/appndxs/app1.jsp; Tanago, E. A., & McAninch, J. W. (Eds.). (2004). *Smith's general urology* (16th ed.). Urological laboratory examination. Retrieved October 15, 2007, from http://www.accessmedicine.com/content.aspx?aID=222712.

Laboratory Values and Medication Administration

Laboratory values and medication administration go hand in hand. Laboratory work may be done to:

- Monitor compliance with medication administration
- Check for therapeutic or toxic levels of medication in the blood

- Evaluate the body's ability to metabolize medications
- Evaluate the need for medications to treat a condition

Whatever the case, it is important that the nurse be aware of the relationship between laboratory values and medication administration.

Medication Blood Levels (Therapeutic Blood Levels)

The amount of medication circulating in the blood can be monitored for some medications. This may include monitoring for blood levels of medications taken on a routine basis or in an emergency situation where drug overdose is suspected. Some medications commonly monitored in the elderly include

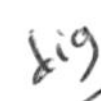

cardiac medications, antiepileptics, and certain antibiotics.

Measuring medication blood levels is important for monitoring the metabolism of the medication so that the correct dosage can be given, at the correct intervals, to obtain the best results without side effects or adverse drug reactions. Metabolism of medications may be altered in the elderly, so this concept is an important one. Some medications are toxic to the body if the level is too high, and may be ineffective if the level is too low.

Compliance with medication administration can also be monitored through this type of testing. Key words associated with measuring the amount of circulating medications are random, trough, and peak.

Random Medication Levels in the Blood

Random levels are not dependent upon the administration time of the medication. The blood level is drawn when the order is received. An example for this type of laboratory work might be a patient who is admitted to the emergency room with altered mental status and a drug overdose is suspected.

Trough Medication Levels in the Blood

Trough levels are dependent upon the administration times of the medication. The trough level is drawn at the time that the blood level is expected to be at its lowest: right before a dose is due. An abnormally high trough level indicates that the time between doses should be adjusted (lengthened); an abnormally low trough level indicates that the time between doses should be shortened. An example of this type of blood work might be an elderly patient who is receiving vancomycin (Vancocin) for an infection, in whom toxic levels must be avoided.

Peak Medication Levels in the Blood

Peak levels are also dependent upon the time of administration. This varies according to the route of administration and for different medications. An abnormally high peak indicates that the dosage needs to be reduced; an abnormally low peak indicates that the dosage should be increased. The peak is typically drawn within a set time after a dose is given, and a trough follows right before the next dose is given. See **Table 8-5** for further information on peak and trough levels from the authors' own facility.

As you can see, it is vitally important that the nurse know the type of level to be drawn (random, peak, or trough) and then draw it at the correct time. The dosage of the drug, the frequency of administration, and the safety of the patient depend on the accuracy of the blood draw.

Toxic blood levels of medications may present in unusual ways in the older population. It is also possible that the older adult will experience side effects at levels that are not considered to be toxic in younger persons. For instance, drug toxicity from digoxin, a cardiac medication, may be evident in symptoms, although the patient's blood level is in the normal range.

Caution must always be used with the interpretation of medication level laboratory results and with dosage adjustments based on a single value. It must be ascertained that the blood was drawn as the order intended, that the preceding medications were given on time with no doses missed, and that there were no unintended drug–drug or food–drug interactions that may have affected the result. Birnbaum et al. (2003) studied a group of 56 elderly nursing home residents whose average age was 80.1 years. All received phenytoin as an antiepileptic drug. All had been on the same dose for at least 4 weeks, and all doses were given, as far as the researchers could tell. Although all of the right parameters were in place, phenytoin levels varied as much as

TABLE 8-5 Serum Levels for Selected Medications

Medication Level	Therapeutic Level	Peak Range	Trough Range	Toxic Levels
Serum amikacin (Amikin)		25–35 mcg/ml	3–10 mcg/ml	Peak: 0.35 mcg/ml Trough: 0.10 mcg/ml
Serum digoxin (Lanoxin)	0.8–1.6 ng/ml			2.4 ng/ml
Serum phenytoin (Dilantin)	10–20 mcg/ml			0.20 mcg/ml
Serum gentamicin (Gentak)		2–8 mcg/ml	0.5–2.0 mcg/ml	Peak: 0.10 mcg/ml Trough: 0.2 mcg/ml
Serum quinidine (Quinaglute)	3.0–6.0 mcg/ml			0.9 mcg/ml
Serum theophylline (Uniphyl)	10–20 mcg/ml			0.20 mcg/ml
Serum tobramycin (Tobrex)		5–10 mcg/ml	0.5–2.0 mcg/ml	Peak: 0.10 mcg/ml Trough: 2.0 mcg/ml
Serum vancomycin (Vancocin)		30–40 mcg/ml	5–10 mcg/ml	Peak: 0.50 mcg/ml Trough: 0.15 mcg/ml

SOURCE: The Laboratory Survival Guide at http://www.utmb.edu/lsg/

two- to threefold for some patients, from 9.7 micrograms per ml to 28.8 mcg per ml. The authors attribute the variability to variations in hydration status and changes in gut motility.

Renal and Hepatic Function

As stated earlier, drugs are metabolized differently in older adults. The kidneys and the liver may not function as well as in younger persons. This can affect how medications are cleared from the body and the likelihood of side effects or toxic levels of medications. Certain medications, such as aminoglycosides, nonsteroidal anti-inflammatory drugs (NSAIDs), ACE inhibitors, and IV contrast materials (used for x-rays) can also affect renal function in the elderly person (Reuben et al., 2004, p. 140). Laboratory tests that are commonly used to monitor the function of the kidneys and the liver, and to help decide the dosage and timing of medications, include the following:

- *Blood urea nitrogen (BUN):* This test is used as a gross measure of glomerular function and the production and excretion of urea (Fischbach, 1996, p. 351). Impairment of kidney function will result in an elevated BUN. The rate at which BUN rises is influenced by the degree of tissue necrosis and the rate at which the kidneys excrete urea nitrogen.
- *Creatinine:* This is a substance removed from the body by the kidneys. Measurement of the creatinine level will give a clue as to the function of the kidneys. For instance, a disorder of the kidneys will increase the level of creatinine in the blood. It is a more specific indicator of kidney disease than the BUN (Fischbach, 1996).

Health care providers commonly use the calculated creatinine clearance rate as a guide when deciding on the proper dosages of medications for older adults. This formula takes into account the patient's weight, gender, age, and renal function:

Creatinine clearance (ml/min) = (140 − age in years) × weight in kg / 72 × serum creatinine (for women, multiply the result by 0.85)

Manufacturers of medications affected by the creatinine clearance rate will help the provider by suggesting appropriate dosages according to the rate.

- *Alkaline phosphatase:* This is an indicator of liver disease. Levels in the blood will rise when excretion of this enzyme is impaired (Fischbach, 1996). Other indicators of liver health or disease are the alanine aminotransferase (ALT), aspartate aminotransferase (AST), albumin, bilirubin, protein, and coagulation factors. See **Table 8-6** for further information about normal laboratory values.

Laboratory Values as Indicators of Need for Medications

Another connection between laboratory values and medications is when laboratory values indicate a need for medications. See **Table 8-7** for some examples of this concept.

The Role of the Nurse

The nurse has several responsibilities regarding laboratory values and medications. These include:

- Being aware of the routes of elimination of medications and the implications of aging on these routes
- Being aware of the effects of aging on the typical signs and symptoms of medication toxicity
- Maintaining knowledge of the signs of medication toxicity in the older adult
- Drawing random, peak, and trough medication levels correctly
- Knowing when to notify the prescriber of an abnormal result

CHALLENGES TO SUCCESSFUL MEDICATION REGIMENS FOR THE OLDER ADULT

For a medication to work properly, the right drug must be taken in the right amount, by the right

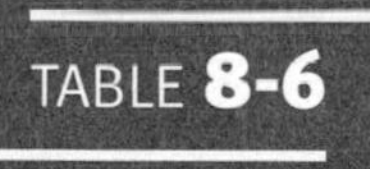

TABLE 8-6 Normal Laboratory Values (serum)

Test	Body System	Normal Levels
Blood urea nitrogen (BUN)	Renal	7–23 mg/dl
Creatinine	Renal	Male, 13 years–adult: 0.7–1.7 mg/dl Female, 13 years–adult: 0.4–1.4 mg/dl
Albumin	Hepatic	3.2–5.2 g/dl
Alkaline phosphatase	Hepatic	34–122 u/l
ALT	Hepatic	9–51 u/l
AST	Hepatic	13–38 u/l
Direct bilirubin	Hepatic	0.0–0.3 mg/dl
Indirect bilirubin	Hepatic	0.1–1.1 mg/dl
Total protein	Hepatic	6.0–8.0 g/dl

ALT: serum alanine aminotransferase
AST: serum glutamine aminotransferase (also called SGOT)

SOURCE: The Laboratory Survival Guide at http://www.utmb.edu/lsg/

TABLE 8-7 **Selected Laboratory Values Indicating a Need for Medication**

Laboratory Test	Normal Values	Abnormal Condition	Selected Examples of Nontreatment	Potential Medications Indicated
Albumin	3.5–5.0 gm/dl	Hypoalbuminemia	Edema	Albumin
Blood culture	Negative	Positive for organisms		Infection antibiotics
Blood glucose	65–110	Hyperglycemia	Polyuria, polydipsia, polyphagia	Hypoglycemic agent
Hemoglobin A1C	4–6%	Chronic hyperglycemia (noncompliance)	Nonhealing wounds	Hypoglycemic agent
Prothrombin time	11–13 seconds	30 seconds	Bruising, bleeding	Vitamin K
Prothrombin time	11–13 seconds	26 seconds	Formation of blood clots in at-risk patient	Warfarin
TSH	0.35–5.5 mc U/ml	Elevated	Primary hypothyroidism	Thyroid hormone
Uric acid	3.6–8.0 mg/dl in men, 2.9–6.0 mg/dl in women	Elevated	Pain from gout	Allopurinol
WBCs	4.5–10.5 $\times 10^3/\mu l$	Elevated	Untreated infection	Antibiotic

TSH: Thyroid stimulating hormone
WBC: white blood cells

route, at the right times, by the right patient. Failure to follow these "five rights" can delay or prevent the outcome intended by the health care provider.

The five rights are important in every setting. In the inpatient setting, such as the hospital or nursing home, the physician, the nurse, and the pharmacist ensure that the five rights are followed. In the outpatient or home setting, it ultimately becomes the patient's responsibility to ensure that they take the right medication by the right route, at the right times, in the right dose. Failure of the patient to follow these requirements is often labeled noncompliance or nonadherence to the recommendations of the health care provider. This section will examine issues related to the older adult in the home setting.

Let's examine these five rights in more detail.

Right Drug

Assuming that the right medication is ordered by the provider and the right drug is filled by the pharmacy, there are still factors that can interfere with the patient receiving the right drug in the home setting. These might include:

- Taking medications prescribed for another person
- Keeping old medications stockpiled and forgetting which ones are currently prescribed
- Receiving prescriptions from two different providers
- Misunderstanding the use of over-the-counter medications

Right Amount

Ensuring that the right amount of drug is taken can be tricky in the home. Confounding factors might include:

- Lack of understanding of the prescribed dosage, number of pills, or amount of liquid medication
- Using teaspoons or other utensils to measure rather than measuring cups, or using the wrong size syringe
- Confusion about medication schedules
- The same prescriptions being ordered by more than one health care provider
- Forgetting which medications have already been taken
- Failing to obtain refills
- Rationing medications so as not to run out

Right Route

Although this might be difficult to imagine, these errors do occur. Examples of failure to administer the medication by the right route might include sublingual medication that is swallowed or a suppository that is chewed.

Right Times

Taking medications at the right times can be very difficult for the older adult, for a multitude of reasons such as:

- Having medications ordered for two, three, or even four times a day

BOX 8-1 Research Highlight

Aim: This survey asked what nurses felt about making and reporting medication errors.

Methods: *Nursing2002* staff surveyed nurses about their attitudes and experiences regarding medication administration and making mistakes. The analysis of the poll was based on 775 responses. The typical respondent was a 42-year-old BSN, RN with 11 years of experience working on a medical/surgical unit of a hospital.

Findings: Seventy-nine percent of nurses felt that most medication errors occurred when nurses did not follow the five rights of administration. Ninety-one percent of nurses felt that thoroughly analyzing incident reports about medication errors was an important step in future prevention of mistakes. Students were more likely to initiate an incident report for another nurse's mistake than were the nurses who worked on the units.

Application to practice: Although responses varied on a number of questions, such as the use of increased technology in medication administration and when and how to report medication errors, the majority of nurses agreed that they were responsible for ensuring safe medication administration to patients and that using the five rights was important for preventing errors.

Source: Cohen, H., Robinson, E. S., & Mandrack, M. (2003). Getting to the root of medication errors: Survey results. *Nursing2003, 33*(9), 36–45.

- Having multiple medications ordered, each at a different time

Right Patient

This one should not be a problem in the home, but it is. It is not unusual for patients in the home setting to "try" medications prescribed for other persons in the household. One recent example from the authors' facility is the case of a woman hospitalized for an unusually prolonged clotting time. It was finally deduced that she disliked the cholesterol medication that was prescribed for her, so she started using her husband's cholesterol pills (which he refused to take). What she didn't know was that her husband's medication was not alright for her, because it interacted with the warfarin she was taking for a heart condition, potentiating the anticoagulant effect and prolonging her clotting time. This type of situation is in no way unusual.

OTHER ISSUES THAT INTERFERE WITH MEDICATION ADMINISTRATION

Other situations may interfere with the ability of the older adult to take the right medication at the right time in the right dose by the right route by the right person.

Function

Impaired **function**, or the inability to perform **activities of daily living**, can interfere with **adherence** to a prescribed medication regimen. For instance, a person with arthritis of the hands or paralysis of the arm can have difficulty opening bottles; a person who has had a stroke can have difficulty walking to get her medications; a person with impaired mobility may have problems getting a glass of water from the kitchen. Swallowing can also be functionally impaired and cause choking, aspiration, and the inability to swallow medications.

Impaired ability to perform **instrumental activities of daily living** can also affect medication regimens. For example, a person who does not drive a car may not be able to get medications from the pharmacy, or a person who cannot manage money may not be able to pay for the medications.

Hearing

The ability to hear instructions given by the health care provider or pharmacist is a very important part of the ability to take medications accurately and safely. The older adult may have a nonfunctioning hearing aid, not have their hearing aid in place, or be hard of hearing and have no hearing aid to use. Thus, it is conceivable that an older adult may not hear instructions given to them by the health care provider to discard all old medications, to take three pills a day, or to call the doctor if they experience certain side effects.

Vision

Vision is another sense that is important to help ensure adherence to prescribed medication regimens. The ability to see to find the medication and read the label can be the difference between adherence and illness. Older adults need to be able to read the literature given to them about their medications, the times to take them, dosages, and side effects.

Reading Ability

Closely associated with vision, the ability to read can affect the medication regimen. If the patient cannot read, can read only at a grade-school level, or cannot read the language in which the instructions are written, the five rights may be missed. Often, written instructions are given to the patient with the best of intentions, but the provider fails to ascertain that the patient can read, and understand, the written words. Also, medication instructions are often written at a high school level, whereas the patient may require instruction at a fifth-grade level.

Memory/Cognition

Impaired memory can be a barrier to adherence with medication routines. Remembering which medications to take and at what times can be difficult if memory is impaired by dementia, delirium, or depression.

Motivation

Motivation is important in adherence to a medication routine. There must be motivation to obtain the medication, to learn about the medication, to take

FIGURE 8-1 **Failure to take medications or attend to other health needs can be a sign that an older adult lacks motivation to adhere to the medication regimen.**

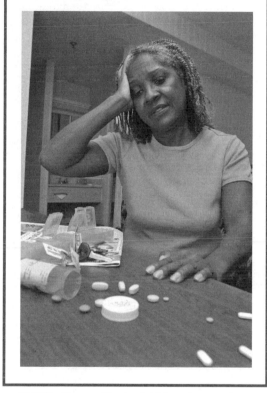

SOURCE: ©Jones and Bartlett Publishers. Courtesy of MIEMSS.

the medication on time, and to report inability to take the medication to the physician. Motivation can be negatively affected by cognitive status, depression, and even societal or family pressures (see **Figure 8-1**).

Funding

Many older adults have difficulty purchasing medications due to costs. Although Medicare has recently added a medication benefit, it will not fully cover the cost of all medications. Supplemental policies purchased by the older adult may help to cover the cost of some medications. Medicaid may supply funds for a limited number of medications, depending upon the state of residence. Persons without insurance, Medicare, or Medicaid may be unable to find the money to purchase needed medications or refills, and thus may go without.

Providers also share the responsibility for the cost of medications. The more medications prescribed, the higher the cost. Also, new, brand-name medications cost much more than those available in a generic form. Medicare D, which concerns prescription benefits, although it makes medications more affordable for some, has made day-to-day living more difficult for others, due to increased dollars taken from monthly Social Security checks to pay for membership in the program and high deductibles. With multiple providers of medications with differing formularies available for the beneficiaries of Medicare, it is yet to be seen if this will be an efficacious program.

One study found that as many as one-third of the chronically ill elders who underuse prescription medications because of the cost never talk to their providers in advance. Many never raise the issue, due to embarrassment or misinterpretation of the provider's feelings. Of those who did not tell a clinician about their inability to pay for medications, 66% reported that no one even asked them about their ability to pay for the prescribed drugs, and 58% thought that the providers could not help them with funding issues. Of those who did talk to their provider about financial concerns, 31% reported that they were not offered less expensive alternatives, 30% were not given information about potential funding sources, and 28% were not given advice on pharmacies that could provide medications for less money (Piette, Heisler, & Wagner, 2004).

NURSING INTERVENTIONS

Nurses in all settings have a responsibility to help ensure that the five rights are followed for each patient. Specific interventions should include:

- *Medication review:* This can take place in the outpatient or the inpatient setting. Ask the patient to bring in all of his or her medications, including over-the-counter (OTC) medications, for review. Compare patient medications to the medical records. Ensure that medications no longer prescribed are discarded. Also discard any expired medications. Be alert for medications ordered by different providers. Inform the physician of any concerns. See **Table 8-8** for further information on medication review.

- *Education:* Ensure that the patient or the person who administers the medications to the patient thoroughly understands the medication instructions. Provide them with a clearly written list that includes:
  - *Name of the medication:* Include both brand name and generic name.
  - *Schedule of administration:* Do not include medical terms such as qid, qd, or bid. Instead, write out "three times a day" or other instructions.
  - *Dosage:* Clearly write out the dosage in full words, such as 10 milligrams or three pills. Instruct them in how to measure out the correct dose of the medication.
  - *Side effects to report:* Instruct the patient about adverse drug reactions and when to seek medical help. Be sure that the patient knows to whom to report adverse drug reactions.
  - *Evaluation of education:* Ask the patient or caregiver to repeat and/or read back instructions you have given them. Ask if they have any questions. Provide them the number of someone they can call if they have questions about their medications.
- *Accommodation:* Note sensory, motor, or cognitive limitations that the patient may have that would interfere with his or her understanding of medication instructions or ability to administer the medications. Ensure glasses and hearing aids are on and in place before educating about medications. Use large-print written resources if necessary. Ask for specially adapted lids on pill bottles from the pharmacy to help facilitate opening lids. For example, Target corporation has redesigned the ordinary pill bottle, making it color coded for each family member, flattening the bottle so the label is easier to read, including a slot for patient instructions, and having a spot to hold oral syringes for liquid medications (see **Figure 8-2**). Obtain weekly pillboxes that can be filled by a health care provider every week. Help the patient investigate the high-tech options on the market to help improve adherence: prompting devices such as beeping pillboxes and talking watches, electronic medication vials, and handheld electronic organizers (McGarry Logue, 2002). Obtain referrals for home health nurses for medication assistance and

TABLE 8-8 Tips for Medication Review

The following tips may serve as a format to use when doing a medication history:

- Current prescription medications
- Current over-the-counter and herbal medications, and frequencies
- Social drug use (e.g., alcohol, tobacco, caffeine)
- Home remedies
- Drug allergies
- Compliance assessment
- Medication administration (need for special devices, patient's mental status, caregiver administration)

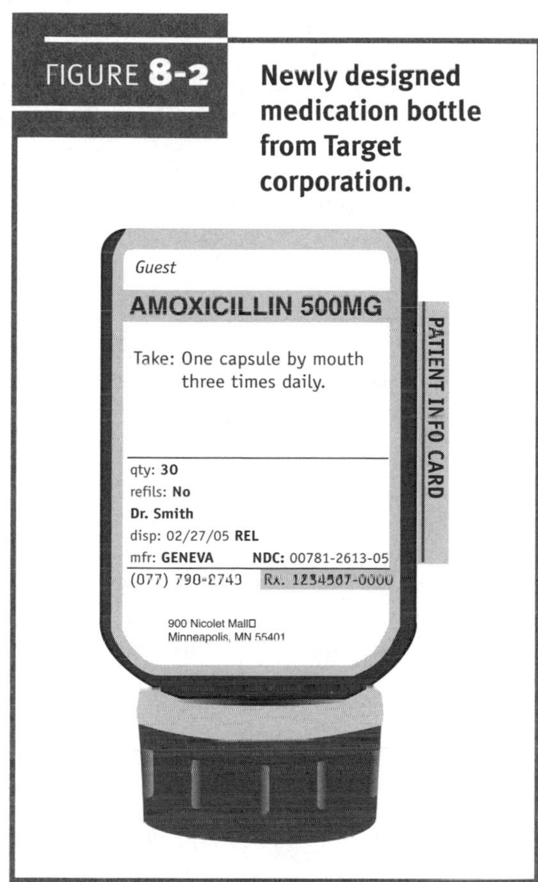

FIGURE 8-2 **Newly designed medication bottle from Target corporation.**

SOURCE: The Institute for Safe Medicine Practices. Online at: http://www.ismp.org/CommunityArticles/Calendar/200505_1.htm

monitoring for persons with severe mobility or cognitive deficits. Ask the ordering provider to try to limit the number and frequency of medications. Occupational therapists and social workers can assist in addressing these types of accommodations.

- *Funding:* Assess the patient's ability to pay for medications—Medicare, Medicaid, supplemental plans, and out-of-pocket expenses. Consult a social worker to help with finding funding sources, if necessary. Ask the ordering provider to try to limit the number of different medications and to use cheaper, generic medications where possible.

A BRIEF OVERVIEW OF SOME MEDICATIONS USED BY THE OLDER ADULT POPULATION

There is not enough space in this chapter to review all medications used by the elderly population, so just three of the more commonly used medication categories will be presented. The reader is referred to the resource list for information on other medications commonly prescribed for older adults.

Medications for Dementia

There are several new drugs on the market for dementia. Although there is as yet no cure, these medications help to slow the progress of the disease. Four medications are commonly used in patients with symptoms of mild to moderate Alzheimer's dementia. Tacrine (Cognex), donepezil (Aricept), rivastigmine tartrate (Exelon), and galantamine (Reminyl) are called cholinesterase inhibitors. They work to increase the brain's levels of acetylcholine, to restore communication between brain cells. Acetylcholine is thought to be important for memory and thinking. Benefits of these medications tend to occur at higher doses; unfortunately, higher doses also have an increased likelihood of side effects (ElderCare Online, 2002; Health-cares.net, 2005).

Aricept is probably the most widely used drug. Although it does not cure Alzheimer's or keep it from getting worse, it does help relieve some of the memory loss. It is most effective in the early stages of the disease. The dosage is typically 5 mg per day to start, increasing to 10 mg, once a day. Side effects include diarrhea, vomiting, nausea, fatigue, insomnia, and weight loss (ElderCare Online, 2002; Health-cares.net, 2005).

Cognex is taken four times a day, has modest benefits, and does not work in patients with the ApoE4 gene. Cognex can potentially affect the liver, so liver enzymes must be closely monitored. Side effects of Cognex include nausea, vomiting, diarrhea, abdominal pain, rash, and indigestion. NSAIDs must be used with caution in combination with this drug (ElderCare Online, 2002; Health-cares.net, 2005).

Reminyl prevents the breakdown of acetylcholine and stimulates nicotinic receptors to release more acetylcholine in the brain. It is taken twice a day. Side effects may include nausea, vomiting, diarrhea, and weight loss. Some antidepressants and other drugs with anticholinergic side effects may cause retention of Reminyl in the body. NSAIDs should be used with caution in combination with this drug (ElderCare Online, 2002).

Exelon is given twice a day. It works by preventing the breakdown of acetylcholine and butyrylcholine in the brain. Side effects may include nausea, vomiting, weight loss, upset stomach, and muscle weakness. NSAIDs should be used with caution in combination with this drug.

Because these four drugs work in a similar way, switching from one drug to another is not expected to improve the outcome. One medication or another may, however, be better tolerated with fewer side effects.

A fifth approved medication is an N-methyl D-aspartate (NMDA) agonist. Memantine (Namenda) is prescribed for the treatment of moderate Alzheimer's disease. It was approved for use in the United States in 2003. It reduces the abnormally high levels of glutamate associated with Alzheimer's-type dementia. The main effect is to slow progression from moderate to severe Alzheimer's disease. The prime advantage may be to maintain certain ADL functions a little longer, and thus maintain independence and decrease caregiver stress (Alzheimer's Disease Education and Referral [ADEAR], 2005).

NSAIDs are currently being studied for their usefulness in slowing the progression of Alzheimer's, as are vitamin E and gingko biloba. Estrogen's effects on Alzheimer's are also of interest to researchers. Selegilene, an anti-Parkinson's drug, appears to slow the onset of Alzheimer's through an antioxidant effect (ADEAR, 2005; Healthcares.net, 2005).

Medications for Osteoporosis

Prevention of osteoporosis is vital in the older adult. Osteoporosis makes the older person more susceptible to fractures and changes posture, thus placing strain and stress on muscles and joints, and it can even affect height. Two main types of drugs

BOX 8-2 Resource List

AgeNet Eldercare Network: http://www.agenet.com
American Geriatrics Society: http://www.americangeriatrics.org
American Geriatrics Society Immunization site:
 http://www.americangeriatrics.org/education/forum/immune.shtml
American Society of Consultant Pharmacists: http://www.ascp.com
Best Practices in Nursing Care to Older Adults from the Hartford Institute for Geriatric Nursing:
 http://www.nursingcenter.com/library/static.asp?pageid=527873
The Institute for Safe Medical Practices Medication Safety Alert: Nurse-Advise ERR:
 http://www.ismp.org/newsletters/default.asp
Medline Plus (National Institutes of Health): http://www.medlineplus.gov
National Guideline Clearinghouse: http://www.guidelines.gov
NeedyMeds.org (a listing of all indigent drug programs for over 900 medications):
 http://www.needymeds.com
RxAssist Patient Assistance Program Center, subsidized by the Robert Wood Johnson Foundation:
 http://www.rxassist.org
RxList (The Internet Drug Index): http://www.rxlist.com

BOX 8-3 Web Exploration

Explore the complete list of medications to avoid in the elderly at http://archinte.ama-assn.org/cgi/reprint/163/22/2716.

are used for prevention and treatment of osteoporosis: antiresorptives and anabolic, or bone-forming, agents.

Antiresorptives slow the rate of bone remodeling, but cannot rebuild bone. Medications in this category include biphosphonates, hormone replacement therapy, and selective estrogen-receptor modulators (SERMs). Anabolic, or bone-forming, agents rebuild bone. Included in this category are parathyroid hormone and fluoride.

Biphosphonates inhibit osteoclast activity (bone resorption), increase bone mass, and are one of the front line classes of drugs for preventing osteoporosis in postmenopausal women and in persons taking corticosteroids or estrogen-suppressing medications. They reduce the risk of both hip and spine fractures. This class includes alendronate (Fosamax) and risedronate (Actonel). Both of these drugs are taken by mouth and should be taken in the morning with plain water, on an empty stomach. Once weekly dosing is possible with both. Studies have documented reduction of hip fracture with these two medications. In one study of 9,331 women, risedronate was found to reduce the 3-year risk of hip fracture by 40% in women with confirmed osteoporosis, and by 60% in a group of women with confirmed vertebral fractures at baseline. Another study showed that alendronate reduced the risk of hip fracture by 51% (Animated Dissection of Anatomy for Medicine {ADAM}, 2002; Kessel, 2004). Etidronate (Didronel) is an older biphosphonate that is sometimes prescribed and is also taken by mouth. Ibandronate (Boniva) was recently approved for use in the United States and is frequently used. Pamidronate (Aredia) is an injectable biphosphonate, as are zoledronic acid (Zometa) and ibandronate. These injectable forms do not cause GI distress as may the oral drugs. Investigative biphosphonates include clodronate and tiludronate, but oral necrosis of the jaw has been associated with use of some biphosphonates such as these (ADAM, 2002).

The National Osteoporosis Foundation's guidelines recommend that women with a below-normal bone density (of 2.5 SD or greater) and who have no history of fractures should take biphosphonates. They recommend consideration of biphosphonates for women with below-normal bone density (of 1 SD or more) with a history of fractures. Alendronate has been approved for use in men with osteoporosis; alendronate and risedronate are also approved for men and women taking corticosteroids. Side effects of this category of drugs include chest pain, heartburn, difficulty swallowing, and ulcers (ADAM, 2002).

Hormone replacement therapy (HRT) increases bone density. HRT consists of estrogen with or without progesterone. It also appears to improve balance and protect against falling. When women stop taking HRT, bone density decreases, and after 5 years off of HRT all protection is lost. Thus, to be of benefit, HRT needs to be taken for life, which is contraindicated due to increased risk for invasive breast cancer, ovarian cancer, heart attacks, strokes, and blood clots. A 2002 study of HRT (by the Women's Health Initiative) was stopped before its scheduled conclusion due to the emergence of these bad outcomes in some women on long-term HRT (ADAM, 2002; Kessel, 2004).

Some drugs have been specially designed to provide the same benefits on bone as HRT without increasing the risk of hormone-related cancers. These selective estrogen-receptor modulators (SERMs) include raloxifene (Evista), which has been approved for prevention of spinal fractures. Raloxifene is also indicated for the prevention and treatment of postmenopausal osteoporosis. Tamoxifen (Nolvadex) may reduce the risk for fractures, but has not been approved for this use. This medication causes increased risk for uterine cancer and blood clots, so its use for osteoporosis may be in question. Tibolone (Livial) is being used outside the United States for improving bone density, especially in the lower spine, with minimal side effects. More study is required on SERMs before they may be deemed useful in the larger population (ADAM, 2002; Kessel, 2004).

Calcitonin also inhibits osteoclastic activity. It is available as a nasal spray (Miacalcin) or an injectable (Calcimar). It is used to *treat* osteoporosis, unlike the above drugs. It may be a viable alternative for those unable to take biphosphonates or SERMs. It also appears to relieve bone pain associated with osteoporosis and fracture. Side effects include headache, dizziness, nausea, anorexia, rash, and edema. The nasal spray can cause nosebleed, sinusitis, and inflammation of the nasal membranes (ADAM, 2002; Kessel, 2004).

Parathyroid hormone in low, intermittent doses can stimulate bone production. It is indicated for use in postmenopausal women who are at high risk for fracture (history of fracture, multiple risk factors for fracture, or intolerant of other treatments). The benefits may persist after the injections have been stopped. Teriparatide (Forteo) has been approved for treatment of osteoporosis in postmenopausal women, but is not yet approved for men. Side effects include nausea, dizziness, and leg cramps (ADAM, 2002).

Calcium and vitamin D supplementation can reduce hip fracture risk. One study of 3,270 women found that 18 months of daily therapy with 1.2 g calcium and 800 IU of vitamin D produced a 43% reduction in hip fracture compared to placebo. Calcium and vitamin D also have been shown to improve femoral neck bone mineral density and reduce the incidence of nonvertebral fractures in both men and women. These two drugs are not considered to be adequate for prevention of fracture in high-risk women (ADAM, 2002; Kessel, 2004).

Several other medications are being studied for their usefulness in osteoporosis. These include osteoprotegerin, which prevents bone breakdown by regulating osteoclasts. Vitamin D derivatives are also being studied, as are statins, dehydroepiandrosterone (DHEA), testosterone, and strontium.

Medications for Anxiety

Several drugs are used to manage anxiety in the older adult. These drugs are appropriate when there is a clear diagnosis of anxiety disorder and a poor response to alternative therapies. As with any medication for the aged, it is recommended that the practitioner start low (dosage) and go slow (make changes slowly).

Benzodiazepines have a long history of use in this age group. Many elders have long-term prescriptions for benzodiazepines such as Valium. In 2003, 18.7% of Texas nursing facility residents age 65 or older were taking benzodiazepines, one-fifth of which were long-acting benzodiazepines (Quality Matters, 2004). Long-acting benzodiazepines, however, should be used with great caution in the older adult due to their long half-life and changes in the metabolism and excretion of drugs in seniors. Short-acting benzodiazepines can be substituted and should be limited to less than 4 months' use. Short-acting benzodiazepines include lorazepam and oxazepam. Paradoxical reactions to benzodiazepines have been reported in the elderly. Symptoms include irritability, anger, and loss of control (Lantz, 2004). Benzodiazepine tapering and withdrawal can be a difficult process and is usually done over 6–12 weeks. Withdrawal symptoms are common and often difficult to differentiate from anxiety symptoms (Gliatto, 2000). As mentioned earlier in this chapter, benzodiazepines are on the Beers list of inappropriate drugs for the elderly. Although short-acting benzodiazepines may be used short term for immediate relief of symptoms, they are typically used until the slower-onset medications have begun to show an effect.

Buspirone can help manage anxiety, does not lead to cognitive impairment, and has no addictive potential or sedative effect. It can cause paradoxical agitation in persons with dementia, however, and it may actually worsen symptoms of cognitive impairment. Persons who have used benzodiazepines extensively in the past are unlikely to benefit from buspirone. Buspirone can take 3–5 weeks before maximal effect is seen (Aparasu, Mort, & Aparasu, 2001; Quality Matters, 2004).

Antidepressants may be used as a first-line treatment of anxiety disorders in older adults, particularly the selective serotonin reuptake inhibitors (SSRIs). Long-term use of SSRIs for anxiety has not been well evaluated. Commonly used SSRIs include fluvoxamine, fluoxetine, sertraline, and paroxetine. SSRIs used for anxiety are prescribed at a lower dose than when used for depression. One drawback to use of SSRIs for anxiety is the length of time to onset of relief—it may take weeks for the effects to begin. Paroxetine, which has anticholinergic effects, should be used with caution in the elderly (Quality Matters, 2004).

Anxiety medications must be used with caution in the older adult. Any medication that affects cognition (thinking), memory, or balance and gait is a safety concern in this population.

SUMMARY

Nurses have a unique opportunity to partner with older adults and to contribute to the success of prescribed medication regimens. The biopsychosocial effects of aging can negatively affect the success of a medication routine; nurses have the knowledge and ability to counteract many of these effects in conjunction with the health care team. **Table 8-9** provides a summary of the key concepts related to medications and the older adult.

Don't be afraid to take the lead in reviewing a patient's medications, screening for inappropriate prescriptions, recommending alternatives, and educating the older adult on medications. You may be the only barrier between an older adult and an adverse drug reaction.

TABLE 8-9 Key Concepts in Geriatric Pharmacology

- Older adults make up about 13% of the population, but consume 33% of all prescription medications.
- Older adults have significant physiological changes related to aging that may interfere with medications.
- The elderly are more sensitive to the effects of drug therapy.
- Adverse drug reactions are any noxious, unintended, or undesired effect of a drug that occurs at doses in humans for prophylaxis, diagnosis, or therapy.
- Certain disease states may interfere with optimal drug therapy.
- Polypharmacy is defined as the prescription, administration, or use of more medications than are clinically indicated for a patient.
- Inappropriate prescribing may be very harmful to elderly persons.
- Compliance to drug regimens is essential to improving medical diagnosis and outcomes.

SOURCE: Author.

Critical Thinking Exercises

1. Mr. Lockwood, a 102-year-old man, is admitted to the hospital from home with a diagnosis of hypotension and dizziness. He lives at home with his grandson, who, Mr. Lockwood says, is gone most of the time. You notice that Mr. Lockwood takes at least 10 different medications. What are your concerns for medication compliance with this patient?
2. Ms. Adams is a geriatric patient whom you see in your rounds for a home health agency. You are suspicious that something is wrong, because she continues to complain of back pain, although pain medications have been prescribed. When you check her pill bottle, it is empty. You call the pharmacy, who says that that prescription for 60 pills was filled last week. How might you respond to this situation? Which health care professionals might be of assistance in clarifying the issue?

continues

Critical Thinking (continued)

3. Mrs. Young lives alone in her house. She is 87 years old, and you suspect that she has dementia. Mrs. Young refuses to allow health care workers into her home. When you assist with discharge planning from the acute care hospital for Mrs. Young, you become worried because you doubt that she will take her medications properly. What resources are available to help Mrs. Young have a safe discharge?

Personal Reflections

1. Think about the medications that you have administered to older adults during your time as a nursing student or nurse. How often have you considered drug interactions and the importance of therapeutic levels in the elderly? How important is it to draw peak and trough levels at the correct time?
2. Which team members play a vital role in assisting you as a nurse to help the patients or residents gain the best therapeutic effect from their medication regimens?
3. Which of the topics in this chapter were least familiar to you? Which topics will you pay more attention to in the future?
4. Do you always think about the five rights when you administer medications? Why or why not?
5. What are some solutions for the problem of identifying residents prior to giving medications in long-term care facilities where name bands are not worn?

References

ADAM. (2002). *Osteoporosis.* Retrieved December 5, 2008, from http://adam.about.com/reports/000018_7.htm

Alzheimer's Disease Education and Referral (ADEAR) Center, National Institute on Aging. (2005). *Treatment.* Retrieved June 10, 2005, from http://www.alzheimers.org/treatment.htm

Aparasu, R. R., Mort, J. R., & Aparasu, A. (2001). Inappropriate psychotropic agents for the elderly. *Geriatric Times, 2*(2). Retrieved June 11, 2005, from http://www.geriatrictimes.com/g010321.html

Beers, M. H. (1997). Explicit criteria for determining potentially inappropriate medication use by the elderly. *Archives of Internal Medicine, 157*, 1531–1536.

Beers, M. H., & Berkow, R. (Eds.). (2000). Clinical pharmacology. In *Merck manual of geriatrics* (3rd ed., pp. 54–74). Whitestation, NJ: Merck Research Laboratories.

Birnbaum, A., Leppik, I. E., Conway, J. M., Bowers, S. E., Lackner, T., & Graves, N. M. (2003). Variability of total phenytoin serum concentrations within elderly nursing home residents. *Neurology, 60*(4), 555–559.

Brigden, M. L., & Heathcote, J. C. (2000). Problems in interpreting laboratory tests. *Postgraduate Medicine, 107*(7). Retrieved December 5, 2008, from http://findarticles.com/p/articles/mi_m0FSS/is_4_14/ai_n17210410/pg_7

California Registry. (2004). *Drug prescribing in the elderly.* Retrieved February 9, 2005, from http://www.calregistry.com/dyk/drug.htm

ClinLab Navigator. (2007). *Aging effect on laboratory values.* Retrieved October 15, 2007, from http://www.clinlabnavigator.com

Cohen, H., Robinson, E. S., & Mandrack, M. (2003). Getting to the root of medication errors: Survey results. *Nursing2003, 33*(9), 36–45.

Delafuente, J. C., & Stewart, R. B. (2001). *Therapeutics in the elderly* (3rd ed.) Cincinnati, OH: Harvey Whitney.

Edwards, N., & Baird, C. (2005). Interpreting laboratory values in older adults. *MEDSURG Nursing, 14*(4), 220–239.

ElderCare Online. (2002). *Alzheimer's disease medications fact sheet*. Retrieved June 10, 2005, from http://www.ec-online.net/Knowledge/Articles/admedications.html

Fick, D. M., Cooper, J. W., Wade, W. E., Waller, J. L., Maclean, J. R., & Beers, M. H. (2003). Updating the Beers criteria for potentially inappropriate medication use in older adults: Results of a U.S. consensus panel of experts. *Archives of Internal Medicine, 163*(22), 2716–2724.

Fischbach, F. (1996). *A manual of laboratory and diagnostic tests* (5th ed.). Philadelphia: Lippincott.

Geriatric Medicine in Clinical Practice. (2002). *Laboratory values*. Retrieved October 15, 2005, from http://geriatricsyllabus.com/syllabus/main.jsp?cid=AGE-LAB

Gliatto, M. F. (2000). Generalized anxiety disorder. *American Family Physician*. Retrieved June 14, 2005, from http://www.aafp.org/afp/20001001/1591.html

Goulding, M. R. (2004). Inappropriate medication prescribing for elderly ambulatory care patients. *Archives of Internal Medicine, 164*(3), 305–312.

Hartford Institute for Geriatric Nursing. (n.d.). Beers' criteria for potentially inappropriate medication use in the elderly. *Try This: Best Practices in Nursing Care to Older Adults*, 16. Retrieved on December 6, 2008, from http://www.consultgerirn.org/uploads/File/trythis/issue16_1.pdf

Health-cares.net. (2005). *What medications are used to cure Alzheimer's disease?* Retrieved June 10, 2005, from http://neurology.health-cares.net/alzheimers-disease-medications.php

Kessel, B. (2004). Hip fracture prevention in postmenopausal women. *Obstetrical and Gynecological Survey, 59*(6), 446–455.

Kudoh, A., Takase, H., Takahira, Y., & Takazawa, T. (2004). Postoperative confusion increases in elderly long term benzodiazepine users. *Anesthesia and Analgesia, 99*(6), 1674–1678.

Lantz, M. S. (2004). Chronic benzodiazepine treatment in the older adult: Therapeutic or problematic? *Clinical Geriatrics, 12*(5), 21–24.

McCabe, B. J. (2004). Prevention of food-drug interactions with special emphasis on older adults. *Current Opinion in Clinical Nutrition and Metabolic Care, 7*(1), 21–26.

McGarry Logue, R. (2002). Self-medication and the elderly: How technology can help. *American Journal of Nursing, 10*(7), 51–55.

Merck. (2007). *Merck manual of geriatrics. Appendix 1: Laboratory values*. Retrieved October 15, 2007, from http://www.merck.com/mkgr/mmg/appndxs/app1.jsp

Piette, J. D., Heisler, M., & Wagner, T. H. (2004). Cost-related medication underuse: Do patients with chronic illnesses tell their doctors? *Archives of Internal Medicine, 164*(16), 1749–1756.

Quality Matters. (2004). *Use of anti-anxiety medications*. Retrieved July 11, 2005, from http://mqa.dhs.state.tx.us/qmweb/Anxiety.htm

Reuben, D. B., Herr, K. A., Pacala, J. T., Pollock, B. G., Potter, J. F., & Semla, T. P. (2004). *Geriatrics at your fingertips* (6th ed.). Malden, MA: Blackwell.

Tanago, E. A., & McAninch, J. W. (Eds.). (2004). *Smith's general urology* (16th ed.). *Urological laboratory examination*. Retrieved October 15, 2007, from http://www.accessmedicine.com/content.aspx?aID=222712

Wagner, A. K., Zhang, F., Soumerai, S. B., Walker, A. M., Gurwitz, J. H., Glynn, R. J., et al. (2002). Benzodiazepine use and hip fractures in the elderly: Who is at greatest risk? *Archives of Internal Medicine, 164*(14), 1567–1572.

CHAPTER 9

Teaching Older Adults

Kristen L. Mauk, PhD, RN, CRRN-A, GCNS-BC

LEARNING OBJECTIVES

At the end of this chapter, the reader will be able to:

- Apply key principles of adult learning.
- Discuss how the baby boomers' generation will impact teaching and learning in the next few decades.
- Identify settings where health education for older adults can take place.
- Acknowledge the impact of cultural diversity and health literacy on teaching and learning with older adults.
- Compare the effect of cognitive, affective, sensory, and psychomotor barriers on learning among older adults.
- Discuss strategies for enhancing teaching of older adults.

KEY TERMS

- Adult learning theory
- Andragogy
- Baby boomers
- Cultural diversity
- Gerogogy
- Health disparity
- Health literacy
- Lifelong learning
- Social cognitive theory (SCT)
- Theory of self-efficacy

The U.S. population is living longer as a result of advances in health care, early treatment and diagnosis of chronic illnesses, advanced technology in disease management, and improved treatments and health care delivery methods. Persons reaching age 65 have an average life expectancy of another 18.4 years (19.8 for females, 16.8 for males). By 2030, 71 million people (20% of the U.S. population) will be over age 65 (Centers for Disease Control and Prevention [CDC], 2007; National Institute on Aging and National Institutes of Health [NIA & NIH], 2007). The 85 years and older population is projected to increase to 6.1 million in 2010, making this the fastest growing age group (Administration on Aging, 2007; Agingstats.gov, 2005).

Gender differences also will impact the aging population. Currently, older women outnumber older men (139:100), and the female/male ratio increases with age.

Educating the older adults of the future presents significant challenges to health care providers. Currently, adults in the older age groups may have been born in the 1910s, 1920s, 1930s, or early 1940s-times when many children did not have the advantage of education, either primary or secondary. On the other hand, the next generation of older adults, the **baby boomers**, begin to turn age 65 in 2011 (CDC, 2007; NIA & NIH, 2007). The baby boomer group is considered more affluent, better educated, and healthier (Manheimer, 2002) than the current group of elders. These baby boomers, who were born between 1946 and 1961, are presenting educators and health care providers with specific educational needs that have not been expressed in previous generations.

With the changing demographics of the United States, a more culturally diverse group will also be reaching retirement years. The minority elderly population is increasing. There will be an estimated 8.1 million minority elderly in 2010, which is 20% of the elderly population, and 12.9 million in 2020 (or 23.6% of the elderly population) (Administration on Aging, 2007). Some members of this cohort may have low literacy or poor English language skills.

Nurses in all settings are expected to provide education to patients and families. All of the demographic factors discussed previously influence how health care providers should structure education for older adults. Nurses must refocus on issues of education in gerontology and the impact on outcomes of health care. Health care educators in industry, the community, rural settings, colleges, universities, adult day care centers, senior centers, hospices, continuing care retirement centers, and assisted living centers (to name a few) are now expected to provide topics of interest not only to the older adult, but also to adults or other family members who are anticipating retirement years. Educational topics may include the management of chronic diseases, health promotion, second career choices, exercise, retirement, employment issues, financial management, legal concerns, and quality-of-life issues. The content in this chapter will assist nurses to understand how the demographics of the upcoming older population will affect how we provide education, and also give some strategies about teaching and learning in older adults.

PRINCIPLES OF ADULT LEARNING

Historically, formal education and learning were considered of little value for anyone over 50 years old. With few people living past the retirement age of 65, education was not considered necessary or beneficial. Learning in past decades may have been considered a selfish, self-centered desire. Working past 65 years old was unwarranted unless financial strains dictated it. Attitudes about learning after a certain age were gauged by how much time was left to live after retirement (Crawford, 2005).

Changes in adult learning began in the post–World War II era when the GI Bill of Rights resulted in millions of veterans being given the opportunity to attend college, promoting the notion that college degrees were not only for the wealthy, but also for the common citizen (Sheppard, 2002). This generation began to change the way adults could learn and introduced the **lifelong learning** approach that resulted in an educational culture shift. The increased number of educated adults fostered economic productivity as well as improved quality of life in older adults (Crawford, 2005).

With an increased life expectancy, retirement at age 65 seems to be early in life, with many people living 20 or 30 years beyond the usual retirement age. The baby boomers account for millions of Americans in the workforce. It is predicted that there will be a labor shortage as the baby boomers start to retire, with many reentering the workforce in second career choices. These events may increase the need for education of older adults (Crawford, 2005). Education for the older adult will also be encouraged by the increasing availability of educational offerings, grants and scholarships, and the change in social norms where lifelong learning is socially acceptable and used for a variety of reasons including education, socialization, and training for new skills.

The education needed for this large number of older adults can be done in formal and informal settings, including the community, health care facilities, support groups, colleges/universities, online, and in long-term care facilities. Because lifelong learning and education have been correlated with a delay in cognitive impairments with aging, their importance is relevant not only for those reasons mentioned earlier, but also to maintain quality of life (Diamond, 2001).

Malcolm Knowles's **adult learning theory** (1984), which is commonly used in teaching adults, has motivation and relevance as two key concepts. Using **andragogy** as a common principle for adult learners, adult learning theory applies certain principles to enhance learning in adults over 18 years old who have completed mandatory public education. Adults expect respect; are autonomous, self-directed, independent learners; are goal oriented, and need to know that what they are learning is relevant and practical. They expect to actively participate in learning and build on previous life events. Adults derive much of their self-identity from past experiences, and nurses should use this knowledge when devising teaching strategies. Fear of failure may also be a concern for this group.

A couple of other theories of note may be useful in educating the older adult. The **theory of self-efficacy** sheds some light on the behavior of older adults. Self-efficacy theory suggests that persons' self-efficacy is related to their belief that their actions influence outcomes in their life. This theory states that "self-efficacy and outcome expectations affect behavior, motivational level, thought patterns, and emotional reactions in response to any situation" (Resnick, 2002, p. 1). The concept of self-efficacy includes behavior, cognitive factors, the environment, and the outcomes desired. Self-efficacy theory is based in **social cognitive theory (SCT)** also called social learning theory. SCT suggests that outcome expectations are beliefs that when a person engages in a certain behavior, certain outcomes will result (Billek-Sawhney & Reicherter, 2004). For example, in using SCT in the education of an older adult with a hip fracture, therapists found that a woman attending and participating in physical therapy (the behavior) saw improvement in her physical status that produced a positive belief (cognitive factors) that she could be successful. She continued an exercise class after discharge that was geared toward seniors (the environment), and this further strengthened her belief that her actions made a difference in her health outcomes as she participated and saw positive results in her physical strength and flexibility (Billek-Sawhney & Reicherter, 2004).

Notable Quotes

"Adult learners flourish when their past and current knowledge is valued, when open-mindedness is encouraged, and when learning leads to understanding that produces professional and personal satisfaction. To teach is to change a life, forever."

-Esther H. Condon, PhD, RN, in Barbara K. Penn's *Mastering the Teaching Role: A Guide for Nurse Educators*, 2008, p. 85.

Older adults may need extra encouragement to engage in learning activities. **Gerogogy** involves strategies used when teaching older adults that aim to lead them to higher levels of empowerment and emancipation (Formosa, 2002; Thomas, 2007). Older adults may choose to participate in educational activities as a way to apply knowledge immediately, increase personal satisfaction, and improve socialization (Blacklock, 1985; Reynolds, 2005). Differences may also be seen when older adults benefit from certain adjustments to teaching methodologies that address impairments in the cognitive, affective, sensory, and psychomotor domains (Reynolds, 2005).

In addition, certain preferences for instructional methodologies relate to how individuals feel they learn best. For example, an older adult who is a visual learner may prefer to view posters or bulletin boards with educational information so that they may learn at their own pace (Thomas, 2007). Self-monitoring has been shown to improve the effectiveness of learning, and it reinforces the principle that adults are independent learners (Dunlosky et al., 2007). Conversely, an older adult who learns best through auditory means may prefer listening to a lecture. Someone who relates to learning using a more hands-on method may retain knowledge best when there are experiential activities that require demonstration and return demonstration. Any and all of these means for educating older adults should be considered, keeping in mind that all learners may have unique preferences and learning styles.

OLDER ADULTS AND LIFELONG LEARNING

Recently, attitudes about aging have changed for the positive, related to the fact that there is an increasing number of baby boomers who see aging as a time in which quality-of-life issues are a priority. This is guiding many groups to conduct preretirement education to assist in the transition to retirement. Although older adults still expect the traditional retirement, 69% plan to work postretirement in positions related to teaching, office support, crafts, retail sales, or health care (Brown, 2003). Despite the trends that support postretirement employment, 67% have concerns that age discrimination will be a major barrier in the workplace. If the predicted percentage of baby boomers seek postretirement careers, there will be an increased demand for continuing education.

Older learners prefer teaching methods that are easy to access and require small investments of time and money. They expect learning to begin immediately through direct hands-on experiences. Reading materials such as newspapers, magazines, books, and journals are used by 64% of older adults for learning.

The most requested educational topics from 2000 are listed in **Table 9-1** (Harris Interactive, 2000). According to the current AARP Web site (2008), frequently requested health topics include Alzheimer's disease, breast cancer, COPD, depression, type 2 diabetes, high cholesterol, hypertension, low back pain, obesity, osteoporosis, prostate cancer, and rheumatoid arthritis.

Many colleges and universities offer tuition-free or discounted enrollment in regular courses for older adults. Educational programs are often offered at no charge through alumni organizations, health care facilities, banks, investment companies, museums, labor organizations, recreation centers, and the Internet. Industries are offering workforce-related education and training. In addition, a variety of educational programs is offered for the older adult through national agencies (see **Table 9-2**).

TABLE **9-1** **Educational Topics on Desired Skills**

Diet and nutrition
Exercise and fitness
Weight control
Stress management
Complementary and alternative practices
Career advancement
Basic life skills: reading, writing, math, driving
Hobbies
Community involvement
Volunteering
Arts and culture or personal enrichment
Enjoyment out of life
Educational travel
Spiritual and personal growth
Getting along with others

SOURCE: AARP. (2000). *AARP survey on lifelong learning.* Retrieved April 27, 2005, from http://www.aarp.org/research/reference/publicopinions/Articles/aresearch-import-490.html

BARRIERS TO OLDER ADULTS' LEARNING

Older adults may experience some unique barriers to learning. These include chronic illnesses, normal aging changes occurring with advancing age, **health disparities**, and other factors that may accompany **cultural diversity**.

Chronic illnesses increase with advanced age and can present barriers to learning among older adults. In 1997, more than half of the older population (54.5%) reported having at least one disability of some type (physical or nonphysical) (Administration on Aging [AoA], 2002). In 2005, about 34 million persons reported being limited in their daily activities due to one or more chronic health problems. The National Health Interview Survey of 2005 reported that 44% of adults age 75 years or older felt they had limitations in their usual activities, and nearly one-third of adults over age 75 rated their health as fair or poor (Adams, Dey, & Vickerie, 2007). Arthritis and hypertension are two of the chronic problems blamed for early retirement among Americans (NIA & NIH, 2007). Almost three-fourths (73.6%) of those age 80 and older report at least one disability. Presence of a severe disability is associated with lower income levels and lower educational attainment (AoA, 2002). In order to facilitate learning and overcome obstacles that chronic conditions may cause, health care providers must have insight into the challenges that this group faces (Hatcliffe, 2003).

Specific barriers to education may include cognitive, affective, sensory, and psychomotor barriers. Many adults have unique physical or cognitive difficulties related to learning (Eun-Shim, Preece, Resnick, & Mills, 2004). Physical changes that can affect learning are listed in **Table 9-3**. Cognitive barriers may include illnesses like Alzheimer's dementia or memory loss after a stroke. Ten percent of persons over age 70 have moderate or

TABLE **9-2** **Education Programs for Older Adults**

Program	Web Address	Description
Elderhostel	http://www.elderhostel.org	A nonprofit organization dedicated to providing learning adventures for people 55 and older.
Administration on Aging	http://www.aoa.gov	Provides a comprehensive overview of a wide variety of topics, programs, and services related to aging.
USA.gov for Seniors	http://www.usa.gov/Topics/Seniors.shtml	Official U.S. gateway to all government information specific to the older adult.
OASIS	http://www.oasisnet.org	A national nonprofit educational organization designed to enhance the quality of life for mature adults; offers challenging programs in the arts, humanities, wellness, technology, and volunteer service, and creates opportunities for older adults to continue their personal growth and provide meaningful service to the community.
SeniorNet	http://www.seniornet.org	A 501(c)3 nonprofit organization of computer-using adults (50 and older) whose purpose is to provide older adults education regarding and access to computer technologies to enhance their lives and enable them to share their knowledge and wisdom.
Shepherd's Centers	http://www.shepherdcenters.org	A network of community volunteer organizations that serves the needs of older adults in four areas: life maintenance, life enrichment, life reorganization, and life celebration.

severe cognitive decline (NIA & NIH, 2007). Affective disorders may include depression and mood disorders. Sensory barriers can include hearing loss, glaucoma, and cataracts. Psychomotor barriers may include chronic illnesses or problems such as Parkinson's, stroke, arthritis, and pulmonary diseases that impact the use of teaching tools or computers. Strategies for working with persons with memory problems such as those that occur with dementia are discussed in Chapter 15.

Multidimensional motor sequence learning may be impaired in older adults (**Box 9-1**). Researchers

TABLE 9-3 Physical Changes in the Older Adult That Can Affect Learning

- Reduced vision
- Reduced hearing
- Impaired cognitive function
- Depression
- Stress
- Chronic illnesses
- Dementia

examining task sequencing that involved repeated motor, spatial, and temporal dimensions and retention tests found that the motor element was the most important for motor learning (Boyd, Vidoni, & Siengsukon, 2008). Their results suggested "an age-related impairment in motor learning" (p. 351) that was found among healthy elderly in the study. Older adults did not seem to benefit from practicing a repeated sequence to improve motor performance.

Literacy levels of older adults may be an additional barrier. About 90 million people (or 74% of older American adults) have some problem accessing, reading, interpreting, or using health care information (Billek-Sawhney & Reicherter, 2005; Hixon, 2004). This dynamic will change in the next few decades as the baby boomers become the predominant older cohort.

At the current time, however, literacy levels for two of five persons (40%) over age 65 are less than a fifth-grade level, with 58% of those over age 85 having low literacy skills. The surgeon general has identified health literacy as a major problem in our health care system, costing up to $73 billion per year (Bass, 2005). **Health literacy** has been defined as "the degree to which individuals have the capacity to obtain, process, and understand basic health information and services needed to make appropriate health decisions" (Institute of Medicine, 2004, p. 1).

Low literacy skills are especially prominent in the minority and older adult community. Only 52% of African American older adults and 36% of

BOX 9-1 Research Highlight

Aim: The purpose of this study was to determine which characteristics of multidimensional sequencing most influence motor sequence learning and whether age was a significant factor in this type of learning.

Methods: Younger, middle-, and older-aged adults practiced sequencing with repeated dimensions to the practice for 2 days; retention and interference tests assessed sequence learning. The mean median response time was used to assess motor sequence learning.

Findings: Older adults showed nonspecific learning that suggested an age-related impairment in motor learning that was not found in younger or middle adult groups.

Application to practice: Some research does support the idea that older adults have some age-related impairment in motor learning. This age-related sequence learning deficit suggests that persons undergoing rehabilitation or other motor-related learning involved in activities such as physical therapy may have a more difficult time or require additional assistance with attaining functional goals. Nurses should realize that there are also many aspects and domains of learning that impact an older person's overall performance and health outcomes.

Source: Boyd, L. A., Vidoni, E. D., & Siengsukon, C. F. (2008). Multidimensional motor sequence learning is impaired in older but not younger or middle-aged adults. *Physical Therapy, 88*(3), 351–362.

Hispanic older adults have a high school education, compared to 76% of whites and 70% of Asians (Agingstats.gov, 2005). These statistics indicate that a large portion of minority older adults may have unique teaching and learning needs.

Low literacy is correlated with poorer health status (per self-report) and increased knowledge deficit about health status. Acknowledging low literacy skills can be embarrassing to patients; educators will have to recognize the scope of the problem in their own communities and patient populations and develop culturally sensitive strategies to assist in improving knowledge and enhancing health outcomes. Issues such as noncompliance, incomplete forms, surrogate readers, and vision/hearing problems may be clues to low literacy levels (Schloman, 2004).

For these reasons, it is recommended that nurses currently working with older adults use educational materials that are geared toward the fifth-grade level or lower. Strategies to improve readability of materials for older adults include:

- Keep the format and content simple,
- Use shorter words and sentences (try to substitute 1- to 2-syllable words where possible).
- Increase the use of pictures.
- Use shorter sentences.
- Use the active voice in brochures or pamphlets (Billek-Sawhney & Reicherter, 2005).

However, nurses need to assess the learning needs of the particular person or group with whom they are working in order to tailor teaching appropriately.

TECHNOLOGY FOR OLDER ADULTS' LIFELONG LEARNING

According to a 2008 Pew Internet Survey on older adults and use of the Internet, 70% of those age 50–64 and 38% of adults 65 or older reported using the Internet (Pew Internet and American Life Project, 2008). The fastest growing group of people learning to use the Internet is those 55 and older. Older adults should have the same opportunities to use information technology (Withnall, 2002). The process of aging may present challenges to older adults who wish to use computers to enhance learning (**Case Study 9-1**). Some of the problems

Case Study 9-1

Connie was 70 years old. She always wanted to learn how to speak Spanish and enrolled in the local college, despite the fact that she was beginning to have some hearing problems. She was enjoying her classes as she continued her responsibilities in her home, including caring for her husband who had hypertension. Unfortunately, her husband suffered from a stroke and Connie had to assume the responsibility of primary caregiver for him, causing her to withdraw from the university. She did purchase some audiovisuals to help her practice her Spanish. When her husband recovered from his stroke, Connie was able to reenroll at the university; however, her hearing loss had become worse over time, which made it difficult to continue learning a language in class. Connie decided to continue using books and tapes to learn Spanish, but she also had a new interest in plants and used educational programs on television to learn more about horticulture and working in her yard.

These activities provided Connie with educational activities in the home while continuing to care for her husband, who died 3 years later. After her husband's death, Connie was feeling isolated and decided to go back to the university and continue her learning. She found a cohort of older adults who were also interested in continuing their education in a variety of ways. At this time, Connie was enjoying art and took a class in art history, something she had always wanted to learn more about. Taking this class was not hindered by her hearing loss. She visited art galleries and was involved in group discussions that were run by the class participants. As an older adult, Connie was engaged in a variety of learning experiences that changed over time due to circumstances in her life.

Questions:

1. How has Connie incorporated lifelong learning in the last few years?
2. How has she adapted to the challenges she has faced to overcome barriers and continue her lifelong learning?
3. As an educator, what might you recommend to Connie to enhance her education or meet her lifelong learning needs?

TABLE 9-4 Problems That Can Be Overcome by Older Adults Using Computers

Age Change	Effect on Computer Use	Possible Solutions
Hearing	Sound from computer may not be heard	Use earphones to enhance hearing and eliminate background noise. Speak slowly and clearly.
Vision	Vision declines, need for bifocal glasses, viewing monitor may be difficult, problems with glaucoma and light/colors	Adjust monitor's tilt to eliminate glare. Change size of font to 14. Make sure contrast is clear. Change the screen resolution to promote color perception.
Motor control, tremors	May affect use of keyboard or control of mouse, may not be able to hold the mouse and consistently click correct mouse buttons	Highlight area and press Enter. Avoid double clicking.
Arthritis	May not be able to hold the mouse and consistently click correct mouse buttons	Highlight area and press Enter. Teach how to use options on keyboard.
Attention span	Problems with inability to focus and making correct inferences	Priming—introduce concept early on. Repetition is key to retention. Use cheat sheets.

can be overcome with adjustments to computer technology (see **Table 9-4**) (Bean & Lavin, 2003).

As the baby boomers enter the 65 and older age group, these statistics will obviously change because of their comfort with technology. Prior experience in the use of computers affects attitudes and outcomes of subsequent training, so the learning needs of the computer literate will change over time (Dyck & Smither, 1994). Seniors can often learn about the computer at public libraries and learning centers that provide access for computer use and education. Telemedicine services are another promising option to educate seniors in distant areas (Adler, 2002). These are discussed in detail in Chapter 16.

Many health care agencies have developed their own Web pages to adapt education for older adult viewers (**Box 9-2**). Web pages can bridge the gaps of health information disparity by offering information in a variety of languages (VanBiervliet & Edwards-Schafer, 2004). Web page usability issues related to the older adult include design, font size, colors, and clear instructions. (See Chapter 16 for further information.) Navigation tasks and the format of the Web page may challenge cognitively impaired persons. The organization of the Web

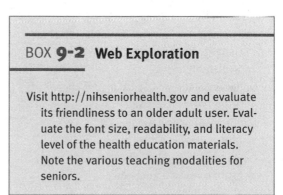

BOX 9-2 Web Exploration

Visit http://nihseniorhealth.gov and evaluate its friendliness to an older adult user. Evaluate the font size, readability, and literacy level of the health education materials. Note the various teaching modalities for seniors.

page should be consistent, with small segments and simple language. Instructions for multimedia should be clearly stated, and plain text should be available as an option (Eun-Shim, Preece, Resnick, & Mills, 2004; National Institute of Aging & National Library of Medicine, 2002). Tips for designing a Web page for older adults are listed in Chapter 16. Application of these principles can be seen at http://nihseniorhealth.gov.

CULTURAL DIVERSITY AND HEALTH DISPARITIES AMONG OLDER ADULTS

The issues of cultural diversity and health disparities cannot be ignored when considering educational issues for older adults. Diversity in terms of age, race, ethnicity, gender, and socioeconomic status is an important factor to consider. By 2050, more than one-third of the elderly population will be composed of African Americans (12%), Hispanics (18%), and Asians (8%) (AgingStats.gov, 2005). Of particular significance is that the proportion of Hispanic individuals age 65 or older is expected to triple in the next decades. Older white Americans are twice as likely to report very good or excellent health as elderly Hispanics or African Americans (NIA & NIH, 2007). Among the Hispanic group, health disparities affecting older adults include new cases of tuberculosis, new cases of AIDS, exposure to particulate matter, and cirrhosis deaths (Keppel, 2007). Diabetes and heart disease are also increased among this group. Strategies found to be effective for educating Hispanic adults with diabetes included educational sessions, written materials in both English and Spanish (especially fact sheets), including family in teaching sessions, and using culturally appropriate interventions (Whittemore, 2007). Nurses will need to become better educated in the cultural norms and health needs of persons from various ethnic groups. A discussion of diversity and health disparities among the major ethnic groups appears in Chapter 18.

These shifts in the diversity of the older population suggest that there may be social and economic issues related to disadvantaged groups that deserve special attention. There are greater disparities in health care delivery and access to care in later life among diverse groups. Culture and race will influence how and what older adults from minority groups will want to learn (Volland & Berkman, 2004). Of great concern is that many minority elderly do not use English as a first language. With this in mind, many educational Web pages now are offered in a variety of languages. Nurses should educate themselves about the literacy and education levels of all elders in the community in which they serve.

BOX 9-3 Recommended Resources

AARP: http://www.aarp.org

American Society on Aging: http://www.asaging.org

Association for Continuing Higher Education: http://www.acheinc.org

Association for Gerontology in Higher Education: http://www.aghe.org

The John A. Hartford Foundation Institute for Geriatric Nursing: http://www.hartfordign.org

National Center for Education Statistics: http://www.nces.ed.gov

National Council on Aging: http://www.ncoa.org

Osher Lifelong Learning Institute: http://www.olli.gmu.edu

IMPLICATIONS FOR GERONTOLOGICAL EDUCATORS

Education must meet the needs of the older adult-and these needs may change over the next several decades. The older adult cohort is not a homogeneous group, but is composed of persons of different cultures, races, education levels, and socioeconomic statuses, all factors that can impact learning. A rapidly growing pool of competent, college-educated adults will soon reach their retirement years. These times will be an exciting period for lifelong learning, which is now viewed as helping older adults improve quality of life and add meaning and creativity to their retirement years (Timmermann, 2003; Withnall, 2002). These needs may also include learning new life skills to manage chronic illnesses (due to increasing longevity), issues related to retirement, health promotion, financial issues, and improving or maintaining quality of life. Educators must also address the diverse cultures and needs of these groups.

Strategies for Teaching Older Adults Individually

Education of older adults must be flexible. Nurses may teach in a variety of settings including one-on-one instruction (**Figure 9-1**) at the bedside in acute care or in the home, or in group settings. Older adults need to have a motivation to learn, so be certain to explain the purpose of your educational session at the beginning. Scheduling teaching time in advance with clear explanations of what will be taught will allow the learner time to mentally prepare and formulate possible questions. Encourage the learner and family members to write down their questions prior to your teaching session.

In one-on-one teaching sessions with older adults, the nurse should remember to apply the principles of adult learning discussed earlier (Shysh, 2000). Condon (2008) suggested "being helpful and respectful as two important aspects of what mature learners expect from their teachers" (p. 77). Establish a rapport with the person. Ask questions about his or her background so that teaching can draw from the learner's past experiences. Evaluate the person's readiness to learn prior to attempting to teach. Avoid providing large amounts of new material when the person is under stress or distracted. Anxiety can interfere with the ability to recall instructions that just took place and thus interfere with learning (Palmer, 2006), so the environment needs to be relaxed and conducive to learning.

During the educational conversation, sit at a comfortable distance facing the older person and be sure that the person's hearing aids, glasses, or other adaptive equipment are being used prior to beginning the teaching session. Have written materials available that are learner-appropriate and literacy-tested (Table 9-2). Consider using a

FIGURE **9-1** **One-to-one instruction as well as involvement of family members are educational strategies for older adults.**

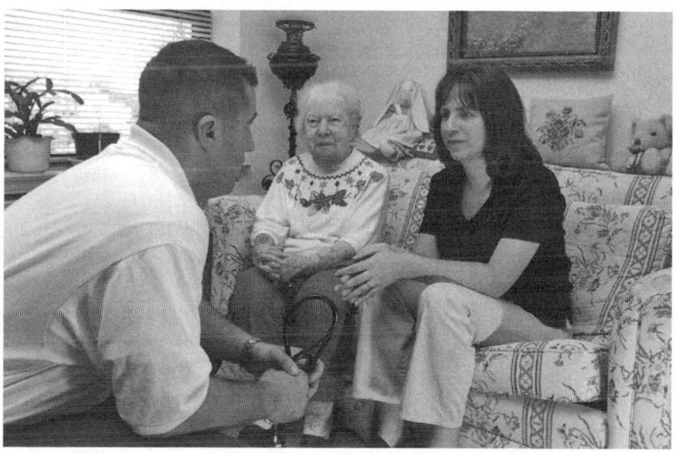

SOURCE: © Jones and Bartlett Publishers. Courtesy of MIEMSS.

memory tool to assist the person in recalling important information later. After discussing the material, allow time for questions and provide clear, concise responses. Follow up with any additional written materials or discussion that may be needed. Document the teaching in the appropriate records.

Strategies for Teaching Older Adults in Groups

Many times gerontological nurses will present to a group of older adults. This may occur in a variety of settings including senior centers, independent living, assisted living, churches, support groups, and other social gatherings. Several steps should be taken to ensure that the listeners will get the most possible out of the discussion. These appear in **Table 9-5.** Advance preparation is needed to ensure that the program presentation and environment are focused on the older adult audience.

In preparing a presentation for a group of older adults, be sure to visit the facility in advance. Ask for a guided tour from a key employee or director at the facility, and ask questions such as: What is the average age of the person who will attend the program? What are the major health concerns of this group? Where will the presentation take place? Will the program conflict with any other activities; if so, how could this be avoided? How will the program be advertised? How many older adults generally attend these types of presentations? Is a microphone available? Are there any other unique aspects of the audience that I should be aware of? Preparing ahead of time by having questions such as these answered will help the nurse to tailor the presentation to each audience so that on the day of the program, participants will gain the most from this interaction.

Be sure to observe the older adults at the facility during your tour. If possible, talk to some of

TABLE 9-5 Preparing a Short Educational Program for Older Adults

1. Visit the location/facility ahead of time and locate the room where you will speak.
2. Talk to the director of the facility to get a sense of what topics would be most valuable to the audience.
3. Talk to older adults at the site when you make a preparatory visit. Ask their opinions about what topics they would like more information on from a geriatric nurse.
4. Arrange the date and time of the presentation several months in advance so that the facility can give seniors adequate notice.
5. Be sure that the date and time do not conflict with regularly planned activities such as Bingo, mealtime, or exercise groups. Try to plan the time around a standing function such as right after dinner (if family members are invited) or right before lunch.
6. Find out how the facility plans to advertise your program. Good suggestions include flyers, community letters, newspapers, announcements at group meetings, signs, and posters.
7. Prepare the material to be presented well in advance. Plan to provide handouts and use multiple audiovisual aids that are elder-friendly.
8. For the educational program itself, employ strategies for teaching older adults (see **Box 9-4**).
9. Be flexible. Allow plenty of time for participants to gather. Realize that the program may not start exactly on time if the audience needs more time to get settled.
10. Build in time for questions, answers, and the opportunity for older adults to share their stories. Take time to personally visit with the participants after the formal program has ended.

them to ascertain interest in the topic you wish to present. Assess and evaluate the learning environment and potential participants during this preparation time. The facility director or educational coordinator may be able to provide topics of interest for the group to which the nurse will make the presentation.

On the day of the presentation, the nurse making the presentation should be sure to arrive early to set up and greet the participants as they enter the room. This makes the audience of older adults feel at ease, and if the presenter is approachable, they will be more likely to ask questions and interact during the presentation. When conducting educational courses, the atmosphere should be conducive to the older adult, including a comfortable temperature, frequent breaks, lack of noise, and accessible bathroom facilities. Use or develop educational materials that are geared toward the fifth-grade level (see previous discussion) unless the educational level of the group is known to be higher. Remember that the general goal of an educational presentation to a group is to provide information and enhance learning about a relevant topic. Having done some background research and asked the appropriate questions in advance, the nurse is already at an advantage by having chosen a topic in which the participants are interested.

Involving learners in the educational process is a good beginning to encouraging participation. Before beginning the presentation, ask a question that requires the audience to answer with yes or no, or give a show of hands. Such an introduction demonstrates an interest on the presenter's part in the opinions and background of the participants and can serve as a way to engage the audience early. Use a variety of teaching modalities such as posters, PowerPoint slides, handouts, games, hands-on experiential learning, and the like (Thomas, 2007)(see Box 9-3). Background information and statistics should be presented in a clear and logical manner. Give sources for the information, using reliable citations that older adults would be familiar with. For example, if the nurse was giving a presentation on stroke prevention, citing statistics and information from the American Heart Association and the American Stroke Association would be recommended.

Working in groups, group discussion, role-playing, and using case studies or simulations may provide methods of engaging older adults in learning. If the audience is known to like games, the presenter(s) may tailor a game such as Bingo to review information on the program topic. For example, if the topic is proper nutrition, the presenter may have a Bingo card that represents the different food groups, vitamins, or the like, and then use this to ask questions about the material discussed in the presentation. Prizes could be awarded for Bingo, such as pieces of fruit or small water bottles, that also emphasize the meaningful aspects of the educational topic.

Additionally, remembering to adapt the topic and the ways in which it is presented to accommodate the physical changes and needs of older adults will result in much better outcomes. Advance preparation is key to any productive talk, workshop, or seminar for the elderly. Be sure to consider the physical changes associated with aging by using a microphone, avoiding glare from lights or windows, and speaking directly to the audience to enhance hearing and comprehension. Box 9-4 summarizes tips for teaching older adults.

SUMMARY

Nurses who are entering the workforce for the first time need to prepare themselves to meet the unique educational needs of this diverse older group, remembering that in the future there may be greater needs for teaching among older women, those over age 85, and minority groups. Older adults need to have a reason to learn that is relevant to their lives and situation. Nurses will need to be flexible and adaptable to meet the needs of the older adult group and use a variety of teaching modalities to make learning appealing and interesting. Advance preparation is an important strategy in preparing an educational program for older adults. Nurses should also consider the physical, cognitive, and sensory changes that occur with normal aging and adapt educational programs and materials to the unique needs of older adults.

BOX 9-4 Strategies for Teaching Older Adults

Use the principles of adult learning theory.

- Assess readiness to learn.
- Involve the audience at the start with questions or stories to which they can relate.
- Draw the participants into the material from the beginning.
- Provide reasons for them to learn by pointing out the significance of the topic using statistics and research.

Use multiple teaching modalities to keep the material interesting and maintain attention.

- PowerPoint slides
- Videos or CDs
- Handouts
- Brochures or pamphlets
- Posters
- Demonstration/equipment
- Quizzes

Remember to accommodate any unique physical needs of older adults.

- Do not stand in front of a window—avoid glare.
- Speak loudly and slowly. Use a microphone if needed. Turn off fans and other distracting noise.
- Face the audience. (Remember that elders often fill in what they cannot hear by lip-reading.)
- Limit programs to about 20–40 minutes.
- Use a room that is large enough to accommodate persons with wheelchairs, walkers, and other adaptive devices.
- Handouts should be in a large font and in black type on white paper for easy readability.
- Keep slides uncluttered; don't provide too much information. Use a large font with an easy-to-see background for slides.
- Control the environment.
- Arrange the room to best suit the particular presentation. Be sure the room is large enough for the expected number of attendees.
- Have a helper to assist with seating late-comers without disrupting the program or to help those who must leave during the presentation for some reason.
- Be sure the room is a neutral temperature—not too hot or cold, and free from drafts.

Make presentations elder-friendly.

- Choose topics of interest to older adults such as living wills, vitamins and minerals, and stroke prevention.
- Create a catchy title for the presentation that will pique interest and curiosity.
- Use lay terms or explain any confusing medical jargon. Define all terms.
- Invite special speakers who are well known in the area to promote attendance.
- Offer prizes, gifts, or some type of take-home item.
- Be sure that handouts are appropriate to the literacy level and cultural background of the group.

Critical Thinking Exercises

1. You have been approached by the director of nursing at a long-term care facility to present an educational program on a "topic of interest" to an expected group of about 10 older adults in assisted living. What topics of interest would you consider? How would you prepare for this presentation? What teaching modalities would you use? How would you adapt the environment to enhance learning for this group? Who would handle advertising of this program?
2. You are a new instructor at a small community college. You have been assigned to develop a service-learning project for an aging class in which the senior BSN students must develop and present a teaching project in local nursing homes. There are 60 students in the class and five facilities available over a 4-month period. How will you divide students into groups and facilities? Would you allow students to choose their own topics, make a list of suggestions, or set this up ahead of time with each facility? What influenced your decision to choose one approach over another for setting up these experiences? How will you evaluate the students' presentations? Is this project reasonable for senior BSN students to undertake? What background and instructions would students need to be successful on this project?
3. On the medical-surgical floor of the hospital where you work as a graduate nurse, the charge nurse asks you to do some one-on-one teaching with a 78-year-old widower who must learn to give himself insulin injections for newly diagnosed diabetes. How long do you think it will take for this patient to learn such a skill? What are the factors you would need to assess prior to beginning your instruction? What strategies will you use to prepare for this teaching session? What tools or teaching aids would be appropriate?

Personal **Reflections**

1. Have you ever cared for an older adult who did not speak English or for whom English was a second language? How did you feel when you tried to explain something to him or her? Did it make you feel frustrated? Did you give up? How was this person's overall health status? How did he or she cope with illness? What could you have done differently to achieve a better long-term health outcome?
2. How do you employ teaching of older adults in your daily nursing care? How important to you is the role of teacher among the nurse's many roles? Have you ever considered a career in gerontological education? If so, how do you visualize yourself 10 years from now in such a position? What type of setting would you most like to work in if your primary job was education relating to older adults?

References

AARP. (2008). *Health conditions.* Retrieved July 25, 2008, from http://www.aarp.org/health/healthguide/

Adams, P. F., Dey, A. N., & Vickerie, J. L. (2007). Summary health statistics for the U.S. population: National Health Interview Survey. National Center for Health Statistics. *Vital Health Statistics, 10*(233).

Adler, R. (2002). *The age wave meets the technology wave: Broadband and older Americans.* Seniornet. Retrieved April 27, 2005, from http://www.seniornet.org/php/default.php?PageID=6694

Administration on Aging. (2002). *Profile of older Americans: Health, health care, and disability.* Retrieved April 27, 2005, from http://www.aoa.gov/prof/Statistics/profile/2005/2005profile.pdf

Administration on Aging. (2007). *A profile of older Americans: 2007.* Retrieved August 12, 2008, from http://www.state.ia.us/elderaffairs/Documents/2007profile.pdf

AgingStats.gov. (2005). *Older Americans 2004: Key indicators of well being.* Retrieved April 27, 2005, from http://www.agingstats.gov

Bass, L. (2005). Health literacy. *Journal of Infusion Nursing, 28*(1), 15–22.

Bean, C., & Lavin, M. (2003). Adapting to seniors: Computer training for older adults. *Florida Libraries, 46*(2), 1–7.

Billek-Sawhney, B., & Reicherter, E. A. (2004). Social cognitive theory: Use by physical therapists in the education of the older adult client. *Topics in Geriatric Rehabilitation, 20*(4), 319–323.

Billek-Sawhney, B., & Reicherter, E. A. (2005). Literacy and the older adult. *Topics in Geriatric Rehabilitation, 21*(4), 275–281.

Blacklock, K. L. (1985). Lifelong learning for the older adult. *Journal of Extension, 23*(3). Retrieved April 29, 2005, from http://www.joe.org/joe/1985fall/a3.html

Boyd, L. A., Vidoni, E. D., & Siengsukon, C. F. (2008). Multidimensional motor sequence learning is impaired in older but not younger or middle-aged adults. *Physical Therapy, 88*(3), 351–362.

Brown, S. K. (2003). *Staying ahead of the curve 2003: The AARP working in retirement study.* Retrieved April 27, 2005, from http://www.aarp.org/research/reference/publicopinions/Articles/aresearch-import-417.html

Centers for Disease Control and Prevention. (2002). *Health, United States, 2004.* Retrieved April 27, 2005, from http://www.cdc.gov/nchs/data/hus/hus04trend.pdf#027

Centers for Disease Control and Prevention & Merck Company Foundation. (2007). *The state of aging and health in America, 2007.* Whitehouse Station, NJ: Merck Company Foundation.

Condon, E. H. (2008). Adults as students; special consideration. In Barbara K. Penn (Ed.), *Mastering the teaching role: A guide for nurse educators* (pp. 77–86). Philadelphia: F. A. Davis.

Crawford, D. L. (2005). *The role of aging in adult learning: Implications for instructors in higher education.* Retrieved April 27, 2005, from http://www.newhorizons.org/lifelong/higher_ed/crawford.htm

Diamond, M. C. (2001, March 10). *Successful aging of the healthy brain.* Paper presented at the Conference of the American Society on Aging and the National Council on the Aging, New Orleans, LA. Retrieved April 27, 2005, from http://www.newhorizons.org/neuro/diamond_aging.htm

Dunlosky, J., Cavallini, E., Roth, H., McGuire, C. L., Vecchi, T., & Hertzog, C. (2007). Do self-monitoring interventions improve older adult learning? *Journals of Gerontology Series B: Psychological Sciences & Social Sciences*, 62 B(special issue 1), 70–76.

Dyck, J., & Smither, J. (1994). Age differences in computer anxiety: The role of computer, experience, gender, and education. *Journal of Educational Computing Research, 10*(3), 239–248.

Eun-Shim, N., Preece, J., Resnick, B., & Mills, M. (2004). Usability of health web sites for older adults: A preliminary study. *Computers, Informatics, Nursing, 22*(6), 326–334.

Formosa, M. (2002). Critical gerogogy: Developing practical possibilities for critical educational gerontology. *Education and Ageing, 17*(1), 73–85.

Fox, S. (2004). *Older Americans and the Internet.* Retrieved April 27, 2005, from http://www.pewinternet.org/pdfs/PIP_Seniors_Online_2004.pdf

Harris Interactive. (2000). *AARP survey on lifelong learning.* Retrieved April 27, 2005, from http://www.aarp.org/research/reference/publicopinions/Articles/aresearch-import-490.html

Hatcliffe, S. (2003). Standing in their shoes. *Journal for Nurses in Staff Development, 19*(4), 183–186.

Hixon, A. (2004). Functional health literacy: Improving health outcomes. *American Family Physician, 69*(9).

Retrieved April 29, 2005, from http://www.aafp.org/afp/20040501/medicine.html

Institute of Medicine. (2004). *Health literacy: A prescription to end confusion.* Retrieved October 26, 2005, from http://www.iom.edu/object.file/master/19/726/0.pdf

Keppel, K. G. (2007). Ten largest racial and ethnic health disparities in the United States based on Healthy People 2010 objectives. *American Journal of Epidemiology, 166,* 97–103.

Knowles, M. (1984). *The adult learner: A neglected species* (3rd ed.). Houston, TX: Gulf.

National Institute on Aging & National Institutes of Health. (2007). *Growing older in America: The health and retirement study.* Retrieved on August 21, 2008, from http://www.nia.nih.gov/NR/rdonlyres/D164FE6C-C6E0-4E78-B27F-7E8D8C0FFEE5/0/HRS_Text_WEB.pdf

National Institute on Aging & National Library of Medicine. (2002). *Making your Web site senior friendly.* Retrieved April 28, 2005, from http://www.nlm.nih.gov/pubs/checklist.pdf

Palmer, J. A. (2006). Nursing implications for older adult patient education. *Plastic Surgical Nursing, 26*(4), 189–194.

Pew Internet and American Life Project. (2008). *Latest trends.* Retrieved on December 1, 2008, from http://www.pewinternet.org/trends.asp.

Resnick, B. (2002). The impact of self-efficacy and outcome expectations on functional status in older adults. *Topics in Geriatric Rehabilitation, 17*(4), 1–10.

Reynolds, S. (2005). Teaching the older adult. *Journal of the American Geriatric Society, 53*(3), 554–555.

Schloman, B. (2004). Health literacy: A key ingredient for managing personal health. *Online Journal of Issues in Nursing.* Retrieved December 1, 2008, from http://www.nursingworld.org/MainMenuCategories/ANAMarketplace/ANAPeriodicals/OJIN/TableofContents/Volume92004/No2May04/HealthLiteracyAKeyIngredientforManagingPersonalHealth.aspx

Sheppard, T. (2002). The learning journey. *Navy Supply Corps Newsletter.* Retrieved April 27, 2005, from http://www.findarticles.com/p/articles/mi_m0NQS/is_3_65/ai_90624361

Shysh, A. (2000). Adult learning principles: You can teach an old dog new tricks. *Canadian Journal of Anesthesia, 47*(3), 837–842.

Thomas, C. M. (2007). Bulletin boards: A teaching strategy for older audiences. *Journal of Gerontological Nursing, 33*(3), 45–52.

Timmermann, S. (2003). Older adult learning: Shifting priorities in the 21st century. *Aging Today, 24*(4). Retrieved April 29, 2005, from http://www.agingtoday.org/at/at-244/Older_Adult.cfm

VanBiervliet, A., & Edwards-Schafer, S. P. (2004). Consumer health information on the Web: Trends, issues, and strategies. *Dermatology Nursing, 16*(6), 519–523.

Volland, P., & Berkman, B. (2004). Education social workers to meet the challenge of an aging urban population: A promising model. *Academic Medicine, 79*(12), 1192–1197.

Whittemore, R. (2007). Culturally competent interventions for Hispanic adults with type 2 diabetes: A systematic review. *Journal of Transcultural Nursing, 18,* 157–166.

Withnall, A. (2002). Three decades of educational gerontology: Achievements and challenges. *Education and Aging, 17*(1), 87–102.

CHAPTER 10

Promoting Independence in Later Life

Luana S. Krieger-Blake, MSW, LCSW

Learning Objectives

At the end of this chapter, the reader will be able to:

- Recognize the importance of self-care in maintaining independence in later life.
- Acknowledge influences of the environment and living situation on the ability to maintain independence.
- Identify strategies to maximize physical and mental function.
- Discuss multiple role changes and transitions that are common to the elderly.
- Develop awareness of preventing complications of existing illness or disease.
- Appreciate the value of rehabilitation.
- Identify the appropriateness of physical and chemical restraints, as well as suitable alternatives when available.
- Describe care options for the elderly and community resources especially suitable to meet their needs.

Key Terms

- Basic activities of daily living (BADLs)
- Frailty
- Functional ability
- Independence
- Instrumental activities of daily living (IADLs)
- Living skills
- Quality of life
- Restraints

This adage, commonly heard, rings true when considering the factors that influence independence in later life. Health, personality, state of mind, and emotional, physical, and spiritual support all have a place in the adjustments one makes to the aging process. Although self-care and health promotion are indeed important in maintaining independence, aging and accompanying health factors often make this a very difficult period of life. As a person moves from the earlier adjustments of aging (65–75 years) to the later ones (75–85 years), circumstances may become even more complex. Although level of physical activity tends to decrease with aging, "many older people can maintain health through social, intellectual, and cultural activities" (Fone & Lundgren-Lundquist, 2003, p. 1051).

Although it is important, high **functional ability** is not absolutely necessary for high **quality of life**. Because many elderly have chronic disabilities, it is important to recognize this distinction and find ways to maximize quality of life through other means—including spirituality, social engagement, environment, and connection—in addition to physical activity programs (Johansson, 2003).

Successful aging has been defined as "the ability to maintain three key behaviors: low risk of disease and disease-related disability, high mental and physical function, and active engagement of life" (Rowe & Kahn, 1998, p. 3). This chapter will discuss the factors that influence these behaviors. The case study interspersed throughout this chapter follows the story of one couple in transition.

Bessie and Sadie, the "Delany Sisters," are famous for remaining physically and mentally active into their second century. They experienced being on the best-seller book list, television talk shows, and national notoriety—all after they became 101 and 103 years of age, respectively! Their comments, advice, and wisdom are quoted periodically throughout this chapter to illustrate their attitudes about living fully.

Notable Quotes

"An ounce of prevention is worth a pound of cure."

—Henry deBracton

"No matter how old you get, you think of yourself as young. In our dreams, we are always young."

—Sadie Delany (Delany & Delany, 1994, p. 40)

"The aging of the U.S. population is one of the major public health challenges we face in the 21st century. One of CDC's highest priorities as the nation's health protection agency is to increase the number of older adults who live longer, high-quality, productive, and independent lives."

—Centers for Disease Control and Prevention (CDC) & Merck Company Foundation. (2007). *The state of aging and health in America, 2007*. Whitehouse Station, NJ: Merck Company Foundation, p. 2.

MAINTAINING INDEPENDENCE

Maintaining maximum **independence** while maintaining maximum quality of life is a balance sought by the elderly, their caregivers, and society in general. Aspects of achieving this balance are often in conflict with each other and are certainly affected by the many factors involved in the aging process (**Figure 10-1**).

Any evaluation of quality of life should include the perceptions of the person being evaluated. Even those with dementia are able to identify mood state, at times with more accuracy than their caregivers. Consideration of the whole person is important, and in so doing, the interdisciplinary team gains important information for developing evaluations, methods, and interventions (Johansson, 2003).

Influences of Environment and Living Situation

Although much emphasis in gerontological nursing is on the physiological aspects of an older person's life, the influences of the environment and the person's living situation can have a significant positive or negative influence on overall health. Living skills, housing, the ability and desire for self-care all influence the general picture of health and wellness.

Living Skills

Remaining in the community for as long as possible is the goal for most Americans, so it is important to be able to evaluate the ability of the person to remain safely in the community while having his or her needs met in an appropriate manner. Such an evaluation might utilize the Kohlman Evaluation of Living Skills (KELS), which has been adapted for the geriatric population and is commonly administered by occupational therapists. It assesses 17 daily **living skills** under five categories—self-care, safety and health, money management, transportation and telephone use, and work and leisure (Zimnavoda, Weinblatt, & Katz, 2002). Other evaluations that can help determine aspects of appropriateness for independent/community living include the Routine Task Inventory (RTI), the Functional Independence Measure (FIM), and the Mini Mental State Examination (MMSE), which screens for dementia—and against which the KELS was tested and compared. The Tinetti Assessment Tool, used by physical therapists, measures gait and balance in evaluating performance-oriented mobility.

Having practical, realistic, and nonsubjective evaluation tools would likely improve an elderly person's ability to identify and reconcile with the need for more care, and would certainly help families who are struggling to identify the level of assistance required by their elderly relatives. For example, a simple evaluation of the ability to use the telephone may help determine the appropriateness of a person remaining in the community.

FIGURE **10-1** **Factors that influence the quality of life of elderly adults.**

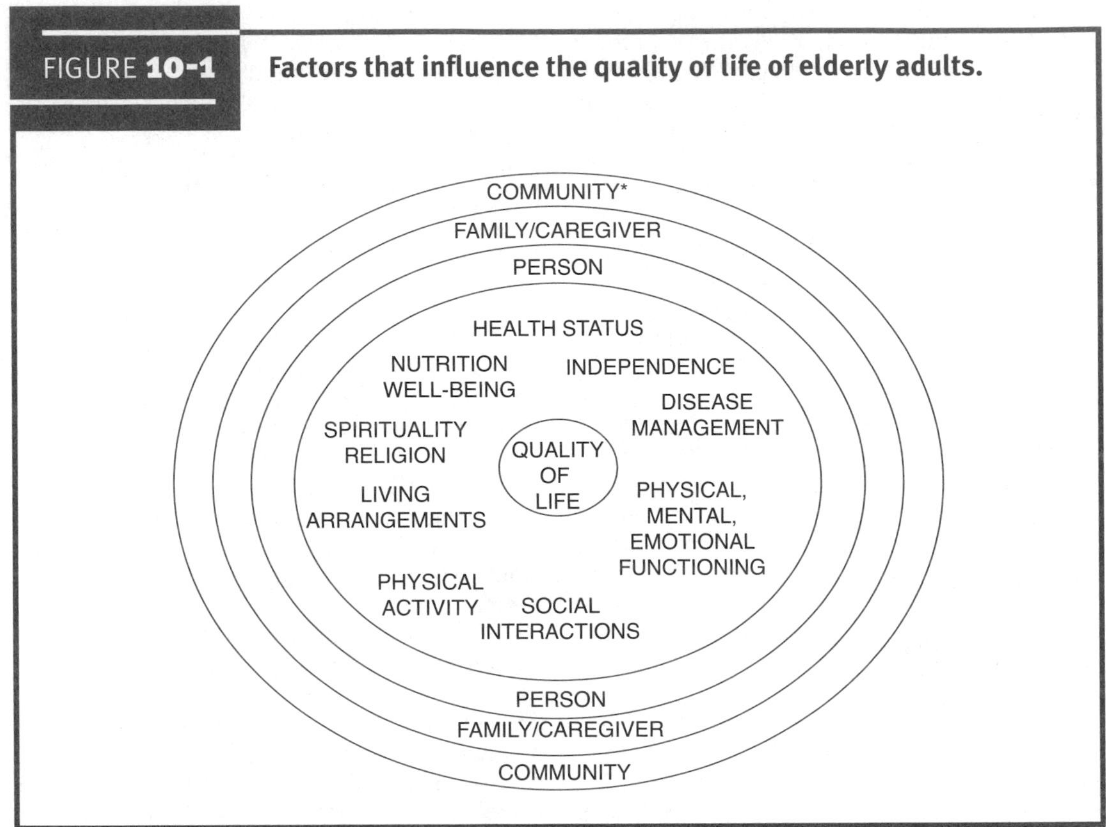

SOURCE: American Dietetic Association. (2005). Nutrition across the spectrum of aging. *Journal of the American Dietetic Association, 105*, 616–633.

Tested on persons with a dementia diagnosis who lived alone, a study found that if a person is unable to reply to a letter requesting a call and if they are unable to use the telephone book, home-alone safety must be questioned. Continuous "practice" in calling frequently used numbers (of family or caregivers) may help for a while, but when a person who lives alone cannot call for assistance or health care, and when even social communication by telephone has become too demanding to cope with, the safety risks of living alone must be considered (Nygard & Starkhammar, 2003).

Housing Influences

The word *home* holds special meanings, usually associated with familiarity as well as security, stability, feelings, memories, a sense of personal identity, and a place where we are in control and have choices. Moving from home to another setting may precipitate a loss of these special meanings and may be a very difficult adjustment—especially if the person is not a part of the planning, decision making, and distribution of belongings. When a move is seen as "something better," adjustment is easier. When it is due to disability and/or the need for additional care, the multiple losses of friends, independence, and control must be acknowledged and grieved. Health care workers and family members need to understand and acknowledge the person's feelings about all these issues and provide assistance and support throughout the adjustment (White, 2003).

Housing choices are greatly influenced by the socioeconomic status and resources of the elderly person. Individuals with more access to quality health care often have better functional abilities and longer life expectancies (Stupp, 2000). Better functional ability and income then affect the number of options and types of living choices available to meet the needs of the elderly, which may, in turn, impact their health. Those with limited incomes may not be able to afford some of the choices that might lead to a healthier living environment.

Housing options include:

- One's own home (independently, or with additional caregiver assistance)
- Family/relative's home
- Senior living complexes/continuing care/supported living retirement communities
- Assisted living facilities
- Paid caregiver homes—licensed or unlicensed
- Extended care facilities

Notable Quotes

"Most folks think getting older means giving up, not trying anything new. Well, we don't agree with that. As long as you can see each day as a chance for something new to happen, something you never experienced before, you will stay young . . . even after a century of living, we haven't tried everything. We've only just started."

—Sadie Delany (Delany & Delany, 1994, p. 11)

"So we do our little bit. Getting involved is satisfying. It keeps us busy and makes us useful. Everyone has something to contribute!"

—Bessie Delany (Delany & Delany, 1994, p. 90)

Carefully designed and implemented retirement communities address the concerns and feelings of displacement that moving from one's home to the unfamiliarity of new surroundings engenders. Some communities provide housing, community life, socialization, transportation, and health care for the elderly. Easily accessible on-site services—which might include recreational activities, social services, spiritual support, banking, and health care—provide a continuum of care that offers an opportunity to "age in place." Other care needs are met with additional services as the needs manifest themselves. Some communities include assisted living and extended care facilities within the community itself. These communities usually require payment of fees and/or monthly service charges (Reicherter & Billek-Sawhney, 2003).

For those who can afford them, retirement communities offer a certain freedom from the stresses of family care, while offering additional security from the risks of neighborhood living. Compared to older people living in the local neighborhood, the retirement community population in one study better maintained their physical and mental health. Peer support, safety and security, and autonomy with inclusion were important factors in maintaining health status. Age-specific shared living can also contribute to enhanced morale while serving as an antidote to age-related prejudice (Kingston, Bernard, Biggs, & Nettleton, 2001).

Self-Care

Maintaining interests or developing new ones is a measure of satisfactory aging. Learning, growing, creating, and enjoying are some of the essential outcomes for measurement of successful aging. Satisfaction and personal growth transcend developmental stages and are dependent on the individual's prior interests, ability to focus on new interests, and availability of and access to additional resources.

For the elderly person with the capacity for activities of some kind, doing for others is another way to measure satisfactory aging. Altruism is high in the elderly; charity giving is proportionately higher for older than for younger age groups (Ebersole & Hess, 1998). Volunteering in various capacities is another way the older person can contribute to his or her community—through peer support, church activities, even maintenance of a small area of an extended care facility. One lady ran a small gift shop of donated items for an hour or two per day in her facility. Another brought her pet bird to visit the residents. These small gestures were activities well within the capabilities of mobility-limited women, but brought them pleasure and contributed to the morale of others as well.

A Canadian study suggests that a uniform concept of **frailty**, relevant to older adults, would have important policy implications, and could improve the planning and distribution of services to those who would benefit. The study recommends a uniform theoretical approach that is multidimensional (not age-related), subjectively defined, and includes both individual and environmental factors (Fried et al., 2001).

Frailty is perceived as a general decline in the physical function of older adults that can increase vulnerability to illness and decline. Defining characteristics include unintentional weight loss of more than 10% in the prior year, feelings of exhaustion, grip strength in the weakest 20% for age, walking speed in the lowest 20% for age, and low caloric expenditure (<270 kcal) per week on physical activity. Neither age nor disability alone makes a person frail, but changes that often occur with age may contribute significantly to its presence. At nearly every age past 65, women commonly experience frailty at a greater percentage than men (Fried et al., 2001).

Notable Quotes

"I'd say one of the most important qualities to have is the ability to create joy in your life. . . . I love my garden so much that I would stay out there all day long if Sadie let me. That's what I mean about creating joy in your life. We all have to do it for ourselves."

—Bessie Delany (Delany & Delany, 1994, pp. 32–33)

"Some people, older people especially, tend to draw into themselves . . . they grow isolated. That's a big mistake! You never know when you might need other people, but you need to earn their help. You have to contribute to your community."

—Bessie Delany (Delany & Delany, 1994, p. 89)

Harvard Women's Health Watch (Forestalling Frailty, 2003) suggests several steps that can be taken to prevent or interrupt the course of frailty:

- Maintain a healthy weight and diet.
- Stay active.
- Practice fall prevention.
- Make connections—maintain relationships with others.
- See medical personnel regularly—physician, eye doctor, dentist.

Role Changes/Transitions

Multiple role changes occur over the course of one's life, and that is no different for the elderly. Changes are sometimes affected by choice, but as people age, their role changes and transitions may increasingly occur outside their control. These changes may be abrupt, crisis-oriented, and undesired, or there may be some time and opportunity for adjustment to the change. Some changes may be very subtle, with a slow shift from one self-concept to another—mostly recognized after the fact. Past skills and a series of adaptations may help prepare for some transitions—like the primary shift from parenting to grandparenting—making them smoother and less stressful. But the shift from functional independence to functional dependence and from health to illness crosses many aspects of life, and likely requires a series of transitional adjustments. These transitions require the freedom of the individual to try various possibilities, as within any other stage of life (see **Case Study 10-1**). Exploration and independence in making adjustments should be encouraged (Ebersole & Hess, 1998).

Retirement

Retirement is perhaps one of the most common role changes faced by the aging person. This is an occurrence that can be planned for and anticipated, or it may be sudden and unexpected (related to illness or injury). Some people find a lack of purpose and fulfillment with this transition, whereas others feel a new sense of personal freedom and time for activities postponed during busier years. Additionally, some find their availability tempered with the need to provide care to those around them, whether older or younger.

Some make the choice to continue to work past "retirement age" because of financial necessity, enjoyment of the challenge, socialization, a need for structure, or the status inherent in the work role. Others, who retire unwillingly, may be at greater risk for unsuccessful adjustments—including alcoholism, depression, and suicide. These people may seek medical intervention, but may not recognize the underlying depression.

Health Transition

The transition from health to illness involves changes in lifestyle, self-concept, and perhaps a lost sense of value and relationships. It is also a change that may occur very subtly, over time, with the development of chronic conditions of increasing disability. Or it may have a sudden onset with a precipitating medical event.

Case Study 10-1

Bill retired at age 65 from a major corporation, where he had been a materials testing engineer. Marge was a homemaker, who worked part time in her church office and a gift shop after their four children were grown and left the house. Bill and Marge were raised during the Depression years and had developed frugal living and financial habits, which enabled them to acquire a sufficient nest egg for their retirement and later years.

They physically worked hard together over the years in building their dream home on a small lake, valuing independence and self-sufficiency as very important quality-of-life indicators. Their relationship of 50 years was frequently contentious, and they often quarreled or verbally sparred as a mode of communication. They were, however, quite committed to each other and Marge did not consider a life without Bill. Marge had been medicated for years for treatment of depression, but had not taken advantage of the recommended counseling support to increase the efficacy of her medication because of Bill's lack of faith in the counseling process and his active ridicule when she attempted it.

At the age of 68, Marge was diagnosed with breast cancer. When their long-time family physician retired the day after her diagnosis, she decided to seek active treatment with an oncologist friend of her daughter who lived in Apex, 3 hours away in the next state. Considerable trust in the physician and ability to maintain some independence in the familiarity of their travel trailer parked in a daughter's driveway made this decision possible. She underwent a left mastectomy at the hospital in Apex.

Critical Thinking: As the discharge nurse at the hospital, what factors influence your suggestions for follow-up protocols/procedures? Consider the traditional release instructions; patient to be 150 miles from the physician with physical assistance from her husband; and the family being less accessible due to distance.

Loss of Spouse

Loss of a spouse causes a profound role change, with numerous transitions. Women who are widowed commonly experience anxiety and fear in the first few years after their loss. Losing the partner in a long, close, and satisfying relationship may feel like the loss of self and one's "core." Even those widows who successfully reorganize their lives and invest in family, friends, and activities find they still profoundly miss their "other half." A new identity, with autonomy and individuation, is often the product of a successful adaptation to widowhood. This adaptation may or may not include remarriage.

Long-term relationships that were markedly unsatisfying may result in a degree of complicated mourning for the widow or widower, accompanied by guilt, anger, or perhaps relief that the relationship has ended. The potential exists that the remaining partner may find other outlets for the negativity they experienced in the relationship. Or they may not have the self-confidence or ability for independent decision making because of a long history of domination by the other. This will likely affect their roles in their families or other support systems, and will certainly affect their adjustment capabilities.

Generally speaking, men who are widowed often hide their grief in a distorted concept of "manliness," in which they carry their pain alone. Until recent years, society has not given men the same explicit permission to grieve as it has afforded to women. Widowers seem to pay less attention to themselves, lose social contacts, and can experience an erosion of self-confidence and sexuality. Widower status in elderly men has been found to be a risk factor for increased dependency in activities of daily living (ADLs) and mobility (van den Brink, 2004). Some men tend to reinvest in new relationships in search of the lost mate, before reconciling to the death of their spouse.

Becoming more common for the elderly, divorce can force a change in roles. The necessity to grieve is similar for this role change, and the need for adjustment may be more devastating if it is unanticipated. There are major individual and generational differences in the expectations for marriage, but even older couples are becoming less likely to remain in unsatisfactory relationships (Ebersole & Hess, 1998).

Individuals with few family or social supports have a more difficult time adjusting to the loss of a spouse than do those with information about the grief process, sufficient support, and permission and time to experience fully their grief.

Role Reversal

Role reversal with a spouse or adult children often occurs for the aging person, as the elder moves from care provider to care recipient through the course of aging. When a very strong and independent elder experiences failing health, the transition to dependency may drain the energies of both the provider and the recipient who are part of the role reversal (see **Case Study 10-2**). If a spouse or adult child is a rather passive or dependent person, he or she may need considerable help in adjusting to the transitions (Ebersole & Hess, 1998).

Some older persons may enjoy the dependency of their failing health, which can create burdens for their families and care providers. Their demanding personalities and failure to maximize their remaining independence can tax the strength, resources, and patience of their caregivers.

Case Study 10-2

Marge's treatment over the next year consisted of 6 months of chemotherapy, CT scans, and oncology appointments. Marge and Bill would travel with their trailer to Apex for each course of treatment as it was scheduled, stay a few days in their daughter's driveway after treatment, and then return to their own home, where Bill cared for her until her treatment reactions subsided. Marge was devastated by her hair loss, and especially by the nausea and vomiting episodes that cumulatively increased with each treatment. Nearing the end of the scheduled treatments, she was begging to forgo the last one.

Critical Thinking: As the oncologist's office nurse, how would you respond to Marge's family who called, relating her tearful refusal to submit to the last chemo treatment, and requesting your advice?

Case Study 10-3

Bill and Marge celebrated their 50th wedding anniversary with a wig and a large party of family, extended family, and friends on the lawn of their beloved lake house. They were able to travel in their trailer for a number of years, even renting their house out for a few years. They spent their time wintering in the south, visiting various family members during the summers, and taking extended travel trips with their travel association. They carried their medical records with them and were treated as needed in the locations where they spent the most time.

Marge had large toe joint replacement while they wintered in Florida and was able to rehab and resume her routine of walking several miles per day. This exercise not only allowed her to be out in the natural beauty of the location, which she cherished, but also kept her in shape and stimulated her ability to sleep better at night, as well as providing some separation from Bill for several hours each day.

During one winter away, Bill was examined for cardiac dysrythmia and palpitations, was diagnosed with tachycardia, and was given medications to control the symptoms he experienced. They returned to life at their home by the lake when Marge began reporting increased confusion in Bill, as well as expressing some fears about his driving, also witnessed by one of the adult children visiting them for a spring break vacation. Another daughter traveled to Florida to drive them and their travel trailer home. Bill voiced much displeasure at the daughter's insistence on driving—insisting he was a far better driver—even though his family had observed confusion in a major intersection, driving the wrong way on a marked street, and other incidents.

After significant family intervention, including individual conversations and a family meeting to discuss the driving concerns, Bill was evaluated by a physician and agreed to psychological testing to determine his ability to continue driving. Probably because of his IQ and propensity for mechanics, Bill placed in the low acceptable percentiles of the test results for his age group and gender. However, the family questioned the test validity because the administrator didn't factor in Bill's history as an engineer and did not take into account the many reports of the decline in Bill's own function vs. the standardized test results. As a result, Bill drove awhile longer, until the physician prohibited his driving some months later after more family reports of increasing safety issues.

With this forced curtailment of driving, Bill became very angry, demonstrating much difficulty in coping with the limitations, and definitely grieving. His negativity and demanding behavior placed increased stress on Marge. He often refused to allow her to drive, making demeaning comments when she did. He further blamed family conspiracy and the physician, challenging suggested medical interventions and the doctor's professional judgment.

Personal Reflection: As a student nurse and a college student now embarking on your own quest for independence, can you relate to losing a major independent activity such as driving? Has anyone in your family faced such a situation? How might you help your parents or your grandparents with the adjustment to giving up driving, a major factor in a person's perception of independence?

Driving

Driving a car is an area of independence with strong emotional and psychological implications, in addition to those of physical capacity. It represents the ability to maintain connections and contribute to the community (Silverstein, Carr, & Kerschner, 2004). Dementia, use of some medications, fractures, cardiac conditions, and poor vision may limit a person's ability to drive, and cessation of driving has been shown to increase symptoms of depression for up to 6 years (Kakaiya, Tisovec, & Fulkerson, 2000).

Safe driving requires not only sound physical and mental capacity, but also alertness, the ability to interpret and judge surroundings, and appropriate reflexes and strength for reaction. The elderly person may be experiencing decline in some of these abilities. The ultimate decision as to whether a person should continue to drive is made by the local licensing authority, but families and patients often look to their physician for help in determining the person's continuing fitness to drive. A number of factors influence the evaluation of fitness to drive, as outlined in **Box 10-1**.

BOX 10-1 Evaluation Factors of Fitness to Drive

- Crash rates per mile driven
- Modification of driving (e.g., fewer miles driven per month; limiting driving to familiar roads, daytime hours, or good weather conditions)
- Driving history (e.g., getting lost in familiar surroundings, near misses, near crashes, traffic violation tickets)
- Medication use
- Visual faculties needed for safe driving (e.g., contraction of visual fields, decline in resistance to glare)
- Cognition assessment instruments (e.g., Mini Mental State Examination, Washington Clinical Rating Scale)
- On-road test by driver's licensing authority
- Effect of terminating patient's right to drive

Source: Kakaiya, R., Tisovec, R., & Fulkerson, P. (2000). Evaluation of fitness to drive: The physician's role in assessing elderly or demented patients. *Postgrad Med*, *107*(3), 229–236.

Instrumental Activities of Daily Living

Instrumental activities of daily living (IADLs), such as cleaning and cooking, shopping, running errands, keeping appointments, maintaining the checkbook, and paying bills, may require the assistance of others. Ability, or not, to maintain these tasks is often defined by functional limitations—sometimes briefly, as during convalescence from a surgery or temporary disability. A precipitating event or advancing illness sometimes makes these role changes more permanent.

Basic Activities of Daily Living

Basic activities of daily living (BADLs) involve personal care, such as bathing, dressing, and feeding. The need for assistance in these activities usually comes subsequent to the need for help with IADLs, unless there is a precipitating factor that causes the need. As physical abilities decrease, need for assistance increases.

Notable Quotes

"Don't depend too much on any one person. If you have a lot of helpers, you can be sure that someone will always be available when you need it. You'll feel a lot more independent. We have different folks who do different things for us—like give us a ride, go to the post office, or buy our vitamins. By spreading out these little favors, we're not a big burden on anyone."

—Sadie and Bessie Delany (Delany & Delany, 1994, p. 126)

Caregiving

As a person requires more and more assistance with IADLs and BADLs, issues of caregiving escalate. At times, the need for caregiver assistance arises long before acceptance of that care. Some elderly may resist recognition of the need for help because that very need exemplifies their increasing limitations and the inability to maintain their independence. Family members may also resist recognizing the need, not wanting to diminish the dignity and freedom of choice for their loved one.

Care Options. A broad spectrum of care options is available when unassisted independent living is no longer possible or appropriate:

Case Study 10-4

Within several years, Marge was diagnosed with Parkinson's disease in its early stages and experienced an increase in her depression, anticipating the expected progressive nature of the disease and demonstrating her fear of a much reduced quality of life. She was embarrassed by the shaking symptoms and tended to isolate herself—declining some dinner and other outing invitations she had previously enjoyed. This tended to separate her from some of her long-standing friends, acquaintances, and church activities. It also kept her at home more in Bill's ongoing negative presence.

Bill's new physician sent him for a cardiac oblation procedure that effectively took care of his symptoms. He was able to discontinue his medications for that problem, and he and his family began seeing a measure of improvement in his confusion and ability to concentrate. Of course, to Bill, this meant he was able to drive again, which he did—to the dismay of his family. Wintering away once again, he re-obtained permission to drive from a doctor-friend from church, who neither invited nor considered any family input. This modest measure of functional improvement also cemented in Bill's mind his perception that the doctors had erred in giving him the cardiac medication in the first place. He did not acknowledge that the medicine had managed his symptoms for several years. It further bolstered his resistance to obtaining medical care for himself while at the same time negating the care Marge was seeking and receiving for her Parkinson's diagnosis and depression.

Living in their hometown placed Bill and Marge 150–250 miles from any of their children. At the ages of 78 and 73, they reluctantly made the decision to give up their dream home of 40 years. Their long-time circle of friends was gradually shrinking. They were no longer able to maintain the rigorous maintenance schedule for their too-large house, and they were experiencing increased physical problems. Although Bill did not perceive the need for himself, he was able to accommodate the decision "for Marge's sake," recognizing she would need increasing help as time passed and her Parkinson's progressed. Marge looked forward to being nearer three of her four children, and in actual proximity to two of them. Bill and Marge sold their home and invested in a condominium near Apex, between two of their daughters.

They also developed their estate plan, completed advance directives, and discussed with their children their desire to remain in their own home throughout their lifetimes. They planned to bring in assistance as needed for meeting their care needs, which they readily verbalized would only increase over time. In fact, their condo could accommodate a live-in caregiver with a separate bedroom, sitting area, and private bathroom.

Bill was diagnosed with benign prostate enlargement and tested several times for cancer because of his high PSA test results and frequent leaks from his bladder. Over a period of months he had a TURP procedure but experienced ongoing difficulty urinating and urinary retention, necessitating Foley catheter placement. His urologist ordered home nursing for catheter care and teaching related to its use. While insisting on being independent with day-to-day ADLs, Bill mostly ignored his need for bathing and grooming—satisfied to wear the same clothes until Marge captured them for the laundry. He could empty his catheter bag by himself, but he apparently did not comprehend the need for clean technique when handling the catheter. When the home care nurse visited, Marge reported that he often let the bag drag by the catheter tubing behind him on the floor when he walked through the house, while he sat at the kitchen table, or went to bed. This did not appear to be painful to him, and he disregarded any family discussion about tight connections, sterile atmosphere, and the social impact of his habit.

Bill was resistant to bathing and shaving—sometimes going for several weeks. He would resent and decline Marge's encouragement and offer of help to do his personal care; he especially resented his family's request for a home health aide to encourage and assist him in bathing.

During this time period, Bill and Marge's family tried a variety of care arrangements to meet their increasing needs, including a housekeeper every week, a cook three times a week to prepare Marge's diabetic meals, prepared meal delivery, and aide assistance for bathing and personal care.

Critical Thinking: As the visiting home care nurse, how would you approach Bill regarding catheter care, personal care, motivation for self-care, Marge's reports of frequent dozing wherever he was, and refusal to eat the meals arranged for by his family?

Are there other possible diagnoses Bill's family should be aware of, alerted to, or educated about?

What other resources may assist them in maintaining some level of independence at home, at this stage of their aging and increasing needs?

Personal Reflection: Imagine that you are 70–80 years old and must decide what to do with your lifetime of belongings, because your new location will accommodate less than half of them. What do you take? What do you do with the rest?

- *Independent living with help:* Cooks, companions, homemaker/cleaning service—formal or informal.
- *Family:* Usually informal; may live in patient's or family member's home.
- *Adult daycare at a facility:* Part-time temporary assistance, frequently for respite or while a family caregiver works; often used for persons with dementia or for the frail elderly needing assistance or at risk for social isolation. Usual discharge is to assisted living or death.
- *Adult daycare at home:* Part-time respite, as above.
- *Senior living complexes/continuing care/supported care retirement communities:* Full range or limited services, depending on the community and level of assistance needed; can be progressive as needs increase.
- *Assisted living:* Homelike setting with more physical and medical care available than in senior complexes.
- *Paid caregiver homes (licensed or unlicensed):* Caregivers accept one or several nonrelatives into their home to receive 24-hour assistance, especially with BADLs, usually on a private-pay basis. In some states, public subsidies may cover adult group/foster home care.
- *Extended care facilities:* Skilled or intermediate care nursing home facilities for rehabilitation or ongoing care; can be paid by Medicare,

Medicaid, or private pay, depending on financial resources. Preadmission screening is usually required by the state regulatory agency.

In planning and making placement for care, it is advisable to request and check provider references. Further discussion of these settings in relationship to nursing care is provided in Chapter 1.

Family caregivers provide the major percentage of informal, in-home care—sometimes at the cost of career advancement, and even the ability to retain employment if the care needs become too great. Family caregivers are challenged by lack of information, lack of practical skills training, and physical and emotional strain. Nurses have the opportunity to impact the care of their patient by giving attention to the family caregivers, remembering that care of the person also means care of the caregiver. In doing this, nurses need to think of the family as the extension of the patient. Several principles apply:

- Provide community resource information for ongoing help to the patient/family.
- Offer anticipatory guidance toward practical and emotional support resources.
- Respect all family caregivers. Assume they are doing the best they can under difficult circumstances.
- Help identify the strengths of the family caregivers, and point them out concretely; give positive reinforcement in all care settings.
- Help family caregivers recognize their own needs and limitations, because they may be at risk for their own health problems (Reinhard, 2001).

In interviews with caregivers, the nurse or interdisciplinary team member may gain additional insight into the patient/caregiver situation from the use of humor by caregivers. Often when relating anecdotes about various aspects of care, the caregiver might use humor to mask discomfort in talking about the issue. Use of humor may also provide caregivers with a face-saving way to explain thoughts and actions in their care provider role. Humor may also provide a clue that the area being discussed may be an area of unresolved conflict or concern, without the caregiver having to say that they are having difficulty. Sensitive probing questions may help identify the need for additional education, revision of treatment plan, or more practical assistance for the patient and caregiver (Sparks, Travis, & Pecchioni, 2000).

> **Notable Quotes**
>
> *"Never lose your sense of humor. The happiest people are the ones who are able to laugh at themselves."*
>
> —Sadie and Bessie Delany (Delany & Delany, 1994, p. 34)

Patients, family members, and caregivers may also use humor as stress relief and to lighten the load of providing care. Humor can provide a welcome relief to the often serious aspects of caretaking.

Caregiver stress may be a factor in whether a person can remain in the home setting. Caregivers who live with their care recipient have a higher level of strain than those who live separately. Financial resources and/or higher education levels do not necessarily mean that the role strain is lessened. The health of the caregiver is important in determining stress levels. When the caregiver's health is poor in addition to that of the care recipient, caregiver stress is likely to be higher (Williams, Dilworth-Anderson, & Goodwin, 2003). Follow-up contacts initiated by agencies receiving a referral for families who need assistance and support enhance the use of those services by the families/caregivers (McCallion, Toseland, Gerber, & Banks, 2004).

Psychosocial and Spiritual Influences

Sometimes the elderly feel they have outlived their meaning, purpose, and usefulness—especially if they are debilitated and must depend on others for care. Ira Byock, in his book, *The Four Things That Matter Most*, suggests that adults tend to think their accomplishments should shield them from the "supposed indignity of physical dependence. This is an illusion," he states (2004, pp. 90–91). He believes that people are inherently dignified, that physical dependence does not detract from their dignity, and that people needlessly suffer from that self-belief. He suggests that providing care fills a need for the caregiver, as well as meeting a need for the care receiver. He encourages the dependent person to allow and accept their family and friends to meet their need to provide care, making a reciprocal relationship—not just a dependent, or one-way, relationship.

Socialization

Relationships provide the structure for social support and connections. These social networks remain important for the elderly, even as physical changes may limit their participation in the network and the network itself may shrink due to the loss of some of its members. Primary relationships are usually with family. For the elderly, these relationships usually provide cross-generational affection and assistance—highly valued evidence of concern and encouragement. As family becomes less available, relationships may be merged with friends and cohabitants of residential facilities.

Socialization is impacted by living arrangements. About 95% of the older adult population lived independently in 2000, of whom about 73% of men and 41% of women lived with their spouse. Several hundred thousand also had grandchildren in their household (American Dietetic Association [ADA], 2002).

Socialization also impacts nutritional intake. Healthy individuals have better food intake—up to 44% greater—when eating with others instead of eating alone (ADA, 2002).

Notable Quotes

"For true happiness, you've got to have companionship—other people . . . in your life. It doesn't have to be a husband or a wife. It can be a friend or, like us, a sister. . . ."

—Sadie Delany (Delany & Delany, 1994, p. 83)

"By now, we've outlived just about everyone we used to know, so many of our friends are much younger than we are. That doesn't matter as long as you care about the same things and, just as important, if you have the same sense of humor. And you know what? Younger people can teach you a lot. They can keep you up to date. So we'll take 'home folks' wherever we find them!"

—Sadie Delany (Delany & Delany, 1994, p. 84)

". . . I cherish most . . . the family traditions, all those little rituals that bind you together . . . like eating meals together, that keep you close. . . . They think it doesn't matter. Well, they're wrong! . . . It was comforting and it was fun."

—Bessie Delany (Delany & Delany, 1994, pp. 19–20)

Spiritual Influences

Spirituality is more than the response to a religion or set of beliefs. It relates to the core of the person's being and his or her connection to the universe. Ultimately, it has to do with one's meaning and purpose in life. As seniors review their lives—often in the presence of disease, disability, and perhaps impending death—their questions may reflect these issues: "Who am I? Did, or do, I make a difference? What is next? Can I handle getting old? What will become of me?" (Taylor, 2001, p. 1). These are spirit-oriented questions, which may indicate a spiritual searching. This searching should be taken into account when helping the patient to identify and achieve his or her goals (Taylor, 2001).

> *People who are facing potentially long-term or debilitating illnesses, confronting acute health crises, or suffering from loss and grief may find themselves re-examining the foundational beliefs they have held since childhood. Usually, at no other time in a person's life is he or she so focused on evaluating the spiritual self than during such crises. . . . (Mauk & Schmidt, 2004, p. 2)*

Ira Byock further encourages resolution of any personal, emotional, and spiritual issues while there is time and opportunity to do so, with the simple but most profound phrases of ". . . please forgive me . . . I forgive you . . . thank you . . . I love you . . . " (Byock, 2004, p. 3).

A Duke University study supported by the National Institute of Aging found that in the over-65 population, people who attend religious services regularly (once or more per week) had a lower incidence of chronic health problems, disabilities, depression, and smoking and alcohol use. They also tended to have less anxiety, lower blood pressure, fewer strokes, fewer suicides, and less depression and substance abuse than less frequent attendees. And they tended to live longer, with a 28% lower chance of dying in the next 6 years (Helm, Hays, Flint, Koenig, & Blazer, 2000). Stress management may be an issue for the elderly, especially as their capacity for adaptation is taxed, at a time when uncontrollable changes may be occurring in their care needs and living circumstances on a regular basis. Some stress management strategies that are effective for other age groups might also be appropriate for the elderly. Being in tune with one's feelings is a starting point from which expression of emotions might be appropriate. Others include exercise, prayer, deep breathing, daydreaming, progressive relaxation, design of a quiet environment, meditation or guided imagery, and developing a clear understanding of the *person's* goals (vs. the stated or implied goals of others in their environment).

Notable Quotes

"You know, when you are this old, you don't know if you're going to wake up in the morning. But I don't worry about dying, and neither does Bessie. We are at peace. You do kind of wonder, when it's going to happen? That's why you learn to love each and every day, child."

—Sadie Delany (Delany & Delany, 1993, p. 205)

"You can't change the past, and too many folks spend their whole lives trying to fix things that happened before their time. You're better off using your time to improve yourself."

—Sadie Delany (Delany & Delany, 1994, p. 19)

"Pride in a job well done is the one kind of pride God allows you to have. I earned that pride. Nothing brings more satisfaction than doing quality work, than knowing that you've done the very best you can. Reach high!"

—Bessie Delany (Delany & Delany, 1994, p. 39)

"It's important to eat healthy, but you won't live a long time unless you indulge yourself every once in awhile!"

—Sadie Delany (Delany & Delany, 1994, p. 114)

Goal Attainment

Old age is often associated with problems involving health and loss of functional ability. Nurses and other health care providers who care for the elderly in any capacity are frequently challenged to promote and maintain quality of life for the persons they serve. However, a goal of their care can rarely be defined as freedom from disease. Rather, we can "help patients to live as good a life as possible, despite their illnesses and decreasing capacities" (Sarvimaki & Stenbock-Hult, 2000, p. 1026). Sarvimaki and Stenbock-Hult's Finnish study to evaluate quality of life in old age found that people who were studied—those who lived in the community—"generally viewed their life as meaningful, intelligible and manageable . . . and seemed to have a strong sense of value or self-worth in terms of self-esteem" (p. 1032). Patients of other cultures and residential settings may have different responses; however, the patient of any culture or in any setting can provide strong clues as to what contributes to his or her own quality of life and goals. These clues can then be incorporated into development of activity programs and exercises.

MAXIMIZING FUNCTION

Preventing Complications of Existing Illness or Disease

Several factors play a role in successful aging. In addition to the discussion in this section, assessment and screenings are described in Chapters 7, 12, and 14.

Nutrition

Physical and mental decline are not necessarily a normal part of the aging process. They can be affected, however, by the person's nutritional status, because nutrition is one of the major determinants of successful aging. "Elderly patients with unintentional weight loss are at higher risk for infection, depression and death" (Huffman, 2002, p. 640). Some causes of involuntary weight loss are depression, cancer, cardiac disorders, gastrointestinal disorders, medications, polypharmacy, and changes in psychotropic medication (Huffman, 2002). Weight loss can also be an indicator of malnutrition or other acute medical conditions. Diagnosis of nutritional problems and appropriate intervention can prevent loss of function and independence (Ennis, Saffel-Shrier, & Verson, 2001). Helpful tips are noted in **Box 10-2**.

Sleep

Although sleep patterns often change as one ages, waking up tired every day and disturbed sleep pat-

BOX 10-2 Nutritional Tips for Older Adults

- Eat breakfast every day.
- Select high-fiber food like whole grain breads and cereals, beans, vegetables, and fruits.
- Have three servings of low-fat milk, yogurt, or cheese a day. Dairy products are high in calcium and vitamin D and help keep your bones strong as you age. Or take a calcium and vitamin D supplement.
- Drink plenty of water. You may notice that you feel less thirsty as you get older, but your body still needs the same amount of water.
- Ask your health care provider about ways you can safely increase the amount of physical activity you do now.
- Fit physical activity into your everyday life. For example, take short walks throughout your day. You do not have to have a formal physical activity program to improve your health and stay active.
- Get enough sleep.
- Stay connected with family, friends, and community.

Source: Weight-Control Information Network, National Institute of Diabetes and Digestive and Kidney Diseases (NIDDK). (2007). *Young at heart: Tips for older adults*. Retrieved January 9, 2008, from http://win.niddk.nih.gov/publications/young_heart.htm

terns are not considered a part of normal aging. Adequate sleep is essential to good health and to quality of life for all persons, including the elderly. Poor sleep contributes to a variety of problems including depression, attention and memory deficits, increased falls at night, increased use of medication to enhance sleep, and daytime sleepiness—all areas of increasing difficulty anyway for elderly folks. Poor sleep can exacerbate these conditions, may be increasingly problematic as a person ages, and can contribute to a poorer quality of life (NIH Senior Health, 2007).

Although short afternoon naps may help restore energy, too much daytime sleep may increase difficulty in sleeping at night. Interventions that may help promote sleep include:

- Maintain a regular routine and sleep-wake schedule every day, including weekends.
- Maintain a regular exercise schedule (finish workout at least 3 hours before bedtime).
- Have a safe and comfortable place to sleep (locks on doors, smoke alarm, easy-on lamp, phone by bed, darkened room, well-ventilated).
- Use the bedroom only for sleeping.
- Get exposure to natural light (sunlight) for several hours per day.
- Reduce the use of caffeine, alcohol, and tobacco, especially late in the day.
- Develop a bedtime routine for each night, to wind down (e.g., read, watch TV news, take a warm bath).
- After turning off the light, allow about 15 minutes to fall asleep; if still awake and not drowsy, get out of bed; go back to bed when you are drowsy (NIH Senior Health, 2007).

Additionally:

- Listening to classical or relaxing music at bedtime can promote relaxation.
- The bedtime routine should be per the patient's needs and wishes, not per a facility schedule.
- Reduce noise levels at night.
- Teach progressive whole-body relaxation techniques.

- Provide an individualized plan for each person.
- Use medication as a last resort (Gaspar, 1998).

Exercise

Participation in a regular exercise program has many benefits for elderly individuals. There are benefits for those with health-related issues such as cardiovascular disease, diabetes, and osteoporosis as well as functional benefits that allow for ongoing independence and activities of daily living. However, regular exercise programs are the key to ongoing positive outcomes. Challenges for nurses and other health care professionals in influencing the exercise capacity of the elderly have to do with education about exercise's ongoing importance, as well as designing interventions that will increase adherence and compliance with these exercise programs (Mazzeo & Tanaka, 2001).

> **Notable Quotes**
>
> *"We get up with the sun, and the first thing we do is exercise. God gave you only one body, so you better be nice to it. Exercise, because if you don't, by the time you're our age, you'll be pushing up daisies."*
>
> —Sadie Delany (Delany & Delany, 1994, p. 11)
>
> *"There's another thing I make Bessie do that she doesn't like too much, and that's exercise. You've got to exercise, not just for your heart and lungs, but to keep from stiffening up. It keeps you limber, and that's important when you get older."*
>
> —Sadie Delany (Delany & Delany, 1994, p. 109)

Basic guidelines for designing exercise programs for the elderly focus more on health and functional capacity than on aerobic fitness. Balance and gait are important aspects of assessments in older adults (see Chapter 7). Interacting elements of an exercise program include:

- *Warm-up:* Gentle stretching of muscles and light movement simulating the actual exercise activities.
- *Low to moderate intensity levels:* To avoid injury and to promote improvement in cardiac risk factors (adapted to tolerance and preferences).
- *Duration:* A longer duration of lower intensity is recommended over the reverse for a minimum of 30 minutes per day; 10 minutes, three times per day is also effective. Gradually increase the duration rather than the intensity.
- *Frequency:* Ideally, low to moderate exercise every day (or most days) of the week; for intense exercise, reduce the frequency.
- *Mode/type of exercise:* Should be based on the participant's fitness level and reflect his or her interests and available resources; walking, cycling, or swimming may be appropriate. Exercise facilities/fitness clubs offer a range of activities that can be combined into one workout (Mazzeo & Tanaka, 2001).

Exercises in water (aquatic therapy) are effective in improving balance and increasing strength and range of motion, especially for those persons with arthritis. The relative density of the person and the water and resulting buoyancy make the flexibility and mobility exercises easier, more effective, and less painful. These benefits then improve the person's balance and stability, which, in turn, helps in reducing falls (Suomi, 2001). For those active older adults who seek underwater adventure, scuba diving may be a sport they can experience and continue to enjoy with their children and grandchildren (**Figure 10-2** and **Figure 10-3**).

Although home exercise programs are helpful, supervised exercise training in a structured, physical therapy–type environment was found to be more beneficial in older physically frail community-dwelling adults. The formalized training reduced physical impairments and improved functional limitations more than the unsupervised home exercise programs. Its benefit was suggested to be "the prevention or postponement of frailty that is severe enough to cause loss of independence" (Binder et al., 2002, p. 1926). The additional socialization of a formal program, as well as the proximity of the university medical center setting, were thought to be additional benefits in this study.

Perhaps more practical, especially for residents of facilities—including assisted living facilities where a study was completed—might be a resident-led walking club. The socialization inherent in such a

FIGURE **10-2** **Active grandparents can share their sense of adventure with grandchildren as they are seen here scuba diving in the Bahamas.**

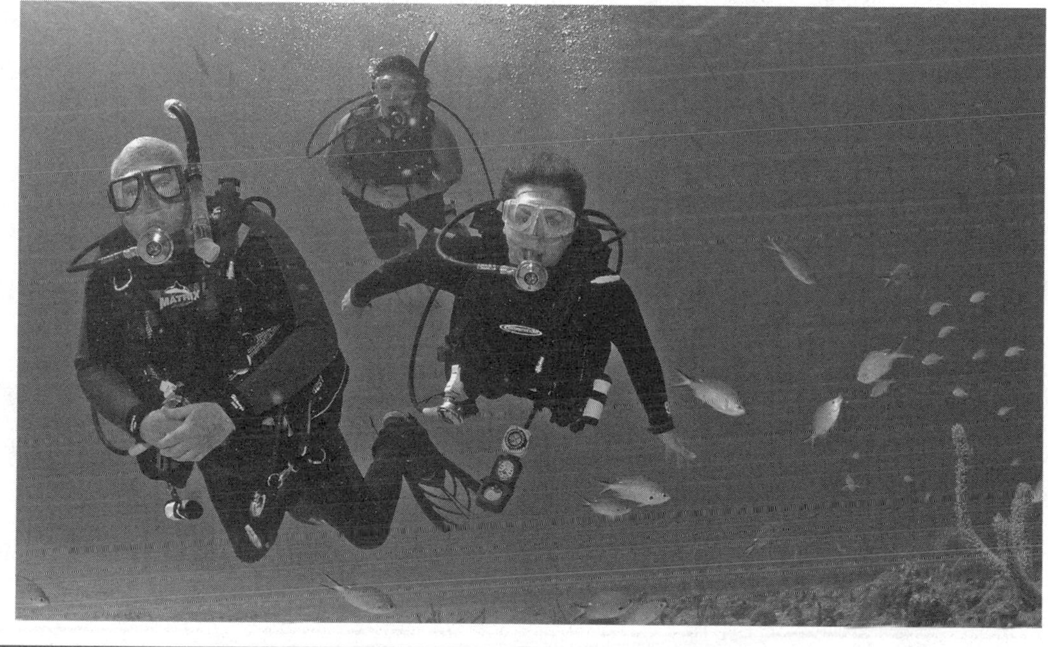

SOURCE: Courtesy of Stuart Cove (www.stuartcove.com)

program helps motivate the participants, which improves compliance. Study participation was voluntary. Daily participation and the distance goals were established by each resident depending on their physical status and endurance. A significant increase in each pretest measurement was noted. Residents found the experience pleasurable, a means to manage current health problems (e.g., arthritic knees), and noted positive physical and emotional benefits from the walking activity (easier to get in and out of an automobile, improved feeling of stability). The program produced benefits for the residents, and required little from the facility in the way of management and staff time (Taylor et al., 2003).

Yoga for exercise or rehabilitation is also appropriate for the elderly. Rather than focusing on the stereotypes of bizarre body positions and Eastern religious practices, the focus should be on the measurable physical and health benefits that result from prolonged practice of the tradition. Over time the practice of yoga, through emphasis on postures, breathing, and meditation, and simple body movements done with mindfulness, can result in increased strength, balance, stamina, flexibility, and relaxation—all areas needing attention from the elderly person (Taylor, 2001).

Fall Prevention

Assessment/Prediction

Numerous studies have determined the importance of evaluation of risk factors for falls, and the impact of physical decline and performance changes. Prevention of falls must take into account the living

FIGURE **10-3** **Active grandparents and grandchildren.**

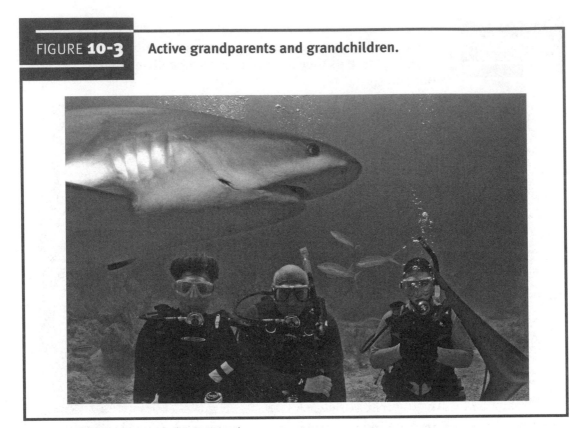

SOURCE: Courtesy of Stuart Cove (stuartcove.com)

situation of the elderly person. Those elderly with a more vigorous functional capacity usually fall due to hazards in their home (e.g., storage problems, clutter, scatter rugs). Falls for the frail elderly are not necessarily related to home hazards, but rather tend to relate to functional changes (e.g., poor depth perception, arthritis). Home modifications should be in place before the person becomes frail (Northridge & Levick, 2002).

Home interventions, which use home visits and a standardized checklist by a team of nurses, therapists, and a social worker, can be helpful in evaluating the potential environmental hazards that might contribute to falls. Suggestions of possible changes to the environment, facilitation of modifications, and training in the use of adaptive equipment were helpful in reducing the number of falls in a group of frail elderly with a history of falls. However, modifications to the environment alone were not sufficient to make the difference. Compliance with the physical changes as well as with the suggested behavioral changes was also important (Nikolaus & Bach, 2003).

Evaluation of physical performance measures may provide easily accessible screening for future risk of hospitalization and estimation of decline in health and function for older adults. Gait speed, chair rise, and balance evaluations provided information that led to prediction of emerging difficulty in physical care and a decline in physical function. Performance measures alone, or in combination with self-report measures, were able to predict outcomes more than self-report alone, suggesting a benefit to the increased use of performance measures as an additional "vital sign" for health-related risk in older adults (Studenski et al., 2003).

Strength (defined as the ability to exert force) is less of a predictor of positive outcomes than muscle power (defined as the ability to exert force quickly) (see **Figure 10-4**). Leg power has been correlated with gait speed, chair-rise time, and stair-climb time. Leg power is a better predictor of physical performance than is leg strength, as studied in community-dwelling, mobility-limited people (Bean et al., 2002).

Technological advances in the medical field have yielded the ability to assess patients for fall risk. Screening and medical products for diagnosing and treating dizziness and balance disorders, which identify those at greater risk for falls due to these causes, are becoming available to physicians, clinics, and facilities for treating the elderly (Vestibular Technologies, 2008).

The Value of Rehabilitation

A decline in quality of life is not necessarily inherent as physical frailty increases with age. Therefore, rehabilitation goals and interventions that affect the outcomes patients may expect to achieve can be developed to optimize each patient's quest for holistic growth. Because medical personnel and family members often place a higher regard on physical problems than the patients themselves do, and

FIGURE 10-4 Borg Category Rating Scale.

Least effort		
6		
7	very, very light effort	
8		
9	very light	
10		
11	fairly light	ENDURANCE
12		TRAINING
13	somewhat hard	ZONE
14		
15	hard	
16		STRENGTH
17	very hard	TRAINING
18		ZONE
19	very, very hard	
20		
Maximum effort		

The Borg category rating scale allows persons to rate their own level of exercise and target their desired level of activity. The numbers on the left allow persons to rate their perception of how hard they are working during an activity. The goal is a total of at least 30 minutes per day on most or every day of the week (NIA, 2008). Effort can be gradually increased, and the goal can be achieved in 10-minute segments to total 30 minutes per day. Strength training is recommended at least twice per week but not for consecutive days with the same muscle group. Persons should work gradually toward their fitness goals and consult with their primary health care provider prior to beginning any exercise program.

SOURCE: National Institute on Aging. (2008). *Exercise: A guide from the National Institute on Aging.* Page last updated 31 January, 2008. Retrieved June 1, 2008, from http://www.nia.nih.gov/HealthInformation/Publications/ExerciseGuide/chapter04.htm

Notable Quotes

"So you want to live to be 100. Well, start with this: No smoking, no drinking, no chewing. And always clean your plate. Well, you can drink a little bit, but not much!"

—Sadie Delany (Delany & Delany, 1994, p. 11)

"We try our best to preserve our health, and one way we do it is to watch what we eat and drink. We start our day by drinking a full glass of water, followed by a teaspoon of cod liver oil and a whole clove of garlic . . . we wash it down with one glass of cold water, then one glass of hot water."

—Bessie Delany (Delany & Delany, 1994, p. 107)

because aging is often seen as the functional losses that occur near the end of one's life, rehabilitation goals are frequently established simply to minimize the progressive losses of function. Rehabilitation goals may also affect one's spirituality and quality of life, in that the elderly may wish to overcome their limitations in search of a wholeness unique to the wisdom, meaning, and life satisfaction they experience. A negotiation of goals to meet the wishes of the elderly patient may provide the most meaningful rehabilitation program for the individual (Johansson, 2003).

Many factors influence the rehabilitation potential of the geriatric population. Coping strategies such as the desire to be in control are helpful, whereas feelings of stress, fear, and anxiety can lead to the helpless feeling of not having control. Returning control to the person in whatever way possible—whether in physical capacities or in a sense of control over one's future—is important in promoting the concept of self-care. Spiritual well-being—manifested by some through prayer and a voiced belief in God—is also a strong component in successful coping (Easton, 1999). Positive social support, providing a sense of stability, security, social interaction, and connectedness, is also important and is associated with better physical outcomes of rehabilitation. Negative social support may undermine the necessary emotional or physical support for the rehab process, and may impair it when family members or friends express a negative attitude toward the person's goals. Family members may also be affected by aging and disability, so family dynamics, resources, and coping strategies should also be considered when evaluating the support systems of the person in rehab. Motivational factors, including goals, humor, caring, encouragement, and power resulting from relationships, were found to be much more motivational than forced compliance or domination.

Self-efficacy, or the degree of confidence possessed by the person that he or she will be successful in performing certain acts, is also important to the success of a rehab program. Self-belief is a powerful predictor of ADL performance months after stroke rehab program completion, indicating the value of incorporating self-efficacy into the assessment and treatment phases (Hellstrom, Lindmark, Wahlberg, & Fugl-Meyer, 2003).

The need for preventive and rehabilitative interventions is particularly important for the oldest-old. Following hospitalization for medical illnesses, the older the patient, the more likely he or she is to lose ADL function during the course of hospitalization. More than half of those over 85 years had worse ADL function following a hospitalization. Discharge outcomes were markedly influenced by functional changes after the hospital admission. This outcome suggests that functional status of the elderly during hospitalization needs to be monitored to promote as much function as possible in order to maintain such function following discharge (Covinsky et al., 2003).

Some studies also indicate that elderly stroke patients who have rehabilitation services at home instead of in the hospital have lower rates of certain medical complications, achieve a better score for rating of depression, and experience lower rates of admission to nursing homes (Bo et al., 2004).

Deterrents

Providing safe care for those with physical and mental limitations is an important concern. There is now convincing evidence that safe care can be provided without unduly restricting freedom and without creating other unnecessary risks (**Box 10-4**). Alternative safety measures, tailored to the individual's specific needs, can help ensure the patient's best possible quality of life (Minnesota Department of Health, 2001). Family members and caregivers may

Notable Quotes

"When you get old, everyone starts to worry about you. They say 'Don't do this, don't do that.' It drives us plumb-jack crazy. Bessie always says, 'If I break my fool neck falling down the stairs while I'm feeding my little dog, well, so be it.' Folks think that because you're old, you're unable to do for yourself. Well, look at us! . . . But you do have to be honest about your limitations. If you don't do that, well, your clock's not ticking right!"

—Sadie Delany (Delany & Delany, 1994, pp. 119–120)

"That's a big problem with some older folks—they have such low expectations of themselves. When they get to a certain age, they just give up. That's a shame! If there's anything I've learned in all these years, it's that life is too good to waste a day. It's up to you to make it sweet."

—Sadie Delany (Delany & Delany, 1994, p. 123 [after fracturing her left hip])

have specific insights that are helpful in determining the patient's habits, likes and dislikes, patterns of behavior, and overall condition. These insights can be used to develop an individualized plan to minimize behaviors that lead to use of physical restraints (see Chapter 14 for further discussion).

Use of Restraints. **Restraint** devices (e.g., belts, vests, pelvic ties, mitts, specialized chairs, bed side rails) are usually considered in order to promote the safety of the recipient—especially those who are forgetful and unsteady. A restraint is defined as "any manual method or physical or mechanical device, material or equipment attached or adjacent to [the resident's] body that the individual cannot remove easily which restricts freedom of movement or normal access to one's body" (Department of Health and Human Services, 1999).

Physical restraints are those applied to the body and a stationary object; chemical restraints are those provided by a medication of some type. It is the restriction of freedom that makes the restraint what it is, whether physical or chemical. Wandering, agitation, lashing out at others, unsteadiness and potential to fall, and pulling at tubing or needles have been common reasons for use of restraints. Because restraints also have the potential for causing falls, injury, or even death and because quality-of-life issues may be affected, there are protocols and stringent rules governing their use. The Omnibus Budget Reconciliation Act (OBRA) mandates that restraints may be used only to treat someone's medical condition, and not for convenience or discipline. Symptoms can be emotional, physical, or behavioral and a danger to the person him- or herself or other people (Frey, 2002).

Restraints may be medically indicated for some situations, such as during procedures that require no movement, following surgery when movement is not advisable, or to keep a patient from pulling out tubes. They should never be used for punishment or for convenience of the caregiver.

Alternatives to Restraints. Since the passage of OBRA in 1987, restraint use in facilities has declined significantly, from an overall prevalence in 1986 of nearly 40% (Strumpf & Evans, 2005), to approximately 13.3% some 10 years later.

Any reduction in use of restraints already in place should be done methodically. There should be a planned substitution of alternative and less restrictive measures to treat the specific symptom necessitating the restraint in the first place, with ongoing monitoring and revision as the plan unfolds. The plan may include one or more of these alternatives:

- Placement of the patient near the nurse's station or oversight personnel
- Use of a call button or alerting device to call a caregiver when needed
- Handy accessibility of necessary items (e.g., tissues, phone, TV remote)
- Physical company of another person (e.g., a "sitter" to monitor and distract as needed)
- Relaxing/calming surroundings (e.g., music, holding a favorite item, home-like features to room)
- Appropriate use of eyeglasses or hearing aids
- Positioning devices (e.g., body pillows, cushions, wedge cushions, tilt-back chair)
- Adequate pain management

Additional fall prevention measures may also help, including a low bed, a night light, clear

BOX 10-3 Additional Resources

Brennan, F. A. (2002). Exercise prescriptions for active seniors. *The Physician and Sports Medicine, 30*(2). Retrieved January 13, 2008, from http://www.physsportsmed.com/issues/2002/02_02/brennan.htm. These tools help identify exercise goals, determine suitability for initiating an exercise program, and evaluate risks for such a program.

Centers for Disease Control and Prevention. (2008). *Healthy aging: Preventing disease and improving quality of life among older Americans*. Retrieved October 4, 2008, from http://www.cdc.gov/nccdphp/publications/aag/aging.htm. This site provides timely and practical information on health and aging for professionals and the public.

Centers for Disease Control and Prevention. (2008). *Injury center: Falls in nursing homes*. Retrieved January 8, 2008, from http://www.cdc.gov/ncipc/factsheets/nursing.htm. This site gives information and statistics on falls in long-term care facilities.

Delany, S., & Delany, A. E., with Hearth, A. H. (1993). *Having our say: The Delany sisters' first 100 years*. New York: Kodansha-America. The Delany sisters have a lot to say about being an older American!

Delany, S. L., with Hearth, A. H. (1997). *On my own: Reflections on life without Bessie*. San Francisco: Harper. Sadie reminisces and adjusts after the death of her lifetime companion.

National Institutes of Health. Retrieved January 13, 2008, from http://www.nihseniorhealth.gov. Aging research at the federal level.

Tinetti, M. E. (2003). *Preventing falls in the elderly*. Retrieved January 9, 2008, from http://www.sgim.org/userfiles/file/handout16TinettiAssessmentTool1.pdf. The Tinetti assessment tool is provided and described here.

University of Pennsylvania. (n.d.). *Gero T.I.P.S. online learning center*. Retrieved September 30, 2007, from http://www.nursing.upenn.edu/centers/hcgne/gero_tips/rfc/3_RFC_Interventions_Falls.htm. Information about falls and fall prevention in the elderly.

pathways in the room, or bed/chair sensor alarms (Healthtouch Online, 2006).

Financial Considerations

Financial resources affect the options available to meet the needs of the elderly. Those with adequate finances have a full range of possibilities open to them for housing, location, and care resources. Others with modest but limited resources can take advantage of a variety of options until their funds are depleted, and then must rely on family or government programs to meet their care needs as they continue to age.

For those with few resources, community and government programs are available to meet needs, and more are developing to meet the anticipated needs of the baby-boomer generation, which is now maturing to older adulthood. Some programs to assist the elderly who have moderate/severe financial limitations include Medicaid waiver, CHOICE, supplemental food banks, food stamps, and assisted living caregivers.

Community Resources

There are many community resources of which nurses should be aware. The yellow pages and some sections in the front of the tele-

BOX 10-4 Alternatives to Restraints

- Personal strengthening and rehabilitation program
- Use of personal assistance devices such as hearing aids, visual aids, and mobility devices
- Use of positioning devices such as body and seat cushions or padded furniture
- Safer physical environment design, including removal of obstacles that impede movement, placement of objects and furniture in familiar places, lower beds, and adequate lighting
- Regular attention to physical and personal needs, including toileting, thirst, hunger, socialization, and activities adapted to current ability and former interests
- Design of physical environment for close observation by staff
- Efforts to increase staff awareness of a person's individual needs, including assignment of staff particularly to the person, in an effort to improve function and decrease difficult behaviors
- Living environment designed to promote relaxation and comfort, minimize noise, provide soothing music, and maintain appropriate lighting
- Provision of massage, art, movement activities, and complementary therapies (e.g., Healing Touch, energy work)
- Use of bed, chair, and door alarms to alert to the need for assistance

Source: Minnesota Department of Health. (2001). http://www.health.state.mn.us/divs/fpc/safety.htm. Accessed January 8, 2008.

phone book may help. Many areas have resource guides published by the community United Way or other organizations. Look for resources such as these:

- *Geriatric case management:* Provides coordination of care and community resource referrals, either through a public agency such as a council on aging or through an entrepreneurial agency (see Chapter 25 for further discussion)
- *Senior transportation options:* Must be available and senior friendly
- *Meals on Wheels, food stamps, senior center meals, etc.:* Government or locally sponsored programs; some have low cost or subsidized funding
- *Caregiver associations and support groups:* National via the Internet; local via social service agencies
- *Respite care agencies:* Provide temporary relief for family members
- *Daycare services for seniors:* Provide therapeutic care and social services during the day for older adults
- *Hospice and palliative care programs:* Through nursing agencies or hospitals
- *Disease-specific support groups and associations:* National or local chapters
- *Eldercare agencies*

BOX 10-5 Web Exploration

Explore a team approach to exercise for older adults. Visit the Web site http://www.physsportsmed.com/issues/2002/02_02/brennan.htm.

- *Center for Medicare and Medicaid Sevices:* Medicare, Medicaid
- *Medicaid waiver programs:* Subsidized home care support; financial criteria for eligibility
- *Local/community health clinics*
- *Medication assistance programs:* Through the medication manufacturer, with the cooperation of the physician or medical care provider

Notable Quotes

"Don't be too proud to accept your limitations. The hardest thing is discovering that you can't do everything the way you used to. We're not happy having folks help us around the house, but we've come to accept it. But make sure you hire folks to do what you want. It's still your house, and you're still the boss!"

—Sadie and Bessie Delany
(Delany & Delany, 1994, p. 126)

IMPLICATIONS FOR NURSING CARE

Nurses in a variety of practice settings have a remarkable opportunity to impact the lives of community-based elderly patients. In the doctor's office, the nurse is usually the first to talk with the patient on a visit. While taking vital signs, the nurse can begin to evaluate eating, sleeping, and socialization factors that might be influencing the patient's condition and ability to remain independent. The nurse can ask about telephone use, social supports, activities, and involvement in the community. If caregivers are present at the appointment, the nurse can ask about patient management, coping mechanisms, and need for respite or relief.

The hospital nurse can also look for and discuss with families/caregivers the safety issues and functional needs and abilities to be considered before a patient is released home (Rose, Bowman, & Kresevic, 2000). Referral to the social services department can provide opportunity for education, counseling, and links to community resources for the patient/caregiver.

Specialty nurses in the clinic, office, or hospital can be on the lookout for those patients and/or families who might benefit from support groups or other referrals particular to their diagnoses or conditions.

Visiting nurse services offer in-home care and support, therapies, and social services that are designed to keep patients functional and community-based for as long as possible, even through end-of-life. Whatever the setting, nurses are important resources for older persons in promoting continued independence into later life.

Personal **Reflections**

1. Consider the value you place on your own level of independence. What measures of independence would be most difficult for you to forfeit if you became increasingly disabled? What accommodations might you want in order to ease the transitions you would encounter? Do these values and wishes differ significantly from those of the elderly people you know?
2. Do you have experiences with elderly family members who have influenced your decision to become a nurse? Elaborate on the personal lessons you have learned from your elderly family members in making your career choice.
3. "But however you do it, you've just got to fight in this life. When you're young, you're busy trying to fight against all the big problems of the world. When you're older, you have to fight to hold on to things like your property and your dignity and your independence. If there's one thing you've got to hold on to, it's the courage to fight!"(Bessie Delany, 1994, p. 125).
   Read the quote above. Do you agree with the Delany sisters' outlook about fighting throughout life? Why or why not?

References

American Dietetic Association. (2002, July 23). *Nutrition across the spectrum of aging*. Retrieved December 1, 2008, from http://www.ncbi.nlm.nih.gov/pubmed/10812387

Bean, J. F., Kiely, D. K., Herman, S., Leveille, S. G., Mizer, K., Frontera, W. R., et al. (2002). The relationship between leg power and physical performance in mobility-limited older people. *Journal of the American Geriatrics Society, 50*, 461–467.

Binder, E. F., Schechtman, K. B., Ehsani, A. A., Steger-May, K., Brown, M., Sinacore, D. R., et al. (2002). Effects of exercise training on frailty in community-dwelling older adults: Results of a randomized, controlled trial. *Journal of the American Geriatrics Society, 50*(12), 1921–1929.

Bo, M., Molaschi, M., Massaia, M., Salerno, D., Amati, D., Tibaldi, V., et al. (2004). Home hospitalization service for acute uncomplicated first ischemic stroke in elderly patients. A randomized trial. *Journal of the American Geriatrics Society, 52*(2), 278–284.

Byock, I. (2004). *The four things that matter most.* New York: Simon and Schuster.

Covinsky, K. E., Palmer, R. M., Fortinsky, R. H., Counsell, S. R., Stewart, A. L., Kresevic, D., et al. (2003). Loss of independence in activities of daily living in older adults hospitalized with medical illness: Increased vulnerability with age. *Journal of the American Geriatrics Association, 51*, 451–458.

Delany, S., & Delany, A. E., with Hearth, A. H. (1993). *Having our say: The Delany sisters' first 100 years.* New York: Kodansha America.

Delany, S., & Delany, A. E., with Hearth, A. H. (1994). *The Delany sisters' book of everyday wisdom*. New York: Kodansha International.

Department of Health and Human Services. (1999). *Survey protocol for long term care facilities. State operations manual, Appendix P.* Retrieved December 1, 2008, from http://www.cms.hhs.gov/manuals/downloads/som107c07.pdf

Easton, K. L. (1999). *Gerontological rehabilitation nursing.* Philadelphia: Saunders/Harcourt Brace, pp. 323–326.

Ebersole, P., & Hess, P. (1998). *Toward healthy aging*. St. Louis: Mosby, pp. 704–741, 900–907.

Ennis, B. W., Saffel-Shrier, S., & Verson, H. (2001). Malnutrition in the elderly: What nurses need to know. *Dimensions of Critical Care Nursing, 20*(6), 28–35.

Fone, S., & Lundgren-Lindquist, B. (2003). Health status and functional capacity in a group of successfully ageing 65–85 year olds. *Disability and Rehabilitation, 25*(18), 1044–1052.

Forestalling frailty. (2003, March). *Harvard Women's Health Watch*, p. 3. Retrieved April 18, 2005, from http://www.health.harvard.edu

Frey, D. (2002). *Physical restraints on the elderly*. Retrieved January 9, 2008, from http://wywy.essortment.com/physicalrestrai_rnrt.htm

Fried, L., Tangen, C. M., Walston, J., Newman, A. B., Hirsch, C., Gottdiener, J., et al. (2001). Frailty in older adults: Evidence for a phenotype. *Journals of Gerontology Series A: Biological Sciences and Medical Sciences, 56*, M146–M157.

Gaspar, P. (1998). Managing basic physiologic needs. In P. Ebersole & P. Hess (Eds.), *Toward healthy aging* (pp. 189–194). St Louis: Mosby.

Healthtouch Online. (2006). *Safe use of restraints for medical management*.

Hellstrom, K., Lindmark, B., Wahlberg, B., & Fugl-Meyer, A. R. (2003). Self-efficacy in relation to impairments and activities of daily living disability in elderly patients with stroke: A prospective investigation. *Journal of Rehabilitative Medicine, 35*(5), 202–208.

Helm, H. M., Hays, J. C., Flint, E. P., Koenig, H. G., & Blazer, D. G. (2000). Does religious attendance prolong survival?: A six year follow-up study of 3,968 older adults. *Journals of Gerontology (Medical), 54*(7), M370–M376.

Huffman, G. B. (2002). Evaluating and treating unintentional weight loss in the elderly. *American Family Physician, 65*(4), 640–651.

Johansson, C. (2003). Rising with the fall: Addressing quality of life in physical frailty. *Topics in Geriatric Rehabilitation, 19*(4), 219–239.

Kakaiya, R., Tisovec, R., & Fulkerson, P. (2000). Evaluation of fitness to drive: The physician's role in assessing elderly or demented patients. *Postgraduate Medicine, 107*(3), 229–236. Retrieved January 9, 2008, from http://www.postgradmed.com/issues/2000/03_00/kakaiya.htm

Kingston, P., Bernard, M., Biggs, S., & Nettleton, H. (2001). Assessing the health impact of age-specific housing. *Health and Social Care in the Community, 94*, 228–235.

Markle-Reid, M., & Browne, G. (2003). Conceptualizations of frailty in relation to older adults. *Journal of Advanced Nursing, 44*(1), 58–68.

Mauk, K. L., & Schmidt, N. A. (2004). *Spiritual care in nursing practice*. Philadelphia: Lippincott Williams & Wilkins.

Mazzeo, R. S., & Tanaka, H. (2001). Exercise prescription for the elderly: Current recommendations. *Sports Medicine, 31*(11), 809–819.

McCallion, P., Toseland, R. W., Gerber, T., & Banks, S. (2004). Increasing the use of formal services by caregivers of people with dementia. *Social Work: A Journal of the National Association of Social Workers, 49*(3), 441–450.

Minnesota Department of Health. (2001). *Safety without restraints: A new practice standard for safe care*. Retrieved January 11, 2008, from http://www.health.state.mn.us/divs/fpc/safety.htm

National Institute on Aging. (2007). *What's new*? Retrieved December 1, 2008, from http://www.nia.nih.gov/NewsAndEvents/

Nikolaus, T., & Bach, M. (2003). Preventing falls in community-dwelling frail older people using a home intervention team (HIT): Results from the randomized falls-HIT trial. *Journal of the American Geriatrics Society, 51*(3), 300–306.

Northridge, M. E., & Levick, N. (2002). Preventing falls at home: Transforming unsafe spaces into healthy places for older people. *Generations, 26*(4), 42–48.

Nygard, L., & Starkhammar, S. (2003). Telephone use among noninstitutionalized persons with dementia living alone: Mapping out difficulties and response strategies. *Scandinavian Journal of Caring Sciences, 17*(3), 239–251.

Reicherter, E. A., & Billek-Sawhney, B. (2003). Use of the social system theory for the analysis of community reintegration of older adults. *Topics in Geriatric Rehabilitation, 19*(4), 298–307.

Reinhard, S. (2001). Nursing's role in family caregiver support. In K. J. Doka & J. D. Davidson (Eds.), *Caregiving and loss: Family needs, professional responses* (pp. 181–190). Washington, DC: Hospice Foundation of America.

Rose, J. H., Bowman, K., & Kresevic, D. (2000). Nurse versus family caregiver perspectives on hospitalized older patients: An exploratory study of agreement at admission and discharge. *Health Communication, 12*(1), 63–80.

Rowe, J. W., & Kahn, R. L. (1998). *Successful aging*. New York: Pantheon.

Sarvimaki, A., & Stenbock-Hult, B. (2000). Quality of life in old age described as a sense of well-being, meaning and value. *Journal of Advanced Nursing, 32*(4), 1025–1033.

Silverstein, N., Carr, D., & Kerschner, H. (2004). *Promoting safety and independence through older driver wellness: Web series 2*. Boston University Institute for Geriatric Social Work. Presented November 10 & 17 and December 9, 2004.

Sparks, B., Travis, S., & Pecchioni, L. (2000). Family caregivers' use of humor in conveying information about caring for dependent older adults. *Health Communication, 12*(4), 361–377.

Strumpf, N. E., & Evans, L. K. (2005). *Individualized restraint-free care.* Retrieved September 30, 2007, from http://www.nursing.upenn.edu/centers/hcgne/restraints.htm

Studenski, S., Perera, S., Wallace, D., Chandler, J. M., Duncan, P. W., Rooney, E., et al. (2003). Physical performance measures in the clinical setting. *Journal of the American Geriatrics Society, 51*, 314–322.

Stupp, H. W. (2000). Area agencies on aging: A network of services to maintain elderly in their communities. *Care Management Journal, 2*(1), 54–62.

Suomi, R. (2001). Pool work helps patients improve balance. *BioMechanics: The Magazine of Body Movement and Medicine.*

Taylor, L., Whittington, F., Hollandsworth, C., Ball, M., King, S., Patterson, V., et al. (2003). Assessing the effectiveness of a walking program on physical function of residents in an assisted living facility. *Journal of Community Health Nursing, 20*(1), 15–37.

Taylor, M. J. (2001). *Yoga for the elderly: Geriatric yoga therapeutics.* Gerinotes. Retrieved January 9, 2008, from http://www.dynamicsystemsrehab.com/item.php?id=133

van den Brink, C. (2004). Effect of widowhood on disability onset in elderly men from three European countries. *Journal of the American Geriatric Society, 52*(3), 353–359.

Vestibular Technologies. (2008). *Fall prevention: Falls risk assessment tools and screening.* Retrieved January 8, 2008, from http://www.preventfalls.com

Weight-Control Information Network, National Institute of Diabetes and Digestive and Kidney Diseases (NIDDK). (2007). *Young at heart: Tips for older adults.* Retrieved December 1, 2008, from http://win.niddk.nih.gov/publications/young_heart.htm

White, L. (2003). *Leaving home.* Retrieved January 9, 2008, from http://www.medrehabconsultants.com/eldercare/articles/movinginlateryears.htm

Williams, S. W., Dilworth-Anderson, P., & Goodwin, P. Y. (2003). Caregiver role strain: The contribution of multiple roles and available resources in African-American women. *Aging and Mental Health, 7*(2), 103–112.

Zimnavoda, T., Weinblatt, N., & Katz, N. (2002). Validity of the Kohlman evaluation of living skills (KELS) with Israeli elderly individuals living in the community. *Occupational Therapy International, 9*(4), 312–326.

SECTION

4

Health Promotion, Risk Reduction, and Disease Prevention

(Competencies 11–12)

CHAPTER 11

PROMOTING HEALTHY AGING

DAVID HABER, PHD

LEARNING OBJECTIVES

At the end of this chapter, the reader will be able to:

- Discuss the promise and limitations of the Healthy People initiatives.
- Apply the health contract technique and nutritional bull's-eye for behavior change.
- Describe several model health promotion programs.
- Explain the concept of re-engagement and provide examples of it.
- Identify the components of Medicare prevention.
- Explain the importance of life review.
- Recognize the importance of exercise and nutrition for healthy aging.
- Discuss the importance of the Green House project to the future of long-term care.

KEY TERMS

- Center for Science in the Public Interest (CSPI)
- Depression
- Exercise
- Green House
- Health behavior change
- Health contract/calendar
- Healthy People initiatives
- Life review
- Medicare prevention
- Mental health
- Model health promotion programs
- Nutrition
- Nutrition bull's-eye
- Re-engagement

Health promotion works, no matter what one's age, and even after decades of practicing unhealthy habits. But it does not work for everyone, all the time. So what needs to be done to increase the odds of promoting healthy aging successfully? Certainly the entire burden cannot be placed on the guilt-ridden backs of individuals. The federal and state governments play a significant role. So do religious institutions, businesses, community centers, hospitals, medical clinics, health professionals, educational institutions, families, neighborhoods, and even shopping malls. In this chapter some of these influences on healthy aging will be explored.

Exercise and **nutrition** are probably the two most widely publicized components of health promotion, and they will be given their due in this chapter as well. We will use a broad definition of health promotion in this chapter, one that includes such diverse topics as self-management through health contracts, promoting mental health through life reviews, promoting **re-engagement** rather than retirement, and promoting the health of frail elders through unique homes rather than through institutions that are merely called (nursing) homes.

One aspect of health promotion lies with the federal government. We'll start by talking about the

Healthy People initiatives and **Medicare prevention.**

HEALTHY PEOPLE INITIATIVES

The federal government has been establishing goals for healthy aging since 1980 when the U.S. Public Health Service published the report *Promoting Health/Preventing Disease: Objectives for the Nation*. This 1980 report outlined 226 objectives for the nation to achieve over the following 10 years. It was referred to by some as Healthy People 1990.

A decade later, in 1990, another 10-year national effort, Healthy People 2000, was initiated by the U.S. Public Health Service in another effort to reduce preventable death and disability for Americans. A third effort is currently under way with the Healthy People 2010 initiative; however, the number of objectives has increased to 467, and these are distributed over 28 priority areas.

There are some notable benefits to the Healthy People initiatives. On the positive side, these initiatives give recognition to health promotion rather than focusing exclusively on wars on diseases (e.g., tabulating the number of deaths from cancer or heart disease, and then organizing a campaign against them). The Healthy People initiatives are health oriented, and as such they recognize the complexity of the socioeconomic, lifestyle, and other nonmedical influences that impact our ability to attain and maintain health.

A second major benefit of the Healthy People initiatives is that they are focused on documenting baselines, setting objectives, and monitoring progress. For instance, according to the *Healthy People 2000 Review, 1998–1999* (National Center for Health Statistics [NCHS], 1999), 15% of the objectives for the year 2000 were met, and 44% demonstrated movement toward the target. However, since the initiative relied mostly on data monitoring and a small amount of publicity—and very little financial support—it is unclear whether Healthy People 2000 contributed directly to this progress. For example, in an area where there was no financial support for encouraging change—being overweight or obese—the trend in America for adults between the ages of 20 and 74 has been in the opposite direction: a steady increase in weight gain for Americans over the decade (NCHS, 1999). There was a similar result with sedentary behavior among Americans. In the absence of financial support for encouraging change in this area, light to moderate physical activity on a near-daily basis between the ages of 18 and 74 had not improved over the decade (NCHS, 1999).

Focusing on those age 65 or over, the Merck Institute on Aging and Health came out with a report card on the Healthy People 2000 initiative (available at www.gericareonline.net) that revealed several failing grades. Older Americans did not reach the 2000 target goals, and in fact fell far short of them in the areas of physical activity, being overweight, and eating fruits and vegetables. Additional failing grades were assigned to the target goals of reducing hip fractures for persons age 65 or over, and fall-related deaths for persons age 85 or over.

In contrast to the mere monitoring of most Healthy People 2000 target goals, financial assistance was provided to older adults through Medicare during the decade for mammogram coverage, pneumococcal vaccination, and influenza vaccination. With this financial support, the percentage of compliance in these three areas doubled among older adults during the decade (Haber, 2002). Consequently, the Healthy People 2000 target goals were met for mammogram screening and influenza vaccination, and fell just short of being met for pneumococcal vaccination.

This raises the question of whether the federal government should be doing more than monitoring data changes when it comes to promoting healthy aging. A comparable question can be asked of state governments. The Healthy People initiatives were supposed to have had a counterpart initiative at each of the state health departments. In this author's experience with several states, however, the initiatives either have been ignored or the state health department has conducted a modest project that was accomplished several years ago, but did not follow up with additional activity. Financing and leadership are needed to make these programs successful. To find out more about the Healthy People 2010 initiative, go to www.health.gov/healthypeople/state/toolkit.

MEDICARE PREVENTION

The federal government does more than just establish Healthy People initiatives. It also reimburses

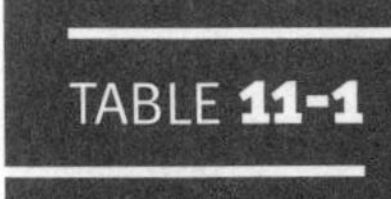

TABLE 11-1 Medicare Prevention

One-Time "Welcome to Medicare Physical"

Within 6 months of initial enrollment; no deductible or copayment.

Physician takes history of modifiable risk factors (coverage makes special mention of depression, functional ability, home safety, falls risk, hearing, vision), height and weight, blood pressure, EKG.

Cardiovascular screening

Every 5 years; no deductible or copayment.

Ratio between total cholesterol and HDL, triglycerides.

Cervical cancer

Covered every 2 years; no deductible, copayment applies.

Pap smear and pelvic exam.

Colorectal cancer

Covered annually for fecal occult blood test; no deductible or copayment.

Covered every 4 years for sigmoidoscopy or barium enema; deductible and copayment apply.

Covered every 10 years for colonoscopy; deductible and copayment apply.

Densitometry

Covered every 2 years; deductible and copayment apply.

Diabetes screening

Annually, those with prediabetes every 6 months; no deductible or copayment.

Not covered routinely, but includes most people age 65+ (if overweight, family history, fasting glucose of 100–125 mg/dl [prediabetes], hypertension, dyslipidemia).

Mammogram

Covered annually; no deductible, copayment applies.

Prostate cancer

Covered annually; no deductible or copayment.

Digital rectal examination and PSA test.

Smoking Cessation

Two quit attempts annually, each consisting of up to four counseling sessions.

Limited to those with tobacco-related diseases (heart disease, cancer, stroke) or drug regimens that are adversely affected by smoking (insulin, hypertension, seizure, blood clots, depression). Clinicians are encouraged to become credentialed in smoking cessation.

Immunization

No deductible or copayment.

Influenza vaccination covered annually; pneumococcal vaccination covered one time, revaccination after 5 years dependent on risk.

Other Coverage

Diabetes outpatient self-management training (blood glucose monitors, test strips, lancets; nutrition and exercise education; self-management skills: 9 hours of group training, plus 1 hour of individual training).

Medical nutrition therapy for persons with diabetes or a renal disease: 3 hours of individual training first year, 2 hours subsequent years.

Glaucoma screening annually for those with diabetes, family history, or African American descent.

Persons with cardiovascular disease may be eligible for comprehensive prevention programs by Drs. Dean Ornish and Herbert Benson: coverage 36 sessions within 18 weeks, possible extension to 72 sessions within 36 weeks.

Frequency and Duration

These are estimates of what researchers recommend, relying most heavily on the U.S. Preventive Services Task Force recommendations, but not exclusively on them.

Blood pressure: Begin early adulthood, annually, ending around age 80.

Cholesterol: Begin early adulthood, every 2–3 years, ending around age 80.

Colorectal cancer: Begin age 50, every 5–10 years for colonoscopy, ending around age 80.

Mammogram: Begin age 40, every year or two; begin age 50 annually; begin age 65 every 2 years; ending around age 80.

Osteoporosis: Begin early adulthood for women (no frequency recommended); every 2–3 years after age 65 for women, less frequently for men.

Pap test: Begin with female sexual activity, two normal consecutive annual screenings, followed by every 3 years; two normal consecutive annual screenings around age 65, then discontinue.

Prostate cancer: Do not do routinely, except if there is a family history or African American heritage.

Definitions

Hypercholesterolemia: LDL above 160/130/100 (depending on risk factors); HDL below 40; ratio (total/HDL) 4.2 or above.

Diabetes: Fasting glucose 126 mg/dl and above; prediabetes, 100–125 mg/dl.

High blood pressure: Over 140/90; between 120/80 and 140/90 is prehypertensive.

Osteopenia: 1–2.5 standard deviations below young-adult peak bone density.

Osteoporosis: 2.5 standard deviations or more below young-adult peak bone density

SOURCE: Permission from D. Haber, *Health Promotion and Aging: Practical Applications for Health Professionals*. New York: Springer Publishing Company, 4th edition, 2007, pp. 100–101.

Medicare recipients for certain prevention activities (see **Table 11-1**). Some of Medicare's reimbursement policies have emerged from the research evidence reviewed by the U.S. Preventive Services Task Force (USPSTF). USPSTF was launched by the U.S. Public Health Service to systematically review evidence of effectiveness of clinical preventive services. This task force periodically updates its research guidelines on a wide variety of screening and counseling recommendations, such as breast cancer screening, colorectal cancer screening, and counseling to promote physical activity.

These updates have been compiled into a two-volume loose-leaf notebook and a CD for the period 2001 to 2006. This notebook, and periodic updates after 2006, can be accesssed by calling the AHRQ Publications Clearinghouse (800) 358-9295, by sending an e-mail to ahrqpubs@ahrq.gov, or by visiting the Web site at www.ahrq.gov/clinic/pocketgd.htm.

If you review the USPSTF recommendations, however, you will notice that they are often out of sync with Medicare reimbursement policies. Some reimbursement policies appear to have been influenced more by medical lobbyists advocating for specific segments of the medical industry (e.g., oncology, urology, orthopedics) than by policy derived from evidence-based medicine (Haber, 2001, 2005).

Although the movement into Medicare prevention—with substantially expanded coverage in 1998 and 2005—undoubtedly benefits older Americans, there is room for considerable improvement in the way the Medicare program promotes health and prevents disease. Lobbyists have promoted medical screenings that are reimbursed too frequently or over too long a period of time. Some screenings may not be worth the expense (e.g., fecal occult blood test, barium enema, sigmoidoscopy, routine prostate cancer screening, baseline EKG). Conversely, Medicare policy is stingy toward risk reduction counseling, which, not surprisingly, has little if any lobbying effort behind it.

Analysts have argued that prevention resources are limited, and we should re-examine policy that is so heavily focused on medical screenings. Perhaps it would be more effective, and cost-effective, to focus on counseling in the areas of sedentary behavior, inadequate nutrition, smoking and tobacco use, and alcohol abuse (Haber, 2001, 2005).

Medical screenings and immunizations are undeniably important tools for disease prevention, but the data collected by the U.S. Preventive Services Task Force (1996) resulted in a surprising conclusion: "Among the most effective interventions available to clinicians for reducing the incidence and severity of the leading causes of disease and disability in the United States are those that address the personal health practices of patients" (p. xxii). Stated another way "conventional clinical activities (e.g., diagnostic testing) may be of less value to clients than activities once considered outside the traditional role of the clinician," namely, counseling and patient education (USPSTF, 1996, p. xxii).

To end this section on an encouraging note, Medicare prevention is moving in positive directions, with coverage for:

- Nutrition therapy for persons with diabetes and kidney disease
- An initial physical examination that includes prevention counseling
- Smoking cessation—for those who have an illness caused by or complicated by tobacco use
- Comprehensive health promotion programs developed by Drs. Dean Ornish and Herbert Benson, for beneficiaries with heart problems

It is important not only to expand these counseling and health education programs, but also to publicize them. Years after implementation, for instance, only a small percentage of seniors eligible for the newly implemented initial physical examination took advantage of this opportunity (Pfizer, 2007).

BOX 11-1 Recommended Readings

Birren, J., & Cochran, K. (2001). *Telling the stories of life through guided autobiography groups*. Baltimore, MD: Johns Hopkins University Press.

Freedman, M. (1999). *Prime time: How baby boomers will revolutionize retirement and transform America*. New York: Public Affairs.

Haber, D. (2007). *Health promotion and aging: Practical applications for health professionals* (4th ed.). New York: Springer.

Lorig, K., Ritter, P., Stewart, A., Sobel, D., Brown, B., Bandura, A., et al. (2001). Chronic disease self-management program: 2-year health status and health care utilization outcomes. *Medical Care, 39*(11), 1217–1223.

Rabig, J., Thomas, W., Kane, R., Cutler, L., & McAlilly, S. (2006). Radical redesign of nursing homes: Applying the Green House concept in Tupelo, Mississippi. *The Gerontologist, 46*(4), 533–539.

Thomas, W. (2004). *What are old people for?* Acton, MA: VanderWyk & Burnam.

HEALTH BEHAVIOR CHANGE

Theories help us understand what influences health behaviors and how to plan effective interventions. A theory of **health behavior change** attempts to explain the processes underlying the learning of new health behaviors. The two most widely cited theories of behavior change are social cognitive theory (Bandura, 1977) and stages of change (Prochaska & DiClemente, 1992). Other theories that have marshaled support are health locus of control (Wallston & Wallston, 1982), health belief model (Becker, 1974), reasoned action (Fishbein & Ajzen, 1975), community empowerment (Wallerstein & Bernstein, 1988), and community-oriented primary care (Nutting, 1987).

The author of this chapter is not an advocate of any single theory. Theories are broad and ambitious, attempting to relate a set of concepts systematically to explain and predict events and activities. Concepts, however, are the primary elements of a theory, and each theory has a concept or two that is particularly well developed and helpful in guiding a risk reduction intervention. Borrowing concepts from different theories can help one plan an intervention.

One behavior-changing tool that borrows concepts from a variety of theories is the health contract/calendar (**Figures 11-1** and **11-2**). The **health contract/calendar** relies on the self-management capability of a client, after initial assistance is provided by a clinician or health educator. The client is helped to choose an appropriate behavior change goal and to create and implement a plan to accomplish that goal. The statement of the goal and the plan of action are then written into a contract format.

A health contract is alleged to have several advantages over verbal communication alone, especially when the communication tends to be limited in direction (i.e., mostly from health professional to client). The alleged advantages of a contract, which still need additional empirical testing, are that it is a formal commitment that not only enhances the therapeutic relationship between provider and client, but also requires the active participation of the client. The contract also:

- Identifies and enhances motivation
- Clarifies measurable and modest goals
- Suggests tips to remember new behaviors
- Provides a planned way to involve support persons such as family and friends

FIGURE **11-1** **Health contract.**

My **health goal** is: ______________________________

____

My **motivation** for my health goal is: 1. ____________ 2. ____________ 3. ____________ My Plan of Action For social or emotional **support** I will... To **remind** me of new behaviors I will...	**Problems** that may interfere with reaching my health goal and **solutions:** ____________ ____________ ____________ ____________ ____________ ____________ ____________ ____________ ____________ My **signature**/ ____ Support person's **signature** ____ date ____ date ____

SOURCE: Permission from D. Haber, *Health Promotion and Aging: Practical Applications for Health Professionals:* NY: Springer Publishing Company, 4th edition, 2007, p. 114.

FIGURE 11-2 **Health calendar.**

Fill in activities and make an X on each day you complete them.

Month:____________________

Backup plan:

Sunday	Monday	Tuesday	Wednesday	Thursday	Friday	Saturday

Weekly Success #days completed/ #days contracted

SOURCE: Permission from D. Haber, *Health Promotion and Aging: Practical Applications for Health Professionals:* NY: Springer Publishing Company, 4th edition, 2007, p. 114.

- Provides a means to problem-solve around barriers that previously interfered with the achievement of a goal
- Suggests ways to design a supportive environment
- Provides incentives to reinforce behaviors

- Establishes a record-keeping system (i.e., a month-long calendar for the health contract/calendar technique)

The health contract/calendar technique includes a set of instructions (see Haber, 2007b) that helps older adults establish a goal, identify motivation, implement a plan of action, identify potential problems, and encourage solutions to overcome these barriers. The contract is signed and dated at the bottom by the older adult and a support person. Progress is typically assessed after one week, and the success of the contract is reviewed at the end of a month. There is also the potential for providing ongoing support.

Health contracts have been applied with varying degrees of success to a wide variety of behaviors, such as drug use, smoking, alcohol abuse, nutrition, and exercise (Berry et al., 1989; Clark et al., 1999; Cupples & Steslow, 2001; Haber, 2007a; Haber & Looney, 2000; Haber & Rhodes, 2004; Jette et al., 1999, Johnson et al., 1992; Leslie & Schuster, 1991; Lorig et al., 1996, 2000; Moore et al., 2000; Neale et al., 1990; Schlenk & Boehm, 1998; Swinburn et al., 1998).

There are many versions of health contracts ranging from the simple to the complex. Here is an example of a simple weight-loss contract developed by Dr. Joseph Chemplavil, a cardiac endocrinologist in Hampton, Virginia:

> *I, (patient's name), hereby promise to myself and to Dr. Chemplavil, that I will make every effort to lose my (agreed-upon) weight, and I will pay $1 to Dr. Chemplavil's Dollar for Pound Fund, for every pound of weight that I gain, on each visit to the office, by cash. I also understand that I will receive $1 from the same fund for each pound of weight that I lose.*

Dr. Chemplavil paid out $1,044 to 118 patients, received $166 from 30 patients, and two patients broke even (Kazel, 2004).

Research on health contracts has been limited and often marred by a lack of random assignment to treatment and control groups, small sample sizes, and lack of replication. In addition, there are several uncertainties about the effectiveness of health contracts in terms of one's ability to identify which components work better than others (e.g., health education, social support, the professional-client relationship, memory enhancement, motivation building, contingency rewards, etc.), whether contracts work better with one type of person than another, and how to determine the content and amount of training that is required for health educators or clinicians to help clients implement health contracts.

Even without a definitive body of research, health contracts are widely used. They are simple to administer, time-efficient, and even cost-effective when medical personnel assign the completion of health contracts to a health educator or trained office worker. The health contract can also be effectively taught to students in the classroom who are interested in health education, risk factor counseling, or program development (Haber, 2007a).

Exercise

The 1996 *Surgeon General's Report on Physical Activity and Health* was an outstanding review of the research on the effects of physical activity on people's health, and it has yet to be improved upon. According to the Surgeon General's report, regular exercise and physical activity improve health in a variety of ways, including a reduction in heart disease, diabetes, high blood pressure, colon cancer, depression, anxiety, excess weight, falling, bone thinning, muscle wasting, and joint pain.

However, 60% of adults did not achieve the recommended amount of physical activity, and 25% of adults were not physically active at all. Inactivity increased with age; by age 75 about one in three men and one in two women engaged in no physical activity. Inactivity was also more common among women and people with lower income and less education.

The most significant component of the Surgeon General's report was its advocacy for several tested exercise principles. First, motivation is very important, and to enhance it requires a large degree of modesty in setting goals and at least a small degree of enjoyment. Hence, the emphasis on being more physically active rather than a narrow adherence to a rigid exercise regimen.

Second, Americans should get at least 30 minutes of physical activity or exercise most days of the week. This statement provided a major perspective shift from previous recommendations by government and exercise leaders. This new message recommended that Americans become more concerned about total calories expended through exercise than about intensity level or duration of continuous exercise. Regarding intensity level, the report stresses the importance of raising respiratory rate and body warmth—physiological changes that are apparent to the participant—but not to be too concerned about raising intensity level to a target heart rate, particularly if the person is sedentary or has a less than active lifestyle.

Regarding duration of continuous exercise, it is no longer deemed essential to obtain 30 consecutive minutes of exercise. For Americans, the large majority of whom are not too active, accumulating shorter activity spurts throughout the day is effective. Taking a brisk walk in a shopping mall or climbing a few stairs in spare minutes can accumulate the benefits of exercise. A review of the research literature concludes that accumulating several 5- or 10-minute bouts of physical activity over the course of the day provides beneficial health and fitness effects (DeBusk et al., 1990; Jakicic et al., 1995; Lee et al., 2000; Murphy et al., 2002; Pate et al., 1995). One study reported that if a person times these bouts of activity correctly they can gain the added benefit of replacing junk food snack breaks (Jakicic et al., 1995).

Regarding exercise itself, it is difficult for adults to go from inactivity to an exercise routine. Thinking about how to accumulate short bouts of activity is a useful way to get started on better health and fitness. For example, nurses can encourage older adults to vacuum the carpet more briskly than normally (even if it means doing it in segments throughout the day), or to put more energy into leaf raking or lawn mowing, gardening with enthusiasm, or dancing to music on the radio. In addition, nurses should not underestimate the ability of older adults to engage in adventurous or unusual sports (**Figure 11-3**).

Finally, the Surgeon General's report urged Americans to be active most days of the week. We should aim for the habit of everyday physical activity or exercise, but should not allow the occasional lapse to discourage us. Making physical activity or exercise a near-daily routine is more likely to become an enduring habit than the previously recommended three-times-per-week exercise routine.

For most older adults, a brisk walking program will provide sufficient intensity for a good aerobics program. An 8-year study of more than 13,000 people indicated that walking briskly for 30 to 60 minutes every day was almost as beneficial in reducing the death rate as jogging up to 40 miles a week (Blair et al., 1989). The authors of a study of 1,645 older adults reported that simply walking 4 hours per week decreased the risk of future hospitalization for cardiovascular disease (LaCroix et al., 1996).

The National Center for Health Statistics (1985) reported that walking has much greater appeal for older adults than high-intensity exercise. A national survey indicated that a smaller percentage of persons age 65-plus (27%) engaged in vigorous activities, in comparison to 41% of the general adult population (41%); however, people of all age groups (41%) were equally likely to walk for exercise.

Many older adults are concerned about unfavorable weather and may abandon their walking routine as a consequence. Prolonged hot or cold spells may sabotage a good walking program. Rather than discontinue this activity because of the weather, adults may choose to walk indoors at their local shopping malls. Many shopping malls—about 2,500 nationwide—open their doors early, usually between 5:30 and 10:00 a.m., for members of walking clubs.

There is also a relationship between one's neighborhood and one's health. Residents who depend on a car to get to most places and have few sidewalks for safe walking are likely to be more obese and have chronic medical conditions that impact on health-related quality of life (Booth et al., 2005; Sturm & Cohen, 2004). For every extra 30 minutes commuters drive each day they have a 3% greater chance of being obese; in contrast, people who live within walking distance of shops are 7% less likely to be obese (Frank et al., 2004). Older persons who believe their neighborhoods are favorable for walking are up to 100% more physically active (King et al., 2003; Li et al., 2005). People at high risk for inactivity may increase their physical activity when they have access to walking trails (Brownson et al., 2000).

A sedentary person is estimated to walk about 3,500 steps a day, and the average American about

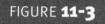

FIGURE **11-3** **Older adults may continue sporting activities well into later life and share them with their grandchildren. These grandparents took their adult grandchildren on a trail ride in the Colorado Rockies.**

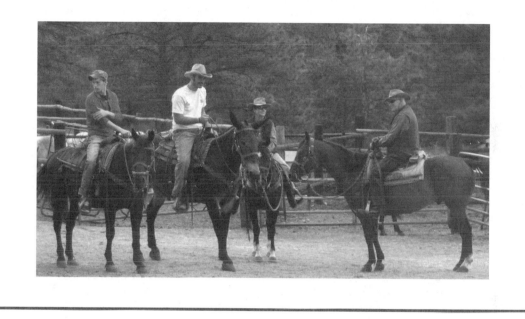

5,130 steps. Many advocates believe Americans should aim for 10,000 steps a day, or about 5 miles. Workplace physical activity, particularly among blue-collar occupations, helps many people reach the 10,000-step target, leaving older adults (and overweight office workers) most likely to be at risk (McCormack et al., 2006).

Pedometers are small devices that count steps, and are typically attached at the waist. They first appeared in Japan in 1965 under the name Manpometer—*manpo* in Japanese means 10,000 steps. Their introduction into America took another few decades, but they have been rapidly increasing in popularity—even McDonald's distributed them for a while as part of an adult Happy Meal called Go Active (salad, bottled water, and a pedometer for $4.99). Studies, though, have been equivocal about the benefits of using a pedometer to motivate individuals.

One study, for instance, reported that pedometers added no additional benefit to a coaching intervention (Engel & Lindner, 2006), whereas another publication noted that it increased the frequency of short walking trips (Stovitz et al., 2005). One study reported that cheap pedometers are likely to overestimate the actual number of steps taken (De Cocker et al., 2006). There are many ways in addition to the use of a pedometer to add steps to a daily routine. For information and guidelines on this topic, contact America on the Move, at www.americaonthemove.org.

Another option for older adults is to join a noncompetitive walking or hiking club, or to participate in a nearby walking or hiking event. Two opportunities in this regard are the American Volkssport Association at 800-830-9255 or www.ava.org, and the local Sierra Club at www.sierraclub.org. If you want to add a mind-body dimension to walking, try ChiWalking, which combines walking with the principles of tai chi (www.chiwalking.com).

Traveling to another city can also be an excuse not to exercise. Or it can be an opportunity to gather information from the local newspaper or chamber of commerce about a walking tour for an enjoyable way to get exercise and a unique way to learn about offbeat aspects of a city's history. Most if not all big cities have walking tours, and some sound particularly intriguing (such as Oak Park, Illinois's self-guided walking tours of Frank Lloyd Wright homes and the Big Onion walking tours of New York City's ethnic communities and restaurants [www.bigonion.com]).

There are many other aspects of exercise besides aerobics that are important for older adults to know about, including strength building, flexibility, and balance. There are also many important topics that need to be considered, such as safety, qualified exercise leaders for older adults, fitness clubs that motivate older adults, and the compatibility of an exercise routine with the medical status of an individual. For a detailed description of a model exercise program and related exercise topics, see Haber (2007b).

NUTRITION

Nutrition is only one component in the development and exacerbation of disease (heredity, environment, medical care, social circumstances, and other lifestyle risk factors also play a part), but eating and drinking habits have been implicated in 6 of the 10 leading causes of death—heart disease, cancer, stroke, diabetes, atherosclerosis, and liver disease—as well as in several debilitating disorders like osteoporosis and diverticulosis.

Older adults are in a particularly precarious position because they are more vulnerable to both obesity and malnutrition than other age groups. The highest percentage of obese adults is in the age group 50–69, with those ages 70–79 the next most obese (Squires, 2002). Also, older adults are at the highest risk of being malnourished (Beers & Berkow, 2000). Social isolation, dental problems, medical disease, and medication usage are among the risk factors for malnourishment in older adults.

Older adults are more conscientious about nutrition than other age groups, according to one national study (Harris et al., 1989). In this sample, a higher percentage of those over age 65 (approximately two-thirds) than of those in their 40s (one-half) reported trying "a lot" to limit sodium, fat, and sugar; eat enough fiber; lower cholesterol; and consume enough vitamins and minerals.

If older adults are paying more attention to their nutritional habits, one can only speculate that they may be motivated by more immediate feedback (heartburn, constipation, and so forth), or by feelings of greater vulnerability (higher risk of impairment from disease and of loss of independence). The next cohort of older adults—today's baby boomers—bring more than motivation to the table. They also bring a higher formal education level, including a strong interest in health education.

The federal government provides a modest amount of nutrition education for older adults and the rest of the American public. The 2005 *Dietary Guidelines for Americans* includes a 70-page blueprint for nutritional policy; a revised Food Guide Pyramid, dubbed MyPyramid; and a Web site, www.mypyramid.gov. The guidelines are redrafted every 5 years by the U.S. Department of Agriculture (USDA) and the Department of Health and Human Services (DHHS). The Food Guide Pyramid, however, had not been updated for 13 years, and the Web site was a brand new initiative. The entire update was billed as an interactive food guidance system rather than a one-size-fits-all initiative.

The guidelines basically encourage Americans to eat fruits, vegetables, whole grains, and low-fat or fat-free dairy products, and there is much more detail on the consumption of these foods than was provided by previous guidelines. Fruits and vegetables are increased to 5 to 13 servings per day. Salt guidelines are specific for the first time, limiting it to one level teaspoon a day. Trans fat is identified for the first time, and the advice is to keep intake as low as possible. Saturated fat limitations have become specific, keeping it to 10% of calories or less. Cholesterol level is to be less than 300 milligrams. Added sugars or sweeteners are discouraged for the first time, particularly in drinks. Whole grains are differentiated from the broad category of carbohydrates, and the recommendation is half the grain servings should be whole grains.

The Web site offers people specific dietary recommendations on grains, vegetables, fruit, milk, meat and beans, total fat, saturated fat, cholesterol, sodium, oils, and fats/sugars. Types and duration of physical activity are assessed as well, with specific recommendations. The Web site is interesting and informative.

Another educational tool is the **nutrition bull's-eye** developed by Covert Bailey (1996). The goal of the bull's-eye is for people to consume the nutritious foods that are listed in the center of it. These foods are low in saturated fat, sugar, and sodium, and high in fiber. They include skim milk, nonfat yogurt, most fruits and vegetables, whole grains, beans and legumes, and water-packed tuna. As you move to the foods listed in the rings farther away from the bull's-eye, you eat more saturated fat, sugar, sodium, and low-fiber foods. In the outer ring of the bull's-eye, therefore, are most cheeses, ice cream, butter, whole milk, beef, cake, cookies, potato chips, and mayonnaise.

Unlike the Food Guide Pyramid, Bailey's bull's-eye is focused on making distinctions *within* food categories. Whole-wheat products, for instance, are in the bull's-eye, whereas products made from refined white flour and those with added sugar are placed in the outer circles. Fresh fruits and vegetables are in the bull's-eye, but juiced vegetables and fruit that lose fiber and that concentrate sugars are placed in a ring just outside of the bull's-eye. Skim milk, low-fat and nonfat cottage cheese, and part-skim mozzarella are in the center ring, whereas whole milk and most cheeses are in the outer circles of the target.

The author has offered older clients a personalized version of the nutrition bull's-eye. In this version, you begin with a blank bull's-eye, and then add food and drink products that you usually consume to each of the rings. The foods and drinks in the personalized nutrition bull's-eye (see **Figure 11-4**) are clearly superior; the second ring is not quite as nutrient dense; the third ring is neutral, products that are not particularly harmful or helpful; and the outer ring includes the least nutritious foods and drinks that should be consumed sparingly.

In the center and innermost ring of the personalized bull's-eye, patients also add the foods and drinks that they are not currently consuming, but that they find sufficiently desirable and are considering adding to their diet (in italics in Figure 11-4). The assignment of food and drink products to each of the rings is likely best done with the aid of a dietitian who can assess their nutritional value. (Darson Rhodes and Mandy Puckett, former nutrition students at Ball State University, identified products for the personalized nutrition bull's-eye in Figure 11-4.)

The **Center for Science in the Public Interest (CSPI)** is the premier educational and advocacy organization for promoting better nutritional habits in the United States. Its educational component consists of the *Nutrition Action Healthletter*, published monthly, which informs more than 800,000 subscribers, including this author. The organization is best known, however, for its advocacy accomplishments, under the leadership of its executive director and cofounder (in 1971), Michael Jacobson.

Jacobson and CSPI staff, for example, have led the fight for nutrition labels on food items in the supermarket; for exposing the hidden fat in Chinese, Mexican, Italian, and delicatessen food; for pressuring movie theaters to stop cooking popcorn in artery-clogging coconut oil; for warning labels on Procter & Gamble's fake fat, Olean, which may interfere with the absorption of nutrients and cause loose stools and cramping; for more accurate labeling of ground beef in supermarkets; and for the listing of trans fat on nutrition labels.

For more information, contact the Center for Science in the Public Interest, at their Web site www.cspinet.org.

MENTAL HEALTH

Neither the average 50% reduction in income at retirement nor the increases in emotional losses, physical losses, and caregiving responsibilities in later life result in a persistent reduction in life satisfaction among most older adults. As sociologist Linda George (1986) notes, "Older adults are apparently masters of the art of lowering aspirations to meet realities" (p. 7).

Life Review

One tool for preserving or enhancing the **mental health** of older adults is the **life review**, which is

FIGURE 11-4 **Personalized nutrition bull's-eye.**

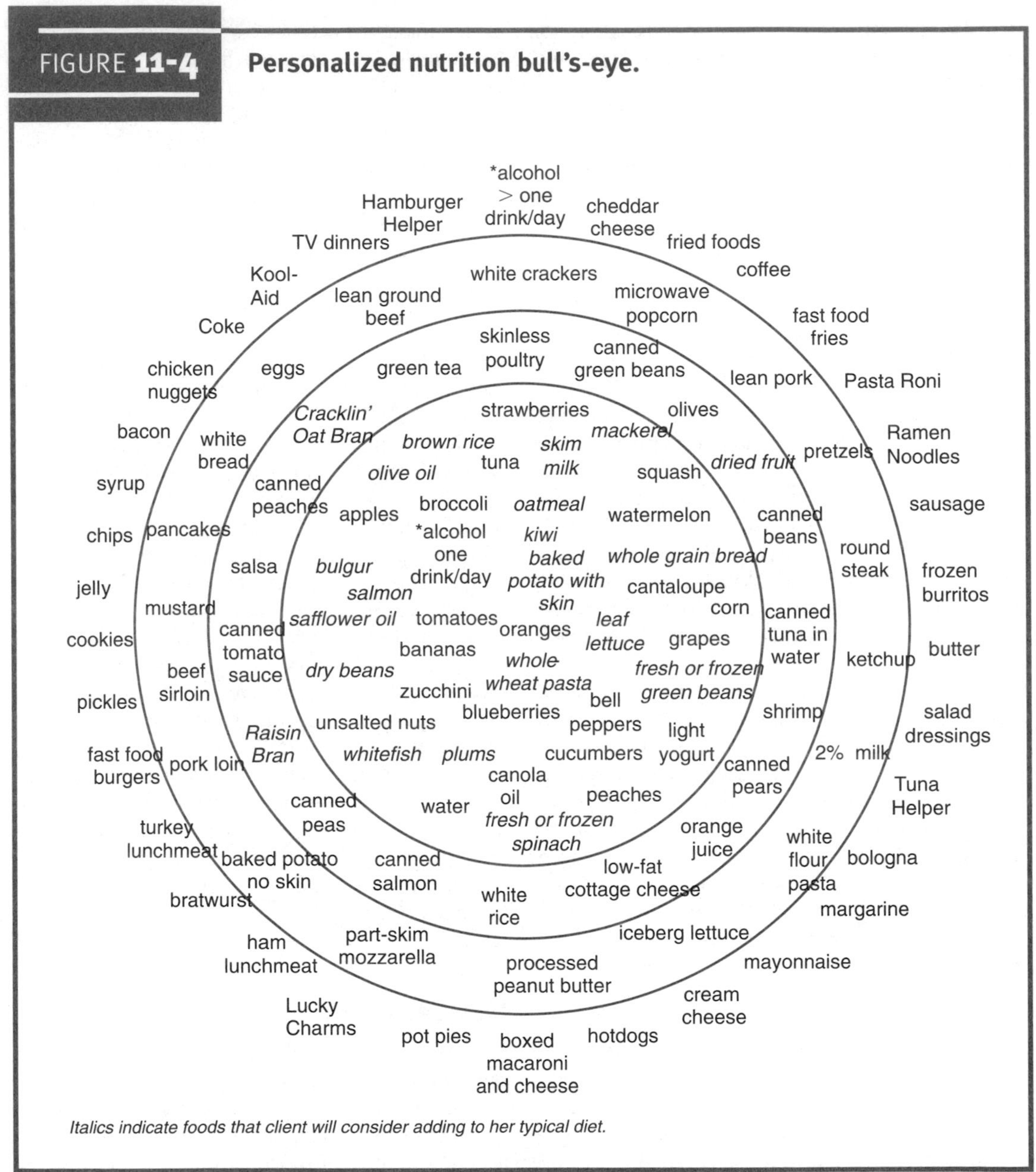

Italics indicate foods that client will consider adding to her typical diet.

SOURCE: Permission from D. Haber, *Health Promotion and Aging: Practical Applications for Health Professionals:* NY: Springer Publishing Company, 4th edition, 2007, p. 191.

an autobiographical effort that can be preserved in print, by tape recording, or on videotape. The review is guided by a series of questions in specific life domains, such as work and family, as well as memories further stimulated through a family photo album, other memorabilia, a genealogy, musical selections from an earlier time, or a trek back to an important place in one's past. It can be conducted by oneself, in a dyad, or as part of a group process. A life review is more likely to be conducted by or with an older adult who is relatively content with his or her life and not seeking therapy than it is to be used therapeutically with an older adult. Nonetheless, life reviews are believed to have therapeutic powers, and they are incorporated into a wide variety of counseling modalities (Haber, 2006).

The psychiatrist Robert Butler first extolled the benefits of the life review process to his colleagues and the public as early as 1961, as a way of incorporating reminiscence in the aged as part of a normal aging process. Dr. Butler described the life review as more comprehensive and systematic than spontaneous reminiscing, and perhaps more important in old age when there may be a need to put one's life in order and to come to an acceptance of present circumstances (Butler, 1995).

Notable Quotes

"To age gracefully requires that we stop denying the fact of aging and learn and practice what we have to do to keep our bodies and minds in good working order through all the phases of life."

—Andrew Weil, MD, from his introduction in his national best-seller *Healthy Aging: A Lifelong Guide to Your Well-Being*, p. 7.

The review of positive and negative past life experiences by older adults has enabled them to overcome feelings of depression and despair (Butler, 1974; Butler et al., 1991; Watt & Cappeliez, 2000). Another study of the life review process reported positive outcomes in terms of stronger life satisfaction, psychological well-being, self-esteem, and reduced depression (Haight et al., 1998).

Although life reviews are usually helpful for improving the mental health of most older adults who are seeking meaning, resolution, reconciliation, direction, and atonement, physicians, nurses, and other clinic personnel find it is too time-consuming to listen to the reminiscences of older clients in this era of medical care. Health professionals can, however, play a key role in referring older clients to appropriate forums or helping them obtain relevant life review materials.

One book, *Aging and Biography*, by the psychologist James Birren and colleagues (1996), helps guide and provide structure for the life review process by suggesting a focus on several themes, such as love, money, work, and family. Birren also suggests in another book, *Telling the Stories of Life Through Guided Autobiography Groups*, that incorporating life reviews into a small-group format can help in the retrieval of memories as well as with the acceptance of memories (Birren & Cochran, 2001).

With careful monitoring, Birren noted that in his years of experience he has not had a group member report becoming depressed as a result of a life review (Birren & Deutchman, 1991). He warned, however, that persons who are already depressed or otherwise needing therapy should be under the supervision of a qualified professional.

Depression

Whether older adults participate in life reviews or not, they are vulnerable to **depression** due to losses that accompany aging such as widowhood, chronic medical conditions and pain, and functional dependence (Lantz, 2002). Not only can these emotional and physical losses lead to depression, but depression in turn can lead to more physical decline (Penninx et al., 1998b).

Although the mechanism is not understood, depression increases the likelihood of mortality from cancer (Penninx et al., 1998a) and heart disease (Frasure-Smith et al., 1995). The mortality rate for depressed patients with cardiovascular disease is twice that of those without depression (Lantz, 2002). Even mild depression can weaken the immune system in older persons if it goes on long enough (McGuire et al., 2002).

Depression also plays a significant role in suicidal behaviors, and older persons have the highest suicide rate of any age group. Older adults account for 25% of all suicide deaths, though they make up only about 13% of the general population. This elevated suicide rate, however, is largely accounted for by white men age 85 or older. The suicide rate of this age/gender category is six times higher than the overall national rate (Centers for Disease Control and Prevention, 1999).

Depression in older adults often goes undetected until it is too late. Between 63% (Rabins, 1996) and 90% (Katon et al., 1992) of depressed older patients go untreated or receive inadequate treatment. One retrospective study of older adults who had committed suicide revealed that 51 of the 97 patients studied had seen their primary care physician within one month of their suicide date. Of these 51, only 19 were even offered treatment, and only 2 of the 51 patients studied were provided adequate treatment (Caine et al., 1996).

Barry Lebowitz (1995) of the National Institute of Mental Health estimated that 15% of Americans age 65 or over suffered from serious and persistent symptoms of depression, but only 3% were reported to be suffering from the clinical diagnosis of major depression. In other words, although depressive disorders that fulfill rigorous diagnostic criteria are relatively rare, subthreshold disorders are considerably more common, infrequently diagnosed or treated with prescribed antidepressants, and because they usually go untreated, are likely to become chronic conditions (Beekman et al., 2002).

Detection of depression is hampered not only by the underreporting of symptoms by older patients, but also by biases on the part of physicians and family members. In one study, 75% of physicians thought that depression was understandable in older persons, that is, a normal facet of old age (Gallo et al., 1999). Family members may also view the signs and symptoms of depression as "normal aging," when in fact the persistence of depressive symptoms is not normal.

MODEL HEALTH PROMOTION PROGRAMS FOR OLDER ADULTS

Although there is no certain method for determining what constitutes a **model health promotion program**, there has been no shortage of attempts to identify them, develop a catalog that includes a summary of these exemplars, and distribute the catalog around the country in order to encourage their replication. Many of these model health promotion programs have been developed over the years with the aid of federal grants and other funding sources, have gone through multiple program evaluations, and can be helpful to health professionals who are interested in launching or improving their own program.

BOX 11-2 Recommended Electronic Newsletter

Human Values in Aging is edited by Harry (Rick) Moody. It is a free, monthly e-newsletter that contains items of interest about humanistic gerontology, including late-life creativity, spirituality, the humanities, arts and aging, and lifelong learning. For a sample copy or free subscription, e-mail hrmoody@yahoo.com.

One of the more recent efforts in this regard has been organized by the Health Promotion Institute (HPI) of the National Council on Aging. HPI started by summarizing 16 model programs or best practices and compiling them into a loose-leaf directory. The summaries included information on the planning process, implementation of the program, and program evaluations. Each year, new best practices have been added to this directory. If interested in obtaining a copy, contact the National Council on Aging, Health Promotion Institute, 300 D St., SW, #801, Washington, DC 20024; 202-479-1200; or www.ncoa.org.

Six model health promotion programs that have focused on older adults and have received national attention are summarized in the following sections. These programs have received federal funding and foundation support to evaluate their effectiveness and to encourage their replication.

Healthwise

The best-known older adult medical self-care program is Healthwise, located in Boise, Idaho. The Healthwise program relies mostly on the *Healthwise Handbook*, which provides information and prevention tips on 190 common health problems, with information periodically updated. The *Healthwise Handbook* (Healthwise, 2006) is now in its 17th edition. This handbook includes physician-approved guidelines on when to call a health professional for each of the health problems it covers. Some Healthwise community programs have supplemented the distribution of the handbook with group health education programs or nurse call-in programs. There is a Spanish language edition of the *Healthwise Handbook*, called *La Salud en Casa*, and a special self-care guide for older adults called *Healthwise for Life*.

With the assistance of a $2.1 million grant from the Robert Wood Johnson Foundation, Healthwise distributed its medical self-care guide to 125,000 Idaho households, along with toll-free nurse consultation phone service and self-care workshops. Thirty-nine percent of handbook recipients reported that the handbook helped them avoid a visit to the doctor (Mettler, 1997). Blue Cross of Idaho reported 18% fewer visits to the emergency room by owners of the guide.

Elements of the Healthwise program have been replicated in the United Kingdom, South Africa, New Zealand, Australia, and Canada. In British Columbia, the *Healthwise Handbook* was distributed to every household, and all 4.3 million residents had potential access to the Healthwise content through a Web site and a nurse call center.

Additional information can be obtained from Donald Kemper or Molly Mettler, at www.healthwise.org.

Chronic Disease Self-Management Program

Kate Lorig, a nurse-researcher at the Stanford University School of Medicine, and her medical colleagues have been evaluating community-based, peer-led, chronic disease self-management programs for more than two decades, beginning with the Arthritis Self-Management Program (Lorig et al., 1986). This program has since evolved into a curriculum that is applicable to a wide array of chronic diseases and conditions.

Typically, each program involves about a dozen participants, led by peer leaders who have received 20 hours of training. The peer leaders, like the students, are typically older and have chronic diseases that they contend with. The program consists of six weekly sessions about 2½ hours long each, with a content focus on exercise, symptom management, nutrition, fatigue and sleep management, use of medications, managing emotions, community resources, communicating with health professionals, problem solving, and decision making. The program takes place in community settings such as senior centers, churches, and hospitals.

The theoretical basis of the program has been to promote a sense of personal efficacy among participants (Bandura, 1997) by using such techniques as guided mastery of skills, peer modeling, reinterpretation of symptoms, social persuasion through group support, and individual self-management guidance. In addition to improving self-efficacy, Lorig and colleagues (2001) reported reduced emergency room and outpatient visits, and decreased health distress, fatigue, and limitations in role function.

The Chronic Disease Self-Management Program is housed at Stanford University's Patient Education Research Center, 1000 Welch Road, #204, Palo Alto, CA 94304; 650-723-7935; http://patienteducation.stanford.edu/programs/cdsmp.html.

Project Enhance

Senior Services of Seattle/King County began the Senior Wellness Project (later renamed Project Enhance) in 1997 at the North Shore Senior Center in Bothell, Washington. It was a research-based health promotion program that included a component of chronic care self-management that was modeled after Kate Lorig's program (Lorig et al., 1999). The program also included health and functional assessments; individual and group counseling; exercise programs; a personal health action plan with the support of a nurse, social worker, and volunteer health mentor; and support groups. A randomized controlled study of chronically ill seniors reported a reduction in number of hospital stays and average length of stay, a reduction in psychotropic medications, and better functioning in activities of daily living (Leveille et al., 1998).

Project Enhance is a partnership among a university, an Area Agency on Aging, local and national foundations, health departments, senior centers, primary care providers, older volunteers, and older participants. Versions of this model program are being replicated at senior wellness sites around the country (80+ sites in the United States) and two sites in Sweden to test its effectiveness in a variety of communities, in an assortment of sites, serving a diversity of clientele. Findings have demonstrated higher levels of physical activity and lower levels of depression among its participants (Dobkin, 2002).

Project Enhance is currently divided into two components: Enhance Fitness and Enhance Wellness. Enhance Fitness is an exercise program that focuses on stretching, flexibility, balance, low impact aerobics, and strength training. Certified instructors have undergone special training in fitness for older adults. Classes last an hour, involve 10 to 25 people, and participants can track their progress through a series of functional evaluations.

Participants who completed 6 months of Enhance Fitness improved significantly in a variety of physical and social functioning measures, as well as reporting reduced levels of pain and depression. There was also a reduction in health care costs (Ackerman et al., 2003). The Enhance Fitness program has been replicated in 64 community sites across 6 states.

Enhance Wellness focuses on mental health, with an emphasis on lessening symptoms of depression and other mood problems, developing a sense of greater self-reliance, and lowering the need for drugs that affect thinking or emotions. Enhance Wellness typically consists of a nurse and social worker working with an individual. An analysis of the effectiveness of the program found that it reduced depression one year after the program and improved exercise readiness, physical activity levels, and self-reported health (Phelan et al., 2002).

To learn more about Project Enhance, contact Susan Snyder, Program Director at Senior Services of Seattle/King County at susans@seniorservices.org.

Ornish Program for Reversing Heart Disease

Dr. Dean Ornish, a physician at the University of California at San Francisco and founder of the Preventive Medicine Research Institute, has developed a program for reversing heart disease that has been replicated at several sites around the country. Dr. Ornish (1992) has recommended a vegetarian diet with fat intake of 10% or less of total calories, moderate aerobic exercise at least three times a week, yoga and meditation an hour a day, group support sessions, and smoking cessation.

Dr. Ornish and his colleagues have reported that as a result of their program, blockages in arteries have decreased in size, and blood flow has improved in as many as 82% of their heart patients (Gould et al., 1995). A 5-year follow-up of this program reported an 8% reduction in atherosclerotic plaques, while the control group had a 28% increase. Also during this time, cardiac events were more than doubled in the control group (Ornish et al., 1998).

The applicability of Ornish's program to the average patient is still of uncertain utility. It may take highly motivated individuals (e.g., patients with severe heart disease) and significant medical and health support (requiring significant resources) for the model program to be useful to others. For additional information, contact Dean Ornish, MD, at http://www.pmri.org.

Benson's Mind/Body Medical Institute

Dr. Herbert Benson is a physician affiliated with Harvard Medical School, and best known for his best-selling books on the relaxation response and for popularizing the term *mind/body medicine*. For individuals feeling the negative effects of stress, Benson's program teaches them to elicit the relaxation response, a western version of meditation. The Benson-Henry Institute for Mind/Body Medicine's clinical programs treat patients with a combination of relaxation response techniques, proper nutrition and exercise, and the reframing of negative thinking patterns.

Benson's nonprofit scientific and educational institute conducts research, provides outpatient medical services, and trains health professionals, postdoctoral fellows, and medical students. The Benson-Henry Institute for Mind/Body Medicine can be contacted at www.mbmi.org.

The research results from Benson's and Ornish's programs attracted the attention of Medicare, which funded a demonstration project to evaluate these programs. As a consequence of the demonstration project, in 2006 Medicare began to reimburse eligible patients for participation in the two cardiac wellness programs, Ornish's Reversing Heart Disease and Benson's Mind/Body Medicine. These two programs have expanded the emphasis in Medicare from acute care medicine, rehabilitative medicine, and prevention to the inclusion of comprehensive wellness.

Strong for Life

The Strong for Life program is a home-based exercise program for disabled and nondisabled older adults. It focuses on strength and balance, and provides an exercise video, a trainer's manual, and a user's guide. The program was designed by physical therapists for home use by older adults, and relies on elastic resistive bands for strengthening muscles. The exercise program led to a high rate of exercise adherence among older participants, as well as increased lower extremity strength, improvements in tandem gait, and a reduction in physical disability (Jette et al., 1999).

This program is housed at Boston University's Roybal Center, Sargent College, 635 Commonwealth Ave., Boston, MA 02215; 617 353-2713; www.bu.edu/roybal.

RE-ENGAGEMENT INSTEAD OF RETIREMENT

In 2011, baby boomers begin turning age 65 and start becoming the gerontology boomers. Most of them will not retire, if by retirement is meant a type of disengagement. Why will these gerontology boomers be different from the current crop of retirees?

First, the boomers will be the *longest-lived cohort* of older adults. They may have 25 or 30 years of life to negotiate after giving up their main line of work. How many of them will be comfortable with the idea of a quarter century without additional earnings? How many will be comfortable letting go of education, exploration, and engagement?

The boomers will be the *best-educated cohort* of older adults. Between 1950 and 2000, the percentage of Americans age 65 or over with a high school diploma leaped from 18% to 66%; college graduates jumped from 4% to 15%. In 1991, 17% of Americans age 60–64 were involved in adult education; by 1999 that had jumped to 32%. They say a mind is a terrible thing to waste, not only from the individual's standpoint, but from society's as well. Seventy-six million minds to be precise.

The boomers will be the *healthiest cohort* of older adults. Almost 90% of Americans ages 65–74 report that they have no disability, and the disability rate for older Americans continues to decline. An increasing number of older adults are exercising in late life, with brisk walking for exercise becoming commonplace among the old. Not only is a mind a terrible thing to waste, so is a healthy body.

Also, the boomers may become the *most-engaged cohort* of older adults. Fifty-four percent of boomers say helping others is important to them. A 2002 national survey by Hart Research Associates reported that about 60% of older Americans believe that retirement is a "time to be active and involved, to start new activities and to set new goals." A 2005 survey by Civic Ventures and the MetLife Foundation reported that 58% of leading-edge baby boomers, those between ages 51 and 59, said they want to take jobs that serve their communities.

In addition, the boomers will be the *largest cohort* of retirees ever. The number of Americans age 65 or older will increase from 35 million in 2000 to more than 70 million in 2030. When these boomers came into the world they revolutionized hospitals and health care just through their sheer size. They did the same thing to public schools, the Vietnam War, and then the housing market, spurring a tremendous growth in building. A cohort this large is unlikely to pass into retirement and leave it unchanged. And boomers are unlikely to accept things as they are.

What might older adults do, if they decide to re-engage rather than retire? Here are two possibilities.

Experience Corps

Experience Corps is a foundation-supported program that has placed 2,000 older adults as tutors and mentors with 20,000 low-income children in urban, public elementary schools and after-school programs in 19 cities. These programs not only boost the academic performance of students, but enhance the well-being of the older volunteers in the process (Fried et al., 2004; Rebok et al., 2004; Tan et al., 2006). Much work remains as two-thirds of the nation's fourth graders in major urban areas are reading below basic levels for their grade. For more information, contact Experience Corps at www.experiencecorps.org.

The North Carolina Center for Creative Retirement

The North Carolina Center for Creative Retirement (NCCCR) has implemented a course entitled Creative Retirement in Uncertain Times. Through lectures, case studies, discussion groups, and community activities, older participants explore their image of retirement, their ability to revitalize themselves, and their plan of action.

With the help of a civic engagement grant from the National Council on Aging, NCCCR created a

Leadership Training Program for Older Persons. It enables low-income older adults age 50 or older to gain the skills and confidence necessary to advocate for their peers by becoming effective leaders in community organizations that rarely include representatives from low-income groups.

The North Carolina Center for Creative Retirement can be contacted at www.unca.edu/ncccr. For information about demonstration grants awarded to encourage civic engagement, contact the National Council on Aging, 300 D. St., SW, #801, Washington, DC, 20024; 202-479-1200; www.ncoa.org.

There are hundreds of courses hosted at institutes of higher education targeted toward older adults, some of which are peer-led by retired older adults. Older adults can find out if there are similar educational offerings in their local area by contacting nearby colleges and universities.

GREEN HOUSE

Nursing homes are not homes, they are institutions. No matter how well run they are, they are not places where most of us want to end up. We are at the beginning of revolutionizing the long-term care industry, and no one has been more innovative and successful at this early stage than William Thomas, MD, founder of the **Green House**. Dr. Thomas started out his career as a medical director in a nursing home and was saddened by how regimented and joyless the environment was.

In traditional nursing homes, residents are viewed as sick and dependent, which fosters learned helplessness and induced disability. Staff may encourage wheelchair dependency to serve the needs of staff members who are pressed for time. Dressing, feeding, bathing, and toileting need to be routinized and sped up for aides needing to stay on schedule. A staff member is more likely to rely on incontinence briefs than to take the time to develop individualized toileting routines.

Green Houses, in contrast, look like surrounding homes in a residential community. They are homes, not home-like, though they are bigger than the average home. The first ones were constructed in Tupelo, Mississippi, in 2003, and were 6,400 square feet. The rooms in these homes include extra expense, such as ceiling lifts, but these innovations can save costs over the long term by reducing back injuries, employee turnover, and workers' compensation.

Green House workers are paid more and are better trained than the typical nursing assistant, but the extra costs are offset by employee empowerment that reduces staff turnover and additional training expenses. The annual employee turnover rate in the average nursing home is 75%, whereas it was less than 10% in the first Green House in Tupelo. Moreover, not one staff person left during the house's first 3 years of existence.

About 10 people live in a Green House, each having a private room and bath, and access to a central hearth where cooking and socializing are done. There is a surrounding garden for contemplative walks and for growing vegetables and flowers. Doors can be opened to view the garden and hearth from an individual room or closed for privacy. With the circular nature of the individual rooms, both the garden and the central hearth are within 30 feet. There is strategically placed furniture to help with "cruising" to central areas and to help with gains in mobility (see **Case Study 11-1**).

Green Houses promote autonomy. Residents get up, eat, and go to bed when they want. They decide on which foods to eat, and that may even include pizza, wine, or ice cream. Medications are locked in individual rooms, rather than distributed by a cart that is wheeled from room to room. There are few features that are different from the typical home. If there are unusual features, they are deemphasized, like a ceiling lift that is recessed and used only when needed for transfer. Induction cooking in the kitchen prevents residents from burning themselves on a stove. Stoves have shut-off valves, with pot trappers to prevent hot pots from burning residents. A safety gate around the kitchen can be used when necessary.

People in the first 10 Green Houses were selected from nursing homes and represented a typical nursing home population. Of the first 40 selected, 12 had advanced dementia, and all Green House residents had the typical array of physical and cognitive limitations associated with the average nursing home resident.

Decision making is lodged in residents and workers, unless there are safety or budget issues that can-

Case Study 11-1

Dr. Brown is a retired superintendent of a large public school system in the Midwest. He has been widowed for 5 years and just recently retired at the age of 69 after experiencing a fall down a flight of stairs at his home that resulted in a fractured hip, skull fracture, and broken shoulder for which he has been treated in the hospital and is being discharged soon. Dr. Brown's two adult children have encouraged him to sell his home and move somewhere where there is help available when he needs it. Dr. Brown hates the thought of a nursing home, especially since his wife spent about a year in one before her death. He is not certain whether an assisted living facility would work for him either. The family asks the hospital nurse for assistance in exploring living options for Dr. Brown.

Questions:

1. What questions should the nurse ask of Dr. Brown to help determine his preferences for living situations?
2. What other factors are essential to know about Dr. Brown in order to assist him with proper choices?
3. Are there any other team members who should be consulted within the hospital that could help with this decision? If so, who?
4. Would a Green House be a better option than assisted or independent living for Dr. Brown? Why or why not? What factors must be considered before answering this question?

not be handled at that level. Aides are called shahbazim (derived from the mythical Persian royal falcon that protected the king), with the primary job responsibility to protect, nurture, and sustain.

Ideal staff ratio is 1 for every 5 residents; nurse ratio is 1 for every 2 houses (or 1 per 20 people), and administrator ratio (and one assistant) 1 for every 12 houses (or 1 per 120 people). Staff find replacements for themselves if sick, either through a substitute pool or through overtime (which is managed within the allowable budget).

Workers receive 120 hours of additional training in areas such as CPR, first aid, culinary skills, safe food handling, communication, and dementia care. They are better paid than the average long-term care worker ($11 per hour versus $7.50) and are given rotating responsibility (purchasing food and cooking, housekeeping, scheduling, budget, etc.). Unless the nonclinical work teams endanger safety or overspend budget, administrators cannot overrule their decisions.

Every Green House has been fully staffed so far, with never a day understaffed. Wheelchair use has declined, and the strength of residents has increased. Residents have the option to eat in a group or alone, with an individualized menu and pleasant surroundings—referred to as a convivium. A local cookbook is assembled to cater to the tastes of people born in a region. Shahbazim can eat with residents and participate in activities with them, along with family and friends.

Most of these ideas are summarized in William Thomas's book, *What Are Old People For?* and in a journal article titled, "*Radical Redesign of Nursing Homes*" (Rabig, Thomas, Kane, Cutler, & McAlilly, 2006). In a publication called *CNS SeniorCare*, Thomas (Rabig et al., 2006) sums up his philosophy:

> *Old age, like all the other phases of our lives, should be about life and living. Treating aging as a medical condition that must be managed with the professional distance prescribed by the medical model is wrong and*

BOX 11-3 Web Exploration

Visit the Web site http://www.mypyramid.gov and explore it for helpful tips and resources. Compare the pyramid to the modified and updated pyramid for older adults found at http://nutrition.tufts.edu/docs/pdf/releases/ModifiedMyPyramid.pdf.

leads to terrible suffering. For decades we have organized the life of the elder or disabled individual in a skilled nursing facility around the needs of the institution, rather than individuals who live there. (p. 14)

The Robert Wood Johnson Foundation provided a $10 million grant (from 2006 to 2010) to establish at least 30 Green Houses around the United States and to allow other long-term care owners and administrators to replicate them through training support and up to $125,000 in predevelopment loans.

SUMMARY

Many exciting changes are taking place in the field of health promotion and aging. Perhaps it is time to establish a pro-aging movement—in contrast to the commercial and exploitive anti-aging movement. No longer needing to impress employers, in-laws, or peers, older adults are free to be themselves. Aging people have an opportunity to be freer, wiser, more engaged in helping others, and more willing to be an advocate not only for their own health, but for the well-being of society.

Critical Thinking Exercises

1. Are you in favor of the federal government monitoring goals for healthy aging? If so, how would you improve federal intervention? If not, why?
2. What do you think is the most important health objective that should be set for the Healthy People 2020 initiative, and what should federal and state governments do to help?
3. How familiar are you with the health-promoting resources in your community? Find one that you are unfamiliar with but believe may be important for older persons. Summarize it sufficiently to answer most questions that older adults might have about it.
4. What is your opinion of the existing Medicare prevention coverage? What would you change, and why?
5. Write a health contract/calendar for yourself for one month. At the end of this time explain your success or lack of such with accomplishing your health goal.
6. What has been your major barrier when it comes to engaging in exercise on a regular basis, and have you attempted to overcome it? If so, how?
7. Check out the new Food Guide Pyramid on the Web site http://www.mypyramid.gov, and see what you can learn about nutrition that is interesting to you. Do you have any suggestions for improving this site?
8. Research suggests that older adults are more conscious of their nutritional habits than younger adults. Conduct your own survey of five older adults and five younger adults, asking them to rate how much attention they give to eating what is good for them, using a scale of 1 (not very often) to 10 (all the time). Does your convenience sample corroborate the positive relationship between age and good nutritional habits?

Personal **Reflections**

1. Create your own nutrition bull's-eye, filling in the foods and drinks that you consume or might consider consuming. Use it for a week to guide your eating choices. Take a list of the food products in the center of your bull's-eye to the supermarket with you. Did you find this technique to be helpful?
2. Have you ever conducted a life review with an older adult? If you have, how satisfying was it for you and for them? If not, why not? How do you feel about not having done one with an older family member?
3. Choose one of the model health promotion programs summarized in this chapter and find out something of interest to you about that program that is not mentioned in this chapter.
4. The author believes that if we become more responsive to the health care needs of older adults, we will probably provide better health care for people of all ages in the United States. What do you think is the logic behind this belief?
5. What does this quotation by Henry Wadsworth Longfellow mean to you? "Age is opportunity no less than youth itself, though in another dress, and as the evening twilight fades away, the sky is filled with stars, invisible by day."
6. Describe a geriatric job, or an aspect of a job, that you would enjoy doing (related to nursing or not) and would be an important service for older adults, but is not currently being done.

References

Ackerman, R.. T., Cheadle, A., Sandhu, N., Madsen, L., Wagner, E. H., & LoGerfo, J. P. (2003). Community exercise program use and changes in health care costs for older adults. *American Journal of Preventive Medicine, 25*(3), 232–237.

Bailey, C. (1996). *Smart eating*. Boston: Houghton-Mifflin.

Bandura, A. (1977). *Social learning theory*. Englewood Cliffs, NJ: Prentice Hall.

Bandura, A. (1997). *Self-efficacy: The exercise of control.* New York: W. H. Freeman.

Becker, M. (1974). The health belief model and personal health behavior. *Health Education Monographs, 2*(4), 236.

Beekman, A., et al. (2002). The natural history of late-life depression: A 6-year prospective study in the community. *Archives of General Psychiatry*, *59*(7), 605–611.

Beers, M., & Berkow, R. (2000). *The Merck manual of geriatrics* (3rd ed.). Whitehouse Station, NJ: Merck Research Laboratories.

Berry, M., et al. (1989). Work-site health promotion: The effects of a goal-setting program on nutrition-related behaviors. *Journal of the American Dietary Association*, *89*(3), 914–920.

Birren, J., & Cochran, K. (2001). *Telling the stories of life through guided autobiography groups*. Baltimore, MD: The Johns Hopkins University Press.

Birren, J., & Deutchman, D. (1991). *Guiding autobiography groups for older adults*. Baltimore, MD: Johns Hopkins University Press.

Birren, J., et al. (1996). *Aging and biography: Explorations in adult development*. New York: Springer.

Blair, S., et al. (1989). Physical fitness and all-cause mortality: A prospective study of healthy men and women. *Journal of the American Medical Association*, *262*(17), 2395–2401.

Booth, K., et al. (2005). Obesity and the built environment. *Journal of the American Dietetic Association, 105* (5 Suppl. 1), S110–S117.

Brownson, R., et al. (2000). Promoting physical activity in rural communities: Walking trail access, use, and effects. *American Journal of Preventive Medicine, 18*(3), 235–241.

Butler, R. (1974). Successful aging and the role of the life review. *Journal of the American Geriatrics Society, 22*(12), 529–535.

Butler, R. (1995). Foreword: The life review. In B. Haight & J. Webster (Eds.), *The art and science of reminiscing* (pp. xvii–xxi). Washington, DC: Taylor and Francis.

Butler, R., et al. (1991). *Aging and mental health: Positive psychosocial and biomedical approaches.* Columbus, OH: Charles E. Merrill.

Caine, E., et al. (1996). Diagnosis of late-life depression: Preliminary studies in primary care settings. *American Journal of Geriatric Psychiatry, 4*(1), S45–S50.

Centers for Disease Control and Prevention. (1999). *Suicide deaths and rates per 100,000.* Retrieved December 15, 2008, from http://www.aacap.org/galleries/PracticeParameters/Suictabl.pdf

Civic Ventures and MetLife. (2005). *New faces of work survey.* Retrieved December 14, 2008, from http://civicventures.org/publications/surveys/new_face_of_work/new_face_of_work.pdf

Clark, J., et al. (1999). Case management and behavioral contracting: Components of rural substance abuse treatment. *Journal of Substance Abuse Treatment, 17*(4), 293–304.

Cupples, S., & Steslow, B. (2001). Use of behavioral contingency contracting with heart transplant candidates. *Progress in Transplantation, 11*(2), 137–144.

DeBusk, R., et al. (1990). Training effects of long versus short bouts of exercise in healthy subjects. *American Journal of Cardiology, 65*(15), 1010–1013.

De Cocker, K., et al. (2006, June 21). The validity of the inexpensive "stepping meter" in counting steps in free-living conditions. *British Journal of Sports Medicine* (Epub ahead of print).

Dobkin, L. (2002). Senior wellness project secures health care dollars. *Innovations, 2,* 16–20.

Engel, L., & Lindner, H. (2006). Impact of using a pedometer on time spent walking in older adults with type 2 diabetes. *Diabetes Education, 32*(5), 98–107.

Fishbein, M., & Ajzen, I. (1975). *Belief, attitude, intention and behavior: An introduction to theory and research.* Reading, MA: Addison-Wesley.

Frank, L., et al. (2004). Obesity relationships with community design, physical activity, and time spent in cars. *American Journal of Preventive Medicine, 27*(2), 87–96.

Frasure-Smith, N., et al. (1995). Depression and 18-month prognosis after myocardial infarction. *Circulation, 91*(4), 999–1005.

Fried, L., et al. (2004). A social model for health promotion for an aging population. *Journal of Urban Health, 81*(1), 64–78.

Gallo, J., et al. (1999). Attitudes, knowledge, and behavior of family physicians regarding depression in late life. *Archives of Family Medicine, 8*(3), 249–256.

George, L. (1986, Spring). Life satisfaction in later life. *Generations,* 5–8.

Gould, L., et al. (1995). Changes in myocardial perfusion abnormalities by positron emission tomography after long-term, intense risk factor modification. *Journal of the American Medical Association, 274*(11), 894–901.

Haber, D. (2001). Medicare prevention: Movement toward research-based policy. *Journal of Aging and Social Policy, 13*(1), 1–14.

Haber, D. (2002). Health promotion and aging: Educational and clinical initiatives by the federal government. *Educational Gerontology, 28*(2), 1–11.

Haber, D. (2005). Medicare prevention update. *Journal of Aging and Social Policy, 17*(2), 1–6.

Haber, D. (2006). Life review: Implementation, theory, and future direction. *International Journal of Aging and Human Development, 63*(2), 153–171.

Haber, D. (2007a). Health contract in the classroom. *Gerontology and Geriatrics Education, 27*(4), 41–54.

Haber, D. (2007b). *Health promotion and aging: Practical applications for health professionals* (4th ed.). New York: Springer.

Haber, D., & Looney, C. (2000). Health contract calendars: A tool for health professionals with older adults. *The Gerontologist, 40*(2), 235–239.

Haber, D., & Rhodes, D. (2004). Health contract with sedentary older adults. *The Gerontologist, 44*(6), 827–835.

Haight, B., et al. (1998). Life review: Preventing despair in newly relocated nursing home residents' short- and long-term effects. *International Journal of Aging and Human Development, 47*(2), 119–142.

Harris, L., et al. (1989). *The prevention index '89: Summary report.* Emmaus, PA: Rodale Press.

Hart, P. (2002). *The new face of retirement: An ongoing survey of American Attitudes on Aging.* Retrieved December 13, 2008, from http://www.experiencecorps.org/images/pdf/new_face_survey_results.pdf

Healthwise. (2006). *Healthwise handbook* (17th ed.). Boise, ID: Author.

Jakicic, J., et al. (1995). Prescription of exercise intensity for the obese patient: The relationship between heart rate, VO2 and perceived exertion. *International Journal of Obesity, 19*(6), 382–387.

Jette, A., et al. (1999). Exercise—It's never too late: The Strong for Life program. *American Journal of Public Health, 89*(1), 66–72.

Johnson, C., et al. (1992). Behavioral counseling and contracting as methods for promoting cardiovascular health in families. *Journal of the American Dietetic Association, 92*(4), 479–481.

Katon, W., et al. (1992). Adequacy and duration of antidepressant treatment in primary care. *Medical Care, 30*(11), 67–76.

Kazel, R. (2004, June 28). Dieting for dollars. *American Medical News*, 17–18.

King, W., et al. (2003). The relationship between convenience of destinations and walking levels in older women. *American Journal of Health Promotion, 18*(1), 74–82.

LaCroix, A., et al. (1996). Does walking decrease the risk of cardiovascular disease hospitalization and death in older adults? *Journal of the American Geriatrics Society, 44*(2), 113–120.

Lantz, M. (2002). Depression in the elderly: Recognition and treatment. *Clinical Geriatrics, 10*(2), 18–24.

Lebowitz, B. (1995, Spring). Depression in older adults. *Aging and Vision News, 7*, 2.

Lee, I., et al. (2000). Physical activity and coronary heart disease risk in men. *Circulation, 102*(4), 981–986.

Leslie, M., & Schuster, P. (1991). The effect of contingency contracting on adherence and knowledge of exercise regimen. *Patient Education and Counseling, 18*(3), 231–241.

Leveille, S., et al. (1998). Preventing disability and managing chronic illness in frail older adults: A randomized trial of a community-based partnership with primary care. *Journal of the American Geriatrics Society, 46*(10), 1191–1198.

Li, F., et al. (2005). Improving physical function and blood pressure in older adults through cobblestone mat walking: A randomized trial. *Journal of the American Geriatrics Society, 53*(8), 1305–1312.

Lorig, K., Lubeck, D., Kraines, R. G., Seleznickm, M., Holman, H. R.(1986). Outcomes of self-help education for patients with arthritis. *Arthritis and Rheumatism, 28*(2), 680–685.

Lorig, K., Ritter, P., Stewart, A. L., Sobel, D. S., Brown, B.W.J., Bandura, A., et al. (2001). Chronic disease self-management program. *Medical Care, 39*(11), 1217–1223.

Lorig, K., Sobel, D., Holeman, M. D., Laurent, D., Gonzales, V., & Minor, M. (2000). *Living a healthy life with chronic conditions.* Palo Alto, CA: Bull.

Lorig, K., Sobel, D., & Stewart, A. (1999). Evidence suggesting that a chronic disease self-management program can improve health status while reducing hospitalization: A randomized trial. *Medical Care, 37*(1), 5–14.

Lorig, K., Stewart, A., Ritter, P., Gonzalez, V., Laurent, D., & Lynch, J. (1996). *Outcome measures for health education and other health care interventions*. Thousand Oaks, CA: Sage.

McCormack, G., et al. (2006). Demographic and individual correlates of achieving 10,000 steps/day: Use of pedometers in a population-based study. *Health Promotion Journal of Australia, 17*(1), 43–47.

McGuire, L., et al. (2002). Depressive symptoms and lymphocyte proliferation in older adults. *Journal of Abnormal Psychology, 111*(1), 192–197.

Mettler, M. (1997). Unpublished update on the *Healthwise Handbook* program. Healthwise, Inc., P.O. Box 1989, Boise, ID 83701.

Moore, J., et al. (2000). A randomized trial of a cognitive-behavioral program for enhancing back pain self care in a primary care setting. *Pain, 88*(2), 145–153.

Murphy, M., et al. (2002). Accumulating brisk walking for fitness, cardiovascular risk, and psychological health. *Medical Science and Sports Exercise, 34*(9), 1468–1474.

National Center for Chronic Disease Prevention and Health Promotion. (1999). *Physical activity and health: A report of the Surgeon General.* Retrieved on December 12, 2008, from http://www.cdc.gov/nccdphp/sgr/contents.htm

National Center for Health Statistics. (1985). *National health interview survey.* Hyattsville, MD: U.S. Public Health Service, *Advance Data, 13*.

National Center for Health Statistics. (1999). *Healthy People 2000 review, 1998–1999*. Hyattsville, MD: U.S. Department of Health and Human Services.

Neale, A., et al. (1990). The use of behavioral contracting to increase exercise activity. *American Journal of Health Promotion, 4*(2), 441–447.

Nutting, P. (1987). Community-oriented primary care: From principle to practice. In P. Nutting (Ed.), *Community-oriented primary care.* (pp. xv–xxv). Albuquerque: University of New Mexico Press.

Ornish, D. (1992). *Dr. Dean Ornish's program for reversing heart disease.* New York: Ballantine.

Ornish, D., et al. (1998). Intensive lifestyle changes for reversal of coronary heart disease. *Journal of the American Medical Association, 280*(23), 2001–2007.

Pate, R., et al. (1995). Physical activity and public health. *Journal of the American Medical Association, 273*(5), 402–407.

Penninx, B., et al. (1998a). Chronically depressed mood and cancer risk in older persons. *Journal of the National Cancer Institute, 90*(24), 1888–1893.

Penninx, B., et al. (1998b). Depressive symptoms and physical decline in community-dwelling older persons. *Journal of the American Medical Association, 279*(21), 1720–1726.

Pfizer. (2007). *The health status of older adults*. Retrieved on December 11, 2008, from http://media.pfizer.com/files/products/The_Health_Status_of_Older_Adults_2007.pdf

Phelan, E., et al. (2002). Outcomes of a community-based dissemination of the health enhanced program. *Journal of the American Geriatrics Society, 50*(9), 1519–1524.

Prochaska, J., & DiClemente, C. (1992). Stages of change in the modification of problem behaviors. In M. Herson et al. (Eds.), *Progress in behavior modification* (pp. 184–218). CA: Sage.

Rabig, J., Thomas, W., Kane, R., Cutler, L., & McAlilly, S. (2006). Radical redesign of nursing homes: Applying the Green House concept in Tupelo, Mississippi. *The Gerontologist, 46*(4), 533–539.

Rabins, P. (1996). Barriers to diagnosis and treatment of depression in elderly patients. *American Journal of Geriatric Psychiatry, 4*(1), S79–S83.

Rebok, G., et al. (2004). Short-term impact of Experience Corps participation on children and schools. *Journal of Urban Health, 81*(1), 79–83.

Schlenk, E., & Boehm, S. (1998). Behaviors in type II diabetes during contingency contracting. *Applied Nursing Research, 11*(2), 77–83.

Squires, S. (2002, October 14–20). We're fat and getting fatter. *Washington Post National Weekly Edition*, p. 34.

Stovitz, S., et al. (2005). Pedometers as a means to increase ambulatory activity for patients seen at a family medicine clinic. *Journal of the American Board of Family Practice, 18*(5), 335–343.

Sturm, R., & Cohen, D. (2004). Suburban sprawl and physical and mental health. *Public Health, 118*(7), 488–496.

Swinburn, B., et al. (1998). The green prescription study: A randomized controlled trial of written exercise advice provided by general practitioners. *American Journal of Public Health, 88*(2), 288–291.

Tan, E., et al. (2006). Volunteering: A physical activity intervention for older adults. *Journal of Urban Health, 83*(5), 954–969.

Thomas, W. (2004). *What are old people for?* Acton, MA: VanderWyk & Burnam.

U.S. Preventive Services Task Force. (1996). *Guide to clinical preventive services*. Baltimore: Williams and Wilkins.

Wallerstein, N., & Bernstein, E. (1988). Empowerment education: Freier's ideas adapted to health education. *Health Education Quarterly, 15*(4), 379–394.

Wallston, K., & Wallston, B. (1982). Who is responsible for your health? The construct of health locus of control. In G. Saunders & J. Suls (Eds.), *Social psychology of health and illness*. NJ: Erlbaum.

Watt, L., & Cappeliez, P. (2000). Integrative and instrumental reminiscence therapies for depression in older adults. *Aging & Mental Health, 4*(2), 166–183.

CHAPTER 12

Identifying and Preventing Common Risk Factors in the Elderly

Joan M. Nelson, RN, MS, DNP

LEARNING OBJECTIVES

At the end of this chapter, the reader will be able to:

- Discuss techniques for assessing and treating factors that lead to functional decline in the elderly.
- Describe recommended screening evaluations for the elderly population.
- Cite the expert recommendations for flu and pneumonia vaccines.
- Identify risk factors and signs of abuse in the elderly.
- Explain the protocol for reporting elder abuse.

KEY TERMS

- Activities of daily living (ADLs)
- Adult protective services agency
- Chronic Disease Self-Management Program (CDSMP)
- Contracting
- Dietary Approaches to Stop Hypertension (DASH) diet
- Framingham Heart Study
- Functional decline
- Health promotion
- Health screening
- Healthy People 2010
- Instrumental activities of daily living (IADLs)
- Nutrition Screening Initiative
- Primary prevention
- Secondary prevention
- Tertiary prevention
- U.S. Preventive Services Task Force (USPSTF)

INTRODUCTION

Health promotion activities can help to prevent **functional decline** in the elderly. Scientific evidence supports the fact that functional disability is not caused by aging, per se, but results from illnesses and diseases that are related to unhealthy lifestyle decisions. Up to 70% of the physical disabilities associated with the aging process result from unhealthy behaviors or lifestyles (National Center for Chronic Disease Prevention and Health Promotion, 1999). This creates an exciting opportunity for nurses to improve the quality of life for the elderly client through evidence-based health promotion activities.

In this chapter, we will review the health promotion and disease prevention guidelines recommended by the following:

- ***U.S. Preventive Services Task Force (USPSTF)***: The USPSTF was convened by the U.S. Public Health Service to systematically review the evidence of effectiveness of clinical preventive services. The task force is an independent panel of private-sector experts in primary care and prevention whose mission is to evaluate the benefits of individual services and to create age-, gender-, and risk-based recommendations about services that should routinely be incorporated into primary medical care. Its recommendations can be found at www.ahrq.gov/clinic/uspstfix.htm.

- ***Healthy People 2010***: Healthy People 2010 is an initiative of the U.S. Department of Health and Human Services that utilized the skills and knowledge of an alliance of more than 350 national organizations and 250 state public health, mental health, substance abuse, and environmental agencies to develop a set of health care objectives designed to increase the quality and quantity of years of healthy life of Americans and to eliminate health disparities. Its recommendations can be found at www.healthypeople.gov.

The recommendations presented in this chapter are guidelines for most patients, most of the time. Clinical judgment must be used in applying these guidelines to individual clients; for example, the risks and benefits of colonoscopy will be quite different for a healthy 75-year-old versus a frail 75- year-old with metastatic cancer. Individual variations in health status increase markedly with age, necessitating an individualized approach to health care.

HEALTH PROMOTION AND DISEASE PREVENTION DEFINITIONS

Health promotion activities are those activities in which an individual is able to proactively engage in order to advance or improve his or her health. **Primary prevention** activities are those designed to completely prevent a disease from occurring, such as immunization against pneumonia or influenza. **Secondary prevention** efforts are directed toward early detection and management of disease, such as the use of colonoscopy to detect small, cancerous polyps. **Tertiary prevention** efforts are used to manage clinical diseases in order to prevent them from progressing or to avoid complications of the disease, as is done when beta blockers are used to help remodel the heart in congestive heart failure.

SCREENING

Health screening is a form of secondary prevention and will be a focus of this chapter. In order to endorse screening for a specific disease, the USPSTF considers whether the disease occurs with enough frequency in a population to justify mass screening. The population is more likely to benefit from screening tests for a disease like diabetes, which occurs frequently, than it is to benefit from screening for Addison's disease, which is uncommon. In order to justify the costs and inconvenience of screening we must be able to detect the condition being screened at a relatively early stage, and have effective treatments for the condition. Early detection of the disease has to result in improved clinical outcomes. The screening tests should be relatively noninvasive and acceptable to patients, cost effective and available, and highly sensitive and specific (see **Case Study 12-1**).

Screening recommendations are graded by expert panels according to the strength of the supporting evidence and the net benefit. The USPSTF uses the following rating scale:

- *Level A:* The USPSTF strongly recommends screening based on good evidence that screening improves health outcomes and the benefits outweigh screening risks.
- *Level B:* The USPSTF recommends screening based on fair evidence that health outcomes and benefits outweigh screening risks.
- *Level C:* The USPSTF makes no recommendation for or against screening because the balance of benefit and risk is too close to justify a general recommendation.
- *Level D:* The USPSTF recommends against screening because there is at least fair evidence that screening is either ineffective or harmful.
- *Level I:* The USPSTF makes no recommendation based on insufficient evidence or research.

THE FOCUS OF HEALTH PROMOTION EFFORTS

A major focus of health promotion efforts for the elderly is to minimize the loss of independence associated with illness and functional decline. Healthy People 2010 and the USPSTF suggest the

Case Study 12-1

You are working as an RN for a managed care organization. Physicians have complained about their inability to adequately care for their elderly patients given the time constraints imposed by the 20-minute office visit. An innovative strategy—in which RNs meet with all clients over the age of 65 on an annual basis, prior to the physician visit, in order to ensure that recommended screening tests are performed—has been instituted by the HMO.

You are visiting with Hilde M., an 82-year-old woman, who is accompanied by her daughter, Roxanne. Roxanne has called you prior to the visit to inform you about her concerns about her mother's ability to live safely alone at home. She confides that her mother is forgetting many appointments and has fallen at least twice in the past 3 months. Although Hilde had a minor stroke 3 years ago, she has not been into the office for the past year because she lacks transportation since she gave up driving 2 years ago due to her poor vision. Roxanne has encouraged her mother to move into an assisted living facility, but Hilde is loathe to sell her home of 50 years and to give up her independence.

What screening tests are appropriate for Hilde at this time? Justify your choices. What instruments will you use to perform the appropriate screening tests? What counseling will you provide for Mrs. M. and her daughter, based on the limited information you have been provided?

following focus areas for nurses in order to promote health and prevent disability in the elderly client:

- Physical activity
- Nutrition
- Tobacco use
- Safety
- Immunization

Many of these foci show considerable overlap with recommendations for younger adults, but some, like injury prevention and hearing and vision screening, are unique to older adults. It is important to consider the impact of health conditions on physical functioning and on quality of life in the older client. This is different from the younger adults' focus on treatment and cure of a single, acute condition. Multiple chronic illnesses are common in the elderly, and cure is often an unrealistic and inappropriate goal. These chronic illnesses can lead to disability and dependency. In fact, almost 15% of Americans over 65 years of age require help with bathing, dressing, meal preparation, or shopping (CDC and the Merck Company Foundation, 2007). Symptoms that impact functional status should be the focus of interventions with this population. Maintaining independence in **activities of daily living (ADLs)** is an important goal for health promoting activities.

By the time we are 85 years old, one-half of our remaining years of life are expected to be lived dependently, often in a nursing home. About 2.3 million elderly Americans have some functional limitation, and half of elderly clients hospitalized for medical illness were found to have some deficiency in ADLs (American Academy of Family Physicians [AAFP], 2004). Some of the preventive strategies that will be discussed in this chapter, like smoking cessation, immunization, physical activity, weight control, blood pressure control, and arthritis and diabetes self-management programs, are known to be effective in lessening disability.

Assessment of functional status requires a multipronged approach. The ADL scale and the **instrumental activities of daily living (IADLs)** scale are valid and reliable self-report tools to assess functional status (Lawton & Brody, 1969). Nurses can use these instruments to identify elderly individuals who are frail and may benefit from an increased level of care or additional in-home support. Fear of being advised to leave their home, however, can cause elderly individuals to deny difficulties. The ADL and IADL scales rely on self-reporting and can fail to detect difficulties when clients are not forthcoming about their limitations.

Performance-based tools, like the Get Up and Go test (Duxbury, 1997), can provide a more objective measurement of functional status and fall risk. This assessment requires clients to rise from a chair, walk 10 feet, turn around, return to the chair, and sit down. These actions are timed and compared with a historic sample of adults without balance problems that were able complete this test in under 10 seconds. Older adults who are dependent in most activities of daily living and have poor balance and gait may take more than 30 seconds to complete the task. Clients are observed for sitting balance, transfers, gait, and ability to maintain balance while turning. If a gait abnormality is detected, weight-bearing exercise and physical rehabilitation may prevent further decline and lessen the risk of falls.

The Study of Osteoporotic Fractures Index (Ensrud et al., 2008) recently has been demonstrated to be an effective predictor of falls and functional decline. It is simple to administer in clinical practice. See the Research Highlight in **Box 12-23** for more information about this tool.

SELF-MANAGEMENT

What can nurses do to encourage clients to adopt health-promoting behaviors and manage their chronic illnesses? Kate Lorig, MD, has been instrumental in developing the concept of self-management and outlining the role of the health care provider in fostering the client's self-management of his or her chronic condition (Lorig & Holman, 2000). Her research, which was sponsored by the Agency for Healthcare Research and Quality (AHRQ), supported the effectiveness of chronic disease self-management in preventing or delaying disability from chronic diseases. She has described how the self-management concept also may be applied to health promotion activities.

The **Chronic Disease Self-Management Program (CDSMP)** is a 17-hour course for patients with chronic diseases that is taught by trained laypeople. The course goal is to teach patients to improve symptom management, maintain functional ability, and adhere to their medication regimens. The proven effectiveness of the intervention is, at least in part, attributable to the improved self-efficacy of clients who participate in the program. Clients come to believe that they can succeed in managing their illness and preventing disability.

Critical to the concept of self-management is an assessment of the client's goals and concerns, which may be different from the health care professional's goals and concerns. The nurse may feel that exercise will help lower her client's blood pressure, which may decrease stroke risk, certainly an important goal. The client's focus, however, may be that he does not want to go shopping for new clothes, as a result of his recent weight gain, and his goal is to continue to be able to use his current wardrobe. He will assess the value of his new exercise program in terms of his clothing budget, not in relation to his blood pressure readings.

Lorig has identified five key elements of self-management programs: problem solving, decision making, resource utilization, forming a health care professional/client partnership, and taking action. In the problem-solving phase, a client may identify several barriers to initiating an exercise program and then list strategies for overcoming each barrier, to arrive at a workable strategy. Decision making helps to arm clients with the information needed to make the decisions they need to make on a daily basis. "How do I know when I am exercising too hard?" "Should I exercise when I don't feel well?" The provider plays an important role in providing accurate and sufficient information for clients to make informed decisions. Providers also teach clients to access and evaluate appropriate resources and to create plans that are easily accomplished, limited in scope, and easily evaluated for success. A technique that has proven successful is to ask the client how confident they are on a scale of 1–10 (10 being maximally confident) that they will accomplish their objective. If the score is less than 7, encourage them to set a more realistic goal.

Contracting for health promoting behaviors is another useful strategy. A successful contract for behavior change is very specific. The contract may begin with the overall behavioral goal ("I wish to lose 20 lbs over the next year in order to improve my overall health, strength, and stamina"). The client determines his or her own short-term goal and means of achieving that goal for the next week ("I will exercise for 20 minutes, three times this week"). The nurse helps the client to pinpoint exactly how and when that will occur. The client is encouraged to write the exact time that the exercise will occur on his or her calendar, and the exact form the exercise will take ("I will walk around my subdivision, which is 1¼ miles in length, at 10 a.m. on Tuesday, Thursday, and Saturday"). Ideally, the client and nurse will meet at the end of that time period to evaluate and modify the plan for the next week or so. Barriers to implementing the plan are reviewed and taken into consideration in order to rewrite the following week's contract.

Self-management classes and contracting are strategies that can be incorporated through individual sessions or in group meetings, to help implement the health promotion and disease prevention ideas discussed in this chapter.

PHYSICAL ACTIVITY

Functional decline in the elderly is attributable, at least in part, to physical inactivity. A significant number of deaths in the United States have been traced to insufficient activity and inadequate nutrition (Buchner, 1997; McGinnis & Foege, 1993). Despite the well-documented benefits of exercise in reducing blood pressure and cholesterol, improving insulin resistance, reducing weight, strengthening bones, and reducing falls, two-thirds of adults between 65 and 75 years of age are inactive. Thirty minutes of moderate activity, like brisk walking, can have dramatic, positive effects on health and well-being, but only 12% of Americans 75 years of age or older perform this level of activity.

Physical inactivity causes increased health care costs to our nation. In fact, a Centers for Disease Control and Prevention (CDC) study has shown that the direct medical costs of inactive Americans are markedly higher than the costs for active Americans. The direct medical costs associated with physical inactivity were nearly $76.6 billion in 2000 (National Center for Chronic Disease Prevention and Health Promotion, 2004).

Scientific evidence supports the effectiveness of moderate physical activity in:

- Decreasing overall mortality
- Decreasing coronary heart disease, the leading cause of death in the United States
- Decreasing colon cancer
- Decreasing the incidence and improving the management of diabetes mellitus
- Decreasing the incidence and improving the management of hypertension
- Decreasing obesity
- Improving depression
- Improving quality of life
- Improving functional status
- Decreasing falls and injury

Moderate exercise is defined as 30 or more minutes of brisk walking on 5 or more days per week. Tai chi and yoga are helpful for improving balance and flexibility. Modified exercises, such as armchair exercises, can be helpful for the frail elderly or those with mobility restrictions. Sporadic, vigorous exercise should be discouraged.

Barriers to physical exercise that have been identified by the elderly include lack of access to safe areas to exercise, pain, fatigue, and impairment in sensory function and mobility. These barriers underscore the need to individualize your approach to helping clients develop an exercise regimen tailored to their unique needs and to participate in community efforts to create environments that foster healthy lifestyles. The Partnership for Prevention (2002) developed an excellent community assessment guide with a list of strategies for communities to overcome barriers encountered by older adults to physical activities. This guide, called "Creating Communities for Active Aging," is accessible on the Web at http://www.prevent.org/images/stories/Files/publications/Active_Aging.pdf.

What can be done to foster participation in physical exercise? Individuals can increase their chances of beginning, and sticking with, an exercise program if they identify activities that can be a regular part of their daily routine and identify individuals who can participate in the exercise with them. Nurses can help clients to assess their current level of activity and barriers that prevent them from exercising. The nurse then can help the client with goal setting, write a prescription for exercise, work with the

BOX 12-1 Physical Activity Counseling

Level I recommendation: The USPSTF found insufficient evidence to determine whether encouraging or counseling patients to begin an exercise program actually led to improvements in their level of physical activity. There is strong evidence, however, to support the effectiveness of physical activity in reducing morbidity and mortality from chronic illness.

client to develop an exercise program individually tailored to the client's unique needs, and follow up by telephone at regular intervals to assess progress and barriers. Follow-up phone calls can also be used to assess how well the client has done with accessing community resources.

NUTRITION

Four of the 10 leading causes of death in the United States (cancer, diabetes, coronary heart disease, and cerebral vascular accidents) are associated with unhealthy dietary patterns. More than 80% of Americans do not eat enough fruits or vegetables and eat too much fat. Elderly clients may be at increased risk for poor nutrition due to the fact that they have multiple chronic illnesses, may have tooth or mouth problems that may interfere with their ability to eat, may be socially isolated, may have economic hardship, may be taking multiple medications that can cause changes in appetite or gastrointestinal symptoms, and may need assistance with self-care. Weight gain or loss may signal nutritional problems.

The USPSTF found good evidence that medium to high counseling interventions can produce significant changes among elderly clients who are at increased risk for diet-related chronic illness. This risk can be assessed with the following assessment tests:

- *DETERMINE Your Nutritional Health Checklist:* A tool created by the **Nutrition Screening Initiative**, a collaborative project of health, medical, and aging organizations. The nutrition checklist can be ordered from the initiative's Web site (http://www.fiu.edu/~gn/Resources/NSIOrderForm.htm) for a nominal fee.
- *Serum albumin:* Less than 3.5 g/dl is associated with malnutrition and increased morbidity and mortality.
- *Body mass index (BMI):* The Nutrition Screening Initiative suggests that a BMI of 22–27 is considered normal. Values above or below this range suggest over- and underweight, respectively. Unintended weight loss is a nutritional risk that requires additional assessment. Obesity is a problem for many older Americans, just as it is for younger adults. The Obesity Education Initiative of the National Heart, Lung, and Blood Institute (2005) has provider guidelines and patient education materials (http://www.nhlbi.nih.gov/about/oei/index.htm).
- *Adult Treatment Panel (ATP III) Cholesterol Guidelines:* An unintended decrease in cholesterol to less than 150 mg/dl is a nutritional risk (http://www.nhlbi.nih.gov/guidelines/cholesterol/index.htm).
- *ADL and IADL measures:* These can assess a client's ability to eat and prepare food and to do the shopping and transportation necessary for good nutrition.
- *Dietary Reference Intakes and Recommended Daily Allowances:* These can be compared with food diaries from a 24- to 48-hour period to assess marked deviation from these guidelines. Clients who use many vitamin and nutritional supplements may be at risk for toxicities.
- *Depression and dementia:* Both are risk factors for nutritional compromise.

The Nutrition Screening Initiative has booklets for clients and providers that are helpful in teaching about screening and treating nutritional problems related to chronic illnesses.

General guidelines for dietary counseling include:

- Limit alcohol to one drink a day for women, two daily for men.
- Limit fat and cholesterol.
- Maintain a balanced caloric intake.
- Ensure adequate daily calcium, especially for women.
- Older adults should consume vitamin B_{12} in crystalline form, which can be derived from fortified cereals and supplements.

BOX 12-2 Nutrition Counseling

Level B recommendation: The USPSTF found good evidence to support counseling interventions among adults at risk for diet-related chronic disease. Interventions that have proven to stimulate healthy dietary changes combine nutrition education with behavioral counseling.

- Older adults who have minimal exposure to sunlight or who have dark skin need supplemental vitamin D. Daily vitamin D intake should be 400–600 IU and can be derived from fortified foods or supplements.
- Include adequate whole grains, fruits, and vegetables.
- Drink adequate water.

TOBACCO USE

It is estimated that 4.5 million Americans age 65 or older smoke cigarettes, and that smoking accounts for one out of every five U.S. deaths. Elderly Americans are just as likely to benefit from quitting smoking as are younger adults. Quitting smoking can decrease the chance of having a myocardial infarction or dying from lung cancer or heart disease. Nonsmokers have improved wound healing, recovery from illness, and cerebral circulation.

A practice guideline to guide clinicians to help their patients quit smoking has been developed through the Public Health Service (AHRQ, 2000) and is available online at http://www.ahrq.gov/clinic/tobacco/whatisphs.htm. The task force stresses that the most important step in helping a client to quit smoking is to screen for tobacco use and assess the client's willingness to quit. It outlines two different interventions—the 5 As, for clients who are ready to quit smoking, and the 5 Rs, for those who need additional motivation before they are ready to quit.

BOX 12-3 Tobacco Cessation Counseling

Level A recommendation: The USPSTF found good evidence that screening, brief behavioral counseling, and pharmacotherapy are effective in helping clients to quit smoking and remain smoke-free after one year. There are good data to support that smoking cessation lowers the risk for heart disease, stroke, and lung disease.

The 5 As

Ask about smoking status at each health care visit.

Advise client to quit smoking.

Assess client's willingness to quit smoking at this time.

Assist client to quit using counseling and pharmacotherapy.

Arrange for follow-up within one week of scheduled quit date.

The 5 Rs

Relevance: Ask the client to think about why quitting may be personally relevant for him or her.

Risks of smoking are identified by the client.

Rewards of quitting are identified by the client.

Roadblocks or barriers to quitting are identified by the client.

Repetition of this process at every clinic visit. Most people who successfully quit smoking require multiple attempts.

SAFETY

Many of the safety recommendations for older adults are similar to those for younger people: use lap and shoulder belts in motor vehicles, avoid driving while intoxicated, use smoke detectors in the home, maintain hot water heaters at or below 120 degrees Fahrenheit. Falls, however, are a safety risk that is relatively unique to the elderly.

Falls are the leading cause of unintentional injury death in older adults in this country. Approximately one-half of elderly adults living in institutions and one-third of community-dwelling elders fall every year (Roman, 2004). Between 5% and 11% of these falls result in serious injuries, including fractures. Twelve thousand Americans die as a result of a fall each year. Elderly adults are susceptible to falls as a result of postural instability, decreased muscle strength, gait disturbances and decreased proprioception, visual and/or cognitive impairment, and polypharmacy. Environmental conditions that contribute to falls are slippery surfaces, stairs, irregular surfaces, poor lighting, incorrect footwear, and obstacles in the pathway.

Patients who fall more than twice in a 6-month period require fall risk assessment and intervention. An easy-to-administer fall risk assessment tool is one that uses the mnemonic "I HATE FALLING." It is described in **Box 12-4**.

Balance and strengthening exercises, home safety modifications, and elimination of high-risk medications have been the focus of fall-risk prevention strategies. There are strong data to support the effectiveness of balance and strengthening exercises for fall reduction (Mitty & Flores, 2007), as well as research to support physiologic and environmental risk factor reduction. At this point, however, the intensity of intervention required to make a difference is not clear. We do not know whether discussing the need to exercise and providing some home safety and medication recommendations during a brief office visit will be effective in reducing falls, or whether a more intensive intervention is necessary. There is evidence to support the latter, intensive approach in community-dwelling elders age 75 or older or in clients 70–74 years of age who use antihypertensive or psychoactive medications, who use four or more prescription medications, or who have cognitive impairment or impairment of gait, strength, or balance (USPSTF, 2004).

BOX 12-4 I Hate Falling

Inflammation of joints or joint deformity

Hypotension (orthostatic blood pressure change)
Auditory and visual abnormalities
Tremor
Equilibrium problems

Foot problems
Arrhythmias, heart block, valvular disease
Leg-length discrepancy
Lack of conditioning (generalized weakness)
Illness
Nutrition (poor, weight loss)
Gait disturbance

Source: Adapted with permission from Sloan, J. P. 1997. Mobility failure. In J. P. Sloan (Ed.), *Protocols in primary care geriatrics* (pp. 33–38). New York: Springer.

BOX 12-5 Fall Prevention Counseling

Level B recommendation: Balance and strengthening exercise programs, home safety assessment, and training and medication monitoring and adjustment are recommended in order to reduce fall risk.

POLYPHARMACY AND MEDICATION ERRORS

Elderly adults are at increased risk of adverse drug effects compared to younger adults, as a result of the fact that they take more medications and due to the biologic effects of aging and chronic diseases. Medication under- and overutilization by this population has been shown to increase the number of hospitalizations and emergency room visits, to worsen cognitive functioning, and to contribute to falls.

The Agency for Healthcare Research and Quality (AHRQ) has appointed a Task Force on Aging to investigate important health issues related to the elderly population. This task force has made enhanced patient safety through reduction of medication errors in the elderly population one of its priorities for clinical practice improvement (Task Force on Aging, 2001). The United States Pharmacopeia (USP, 2004) has created a Personal Medication Organizer to help seniors play an active role in keeping track of their own medications. The organizer is available at http://www.usp.org/pdf/EN/patientSafety/personalMedOrg.pdf.

Adults over 65 years of age take an average of 4.5 prescription and 2 over-the-counter medications at any one time. This number is markedly higher for hospitalized patients or those living in nursing homes or assisted living facilities. Polypharmacy is not always inappropriate in this population of clients who have multiple chronic illnesses, but increased numbers of medications carry increasing risks. Frail elderly adults are more likely than healthier age-mates to suffer adverse drug reactions.

It is estimated that one-fifth of community-dwelling elderly clients are prescribed medications that are not recommended for use in this population (Fick et al, 2003). These medications include long-acting benzodiazepines, sedative or hypnotic agents, long-acting oral hypoglycemics, analgesics, antiemetics, and gastrointestinal antispasmodics. Elderly clients who require home care services and are, therefore, among the more disabled, are prescribed these medications even more often than the healthier members of their cohort. The Beers List of medications to be avoided in the elderly has become a national guideline for prescribers and pharmacists in the United States (Fick etal., 2003).

IMMUNIZATIONS

Annual vaccination against influenza is recommended for all adults 65 years of age or older because more than 90% of the deaths from influenza occur in this population. Several studies suggest that flu vaccination is beneficial in preventing illness, hospitalization, and mortality in both community-dwelling and institutionalized elderly individuals.

Older adults, especially those with chronic illnesses or who live in nursing homes, are susceptible to pneumococcal pneumonia, which results in death in over one-third of clients over 65 years of age who acquire the disease. The emergence of drug-resistant strains of pneumococcal pneumonia underscores the importance of acquired immunization against the illness. Pneumococcal vaccine is given once for clients who are 65 years of age or older. There is evidence to support one-time-only revaccination for clients 75 years or older who have not been vaccinated in 5 or more years.

Tetanus and diphtheria are uncommon diseases in the United States, but only 28% of adults age 70 or older are immune to tetanus. It is these adults who account for the majority of tetanus, a disease that results in death in more than one-quarter of cases. The tetanus and diphtheria (Td) vaccine is highly efficacious against tetanus, but immunity may wane after 10 years. Periodic boosters of tetanus vaccine, traditionally given every 10 years in the United States, are recommended for older adults by the USPSTF.

BOX 12-6 Vaccination Recommendations

Annual influenza vaccination: Level B recommendation

Amantadine or rimantadine prophylaxis: Level B recommendation

MENTAL HEALTH SCREENING

Mental health enables individuals to participate in productive activities and relationships and to adjust to change and loss. Mental disorders are characterized by alterations in mood, behaviors, or cognition and are associated with impaired functioning and/or distress. Mental disorders have been associated with complications resulting in disability or death, and they profoundly affect family members as well as patients. Mental disorders are as common in late life as they are during other stages of the life span, but some disorders are relatively unique to elderly clients.

Depression

Although estimates of depression vary widely, up to 37% of community-dwelling older adults are

BOX 12-7 Vaccination Recommendations

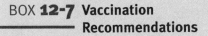

Pneumococcal vaccine: Level B recommendation

> **BOX 12-8 Vaccination Recommendations**
>
> *Tetanus vaccination:* Level A recommendation

depressed. Depression rates increase markedly among clients who have a chronic illness or disability and have been found to be 12% for hospitalized geriatric clients and up to 25% for nursing home residents (Adams, Dey, & Vickerie, 2007). Elderly men have the highest rates of suicide in the nation.

There is good evidence to support screening for depression in adults, including older adults. Screening can improve identification of depressed elders and improve outcomes. Screening efforts must be coordinated with effective treatment and follow-up in order to have maximal benefit. Initial screening may be accomplished by asking two questions about mood and anhedonia: "Over the past 2 weeks, have you felt down, depressed, or hopeless?" and "Over the past 2 weeks, have you felt little interest or pleasure in doing things?" A positive response to this initial screen may be followed with the Geriatric Depression Scale (see **Figure 12-1**), which has been found to have a 92% sensitivity and 89% specificity for detecting depression in elderly adults (Kurlowicz & Greenberg, 2007). A positive depression screen should be followed with an assessment of suicide risk and substance abuse.

Dementia

Dementia affects almost half of elderly Americans 85 years of age or older. Alzheimer's disease (AD) accounts for 60–70% of all cases of dementia and is associated with doubling of the death rate, compared to clients who are free from AD, and markedly increased rates of nursing home admissions. AD prevalence rates double every 5 years after the age of 65. Multi-infarct dementia accounts for 20–30% of dementias and is the second leading cause of dementia in the United States. Dementia is a chronic and progressive illness characterized by behavioral and cognitive changes that affect memory, problem solving, judgment, and speech and that cause deficits in functional abilities.

> **BOX 12-9 Depression**
>
> Level B recommendation to support screening: The USPSTF found good evidence that screening effectively identifies depressed patients and that treatment of depression improves clinical outcomes.

Unfortunately, there is insufficient evidence at this time to suggest that population-wide screening of Americans 65 years and older for dementia is beneficial. We do know that it is difficult to recognize early AD and, in fact, one study demonstrated that primary care physicians failed to detect AD 24–72% of the time. Failure to diagnose early AD may severely compromise client safety as a result of household accidents and motor vehicle accidents. These clients are susceptible to financial losses through errors and scams that prey on the elderly. There is sufficient evidence to support the fact that medication delays the rate of cognitive impairment associated with AD, which can lead to improved quality of life for individuals and families and decreased costs of care for our nation. Experts do recommend thorough screening for clients in whom cognitive impairment is suspected or when concerns are expressed by family members or friends.

Three screening tests are commonly used for all forms of dementia. The Mini Mental State Examination (MMSE) is considered the "gold standard" diagnostic test to detect dementia. It has reasonable sensitivity and specificity, and can be made more sensitive or specific depending on the cut-point used to diagnose dementia (Folstein, Folstein, & McHugh, 1975). The clock-drawing test, in which the client is asked to draw a clock face and indicate a particular time, is a sensitive but nonspecific screening test (Sunderland et al., 1989). The use of informant reporting of an individual's cognitive status has been found to be a useful screening tool, as well.

It is important to distinguish between screening tools and tests used for the differential diagnosis

FIGURE 12-1 Geriatric depression scale (gds), short form.

Choose the best answer for how you have felt over the past week:

1. Are you basically satisfied with your life? YES / **NO**
2. Have you dropped many of your activities and interests? **YES** / NO
3. Do you feel that your life is empty? **YES** / NO
4. Do you often get bored? **YES** / NO
5. Are you in good spirits most of the time? YES / **NO**
6. Are you afraid that something bad is going to happen to you? **YES** / NO
7. Do you feel happy most of the time? YES / **NO**
8. Do you often feel helpless? **YES** / NO
9. Do you prefer to stay at home, rather than going out and doing new things? **YES** / NO
10. Do you feel you have more problems with memory than most? **YES** / NO
11. Do you think it is wonderful to be alive now? YES / **NO**
12. Do you feel pretty worthless the way you are now? **YES** / NO
13. Do you feel full of energy? YES / **NO**
14. Do you feel that your situation is hopeless? **YES** / NO
15. Do you think that most people are better off than you are? **YES** / NO

Scoring: One point for each of these answers. Normal, 0–5; suggests depression, above 5. For additional information on administration and scoring, refer to the following reference.

SOURCE: Sheikh, J. I., & Yesavage, J. A. (1986). Geriatric Depression Scale (GDS): Recent evidence and development of a shorter version. *Clinical Gerontologist*, *5*, 165–172. (Reprinted with permission from Hawthorn Press, Inc.)

of dementia. A thorough dementia evaluation involves systematic history and examination, laboratory testing, and brain imaging.

ALCOHOL ABUSE

The prevalence of alcohol abuse by community-dwelling elderly in the United States is largely unknown, but 6% to 11% of elderly adults admitted to hospitals are found to have problems with alcohol (National Institute of Alcohol Abuse and Alcoholism, 1998). It is very difficult to diagnose alcohol problems in the elderly for several reasons. Retired people do not have the lifestyle disruptions caused by heavy alcohol use that are commonly encountered in younger adults. They are less likely to be arrested due to disorderly conduct or aggression related to their drinking. Alcoholics over the age of 65 are more likely to be living alone and drinking alone, than younger adults. On the other hand, the older drinker is more likely to honestly report his or her drinking to the health care provider and is more likely to comply with treatment strategies.

Elderly clients have alcohol-related complications that are not generally seen in younger adults, such as increased rates of hip fractures due to falls and medication reactions due to alcohol's effects on liver enzyme systems.

There is some evidence to suggest that light to moderate alcohol consumption in older adults may reduce the risk of coronary heart disease. The National Institute on Alcohol Abuse and Alcoholism recommends no more than one drink per day for this purpose. More than 7 drinks per week for women, or 14 drinks per week for men, has been defined as "risky" or "hazardous."

> **BOX 12-10 Dementia Screening**
>
> Level I recommendation: The USPSTF found the clinical evidence to be insufficient to recommend screening for all elderly clients in a primary care setting. Most expert panels agree that clients who are suspected of having cognitive impairment or whose families express concern about their cognitive functioning should be screened.

Several screening tools are commonly used to screen for alcohol abuse. The CAGE questionnaire is a self-report screening instrument that is easy and quick to administer (Ewing, 1984). It asks four yes/no questions and requires approximately 1 minute to complete. CAGE is a mnemonic for the four key screening questions:

- *Cut down:* Refers to attempts by the client to cut down on drinking
- *Annoyance:* Related to suggestions by friends or family to cut down on drinking
- *Guilt:* Relates to client guilt about drinking
- *Eye opener:* Relates to the need for a drink in the morning to get going

The CAGE questionnaire has been found to have a 75% sensitivity and a 96% specificity. The 5 As and 5 Rs strategies, defined under the section on tobacco abuse in this chapter, are also suggested strategies for reducing alcohol consumption.

Another screening tool, the Alcohol Use Disorders Identification Test (AUDIT), is a 10-item screening test developed by the World Health Organization and is sensitive for detecting alcohol dependence and abuse (Babor, Higgins-Biddle, Saunders, & Monteiro, 2001). You can learn more about this screening tool at http://whqlibdoc.who.int/hq/2001/WHO_MSD_MSB_01.6a.pdf.

ELDER ABUSE AND NEGLECT

Unfortunately, it is difficult to estimate the prevalence of elder abuse and neglect in this country due, at least in part, to the lack of appropriate screening instruments and consequent underreporting of abuse and neglect by health care professionals. Reporting of elder abuse to the **adult protective services agency** is mandatory in almost all states, but it is estimated that only 1 in 10 cases of elder abuse and neglect is actually reported. There is a paucity of studies to determine the effectiveness of interventions in decreasing abuse. Studies directed toward identification of both abuse victims and perpetrators are needed.

Elder abuse may include physical, sexual, psychological, and financial exploitation, neglect, and violation of rights. Physical abuse includes shaking, restraining, hitting, or threatening with objects. Sexual abuse includes unwanted contact with the genitals, anus, or mouth. Clients who are psychologically abused experience threats, insults, or harassment, or are recipients of harsh commands. Financial abuse occurs in the form of scams or can be done by family members who try to misuse a client's money or possessions. Neglect may be intentional or unintentional and occurs when required food, medication, or personal care is not provided. Abandonment is a form of neglect where someone who has agreed to provide care for an elderly client deserts that client. Clients who are denied the right to make their own decisions, even though they are competent to do so, or are not provided privacy or the right to worship are suffering from a violation of their inalienable rights.

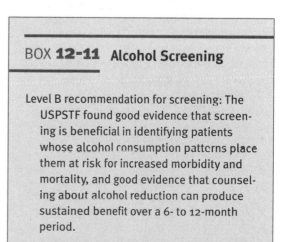

> **BOX 12-11 Alcohol Screening**
>
> Level B recommendation for screening: The USPSTF found good evidence that screening is beneficial in identifying patients whose alcohol consumption patterns place them at risk for increased morbidity and mortality, and good evidence that counseling about alcohol reduction can produce sustained benefit over a 6- to 12-month period.

Most cases of elder abuse are perpetrated by a family member, and reasons for the abuse include caregiver burnout and stress, financial worries, transgenerational violence, and psychopathology in the abuser. Women and dependent elders tend to be the most vulnerable to abuse.

Assessment of abuse can be very difficult because the victim may be cognitively impaired and unable to describe the abuse. It is not unusual for elderly clients to have multiple bruises due to poor balance and loss of subcutaneous fat. Clues to abuse may include:

- The presence of several injuries in different stages of repair
- Delays in seeking treatment
- Injuries that cannot be explained or that are inconsistent with the client's history
- Contradictory explanations by the caregiver and the patient
- Bruises, burns, welts, lacerations, or restraint marks
- Dehydration, malnutrition, decubitus ulcers, or poor hygiene
- Depression, withdrawal, or agitation
- Signs of medication misuse
- A pattern of missed or cancelled appointments
- Frequent changes in health care providers
- Discharge, bleeding, or pain in the rectum or vagina or a sexually transmitted disease
- Missing prosthetic device(s), such as dentures, glasses, or hearing aids

Notable Quotes

"Elders who are victim to physical abuse, caregiver neglect, or self-neglect have triple the mortality of those never reported as abused. Early detection and intervention by healthcare professionals in elder abuse cases may lead to decreased morbidity and mortality. Healthcare provider involvement is paramount, as studies have shown that only 1 in 6 victims are likely to self-report mistreatment to the appropriate legal authorities"

—Monique I. Sellas, MD, Staff Physician, Department of Emergency Medicine, Harvard Medical School, Brigham and Women's Hospital/Massachusetts General Hospital, as quoted in her 2006 article "Elder Abuse" from http://www.emedicine.com/EMERG/topic160.htm.

The USPSTF decided that there is insufficient evidence to support mass screening of asymptomatic elderly clients for abuse or for the potential for abuse. Suspected abuse should be evaluated through a thorough history with patients, caregivers, and other significant informants, taken separately. Home visits also can yield important clues to the situation. Physical examination, including mental status and evaluation of mood, is critical. Laboratory and imaging studies can support suspicions of dehydration, malnutrition, medication abuse, and fractures or other injuries.

Several assessment tools may help the nurse to determine whether a client is being abused or is at risk for abuse, although none have been adequately tested for validity, reliability, and generalizability, according to the National Center on Elder Abuse (Wolf, 2007). The Hwalek-Sengstock Elder Abuse Screening Test (H-S/EAST) (Neale, Hwalek, Scott, Sengstock, & Stahl, 1991) and the Vulnerability to Abuse Screening Scale (Schofield & Mishra, 2003) are commonly used screening instruments that are completed by the older adult.

If suspicions are strengthened through this assessment, a collaborative approach to management and prevention is required. Team members include the adult protective services agency, social workers, psychiatrists, lawyers, and law enforcement officials. It is important to ascertain whether the client is in immediate danger, in which case law enforcement will be helpful in removing the client from the dangerous situation. The approach to any abuse case should be coordinated with the adult protective services agency, as mandated by law. Abuse and neglect should be reported within 48 hours of the time that you become aware of the situation. Elder abuse that occurs in nursing homes and assisted living facilities must be reported to the Long-Term Care Ombudsman Program in most states.

In summary, guidelines for elder abuse treatment recommend that you 1) report abuse and neglect to adult protective services or other state-mandated agencies; 2) ensure that there is a safety plan and assess safety; 3) assess the client's cognitive, emotional, functional, and health status; and 4) assess the frequency, severity, and intent of abuse. It is

> **BOX 12-12 Elder Abuse Screening**
>
> Level I evidence: Insufficient evidence to support mass screening based on insufficient research to support the use of any particular screening tool, and lack of evidence to support that identification of risk changes outcomes.

important that the nurse's involvement does not end with the referral, but includes an ongoing plan of care because elderly persons referred to adult protective services are at increased risk of mortality in the decade following the referral.

HEART AND VASCULAR DISEASE

Coronary heart disease (CHD) is the leading cause of death in the United States. Every year over 1 million Americans have a new or recurrent myocardial infarction (MI) or die from coronary heart disease. Over 25% of patients who suffer MI or sudden death have no prior warning symptoms (Greenland, Smith, & Grundy, 2001). Most of these unexpected cardiac events and cases of sudden death occur in patients over 65 years of age. For this reason, identification of clients at risk for MI, who may be able to benefit from primary prevention strategies, is desirable. National Health and Nutrition Examination Survey (NHANES) III data (National Center for Health Statistics, 2004) suggest that approximately 25% of U.S. adults may be at high risk for a coronary event and may be potential beneficiaries of primary prevention strategies. The **Framingham Heart Study** has elucidated many of the risk factors associated with coronary heart disease. This study began with over 5,000 male and female subjects about 50 years ago in order to study cardiovascular risk factors. As a result of decades of epidemiologic work, the following risk factors have been identified:

- Age greater than or equal to 50 for men and 60 for women
- Hypertension
- Smoking
- Obesity
- Family history of premature CHD
- Diabetes (considered to be a CHD risk-equivalent, i.e., carries the same risk of a coronary event as known CHD)
- Sedentary lifestyle
- Abnormal lipid levels (Expert Panel on Detection, Evaluation, and Treatment of High Blood Cholesterol in Adults, 2001)

Several emerging risk factors, including homocysteine, lipoprotein(a) [Lp(a)] and infectious agents, are currently under investigation. A risk assessment tool developed as a result of discoveries from the Framingham study can be accessed at http://hin.nhlbi.nih.gov/atpiii/calculator.asp?usertype=prof. The risk factors included in the Framingham calculation of 10-year risk are age, total cholesterol, HDL cholesterol, systolic blood pressure, treatment for hypertension, and cigarette smoking (National Cholesterol Education Program, 2004). Patients who have diabetes or atherosclerotic diseases are known to have a more than 20% chance of a cardiac event in the next 10 years; the tool is not necessary to calculate risk for these patients.

In order to utilize this risk assessment tool, screening for the cardiac risk factors included in the tool must be performed. We will examine these screening guidelines, and the evidence to support these screenings, individually.

Lipids

There is strong evidence to link elevations in total cholesterol (TC) and low-density lipoprotein (LDL-C), and low levels of high-density lipoprotein (HDL-C) with coronary risk. Four large primary prevention trials documented a 30% reduction in cardiac events for clients whose cholesterol was reduced using statin therapy (USPSTF, 2004).

Unfortunately, there were very few subjects older than 65 years of age in these trials, but the USPSTF has determined that the results are generalizable to the elderly population. There is no age at which the task force recommends screening be stopped, but cholesterol levels are unlikely to increase after age 65. For patients who have been tested and found to have normal levels of

BOX 12-13 Lipid Screening

Level A recommendation for screening: There is strong evidence to correlate lipid abnormalities with cardiac risk. A simple blood test is a valid and reliable method of diagnosing lipid abnormalities, and diet and drug therapies are effective remedies.

cholesterol before the age of 65, testing may not be necessary in later years.

The ratios of TC to HDL-C or LDL-C to HDL-C are better predictors of risk than TC alone. It is possible to accurately measure TC and HDL-C on nonfasting venous or capillary blood samples, but fasting blood samples are required for accurate LDL-C measurement. Two separate measurements are required for definitive diagnosis. The optimal interval for lipid testing has not been determined, but most expert guidelines support testing every 5 years, with shorter intervals for people who have elevated lipid levels and who may require therapy.

Hypertension

Fifty million Americans have high blood pressure. Older Americans have the highest prevalence of hypertension and are the least effectively treated. Framingham data suggest that clients who have normal blood pressure at age 55 have a 90% chance of developing hypertension at some time in their life. High systolic blood pressure, which is more strongly correlated with CVAs, renal failure, and heart failure than diastolic blood pressure, is the most common form of hypertension in the elderly and is less likely to be well controlled than diastolic blood pressure. The NHANES study found that among subjects 60 years of age or older, isolated systolic hypertension (systolic 140 mm Hg with diastolic ≥ 90 mm Hg) was present in 65% of cases of high blood pressure.

The Seventh Report of the Joint National Committee on Prevention, Detection, Evaluation, and Treatment of High Blood Pressure (U.S. Department of Health and Human Services, 2004) is a national guideline for blood pressure screening and treatment and can be accessed at www.nhlbi.nih.gov/guidelines/hypertension/. It is important to diagnose and treat hypertension to reduce the incidence of cardiac disease. The correlation of cardiovascular risk and blood pressure is dramatic: Risk doubles with each increment of 20/10 mm Hg after 115/75. Treatment of isolated systolic hypertension in the elderly reduced stroke and coronary heart disease events by 30%, heart failure by 50%, and total mortality by 13%. (U.S. Department of Health and Human Services, 2004).

Blood pressure readings can be accurately determined by a properly calibrated sphygmomanometer using an appropriately sized cuff. (The cuff's bladder needs to encircle at least 80% of the client's arm.) Clients should have been seated in a chair for at least 5 minutes before blood pressure is measured. The client's feet should be uncrossed on the floor and the arm at heart level. Blood pressure measurements should be validated by measuring pressure in the contralateral arm. It is recommended that hypertension be diagnosed only after two or more elevated readings are obtained on at least two visits over a period of one to several weeks.

Lifestyle modifications are effective in preventing hypertension and lowering blood pressure in clients who have hypertension. These lifestyle changes include physical activity, weight loss, reducing dietary sodium, and following the **Dietary**

BOX 12-14 Blood Pressure Screening

Level A recommendation: There is strong evidence that blood pressure measurement can identify adults at increased risk for cardiovascular disease due to high blood pressure. Treatment of hypertension substantially decreases the incidence of cardiovascular disease.

Approaches to Stop Hypertension (DASH) diet, published by the National Institutes of Health (NIH) and downloadable from the Web at http://www.nhlbi.nih.gov/health/public/heart/hbp/dash/new_dash.pdf. This is a comprehensive plan that can be given to patients and includes a summary of the JNC-7 guidelines on hypertension, the results of studies on the DASH eating plan and its effectiveness in lowering hypertension, a diet journal, a tutorial on reading and understanding food labels, and meal plans using the DASH diet.

Aspirin Therapy

Aspirin therapy has long been known to be effective as a secondary prevention strategy for clients with heart disease, but the risks of gastrointestinal bleeding and hemorrhagic stroke associated with aspirin therapy have delayed recommendations of aspirin as a means of primary prevention. A meta-analysis of five primary prevention trials (USPSTF, 2002) that showed a 28% reduction of cardiac disease in subjects (most of whom were older than 50) has led experts to recommend "discussion" about aspirin chemoprophylaxis with clients at high risk for developing CHD. Gastrointestinal bleeding occurred in about 0.3% of subjects given aspirin for 5 years, causing some concerns about the risk versus benefit of aspirin for primary prevention of heart disease in patients who are at low risk for cardiac illness.

BOX 12-15 Aspirin Therapy

Level A recommendation: There is good evidence that aspirin decreases the incidence of CHD in adults who are at increased risk for heart disease, but aspirin increases the incidence of gastrointestinal bleeding and hemorrhagic strokes. The USPSTF concluded that evidence is strongest to support aspirin therapy in patients at high risk of CHD.

STROKE

Cerebrovascular accidents (CVAs) are the third leading cause of death in the United States, with more than two-thirds of stroke occurring in persons age 65 years or older (America Heart Association, American Stroke Association, 2008). The physical, psychological, economic, and social costs of CVAs are enormously high, to clients as well as their families. Strokes are a significant cause of dependency among the elderly.

The primary risk factors for ischemic stroke are similar to those described in the previous section on heart disease: increased age, hypertension, smoking, and diabetes. Clients with coronary artery disease are at increased risk for stroke because atherosclerotic vessel disease is a common etiology for the two diseases. Lifestyle factors associated with CVA risk that have been identified by the National Stroke Association are heavy alcohol use, cigarette smoking, sedentary lifestyle, and a high-fat diet. In addition to these risk factors, atrial fibrillation and asymptomatic carotid stenosis place clients at high risk for cerebrovascular disease.

It is estimated that 36% of strokes suffered by clients 80–89 years of age are as a result of nonvalvular atrial fibrillation (National Stroke Association, 1999). Adequate anticoagulation with warfarin therapy in patients with atrial fibrillation has been found to reduce stroke occurrence by 68%. Aspirin therapy was found to reduce CVAs by only 21%. It is based on these data that National Stroke Association guidelines recommend the use of oral anticoagulation with warfarin for patients older than 75 years of age with nonvalvular atrial fibrillation. Patients 65 to 75 years old with atrial fibrillation as well as other CVA risks should be treated with warfarin, and those without additional risk factors may be treated with warfarin or aspirin. The consensus panel of the Stroke Association underscores the importance of weighing the risk of hemorrhage against the benefit of therapy on an individual patient basis.

Carotid stenosis is an important stroke risk factor. However, there is insufficient evidence to recommend screening asymptomatic persons for carotid artery stenosis, using either physical examination or carotid ultrasound. Screening is justified if early treatment can change clinical outcomes and if there are effective, low risk screening tests. The inability of experts to recommend screening is based on the fact that there is significant debate about the risks and benefits of carotid endarterectomy as a treatment for asymptomatic disease. The American Heart Association (1998) recommends carotid endarterectomy for asymptomatic stenosis when the artery is at least 60% occluded, but the USPSTF does not recommend carotid ultrasound for asymptomatic patients based on remaining questions about the risks and benefits of carotid endarterectomy as a result of varying surgical risks among studies. Physical findings that suggest stenosis, by auscultation of the carotid artery, are a poor predictor of subsequent stroke.

Experts agree that the risk of a stroke can be minimized through treatment of hypertension; using statin therapy after MI for normal and high cholesterol; using warfarin for patients with atrial fibrillation and specific risk factors, and for patients after MI who have atrial fibrillation, left ventricular thrombus, or decreased left ventricular ejection fraction; and modification of lifestyle-related risk factors like smoking, alcohol use, physical activity, and diet.

THYROID DISEASE

The USPSTF has found insufficient evidence to support screening for thyroid disease in adults. Older adults are far more susceptible to thyroid dysfunction than younger adults. Overt disease affects 5% of American adults, but the prevalence of subclinical hypothyroidism (elevated thyroid-stimulating hormone [TSH] with normal levels of thyroid hormone) is 17.4% among women older than age 75 and 6.2% among men over age 65. Approximately 2–5% of these cases of subclinical hypothyroidism will progress to overt hypothyroidism each year (USPSTF, 2004). The American Association of Clinical Endocrinologists (AACE, 2002) has published clinical guidelines for the diagnosis and management of thyroid disease, in which it states that subclinical hypothyroidism may be associated with gastrointestinal disorders, depression, dementia, lipid disorders, increased likelihood of goiter, and overt thyroid disease.

Subclinical hyperthyroidism is far less common in the population, affecting only a little more than 1% of adults over 60 years of age, but it is present in up to 20% of patients taking levothyroxine for hypothyroidism (AACE, 2002).

Untreated hyperthyroidism can lead to atrial fibrillation, congestive heart failure, osteoporosis, and neuropsychiatric disorders. Hypothyroidism can cause constipation and ileus, lipid abnormalities, weight gain, decreased cognition, depression, and negative changes in functional status. The goal of screening would be to decrease the negative effects of overt thyroid disease.

The task force's inability to recommend for or against screening of asymptomatic persons for thyroid disease results from the lack of clarity about the risks of subclinical disease. It is clear that both hypothyroidism and hyperthyroidism cause significant morbidity and need to be treated, but the negative consequences of these diseases appear to be present primarily in patients who present with symptoms of the disease. There are significant costs and risks associated with thyroid replacement, which need to be considered before recommending mass screening. Many patients who receive thyroid hormone replacement develop subclinical hyperthyroidism, which may increase the risk of developing osteoporosis, hip fracture, and atrial fibrillation. The task force recommends that clinicians be cognizant of the signs and symptoms of thyroid disease, and test symptomatic patients; evidence is lacking to justify screening of asymptomatic patients, however. The AACE supports treatment of subclinical hypothyroidism if thyroid antibodies are positive. Thyroid antibodies are elevated in Hashimoto's thyroiditis, the most common cause of subclinical hypothyroidism. Clients with goiters and positive antibodies are more likely than other patients to progress to overt hypothyroidism.

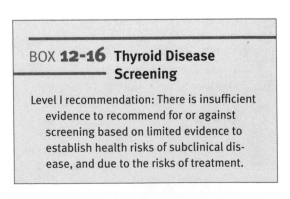

BOX 12-16 Thyroid Disease Screening

Level I recommendation: There is insufficient evidence to recommend for or against screening based on limited evidence to establish health risks of subclinical disease, and due to the risks of treatment.

OSTEOPOROSIS

Half of all postmenopausal women will have a fracture related to osteoporosis at some point in their life. The risk for the development of osteoporosis markedly increases with age, and osteoporosis is responsible for 70% of the fractures that occur in older adults. Women ages 65–69 have 6 times the risk of osteoporosis than younger postmenopausal women, and that rate increases to 14 times in women ages 75–79 (USPSTF, 2004). Age, low body mass index (BMI), and failure to use estrogen replacement are the strongest risk factors for osteoporosis development. Other possible risks include white or Asian race, family history of compression or stress fracture, fall risk or history of fracture, low levels of weight-bearing exercise, smoking, excessive alcohol or caffeine use, and low intake of calcium or vitamin D. Certain medications, such as thyroid medication or prednisone, increase the chances of developing osteoporosis.

Some men are at increased risk for osteoporosis, and decisions about screening may be made on an individual basis. Men with chronic lung disease, low testosterone levels, and who require steroid medications for extended periods of time are at increased risk of bone loss.

There is a strong association between bone mass and fracture risk, which continues into old age. Multiple studies demonstrate that therapies that slow bone loss are effective in reducing fracture risk, even if they are begun in old age.

The risk associated with age alone was high enough that the USPSTF recommends routine screening for all women over the age of 65. If risk factors, especially weight less than 70 kg (about 154 pounds) and no estrogen therapy, are present, the task force suggests screening women at age 60. Bone density testing at the femoral neck by dual energy x-ray bone densitometry is the gold standard screening tool, and the one most closely correlated with hip fracture risk, though heel measurements using ultrasonography are also predictive of short-term fracture risk.

Men are at significantly less risk for osteoporosis development than are women, and there are no recommendations for male screening.

BOX 12-17 Osteoporosis Screening

Level B recommendation: Osteoporosis is common in the elderly and is correlated with fracture risk. There are good screening tests to diagnose osteoporosis and effective treatments for the disease.

VISION AND HEARING

The prevalence of hearing and visual impairment increases with age and has been correlated with social and emotional isolation, clinical depression, and functional impairment. An objective hearing loss can be identified in over one-third of persons age 65 years or older and in up to half of patients age 85 years or older. High-frequency loss is the most important contributor to this increase in hearing loss, though up to 30% of cases may be caused or compounded by cerumen impaction or otitis media, which are easily treated (Ivers, Cumming, Mitchell, Simpson, & Pedulo, 2003).

About 4% of adults ages 65–74 and 16% of those 80–84 years of age have bilateral visual acuity worse than 20/40. Macular degeneration is the most common cause of visual loss in elderly whites, whereas African Americans are more likely to lose vision as a result of cataracts, glaucoma, and diabetes. Visual impairment has been correlated with falls and hip fractures in the elderly (Ivers et al., 2003).

The Snellen eye chart is a useful tool for vision screening. Ophthalmology referral may be useful for clients whose corrected vision is worse than 20/40, or who report visual problems that limit activities such as reading or driving. Many expert panels, including the American Academy of Ophthalmology, the American Optometric Association, and Prevent Blindness America, recommend regular ophthalmologic exams for adults over 65 years of age (40 years of age for African Americans) based on the fact that effective glaucoma screening should be performed by eye specialists with specialized equipment to evaluate the optic disc and measure visual fields. The optimal frequency for glaucoma screening has not yet been determined.

BOX 12-18 Hearing Screening

Level B recommendation: The task force recommends screening older adults for hearing loss by asking them about their hearing, counseling them about hearing aids, and referring them to specialists when abnormalities are detected.

The USPSTF recommends screening for hearing impairment for older adults by periodically questioning about their hearing, counseling about the availability of hearing aid devices, and referring clients with abnormalities. Pure-tone audiometry has a sensitivity of 92% and a specificity of 94% for detecting sensorineural hearing loss. One randomized controlled trial demonstrated a measurable improvement in social, cognitive, emotional, and communication function in a group of elderly veterans with hearing loss when they were fitted for and used hearing aids (Mulrow et al., 1990). It can sometimes be difficult for elderly individuals to adjust to the use of hearing aids, but compliance rates of close to 40–60% have been documented. Hearing aids can improve communication, social function, and emotional well-being.

PROSTATE CANCER

Prostate cancer is both the second most common form of cancer among U.S. men and the second leading cause of cancer death in U.S. men. The risk of developing prostate cancer increases with age and is the second leading cause of death in American men (American Cancer Society, 2008). The disease is most prevalent in African Americans and least prevalent among Asian Americans.

Two tests are commonly used in prostate cancer screening: the digital rectal exam (DRE) and the prostate-specific antigen (PSA) blood test. "The pooled sensitivity, specificity, and positive predictive value for PSA were 72.1%, 93.2% and 25.1%, respectively; and for DRE were 53.2%, 83.6% and 17.8%, respectively" (Mistry & Cable, 2003, p. 95). Benign prostatic hypertrophy is common in older men, and the presence of this disease increases the likelihood of false-positive testing with the PSA. Most prostate cancers are slow-growing and unlikely to be a cause of significant morbidity and mortality in older men. The greatest controversy regarding screening for prostate cancer is the inability to accurately predict which cancers will be aggressive and require treatment, and which are unlikely to metastasize.

Over 80% of cancers detected by PSA and DRE screening are localized to the prostate (Mistry & Cable, 2003). There are two methods to treat these organ-confined cancers: radiation and prostatectomy. There are no large randomized controlled trials that demonstrate the effectiveness of either of these methods compared to "watchful waiting" in treating screening-identified, organ-confined prostate cancer. A large clinical trial sponsored by the National Cancer Institute is currently under way. The Prostate, Lung, Colon and Ovarian (PLCO) Cancer Screening trial is designed to determine whether prostate screening, and early detection of prostate cancer, improves patient outcomes (National Cancer Institute, 2001). The PLCO study's preliminary findings suggest that the frequency of screening may need to be less often than commonly performed. Five-year intervals between PSA/DRE screenings may be sufficient for most men with low levels of PSA.

BREAST CANCER

Breast cancer is the most common cancer among U.S. women, and the prevalence of the disease

BOX 12-19 Prostate Cancer Screening

Level I recommendation: There is insufficient evidence to recommend screening based on inconclusive evidence that screening with DRE and PSA improves health outcomes. Men with a life expectancy of less than 10 years are unlikely to benefit from prostate screening.

BOX 12-20 Breast Cancer Screening

Screening with mammography (with or without clinical breast exam): Level B evidence: There is fair evidence to support benefit from breast cancer screening for older women by mammogram every 1–2 years. There is no age at which screening should be discontinued, but the task force agrees that screening would have no benefit when life expectancy is significantly limited by dementia or other serious, life-limiting chronic illnesses.

Clinical breast exam screening: Level I evidence.

Self breast exam screening: Level I evidence.

increases with age. According to the CDC (2008), 3–4% of women who are 60 years old today will get breast cancer by the age of 70. Other risk factors for the disease include family history of breast cancer, atypical hyperplasia in breast tissue, and birth of a first child when a woman is over 30 years of age. The USPSTF examined whether breast cancer screening, by mammography, was beneficial in older women. Although disease prevalence is high in this population, the task force wondered whether early detection of disease would improve health outcomes in a population that also has a higher incidence of other chronic illnesses. They wondered if there was an upper age limit at which breast cancer screening would no longer be beneficial. There have been no studies that analyzed screening for women over 74 years of age, but the task force concluded that, unless a woman has significant comorbidity that will significantly limit her life expectancy, screening is warranted based on the high mortality from the disease in older women.

Screening tests used to detect breast cancer include mammography, clinical breast exam by a health care provider, and self breast exam. The sensitivity of mammography to detect breast cancer varies widely, depending on a woman's age, whether she takes hormonal replacement, the technical quality of the testing equipment, and the skill of the radiologist. Overall, the test is more sensitive for older women than for younger women. Unfortunately, there are many false-positive tests, and up to one-quarter of women who have annual mammograms may need to undergo unnecessary, invasive follow-up testing as a result of false-positive tests from mammography at some point in their lives. No studies have looked at the effectiveness of clinical breast exam without concurrent mammography to detect breast cancer. Self breast exam has not been found to decrease breast cancer morbidity or mortality, but there have not been enough studies to evaluate the issue.

COLORECTAL CANCER SCREENING

Colorectal cancer is both the third most common cancer in the United States and the third leading cause of cancer death in the United States. The prevalence of the disease increases with age, and over 90% of colorectal cancer is diagnosed in clients over the age of 50 (American Cancer Society, 2008).

There are several good screening methodologies to detect early colon cancer: fecal occult blood testing (FOBT), sigmoidoscopy, and colonoscopy. Choice of screening test is determined based on client risk factors and preference. Patients who have a history of adenomatous polyps or inflammatory bowel disease, or a family history of

BOX 12-21 Colorectal Screening

Level A recommendation: The task force strongly recommends colorectal screening by FOBT, FOBT + sigmoidoscopy, or sigmoidoscopy alone for clients with average risk of developing colorectal cancer. The task force was unable to determine whether the increased sensitivity of colonoscopy compared with the other screening methods outweighed the costs, risks, and inconvenience of the procedure.

BOX 12-22 Web Exploration: Clinical Practice Guidelines

Behavioral Counseling in Primary Care to Promote a Healthy Diet: Recommendations and Rationale (USPSTF, independent expert panel, revised 2003):

http://www.guideline.gov/summary/summary.aspx?doc_id=3494&nbr=002720&string=osteoporosis+AND+prevention

Clinical Practice Guidelines for the Assessment and Prevention of Falls in Older People (National Institute for Clinical Excellence, London, 2004):

http://www.guideline.gov/summary/summary.aspx?doc_id=6118&nbr=003968&string=osteoporosis+AND+prevention

Elder Abuse Prevention (University of Iowa Gerontological Nursing Interventions Research Center, 2004):

http://www.guideline.gov/summary/summary.aspx?doc_id=6829&nbr=004196&string=elder+AND+abuse

colorectal cancer or adenomatous polyps, should receive colonoscopy. Screening for these high-risk clients is begun before age 50.

Colonoscopy is the most sensitive of the screening methodologies but is associated with the highest costs and risks. These risks include a small risk of perforation and bleeding and the risks associated with sedation, which is required for the procedure.

Commonly used screening strategies for clients of average risk include annual FOBT, sigmoidoscopy performed every 5 years, or a combination of FOBT performed annually with sigmoidoscopy every 5 years when FOBT testing is negative. If the results of this test are positive, clients are sent for colonoscopy or double contrast barium enema combined

BOX 12-23 Research Highlight

Aims: This prospective cohort study compared two different frailty indexes (the Cardiovascular Health Study Index [CHSI] and the Study of Osteoporotic Fractures Index [SOFI]) for their ability to predict falls, disability, fractures, and death in elderly women. This study is important because many frailty indexes are difficult to administer in the office, but the SOFI is very simple to perform because it uses only weight loss, a yes/no question about energy from the Geriatric Depression Scale, and an assessment of the client's ability to rise from a chair without using his or her arms.

Methods: 6,701 community-dwelling women 69 years or older were identified as robust, intermediate or prefrail, or frail, based on two different frailty assessments. Self-reports of falls or fracture were reported every 4 months for 2 years; functional status was measured at 1 and at 4.5 years postinitial exam. Fracture reports were confirmed radiographically. A logistic regression was used to determine whether the two frailty scales were equally beneficial in predicting falls, fracture, death, and functional decline.

Findings: There was no difference between the CHSI and the SOFI in predicting falls, disability, fracture, or death.

Application to practice: The SOFI may be a good, easy to administer clinical tool to identify frailty and morbidity among elderly women.

Source: Ensrud, K., Ewing, S., Taylor, B., Cawthon, P., Stone, K., Hillier, T. et al. (2008). Comparison of two frailty indexes for prediction of falls, disability, fractures, and death in older women. *Archives of Internal Medicine, 168*(4), 382–389.

with sigmoidoscopy, in cases where colonoscopy is not available. The best methodology for FOBT is the three consecutive stool samples that are collected at home by the patient on an annual basis. These tests should be examined without rehydration due to the decreased specificity of the test that is associated with rehydration of the samples. A single guiaic test, performed in the office with DRE, is not recommended as an adequate screening test (National Guideline Clearinghouse, 2005).

There is strong evidence to support colorectal screening for men and women age 50 or older, but insufficient evidence to determine which of the various screening options is the preferred method for screening.

SUMMARY

In summary, there are many effective screenings for various diseases common to the elderly population. Nurses should utilize the appropriate resources to obtain and put into practice screening of aged patients according to the USPSTF guidelines. (**Table 12-1** contains a summary of guidelines.) Proper screening of older adults can save lives.

TABLE 12-1 Summary of USPSTF Screening Recommendations for Older Adults

Screening Test	Recommendation	Level of Evidence
Physical activity	Physical activity has a positive impact on health but we don't know whether counseling about exercise is effective in helping people to begin exercising.	Level I
Nutrition	Counseling clients with chronic illnesses about nutrition is beneficial. Information should be geared to the chronic illness.	Level B
Tobacco use	Screening is helpful in identifying tobacco use, and counseling is effective in helping people quit smoking.	Level B
Safety	Falls can be prevented by medication monitoring, balance and strength exercises, and home safety evaluation.	Level B
Immunizations	Annual flu vaccine	Level B
	Pneumococcal vaccine once after age 65 and one-time revaccination for clients over age 75 who've not been vaccinated in 5 years	Level B
	Td vaccine every 10 years	Level A
Depression	Screening is effective in identifying depression and treatments are effective.	Level B
Dementia	Insufficient evidence to support mass screening of elders for dementia, but good evidence to suggest screening to follow up on family or client's concerns about memory loss.	Level I
Alcohol abuse	Screening is beneficial and treatment is effective.	Level B
Elder abuse and neglect	No evidence that either screening or interventions are effective.	Level I

(continues)

TABLE **12-1** **Summary of USPSTF Screening Recommendations for Older Adults (continued)**

Screening Test	Recommendation	Level of Evidence
Lipids	Good evidence to support that treatment and screening are effective.	Level A
Hypertension	Good evidence to support that treatment and screening are effective.	Level A
Aspirin therapy	Good evidence to support aspirin therapy in clients at high risk for CV disease.	Level A
Cerebrovascular disease	Insufficient evidence for use of carotid ultrasound to screen for carotid stenosis as a CVA risk factor.	Level I
Thyroid disease	Insufficient evidence to support screening for thyroid disease.	Level I
Osteoporosis	Screening is recommended for all women over 65 years of age.	Level B
Vision and hearing	Hearing screening is recommended for older adults. Glaucoma testing by an ophthalmologist is recommended for adults at risk of developing glaucoma.	Level B
Prostate cancer	Insufficient evidence to recommend screening.	Level I
Breast cancer	Mammography is recommended every 2 to 3 years as a screening for breast cancer for older women.	Level B
Colorectal cancer	Screening for colorectal cancer by FOBT, sigmoidoscopy, or FOBT + sigmoidoscopy is recommended.	Level A

Critical Thinking *Exercises*

1. Iola R., a 72-year-old, overweight woman, tells you that she wishes that she could exercise, but that she can never bring herself to begin an exercise program. She knows that her hypertension, diabetes, and high cholesterol would benefit from regular exercise. She is caring for her grandchildren 3 days per week and can't find the time to engage in regular exercise. She is not sure if it is safe to walk alone around her neighborhood, anyway. Explain how you could use the concepts of self-management of chronic illness and contracting to help Iola begin an exercise program. What benefits might she obtain through regular exercise? How frequently should she plan to exercise?

continues

Critical Thinking (continued)

2. Mr. Gottlieb complains that he has been falling a lot recently. He can remember at least three falls in the past 6 months, but luckily, none have resulted in injury yet. His friend is living in a nursing home as a result of complications and debility that followed a hip fracture, and Mr. Gottlieb does not want the same fate for himself. Describe how you will assess and manage Mr. Gottlieb's fall risk.
3. Mrs. Hall is a 94-year-old woman with Alzheimer's disease. Her daughter is her primary caregiver and calls to report that caring for her mother has become intolerable. "I can't make her eat, drink, or stop her incessant whining." You notice that Mrs. Hall has not been in to see her primary care doctor in over 3 years, but that she has been in to the emergency department four times in the past year for dehydration, urinary tract infections, and behavior management. You want to assess the home situation for safety and provide caregiver support to the patient's daughter. What signs of abuse and neglect might you look for through a chart review? Through a clinic visit and evaluation of the client? Through laboratory testing? How could you get a better assessment of the actual home situation? If your suspicions are strengthened, how will you proceed to intervene with this case of suspected elder abuse and neglect?

Personal Reflections

1. In the case described in #3 of the Critical Thinking Exercises, which of the two clients described, Mrs. H. or her daughter who initially called you, is your primary patient? Do you have loyalties to both? How could you address the care needs of Mrs. H.'s daughter?
2. Do you feel that you can counsel a client about health promotion if you do not adopt these behaviors yourself?
3. Mr. J., an 88-year-old gentleman, had a colonoscopy 6 years ago in which an adenomatous polyp was removed. His gastroenterologist has asked for your help in bringing Mr. J. back for follow-up testing. You call the patient who tells you that, although he recognizes the risk, he is not willing to undergo the procedure again. He believes his life expectancy is limited anyway and would prefer not to know if he has another polyp because he would not want to undergo surgery anyway. What do you do?

References

Adams, P. F., Dey A. N., & Vickerie J. L. (2007). *Summary health statistics for the U.S. population: National Health Interview Survey*. National Center for Health Statistics. Vital Health Statistics, 10(233).

Agency for Healthcare Research and Quality. (2000). *Treating tobacco use and dependence: PHS clinical practice guideline*. Retrieved January 27, 2005, from http://www.ahrq.gov/clinic/tobacco/whatisphs.htm

American Academy of Family Physicians. (1998). *Nutrition and health.* Retrieved May 17, 2008, from http://www.aafp.org/afp/980301ap/edits.html

American Academy of Family Physicians. (2004). *Aging and health issues: The family physician's role.* (Video CME program). Leawood, KS: Author.

American Association of Clinical Endocrinologists Task Force. (2002). American Association of Clinical Endocrinologists medical guidelines for clinical practice for the evaluation and treatment of hyperthyroidism and hypothyroidism. *Endocrine Practice, 8*(6), 457–467.

American Cancer Society. (2008). *What are the risk factors for colorectal cancer?* Retrieved on December 20, 2008, from http://www.cancer.org/docroot/CRI/content/CRI_2_4_2X_What_are_the_risk_factors_for_colon_and_rectum_cancer.asp

American Heart Association. (1998). Guidelines for carotid endarterectomy. A statement for healthcare professionals from a special writing group of the Stroke Council, American Heart Association. *Circulation, 97*, 501–509.

American Heart Association, American Stroke Association. (2008). *Heart disease and stroke statistics.* Retrieved December 15, 2008, from http://www.americanheart.org/downloadable/heart/1200082005246HS_Stats%202008.final.pdf

Babor, T. F., Higgins-Biddle, J. C., Saunders, J. B., & Monteiro, M. G. (2001). *The alcohol use disorders identification test* (2nd ed.). World Health Organization. Retrieved January 27, 2005, from http://whqlibdoc.who.int/hq/2001/WHO_MSD_MSB_01.6a.pdf

Buchner, D. M. (1997). Preserving mobility in older adults. *Western Journal of Medicine, 167*(4), 258–264.

Centers for Disease Control and Prevention. (2008). *Risk of breast cancer by age.* Retrieved on December 20, 2008, from http://www.cdc.gov/cancer/breast/statistics/age.htm

Centers for Disease Control and Prevention (CDC) & the Merck Company Foundation. (2007). *The state of aging and health in America, 2007*. Whitehouse Station, NJ: The Merck Company Foundation.

Duxbury, A. S. (1997). Gait disorders in the elderly: Commonly overlooked diagnostic clues. *Consultant, 37*, 2337–2351.

Ensrud, K., Ewing, S., Taylor, B., Cawthon, H., Stone, P., Hillier, K., et al. (2008). Comparison of two frailty indexes for prediction of falls, disability, fractures, and death in older women. *Archives of Internal Medicine, 168*(4), 382–389.

Ewing, J. A. (1984). Detecting alcoholism. The CAGE questionnaire. *Journal of the American Medical Association, 252*, 1905–1907.

Expert Panel on Detection, Evaluation, and Treatment of High Blood Cholesterol in Adults. (2001). Executive summary of the third report of the National Cholesterol Education Program (NCEP) Expert Panel on Detection, Evaluation, and Treatment of High Blood Cholesterol in Adults (Adult Treatment Panel III). *Journal of the American Medical Association, 285*(19), 2486–2497.

Fick, D. M., Cooper, J. W., Wade, W. E., Waller, J. L., Maclean, R., & Beers, M. (2003). Updating the Beers criteria for potentially inappropriate medication use in older adults. *Archives of Internal Medicine, 163*(27), 2716–2724.

Folstein, M. F., Folstein, S. E., & McHugh, P. R. (1975). "Mini-mental state." A practical method for grading the cognitive state of patients for the clinician. *Journal of Psychiatric Research, 12,* 189–198.

Greenland, P., Smith, S. C. Jr., & Grundy, S. M. (2001). Improving coronary heart disease risk assessment in asymptomatic people: Role of traditional risk factors and noninvasive cardiovascular tests. *Circulation, 104*, 1863.

Healthy People 2010. (2005). *Dietary guidelines for Americans 2005.* Office of Disease Prevention and Health Promotion, U.S. Department of Health and Human Services. Retrieved January 27, 2005, from http://www.healthypeople.gov

Ivers, R. Q., Cumming, R. G., Mitchell, P., Simpson, J. M., & Peduto, A. J. (2003). Visual risk factors for hip fracture in older people. *Journal of the American Geriatric Society, 51*, 356–363.

Kurlowicz, L., & Greenberg, S. (2007). The geriatric depression scale (GDS). *Hartford Institute for Geriatric Nursing, 4*. Retrieved December 20, 2008, from http://www.consultgerirn.org/uploads/File/trythis/issue04.pdf

Lawton, M. P., & Brody, E. M. (1969). Assessment of older people: Self-maintaining and instrumental activities of daily living. *Gerontologist, 9,* 179–186.

Lorig, K., & Holman, H. (2000). *Self management education: Context, definition and outcomes and mechanisms.* Australian Government Department of Health and Ageing. Retrieved January 27, 2005, from http://www.chronicdisease.health.gov.au/pdfs/lorig.pdf

McGinnis, J. M., & Foege, W. H. (1993). Actual causes of death in the United States. *Journal of the American Medical Association, 270*(18), 2207–2220.

Mistry, K., & Cable, G. (2003). Meta-analysis of prostate-specific antigen and digital rectal examination as screening tests for prostrate carcinoma. *Journal of the American Board of Family Practice, 16*, 95–101.

Mitty, E., & Flores, S. (2007). Fall prevention in assisted living: Assessment and strategies. *Geriatric Nursing, 28*(6), 349–357.

Mulrow, C. D., Aguilar, C., Endicott, J. E., Tuley, M. R., Velez, R., Charlip, R. S., et al. (1990). Quality of life changes and hearing impairment: Results of a randomized trial. *Annals of Internal Medicine, 113,* 188–194.

National Cancer Institute. (2001). *Prostate, lung, colorectal and ovarian cancer screening trial (PLCO).* U.S. National Institutes of Health. Retrieved December 20, 2008, from http://prevention.cancer.gov/programs resources/groups/ed/programs/plco/about

National Center for Chronic Disease Prevention and Health Promotion. (1999). *Chronic disease overview.* Centers for Disease Control and Prevention. Retrieved January 27, 2005, from http://www.cdc.gov/nccdphp/overview.htm

National Center for Chronic Disease Prevention and Health Promotion. (2004). *Improving nutrition and increasing physical activity.* Centers for Disease Control and Prevention. Retrieved December 20, 2008, from http://www.cdc.gov/nccdphp/publications/factsheets/Prevention/pdf/obesity.pdf

National Center for Health Statistics. (2004). *Third National Health and Nutrition Examination Survey (NHANES III) public-use data files.* Retrieved January 29, 2005, from http://www.cdc.gov/nchs/products/elec_prods/subject/nhanes3.htm

National Cholesterol Education Program. (2004). *Risk assessment tool for estimating 10-year risk of developing hard CHD (myocardial infarction and coronary death).* Retrieved January 29, 2005, from http://hin.nhlbi.nih.gov/atpiii/calculator.asp?usertype=prof

National Guideline Clearinghouse. (2005). *Colorectal cancer screening and surveillance: Clinical guidelines and rationale—update based on new evidence.* AHRQ. Retrieved February 5, 2005, from http://www.guideline.gov/summary/summary.aspx?doc_id=3686&nbr=2912

National Heart, Lung, and Blood Institute. (2004). *Third report of the Expert Panel on Detection, Evaluation, and Treatment of High Blood Cholesterol in Adults (Adult Treatment Panel III). National Cholesterol Education Program.* Retrieved January 27, 2005, from http://www.nhlbi.nih.gov/guidelines/cholesterol/index.htm

National Heart, Lung, and Blood Institute. (2005). *Obesity education initiative.* Retrieved January 27, 2005, from http://www.nhlbi.nih.gov/about/oei/index.htm

National Heart, Lung, and Blood Institute & Boston University. (2007). *About the Framingham heart study.* Retrieved May 17, 2008, from http://www.framinghamheartstudy.org/about/index.html

National Institute on Alcohol Abuse and Alcoholism. (1998). *Alcohol and aging, alcohol alert #40.* Retrieved December 20, 2008, from http://pubs.niaaa.nih.gov/publications/aa40.htm

National Stroke Association. (1999). Prevention of a first stroke: A review of guidelines and a multidisciplinary consensus statement from the National Stroke Association. *Journal of the American Medical Association, 2851*(12), 1112–1120.

Neale, A. V., Hwalek, M. A., Scott, R. O., Sengstock, M. C., & Stahl, C. (1991). Validation of the Hwalek-Sengstock elder abuse screening test. *Journal of Applied Gerontology, 10*(4), 406–418.

Partnership for Prevention. (2002). *Creating communities for healthy aging.* Retrieved December 20, 2008, from http://www.prevent.org

Roman, M. (2004). Falls in older adults. *AACN ViewPoint, 26*(2), 1–7.

Schofield, M. J., & Mishra, G. D. (2003). Validity of self-report screening scale for elder abuse: Women's Health Australia Study. *The Gerontologist, 43*(1), 110–120, Table 1.

Sloan, J. P. (1997). Mobility failure. In J. P. Sloan (Ed.), *Protocols in primary care geriatrics* (pp. 33–38). New York: Springer.

Sunderland, T., Hill, J. L., Mellow, A. M., Lawlor, B. A., Gundersheimer, J., Newhouse, P. A., et al. (1989). Clock drawing in Alzheimer's disease. A novel measure of dementia severity. *Journal of the American Geriatric Society, 7*(8), 725–729.

Task Force on Aging. (2001). *Improving the health care of older Americans.* AHRQ. Retrieved January 27, 2005, from http://www.ahrq.gov/research/olderam/

Teaser, P., Dugar, T., Mendiondo, M., Abner, E., & Cecil, K. (2006). *The 2004 survey of state adult protective services: Abuse of adults 60 years of age and older.* Retrieved May 17, 2008, from http://www.ncea.aoa.gov/ncearoot/Main_Site/pdf/2-14-06%20FINAL%2060+REPORT.pdf

U.S. Department of Health and Human Services, National Institutes of Health, & National Heart, Lung, and Blood Institute. (2004). *The seventh report of the Joint National Commission on the prevention, detection, evaluation, and treatment of high blood pressure.* Retrieved December 14, 2008 from http://www.nhlbi.nih.gov/guidelines/hypertension/jnc7full.pdf

U.S. Department of Health and Human Services, National Institutes of Health, & National Heart, Lung, and Blood Institute. (2006). *DASH eating plan: Lower your blood pressure.* Retrieved May 17, 2008, from http://www.nhlbi.nih.gov/health/public/heart/hbp/dash/new_dash.pdf

U.S. Pharmacopeia. (2004). *Personal medication organizer.* Retrieved January 27, 2005, from http://www.usp.org/pdf/patientSafety/personalMedOrg.pdf

U.S. Preventive Services Task Force. (2002). Aspirin for the primary prevention of cardiovascular events: Summary of the evidence. *Annals of Internal Medicine, 136*(2), 161–172.

U.S. Preventive Services Task Force. (2004). *Recommendations.* AHRQ. Retrieved January 27, 2005, from http://www.ahrq.gov/clinic/uspstf/uspstopics.htm

Wolf, R. (2007). *Risk assessment instruments.* NCEA. Retrieved July 31, 2007, from http://www.elderabusecenter.org/print_page.cfm?p=riskassessment.cfm

SECTION

5

ILLNESS AND DISEASE MANAGEMENT

(Competencies 13–15)

CHAPTER 13

Management of Common Illnesses, Diseases, and Health Conditions

Kristen L. Mauk, PhD, RN, CRRN-A, GCNS-BC
Patricia Hanson, PhD, APRN, GNP

LEARNING OBJECTIVES

At the end of this chapter, the reader will be able to:

- Name the major risk factors associated with cardiovascular disease (CVD).
- Discuss the impact of the major CVDs seen in older adults on the health of the U.S. population.
- Recognize signs of myocardial infarction that may be unique to the older adult.
- Utilize resources and research to promote heart-healthy lifestyles in older adults.
- State the warning signs of stroke.
- Apply the Mauk model for poststroke recovery to the care of stroke survivors.
- Identify common treatments for pneumonia, tuberculosis (TB), and chronic obstructive pulmonary disease (COPD).
- Discuss how to minimize risk factors for common gastrointestinal problems in the elderly.
- Describe nursing interventions for patients dealing with gastroesophageal reflux disease (GERD).
- Identify signs, symptoms, and treatments for benign prostatic hyperplasia (BPH) and vaginitis.
- Recognize common treatments for several cancers in older adults: bladder, prostate, colorectal, cervical, and breast.
- List several medications that can contribute to male impotence.
- Recognize the clinical treatments for persons with Parkinson's disease (PD).
- Devise a nursing care plan for someone with Alzheimer's disease (AD).
- Discuss possible causes and solutions for dizziness in the elderly.
- List the modifiable risk factors for osteoporosis.
- Distinguish between osteoarthritis and rheumatoid arthritis in relation to typical presentation, treatment, and long-term implications.
- Contrast rehabilitative care for older adults with hip and knee replacement surgery.
- Describe the most effective way to condition a stump to promote use of a prosthesis.
- Distinguish the signs and symptoms of cataracts, glaucoma, macular degeneration, and diabetic retinopathy.
- Contrast management of the four most common eye disorders seen in the elderly.
- Distinguish among the three major types of skin cancer.
- Identify signs and symptoms of herpes zoster appearing in the elderly.
- Review prevention of the most common complications of diabetes in older adults.

- Devise a plan for good foot care for older adults with diabetes.
- Synthesize knowledge about hypothyroidism into general care of the older adult.
- Discuss the causal factors, symptoms, and management of delirium in older adults.

KEY TERMS

- Activities of daily living (ADLs)
- Age-related macular degeneration (ARMD)
- Alzheimer's disease (AD)
- Angina
- Atherosclerosis
- Benign paroxysmal positional vertigo (BPPV)
- Benign prostatic hyperplasia (BPH)
- Bone mineral density (BMD)
- Cardiovascular disease (CVD)
- Cataracts
- Cerbrovascular accident (CVA)
- Chronic bronchitis
- Chronic obstructive pulmonary disease (COPD)
- Congestive heart failure (CHF)
- Continuous bladder irrigation (CBI)
- Corneal ulcer
- Coronary artery disease (CAD)
- Coronary heart disease (CHD)
- Cystectomy
- Delirium
- Diabetic retinopathy
- Diverticulitis
- Dysphagia
- Emphysema
- Erectile dysfunction (ED)
- Gastroesophageal reflux disease (GERD)
- Glaucoma
- Gonioscopy
- *Helicobacter pylori (H. pylori)*
- Hemiparesis
- Hemiplegia
- Herpes zoster
- Histamine 2 (H_2) blockers
- Hypertension (HTN)
- Incontinence
- Instrumental activities of daily living (IADLs)
- Intraocular pressure (IOP)
- Mauk model for poststroke recovery
- Meniere's syndrome
- Mini Mental State Examination (MMSE)
- Myocardial infarction (MI)
- Osteoporosis
- Otoconia
- Parkinson's disease (PD)
- Peripheral artery disease (PAD)
- Peripheral vascular disease (PVD)
- Phantom limb pain
- Proliferative retinopathy
- Prostate-specific antigen (PSA)
- Proton pump inhibitors (PPIs)
- Radical prostatectomy
- Retinal detachment
- Scatter laser treatment
- Stroke
- Tinnitus
- Tonometer
- t-PA (tissue plasminogen activator)
- Transient ischemic attack (TIA)
- Transurethral resection of the prostate (TURP)
- Tuberculosis (TB)
- Urostomy
- Vitrectomy

The purpose of this chapter is to present basic information related to common diseases and disorders experienced by older adults. It is assumed that the reader of this text has fundamental nursing knowledge and will study disease processes more in depth in other courses. Extensive discussion of the nursing care and treatment of each disease is beyond the scope of this book, but nurses are encouraged to refer to traditional medical-surgical textbooks for further reading. The discussion in this chapter will use a systems approach to provide a "snapshot" of essential information regarding background, risk factors, signs and symptoms, diagnosis, and usual treatment, while emphasizing any important aspects unique to care of the elderly with each disorder. Chapter 14 provides a thorough discussion of some additional common problems.

CARDIOVASCULAR PROBLEMS

Several conditions and diseases related to the cardiovascular system are common in older adults. The specific conditions discussed in this section include **myocardial infarction (MI)**, **hypertension**, **angina**, **congestive heart failure (CHF)**, **coronary artery disease (CAD)**, **stroke**, and **peripheral vascular disease**.

Although the death rate from cardiovascular disease has decreased in the last 40 years, the rate still remains high. More than 27 million American adults age 65 or older have some form of **cardiovascular disease (CVD)**, making it a significant health problem among the elderly. In the United States, 32% of all deaths in 2008 were attributed to CVD (American Heart Association [AHA], 2008c). In Canada, 34% of all male deaths and 36% of all female deaths in 2000 were due to heart disease and stroke (Heart and Stroke Foundation of Canada, 2005). The AHA lists the following as the major cardiovascular diseases: hypertension (HTN), **coronary heart disease** (**CHD**; includes myocardial infarction and angina), congestive heart failure (CHF), and stroke. These will be discussed in the following sections.

BOX 13-1 Resources About Cardiovascular Disease

American Heart Association
1-800-AHA-USA1
http://www.americanheart.org

American Society of Hypertension (ASH)
http://www.ash-us.org

American Stroke Association
1-888-4-STROKE
http://www.strokeassociation.org

Heart and Stroke Foundation of Canada
http://www.heartandstroke.ca

Heart and Stroke Foundation of Alberta, Canada
http://www.heartandstroke.ab.ca

National Emergency Medicine Association
http://www.nemahealth.org

National Institute of Neurological Disorders and Stroke
http://www.ninds.nih.gov

National Stroke Association
http://www.stroke.org

South African Heart Association
http://www.saheart.org

Hypertension

In 2004, 63.6% of men and 73.9% of women ages 65–74 were diagnosed with HTN; of those age 75 or older, 69.5% of men and 83.8% of women had HTN. African Americans continue to have a 1.8 times greater risk than whites of having a fatal stroke, and a 4.2 times greater chance of developing end stage renal disease (AHA, 2008d).

Blood pressure is determined by many factors, some of which, such as the condition of the heart and blood vessels, are influenced by age. Over 95% of hypertension is called "essential" hypertension; that is, it has no known cause (National Institutes of Health, 2005). High blood pressure may also result from disease processes. Additionally, those with prehypertension, a systolic blood pressure between 120 and 139 or a diastolic blood pressure between 80 and 89 on multiple readings, should receive a recommendation to make lifestyle changes, because they often develop hypertension. Diagnosis of hypertension should be based on several readings at different times or visits to the primary health care provider.

Risk factors for hypertension include family history, ethnicity, poor diet, being overweight, excessive alcohol intake, a sedentary lifestyle, and certain medications (**Table 13-1**). A blood pressure consistently under 120/80 is desirable. As persons age, the systolic blood pressure (the measure of the heart at work) tends to rise, but because of the significant risk of stroke associated with hypertension, older adults are being treated earlier and more aggressively than in years past. Although some clinicians may consider HTN in the elderly as a blood pressure greater than 160/90, because of the rise in systolic blood pressure with age, those with isolated systolic HTN (i.e., a systolic BP over 140 and a

TABLE 13-1 Risk Factors for Hypertension

Risk Factors for Hypertension
Heredity
Race (African American)
Increased age
Sedentary lifestyle
Male gender
High sodium intake
Diabetes or renal disease
Heavy alcohol consumption
Obesity
Pregnancy
Some oral contraceptives
Some medications

SOURCE: AHA, 2005.

diastolic BP less than 90) should be aggressively treated (Reuben et al., 2004). Complete information about the Joint National Committee's seventh report (JNC 7) for control of high blood pressure can be found at http://www.nhlbi.nih.gov/guidelines/hypertension/.

Lifestyle modifications may help older adults to control blood pressure. **Table 13-2** lists recommended strategies for older adults. Several medications may be used to treat hypertension in the elderly (**Table 13-3**). The goal of medical treatment in older adults is to lower the blood pressure to 120/80 or below. Thiazide diuretics or beta blockers are often used as drugs of choice for those elderly who do not have other coexisting medical conditions. It is not uncommon for older adults to require more than one and even up to several medications to achieve adequate control. In fact, combination therapy for older adults "allows for smaller doses of each drug and thus avoids unpleasant side effects" (Tully, 2002, p. 36). The most common combinations are a thiazide diuretic with either a potassium-sparing diuretic, a beta blocker, a calcium channel blocker, angiotensin-converting enzyme inhibitors (ACEIs), or angiotensin receptor blockers (ARBs) (National Institutes of Health [NIH], 2008).

Older adults should work with their physicians and nurses to achieve good control of their blood pressure, because it is a risk factor and contributor to many other serious health conditions including heart disease, stroke, and renal disease. Nurses may need to do extensive teaching about lifestyle modifications to assist older adults with smoking cessation and appropriate dietary choices. Remember that in addition to promoting nutrition, nurses should teach patients to read labels, avoid processed foods, prepare foods appropriately, and drink adequate amounts of fluids to stay hydrated.

TABLE 13-2 Strategies to Help Older Adults Control High Blood Pressure

Strategies to Help Older Adults Control High Blood Pressure
Limit alcohol intake to one drink per day.
Limit sodium intake.
Stop smoking.
Maintain a low fat diet that still contains adequate vitamins and minerals by adding leafy green vegetables and fruits.
Do some type of aerobic activity nearly every day of the week.
Lose weight. (Even 10 pounds may make a significant difference.)
Have blood pressure checked regularly. Report any significant rise in blood pressure to the physician.
Take medications as ordered. Do not skip doses.

TABLE 13-3 Some Types of Medications Used to Treat Cardiovascular Disease

Classification	Action	Example
+Diuretics	Decrease water and salt retention	Furosemide (Lasix)
+Beta-blockers	Lower cardiac output and heart rate	Atenolol (Tenormin)
+ACE inhibitors	Block hormone that causes artery constriction	Captopril (Capoten)
+Central alpha agonists	Block constriction of vessels	Clonidine (Catapres)
+Calcium channel blockers	Relax blood vessels to the heart	Amlodipine (Norvasc)
+Angiotensin II receptor blockers	Relax blood vessels by blocking angiotensin II	Irbesartan (Avapro)
+Vasodilators	Relax the walls of the arteries	Hydralazine (Apresoline)
*Digitalis	Strengthens and slows the heart	Digoxin (Lanoxin)
*Potassium	Helps control heart rhythm	K-Dur, K-Tab
*Blood thinners	Prevent clots	Warfarin (Coumadin); Heparin

+Medications used for both CHF and HTN
*Medications used for CHF

Coronary Heart Disease

Coronary heart disease (CHD), also called coronary artery disease (CAD) or ischemic heart disease, affects millions of people each year in many countries. This condition is caused by hardening and narrowing of the blood vessels of the heart (**atherosclerosis**), resulting in an impaired blood supply to the myocardium. Thirteen million Americans are affected each year. The rates for older females after menopause are more than twice that of older females prior to menopause. Over 82% of people who die with CHD are age 65 years or over (AHA, 2008c). Angina and myocardial infarction are two results of CHD that will be discussed here.

Angina

Angina pectoris is chest pain that results from lack of oxygen to the heart muscle. A small number of deaths are attributed to this cause each year, but mortality statistics related to angina are often included with CHD reports. Only about 20% of heart attacks are preceded by diagnosed angina. Among Americans ages 40–74, the prevalence of angina is slightly higher for females, significantly higher for Mexican American males and females, and slightly higher, though not significantly so, for African American females (AHA, 2005a). According to the AHA, the incidence of angina per 1,000 people is highest for nonblack males (28.3), followed by black males (22.4), black females (15.5), and nonblack females (14.1) (AHA, 2008a).

Angina is usually the first symptom of CAD in the older adult. It is classified as stable or unstable. Although the symptoms of angina may be similar to myocardial infarction, there are several notable differences. Angina often occurs related to exercise or stress and is relieved by rest and/or nitroglycerin. The associated chest pain is generally shorter (less than 5 minutes) than MI, though the classic presentation is squeezing pain or pressure in the sternal area. Older adults with angina may first complain of dyspnea, dizziness, or confusion versus classic chest pain (Tully, 2002). In addition to a thorough history and checking vital signs, a 12-lead EKG and lab tests will help rule out or confirm an MI.

Treatment is ongoing for angina. Unstable angina may require hospitalization, whereas stable angina can be managed with medication and lifestyle modifications aimed at reducing the workload on the heart and the accompanying oxygen demand. Teaching of patients and families will include weight management, stress management, limiting caffeine, smoking cessation, an exercise regimen that considers the person's myocardial capacity, control of hypertension, and medical management of any coexisting endocrine disorder (such as hyperthyroidism). Beta blockers and calcium channel blockers are often prescribed to decrease the oxygen demand on the heart. Patients should be alerted to side effects from these medications such as fatigue, drowsiness, dizziness, and slow heart rate.

Myocardial Infarction

Each year there are over 1.5 million incidences of myocardial infarction and between 500,000 and 700,000 deaths (Garas & Zafari, 2006). The risk of MI increases with age; men have the highest incidence of MI until approximately age 70, when the incidences of MI converge and the rate of MI for men and women equalizes (Garas & Zafari, 2006).

Risk factors for MI include hypertension, race (especially African American males with HTN), high-fat diet, sedentary lifestyle, diabetes, obesity, high cholesterol, family history, cigarette smoking, excessive alcohol intake, and stressful environment. Many of these risk factors are modifiable or controllable. Warning signs of MI are listed in **Table 13-4**. It is important to note that the warning signs are often very different for women than they are for men. Women often do not have the substernal chest pain, but more often experience sharp pain, fatigue, weakness, and other nonspecific symptoms (Garas & Zafari, 2006).

"Thrombolytic therapy, if administered early in the course of MI, significantly reduces the morbidity and mortality associated with MI" (Tully, 2002, p. 40). The following steps are recommended, if possible, while awaiting emergency treatment:

1. Have the patient rest.
2. Provide supplemental oxygen.
3. Give nitroglycerin sublingually every 5 minutes times three and monitor vital signs.
4. Give aspirin if not contraindicated.

Some nurses use the mnemonic MONA (morphine, oxygen, nitroglycerin, aspirin) to remember the steps in acute care treatment of MI. If neither oxygen nor nitroglycerin is available, proceed with giving aspirin.

TABLE 13-4 Warning Signs of Heart Attack

Chest pain appearing as tightness, fullness, or pressure
Pain radiating to arms
Unexplained numbness in arms, neck, or back
Shortness of breath with or without activity
Sweating
Nausea
Pallor
Dizziness
*Unexplained jaw pain
*Indigestion or epigastric discomfort, especially when not relieved with antacids

*Of particular significance in the elderly

Diagnosis may include a variety of tests including electrocardiogram (ECG) and angiogram or cardiac catheterization to visualize any areas of blockage. **Figure 13-1** shows the results of an angiogram with some degree of blockage in a major heart vessel. Such procedures are generally done in a special catheterization lab within a heart center or hospital by a cardiologist. Important nursing interventions after these procedures include keeping the leg straight with pressure on the femoral artery entry site per the facility's protocol. Instruction of the patient and family after this outpatient procedure should include emphasis on the importance of monitoring the entry site. Patients should be taught that bleeding at the site is considered an emergency and that firm, direct pressure must be applied to the site immediately. It is common for bruising to occur, and limits to lifting and driving should be strictly followed after the procedure to prevent complications.

Usual medical treatment of MI includes several options, depending on the results of the diagnostic tests and extent of damage and blockage.

FIGURE **13-1** **Coronary angiogram illustrating segmental narrowing (arrows).**

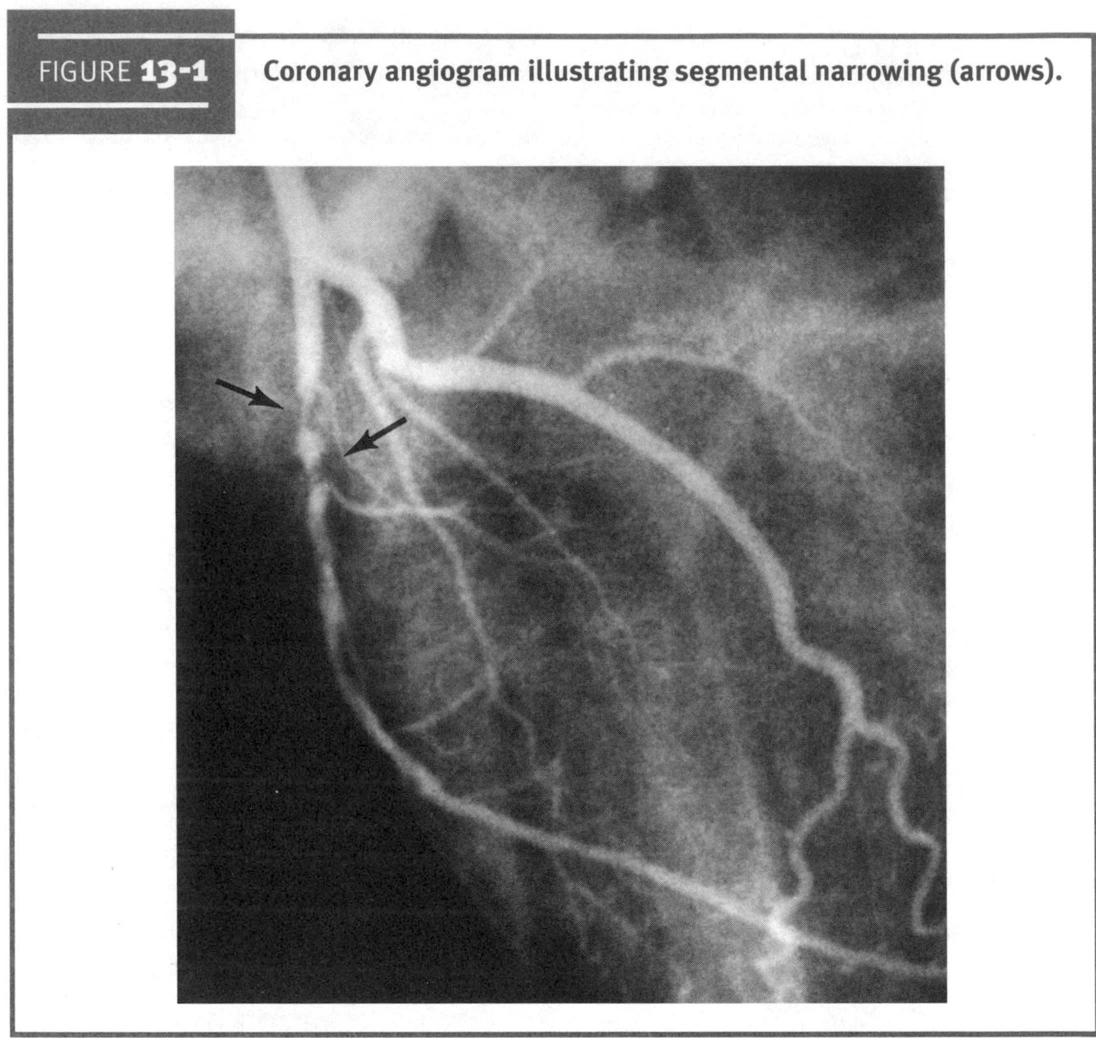

SOURCE: Leonard Crowley, *Introduction to Human Disease* (6th ed.). Sudbury, MA: Jones and Bartlett Publishers, 2005.

Angioplasty (**Figure 13-2**) is a common procedure that uses a balloon or other device to open the blocked vessel. Coronary artery bypass graft (CABG), commonly known as open heart surgery, is often used for those with several major arteries blocked, in order to restore blood flow (**Figure 13-3**). Pharmacological treatment may include beta blockers, angiotensin-converting enzyme (ACE) inhibitors, and antihypertensives, to name a few. The recovery period will include careful monitoring in cardiac intensive care, then progression to cardiac rehabilitation in which patients will be closely monitored after discharge and assisted by specialized nurses to make lifestyle modifications to promote maximal recovery and return to function. Patients are discharged from the hospital as early as possible; therefore, the cardiac rehabilitation will likely occur on an outpatient basis. It is important to encourage patients to follow through with cardiac rehabilitation even though they may be feeling well.

Persons surviving a heart attack should be dedicated to reducing risk factors associated with heart

FIGURE 13-2 **Coronary angioplasty. A, Severely narrowed coronary artery (arrow) shown by angiogram. B, Same artery after successful dilation by angioplasty.**

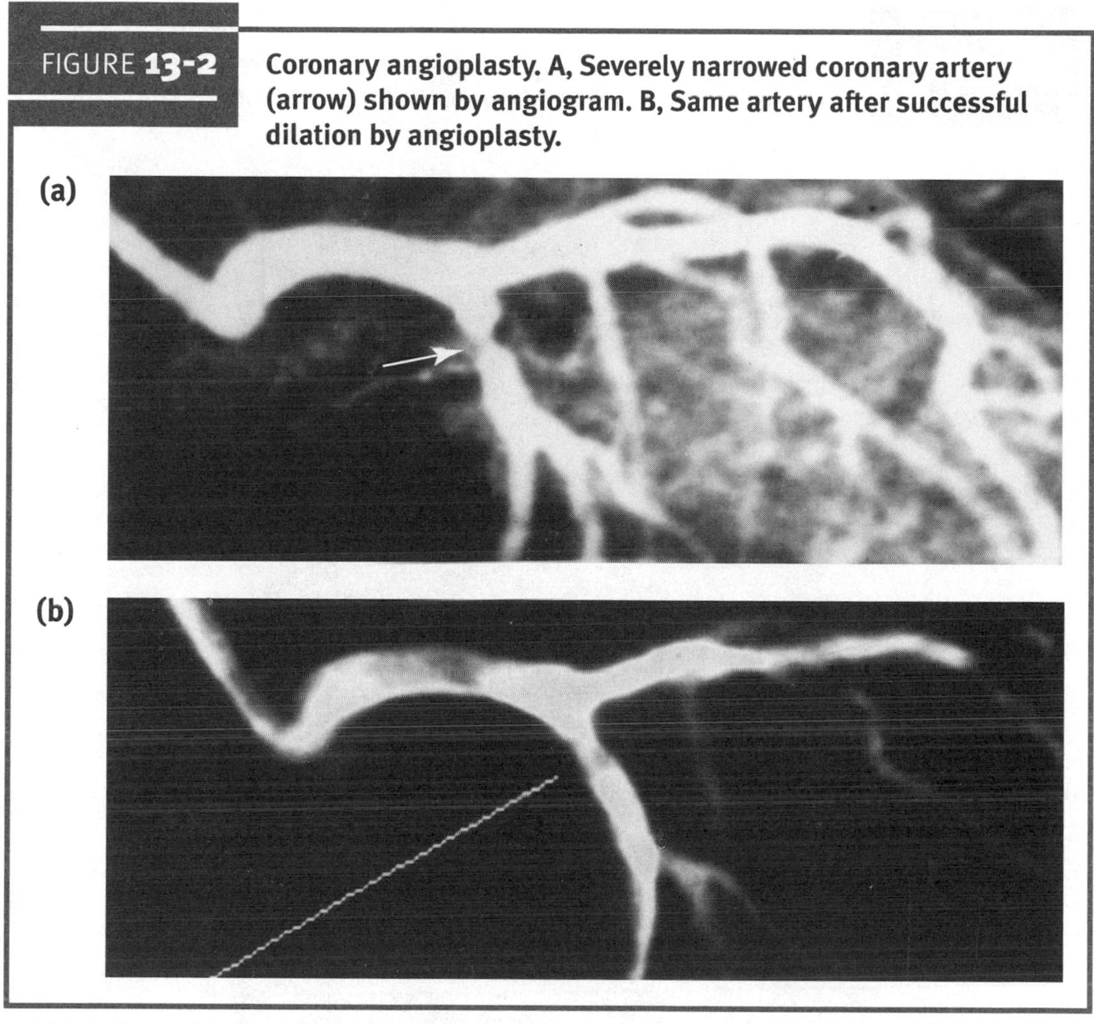

SOURCE: Leonard Crowley, *Introduction to Human Disease* (6th ed.). Sudbury, MA: Jones and Bartlett Publishers, 2005.

disease. **Table 13-5** lists several strategies for older adults to prevent a first or recurring heart attack. Nurses should encourage patients to attend cardiac rehabilitation programs during the posthospitalization period. Zucker (2002) stated that "unless patients are consistently referred to cardiac rehabilitation or are followed closely after discharge, they have little support as they attempt to incorporate and maintain new, healthier behaviors" (p. 187). Support groups for survivors and families may also be helpful. Family members, particularly spouses, should be included in the rehabilitation process (**Case Study 13-1**).

Congestive Heart Failure (CHF)

The incidence of congestive heart failure (CHF) varies among races and across age groups. For example, white men have an incidence of 15.2 per 1,000 between the ages of 65 and 74, 31.7 per 1,000 between the ages of 75 and 84, and 65.2 per 1,000 when greater than 85 years of age. Considering these same age ranges, the incidence of heart

FIGURE **13-3** **Vein graft extending from aorta above the origin of the coronary arteries to the anterior interventricular (descending) coronary artery distal to the site of arterial narrowing.**

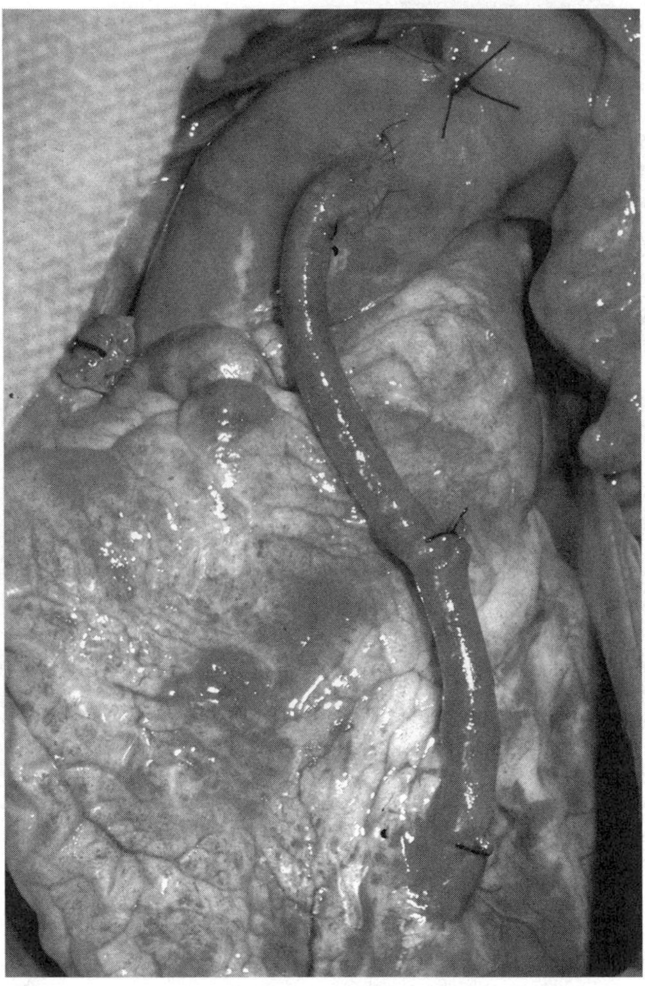

SOURCE: Leonard Crowley, *Introduction to Human Disease* (6th ed.). Sudbury, MA: Jones and Bartlett Publishers, 2005.

failure for white women is 8.2, 19.8, and 45.6, respectively; for black men 16.9, 25.5, and 50.6, respectively; and for black women, 14.2, 25.5, and 44.0, respectively (AHA, 2008b). The lifetime risk for someone to have CHF is 1 in 5. The risk of CHF in older adults doubles for those with blood pressures over 160/90. Seventy-five percent of those with CHF also have hypertension (AHA, 2005a). The major risk factors for CHF are diabetes and MI. CHF often occurs within 6 years after a heart attack.

TABLE 13-5 Strategies for Older Adults to Reduce Risk of Heart Attack

Exercise regularly.
Do not smoke.
Eat a balanced diet with plenty of fruits and vegetables; avoid foods high in saturated fats.
Maintain a healthy weight.
Manage stress appropriately.
Control existing diabetes by maintaining healthy blood sugars and take medications as prescribed.
Limit alcohol intake to one drink per day for women and two drinks per day (or less) for men.
Visit the doctor regularly.
After a heart attack, participate fully in a cardiac rehabilitation program.
Involve the entire family in heart-healthy lifestyle modifications.
Report any signs of chest pain immediately.

Signs and symptoms of heart failure are many; these appear in **Table 13-6**. It is essential that older adults diagnosed with CHF recognize signs of a worsening condition and report them promptly to their health care provider. Older adults may present with atypical symptoms such as decreased appetite, weight gain of a few pounds, or insomnia (Amella, 2004). For in-home monitoring, daily weights at the same time of day with the same clothes on the same scale are essential. The physician or primary care provider will give guidelines for the patient to call if the weight exceeds his or her threshold for weight gain. This is usually between 1 and 3 pounds. In the office or long-term care setting, O_2 saturation levels can be easily monitored. An O_2 saturation of less than 90% in an older person is cause for concern and further investigation.

Treatment for CHF involves the usual lifestyle modifications discussed for promoting a healthy heart (Table 13-5), as well as several possible types of medications. These include ACE inhibitors, diuretics, vasodilators, beta blockers, blood thinners, angiotensin II blockers, calcium channel blockers, and potassium. Digoxin, once a mainstay in the treatment of CHF, is rarely used now, although it may be seen on occasion. Most CHF is managed with lifestyle modifications and medications; however, in extreme cases, surgery may be a treatment option if valvular repair/replacement or heart transplant becomes necessary.

In addition, nurses should teach older adults about lifestyle modifications that can decrease

Case Study 13-1

Mr. Jones is a 62-year-old man who lives next door to you. He comes over while you are out in your yard and says, "You're a nurse, so I have this question for you. I have had this annoying heartburn all day that just doesn't go away no matter what I do." He points to his epigastric area. "It just feels like this pressure right here and makes me a little sick to my stomach." Mr. Jones looks pale and a bit diaphoretic.

Questions:

1. What is your best response to this situation?
2. What could these signs and symptoms indicate?
3. What would you expect Mr. Jones to do at this point?
4. Are there any other questions you could ask that would provide additional information about the potential seriousness of his complaint?

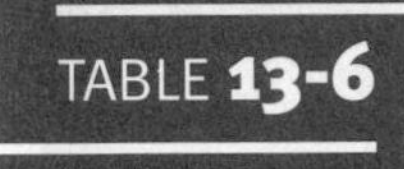

TABLE 13-6 Signs and Symptoms of Heart Failure

Shortness of breath
Edema
Coughing or wheezing
Fatigue
Lack of appetite or nausea
Confusion
Increased heart rate

SOURCE: AHA, 2005.

and/or help manage the workload on the heart. To minimize exacerbations, patient and family counseling should include teaching about the use of medications to control symptoms and the importance of regular monitoring with a health care provider (Johnson, 1999). These teaching points appear in **Table 13-7**. With a proper combination of treatments such as lifestyle changes and medications, many older persons can still live happy and productive lives with a diagnosis of heart failure, and minimize their risk of complications related to this disease.

Stroke

Stroke, also known as **cerebrovascular accident (CVA)** or brain attack, is an interruption of the blood supply to the brain that may result in devastating neurological damage , disability, or death. Approximately 780,000 people in the United States have a new or recurrent stroke each year (American Stroke Association [ASA], 2008). Stroke accounted for 1 in 16 deaths in 2004, making it the third leading cause of death. In Canada, stroke is the fourth leading cause of death, affecting 50,000 people each year (Heart and Stroke Foundation of Canada, 2005).

Assessment and Diagnosis

There are two major types of stroke: ischemic and hemorrhagic. The vast majority of strokes are caused by ischemia (88%), usually from a thrombus or embolus. The symptoms and damage seen depend on which vessels in the brain are blocked. Carotid artery occlusion is also a common cause of stroke related to stenosis (**Figure 13-4**).

Some risk factors for stroke are controllable and others are not. These risk factors appear in **Table 13-8**. The most significant risk factor for stroke is hypertension. Controlling high blood pressure is an important way to reduce stroke risk. Those with a blood pressure of less than 120/80 have half the lifetime risk of stroke as those with hypertension

TABLE 13-7 Lifestyle Modifications to Teach Older Adults with Heart Failure

Limit or eliminate alcohol use (no more than 1 oz. ethanol per day = one mixed drink, one 12 oz. beer, or one 5 oz. glass of wine).
Maintain a healthy weight. Extra pounds put added stress and workload on the heart. Weigh daily and report weight gains of 5 pounds or more to health care provider.
Stop smoking (no tobacco use in any form).
Limit sodium intake to 2–3 g per day—read the labels: avoid canned and processed foods. Take care with how foods are cooked or prepared at home (e.g., limit oils and butters).
Take medications as ordered—do not skip doses. Report any side effects to the physician.
Exercise to tolerance level—this will differ for each person. Remain active without overdoing it.
Alternate rest and activity. Learn energy conservation techniques.

FIGURE 13-4 **Angiogram showing narrowed carotid artery.**

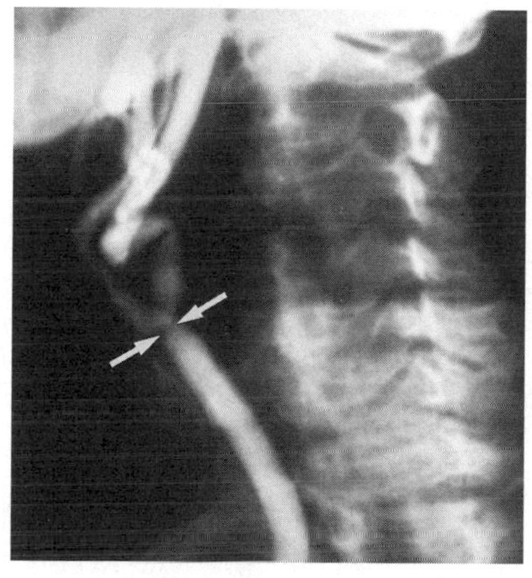

SOURCE: Leonard Crowley, *Introduction to Human Disease* (6th ed.). Sudbury, MA: Jones and Bartlett Publishers, 2005.

(ASA, 2008). Although the American Stroke Association and the National Stroke Association have funded national campaigns to promote education about the warning signs of stroke, in persons age 75 or older, blacks and males were found to be the least knowledgeable about these signs (ASA, 2008), emphasizing the continued need for education among older age groups. Smoking 40 or more cigarettes per day (heavy smoking) increases the stroke risk to twice that of light smokers. If a person quits smoking, their risk after 5 years mirrors that of a nonsmoker, so older adults should be particularly encouraged to stop smoking.

Several warning signs are common with stroke (**Table 13-9**). Thromboembolic strokes are more likely to show classic signs than hemorrhagic strokes, which may appear as severe headaches but with few other prior warning signs. A quick initial evaluation for stroke can be summed up by assessing for three easy signs: facial droop, motor weakness, and language difficulties.

TABLE 13-8 **Risk Factors for Stroke**

Controllable	Uncontrollable
Hypertension High cholesterol Heart disease Smoking Obesity Stress Diabetes Depression Atrial fibrillation	Advanced age Gender (males more than females until menopause) Race (African Americans more than whites) Heredity

Other warning signs of stroke include a temporary loss of consciousness or the appearance of the classic warning signs that go away quickly (**Case Study 13-2**). **Transient ischemic attacks (TIAs)** are defined as those symptoms similar to stroke that go away within 24 hours (and usually within minutes) and leave no residual effects. Most TIAs in whites are from atherothrombotic disease, with another 20% from cardiac emboli and 25% from

TABLE 13-9 **Warning Signs of Stroke**

- Sudden numbness or weakness of face, arm, or leg, especially on one side of the body
- Sudden confusion; trouble speaking or understanding
- Sudden trouble seeing in one or both eyes
- Sudden trouble walking, dizziness, loss of balance or coordination
- Sudden severe headache with no known cause

SOURCE: NSA, 2005, p. 1.

Case Study 13-2

Your grandfather is 85 years old and tells you at a family gathering that yesterday he had some blurred vision and numbness down his right arm. He didn't tell his wife or anyone else because the symptoms went away within 10 minutes, but he wanted to tell you just in case he should have it checked out.

Questions:

1. What should you tell your grandfather? What do his symptoms possibly indicate?
2. What risk factor does he have for stroke?
3. What other questions should you ask to gain more information?
4. What is the next step of action that your grandfather should take?
5. Should anything be discussed with his wife? If so, what?
6. Are there specific topics that should be taught at this point to your grandfather?

occlusion of smaller vessels (Warlow, Sudlow, Martin, Wardlaw, & Sandercock, 2003). At least 10% of those having a TIA will go on to have a stroke within a year (ASA, 2008).

Older adults experiencing the warning signs of stroke should seek immediate treatment by activating the emergency response system in their area. Transport to an emergency medical facility for evaluation is essential for the best array of treatment options. A history and neurological exam, vital signs, as well as diagnostic tests including electrocardiogram (ECG), chest x-ray, platelets, prothrombin time (PT), partial thromboplastin time (PTT), electrolytes, and glucose are routinely ordered. Diagnostic testing may include computed tomography (CT) without contrast, magnetic resonance imaging (MRI), arteriography, or ultrasonography to determine the type and location of the stroke.

Acute Management

The first step in treatment is to determine the cause or type of stroke. A CT scan or MRI must first be done to rule out hemorrhagic stroke (**Figure 13-5**). Hemorrhagic stroke treatment often requires surgery to evacuate blood and stop the bleeding.

The gold standard at present for treatment of ischemic stroke is **t-PA (tissue plasminogen activator)**. At this time, t-PA must be given within 3 hours after the onset of stroke symptoms. This is why it is essential that older adults seek treatment immediately when symptoms begin. T-PA is generally ineffective after the 3-hour window. New treatments are being explored to extend this window, including the use of a synthetic compound derived from bat saliva that contains an anticoagulant-type property. The major side effect of t-PA is bleeding. T-PA is not effective for all patients, but may reduce or eliminate symptoms in over 40% of those who receive it at the appropriate time (Higashida, 2005). Other much less common procedures such as angioplasty, laser emulsification, and mechanical clot retrieval may be options for treatment of acute ischemic stroke.

Additionally, the use of cooling helmets to decrease the metabolism of the brain is thought to preserve function and reduce ischemic damage. The roles of hyperthermia, hyperglycemia, and hypertension are all being further explored, as these are known to be associated with mortality and other poor outcomes related to ischemic stroke.

To prevent recurrence of stroke, medications such as aspirin, ticlopidine (Ticlid), clopidogrel (Plavix), dipyridamole (Persantine), heparin, warfarin (Coumadin), and enoxaparin (Lovenox) may be used to prevent clot formation. Once the stroke survivor has stabilized, the long process of rehabilitation begins. Each stroke is different depending on location and severity, so persons may recover with little or no residual deficits or an entire array of devastating consequences.

The effects of stroke vary, but may include **hemiplegia**, **hemiparesis**, visual and perceptual deficits, language deficits, emotional changes, swallowing dysfunction, and bowel and bladder problems. Although the deficits that present themselves depend on the area of brain damage, it is sometimes helpful to picture most strokes as involving one side of the body or the other. A person with left brain injury presents with right-sided weakness or paralysis, and a person with right-sided stroke presents with left-sided weakness or paralysis. **Table 13-10** lists common deficits caused by stroke, seen

FIGURE **13-5** **CT scan showing cerebral hemorrhage.**

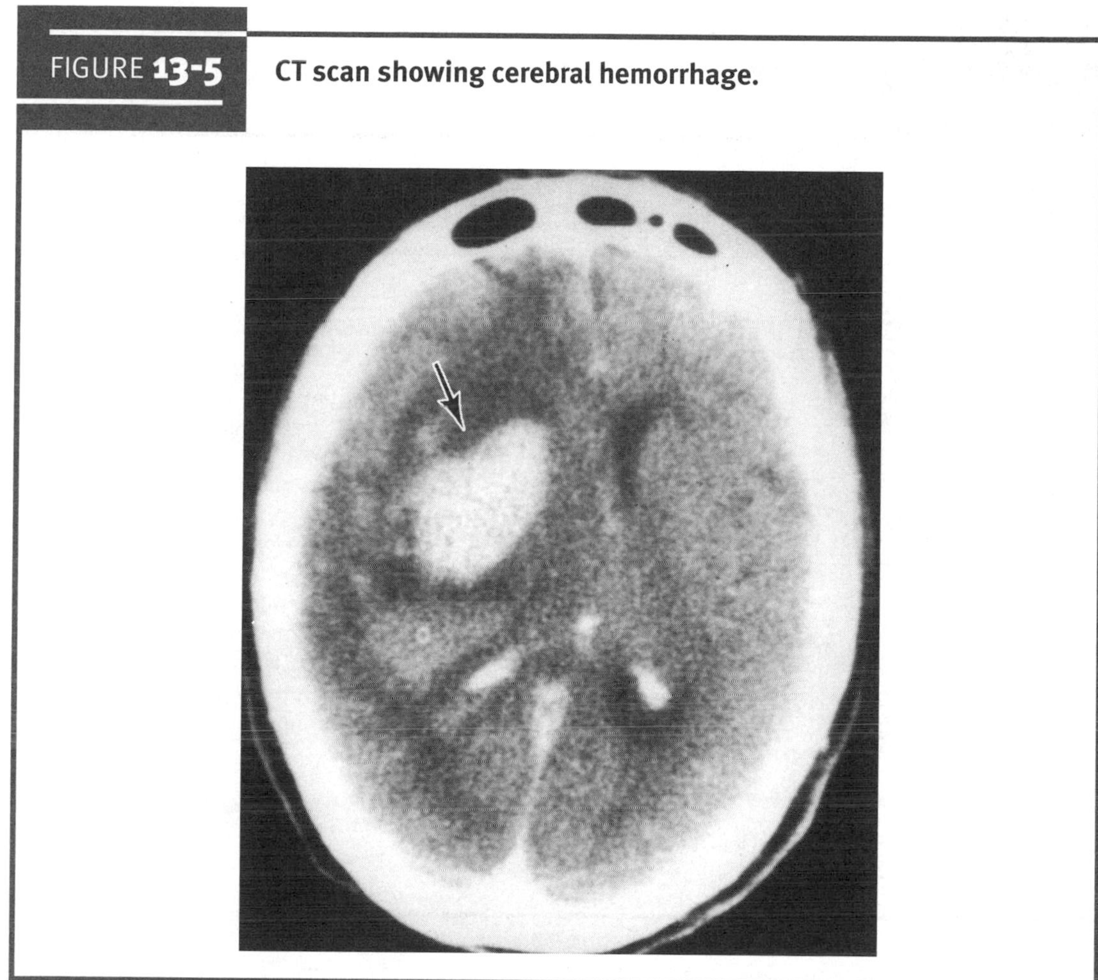

SOURCE: Leonard Crowley, *Introduction to Human Disease* (6th ed.). Sudbury, MA: Jones and Bartlett Publishers, 2005.

in varying degrees, and some common problems associated with strokes on one side of the brain versus the other.

Poststroke Rehabilitation

Rehabilitation after a stroke focuses on several key principles. These include maximizing functional ability, preventing complications, promoting quality of life, encouraging adaptation, and enhancing independence. Rehabilitation emphasizes the survivor's abilities, not disabilities, and helps him or her to work with what he or she has while acknowledging what was lost.

If significant functional impairments are present, evaluation for transfer to an intensive acute inpatient rehabilitation program is recommended. Inpatient rehabilitation units offer the survivor the best opportunity to maximize recovery, including functional return. An interdisciplinary team of experienced experts including nurses, therapists, physicians, social workers, and psychologists will help the survivor and the family to adapt to the changes resulting from the stroke. Although the goal of rehabilitation will usually be discharge back to the previous home environment, this is not always possible. Advanced age and functional capacity, particularly

TABLE 13-10 Common Deficits Caused by Stroke

Common Characteristics Associated with Stroke of Either Side	Right Hemisphere Stroke	Left Hemisphere Stroke
Weakness/paralysis Fatigue Depression Emotional lability Some memory impairment Sensory changes Social isolation Altered sleep patterns	Left hemiparesis or hemiplegia Left homonymous hemianopsia Difficulty with cognitive tasks such as spatial-perceptual tasks, sequencing, following multi-step instructions, and writing Memory deficits related to performance May not recognize or accept limitations or deficits Overestimating abilities Impulsive Quick movements Anosognosia or other forms of left-sided neglect Impaired judgment Inappropriately low anxiety Higher risk for falls due to lack of safety awareness Deficits less easily recognized by others	Right hemiparesis or hemiplegia Right homonymous hemianopsia Aphasia (especially expressive type) Reading/writing problems Dysarthria Dysphagia Anxiety when trying new tasks Tendency to worry and be easily frustrated Slow, cautious Memory deficits related to language

SOURCE: Adapted from Easton, 1999, p. 198, with permission of author.

ambulatory ability, may be predictors of discharge to a nursing home (Lutz, 2004).

Research by Easton (Mauk) (1999, 2001) demonstrated through grounded theory development that stroke survivors seem to go through a common process of recovery (**Box 13-2**). The **Mauk model for poststroke recovery** can help guide nursing practice by suggesting focused interventions for each of the six phases of stroke recovery. **Tables 13-11** and **13-12** list the major concepts and subconcepts of the model (**Figure 13-6**) and the major tasks for survivors and nurses.

Many survivors will need time to work through the first two phases of stroke recovery: agonizing and fantasizing. During this time, the person may be in denial about the consequences of the stroke and feel that soon everything will go back to "normal." Family members also may express these feelings. Survival and ego protection are the main goals of these early phases. The length of time a survivor spends in these early phases of recovery may be buffered by certain factors, as presented in the model. For example, older adults may spend less time agonizing over what has happened because they expected some health problems would come with advanced age, whereas younger persons may struggle more with the realities of stroke before being able to move on with rehabilitation.

As suggested by the Mauk model, once a stroke survivor has been medically stabilized and realizes

BOX 13-2 Research Highlight

Aim: To discover the process of recovery after stroke

Methods: Using grounded theory development, a concept analysis, concept synthesis, and subsequent theory synthesis were done. The researcher reviewed the literature on the writings as well as videotapes of stroke survivors as initial data. From this theoretical work, a model with six phases of post-stroke recovery emerged. The researcher then conducted face-to-face interviews with stroke survivors until data saturation ($n = 18$) was reached, refining concepts and subconcepts of the model.

Findings: The six phases of poststroke recovery emerging from the data were labeled in a model: agonizing, fantasizing, realizing, blending, framing, and owning. Assumptions and relational propositions were suggested by the model. The researcher further identified essential tasks for each phase (Table 13-12). These phases describe the process of poststroke recovery. Certain factors seemed to facilitate the recovery process including social and spousal support, expectations related to health, advanced age, faith in God, life experience in dealing with losses, and knowing the cause of the stroke.

Application to practice: By using the Mauk model for poststroke recovery, nurses can more efficiently target their care by focusing nursing interventions unique to the phase of recovery in which survivors are. Nurses should assess the phase of recovery and focus on care interventions related to the essential tasks for each phase.

Source: Easton-Mauk, K. L. (2001). The poststroke journey: From agonizing to owning. Doctoral dissertation. Wayne State University, Detroit, MI: Author.

the reality of the stroke situation, the focus of care will shift from survival to adaptation and adjustment. Nursing diagnoses common to stroke rehabilitation appear in **Table 13-13**. The Mauk model suggests that survivors do not fully participate in the recovery or rehabilitation process until they work through the realizing phase in which they begin to acknowledge that the effects of the stroke may not just go away. During this time, strong emotions such as anger and depression may surface. Depression is common after stroke and may be decreased by interventions that support the older adult's right to make choices and be supported in self-determination activities that enhance autonomy (Castellucci, 2004). As stroke survivors continue to receive support and appropriate interventions to facilitate the recovery process, they move into the last three phases of blending the old life with the new (after stroke), framing the experience in light of past and familiar experiences, and owning the fact that the stroke occurred and they will accept it and go on with a productive life. A qualitative, longitudinal study of patient expectations of recovery after stroke showed that stroke survivors maintained high expectations for recovery during the first 3 months (Anderson & Marlett, 2004; Rochette, Korner-Bitensky, & Lavasseur, 2006; Wiles, Ashburn, Payne, & Murphy, 2002, 2004). Realistic expectations can be reinforced by therapists and nurses, but it is important not to destroy hope of an increased quality of life.

Patient and Family Education

A large amount of teaching is often done by stroke rehabilitation nurses who work with older survivors. Training informal caregivers has been

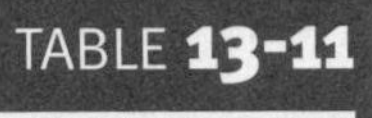

TABLE 13-11 The Six Phases (Concepts) of the Poststroke Journey with Characteristics

Phase/ Concept	Characteristics/ Subconcepts
Agonizing	Fear, shock/surprise, loss, questioning, denial
Fantasizing	Mirage of recovery, unreality
Realizing	Reality, depression, anger, fatigue
Blending	Hope, learning, frustration, dealing with changes
Framing	Answering why, reflection
Owning	Control, acceptance, determination, self-help

SOURCE: Easton, K. L. (2001). The poststroke journey: From agonizing to owning. Doctoral dissertation. Wayne State University. Detroit, MI: Author.

shown to improve quality of life for stroke survivors and their caregivers, and to decrease costs over time (Kalra et al., 2004). Many topics may need to be covered, depending on the extent of brain damage that has occurred. Some topics should be addressed with all survivors and their families. These include knowing the warning signs of stroke and how to activate the emergency response system in their neighborhood, managing high blood pressure (and how hypertension is the number one risk factor for stroke), understanding what medications are ordered as well as how often to take them and why, the importance of regular doctor visits, preventing falls and making the home environment safe, available community education and support groups, and the necessity of maintaining a therapeutic regimen and lifestyle to decrease the risk of complications and recurrent stroke. All survivors will need assistance in re-integrating into the community. This is generally begun in the rehabilitation setting.

Family caregivers of stroke survivors must also deal with many issues. A classic study by Mumma (1986) revealed that stroke patients and their spouses perceived losses in such areas as mobility, traveling, the ability to do certain desired activities, and independence. A study by Pierce, Gordon, and Steiner (2004) revealed that families dealing with stroke survivors identified five top self-care needs that they wished to have information about: preventing falls, maintaining adequate nutrition, staying active, managing stress, and dealing with emotional and mood changes. Conversely, nurses chose topics such as understanding the disease process, preventing pressure ulcers, demonstrating safe transfer technique, preventing aspiration, and dealing with communication and social interaction problems as being more important. These differing

TABLE 13-12 Summary of Major Survivor and Nursing Tasks for Each Phase of the Poststroke Journey

Phase	Survivor Task	Nursing Task
Agonizing	Survival	Protection and physical care
Fantasizing	Ego protection	Reality orientation and emotional support
Realizing	Facing reality	Emotional and psychosocial support
Blending	Adaptation	Teaching
Framing	Reflection	Listening; providing reason for the stroke
Owning	Moving on	Enhancing inner and community resources

SOURCE: Easton, K. L. (2001). The poststroke journey: From agonizing to owning. Doctoral dissertation. Wayne State University. Detroit, MI: Author.

FIGURE 13-6 The Mauk model of poststroke recovery.

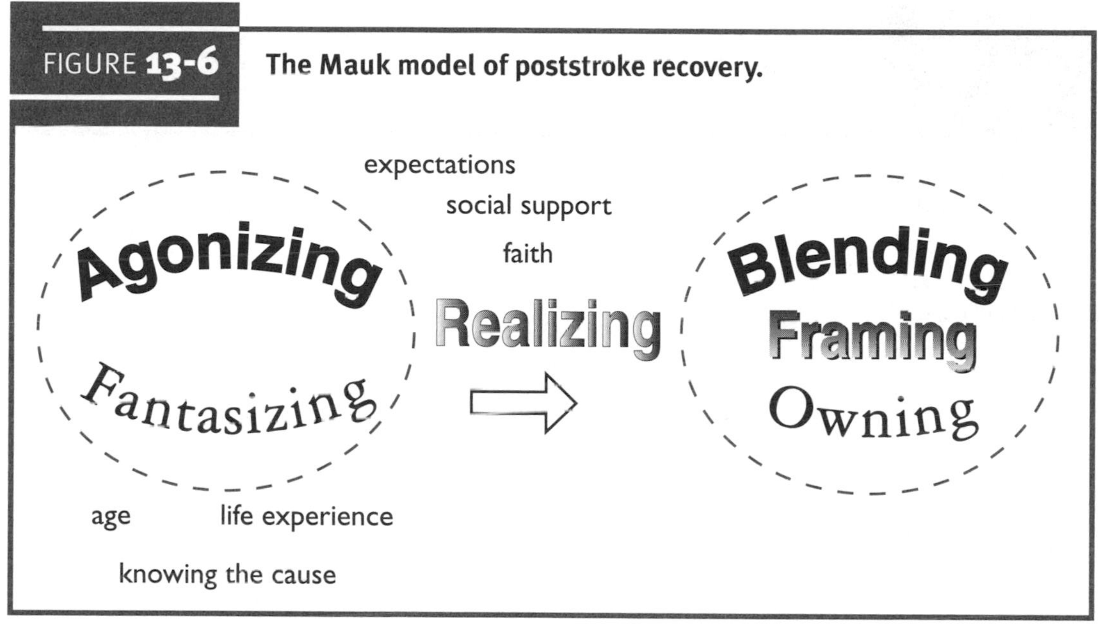

results demonstrate a need for teaching that goes beyond what is taught in the traditional hospital setting. Pierce, Steiner, Govoni, et al. (2004) also found that using an Internet-based support group for rural caregivers produced positive responses and suggested common problems that caregivers face. These include such things as changing roles, problem solving, feeling connected with the family and survivor, using spirituality to cope, and balancing feelings of success in adapting with losses that have occurred. Other studies have supported the need for family caregivers to have extensive support as the stroke victim and his or her family members transition from the acute care setting to home (Cameron & Gignac, 2008; Lefebure, Levert, Pelchat, & Lepage, 2008; Steiner et al., 2008). Ninety percent of all **dysphagia** results from stroke (White, O'Rourke, Ong, Cordato, & Chan, 2008). Stroke survivors with dysphagia may return home on a feeding tube, so teaching about nutritional requirements, tube management, and administering medications via the tube will be important. (See Chapter 14 for further discussion of dysphagia.) Many survivors will continue to benefit from outpatient therapies in occupational therapy, physical therapy, and/or speech therapy. Some will need referrals to vocational counseling if they wish to return to work. Others may need to follow up with an orthotist for splints or other orthotic devices.

Outcomes for geriatric stroke survivors are enhanced by intensive rehabilitation programs, whether offered in rehabilitation units or in skilled nursing facilities (Jett, Warren, & Wirtalla, 2005). **Table 13-14** presents general approaches to care for stroke survivors. Generally, advanced age is considered to be a negative factor in recovery from stroke, but factors such as motivation and hope must also be considered in the rehabilitation process. In addition, much of the research literature regarding functional level of recovery after stroke suggests that return of function peaked and did not significantly progress much after the 3- to 6-month mark poststroke. However, Easton's (Mauk's) research (1999b, 2001) as well as other emerging research suggest that survivors can and do continue to make improvements in daily function even years after their strokes. Much of this improvement may be in the area of **instrumental activities of daily living (IADLs)**, or home activities that the survivor wished to resume after the stroke. New research

TABLE 13-13 Common Problems Related to Stroke

Common Potential Nursing Diagnoses Related to Stroke	Common Medical Complications After Stroke
Activity intolerance	Depression
Aspiration, risk for	Deep vein thrombosis
Body image, disturbed	Dysphagia (sometimes resulting in aspiration)
Communication, impaired verbal	Pressure ulcers
Constipation, risk for	Neurogenic bowel
Coping, ineffective	Neurogenic bladder
Disuse syndrome, risk for	Shoulder subluxation
Fall, risk for	Spasticity
Fatigue	
Fear	
Grieving	
Hopelessness	
Injury, risk for	
Knowledge, deficiency	
Mobility: physical, impaired	
Nutrition, imbalanced: less than body requirements	
Self-care deficit: bathing/hygiene	
Self-care deficit: dressing/grooming	
Self-care deficit: feeding	
Self-care deficit: toileting	
Sensory perception, disturbed (tactile,visual)	
Sexual dysfunction	
Skin integrity, risk for impaired	
Social isolation	
Spiritual distress, risk for	
Tissue integrity, risk for impaired	
Tissue perfusion, ineffective, cerebral	
Unilateral neglect	
Urinary elimination, impaired	
Walking, impaired	

out of the Cincinnati College of Medicine in Ohio suggests that even mental practice of upper arm mobility may have a significant and positive impact on a stroke survivor's ability to use the affected upper limb (Morris, 2006; Page, Levine, & Leonard, 2005).

In summary, stroke is a condition that affects millions of Americans and can lead to significant chronic functional limitations and decreased quality of life. It is hopeful for survivors, however, that stroke is not a degenerative or chronic disease. Improvements can be seen after many years in

TABLE **13-14** **General Approaches to Traditional Nursing of the Stroke Survivor**

Common Characteristics Associated with Stroke of Either Side	Right Hemisphere Stroke	Left Hemisphere Stroke
When working with the patient, encourage use of the affected side to reduce neglect. When the person is alone, place items (such as the call light, tissues, and other personal items) on the unaffected side to promote self-care and safety and to avoid isolation. Use a variety of teaching modalities during educational sessions to promote learning. Minimize distractions during educational sessions. Keep these teaching items short and relevant. Use terms such as *affected/unaffected* side or *weak/strong* side instead of *good/bad*. Use critical pathways or care plans to promote consistency of care, but remember that each survivor is unique and be sure to adapt nursing care accordingly. Alternate rest and activity. Build endurance slowly. Remember that a stroke is exhausting to the entire body. Include the person and family in the plan of care. Assist the patient and family in setting reasonable goals. Make early referrals to stroke services or the specialized stroke team. Connect the family with a stroke support group or club. Use a discharge follow-up plan.	Foster a calm and unhurried care environment. Break tasks into simple steps. Be especially attentive to safety issues that may arise from poor judgment and lack of safety awareness. Protect the patient from injury. Be alert for possible deficits that may not be overt. Avoid overstimulation.	Speak slowly and distinctly. Use simple sentences for those with aphasia. Encourage all forms of communication. Use a variety of communication techniques: gesturing, cues, pointing, writing, communication boards, yes/no questions (if appropriate). Find what is most effective for each person. Allow time for the person to respond to questions. Provide teaching in a quiet, structured environment. Monitor the patient for swallowing difficulties. Promote a positive self-image by attention to good grooming, personal hygiene, and positive reinforcement.

SOURCE: Adapted from Easton, 1999b, p. 196, with permission of author.

areas that enhance quality of life for survivors and their families. Nurses should continue to follow research trends related to treatment of acute stroke and to educate survivors and their families about the recovery process.

Peripheral Artery Disease (PAD)

Peripheral artery disease (PAD), the most common type of peripheral vascular disease (PVD), affects 8–12 million Americans, 12–20% of those over the age of 65. The risk factors for PAD are the same as those for CHD, with diabetes and smoking being the greatest risk factors (AHA, 2005b). According to the American Heart Association, only 25% of those older adults with PAD get treatment.

The most common symptoms of PAD are leg cramps that worsen when climbing stairs or walking, but that dissipate with rest, commonly called intermittent claudication (IC). The majority of persons with PAD have no symptoms (AHA, 2005b). PAD is a predictor of CHD and makes a person more at risk for heart attack and stroke. Left untreated, PAD may eventually lead to impaired function and decreased quality of life, even when no leg symptoms are present. In the most serious cases, PAD can lead to gangrene and amputation of a lower extremity. Most cases of PAD can be managed with lifestyle modifications such as those discussed previously for heart-healthy living. Nurses should also encourage patients with PAD to discuss their symptoms with both their health care provider and a physical therapist, because some patients find symptom relief through a combination of medical and therapy treatments (Aronow, 2007).

RESPIRATORY PROBLEMS

Respiratory problems are common among older adults and a leading contributor to mortality and morbidity. This section will present information on pneumonia, chronic obstructive pulmonary diseases (COPDs), and tuberculosis. There are many nursing interventions to enhance quality of life for older adults with breathing problems. These will also be reviewed.

Pneumonia

Pneumonia is a leading cause of death among the elderly. Many statistics related to the number of cases of pneumonia are outdated, but in 2005 there were 651,000 hospital discharges of males diagnosed with pneumonia and 717,000 discharges of females, with greater than 62,000 deaths attributed to pneumonia (American Lung Association [ALA], 2008). The majority of these cases occurred in those age 65 or over, with older adults having 5–10 times the risk of death from pneumonia as younger adults (Kennedy-Malone, Fletcher, & Plank, 2004).

Pneumonia is an inflammation or infection in the lungs that can be caused by a variety of factors including bacteria, viruses, and aspiration. The elderly are considered at particularly high risk for pneumonia, and even more so if they suffer from **chronic obstructive pulmonary disease (COPD)**, CHF, or any immune-suppressing diseases such as AIDS. The incidence of community-acquired pneumonia among those age 65 or greater is 221.3 per 10,000 (ALA, 2008).

Diagnosis is made through chest x-ray, complete blood count, and/or sputum culture to determine the type and causal agents (if bacterial). A thorough history and physical should also be obtained. Crackles may be heard in the lungs through auscultation, and chest pain with shortness of breath is a common complaint.

Cases of viral pneumonia account for about half of all types of pneumonia and tend to be less severe than bacterial pneumonia. Symptoms of viral pneumonia include fever, nonproductive hacking cough, muscle pain, weakness, and shortness of breath. The onset of bacterial pneumonia can be sudden or gradual, but older adults may not present with the typical symptoms of chills, chest pain, sweating, productive cough, or dyspnea. Confusion, disorientation, or delirium may be additional signs in the elderly.

Bacterial pneumonia can often be treated successfully when detected early, and viral pneumonia generally heals on its own (antibiotics are not effective if pneumonia is caused by a virus), though older adults may experience a greater risk of complications than younger adults. Oral antibiotics will significantly help most patients with bacterial pneumonia, and even though many older persons may require hospitalization, intravenous (IV) antibiotics have not been shown to be necessarily more effective than oral types, with IV treatment resulting in longer hospital stays and more hospital-acquired problems (Loeb, 2002).

Aspiration pneumonia is caused by inhalation of a foreign material, such as fluids or food, into the lungs. This occurs more often in persons with impaired swallowing (see Chapter 14 for a discussion on dysphagia) and those who have esophageal reflux disease or who are unconscious. One particular danger to which nurses should be alert is those older adults receiving tube feedings. Care must be taken to avoid having the person in a laying position during and immediately after tube feeding because aspiration can occur. Having the head of the bed elevated or, even better, the person in a sitting position when eating or receiving enteral nutrition helps to avoid the potential complication of pneumonia related to aspiration.

When recovering from pneumonia, the older adult should be encouraged to get plenty of rest and take adequate fluids to help loosen secretions (with accommodations made to support the added need to urinate due to the increased fluid intake, a common reason why elderly people will not drink adequate fluids). Tylenol or aspirin (if not contraindicated by other conditions) can be taken to manage fever as well as aches and pains. Exposure to others with contagious respiratory conditions should be avoided. Respiratory complications are often what lead to death in the elderly, so older adults should be cautioned to report any changes in respiratory status such as increased shortness of breath, high fever, or any other symptoms that do not improve.

Prevention of pneumonia is always best. Adults over the age of 65 are advised to get a pneumonia vaccine (pneumococcal polysaccharide vaccine, PPV), although its effectiveness may be somewhat diminished in higher risk groups than in healthy younger adults (ALA, 2008). This vaccine is generally given one time, though sometimes a revaccination is recommended after about 6 years for older adults with higher risk. A yearly flu vaccine is also recommended for older adults, because pneumonia is a common complication of influenza in this age group. Medicare will cover these vaccines for older persons, so cost should not be a prohibiting factor in prevention.

Chronic Obstructive Pulmonary Disease (COPD)

COPD refers to a group of diseases resulting from obstructed airflow. The most common of these diseases in older adults are **emphysema** and **chronic bronchitis**, often occurring together with the preferred label of COPD.

COPD is the fourth leading cause of death in the United States, accounting for about 118,171 deaths in 2004. It is estimated that nearly 24 million U.S. adults have some type of impaired lung function. Slightly more females than males are affected, with female smokers having a 13 times greater chance of death from COPD than nonsmoking females (ALA, 2004).

The major risk factor for COPD is smoking, which causes 80–90% of COPD deaths. Other risk factors appear in **Table 13-15**. Alpha-1-antitrypsin deficiency is a rare cause of COPD, but can be ruled out through blood tests. Although "COPD is almost 100% preventable by avoidance of smoking" (Kennedy-Malone et al., 2003), environmental factors play a strong role in the incidence of COPD. Approximately 19.2% of people with COPD can link the cause to work exposure, and 31.7% have never smoked (ALA, 2008).

Persons with COPD often experience a decrease in quality of life as the disease progresses. Shortness of breath so characteristic of these diseases impairs the ability to work and do usual activities. According to a recent survey by the American Lung Association, "half of all COPD patients (51%) say their condition limits their ability to work . . ." and ". . . limits

TABLE 13-15 Risk Factors for COPD

Smoking
Air pollution
Second-hand smoke
Heredity
History of respiratory infections
Industrial pollutants
Environmental pollutants
Excessive alcohol consumption
Genetic component (alpha-1-antitrypsin deficiency)

them in normal physical exertion (70%), household chores (56%), social activities (53%), sleeping (50%), and family activities (46%)" (2004, p. 3).

Chronic Bronchitis

Chronic bronchitis is a common COPD among older adults. It results from recurrent inflammation and mucus production in the bronchial tubes. Repeated infections produce blockage from mucus and eventual scarring that restricts airflow. The American Lung Association stated that about 8.5 million Americans had been diagnosed with chronic bronchitis as of 2005. Females are twice as likely as males to have this problem.

The signs and symptoms of chronic bronchitis include increased mucus production, shortness of breath, wheezing, decreased breath sounds, and chronic productive cough. Chronic bronchitis can lead to emphysema.

Emphysema

Emphysema results when the alveoli in the lungs are irreversibly destroyed. As the lungs lose elasticity, air becomes trapped in the alveolar sacs, resulting in carbon dioxide retention and impaired gas exchange. More males than females are affected with emphysema, and most (91%) of the 3.8 million Americans with this disease are over the age of 45 (ALA, 2004). Signs and symptoms of emphysema include shortness of breath, decreased exercise tolerance, and cough. Diagnosis is made through pulmonary function and other tests, and a thorough history and physical.

Treatment for COPD

Although there are no easy cures for COPD, older adults can take several measures to improve their quality of life by controlling symptoms and minimizing complications. These include lifestyle modifications, medications, respiratory therapy, and pulmonary rehabilitation (see **Table 13-16**). Oxygen therapy is usually required as the disease progresses.

Medications are used to help control symptoms, but they do not change the downward trajectory of COPD that occurs over time as lung function worsens. Typical medications given regularly include bronchodilators through oral or inhaled routes. Antibiotics may be given to fight infections and systemic steroids for acute exacerbations.

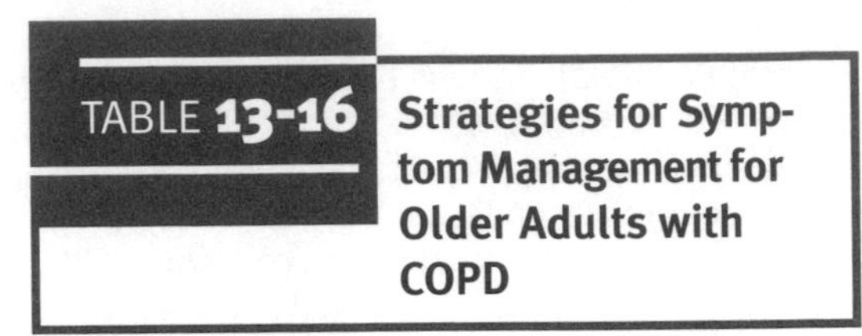

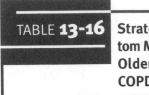

TABLE **13-16** **Strategies for Symptom Management for Older Adults with COPD**

Do not smoke.
Avoid second-hand smoke.
Avoid air pollutants and other lung irritants.
Exercise regularly as tolerated or prescribed.
Maintain proper nutrition.
Maintain adequate hydration—especially water intake.
Take medications as ordered: bronchodilators (antibiotics and steroids for exacerbations).
Use energy conservation techniques.
Alternate activities and rest.
Learn and regularly use breathing exercises.
Learn stress management and relaxation techniques.
Recognize the role of supplemental oxygen.
Receive yearly pneumonia and influenza vaccines to avoid serious infections.
Investigate pulmonary rehabilitation programs.
Join a support group for those with breathing problems and their families.
Explore any possible surgical options with the physician.

In extreme cases, lung transplantation or lung volume reduction surgery may be indicated. Older persons with severely impaired lung function related to emphysema may be at higher risk of death from these procedures and have poorer outcomes.

Nurses working with older adults with COPD will find it challenging to assist them with a home maintenance program that addresses their unique needs with this chronic disease. Teaching should involve the patient and family and should plan for the long term. Reducing factors that contribute to symptoms, use of medications, alternating rest and activity, energy conservation, stress management, relaxation, and the role of supplemental oxygen should all be addressed. Many older adults with COPD find it helpful to join a support group for those who are living with similar problems.

Tuberculosis (TB)

Tuberculosis (TB), or *Mycobacterium tuberculosis*, is an infection that can attack any part of the body, but particularly targets the lungs. TB is spread through the air by coughing, sneezing, laughing, or other activities in which particles may become airborne.

According to the American Lung Association, the number of new cases of TB in the United States has steadily decreased over the past 10 years. In 2006, there were 13,767 new cases in the United States. TB is seen more often in (in descending order) Asian Americans, Pacific Islanders, African Americans, American Indians, and Hispanics than whites. The rate of TB cases among those from other countries is eight times greater than for those born in the United States (ALA, 2005). The AIDS epidemic has contributed to the spread of TB, particularly in less developed countries, due to the suppression of the immune system associated with those who are infected with HIV.

Nursing home residents are considered an at-risk group due to the typically higher rates found in this population. General guidelines from the Advisory Committee for Elimination of Tuberculosis (Centers for Disease Control and Prevention [CDC], 1990) set a concrete strategy for prevention and management of TB in nursing homes to decrease the spread among this institutionalized and vulnerable population. Thus, older adults who may be discharged from acute care facilities to a nursing home will generally undergo TB skin testing prior to discharge.

Screening for TB is simple and can be done at the local health department, clinic, or doctor's office. A Mantoux test is an intradermal injection that is read for results in 48–72 hours after administration. A result of 11 mm or greater of induration (not redness, but swelling) is considered a positive result. It is recommended that older adults undergo a two-step screening wherein the test is given again, because there are many false results in the elderly. A positive TB skin test should be followed up with a chest x-ray to rule out active disease.

It must be noted that persons who received a vaccine for TB may have a positive reaction. A TB vaccine is commonly given in many countries outside the United States.

A person can be infected with TB and have no symptoms. This means they may have a positive skin test, but cannot spread the disease. Such a person can develop TB later if left untreated. Those with active TB can spread the disease to others and should be treated by a physician. The signs and symptoms of TB appear in **Table 13-17**.

For older adults born in the United States, a positive skin test may prompt the physician to initiate preventative treatment. The medication isoniazid (INH) is generally given to kill the TB bacteria. Treatment with INH often lasts at least 6 months. Few adults have side effects from the medication, but those that are possible include nausea, vomiting, jaundice, fever, abdominal pain, and decreased appetite. Patients taking INH should be cautioned not to drink alcohol while on the medication.

Patients with active TB can be cured, but the medication regimen is complex, with several different drugs taken in combination. Caution should be taken to avoid spread of the disease. This generally means isolation for patients in the hospital with active TB. In 1998, the FDA approved a new medication, rifapentine (Priftin), to be used with other drugs for TB. Medications should be strictly taken for the entire period of time (many months)

TABLE 13-17 Signs and Symptoms of Tuberculosis (TB)

A severe cough that lasts more than 2 weeks
Chest pain
Bloody sputum
Weakness
Fatigue
Weight loss
*Chills
*Fever
*Night sweats

*May not be present in the elderly.
SOURCE: CDC, 1999.

to kill all of the bacteria. Older adults may need assistance with keeping track of these medications. The use of a medication box set up by another competent and informed family member to ensure compliance with the medication regimen may be helpful, because it can be overwhelming for some persons. Adequate rest, nutrition, and hydration as well as breathing exercises may help with combating the effects of TB. Since over half of all patients with actively diagnosed TB have come to the United States from other countries, language may be a barrier. Education requires understanding and may necessitate an interpreter to ensure understanding of the complex regimens required to eradicate the bacteria.

GASTROINTESTINAL DISORDERS

Gastrointestinal problems are among the most frequent complaints in older adults. Several of the more common disorders will be discussed here, including gastroesophageal reflux, peptic ulcer, **diverticulitis**, constipation, and several types of cancers.

Gastroesophageal Reflux Disease (GERD)

Gastroesophageal reflux disease (GERD) is thought to occur in 5–7% of the world's population and 21 million Americans (International Foundations for Functional Gastrointestinal Disorders, 2008), affecting men, women, and children. It results when acid or other stomach contents back up into the esophagus. Many children outgrow this problem by the age of about 1 year, but for older adults, GERD can be a chronic disorder that affects quality of life.

GERD may be related to several factors including decreased lower esophageal sphincter (LES) tone and increased pressure in the stomach or abdomen. Decreased peristalsis and delayed emptying of the stomach may also play a role. GERD causes esophageal irritation and many of the common symptoms associated with this disorder.

Factors related to GERD include pregnancy, obesity, and activities that increase intra-abdominal pressure such as wearing tight clothing, bending over, or heavy lifting (MedlinePlus, 2005a).

The most common symptom of GERD is heartburn. In patients with GERD this may occur daily to weekly. Chest pain, difficulty swallowing, a hoarse voice, coughing, and respiratory problems such as asthma or wheezing may also result (Edwards, 2002). It is important for older adults to have proper diagnosis and treatment, because continued reflux can result in esophagitis, and over time abnormal cells may develop (Barrett's esophagus) that can increase the risk for cancer of the esophagus.

Diagnosis is made through a history and physical. Many cases of GERD can be treated with lifestyle modifications and medication. Persistent symptoms of GERD should be referred to an internist or gastroenterologist. This is particularly true of older adults, who may not present with typical symptoms, or who may present with vague symptoms that might be attributed to other causes. The physician may wish to do a series of tests, one of the most reliable being examining the esophagus and stomach through a fiber-optic scope while the person is under conscious sedation. This allows the doctor to visualize the entire area, view damage, and take biopsies if needed. A common cause of GERD is ***Helicobacter pylori (H. pylori)***, and this can be diagnosed through biopsy. GERD can be treated with a combination of medications that includes antibiotics and drugs to inhibit gastric secretions.

Treatment involves lifestyle modifications aimed at decreasing causal factors. Patients should be instructed to avoid offending foods such as caffeine, chocolate, nicotine, alcohol, and peppermint. These substances decrease the LES tone and allow the sphincter to become floppy, letting acid creep up into the esophagus. Certain medications may have the same affect, particularly anticholinergics, some hormones, calcium channel blockers, and theophylline. The older person's medication list should be carefully reviewed and offending medications modified. Additional lifestyle modifications include avoiding spicy and tomato-based foods, acidic products, carbonated beverages, and stress that can trigger increased acid production. Patients should be instructed to avoid eating or drinking 3–4 hours prior to bedtime and to elevate the entire head of the bed on 6- to 8-inch blocks. Some persons feel better sleeping in a recliner chair with the head elevated during flare-ups of heartburn symptoms. Additionally, more frequent but smaller meals will help minimize the pressure in the stomach and should decrease reflux.

BOX 13-3 Resources for Those with GERD

American College of Gastroenterology (ACG)
4900-B South 31st Street
Arlington, VA 22206-1656
703-820-7400
http://www.acg.gi.org

American Gastroenterological Association (AGA)
4930 Del Ray Avenue
Bethesda, MD 20814
301-654-2055
http://www.gastro.org

Medications play an important role in the treatment of GERD. Antacids are usually used in conjunction with **histamine 2 (H_2) blockers** such as Tagamet, Zantac, Pepcid AC, and Axid for mild GERD. If those are ineffective in controlling symptoms, the **proton pump inhibitors (PPIs)** are the drugs of choice. These include the popularly advertised medications Nexium, Prevacid, and Protonix.

GERD is a potentially serious condition. GERD is a common upper gastrointestinal problem, and although elderly patients have fewer complaints of heartburn, the actual disease is usually more severe and has more complications (Chait, 2005). Older persons displaying symptoms should be thoroughly evaluated and aggressively treated. The key nursing interventions center around teaching lifestyle modifications and proper use of medications. Most medications used in GERD can have antacids taken with them between meals and before bed to help control heartburn symptoms. Most of the medications for this disorder are also taken in the morning prior to breakfast (on an empty stomach). H_2 blockers are sometimes ordered twice per day. PPIs, usually taken once per day but sometimes in a divided dose (morning and evening), should be taken on an empty stomach. With most such medications, the person then should remember to eat one hour after taking the medication in order for it to be most effective. In order to prevent associated complications, remember that management of GERD poses significant challenges to the health care team.

Peptic Ulcer

The actual incidence of peptic ulcer disease is hard to determine; however, the American Gastroenterology Association (2008) estimates that there are 350,000–500,000 new cases per year, with more than 1 million peptic ulcer–related hospitalizations yearly. The direct cost to the health care system exceeds $2 billion per year, and the indirect costs, such as time lost from work or unproductive time, exceeds $500,000 yearly. The incidence increases with age and occurs more often in Hispanics and African Americans than whites. The two most common causes of peptic ulcer disease are the use of nonsteroidal anti-inflammatory drugs (NSAIDs) for comorbidities and *Helicobacter pylori* infection (Zullo, Hassan, Campo, & Morini, 2007). As with many such problems, early symptoms may not be seen in the elderly, but when the disease presents itself, the patient is often severely ill due to the overall reduction in defensive mechanisms in the GI mucosa and the increased susceptibility to gastrointestinal bleeding (Zullo et al., 2007). An increase in stress, such as occurs with COPD, can trigger an ulcer as a complication, so many older adults with chronic respiratory problems are prescribed prophylactic medications during hospitalization. Additionally, the increased use of aspirin and NSAIDs for the treatment of arthritic diseases and other comorbidities has contributed to a higher incidence of peptic ulcer in the general population. These medications contribute to ulcer development by causing a further decrease in the protection of the gastrointestinal mucosa.

Risk factors for peptic ulcer disease include smoking, drinking alcohol, caffeine, stress, and *Helicobacter pylori* (*H. pylori*) infection. Signs and symptoms of peptic ulcer include continued epigastric pain, particularly after meals; bowel changes; bloating; and eventually anorexia. In older adults, it is essential to distinguish between ulcer pain and cardiac pain, because both may present as "indigestion."

Diagnosis of peptic ulcer is made through a thorough history and physical. The physician or primary care provider must first determine the type of ulcer. Edwards (2002) stated that "90–100% of individuals with duodenal ulcers are infected with *H. pylori* and this is as accurate as any diagnostic test" (p. 204). Barium contrast testing is an initial diagnostic tool, followed by endoscopy and biopsy, if needed, keeping in mind that less invasive and more inexpensive methods of diagnosis should be tried first.

Treatment of ulcers involves antibiotics, antacids and other medication to control acid production, diet, avoidance of risk factors, and combination therapy if *H. pylori* is the cause. Nurses will need to engage in patient education for treatment to have the best outcome. The medication regimen to treat *H. pylori* is challenging for older patients, yet will eradicate the problem in many cases. Nurses should emphasize that *H. pylori* is considered a toxin to the body, because it can predispose a person to cancer (Edwards, 2002). Stress management may be helpful to some people, and dietary issues such as avoidance of caffeine, alcohol, and milk products while the ulcer is healing is recommended. Patients who smoke should stop, because this is an associated risk factor. Serious complications such as bleeding can result if patients neglect treatment.

Diverticulitis

Diverticulitis is inflammation or infection of the pouches of the intestinal mucosa. Sixty-five percent of older adults will develop diverticulosis ("pouches of the intestinal mucosa in the weakened muscle wall of the large bowel" [Eliopoulos, 2005, p. 332]) (**Figure 13-7**) by age 85, with some going on to develop diverticulitis (Kennedy-Malone et al., 2004). Most persons developing diverticulitis are elderly men.

Risk factors for diverticulitis include obesity, chronic constipation, and hiatal hernia. A diet low in fiber also is thought to contribute to this problem. Older persons may not present with the typical symptoms of pain in the left lower quadrant, nausea, and fever. During bouts of this disorder, the person may experience constipation, diarrhea, and mucus and/or blood in the stools. Certain foods may irritate the condition, especially those with seeds such as berries or pickles that are not easily digested.

Diagnosis is made through barium enema. Nurses should be sure that after this exam is done, the patient is taught to take the prescribed medications to empty the bowel so that the barium does not harden inside and cause constipation and other difficulties.

Treatment is generally with antibiotics, and if hospitalization is necessary, intravenous fluids will be given. The person should be taught to avoid irritating foods. In extreme cases diverticulitis may result in bowel obstruction leading to a colostomy. In certain circumstances of advanced disease, patients may elect to undergo removal of the diseased bowel to prevent emergency surgery for bowel obstruction.

Cancers

According to Edwards (2002), GI cancers account for greater than 25% of all cancer deaths in older adults, making them the number two cause of cancer next to lung disease. It is encouraging to note that in 2004 the data reported showed that the incidence of colorectal cancers had decreased between 1% and 4% across the various federally defined populations (NIH, Senior Health, 2008).

Esophagus

The two most common types of cancers of the esophagus are squamous cell carcinoma and adenocarcinoma. Of the squamous cell type, black males with a history of alcoholism and heavy smoking comprise the group with the highest risk and incidence. Adenocarcinoma is being seen more often in white males, particularly resulting from Barrett's epithelium (a complication of GERD, as discussed earlier) (Edwards, 2002). Over the last 10 years the rates of esophageal cancer have decreased across all races and genders (National Cancer Institute [NCI], 2008b).

Early detection of esophageal cancer is key, because prognosis for either type is rather poor. Esophagoscopy is a major diagnostic test. Major symptoms of esophageal cancer include weight loss and trouble swallowing. In older adults, symptoms may not appear until the cancer is advanced and perhaps already metastasized. It responds poorly to radiation and may be inoperable. Nurses should instruct older persons with these symptoms to be checked by a physician. Nurses can help with primary prevention of this type of cancer by being proactive in smoking cessation groups and by encouraging limitation of

FIGURE 13-7 **Diverticula.**

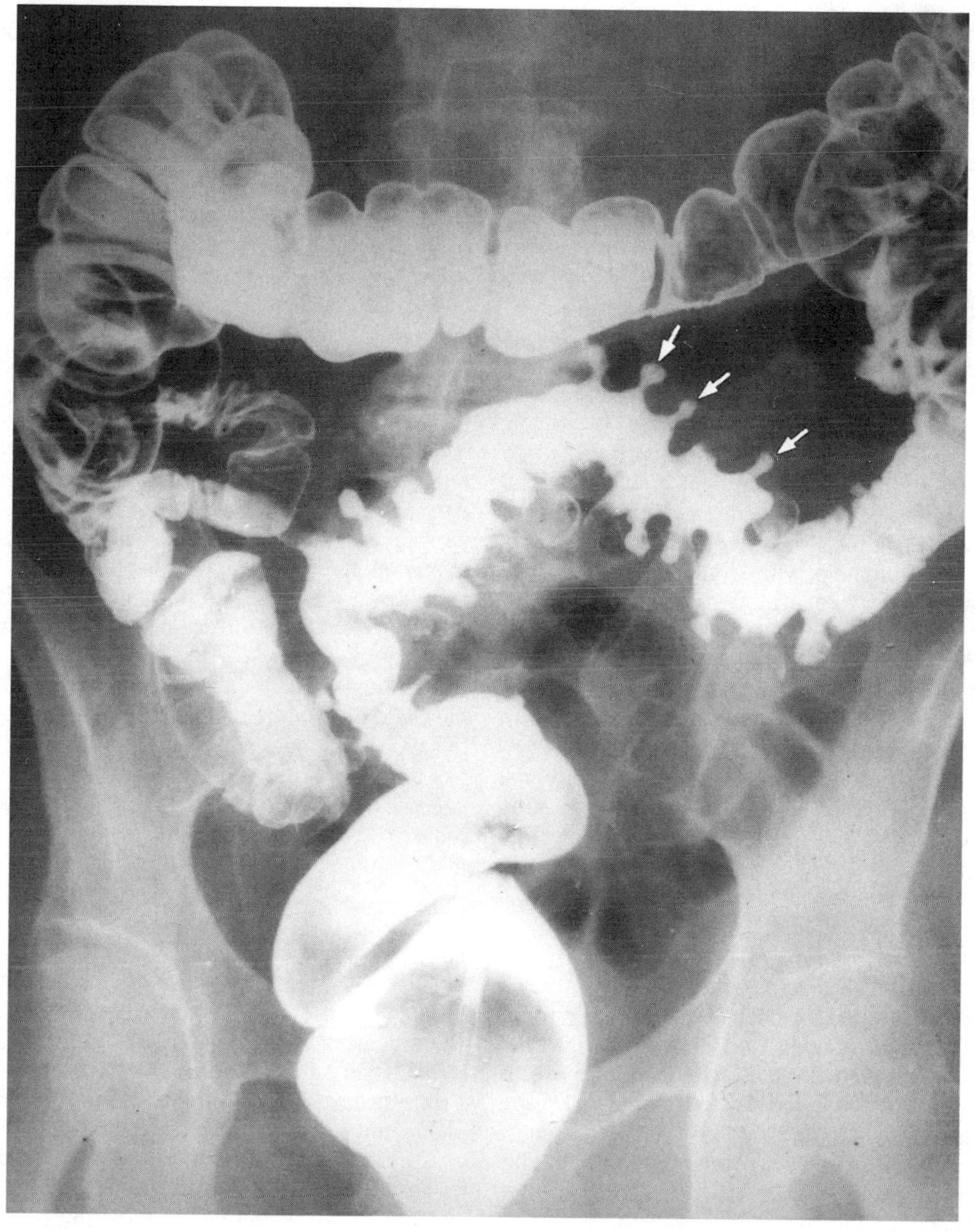

SOURCE: Leonard Crowley, *Introduction to Human Disease* (6th ed.). Sudbury, MA: Jones and Bartlett Publishers, 2005.

alcohol intake (a maximum of one drink per day for females, and two for males).

Stomach

Stomach cancer is most often seen in older men ages 65–74 (Eliopoulous, 2005). There is a greater incidence among Hispanics, African Americans, and Asians/Pacific Islanders than whites. Rates also are high among Japanese men living in Japan (American Cancer Society, 2005c). Men have twice the risk of women.

When detected early, there is a good prognosis, but once a tumor has advanced, patients may deteriorate quickly. Early signs may not be present in older persons, but may include epigastric pain, anorexia, nausea, and difficulty with swallowing. Surgery, radiation, and chemotherapy are options for treatment (and often used in combination), but not all of these methods are equally successful with each type of tumor.

H. pylori infection can be a contributing factor to stomach tumors, and treatment of the bacterial infection may be more effective in cancer treatment than treatment for other unknown causes.

Nurses can help with primary prevention of stomach cancer by educating older adults as to risk factor reduction and early recognition of symptoms. Dietary changes are a significant way to reduce risk. A diet lower in red meats (risk doubles if eating red meat more than 13 times per week) and higher in antioxidants has a protective effect (American Cancer Society, 2005c). Additionally, regular physical exams and reporting suspicious symptoms for early testing can help increase chances of survival. Men, particularly those of the at-risk ethnic groups, should be especially alerted to these factors.

Colorectal

Colorectal cancer is one of the most common yet treatable forms of cancer. The vast majority of this type of cancer is adenocarcinomas arising from polyps. Although most polyps do not become malignant, the risk of cancer increases as polyp size increases (Edwards, 2002). Thus, routine screening for this type of cancer is recommended in middle age, and certainly in those with a family history. (See Chapter 12 for screening guidelines.)

Colorectal cancer is the second leading cause of cancer deaths in both men and women. Hispanics and African Americans are at higher risk than whites. About 145,290 persons were diagnosed in 2005, with 56,290 deaths resulting from this type of cancer (Cancer Research and Prevention Foundation, 2005). It was estimated that there would be approximately 108,070 new cases of colon cancer and 40,740 new cases of rectal cancer in 2008, as well as 40,960 deaths from colon and rectal cancer in 2008. The median age for colon/rectal cancer diagnosis is 77.1 years (NCI, 2008a). The 5-year survival rate when detected in early stages is greater than 90% (American Cancer Society, 2005a).

Risk factors for colorectal cancer include upper socioeconomic groups, high fat intake, alcohol consumption, cigarette smoking, sedentary lifestyle, and exposure to environmental toxins. Symptoms depend on location of the lesion, but may include rectal bleeding, anemia, fatigue, abdominal cramping, and change in bowel patterns. Diagnosis is made through history and physical as well as diagnostic tests such as hemoccult, barium enema, and endoscopic exams. The flexible sigmoidoscopy is currently thought to be the best test for detecting early problems. Surgery is the best option for treatment of early malignant polyps.

Colorectal cancers are largely preventable, so nurses need to focus interventions on educating the public about this problem. Nurses should teach their patients and clients that adding fruits, vegetables, and fiber to the diet may help protect against this type of cancer. Increasing activity levels while avoiding smoking, obesity, high-fat foods, high-sucrose foods, and excess alcohol are all ways to reduce risk (Cancer Research and Prevention Foundation, 2005; Edwards, 2002).

Pancreas

Pancreatic cancer is found more often in older adults and is a leading cause of death for this age group. It generally strikes those between 60 and 80 years of age and the incidence is 10 times greater in men over age 75 (Kennedy-Malone et al., 2004). Cigarette smoking, family history, and diabetes are significant risk factors. In fact, the American Cancer Society (2005c) estimates that 3 in 10 cases of pancreatic cancer are attributed to smoking.

Cancer of the pancreas generally progresses rapidly and carries a poor prognosis. Early detection is not always possible due to lack of symptoms.

Early symptoms may include nausea, vomiting, anorexia, weight loss, depression, and excessive belching. Jaundice and itching occur with progression of the cancer (ACS, 2008e; Kennedy-Malone et al., 2004).

Treatment is usually palliative, particularly for advanced cancer in the older adult. Surgery is an option in some types/locations of tumors, but given the poor prognosis in the elderly, interventions will focus on comfort measures such as pain control. Narcotic analgesics and antihistamines for itching are standard treatment. Hospice services should be obtained as early as possible when the prognosis is terminal.

Constipation

Constipation is the most common bowel problem in older adults. Bowel function is not a topic generally discussed in most societies. Because of the private nature of elimination activities, older adults may experience difficulties in bowel function and not let the problem be known until it is serious enough to interfere with normal daily functioning. Normal bowel function is considered a bowel movement anywhere from three times per day to three times per week, so patterns vary widely among individuals. In most hospital settings, constipation is considered to be present in a patient when there has been no bowel movement for more than 2 days.

The results of normal aging contribute to this disorder through the slowing of intestinal peristalsis and the decrease in thirst mechanism, resulting in less fluid intake. Other causes include dehydration, decreased activity, lack of fiber in the diet, side effects of medications, and neurogenic bowel or other disease. Constipation can lead to fecal impaction and even bowel obstruction in the most severe cases.

Generally, constipation is a manageable problem that is often best remedied by carefully planned nursing interventions. The interventions depend on the cause. There are several factors to be considered (see **Table 13-18**). Factors that cannot be controlled related to bowel function include a family history of disease or presence of neurogenic bowel or another disorder. However, there are many factors that can be modified to assist with prevention of constipation and maintenance of an effective bowel program. These include diet, fiber, fluids, timing, activity, exercise, positioning, and medications (Mauk, 2005).

The method of treatment and subsequent prevention of constipation depend on the cause. General principles (**Table 13-19**) are to use all natural means first and start with a clean bowel. That is, if impaction is present, manually remove the stool if possible and administer prescribed medications to cleanse the bowel prior to beginning any bowel program. Bowel management focuses on modification of the controllable factors. First, the person should be encouraged to consume a diet high in fiber. This includes foods such as whole grains, bran cereal, beans, pulpy fruits, and root vegetables. Although popcorn and nuts are high in fiber, they pose a problem for older adults with dysphagia or diverticulitis, so care should be taken when recommending certain foods. Patients should drink plenty of fluids, and water is the best choice. Generally, between 1,500 and 2,000 cc (or 1½–2 liters) per day is a good intake for older adults.

Timing is another important factor in treatment. Persons should take advantage of their usual bowel patterns; that is, if they usually defecate first thing in the morning, then that time should be tried first. If this fails, the person should attempt to move the bowels shortly after breakfast, because this is when the gastrocolic reflex is strongest. Sitting up, not on the bedpan or lying in bed, is best to allow gravity

TABLE 13-18 Factors to Consider in Bowel Management

Uncontrollable Factors	Controllable Factors
Family history	Diet
Presence of neurogenic bowel	Fiber
Existence of prior bowel disease	Fluids
	Timing
	Activity
	Positioning
	Medications

TABLE 13-19 Principles of Bowel Programs to Prevent Constipation

- Start with a clean bowel. (Administer needed medications or enemas to cleanse the bowel prior to initiating a program or protocol.)
- Try all natural means first: fiber, fluids, activity, timing, positioning.
- Be sure the person is taking adequate fiber and fluids before adding medications.
- Change only one item at a time in the program. Allow several days to pass before evaluating the effectiveness of the change. If needed, add another intervention.
- Stool softeners are given for hardened stool, and the person must drink at least a liter of fluid per day for them to be effective.
- Peristaltic stimulators are useful when the person is unable to move the stool down into the rectum.
- Use the least caustic type of suppository that is effective for the older person.
- Avoid the use of bedpans—have the person sit upright on the toilet or commode.
- Avoid the regular use of enemas.

to assist and to promote a feeling of normalcy. Even those who cannot ambulate to the toilet can use a bedside commode. Increasing activity will help to stimulate peristalsis and decrease constipation. One way to look at activity is to consider the following: If the patient normally is in bed all day, have them sit up; if they sit up most of the time, assist them to stand; and if they can stand, assist them to walk. All of these methods are employed in a bowel maintenance program.

Last, medications may play a role for those patients with constipation that is due to disease or disorders such as stroke, brain injury, or spinal cord injury. Oral medications fall into many categories including bulk formers (Fibermed, Metamucil), which require large amounts of water intake to be successful; stool softeners (Docusate/Colace); and peristaltic stimulators (Pericolace or Senna), to name a few. Oral medications such as Colace are the most common. Nurses must instruct patients to drink at least 1,000 cc (1 liter) of water per day for Colace to be effective. Ironically, for some persons, increasing fluids to this level may preclude the need for medication to treat constipation.

Rectal medications include several types of suppositories: glycerin suppositories (mild), bisacodyl (Dulcolax) suppositories (strong but effective, and can cause cramping), CEO-2 suppositories (work by releasing gas and distending the rectum), and combinations such as the Therevac mini-enema (melted glycerin, Colace, and soap in a plastic dispenser). The Therevac mini-enema may produce results more quickly because the medication is already liquefied and more readily absorbed. One drawback of Therevac is that the tip of the plastic dispenser that is inserted into the rectum can cause small tears without adequate care and lubricant.

Important to remember in administering suppositories is that the typical suppository works by acting as an irritant to the rectal mucosa, so it must be placed next to the rectal wall in order to work. Placing suppositories into impacted stool will be ineffective. When inserting the suppository, the person should be laid on their left side to position the bowel in the most correct way for effectiveness. Products such as the Therevac mini-enema are quite effective in older adults and take little time for results. Waxy suppositories may take 15–60 minutes to melt and produce results.

Digital stimulation is used in some instances, particularly in those with spinal cord injury, in combination with suppository therapy as a daily bowel program. However, as a rule, digital stimulation should be avoided in the elderly due to the potential for vaso-vagal stimulation that can cause heart and blood pressure changes. Other methods, as discussed earlier, are generally more effective and safer in older adults, except for those with certain types of spinal injury.

Enemas should also be avoided as part of a routine bowel program. Enema use should be restricted to cleansing of the bowel for presurgical preparation or for impaction. In older adults, making enemas part of the regular bowel program may result in a distended, lazy bowel and dependence on enemas for evacuation. Likewise, over-the-counter laxatives should be used only when needed, and older persons should be educated on their appropriate use.

Finally, special bowel programs may be needed for those with neurogenic bowel function. Patients with problems in the brain and/or spinal cord, such as those with stroke, dementia, Parkinson's disease (PD), multiple sclerosis, traumatic brain injury, or spinal cord injury, will need the expertise of rehabilitation nurses to develop a comprehensive and realistic plan for bowel management and the prevention of constipation.

GENITOURINARY PROBLEMS

The elderly can have several major problems related to reproductive and urinary systems. This section will discuss these common problems, including bladder cancer, vaginitis, breast and cervical cancer, and **benign prostatic hyperplasia (BPH)**.

Bladder Cancer

The American Cancer Society estimated that in 2008 there would be approximately 68,810 new cases of bladder cancer in the United States, about 51,230 men and 17,580 women. The ACS also estimated about 14,100 deaths from bladder cancer during 2008, about 9,950 men and 4,150 women (ACS, 2008b). "It is the fourth most common type of cancer in men and the eighth most common in women" (NCI, 2005). The incidence increases with age, with an average age at diagnosis of 68 or 69 (Mayo Clinic, 2004). Men are three times as likely to get cancer of the bladder as women (American Foundation for Urologic Disease, 2008). Risk factors include chronic bladder irritation and cigarette smoking, the latter contributing to over half of cases (**Case Study 13-3**).

Case Study 13-3

Dr. Johnson is a 62-year-old dentist who runs a busy practice in a large suburb of Chicago. He had been a smoker for over 30 years but recently quit. For some time he has noted little spots of blood in his urine, but he did not have pain, so he attributed it to some prostate problems he has had in the past. Dr. Johnson hears a couple of his patients discussing a mutual friend with bladder cancer who has similar symptoms, and this prompts him to visit his family physician for a checkup. After several tests and a cystoscopy, Dr. Johnson is diagnosed with early stage bladder cancer.

Questions:

1. What risk factors did Dr. Johnson have for bladder cancer?
2. What primary sign did he exhibit?
3. Since his cancer was detected early, what treatments might be options in his case?
4. If Dr. Johnson's cancer becomes invasive, what other options are available for treatment?
5. Describe the nursing implications and care required if Dr. Johnson needed to have a cystectomy.
6. How would you explain this procedure to his family?

The classic symptom of bladder cancer is painless hematuria, which may be a reason that older adults sometimes do not seek treatment right away. They may attribute the bleeding to hemorrhoids or other causes and feel that because there is no pain, it could not be serious. Diagnosis may involve several tests including an intravenous pyelogram (IVP), urinalysis, and cystoscopy (in which the physician visualizes the bladder structures through a flexible fiber-optic scope).

Once diagnosed, treatment depends on the invasiveness of the cancer. Treatments for bladder cancer include surgery, radiation therapy, immunotherapy, and chemotherapy (ACS, 2008b). Specifically, a transurethral resection (TUR) may involve burning superficial lesions through a scope. Bladder cancer may be slow to spread, and less invasive

BOX 13-4 Resources for Those with Common Cancers

American Cancer Society (all forms of cancer)
I Can Cope (community support groups)
1599 Clifton Road, N.E.
Atlanta, GA 30329
1-800-ACS-2345
http://www.cancer.org

American Urological Association
Online patient information resource
http://www.urologyhealth.org
Bladder Health Council
c/o American Foundation for Urologic Disease
1000 Corporate Boulevard, Suite 410
Linthicum, MD 21090
800-828-7866

National Breast Cancer Foundation
http://www.nationalbreastcancer.org

treatments may continue for years before the cancer becomes invasive, if ever. Certainly chemotherapy, radiation, and immune (biological) therapy are other treatment options, depending on the extent of the cancer. Immune/biological therapy includes Bacillus Calmette-Guérin (BCG) wash, an immune stimulant that triggers the body to inhibit tumor growth. Treatments are administered directly into the bladder through a catheter for 2 hours once per week for 6 or more weeks (Mayo Clinic, 2004). However, in 90% of the cases, surgery is involved as a standard treatment (ACS, 2004).

If the cancer begins to invade the bladder muscle, then removal of the bladder (**cystectomy**) is indicated to prevent metastasis. Additional diagnostic tests will be performed if this is suspected, including CT scan or MRI. Chemotherapy and/or radiation may be used in combination with surgery. When the cancerous bladder is removed, the person will have a **urostomy**, a stoma from which urine drains into a collection bag on the outside of the body, much like a colostomy does. Nursing care includes assessment and care of the stoma, emptying and changing collection bags as needed, and significant education of the patient related to intake/output, ostomy care, appliances, and the like.

Female Reproductive System

Several problems common among older females will be discussed here. These include vaginitis and cervical and breast cancer.

Vaginitis

Normal aging changes in the female reproductive system (see Chapter 6) make elderly women more at risk for infection. The vaginal canal becomes more fragile with age due to atrophy. Less vaginal lubrication and more alkaline pH due to lower estrogen levels put elderly women at increased risk of vaginitis. Symptoms of vaginitis may be similar to those of a urinary tract infection (UTI) or yeast infection and may include itching and foul-smelling discharge.

Vaginitis is treated with topical estrogen creams or estrogen replacement therapy. Women should be instructed to avoid douching and feminine deodorant sprays or perfumes. Wearing cotton undergarments may also help. A water-soluble lubricant such as K-Y gel should be used during intercourse if vaginal dryness is a problem, because the use of other lubricants such as Vaseline contributes to cases of vaginitis.

Cervical Cancer

Cervical cancer incidence peaks in women ages 50 to 60, with women over age 65 accounting for a significant number of new cases and deaths each year. Healthy People 2010 initiatives have helped to raise awareness among health care providers and the general public about the need for screening for cervical cancer. However, even with heightened awareness, studies indicate that older patients are generally treated less aggressively (radiation versus surgery) and have poorer outcomes than younger patients, with some older women refusing treatment altogether (Rissner & Murphy, 2005). Additionally, late-stage cancer diagnoses and subsequent death are more common among women over 65 than among those in younger age groups (Bradley, Given, & Roberts, 2004).

The current American Cancer Society guidelines state that women should have annual Pap smears until age 70. After age 70, with no history of abnormal smears, women may elect to have the screening done every 2–3 years. Those age 70 or older may choose to stop screening entirely if they have had no abnormal results in the past three smears and no abnormal results within 10 years' time prior to age 70 (Smith, Cokkinides, & Eyre, 2003).

Risk factors include smoking, onset of sexual intercourse prior to age 18, and multiple sexual partners. Screening offers the opportunity of early treatment. A new vaccine is now available using the human papillomavirus to prevent cervical cancer. It is given between the ages of 11 and 26, and may help to decrease the number of women with cervical cancer among the geriatric population in future decades.

The symptoms of cervical cancer are not usually evident in early stages, but may include vaginal bleeding, generally without pain until later stages. Any vaginal bleeding after menopause should be investigated. Prognosis is good for cervical cancer if detected early. Most early precancerous lesions can be successfully treated with laser or cryotherapy. Traditional treatment for cancer generally includes radiation and/or surgery, depending on the stage of progression.

Breast Cancer

Breast cancer is the second leading cause of death for women. The method of estimating all cancers, including breast cancer, has changed to reflect more accurate predictions. In 2007 it was estimated that 178,480 new cases of invasive breast cancer would be diagnosed, as well as 62,030 cases of new *in situ* cancer in women and about 2,030 cases of breast cancer in men. It was also estimated that 40,460 women would die from breast cancer in 2007 (ACS, 2008c). The incidence of breast cancer in women over age 50 has begun to decrease in recent years, while the incidence in women over age 50 has remained stable. Half of all breast cancers are diagnosed in women over the age of 65 (National Breast Cancer Foundation, 2005). White women have a higher incidence of breast cancer after age 40, while African American women have a higher incidence rate prior to age 40 and a higher likelihood of dying from breast cancer at any age (ACS, 2008c). Men may also develop breast cancer, though this is much less frequent, and they should not be excluded from education about the disease.

Screening guidelines for older women include mammography, yearly clinical breast exam (CBE), and monthly self breast exam (SBE). Starting at age 40, women should have mammography yearly until age 75, and then every 2–3 years thereafter, assuming there have been no abnormalities.

There are several risk factors for breast cancer, some controllable, some not. These include family history, late menopause, having the first child after age 30, high fat intake, and alcohol consumption. Of course, primary nursing care focuses on those factors that can be modified. Geriatric nurses should be particularly aware of the importance of early detection among those older women who are at higher risk.

Signs and symptoms of breast cancer include a breast mass or lump, breast asymmetry, dimpling of the skin or "orange peel" appearance, and nipple changes (Kennedy-Malone et al., 2003). Mammography and biopsy, in addition to lab tests, chest x-ray, and bone scans, are indicated for diagnosis (**Case Study 13-4**).

There are various stages of breast cancer. Stage I has a 98% survival rate at 5 years, whereas Stage IV has a 16% survival rate at 5 years (National Breast Cancer Foundation, 2005). Treatment for breast cancer depends on stage, but includes any combination of radiation, chemotherapy, and/or surgery. Depending on the type of tumor, hormone therapy may also be effective.

Nursing care is important at all levels of prevention. Nurses working with older adults should encourage appropriate screening according to recommended guidelines. The elderly should be taught proper technique for self breast exam and encouraged to have regular checkups with their physician. Although controversy exists over the use of mammography, it remains an effective means to detect many cancerous tumors at an earlier stage with minimal risk to the person.

Older women undergoing mastectomy as treatment for breast cancer may require more time for recovery. Promotion of the return of full range of motion of the arm on the operative side is essential. This may require physical therapy in addition to the psychosocial and emotional support involved in rehabilitation. "The National Cancer Institute estimates that approximately 2.4 million women with a history of breast cancer were alive in 2004" (ACS, 2008c).

Case Study 13-4

Dr. Johnson is a 62-year-old dentist who runs a busy practice in a large suburb of Chicago. He had been a smoker for over 30 years but recently quit. For some time he has noted little spots of blood in his urine, but he did not have pain, so he attributed it to some prostate problems he has had in the past. Dr. Johnson hears a couple of his patients discussing a mutual friend with bladder cancer who has similar symptoms, and this prompts him to visit his family physician for a checkup. After several tests and a cystoscopy, Dr. Johnson is diagnosed with early stage bladder cancer.

Questions:

1. What risk factors did Dr. Johnson have for bladder cancer?
2. What primary sign did he exhibit?
3. Since his cancer was detected early, what treatments might be options in his case?
4. If Dr. Johnson's cancer becomes invasive, what other options are available for treatment?
5. Describe the nursing implications and care if Dr. Johnson needed to have a cystectomy?
6. How would you explain this procedure to his family?

Male Reproductive System

The most common disorders related to the reproductive system among older men include benign prostatic hyperplasia (BPH), cancer of the prostate, and **erectile dysfunction (ED)** or impotence.

Benign Prostatic Hyperplasia (or Hypertrophy) (BPH)

BPH, also known as prostatism, results from a noncancerous enlargement of the prostate gland that is associated with advanced age. This condition affects 50% of men ages 51–60 and up to 90% of men over 80 years (American Urological Association, 2005a). Although the enlargement is benign, it is sometimes associated with prostate cancer, so men with this condition should be carefully monitored.

BPH occurs when the enlarged prostate squeezes the urethra it encompasses and causes related symptoms. The symptoms include a decreased urinary stream, increased frequency, increased urgency, nocturia, incomplete emptying, dribbling, a weak urine stream, and urinary **incontinence** (**Table 13-20**). The urge to void may be so frequent in men with BPH (every 2 hours) that it can interfere with sleep and activities of daily living. Risk factors for BPH include advanced age and family history.

Diagnosis is made using any number or combination of tests and studies including urinalysis, postvoiding residual, **prostate-specific antigen (PSA)**, urodynamic studies, ultrasound, and cystoscopy. Medical treatment generally includes medications and surgery. The two most frequently used types of medications are alpha-blockers and 5-alpha-reductase inhibitors. Alpha-blockers such as doxazosin (Cardura), terazosin (Hytrin BPH), and tamsulosin (Flomax MR) work to relieve symptoms of BPH by relaxing the smooth muscle of the prostate and bladder neck to allow urine to flow more easily. A 5-alpha-reductase inhibitor such as finasteride (Proscar) works differently by shrinking the prostate to promote urine flow, but has sexual side effects such as impotence (American Urological Association, 2005a; Mead, 2005).

A common surgical intervention for BPH is a **transurethral resection of the prostate (TURP)**. During this procedure, the urologist resects the enlarged prostate gland through a cystoscope (**Figure 13-8**). Older men sometimes call this the "Rotor

TABLE 13-20 Signs and Symptoms of BPH

Decreased urinary stream
Urinary frequency
Urinary urgency
Nocturia
Urinary incontinence
Incomplete bladder emptying
Urinary dribbling
Feelings of urge to void but difficulty starting urine stream
Decreased quality of life related to symptoms
Altered sleep patterns related to nocturia

FIGURE 13-8 TURP.

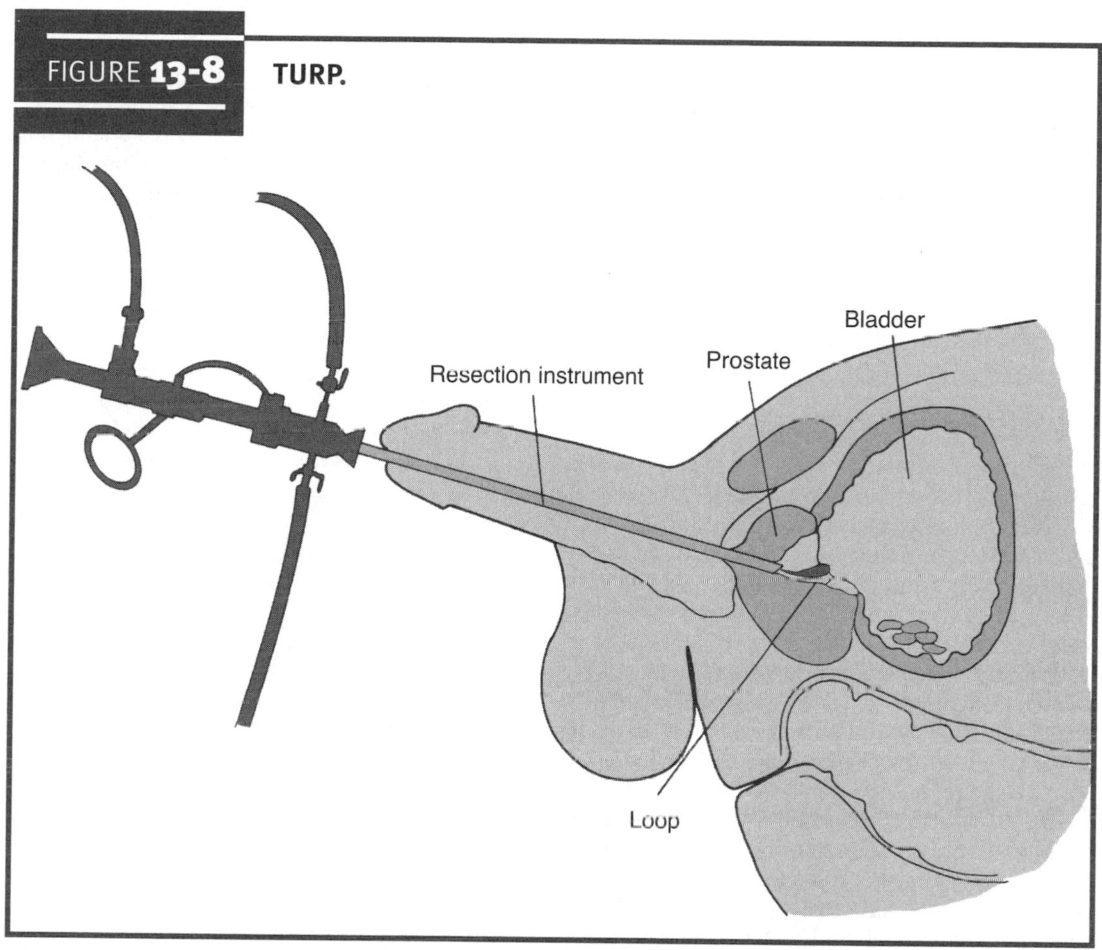

SOURCE: Leonard Crowley, *Introduction to Human Disease* (6th ed.). Sudbury, MA: Jones and Bartlett Publishers, 2005.

Rooter" surgery. Nursing care after this procedure is essential to avoid complications related to the heavy bleeding that may occur. The patient will have an indwelling urinary catheter with three ports. Postoperatively, **continuous bladder irrigation (CBI)** must be maintained to prevent dangerous clotting of the blood. The nurse is responsible for assessing the color of the urine draining from the catheter. The urine in the tube should be charted with specific terms such as bright red, brick red, tea colored, amber, yellow, or clear. The number and size of clots draining from the catheter should be described. The goal of the CBI is to flush the bladder, so the nurse must regulate the rate of the fluid to keep the urine yellow or as clear as possible. CBI will continue postoperatively until the bleeding stops. Bleeding complications may result if the CBI is allowed to go dry or the catheter is removed too soon after surgery. In the event that the patient is unable to void after removal of the catheter post-TURP, the catheter may need to be reinserted. If the nurse is unable to reinsert the catheter, the physician may need to be called in to do this. Nurses should be particularly alert to the potential for complications in older men after this procedure.

Prostate Cancer

Prostate cancer is the second leading cause of cancer death in U.S. males, with an estimate of over

186,320 new cases and 28,669 deaths in 2008 (NCI, 2008a). One in 6 men will have prostate cancer in his lifetime, but mortality (1 in 33) has declined (ACS, 2008d; NCI, 2008a). When found in the local and regional stages, 9 out of 10 men with prostate cancer have the same 5-year survival rate as a man without prostate cancer (ACS, 2008d). The incidence of prostate cancer increases with age. Over half of men 70 and older show some histologic evidence, though only a small percentage die from this disease.

Older men with prostate cancer may be asymptomatic, so screening is still recommended. If present, symptoms of prostate cancer may include urinary urgency, nocturia, painful ejaculation, blood in the urine or semen, and pain or stiffness in the back or thighs (Medline Plus, 2005b; NCI, 2008a). Risk factors for prostate cancer include advanced age, a diet high in saturated fats, family history, and race/ethnicity (African Americans slightly higher than whites, and low incidence among Asian males) (ACS, 2008d; Bradway & Yetman, 2002).

Diagnosis of prostate cancer begins with a digital rectal exam and PSA test. The rectal exam may detect malignancy in the form of a hard, nodular prostate. A PSA of less than 4 ng/ml is considered normal for ages 60–69 years, whereas 7 ng/ml may be normal in the 70–79 age group, because PSA rises with age. Sixty percent of men with a PSA above 10 ng/ml have prostate cancer (Bradway & Yetman, 2002; Mead, 2005). Diagnosis can only be confirmed through biopsy, however. Although recently the PSA test has been questioned as a reliable screening test, many urologists believe it is "still the best tool for early diagnosis" (Crawford, 2005, p. 1450). A series of PSA tests is the most effective means of screening, because a rise of 20% over a year (greater than 0.75 ng/ml per year) generally indicates cancer (Mead, 2005).

Treatment depends on the stage of cancer growth, but for more localized cancers generally includes three major options: **radical prostatectomy**, radiation therapy, and surveillance. Surgery is considered the best option when the cancer is caught early; however, because a radical prostatectomy is major surgery and carries some inherent risks, all options should be considered with the older patient. The major problems after surgery to remove the prostate include urinary incontinence (which is often temporary) and impotence. The skill and experience of the surgeon can decrease the risk of urinary incontinence after surgery to 2–5% (American Urological Association, 2005b).

A holistic approach to care may include dietary changes such as a low fat diet and the addition of vitamin E, selenium, and soy protein (Bradway & Yetman, 2002). It is important that a patient not adopt complementary medicine treatments without talking with his doctor.

Nursing care surrounding treatment for prostate cancer will involve helping families to explore the options, linking them to community resources, and providing education related to managing postoperative complications if surgery is indicated. Geriatric nurses should be informed as to the various options available for treatment of impotence that accompanies this type of surgery. Couples should be provided with support group information as well as information on penile implants and other devices that patients may wish to consider after recovery.

Erectile Dysfunction (ED)

Erectile dysfunction, also known as impotence, is defined as the inability to achieve and sustain a sufficient erection for intercourse. ED is prevalent in approximately 70% of men age 70 or over (Reuben et al., 2004). One in every 6 American men is affected by ED (10–20 million)(Hatzimouratidis & Hatzichristou, 2005). The incidence of ED increases with age, but it is not inevitable and is highly treatable in many cases. The causes of ED may be many, including diabetes, hypertension, multiple sclerosis, spinal cord injury, thyroid disorders, alcoholism, renal failure, hypogonadism, other diseases, medications (**Table 13-21**), and psychological factors.

Treatment options for ED fall into several categories including oral medications, vacuum pump devices, penile implants, and drugs injected into the penis. Sildenafil (Viagra) is an oral medication that is taken 1 hour prior to sexual activity. It is contraindicated in those with heart disease and may result in some cardiovascular-related side effects including headache, flushing, and nasal congestion. Other oral products on the market (Cialis, Levitra) are based on similar principles. A recent complaint about Viagra is the possibility of irreversible visual impairment in some men, but screenings for those at increased risk of this complication (those with

TABLE 13-21 Medications That May Affect Sexual Function

Anticholinergics
Antidepressants
Antihypertensives
Digoxin
Hypnotics
Sedatives
Sleeping medications
Tranquilizers

certain characteristics in the inner eye being at higher risk) can be done by most primary care physicians or ophthalmologists.

Vacuum devices have a good acceptance in the elderly population, with a 70–90% success rate (Reuben et al., 2004). These devices work in various ways to pump or draw blood into the penis and use another mechanism such as a ring around the base of the penis to help sustain the erection for intercourse. Risks from use of this device would include bruising or bleeding (in extreme cases). Nursing instruction to couples on the use of such a device is essential to prevent harm. Other treatments for ED include medications that may be injected directly into the penis to cause temporary erection, and some persons may opt for having surgery to insert a penile implant. There are two types of penile implants, one that results in permanent erection and one that may be pumped to cause erection and then released. All options should be explored with persons wishing information on treatment of ED.

NEUROLOGICAL DISORDERS

Several neurological disorders are common to the elderly, including diseases and conditions that are often secondary to common diseases. Two of the most frequently occurring neurological diseases in the elderly will be discussed here: **Parkinson's disease (PD)** and **Alzheimer's disease (AD)**. Stroke may also be considered a neurological disorder, but was discussed previously in the section on circulation problems. Complications that affect the neurological system as a result of a variety of causes may include seizures, tremor (see discussion on PD), peripheral neuropathy (see discussion on diabetes), and dizziness.

Alzheimer's Disease (AD)

Alzheimer's disease (AD) is the most common type of dementia seen in older adults. Other forms of dementia include vascular dementia, dementia with Lewy bodies, and Parkinson's dementia. Care of the person with AD provides an example of nursing interventions for all persons with dementia. Advanced age is the single most significant risk factor for AD.

> *An estimated 5.2 million Americans of all ages have Alzheimer's disease in 2008. This figure includes 5 million people age 65 and over. Two hundred thousand individuals under age 65 have younger-onset Alzheimer's. The number of people age 65 and over with Alzheimer's disease is estimated to reach 7.7 million in 2030, a greater than 50 percent increase from the 5 million age 65 and over who are currently affected. By 2050, the number of individuals age 65 and over with Alzheimer's could range from 11 million to 16 million unless science finds a way to prevent or effectively treat the disease. By that date, more than 60 percent of people with Alzheimer's disease will be age 85 or older. (Alzheimer's Association, 2008, p. 21)*

Those affected with AD may live from 3–20 years or more after diagnosis, making the life span with this disease highly variable. Seventy percent of people with AD live at home until the latest stages, being cared for mainly by family members (Alzheimer's Association, 2005). Currently the annual cost of AD in health care services, lost productivity, and strain on family is approximately $61 billion. Considering the increasing number of people expected to develop AD, these costs are expected to exceed $163 billion per year by 2050 (National Conference of Gerontological Nurse Practitioners & National Gerontological Nursing Association, 2008a). These statistics reveal that AD has and will continue to have a great impact on our society.

AD is characterized by progressive memory loss. It is a terminal disease that over its course will eventually leave a person completely dependent upon others for care. Initially the clinical progression of the disease is slow with mild decline; however, deterioration increases the longer the person lives, with an average life span of 8 years after diagnosis (Cotter, 2002; Fletcher, Rapp, & Reichman, 2007). The underlying pathology is not clear, but a growth of plaques and fibrillary tangles, loss of synapses, and neuronal cell loss are key hallmarks of AD that interfere with normal cell growth and the ability of the brain to function. Absolutely definitive diagnosis is still through autopsy, although clinical guidelines make diagnosis easier than decades ago when less was known about the disease.

The clinical course of AD is divided into several stages, depending on the source consulted. For the purposes of this text, early, middle, and late phases will be described; however, it should be noted that the Alzheimer's Association lists seven stages for AD, ranging from no symptoms to mild symptoms and diagnosis occurring in the first three phases.

In the early course of AD, the person may demonstrate a loss of short-term memory. This involves more than common memory loss such as where the keys were put, and may involve safety concerns such as forgetting where one is going while driving. The inability to perform math calculations and to think abstractly may also be evident. In the middle or moderate phase, many bodily systems begin to decline. The person may become confused as to date, time, and place. Communication skills become impaired and personality changes may occur. As cognitive decline worsens, the person may forget the names of loved ones, even their spouse. Wandering behavior as well as emotional changes, screaming, delusions, hallucinations, suspiciousness, and depression are common. The person with AD is less able to care for her- or himself and personal hygiene suffers. In the most severe and final phase, the person becomes completely dependent upon others, experiences a severe decline in physical and functional health, loses communication skills, and is unable to control voluntary functions. Death eventually results from body systems shutting down and may be accompanied by an infectious process.

Notable Quotes

"My father started growing very quiet as Alzheimer's started claiming more of him. The early stages of Alzheimer's are the hardest because that person is aware that they're losing awareness. And I think that that's why my father started growing more and more quiet."

—Patti Davis regarding her father, President Ronald Reagan

Although there is no single test, and the diagnosis may be one of exclusion, early diagnosis is important to maximize function and quality of life for as long as possible. Persons experiencing recurring and progressing memory problems or difficulties with daily activities should seek professional assistance from their physician. Warning signs of Alzheimer's are listed in **Table 13-22**.

Treatment for AD is difficult. There are several medications (such as Aricept, Namenda, Razadyne, and Exelon) that may help symptoms (such as memory), but they do not slow the course of the disease. There is currently no cure; however, research continues to occur in pharmacology, nonpharmacology, and the use of stem cells to manage symptoms and perhaps one day eradicate the disease.

Nursing care will focus on symptom management, particularly in the areas of behavior, safety, nutrition, and hygiene. Dealing with behavioral issues such as wandering and outbursts poses a constant challenge. Many long-term care facilities

TABLE 13-22 Ten Warning Signs of Alzheimer's Disease

Memory loss
Difficulty performing familiar tasks
Problems with language
Disorientation to time and place
Poor or decreased judgment
Problems with abstract thinking
Misplacing things
Changes in mood or behavior
Changes in personality
Loss of initiative

SOURCE: Alzheimer's Association, 2005.

have instituted special units to care for Alzheimer's patients from the early to late stages of the disease. These units provide great benefits such as consistent and educated caregivers with whom the patient or resident will be familiar, a safe and controlled environment, modified surroundings to accommodate wandering behaviors, and nursing care 24 hours a day. Additionally, nurses are present to manage medications and document outcomes of therapies. However, many family members wish to care for their loved ones at home for as long as possible.

Thus, another important aspect of care in AD is care for the caregivers. Howcroft (2004) suggested that "support from carers is a key factor in the community care of people with dementia, but the role of the caregiver can be detrimental to the physical, mental, and financial health of a carer" (p. 31). She goes on to say that the caregivers of persons with AD would benefit from training in how to cope with behaviors that arise in these patients and how to cope with practical and legal issues that may occur.

Research from Paun, Farran, Perraud, and Loukissa (2004; see also Mannion, 2008a, 2008b) showed that ongoing skills were needed by family caregivers to deal with the progressive decline caused by AD. In fact, "a 63% greater risk of mortality was found among unpaid caregivers who characterized themselves as being emotionally or mentally strained by their role versus non-caregivers" (National Conference of Gerontological Nursing Practitioners & National Gerontological Nursing Association, 2008b, p. 4). Adapting to stress, working on time management, maximizing resources, and managing changing behavior were all skills caregivers needed to develop in order to successfully manage home care of their loved ones. Caregivers needed not only to acquire knowledge and skills, but also to make emotional adjustments themselves to the ever-changing situation. Such findings suggest that nurses should focus a good deal of time on educating caregivers of persons with AD to cope with, as Nancy Reagan put it, "the long good-bye."

Notable Quotes

"The memories stayed with him for so long, and stayed vivid. And it didn't matter to me that he'd already repeated that before. I could hear it forever."

—Patti Davis regarding her father, President Ronald Reagan

Scientists continue to explore the causes of AD and hope in the near future to be able to isolate the gene that causes it. In the meantime, results from a fascinating study (called the nun study) on a group of nuns who donated their brains to be examined and autopsied after death has suggested that there is a connection between early "idea density" and the emergence of AD in later life. That is, essays the nuns wrote upon entry to the convent were analyzed and correlated with those who developed AD. It was found that those with lower idea density (verbal and linguistic skills) in early life had a significantly greater chance of developing AD (Snowden, 2004). The nun study has allowed researchers to examine about 500 brains so far in nuns who died between 75 and 107 years of age and discover other important facts such as a relationship between stroke and the development of AD in certain individuals, and the role of folic acid in protecting against development of AD (Snowden, 2004). Scientists from a number of fields continue to research the causes and possible treatments for AD. Snowden's research suggests that early education, particularly in verbal and cognitive skills, may protect persons from AD in later life.

Parkinson's Disease (PD)

PD is one of the most common neurological diseases. "Parkinson's disease (PD) affects at least 500,000 people in the United States, with approximately 50,000 new cases reported annually. PD usually affects people over the age of 50, and the likelihood of developing PD increases with age" (National Institute of Neurological Disorders, 2008). It affects both men and women, particularly those over the age of 50 years (American Parkinson Disease Foundation, 2005). PD was first described by Dr. James Parkinson as the "shaking palsy," so named to describe the motor tremors witnessed in those experiencing this condition.

A degenerative, chronic, and slowly progressing disease, PD has no known etiology, though several causes are suspected. There is a family history in 15% of cases. Some believe a virus or environmental factors play a significant role in the development of the disease. A higher risk of PD has been noted in teachers, medical workers, loggers, and miners, suggesting the possibility of a respiratory virus being to blame. More recent theories blame herbicides or pesticides. An emerging theory discusses PD like an injury related to an event or exposure to a toxin versus a disease. Interestingly, coffee drinking and cigarettes are thought to have a protective effect in the development of PD (Films for the Humanities and Sciences, 2004).

PD is a disorder of the central nervous system in which nerve cells in the basal ganglia degenerate. A loss of neurons in the substantia nigra of the brainstem causes a reduction in the production of the neurotransmitter dopamine, which is responsible for fine motor movement. Dopamine is needed for smooth movement and also plays a role in feelings and emotions. One specific pathological marker is called the Lewy body, which under a microscope appears as a round, dying neuron. There is no one specific test to diagnose PD.

The signs and symptoms of PD are many; however, there are four cardinal signs: bradykinesia (slowness of movement), rigidity, tremor, and gait changes. A typical patient with PD symptoms will have some distinctive movement characteristics with the components of stiffness, shuffling gait, arms at the side when walking, incoordination, and a tendency to fall backward. Not all patients exhibit resting tremor, but most have problems with movement, such as difficulty starting movement, increased stiffness with passive resistance, and rigidity as well as freezing during motion (National Institute of Neurological Disease and Stroke [NINDS], 2005). Additional signs, symptoms, and associated characteristics of PD appear in **Table 13-23**. Advanced PD may result in Parkinson's dementia.

Nurses should note that several other conditions may cause symptoms similar to PD, such as the neurological effects of tremor and movement disorders. These may be attributed to the effects of drugs or toxins, Alzheimer's disease, vascular diseases, or normal pressure hydrocephalus, and not be true PD.

Management of PD is generally done through medications. Levodopa, a synthetic dopamine, is an amino acid that converts to dopamine when it crosses the blood–brain barrier. Levodopa helps lessen most of the serious signs and symptoms of PD. The drug helps at least 75% of persons with PD, mainly with the symptoms of bradykinesia and rigidity (NINDS, 2005). One important side effect to note is hallucinations. A more common treatment, and generally the drug of choice, involves a medication that combines levodopa and carbidopa (Sinemet), resulting in a decrease in the side effect of nausea seen with levodopa therapy alone, but with the same positive control of symptoms, par-

TABLE 13-23 Signs, Symptoms, and Associated Problems Seen in Persons with PD

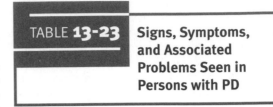

Bradykinesia
Rigidity
Tremor
Pill rolling
Incoordination
Shuffling gait, arms at side
Freezing of movements
Balance problems (tendency to fall backward)
Vocal changes; stuttering
Swallowing problems
Drooling
Visual disturbances
Bowel and bladder dysfunction
Sexual dysfunction
Dizziness
Sweating
Dyskinesias
Sleep pattern disturbances
Dementia
Memory loss
Emotional changes
Confusion
Nightmares
Twitching
Handwriting changes
Depression
Anxiety
Panic attacks
Hallucinations
Psychosis

ticularly with relation to movement. Patients should not be taken off of Sinemet precipitously, so it is important to check all of a patient's medications if they are admitted to either acute or long-term care. Selegiline is another medication that interferes with one of the enzymes that breaks down dopamine. Dopamine receptor agonists such as Permax and Parlodel are synthetic compounds that mimic the effect of dopamine, but are not as powerful as levodopa. The earliest drugs used were anticholinergics such as Artane and Cogentin, and newer medications are being examined in clinical studies. Medications such as Sinemet show a wearing off effect, generally over a 2-year period. During this time, the person must take larger doses of the medication to achieve the same relief of symptoms that a smaller dose used to bring. For an unknown reason, if the medication is stopped for about a week to 10 days, the body will reset itself and the person will be able to restart the medication at the lower dose again until tolerance is again reached. This taking off time from the medication is called a "drug holiday" and is a time when the person and family need extra support, because the person's symptoms will be greatly exacerbated without the medication.

There are many other treatments for Parkinson's disease being explored. These include deep brain stimulation (DBS), with electrode-like implants that act much like a pacemaker to control PD tremors and other movement problems. The person using this therapy will still have the disease and generally uses medications in combination with this treatment, but may require lower doses of medication (NINDS, 2005). Thalamotomy, or surgical removal of a group of cells in the thalamus, is used in severe cases of tremor. This will manage the tremors for a period of time, but is a symptomatic treatment, not a cure. Similarly, pallidotomy involves destruction of a group of cells in the internal globus pallidus, an area where information leaves the basal ganglia. In this procedure, nerve cells in the brain are permanently destroyed.

Fetal tissue transplants have been done experimentally in Sweden with mild success in older adults and more success among patients whose PD symptoms were a result of toxins. Stem cell transplant uses primitive nerve cells harvested from a surplus of embryos and fetuses from fertility clinics. This practice, of course, poses an ethical dilemma and has been the source of much controversy and political discussion.

A more recent promising development includes the use of adult stem cells, a theory that is promising but not yet well researched. Cells may be taken from the back of the eyes of organ donors. These epithelial cells from the retina are micro-carriers of gelatin that may have enough cells in a single retina to treat 10,000 patients (Films for the Humanities and Sciences, 2004). This is a more practical and ethically pleasing source of stem cells than embryos.

Much of the nursing care in PD is related to education. Because PD is a generally chronic and slowly progressing disorder, patients and family members will need much instruction regarding the course of the disease and what to anticipate. Instruction in the areas of medications, safety promotion, prevention of falls, disease progression, mobility, bowel and bladder, potential swallowing problems, sleep promotion, and communication is important. Most of the problems seen as complications of PD are handled via the physician as an outpatient, but certainly complications such as swallowing disorders as the disease progresses may require periods of hospitalization. When persons suffer related dementia in the last phases of the disease, they are often cared for in long-term care facilities that are equipped to handle the challenges and safety issues related to PD dementia. Areas for teaching appear in **Table 13-24**. In addition, access to resources and support groups is essential. A list of helpful resources and agencies is provided in **Box 13-5**.

Dizziness

Dizziness is quite common in older adults, affecting about 30% of those over age 65. It represents about 2% of the consultations in primary health care (Hansson, Mansson, & Hakanson, 2005) and is the most common complaint in those over 75 who are seen by office physicians (Hill-O'Neill & Shaughnessy, 2002). There are four major types of dizziness according to Hill-O'Neill and Shaugh nessy: vertigo, presyncope (light-headedness), disequilibrium (related to balance), and ill-defined (i.e., it does not fit in any other categories).

Vertigo—a false sense of motion or spinning—may be caused by **benign paroxysmal positional vertigo (BPPV)**, which is brought on by normal calcium carbonate crystals breaking loose and

TABLE 13-24 Client/Family Teaching Regarding PD Key Areas

Medication therapy (side effects, wearing off, drug holidays, role of diet in absorption)
Safety promotion/fall prevention
Disease progression
Effects of disease on bowel and bladder, sleep, nutrition, attention, self-care, communication, sexuality, and mobility
Swallowing problems
Promoting sleep and relaxation
Communication
Role changes
Caregiver stress/burden—need for respite
Community resources

SOURCE: Adapted from Easton, 1999b, with permission of author.

falling into the wrong part of the inner ear. It can also be caused by inflammation in the inner ear, **Meniere's syndrome**, vestibular migraine, acoustic neuroma, rapid changes in motion, or more serious problems such as stroke, brain hemorrhage, or multiple sclerosis.

Presyncope is when the older person complains of feeling faint or light-headed. It is associated with a drop in blood pressure such as occurs when the person sits up or suddenly changes to a standing position, or with an inadequate output of blood from the heart. It can also be caused by medications that induce orthostatic hypotension, hypovolemia, low blood sugar, or some other cause of lack of blood flow to the brain.

Disequilibrium is a loss of balance or the feeling of being unsteady when walking. Causes of disequilibrium include vestibular problems, sensory disorders, joint or muscle problems, or medications.

The fourth category is really a "catch all" for possible causes of dizziness not included in the first three categories. Problems in this category include such things as other inner ear disorders, anxiety disorders, hyperventilation, cerebral ischemia, side effects of medications, Parkinsonian symptoms, hypotension, low blood sugar, and benign positional vertigo.

Dizziness is generally treatable by addressing the cause. However, in some cases, such as dizziness associated with poststroke, it can be a permanent impairment.

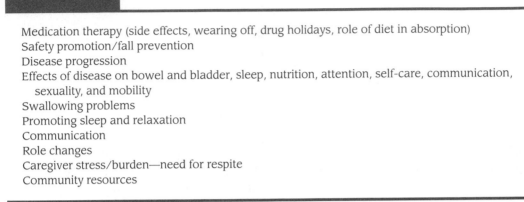

BOX 13-5 Resources for Those with PD

American Parkinson Disease Association
800-223-2732
http://www.apdaparkinson.org

Michael J. Fox Foundation for Parkinson's Research
212-509-0995
http://www.michaeljfox.org

National Institute of Neurological Disorders and Stroke (NINDS)
800-352-9424
http://www.ninds.nih.gov

National Parkinson Foundation
800-327-4545
http://www.parkinson.org

Parkinson's Disease Foundation
800-457-6676
http://www.pdf.org

Otological dizziness (a major classification in the elderly, according to Hain and Ramaswamy [2005]) refers to vertigo caused by changes in the vestibular system. The most common types in the elderly are Meniere's syndrome and benign paroxysmal positional vertigo (BPPV). These two major causes of dizziness will be discussed in the following sections.

Meniere's Syndrome

Meniere's syndrome is common in those over age 50. The cause is unknown, though it is often attributed to a virus or bacterial infection. Signs and symptoms include a rapid decrease in hearing, a sense of pressure or fullness in one ear, accompanied by loud **tinnitus** (ringing in the ears) and then vertigo (Hain & Ramaswamy, 2005; Hill-O'Neill & Shaughnessy, 2002). It may involve the excessive buildup of fluid in the inner ear, which is the cause of the feeling of fullness in the ear. A feeling of being unsteady or dizzy may last for as little as 30 minutes or for days after the episode (Mayo Clinic, 2008).

Benign Paroxysmal Positional Vertigo (BPPV)

As mentioned previously, BPPV is the most common cause of dizziness in the older age group, accounting for as much as 50% of all dizziness, with an increasing incidence with age (Hain, 2003). BPPV occurs when debris called **otoconia** ("rocks in the ears") becomes dislodged from their usual place in the ear and get stuck elsewhere in the vestibular system. Although in most cases the underlying cause of BPPV is not known, the degeneration of the vestibular system in the inner ear that occurs with normal aging is thought to play a major role. In cases of vertigo that do not respond to traditional medication for dizziness (such as Antivert), BPPV should be suspected.

Signs and symptoms of BPPV include dizziness, presyncope, feelings of imbalance, and nausea. The symptoms begin when the person changes head position, even something as usual as tipping the head back or turning the head in bed. A key to diagnosis is Hallpike's maneuver, in which the patient is laid down quickly from a sitting position, with the head turned to the side and hung over the back of the exam table. This will produce a characteristic nystagmus if the cause is BPPV.

BPPV can be treated in the office by the physician, advanced practice nurse, or even a physical therapist with knowledge of the proper maneuvers. The Epley maneuver is a technique by which the patient is put into a serious of specific positions and head turns to promote return of the otoconia to their proper place in the ear. After this treatment, the patient must stay in the office for 10 minutes and then sleep in a recliner chair at 45 degrees for the following two nights. They should also be instructed to avoid head positions that cause BPPV for at least another week (Hain, 2003). Other maneuvers and even surgical treatment may be necessary in rare variations of BPPV. These would be recommended by the physician on a case-by-case basis.

Dizziness, whatever the cause, can be particularly distressing to the older adult. It can interfere with activities of daily living, the ability to drive, and the maintenance of independence. Elders may decrease activities and spend more time at home due to the fear of dizzy spells or of falling. It is a leading cause of elderly persons discontinuing driving, which may be depressing to them and limit their social activity. In other cases the fear of having to stop driving will keep a person from seeking medical attention. Early diagnosis of the cause of dizziness can result in better outcomes by addressing treatment sooner and avoiding complications that can result from bouts of syncope or vertigo. Nurses should encourage older adults with complaints of dizziness to seek medical help. Treatment may be with medication, simple maneuvers, or lifestyle changes. Emotional support during diagnosis and testing, and reassurance that most causes of dizziness are treatable, can be a comfort to the older adult with this problem.

Seizures

Once thought to be mainly a disorder of children, recurrent seizures or epilepsy is thought to be present in about 7% of older adults (Spitz, 2005) and is usually related to one of the common comorbidities found in older adults (Bergey, 2004; Rowan & Tuchman, 2003). Epilepsy affects up to 3 million Americans of all ages (Velez & Selwa, 2003).

Seizures can be caused by a variety of conditions in older persons, but "the most common cause of new-onset epilepsy in an elderly person is arteriosclerosis and the associated cerebrovascular disease" (Spitz, 2005, p. 1), accounting for 40–50%

of seizures in this age group (Rowan & Tuchman, 2003). Seizures are associated with stroke in 5–14% of survivors (Spitz, 2005; Velez & Selwa, 2003). Other common causes of epilepsy in the elderly include Alzheimer's disease and brain tumor. A list of potential causes of seizures in older adults appears in **Table 13-25**.

There are three major classifications of epilepsies. Generalized types are more common in young people and associated with grand mal or tonic-clonic seizures. A number of cases have an undetermined origin and may be associated with certain situations such as high fever, exposure to toxins, or rare metabolic events. In older adults, localized (partial or focal) epilepsies are more common, particularly complex partial seizures. In contrast to young adults, Rowan and Tuchman (2003) cite other differences in seizures in the elderly: low frequency of seizure activity, easier to control, high potential for injury, a prolonged postictal period, and better tolerance with newer antiepileptic drugs (AEDs). Additionally, older adults may have coexisting medical problems and take many medications to treat these problems.

The most obvious signs and symptoms of epilepsy are seizures, although changes in behavior, cognition, and level of consciousness may be other signs. Diagnosis is made by careful description of the seizure event, a thorough history and physical, complete blood work, chest x-ray, electrocardiogram (ECG), and electroencephalogram (EEG) to help determine the type of seizure.

TABLE 13-25 Possible Causes of Seizures in the Elderly

Stroke or other cerebrovascular disease
Arteriosclerosis
Alzheimer's disease
Brain tumor
Head trauma
Intracranial infection
Drug abuse or withdrawal
Withdrawal from antiepileptic drug

Treatment for epilepsy is aimed at the causal factor. The standard treatment for recurrent seizures is AEDs. The rule of thumb "start low and go slow" for medication dosing in older adults particularly applies to AEDs. The elderly tend to have more side effects, adverse drug interactions, and problems with toxicity levels than younger people.

Recent research has suggested that older adults may have better results with fewer side effects with the newer AEDs than the traditional ones, though about 10% of nursing home residents are still medicated with the first-generation AEDs (Mauk, 2004). The most common medications used to treat seizures include barbiturates (such as phenobarbital), benzodiazepines (such as diazepam/Valium), hydantoins (such as phenytoin/Dilantin), and valproates (such as valproic acid/Depakene) (Deglin & Vallerand, 2005). Several newer drugs are also used, depending on the type of seizure. These newer medications include carbamazapine (Tegretol), oxycarbazepine (Trileptal), and topiramate (Topamax) (Uthman, 2004). Each of these medications has specific precautions for use in patients with certain types of medical problems or for those taking certain other medications. When assessing for side effects in older patients, be sure to be alert to potential GI, renal, neurological (ataxia), and hepatic side effects. Additionally, some newer extended-release AEDs are thought to be better tolerated and have a lower incidence of systemic side effects (such as tremors) (Uthman, 2004).

MUSCULOSKELETAL DISORDERS

Among older adults, there are several significant musculoskeletal problems that can significantly impact quality of life. Osteoporosis can lead to fractures. Arthritis is a major source of pain among older adults, and those who experience related decreased range of motion may have joint replacement surgery. Some of these common disorders will be discussed in this section.

Osteoporosis

Osteoporosis is a bone disorder characterized by low bone density or porous bones. Over 44 million Americans including 55% of adults age 50 or over have this disease. Although often thought of as a woman's disease, 80% of cases are women and 20% are men (National Osteoporosis Foundation, 2008). Older persons of all ethnic backgrounds may experience osteoporosis, though it is more common among whites and Asians. The risk factors for this disorder are many and appear in **Table 13-26**.

A major complication of osteoporosis is fractures. These are especially common in the vertebral spine, hips, and wrists. The cost in 2002 related to osteoporotic hip fractures alone was more than $19 billion, with an estimated cost by 2025 to be $25.3 billion (National Osteoporosis Foundation, 2005). Because there are sometimes no signs or symptoms during the early course of bone deterioration, osteoporosis is often undiagnosed and untreated until fracture occurs. Such fractures may lead to pain, immobility, and other complications. If signs and symptoms are present besides fractures, they may take the form of pain and kyphosis (**Figure 13-9**). Diagnostic testing would reveal decreased bone density and any pathological fractures present via x-ray. On occasion hairline fractures do not manifest themselves with the initial x-ray, but appear 5–10 days after the initial assault.

Because this is a highly treatable and often preventable disease when detected early, all women over the age of 65 years should have **bone mineral density (BMD)** or bone mass measurement done. Steps can be taken to prevent osteoporosis by habits that help build strong bones before the age of 20, when bones are fully developed. Preventing osteoporosis in adolescent years would include eating a well-balanced diet with plenty of calcium and vitamin D, no smoking or excessive alcohol intake, plenty of weight-bearing exercise, and discussing any needed treatments with the physician to minimize the risk of the disease. It should be noted that most of the calcium in the diet of American children comes from milk, though yogurt, broccoli, and certain enriched cereals may provide additional

TABLE 13-26 Risk Factors for Osteoporosis

Personal history of fracture after age 50
Current low bone mass
History of fracture in a first-degree relative
Being female
Being thin and/or having a small frame
Advanced age
A family history of osteoporosis
Estrogen deficiency as a result of menopause, especially early or surgically induced
Abnormal absence of menstrual periods (amenorrhea)
Anorexia nervosa
Low lifetime calcium intake
Vitamin D deficiency
Use of certain medications, such as corticosteroids and anticonvulsants
Presence of certain chronic medical conditions
Low testosterone levels in men
An inactive lifestyle
Current cigarette smoking
Excessive use of alcohol
Being white or Asian, although African Americans and Hispanic Americans are at significant risk as well

SOURCE: From the National Osteoporosis Foundation, 2005, p. 1.

FIGURE 13-9 **Kyphosis.**

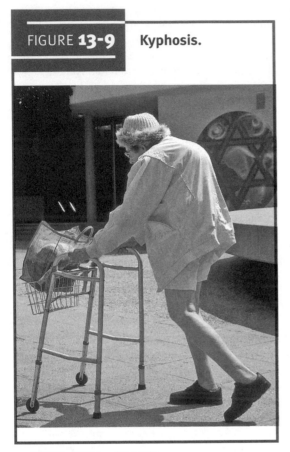

SOURCE: © Bill Aron/PhotoEdit

sources. Nurses can be active in primary prevention of osteoporosis through educating children in the schools about the effects of this disease in later life and how to prevent it.

Treatment of existing osteoporosis takes many forms. Postmenopausal women are often prescribed biphosphonates (such as Fosamax), calcitonin (Miacalcin), or estrogen/hormone replacement medications (such as Estratab or Premarin). Some of these medications are aimed at promoting adequate amounts of calcium in the bones, whereas the hormone replacement therapies replace estrogen not being produced after menopause to create more of a balance between the delicate hormones that guide bone reabsorption and demineralization. The use of estrogen replacement therapy has been shown to decrease the incidence of serious fractures in postmenopausal women, though there are side effects that should be discussed with the physician before a woman uses this option. Weight-bearing exercises and getting enough calcium in the diet or through supplementation are other treatments to consider. If vitamin supplementation is used, it is essential that the patient take not only calcium but also vitamin D to promote the absorption of the calcium. Nurses should encourage patients to discuss all treatment options with their physicians. Nutritional counseling and the role of sunlight (a source of vitamin D) and exercise should also be addressed. One potential exercise that is being explored for its benefit for both balance and promoting bone health is tai chi, a form of Eastern martial arts. One randomized controlled trial demonstrated that the tai chi group increased the effectiveness of a balance activity (Maciaszek, Osinski, Szeklicki, & Stemplewski, 2007).

Arthritis

Arthritis, or inflammation of the joint, is the number one chronic complaint and cause of disability in the United States (Arthritis Foundation, 2008; Mayo Clinic, 2005), affecting nearly 46 million people (nearly 1 in 5 adults, or 20% of the U.S. population) with a cost of $138 billion per year (Arthritis Foundation; CDC, 2008). There are over 100 types of arthritis, with the two most common being osteoarthritis (OA) and rheumatoid arthritis (RA). These will be discussed here in relationship to their impact on the lives of older adults.

Osteoarthritis

Osteoarthritis (OA) is also called degenerative joint disease, osteoarthrosis, hypertrophic arthritis, and degenerative arthritis (Arthritis Foundation, 2008). OA affects about 13.9% of the U.S. population age 25 or older and 33.6% of those 65 or older, which equals an estimated 26 million adults (CDC, 2008). This disease is characterized by chronic deterioration of the cartilage at the ends of the bones that eventually results in bones at the joint becoming inflamed due to cartilage breakdown, causing cytokines (inflammation proteins) and enzymes that further damage the cartilage. This results in a change in the shape and make-up of the joint so that it will not function smoothly. Bone fragments and cartilage may float in what joint fluid there is, causing irritation and pain, and often resulting in bone spurs (osteophytes) forming near the end of the bone (Arthritis Foundation, 2008).

The cause of OA is unknown, but it affects females more often than males, and risk increases with certain factors. Modifiable risks include obesity, joint injury, occupation, structural alignment, and muscle weakness. Nonmodifiable risks include gender (women are more at risk), age, race (white and Asian people are at higher risk), and genetic predisposition (CDC, 2008). At this point, it is unknown whether smoking increases risk.

Signs and symptoms of OA include pain, stiffness (especially in the morning), aching, some joint swelling, and inflammation. OA targets joints such as the fingers, feet, knees, hips, and spine (Yurkow & Yudin, 2002). Heberden's nodes (bony enlargements at the end joints of the fingers) and Bouchard's nodes (bony enlargements at the middle joints of the fingers) are common (**Figure 13-10**). Radiographs would show increased heat at the site of inflammation as well as bone deterioration. As OA progresses, the individual may experience crepitus, limping, limited range of motion, increased pain, and even fractures. Diagnosis is made through various lab tests, x-rays, MRIs, or CT scans to visualize areas of damage.

FIGURE **13-10** **Bouchard's and Herberden's nodes.**

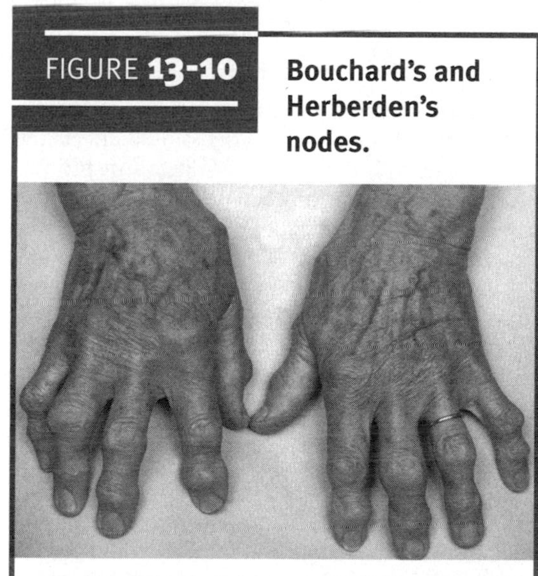

SOURCE: © Visuals Unlimited

The most common associated complication of OA is pain. Although there is no cure for OA, treatment is generally aimed at symptom reduction through lifestyle modifications, nonpharmacological therapies, and medication. For example, risk factors that can be modified such as excessive stress to the joint (perhaps caused by sports or obesity) should be addressed with exercise programs for strengthening muscles and weight loss (**Case Study 13-5**). Exercise programs that are holistic and interdisciplinary, particularly those offered in rehabilitation units, may help individuals cope with pain and increase functional levels. In addition, many persons use alternative methods of pain control in combination with medications. **Table 13-27** provides a summary of common treatments for pain for those with OA.

Medications used for treatment of OA include acetaminophen (Tylenol), aspirin, nonsteroidal

Case Study 13-5

Mrs. Valdez is a 65-year-old woman who comes to the physician's office after experiencing enlargement of her right breast upon self-exam. The nurse observes during the physician's physical examination that Mrs. Valdez's right breast is twice as large as the left one and has a puckered appearance. The physician tells Mrs. Valdez that she will need to have some tests and a biopsy and then he leaves the room. Mrs. Valdez looks at the nurse and asks "What does he mean? What is wrong with me?"

Questions:

1. What should the nurse explain to Mrs. Valdez at this point? What educational materials might she need?
2. What tests would the nurse expect the physician to order?
3. Are there possible risk factors for breast cancer that Mrs. Valdez might have? If so, what are they?
4. Given the physical observations, what would the nurse expect to see done for this patient?

TABLE 13-27 **Treatments for Pain Associated with Osteoarthritis**

Pharmacological	Nonpharmacological
Acetaminophen	Moist heat
Aspirin	Warm paraffin wraps
NSAIDs	Stretch gloves or stockings
Capsaicin (topically, with other therapies)	Range of motion exercises
Nabumetone	Upper extremity activities (such as piano playing, typing, card-playing)
	Swimming
	Adaptive equipment
	Heat/cold applications
	Warm bath (limit to 20 minutes)
	Good posture
	Supportive shoes
	Well-balanced diet
	Maintenance of appropriate weight

SOURCE: From Easton, 1999b, p. 292; adapted with permission.

anti-inflammatory drugs (NSAIDs) such as ibuprofen and naproxen, COX-2 inhibitors (such as celecoxib/Celebrex), tramadol (Ultram), and antidepressants. Other therapies include injection of steroids into the joint to decrease inflammation or injection of synthetic material (such as Synvisc) that acts as a lubricant in the absence of synovial fluid to provide comfort. Other therapies to preserve motion and decrease pain include heat or cold, splints, adaptive equipment, aquatic therapy, and nutrition. In cases of severe dysfunction and pain, surgery with joint replacement may be an option.

Important for any nurse caring for older persons taking NSAIDs is the awareness of common side effects. The most common adverse effects of NSAIDs include gastrointestinal symptoms such as stomach upset, nausea, vomiting, and more seriously, gastric ulcers. COX-2 drugs were thought to minimize these effects, although more recently Vioxx and Celebrex as well as other medications in this classification have come under scrutiny due to rare reports of serious side effects such as MI and stroke (Moore, Derry, Makinson, & McQuay, 2005). Vioxx was removed from the market, but Celebrex is still presently available.

Rheumatoid Arthritis (RA)

RA is characterized by remissions and exacerbations of inflammation within the joint. It affects the fingers, wrists, knees, and spine. In contrast to OA, RA is due to chronic inflammation that can cause severe joint deformities and loss of function over time (**Figure 13-11**).

RA affects over 2 million Americans and is more common in women than men. RA is generally diagnosed between the ages of 20 and 50 and can cause significant disability for adults who live into old age with this disorder (Mayo Clinic, 2005). Although the cause is unknown, researchers believe it may be due to a virus or hormonal factors.

Risk factors for RA include being female, having a certain predisposing gene, and exposure to an infection. Advanced age is a risk factor until age 70, after which incidence decreases. Cigarette smoking over a period of years is another risk factor.

FIGURE 13-11 **Rheumatoid arthritis.**

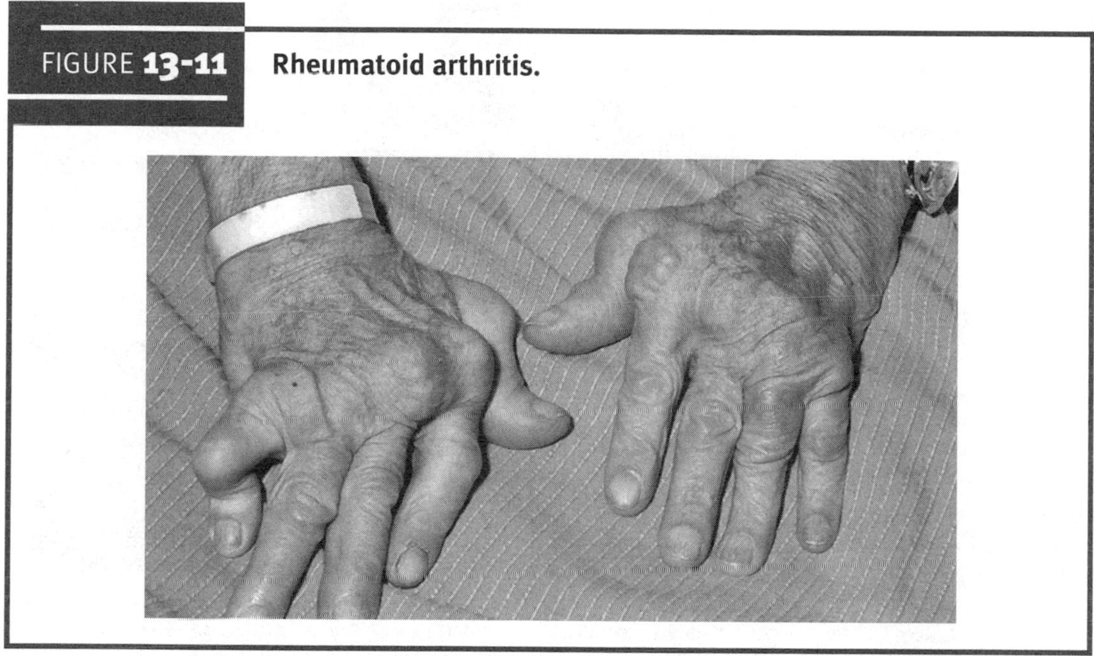

SOURCE: Leonard Crowley, *Introduction to Human Disease* (6th ed.). Sudbury, MA: Jones and Bartlett Publishers, 2005.

Signs and symptoms of RA are systemic and include malaise, fatigue, symmetrical patterns of joint inflammation, pain, stiffness, swelling, gelling (joints stiff after rest), elevated sedimentation rate, presence of serum rheumatoid factor, and elevated white blood cell count (WBC) in the synovial fluid of the inflamed joint. Radiographs will show erosion of the bone. Pain is more prevalent in RA, and joint deformities can cause more debilitation than is generally seen with OA. In addition, RA often strikes in young to middle adulthood, with more degeneration seen over time than with OA.

The treatment for RA is similar to OA with the exception that anti-inflammatory and immune-suppressing drugs may play a more important role. DMARDs (disease-modifying anti-rheumatic drugs) are also used in RA. Historically these drugs were not used until all other medications had been tried. Now, however, the DMARDs are often used within 3 months of diagnosis, the intention being to modify the disease process and prevent the deformities and pain associated with the disease. These medications may not show results for several months, and nurses should teach patients to recognize signs of infections such as chills, pain, and fever.

Nurses should expect to see many complications associated with arthritis. Some potential nursing diagnoses are pain, impaired physical mobility, fatigue, decreased endurance, powerlessness, self-care deficits, sleep pattern disturbance, depression, impaired coping, social isolation, fear, anxiety, and body-image disturbance. Goals for care include promoting independence within limitations, pain management, and education.

Educational programs for persons with arthritis should include exercise and mobility, education, counseling, individual PT and OT, and a focus of independence in **activities of daily living (ADLs)** with self-care. These types of programs help decrease disability, pain, and the need for assistance, as well as reduce joint tenderness. Pain coping and exercise training may also enhance pain control.

Joint Replacement

Joint replacement is used for several different purposes including fracture, immobility, and intractable pain. The two most commonly performed joint replacement surgeries are total hip arthroplasty and total knee arthroplasty. Knee replacements are mainly related to advanced arthritis that causes severe pain and decreased function. Hip replacements may also be done related to arthritis or due to fracture, usually from falling.

Dunlop, Song, Manheim, and Chang (2003) reported significantly fewer joint replacements done on Hispanics and blacks than whites, due to reasons beyond access and financial resources. The researchers suggested that cultural differences, values, and attitudes may also play a role in seeking joint replacement.

Total Hip Arthroplasty/Replacement

Hip replacement surgery may be indicated when an older person demonstrates lack of function, trouble with ADLs, and continued pain that is not sufficiently addressed with traditional medical therapy. Certainly those with certain types of hip fractures will be candidates for this surgery also. In women, body weight and older age have been found to be risk factors for needing hip replacement due to OA (National Institute of Arthritis and Musculoskeletal and Skin Diseases, 2003).

During hip replacement, a prosthetic device made of metal, plastic, ceramic, or various other substances is substituted for the worn-out, damaged, or fractured portions of the hip. The implant is made of a ball-type device on a stem that fits into the femur. The socket of the pelvis helps hold the ball that is articulated onto the joint (**Figure 13-12**). During surgery, physicians may choose to cement the prosthesis into the femur or not. Staples are generally used to close the wound, with a nonstick dressing applied. Staples are usually removed 7–10 days after surgery, depending on healing of the wound. Sometimes physicians will order half of the staples removed initially and the other half later. Steri strips may be applied to assist with wound edge approximation.

Postoperatively, the person will remain in acute care for several days to a week, and then many older adults may need rehabilitation services as inpatients or outpatients, depending on comorbidities, physical condition, and family support. Weight bearing is progressive and depends upon the physician's orders based on the condition of the bones observed during surgery. It is essential that the nurse and other team members strictly observe weight-bearing instructions (such as toe-touch, partial, or full) to avoid injury to the healing hip. Dislocation of the prosthesis can also result from not following routine hip precautions after surgery. Routine hip precautions include not crossing the legs at the knees or ankles, not bending in a chair more than 90 degrees, keeping a pillow between the knees (to maintain abduction) until determined by the physician, and avoiding lying on the operative side until the physician gives permission to do so.

FIGURE **13-12** **Total hip prosthesis.**

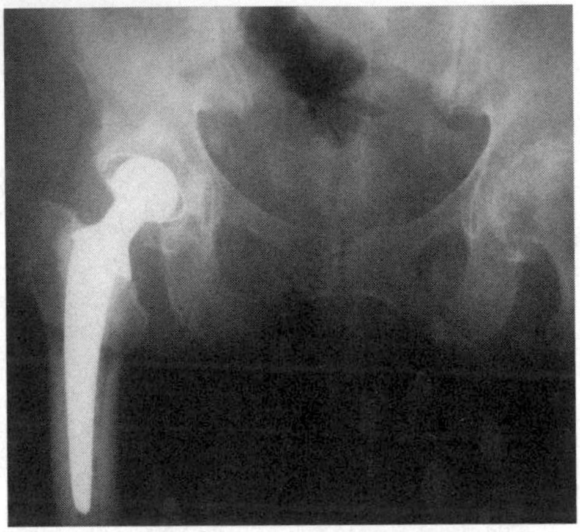

SOURCE: Leonard Crowley, *Introduction to Human Disease* (6th ed.). Sudbury, MA: Jones and Bartlett Publishers, 2005.

Nursing instruction to patients and family members should include watching for signs and symptoms of wound infection. Patients should report any redness, swelling, drainage, or odor from the operative site. A small amount of brownish drainage from the site a few days postoperatively is normal. Fever or malaise could also be signs of infection and should be promptly reported to the physician.

Additionally, reminders about routine hip precautions, exercises, and ambulation as indicated by the physical therapist, as well as traveling implications, should be given. Some prostheses will cause the alarm at airport security to go off. Teach patients to inform security personnel of their hip prosthesis prior to entering the security gate.

Dr. Robert Zann, an orthopedic specialist, stated that recovery from hip replacement surgery generally takes longer than many patients think: "It is interesting that patients undergoing hip replacement surgery will uniformly reach their maximum improvement between 1–2 years" (2005, p. 1). Physicians attribute this to the need for tissue healing (of which 90% occurs in the first 3 months) and return of muscles to normal function and strength, which takes longer.

Total Knee Arthroplasty/Replacement

Similar to hip replacement, knee replacement is done when a person is experiencing decreased range of motion, trouble walking or climbing stairs, and increased degeneration of the joint so as to impair quality of life. This most often occurs as a result of arthritis (either osteo- or rheumatoid arthritis).

Knee replacement surgery involves resurfacing or removing the distal portion of the femur that articulates with the end of the shin bone. The prosthesis consists of metal and plastic or similar materials that are cemented onto the newly resurfaced areas of the articulating bones. Although often done under general anesthetic, this surgery can also be performed under spinal anesthesia. Sometimes blood loss is significant, so patients may be asked to donate their own blood ahead of time to be given back to them in the event it is needed. In addition, a growing trend is toward bilateral knee replacement in those persons requiring both knees to be surgically repaired. The benefits of this are the one-time operative anesthetic and room costs, and many physicians feel recovery from bilateral replacement is similar to single replacement. However, the pain and lack of mobility, as well as the significant increase in the assistance needed after surgery when a bilateral replacement is done, may make this less than ideal for most older patients.

Discomfort after knee surgery is generally severe in the first few days. Nurses should encourage patients to use cold packs on the operative area for the first day and take pain and sleeping medications as ordered. In addition, alternative therapies such as guided imagery have been shown to help with pain management (Antall & Kresevic, 2004). Many joint replacement patients feel a loss of control and independence. Nurses can help the recovery process by maintaining a professional therapeutic relationship with patients. This has been shown to assist older persons in regaining their sense of independence (Loft, McWilliam, & Ward-Griffin, 2003).

Therapy will begin immediately in the acute care hospital. Although weight bearing does not usually occur until 24 hours after surgery, sitting in a chair and using a continuous passive motion machine (CPM) (if ordered) will ease recovery. The use of a CPM is generally based on the surgeon's preference. There is research to support it, as well as studies indicating that walking soon after surgery has an equal effect and makes the CPM unnecessary. However, in cases of an older person who may not have the mobility skills initially after surgery that a younger person would, a CPM may be beneficial to keep the joint flexible and decrease pain.

Dr. Zann (2005) indicated that "patients undergoing total knee replacement do not achieve their maximum improvement until 2–4 years" (p. 1). This is attributed to the lack of muscular structures that surround and protect the knee and the need for the ligaments and tendons to adapt to the indwelling prosthesis. Recovery times vary and depend upon a number of variables, including the patient's overall health, age, comorbidities, and motivation. Patients report that the new knee joint never feels normal even years after the surgery, but they do experience an increase in function and generally much less pain than before.

Nursing implications include teaching the patient about signs and symptoms of infection, care of the surgical site (if staples are still present), pain management, and expectations for recovery. A range of motion from 0–90 degrees is the minimum needed for normal functioning. Most prostheses will allow up to about 120 degrees of flexion, though 110 degrees is considered good range of motion after knee replacement. After discharge, a walker is usually used in the first few weeks, followed by light activities 6 weeks after surgery. In addition, the patient's spouse may experience feelings of being overwhelmed due to role transitions that occur after surgery and during the recovery period. Nurses can help facilitate this transition by providing education and discussing realistic expectations (Showalter, Burger, & Salyer, 2000).

Amputation

Amputation is an acquired condition that results in the loss of a limb, typically from disease, injury, and/or associated surgery. There are approximately 135,000 new amputees each year in the United States (University of Utah, 2008). Two-thirds of these cases are from circulatory problems, particularly PVD related to diabetes. Most of the rest are attributed to trauma.

Most amputations involve the lower extremities, above or below the knee. The greatest risk factor for amputation is diabetes with accompanying peripheral vascular disease, with African American men having a 2.3 times greater rate of amputation than whites with diabetes. Advanced age and the incidence of diabetes in the elderly make this a potential problem in the older age group. Additionally, a recent study showed that HgbA1c level was a significant predictor of foot amputation (Watts et al., 2001).

In the acute phase of recovery after surgery, it is important to prevent contractures of the knee joint (if present) and attempt to maintain normal muscle power and range of motion in remaining joints. The limb should not be hung over the bedside or placed in a dependent position. Both in acute care and rehabilitation, the stump should be conditioned to prepare for the wearing of a prosthesis. In certain circumstances, an older person may choose, in consultation with the physician, not to wear a prosthesis. This generally occurs when there are other health issues such as poor balance from another disease or disorder that would make falling and injury more likely with prosthetic use.

Initially, there may be drainage from the surgical site, and a sterile dressing will be kept in place and changed at least daily. Eventually, the staples or sutures will be removed and a thick, black eschar will form at the amputation site and gradually come off. An Ace wrap or stump shrinker sock (elastic) is used to help prepare the stump for wearing the prosthesis. Several factors should be considered when preparing the stump to wear a prosthesis. These include a movable scar, lack of tenderness/sensitivity, a conical shape, firm skin, and lack of edema. All of these can be achieved by proper wrapping of the stump to maximize shrinkage and minimize swelling. The prone position, if tolerable, is an excellent way to promote full extension of the residual limb.

It is also important for the person to begin therapy right away. The *Merck Manual of Geriatrics* (Beers, 2005) states that "ambulation requires a 10 to 40% increase in energy expenditure after below-the-knee amputation and a 60 to 100% increase after above-the-knee amputation. To compensate, elderly amputees generally walk more slowly" (p. 284). When using the prosthesis at first, an older adult may tire easily. Be sure to take into account any coexisting problems such as cardiopulmonary disease when considering energy expenditure. The newest technologies allow prosthetics to be light, durable, and more comfortable.

Nurses will need to teach patients and families about stump care, mobility, adaptation, coping, and self-care. Home maintenance, dealing with complications and/or additional health problems, wear and tear on non-weight-bearing joints, adapting to the environment, accessibility, stigma, depression, role changes, decreased energy, and chronic pain are all issues to be aware of related to amputation. It is likely that the person with lower extremity amputation will experience some shoulder problems over time due to the additional stress on this non-weight-bearing joint. Remember that alteration in body image is a significant hurdle to overcome for some individuals. **Phantom limb pain**, or pain sensations in the nonexistent limb, is more common after traumatic amputations and may last for weeks after amputation. Massage and medications may help with this type of pain control (Beers, 2005). Additionally, proper wrapping of the stump (in a figure-eight wrap) may help decrease the chance of phantom limb pain later (Easton, 1999b).

In general, older persons with amputation may return to a normal quality of life with some adaptations. The care provided by nurses and physicians in rehabilitation after amputation may make the difference in the person's ability to cope with the changes that result after surgery. Geriatric nurses can facilitate the transition back into the community after amputation by educating patients and families about resources to assist with adaptation.

SENSORY IMPAIRMENTS

Although many normal aging changes occur in the sensory system, most of the common abnormalities seen in the elderly are related to vision. According to Lighthouse International, a leading resource on vision impairment and visual rehabilitation, the most common age-related vision problems are cataracts, glaucoma, macular degeneration, and diabetic neuropathy (2005). This section will discuss these impairments and others. Diseases related to the senses of touch, hearing, and taste are rare, though neuropathy will be addressed in a different section as related to diabetes. The other most common sensory problem in older adults is chronic sinusitis. This will also be discussed.

Cataracts

Cataracts are so common in older adults that some almost consider them an inevitable consequence of old age. According to the University of Washington, Department of Ophthalmology (2008), 400,000 new cases of cataract development are diagnosed each year, 1,350,000 cataract extractions are currently performed each year, 3,700,000 visits to an MD related to cataracts occur each year, and 5,500,000 people have visual obstruction due to cataracts. The etiology is thought to be from oxidative damage to lens protein that occurs with aging. Although about half of people between 65 and 75 years of age have cataracts, they are most common in those over age 75 (70%), and there are no ethnic or gender variations (Trudo & Stark, 1998, p. 2). The two most common causes are advanced age and heredity, though contributing factors also include diabetes, poor nutrition, hypertension, excessive exposure to sunlight (ultraviolet radiation), cigarette smoking, high alcohol intake, and eye trauma (Lighthouse International, 2005).

Cataracts cause no pain or discomfort, but persons will present with a gradual loss of vision that may begin with complaints of vision being fuzzy, sensitivity to glare, and noticing a halo effect around lights. Decreased night vision and a yellowing of the lens, as well as trouble distinguishing colors, may also be noted. Eventually the pupil changes color to a cloudy white (**Figure 13-13**). Generally, the most common objective finding is decreased visual acuity, such as that measured with a Snellen eye chart.

FIGURE **13-13** **A cataract.**

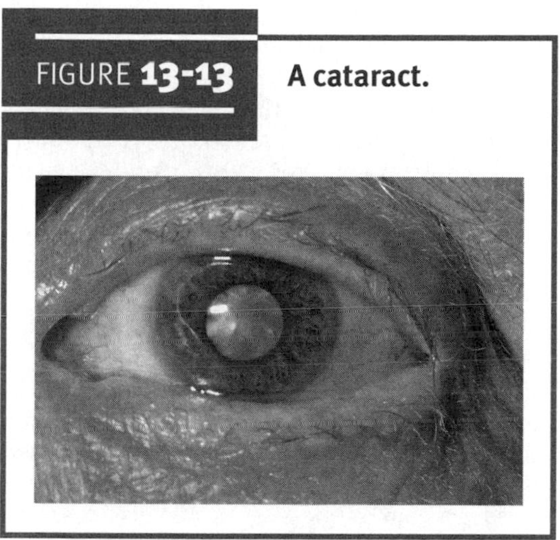

SOURCE: © Dr. P. Marazzi/Science Photo Library/Custom Medical Stock Photo.

Although changes in eyeglasses are the first option, when quality of life becomes affected, the most effective treatment for cataracts is surgery. This is the most common operation among older adults, and more than 95% of them have better vision after surgery (Trudo & Stark, 1998). The benefits of surgery include improved visual acuity, depth perception, and peripheral vision, leading to better outcomes related to ADLs and quality of life. Complications associated with surgery are rare but include retinal detachment, infection, and macular edema. Surgery is relatively safe and usually done as an outpatient procedure. The lens is removed through an incision in the eye and an intraocular lens is inserted. The surgical incision is either closed with sutures or can heal itself. After surgery, patients will need to avoid bright sunlight; wear wrap-around sunglasses for a short time; and avoid straining, lifting, or bending. Cataract surgery today offers a safe and effective treatment to maintain independence and improve quality of life for older adults.

Glaucoma

Glaucoma is a group of degenerative eye diseases in which the optic nerve is damaged by high **intraocular pressure (IOP)** resulting in blindness due to nerve atrophy (Podolsky, 1998). Glaucoma is a leading cause of visual impairment, responsible for 10–20% of all blindness in the United States, and occurs more often in those over 40, with an increased incidence with age (3% to 4% in those over age 70) (Kennedy-Malone et al., 2000; Podolsky, 1998).

Unlike cataracts, there are some ethnic distinctions with the development of glaucoma. African Americans tend to develop it earlier than whites, and females more often than males. Glaucoma is more common in African Americans, Asian Americans, and Alaska Natives. Other contributing factors include eye trauma, small cornea, small anterior chamber, family history, cataracts, and some medications (Eliopoulos, 2005; Kennedy-Malone et al., 2000).

Although the cause is unknown, glaucoma results from pupillary blockage that limits flow of aqueous humor, causing a rise in intraocular pressure (IOP). Two major types are noted here: acute and chronic. Acute glaucoma is also called closed angle or narrow angle. Signs and symptoms include severe eye pain in one eye, blurred vision, seeing colored halos around lights, red eye, headache, nausea, and vomiting. Symptoms may be associated with emotional stress. Acute glaucoma is a medical emergency and the patient should seek emergency help immediately. Blindness can occur from prolonged narrow angle glaucoma.

Chronic glaucoma, also called open angle or primary open angle, is more common than acute (90% of cases are this type), affecting over 2 million people in the United States. One million people probably have glaucoma and don't know it, and 10 million people have above normal intraocular pressure that may lead to glaucoma if not treated (University of Washington, Department of Ophthalmology, 2008).

This type of glaucoma occurs gradually. Peripheral vision is slowly impaired. Signs and symptoms include tired eyes, headaches, misty vision, seeing halos around lights, and worse symptoms in the morning. Glaucoma often involves one eye, but may occur in both.

Early detection and treatment are essential in preventing loss of vision, because once vision has been lost to glaucoma, it cannot be restored. Diagnosis is made using a **tonometer** to measure IOP. Normal IOP is 10–21 mm Hg. Ophthalmologic examination will reveal changes in the color and contour of the optic nerve when glaucoma is present. **Gonioscopy** (direct exam) provides another means of evaluation.

Treatment is aimed at reducing IOP. Medications to decrease pressure may be given, and surgical iridectomy to lower the IOP may prevent future episodes of acute glaucoma. In chronic glaucoma, there is no cure, so treatment is aimed at managing IOP through medication and eyedrops. Nurses should monitor patients for response to medications and to verify that eyedrops are being taken regularly and properly. In addition, older adults should be assessed for safety related to visual changes and also reminded to keep regular visits with their eye doctor.

Macular Degeneration

Age-related macular degeneration (ARMD) is the most common cause of blindness for those over age 60, affecting about 12 million Americans over the age of 40 and more than 1 out of every 3 people over age 75 (Seftel, 2005; Starr, Guyer, & Yannuzzi, 1998). Macular degeneration occurs in approximately 10% of long-term care residents ages 66–74 and increases to 30% for those residents ages 75–85 (Stefanacci, 2007). Risk factors for this sensory problem include high cholesterol, hypertension, diabetes, smoking, overexposure to ultraviolet light, and heredity.

Macular degeneration results from damage or breakdown of the macula and subsequent loss of central vision. Generally associated with the aging process, it can also result from injury or infection. Two types are noted: dry (nonexudative) and wet (exudative). Dry macular degeneration affects 90% of those with the disease (Lighthouse International, 2005) and has a better prognosis. The dry type progresses slowly with more subtle changes in vision than the wet type, which comes on suddenly and may cause more severe loss in vision. The signs and symptoms of ARMD are decreased central vision, seeing images as distorted, decreased color vision, and sometimes a central scotoma (a large, dark spot in the center of vision).

Although there is no cure for macular degeneration, some new therapies show promise (**Case Study 13-6**). Photodynamic therapy uses a special laser to seal leaking blood vessels in the eye. Antioxidant vitamins (C, D, E, and beta-carotene) and zinc also seem to slow the progress of the disease (Age-Related Eye Disease Study Authors [AREDS], 2001). Retinal cell transplantation or regeneration works by harvesting cells from the body and injecting them into diseased macular sites

Case Study 13-6

Mrs. Chiu is a small, 100-pound, 90-year-old Chinese woman with fractures of the vertebral spine. Because of kyphosis and pain associated with os teoporosis, Mrs. Chiu has been bedbound in a nursing home for several months. Her family visits regularly and has many questions about her con dition, especially if it is something that her teenage granddaughters might develop.

Questions:

1. What are Mrs. Chiu's known risk factors for osteoporosis and resulting fractures?
2. How should you answer the family's questions?
3. Are the granddaughters at risk because Mrs. Chiu has osteoporosis? If so, what can they do to prevent it?
4. What teaching should be done with this family?

in the hope that new and healthy cells will grow, thus reversing the damage caused by ARMD (Macular Degeneration Foundation, 2005).

New medications have been approved for the treatment of macular degeneration. Ranibizumab (Lucentis) was approved in 2006, and not only has it shown promise in stopping the progression of macular degeneration, but approximately 50% of the patients taking the medication have shown an improvement in their vision to 20/40. It is given by injection into the eye by an ophthalmologist every 4 weeks for 2 years. Bevacizumab (Avastin) has been used in the treatment of wet macular degeneration and was widely used prior to the advent of ranibizumab. Pegaptanib (Macugen) was approved in 2004 for the treatment of neovascular macular degeneration. It is also injected directly into the eye and targets endothelial growth factor (Stefanacci, 2007).

Chances are that most gerontological nurses will care for older adults with ARMD. Initially, small changes in the environment should be encouraged, such as better lighting in hallways, minimizing glare from lamps or shiny floors, and decorating living spaces in contrasting colors (McGrory & Remington, 2004). Visual adaptive devices such as magnifying glasses and reading lamps may provide temporary help as vision worsens. Auditory devices such as books on tape and adaptation of the environment to the visual impairment may help maintain independence. Nurses should be aware of the treatments being researched and can assure patients that although there is no cure at present, there is hope for the future. In addition, nurses should teach the elderly that the modification of any controllable risk factors, such as smoking cessation, can decrease risk of developing ARMD. It is crucial to remind patients not to just assume that visual changes are "due to aging," but that they may be treatable. Many people avoid seeking treatment for fear that nothing can be done and that they could lose their driver's license.

Diabetic Retinopathy

Diabetic retinopathy is a leading cause of blindness among older adults, resulting from breakage of tiny vessels in the retina as a complication of diabetes. It generally affects both eyes. The longer a person has diabetes, the more likely he or she is to suffer visual impairment (Eyecare America, 2005). Currently approximately 7 million diabetics suffer from diabetic retinopathy, 700,000 are at risk for blindness, and 16 million are prime targets for blinding disorders (University of Washington, Department of Ophthalmology, 2008). Early diagnosis and treatment can prevent much of the blindness that occurs from this disorder.

There are four stages of diabetic retinopathy. These appear in **Table 13-28**. Of the four stages, **proliferative retinopathy** is the most severe and accounts for 64% of vitreous hemorrhage in non–type 1 diabetic patients and for 89% of vitreous hemorrhage in type 1 diabetics (Manuchehri & Kirkby, 2003). As new fragile and abnormal blood vessels grow to compensate for the blocked vessels in the retina, these vessels may leak blood into the eye, causing swelling of the macula and blurred vision. This is what causes much of the blindness seen with diabetic retinopathy.

There are no early warning signs of diabetic retinopathy, so it is essential that older adults with diabetes have a dilated eye exam each year. During the eye exam the eye care professional will do a visual acuity test, a dilated eye exam, and tonometry. If a person complains of seeing spots floating in

BOX 13-6 Resources for Those with Visual Impairments

American Academy of Ophthalmology
P.O. Box 7424
San Francisco, CA 94120-7424
415-561-8500
http://www.aao.org

American Council of the Blind
1155 15th Street, NW, Suite 720
Washington, DC 20005
http://www.acb.org

American Printing House for the Blind
P.O. Box 6985
1839 Franklin Avenue
Louisville, KY 40206
http://www.aph.org

EyeCare America
A Public Service Foundation of the American Academy of Ophthalmology
1-877-887-6327
1-800-222-3937
http://www.eyecareamerica.org

Lighthouse International
111 East 59th Street
New York, NY 10022-1202
1-800-334-5497
1-800-829-0500
http://www.lighthouse.org

Macular Degeneration Foundation
http://www.eyesight.org

National Eye Institute
31 Center Drive MSC 2510
Bethesda, MD 20892-2510
301-496-5248
http://www.nei.nih.gov

the visual field, bleeding may be occurring and the person should see an eye doctor as soon as possible.

The first three stages of diabetic retinopathy are not treated. The first priority in treating proliferative retinopathy is to treat the cause of the vitreous hemorrhage itself. This is followed by a treatment using a procedure called **scatter laser treatment** that helps shrink the abnormal vessels (Manuchehri & Kirkby, 2003). This procedure may require at least two visits, because multiple areas away from the retina are burned with a laser in order to shrink abnormal vessels. Although patients may note some loss of peripheral sight, and/or color vision with this procedure, it is the standard for preserving the majority of central and essential vision.

For more severe cases of bleeding in the eye, a **vitrectomy** may be needed. When blood collects in the center of the eye, a vitrectomy allows removal of the vitreous gel that has blood in it through a small incision in the eye. The blood-contaminated vitreous gel is replaced with a saline-type solution. This is often done as an outpatient procedure. The patient will need to wear an eye patch for days to weeks and use medicated eyedrops to prevent infection. After a vitrectomy, the person's eye may be red and sensitive for some time.

The most important nursing consideration in caring for older persons who may be at risk for diabetic retinopathy is to emphasize prevention of this complication. Treatment becomes necessary with more severe cases, so the best treatment is prevention through regular eye exams, good control of blood sugars, monitoring hypertension, and controlling cholesterol levels. The nurse should encourage the older adult with diabetes to develop a good working relationship with a trusted eye care professional.

Retinal Detachment

Although not as common as the other visual problems discussed, **retinal detachment** may occur in the older adult. It can be the result of trauma to the eye. Symptoms may be gradual or sudden and may look like spots moving across the eye, blurred vision, light flashes, or a curtain drawing. If an older person presents with such symptoms, he or she should seek immediate medical help. Keep the person quiet to minimize further detachment. Surgery may be required to save vision.

Corneal Ulcer

Corneal ulcers are more common in the elderly than in younger age groups due to decreased tearing that occurs with normal aging. Also, many el-

TABLE 13-28 Four Stages of Diabetic Retinopathy

Stage	Description	Pathophysiology
Stage 1	Mild nonproliferative retinopathy	Microaneurysms in retina
Stage 2	Moderate nonproliferative retinopathy	Blockage of some blood vessels supplying retina
Stage 3	Severe nonproliferative retinopathy	Blockage of many blood vessels supplying retina; retina is deprived of needed circulation
Stage 4	Proliferative retinopathy	Advanced stage; new blood vessels that are abnormal and easily breakable form to compensate for blockage of circulation to retina; these vessels may break and leak to cause macular edema and blurred vision

SOURCE: National Eye Institute, 2005.

derly patients have worn contact lenses, either for a very long time or as a result of cataract surgery. Improper cleaning or accidents can occur when placing the lenses, which can cause corneal abrasions. The ulcers may also result from inflammation of the cornea related to stroke, fever, irritation, dehydration, or a poor diet. Corneal ulcers are difficult to treat and may leave scars that affect vision. Signs of corneal ulcer may include bloodshot eye, photophobia, and complaint of irritation. The nurse should encourage the older person to seek prompt assistance from an eye care professional.

Chronic Sinusitis

Consistently one of the top 10 chronic complaints of the elderly is chronic sinusitis (Eliopoulos, 2005). Over 15% of older persons report having this condition (Stotts & Deitrich, 2004). This results from irritants blocking drainage of the sinus cavities, leading to infection. When symptoms continue over a period of weeks and up to 3 months and are often recurring, chronic sinusitis should be suspected. Symptoms include a severe cold, sneezing, cough (that is often worse at night), hoarseness, diminished sense of smell, discolored nasal discharge, postnasal drip, headache, facial pain, fatigue, malaise, and fever (Kelley, 2002). Upon physical examination, the person may complain of pain on palpation of the sinus areas, and edema and redness of the nasal mucosa may be evident. Allergies, common cold, and dental problems should be ruled out for differential diagnosis. A CT scan of the sinuses will show areas of inflammation.

Treatment for chronic sinusitis is with antibiotics, decongestants, and analgesics for pain. Inhaled corticosteroids may be needed to reduce swelling and ease breathing. Irrigation with over-the-counter normal saline nose spray is often helpful and may be done two to three times per day The person with chronic sinusitis should drink plenty of fluids to maintain adequate hydration and avoid any environmental pollutants such as cigarette smoke or other toxins. Chronic sinusitis is a condition that many older adults wrestle with their entire life. Avoidance of precipitating factors for each individual should be encouraged.

BOX 13-7 Web Exploration

Visit Lighthouse International at http://www.lighthouse.org and read about new software that may assist persons with visual problems.

INTEGUMENTARY PROBLEMS

Many changes occur in the integumentary system with normal aging. These are discussed in Chapter 6. One of the most common problems in the elderly is a skin breakdown due to pressure ulcers. The treatment of pressure ulcers is discussed at length in Chapter 14. Skin cancer and herpes zoster infection (shingles) are also common ailments. These two disorders will be briefly addressed here.

Skin Cancers

There are three major types of skin cancer: basal cell, squamous cell, and malignant melanoma (MM). The major risk factor for all types of skin cancer is sun exposure.

Basal cell carcinoma (**Figure 13-14**) is the most common skin cancer, accounting for 65–85% of cases (Kennedy-Malone et al., 2000). According to the American Cancer Society (2008a), this means that about 800,000–900,000 cases of basal cell carcinoma are diagnosed each year. It is often found on the head or face, or other areas exposed to the sun. When treated early, it is easily removed through surgery and is not life threatening, though it is often recurring.

Squamous cell carcinoma is more common in African Americans and is also less serious than malignant melanoma. It accounts for approximately 200,000–300,000 new cases yearly. Malignant melanoma accounts for only 3% of all skin cancers, but it is responsible for the majority of deaths from skin cancer. About 8,420 people were estimated to die from malignant melanoma in 2008. The American Cancer Society (2008a) estimated that in 2008 there would be 62,480 new cases in the United States. Surgical treatment is required in malignant melanoma (**Figure 13-15**), with chemotherapy and radiation. The prognosis for MM depends on the extent and staging of the tumor, but when caught very early, the cure rate is nearly 100%.

The best treatment for skin cancer in the elderly is prevention. All older persons, especially those with fair skin who are prone to sunburn, should wear sunblock and protective clothing. Annual physical examinations should include inspection of the skin for lesions. Older adults should be taught to report any suspicious areas on their skin to the physician. Persons should particularly look for changes in shape, color, and whether a lesion is raised or bleeds. Most skin cancers, when treated early, have a good prognosis.

FIGURE **13-14** **Basal cell carcinoma.**

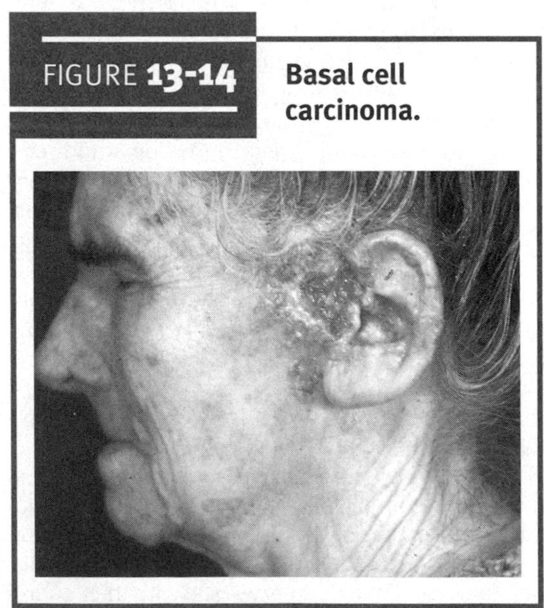

SOURCE: Leonard Crowley, *Introduction to Human Disease* (6th ed.). Sudbury, MA: Jones and Bartlett Publishers, 2005.

FIGURE **13-15** **Malignant melanoma.**

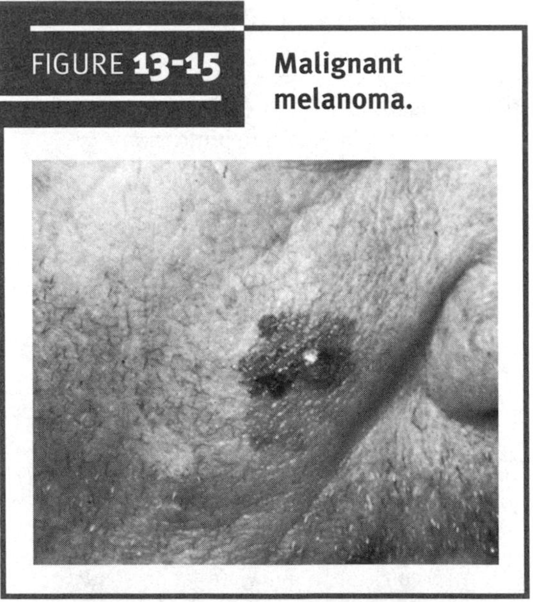

SOURCE: Leonard Crowley, *Introduction to Human Disease* (6th ed.). Sudbury, MA: Jones and Bartlett Publishers, 2005.

Herpes Zoster (Shingles)

Commonly known as shingles, **herpes zoster** is the reactivation of the virus that causes chicken pox (**Case Study 13-7**). Older persons may be infected with this latent varicella virus after initial exposure to it in the form of chicken pox. The virus then lays dormant in the neurons until it is reactivated, often due to immunosuppression, when it appears in the form of painful vesicles along the sensory nerves. This reactivation tends to occur only once in a lifetime, with repeat attacks occurring about 5% of the time (Flossos & Kostakou, 2006). Herpes zoster occurs in both men and women equally, with no specific ethnic variations, but is more common in the elderly.

Risk factors for developing shingles are age over 55 years, stress, and a suppressed immune system. For many older women particularly, emotional or psychological stress can trigger reactivations.

Signs and symptoms of herpes zoster include painful lesions that erupt on the sensory nerve path, usually beginning on the chest or face. These weepy vesicles get pustular and crusty over several days, with healing occurring in 2–4 weeks (Kennedy-Malone et al., 2003). Diagnosis can be made by clinical appearance of the lesions and a history of onset. A scraping will confirm some type of herpes virus. The most common complaint of those with herpes zoster is severe pain that usually subsides in 3–5 weeks (NINDS, 2005). Postherpetic neuralgia, a complication of herpes zoster, may last 6–12 months after the lesions disappear and may involve the dermatome, thermal sensory deficits, allodynia (the perception of pain where pain should not be), and/or severe sensory loss, all of which can be very distressing for the patient (Flossos & Kostakou, 2006).

Anitviral medications such as acyclovir are used to treat shingles, but must be given within 48 hours of the eruption of the lesion. Topical ointments may help with pain and itching. Pain medications, particularly acetaminophen, are appropriate for pain management in older adults. Persons with pain that lasts past 6 weeks after the skin lesions are gone and that is described as sharp, burning, or constant require re-evaluation by a physician. Postherpetic neuralgia usually disappears within a year (NINDS, 2005).

Nursing interventions for the older adult with shingles are largely to recommend rest and comfort. The patient should be advised to seek medical attention as soon as he or she suspects shingles, in order to receive the best results from acyclovir. The virus will run its course, but the person is contagious while vesicles are weepy. Persons should not have direct contact (even clothing) with pregnant women, people who have not had chicken pox, other elderly persons, or those with suppressed immune systems. The older person with shingles may experience concerns with pain management and feel a sense of isolation, particularly if they live alone. Arranging for a family member or friend who does not have a high risk of infection to check on the older person at home is advisable. Recently, Zostavax, a vaccine for shingles, has become available, and it is recommended for all persons age 60 or older. At this time it is covered by Medicare. (**Case Study 13-8**)

Case Study 13-7

Mrs. Booker has recently been diagnosed with ARMD. She is distressed to feel she is going blind and there is nothing she can do about it. She expresses these frustrations to the nurse and asks for help.

Questions:

1. What should the nurse's response be?
2. What initial adaptations need to be made early in the disease process?
3. Are there any things that Mrs. Booker can do now to help modify her environment for this progressive vision loss? What would those things be?
4. To which resources should the nurse refer Mrs. Booker for further information and support?

ENDOCRINE/METABOLIC DISORDERS

Two of the most common disorders in this category among older adults are diabetes and hypothyroidism. These will be discussed in this section.

Diabetes Mellitus

Diabetes mellitus (DM) is a disorder in which the body does not make enough insulin or cannot

Case Study 13-8

Eloise Mitchell is a 90-year-old female who lives alone in a senior living apartment. She has three children, none of whom live nearby. Although she has been in good health, Ms. Mitchell has recently experienced weight loss and frequent "colds." She was recently diagnosed with shingles and comes to you, the nurse for the senior living complex, for some help. How would you respond to the following questions from Ms. Mitchell?

Questions:

1. What caused the shingles?
2. The doctor says it's like chicken pox, but I wasn't exposed to that, so how did I get it?
3. Why is there so much pain with this problem? Is there anything I can do to get relief? The medication doesn't help that much.
4. Can I really have sores on the bottom of my feet and in my mouth?
5. How long am I contagious?
6. When will I start to feel better? I had a friend who was under the weather for months! Is that usual?
7. Can I ever get this again? If so, how can I prevent it? It's awful!

effectively use the little insulin that it does produce. There are two major types of diabetes: type 1 (insulin-dependent diabetes mellitus, IDDM) and type 2 (often referred to as non-insulin-dependent diabetes mellitus). Type 1 generally occurs in children and used to be known as juvenile onset diabetes. It is characterized by hyperglycemia and little or no insulin production. Type 2 is seen in the vast majority of those with diabetes and is managed more often by diet, exercise, and oral medications. Patients with type 2 diabetes may need to take insulin to supplement their oral medication even though they are classified as non-insulin-dependent diabetic patients. Type 2 is most common in those over 30 and is characterized by hyperglycemia and insulin resistance.

DM is the seventh leading cause of death among older adults. The risk of diabetes increases with age, as does mortality from this disease. Risk factors include family history, obesity, race (African Americans, Hispanics, Native Americans, Asian Americans, Pacific Islanders), age over 45, hypertension (greater than or equal to 140/90), less "good" cholesterol (less than 35 mg/dl), and for women, having a history of large babies (Maschak-Carey, Bourne, & Brown-Gordon, 2002).

It is estimated that 11.5 million women and 12.0 million men over the age of 60 have diabetes, but many do not know it. Type 2 is the most common type in older women (CDC, 2007). The Indian Health Service reported via the National Diabetes Survey of 2007 that of the 1.4 million Native Americans and Alaska Natives, 14.2% age 20 or older have diagnosed diabetes. Rates vary by region, from 6.0% of Alaska Natives to 29.3% of the Native Americans in southern Arizona (CDC, 2007). The risk of death from DM is significantly higher among older Mexican American, African American, and Native American women when compared to whites. The Centers for Disease Control (2005) names obesity, weight gain, and physical inactivity as the major risk factors for DM among women.

Early diagnosis is difficult in the elderly, because they may not present with the typical classic symptoms of polydypsia, polyuria, and polyphagia (Amella, 2004). Glucose intolerance may be an initial sign in the elderly; however, diagnosis is made through lab tests and patient history. Due to the increased incidence with age, screening is recommended every 3 years with a fasting blood sugar for those over 45 years of age.

Management is successful when a balance is achieved among exercise, diet, and medications. Medications may be oral hypoglycemics or insulin injection (needed in type 1 and sometimes in type 2). Nurses will need to do a significant amount of teaching (**Tables 13-29** and **13-30**) regarding the signs and symptoms of hyper- and hypoglycemia and the role of medications in managing blood sugar.

Although much of the teaching done with older adults is usually in the acute care hospital or rehabilitation setting, telephone follow-up calls have been shown to improve patient adherence to diet. Additionally, a significant finding of Kim and Oh's (2003) research was that patients receiving phone calls from the nurse about adherence to the prescribed regimen for diabetes management showed

TABLE 13-29 The National Diabetes Education Program's Seven Principles for Management

Principle 1: Find out what type of diabetes you have.
Principle 2: Get regular care for your diabetes.
Principle 3: Learn how to control your diabetes.
Principle 4: Treat high blood sugar.
Principle 5: Monitor your blood sugar level.
Principle 6: Prevent and diagnose long-term diabetes problems.
Principle 7: Get checked for long-term problems and treat them.

SOURCE: National Diabetes Education Program, 2005, p. 1.

TABLE 13-30 Key Areas for Nursing Teaching of Older Persons with Diabetes

Proper nutrition
Exercise
Medications
Signs and symptoms of hyper- and hypoglycemia
Meaning of lab tests: FBS, blood glucose, HgbA1c
Use of a glucometer
Foot care
Importance of adherence to therapeutic regimen
Possible long-term complications
Prevention of complications
Develop a plan of action for when illness occurs

an improved HgbA1c over those who did not have follow-up phone calls.

Thorough evaluation of readiness to learn and of the ability of an older person to manage his or her medications must be done. Older adults who need to give themselves insulin injections may experience anxiety about learning this task. Demonstration, repetition, and practice are good techniques for the older age group. Adaptive devices such as magnifiers may help if the syringes are hard to read. A family member should also be taught to give the insulin to provide support and encouragement, although the older adult should be encouraged to remain independent in this skill if possible. Williams and Bond's (2002) research suggested that programs that promote confidence in self-care abilities are likely to be effective for those with diabetes. A plan for times of sickness and the use of a glucometer to monitor blood sugars will also need to be addressed. Additionally, the dietician may be consulted to provide education for the patient and family on meal planning, calorie counting, carbohydrate counting, and nutrition. Many patients benefit from weight loss, so the nutritionist can assist with dietary planning in this regard also.

Due to the increased risk of infection and slow healing that result from diabetes, foot care is an essential component in teaching older adults to manage DM. Some experts believe that good preventive foot care would significantly reduce the incidence of amputation in the elderly. Older persons with DM should never go barefoot outside. Extremes in temperature should be avoided. Shoes should be well fitting and not rub. Socks should be changed regularly. Elders should be taught to inspect their feet daily, with a mirror if needed. Corns and ingrown toenails should be inspected and treated by a podiatrist, not by the patient. Older persons should see their podiatrist for a foot inspection at least yearly. Patients should be cautioned that even the smallest foot injury such as a thorn or blister can go unnoticed and unfelt—and often results in partial amputations that lead to a cascade of lower extremity problems.

Complications from DM are many. The most commonly seen in older adults are heart disease, stroke, kidney failure, nerve damage, and visual problems. A key to successful long-term management of diabetes in older adults is prevention of complications. This is best achieved by a careful balance of diet, exercise, and medication. Oral hypoglycemics or insulin help to keep blood sugar under control. The best measure of good blood glucose management and controlled blood sugars is HgbA1c levels (glycosylated hemoglobin). This measure of hemoglobin provides insight into the previous 3 months of blood sugar control. If HgbA1c is elevated, it indicates that the blood sugar has been high over time. Treatment is aimed at helping patients to maintain a normal level to decrease risk of complications. There is some controversy that HgbA1c may not be reliable in the elderly. However, Watts et al. (2001) found that HgbA1c was a predictor of foot amputation in patients with diabetes.

Most of the complications of DM seen in the elderly have been discussed elsewhere in this chapter. These include MI, stroke, ESRD, diabetic retinopathy, and PVD. Peripheral neuropathy, seen so commonly in older persons with diabetes, is most often the result of PVD. Peripheral neuropathy presents as uncomfortable, painful sensations in the legs and feet that are difficult to treat. A lack of sensation may also be present and contribute to the risk of falls. There is no cure for peripheral neuropathy, and it tends to be a complication that patients struggle with continually. A combination of medication to address pain and interventions by a physical therapist seem to be the best current treatment.

Hypothyroidism

Hypothyroidism results from lack of sufficient thyroid hormone being produced by the thyroid gland. Older adults may have subclinical hypothyroidism, in which the TSH (thyroid-stimulating hormone) is elevated and the T4 (thyroxine or thyroid hormone) is normal; 4.3–9.5% of the general population has this problem (Woolever & Beutler, 2007). In this condition, the body is trying to stimulate production of more thyroid hormone. Some older adults with this condition will progress to have primary or overt hypothyroidism. This is when the TSH is elevated and T4 is decreased. Hashimoto's disease is the most common cause and represents 90% of all patients with hypothyroidism (American Association of Clinical Endocrinologists [AACE], 2005; Woolever & Beutler, 2007), though certain pituitary disorders, medications, and other hormonal imbalances may be causal factors.

Older adults may present an atypical picture, but the most common presenting complaints are fatigue and weakness. **Table 13-31** provides additional classic signs and symptoms. Diagnosis should include a thorough history and physical; bradycardia and heart failure are often associated factors. Lab tests should include thyroid and thyroid antibody levels (common to Hashimoto's), and lipids, because hyperlipidemia is also associated with this disorder.

Treatment centers on returning the thyroid hormone level to normal. This is done through oral thyroid replacement medication, usually L-thyroxine. Whenever a patient is started on this medication, checks should be done at 3, 6, and 12 months to monitor effectiveness and blood levels, because hyperthyroidism is a side effect of this therapy and can have serious implications on the older person's health.

Nurses should teach patients about the importance of taking thyroid medication at the same time

TABLE 13-31 Signs and Symptoms of Hypothyroidism

*Weakness
*Fatigue
Dry skin
Brittle hair
Hair loss
Weight gain (7–20 pounds)
Cold sensitivity
Puffy face
Headache
Difficulty sleeping
Goiter
Trouble breathing or swallowing
Constipation
Ataxia
Depression
Bradycardia
Anorexia

*Primary signs in the elderly; others may or may not be present.

SOURCE: AACE, 2005; Freil & Cotter, 2002; Reuben et al., 2003.

each day without missing doses. Sometimes older adults have other problems associated with hypothyroidism such as bowel dysfunction and depression. Any signs of complicating factors should be reported to the physician, and doctors' appointments for monitoring should be religiously kept. Strategies for managing fatigue and weakness should also be addressed, because some lifestyle modifications may need to be made as treatment is initiated.

OTHER DISORDERS OR SYNDROMES

There are several notable conditions commonly seen in older adults that may be the result of a variety of factors, not just one physical problem or disease. These include depression, anxiety, delirium, dementia, and insomnia. Depression, anxiety, and insomnia are all discussed at length in Chapter 14. Dementia of the Alzheimer's type was addressed earlier in this chapter. Delirium and sundowner's syndrome will be discussed here.

Delirium

Delirium, also called acute confusion, is frequently seen in older adults. "It is important to remember that it is a medical/surgical diagnosis with psychiatric manifestations. This means that the treatment of delirium requires the diagnosis and treatment of the underlying physiological problem while using pharmacologic and non-pharmacologic interventions to maintain patient safety and return the patient to the pre-delirium state" (Wiesenfeld, 2008). It occurs in 22–38% of older patients in the hospital and in as many as 40% of long-term care residents (Kurlowicz, 2002). Because it can present itself with either hyperactivity, hypoactivity, or a combination of both, the diagnosis is missed in the vast majority of cases (Waszynski, 2001; Wiesenfeld, 2008). Delirium should be addressed in the elderly, because it is associated with increased length of stay in the hospital and higher mortality rates, not to mention distress for the patient as well as the family and other caregivers.

This condition has several distinguishing traits, but especially cognitive-perceptual difficulties and altered level of consciousness. Other characteristics of delirium appear in **Table 13-32**. Delirium is a temporary, reversible condition that may have many different causes, including those listed in **Table 13-33**. Persons' lucidity and confusion may fluctuate hourly but worsen at night. A short attention span, disorganized thinking, and disturbed sleep patterns are also common.

TABLE 13-32 Characteristics of Delirium in the Elderly

Abrupt onset
Time limited
Often associated with a change in environment or unfamiliar surroundings
Often associated with an acute illness such as urinary tract infection
May be associated with a change in medications or dosing
Altered level of consciousness
Fluctuates during the day
Disturbed sleep patterns
Disorientation
Short attention span; easily distracted
Physiological changes
Disorganized thinking
Cognitive-perceptual changes
Impaired memory
Loud or incoherent speech

The symptoms of delirium are disorientation to time and place, altered attention, impaired memory, mood swings, poor judgment, altered level of consciousness, and a decreased **Mini Mental State Examination (MMSE)** score. A score of 23 (out of 30) or less on the MMSE indicates cognitive disturbance, but the MMSE does not distinguish delirium from dementia. All possible causes should be considered. Delirium symptoms tend to have a sudden onset, but may be associated with any of the causes listed in Table 13-32. The subtypes of delirium are hyperactive, hypoactive, and mixed, indicating that a variety of behaviors may be seen within delirium, from increased activity to lethargy or a combination of both.

Delirium can be detected promptly by a good history and physical examination. MMSEs, the confusion assessment method (CAM), and geriatric depression screenings are good tools to assist with

TABLE **13-33** **Potential Causes of Delirium**

Fluid and electrolyte imbalances
Infection
CHF
Certain medications or polypharmacy
Pain
Impaired cardiac or respiratory function
Emotional stress
Unfamiliar surroundings
Malnutrition
Anemia
Dehydration
Alcoholism
Hypoxia

differential diagnosis. Lab tests such as a complete blood count, electrolytes, liver and renal function tests, serum calcium and glucose, urinalysis, chest x-rays, ECG, and oxygen saturation will all help determine the underlying cause (Reuben et al., 2004). Resnick (2005) advises nurses to first check for medical causes of delirium such as infection, medications, or change in oxygenation.

The stress of hospitalization may add to the risk of delirium in older adults. Other risk factors for delirium include dementia, advanced age, sleep deprivation, immobility, dehydration, and sensory impairment (Reuben et al., 2004). Kurlowicz (2002) lists common causes in elderly hospitalized patients as medication, pain, dehydration, electrolyte imbalances, and infection. Evaluation of delirium can be done using the IN-OUT approach. First you look at the IN and OUT of the brain. What could have happened IN the brain to bring on the delirium (stroke, brain injury, infection such as meningitis) and what could have happened physiologically OUTside of the brain (endocrine dysfunction, organ failure, urinary tract infection, dehydration, etc.)? Next evaluate what could have been taken IN by the patient (medications such as opiates, benzodiazapines, anticholinergics, steroids), and what might be going on OUTside of the body (such as alcohol withdrawal, or withdrawal from any psychoactive medication such as antidepressants, sedatives, etc.) (Wiesenfeld, 2008).

Treatment of delirium depends on the cause. Symptoms of delirium should not be accepted as normal nor dismissed as a part of old age. Treatment requires almost an obsessional attention to the patient. Wiesenfeld (2008) suggests the ADVISE model be used. A stands for advocacy, meaning someone has to speak up for the patient because they can't speak for themselves when they are delirious. D stands for diligence in exploring what could be causing the problem and an assumption that this is not normal, something has to be wrong. V stands for vigilance to make sure that once the cause of the delirium is found that it is discontinued; for example, if a medication is the culprit, it must not be given again. I stands for integration, meaning that all care providers from all disciplines for the patient must be alerted to what is happening and understand that the delirium is likely temporary and to treat the person gently, optimizing their return to their baseline state. S stands for support. The patient and his or her family are likely experiencing emotional pain because of this disorienting episode. They need support to get through it. Last, E stands for education. This extends to family and care providers as well as the patient once he or she is able. Once the trigger for the delirium is identified, everyone needs to know so that it won't happen again.

Interventions to treat the causal factor should be implemented. For example, if the person is found to have a urinary tract infection, it should be actively treated. If numerous medications may be to blame, the medication regimen must be re-examined. If the person has hypoxia, improved oxygenation is the remedy.

To manage the symptoms of delirium such as confusion, disorientation, and lack of attention while the cause is being addressed, nurses should initiate several measures. First, the person must be kept safe from harm when confused. Having a family member stay at the bedside with the person may be helpful. Reorientation to surroundings, person, time, and place should be consistent and reinforced by all team members; however, if this increases the agitation of the patient, it is doing more harm than good and need not be continued. Adequate hydration and nutrition are essential to maintain electrolyte balances. Familiar items such as pictures, favorite blankets, or clothing should be provided for comfort. The environment should be conducive to sleep, and interruptions limited. Cognitively stimulating activities such as reminiscence, word games, or cards should be provided during waking hours. In addition, during the period of delirium, care should be taken to avoid complications, such as the hazards of immobility.

Medications that contribute to the problem should be discontinued or decreased to minimal doses. Low-dose neuroleptics such as haloperidol (Haldol) have been traditionally used to treat delirium, but they have a significant risk for serious side effects. Newer antipsychotics such as risperidone (Risperdal) have a lower incidence of side effects and may be a better alternative to Haldol. Other antipsychotics such as chlorpromazine (Thorazine) or thioridazine (Mellaril) should be avoided due to potential cardiac side effects (Reuben et al., 2004).

Generally, delirium should be short in duration, resolving with treatment in a month or less. Early detection and treatment can assist in preventing complications that are often associated with this condition.

Sundowner's Syndrome

Also referred to as sundowning, sundowner's syndrome is a form of delirium and refers to behavior problems that are sometimes seen, particularly in persons with dementia, in the late afternoon or early evening when the sun sets. This behavior may include disorientation, emotional upset, or confusion. There is no exact explanation as to why this occurs in some older persons, but ideas include the lack of light that contributes to disorientation with their surroundings, boredom at that time of day, or stress (Alzheimer's Association, 2005).

Some suggestions for minimizing the occurrence of this syndrome include keeping the person busy and active during the day to avoid napping so that normal sleep patterns will be maintained. Brisk walks and increased exercise during the day may minimize wandering or walking behaviors at night. Keeping the lights on in the room to minimize confusion as the sun sets until bedtime is thought helpful by some. Make bedtime a quiet and stress-free experience by eliminating excess noise and providing a routine such as snack and television or reading. Maintaining a calm and pleasant environment while continually reorienting those affected by sundowner's syndrome may minimize the emotional stress experienced by these older persons. Additionally, discuss the possibility of sleeping medications for those who are continually restless at night. Whatever strategies are used to manage behaviors associated with sundowning, the nurse and caregivers should remain calm, reassuring, and flexible while maintaining a safe environment for the older adult

SUMMARY

In summary, this chapter provided brief and concise snapshots of illnesses, diseases, and health conditions common to older adults. Students and health professionals may learn additional information about these problems in greater detail from other courses or sources. This chapter focused on a review of basic knowledge but added specific information related to older adults who may require interventions related to certain common conditions.

Critical Thinking Exercises

1. This chapter discusses a great deal of content. Choose one health condition or disease that interests you most and search the Internet site of the organization dedicated to that cause. What resources are available for persons with this problem?
2. Volunteer through your local hospital to help with stroke and/or blood pressure screenings of older adults. Note any common risk factors you observe among the persons that are being screened.
3. Visit a support group related to one of the long-term conditions discussed in this chapter. It might be a stroke survivor's meeting, the breather's club, or a Parkinson's disease group. Listen to the participants and their family members. Write down anything new you learned about how people live with and manage this condition. Talk personally with a family who is living with the condition that you are further investigating.participants and their family members. Write down anything new you learned about how people live with and manage this condition. Talk personally with a family who is living with the condition that you are further investigating.
4. Go to your local mall, church, shopping center, restaurant, or other place where seniors living in the community might gather. Listen to casual conversations between older adults. What types of health problems and concerns do they express?
5. Talk to a nurse who works in the emergency room, or to a local cardiologist. Ask what symptoms they have seen in older adult patients who were diagnosed with myocardial infarction. How are these symptoms different from or similar to a classic presentation?

Personal **Reflections**

1. Of the disorders presented in this chapter, which are the most familiar to you? Which do you feel you need to do more reading about? Have you ever cared for an older patient with any of these problems? Did the information in the text present what you saw as signs and symptoms in this patient?
2. Which of the diseases in this chapter do you feel are most common in the people you take care of? Have you noticed any ethnic or cultural differences in the geographic area where you work?
3. If an older person came to you and wanted to know about one of the diseases in this chapter, what would you tell the person? How is your comfort level with what needs to be taught for each of the disorders in this chapter?
4. Make a list of three diseases that you are least knowledgeable about and re-read that section of this chapter. Memorize the signs and symptoms, and think about the nursing interventions you should use.

References

Age-Related Eye Disease Study Authors. (2001). A randomized, placebo-controlled, clinical trial of high-dose supplementation with vitamins C and E, beta carotene, and zinc for age-related macular degeneration and vision loss. *Archives of Ophthalmology, 119*, 1417–1436.

Alzheimer's Association. (2005). *Alzheimer's facts and figures*. Retrieved October 13, 2005, from http://www.alz.org/AboutAD/statistics.asp

Alzheimer's Association. (2008). Alzheimer's disease. Incidence and prevalence. Retrieved June 22, 2008, from http://www.alz.org

Amella, G. J. (2004). Presentation of illness in older adults. *American Journal of Nursing, 104*(10), 40–51.

American Association of Clinical Endocrinologists. (2005). *Hypothyroidism*. Retrieved March 7, 2005, from http://www.aace.com/clin/guidelines

American Cancer Society. (2004). *How is bladder cancer treated?* Retrieved April 1, 2005, from http://www.cancer.org

American Cancer Society. (2005a). *All about colon and rectum cancer.* Retrieved June 11, 2005, from http://www.cancer.org

American Cancer Society. (2005b). *Making strides against breast cancer.* Retrieved April 27, 2005, from http://www.cancer.org

American Cancer Society. (2005c). *Stomach cancer*. Retrieved June 11, 2005, from http://www.cancer.org

American Cancer Society. (2008a). *Basal cell carcinoma statistics*. Retrieved June 26, 2008, from http://www.cancer.org

American Cancer Society. (2008b). *Bladder cancer statistics*. Retrieved June 24, 2008, from http://www.cancer.org

American Cancer Society. (2008c). *Information about breast cancer.* Retrieved June 24, 2008, from http://www.cancer.org

American Cancer Society. (2008d). Overview: Prostate cancer. Retrieved December 28, 2008, from http://www.cancer.org/docroot/CRI/CRI_2_1x.asp?dt=36

American Cancer Society. (2008e). *Pancreatic cancer.* Retrieved June 25, 2008, from http://www.cancer.org

American Foundation for Urologic Disease (AFUD). (2008). *Bladder cancer*. Retrieved on December 29, 2008, from http://www.urologyhealth.org/search/index.cfm?topic=37&search=bladder%20AND%20cancer%20AND%20treatment&searchtype=and

American Gastroenterology Association. (2008). *Gastroesophageal reflux disease.* Retrieved December 28, 2008, from http://www.gastro.org/wmspage.cfm?parm1=848#GERD?

American Heart Association. (2005). *PAD quick facts*. Retrieved May 18, 2005, from http://www.americanheart.org

American Heart Association. (2008a). *Angina*. Retrieved June 24, 2008, from http://www.americanheart.org

American Heart Association. (2008b). *Congestive heart failure*. Retrieved June 24, 2008, from http://www.americanheart.org

American Heart Association. (2008c). *Heart disease and stroke statistics: 2008 update*. Brochure: Author.

American Heart Association. (2008d). *Am I at risk?* Retrieved on December 29, 2008, from http://www.americanheart.org/presenter.jhtml?identifier=2142

American Lung Association. (2004). *Chronic obstructive pulmonary disease (COPD) fact sheet*. Retrieved May 23, 2005, from http://www.lungusa.org

American Lung Association. (2005). *Tuberculosis fact sheet.* Retrieved May 23, 2005, from http://www.lungusa.org

American Lung Association. (2008). *Pneumonia fact sheet*. Retrieved June 25, 2008, from http://www.lungusa.org

American Parkinson Disease Association. (2005). *Patient information*. Retrieved October 12, 2005, http://www.apdaparkinson.org/userND/index.asp

American Stroke Association. (2008). *Warning signs*. Retrieved June 24, 2008, from http://www.strokeassociation.org

American Urological Association. (2005a). *BPH*. Retrieved April 28, 2005, from http://www.urologyhealth.org

American Urological Association. (2005b). *Prostate cancer*. Retrieved April 28, 2005, from http://www.urologyhealth.org

Anderson, S., & Marlett, S. (2004). The language of recovery: How effective communication of information is crucial to restructuring post-stroke life. *Topics in Stroke Rehabilitation, 11*(4), 55–67.

Antall, G. F., & Kresevic, D. (2004). The use of guided imagery to manage pain in an elderly orthopaedic population. *Orthopaedic Nursing, 23*(5), 335–340.

Aronow, W. S. (2007). Recognition of aortic stenosis in the elderly. *Geriatrics, 62*(12), 23–32.

Arthritis Foundation. (2005). *The facts about arthritis.* Retrieved October 11, 2005, from http://www.arthritis.org/resources/getting started

Arthritis Foundation. (2008). *Osteoarthritis.* Retrieved June 8, 2008, from http://www.arthritis.org/

Beers, M. H. (Ed.). (2005). *Merck manual of geriatrics.* Whitehouse Station, NJ: Merck Research Laboratories.

Bergey, G. E. (2004). Initial treatment of epilepsy: Special issues in treating the elderly. *Neurology, 63*(10), S40–S48.

Bradley, C., Given, C. W., & Roberts, C. (2004). Health care disparities and cervical cancer. *American Journal of Public Health, 94*(12), 2098–3002.

Bradway, C. W., & Yetman, G. (2002). Genitourinary problems. In V. T. Cotter & N. E. Strumpf (Eds.), *Advanced practice nursing with older adults: Clinical guidelines* (pp. 83–102). New York: McGraw-Hill.

Cameron, J., & Gignac, M. A. M. (2008). "Timing it right": A conceptual framework for addressing the support needs of family caregivers to stroke survivors from the hospital to home. *Patient Education and Counseling, 70*(3), 305–314.

Cancer Research and Prevention Foundation. (2005). *About colorectal cancer.* Retrieved June 11, 2005, from http://www.preventcancer.org

Castellucci, D. R. (2004). Perceptions of autonomy in post-stroke elderly clients. *Rehabilitation Nursing, 29*(1), 24–29.

Centers for Disease Control and Prevention. (1990). *Prevention and control of tuberculosis in facilities providing long-term care to the elderly: Recommendations of the Advisory Committee for Elimination of Tuberculosis.* Retrieved May 23, 2005, from http://www.cdc.gov/niosh/topics/tb/

Centers for Disease Control and Prevention. (2005). *Diabetes and women's health across the life stages: A public health perspective.* Retrieved June 12, 2005, from http://www.cdc.gov

Centers for Disease Control and Prevention. (2007). *National diabetes fact sheet 2007.* Retrieved December 28, 2008, from http://www.cdc.gov/diabetes/pubs/pdf/ndfs_2007.pdf

Centers for Disease Control and Prevention. (2008a). *Tuberculosis: Learn the signs and symptoms of TB disease.* Retrieved on December 28, 2008, from http://www.cdc.gov/Features/TBsymptoms/

Centers for Disease Control and Prevention. (2008b). *Osteoarthritis statistics.* Retrieved June 20, 2008, from http://www.cdc.gov

Chait, M. (2004). Gastroesophageal reflux disease in the elderly. *Clinical Geriatrics, 12*(4), 39–47.

Cotter, V. T. (2002). Dementia. In V. T. Cotter & N. G. Strumpf (Eds.), *Advanced practice nursing with older adults: Clinical guidelines* (pp.183–200). New York: McGraw-Hill.

Crawford, E. D. (2005). PSA testing: What is the use? *Lancet, 365*(9469), 1447–1450.

Deglin, J. H., & Vallerand, A. H. (2005). *Davis's drug guide for nurses.* Philadelphia: F. A. Davis.

Dunlop, D. D., Song, J., Manheim, L. M., & Chang, R. W. (2003). Racial disparities in joint replacement use among older adults. *Med Care, 41*(2), 288–298.

Easton, K. L. (1999a). *Gerontological rehabilitation nursing.* Philadelphia: W. B. Saunders.

Easton, K. L. (1999b). The post-stroke journey: From agonizing to owning. *Geriatric Nursing, 20*(2), 70–75.

Easton, K. L. (2001). *The post-stroke journey: From agonizing to owning.* Doctoral dissertation. Wayne State University.

Edwards, W. (2002). Gastrointestinal problems. In V. T. Cotter & N. E. Strumpf (Eds.), *Advanced practice nursing with older adults: Clinical guidelines* (pp. 201–216). New York: McGraw-Hill.

Eliopoulos, C. (2005). *Gerontological nursing.* Philadelphia: Lippincott.

Eyecare America. (2005). *Diabetes: An eye exam can save your life.* Brochure: Author.

Films for the Humanities and Sciences. (2004). *The Parkinson's enigma* (DVD). Princeton, NJ: Author.

Fletcher, K., Rapp, M. P., & Reichman, W. R. (2007). Optimal management of Alzheimer's disease: A multimodal approach. Special report published by *Geriatrics.*

Flossos, A., & Kastakou, C. (2006). A review of postherpetic neuralgia. *Internet Journal of Pain Symptom Control & Palliative Care, 4*(2). Retrieved June 27, 2008, from http://web.ebscohost.com/ehost/deliverly?vid=7&hid=112&sid=8ba80619-4e14-896e

Freil, M. A., & Cotter, V. T. (2002). Thyroid disorder. In V. T. Cotter & N. E. Strumpf (Eds.), *Advanced practice nursing with older adults: Clinical guidelines* (pp. 127–139). New York: McGraw-Hill.

Garas, S., & Zafari, A. M. (2006). Myocardial infarction. *eMedicine.* Retrieved June 25, 2008, from http://www.emedicine.com/MED/topic1567.htm

Hain, T. C. (2003). *Benign paroxysmal positional vertigo.* Retrieved March 25, 2003, from http://www.tchain.com

Hain, T. C., & Ramaswamy, T. (2005). *Dizziness in the elderly.* Retrieved June 7, 2005, from http://www.galter.northwestern.edu

Hansson, E. E., Mansson, N.-O., & Hakansson, A. (2005). Balance performance and self-perceived handicap among dizzy patients in primary healthcare. *Scandinavian Journal of Primary Health Care, 23*, 215–220.

Hatzimouratidis, K., & Hatzichristou, D. G. (2005). A comparative review of the options for treatment of erectile dysfunction: Which treatment for which patient? *Drugs, 65*(12), 1621–1650.

Heart and Stroke Foundation of Canada. (2005). *Stroke statistics*. Retrieved October 12, 2005, from http://www.heartandstroke.on.ca

Higashida, R. (2005). *Nonpharmacologic therapy for acute stroke*. Paper presented at the American Stroke Association International Stroke Conference 2005, State-of-the-Art Stroke Nursing Symposium, New Orleans, Louisiana

Hill-O'Neill, K. A., & Shaughnessy, M. (2002). Dizziness and stroke. In V. T. Cotter & N. E. Strumpf (Eds.), *Advanced practice nursing with older adults: Clinical guidelines* (pp. 163–182). New York: McGraw-Hill.

Howcroft, D. (2004). Caring for persons with Alzheimer's disease. *Mental Health Practice Journal, 7*(8), 31–37.

International Foundations for Functional Gastrointestinal Disorders. (2008). *About GERD*. Retrieved on December 28, 2008, from http://www.aboutgerd.org/

Jett, D. U., Warren, R. L., & Wirtalla, C. (2005). The relation between therapy intensity and outcomes of rehabilitation in skilled nursing facilities. *Archives of Physical Medicine and Rehabilitation, 86*(3), 373–379.

Johnson, M. A. (1999). Cardiovascular conditions. In J. T. Stone, J. F. Wyman, & S. A. Salisbury (Eds.), *Clinical gerontological nursing* (pp. 489–514). Philadelphia: W. B. Saunders.

Kalra, L., Evans, A., Perez, I., Melbourne, A., Patel, A., Knapp, M., et al. (2004). Training carers of stroke patients: Randomized controlled trial. *British Medical Journal, 328*, 1099–1103.

Kelley, M. F. (2002). Respiratory problems in older adults. In V. T. Cotter & N. E. Strumpf (Eds.), *Advanced practice nursing with older adults: Clinical guidelines* (pp. 67–82). New York: McGraw-Hill.

Kennedy-Malone, L. D., Fletcher, K. R., & Plank, L. M. (2004). *Management guidelines for nurse practitioners working with older adults*. Philadelphia: F. A. Davis.

Kim, H., & Oh, J. (2003). Adherence to diabetes control recommendations: Impact of nurse telephone calls. *Journal of Advanced Nursing, 44*(3), 256–261.

Kurlowicz, L. H. (2002). Delirium and depression. In V. T. Cotter & N. E. Strumpf (Eds.), *Advanced practice nursing with older adults: Clinical guidelines* (pp. 141–162). New York: McGraw-Hill.

Lefebure, H., Levert, M., Pelchat, D., & Lepage, J. (2008). Nature, sources and impact of information or the adjustment of family caregivers: A pilot project. *Canadian Journal of Nursing Research, 40*(1), 143–160.

Lighthouse International. (2005). *The four most common causes of age-related vision loss*. Retrieved March 30, 2005, from http://www.lighthouse.org

Loeb, M. (2002). Community-acquired pneumonia. *American Family Physician*. Retrieved May 25, 2005, from http://www.aafp.org

Loft, M., McWilliam, C., & Ward-Griffin, C. (2003). Patient empowerment after total hip and knee replacement. *Orthopaedic Nursing, 22*(1), 42–47.

Lutz, B. J. (2004). Determinants of discharge destination for stroke patients. *Rehabilitation Nursing, 29*(5), 154–163.

Maciazek, W., Osinski, W., Szeklicki, R., & Stempliwski, R. (2007). Effect of tai chi on body balance: Randomized controlled trial in men with osteopenia or osteoporosis. *American Journal of Chinese Medicine, 35*(1), 1–9.

Macular Degeneration Foundation. (2005). *As therapy for macular degeneration, regenerating retinal cells moves several steps closer to reality*. Retrieved March 28, 2005, from http://www.eyesight.org

Mannion, E. (2008a). Alzheimer's disease: The psychological and physical effects of the caregivers' role. Part 1. *Nursing Older People, 20*(4), 27–32.

Mannion, E. (2008b). Alzheimer's disease: The psychological and physical effects of the caregivers' role. Part 2. *Nursing Older People, 20*(4), 33–38.

Manuchehri, K., & Kirby, G. R. (2003). Vitreous haemorrhage in elderly patients: Prevention and management. *Drugs & Aging, 20*(9), 655–661.

Maschak-Carey, B. J., Bourne, P. K., & Brown-Gordon, I. (2002). Diabetes mellitus. In V. T. Cotter & N. E. Strumpf (Eds.), *Advanced practice nursing with older adults: Clinical guidelines* (pp. 103–125). New York: McGraw-Hill.

Mauk, K. L. (2004). Pharmacology update: Antiepileptic drugs. *ARN Network, 20*(5), 3, 11.

Mauk, K. L. (2005). Preventing constipation in older adults. *Nursing2005, 35*(6), 22–23.

Mayo Clinic. (2004). *Bladder cancer*. Retrieved April 1, 2005, from http://www.mayoclinic.com

Mayo Clinic. (2005). *Osteoarthritis*. Retrieved October 16, 2005, from http://www.mayoclinic.com.

McGrory, A., & Remington, R. (2004). Optimizing the functionality of clients with age-related macular degeneration. *Rehabilitation Nursing, 29*(3), 90–94.

Mead, M. (2005). Assessing men with prostate problems: A practical guide. *Practice Nurse, 29*(6), 45–50.

Medline Plus. (2005a). *GERD*. Retrieved April 28, 2005, from http://www.nlm.nih.gov/medlineplus/gerd.html

Medline Plus. (2005b). *Prostate cancer*. Retrieved April 28, 2005, from http://www.nlm.nih.gov/medlineplus/prostatecancer.html

Moore, R. A., Derry, S., Makinson, T., & McQuay, H. J. (2005). Tolerability and adverse events in clinical trials of celecoxib in osteoarthritis and rheumatoid arthritis: Systematic review and meta-analysis of information from company clinical trial reports. *Arthritis Research and Therapy, 7*, 644–665.

Morris, H. (2006). Dysphagia in the elderly—A management challenge for nurses. *British Journal of Nursing, 15*(15), 558–562.

Mumma, C. (1986). Perceived losses following stroke. *Rehabilitation Nursing, 11*(3), 19–24.

National Breast Cancer Foundation. (2005). *Breast cancer*. Retrieved October 12, 2005, from http://www.nationalbreastcancer.org

National Cancer Institute. (2005). *General information about bladder cancer*. Retrieved April 1, 2005, from http://www.cancer.gov/cancerinfo

National Cancer Institute. (2008a). *Cancer fact sheet. Colon and rectal cancer*. Retrieved June 30, 2008, from http://www.nci.org

National Cancer Institute. (2008b). *Esophageal cancer*. Retrieved June 22, 2008, from http://www.nci.org

National Conference of Gerontological Nursing Practitioners & National Gerontological Nursing Association. (2008a). Current treatment options and management strategies in Alzheimer's disease and related dementias. *Counseling Points, 1*(1), 4–13.

National Conference of Gerontological Nursing Practitioners & National Gerontological Nursing Association. (2008b). Current treatment options and management strategies in Alzheimer's disease and related dementias. *Counseling Points, 1*(3), 4–12.

National Diabetes Education Program. (2004). *Guiding principles for diabetes care: For health care providers*. Retrieved on December 28, 2008, from http://www.ndep.nih.gov/diabetes/pubs/GuidPrin_HC_Eng.pdf

National Diabetes Survey. (2007). *National diabetes survey*. Retrieved June 27, 2008, from http://www.nationaldiabetessurvey.org

National Eye Institute, U.S. National Institutes of Health. (2005). *Diabetic retinopathy: What you should know*. Retrieved March 30, 2005, from http://www.nei.nih.gov/health/diabetic/retinopathy.asp#1

National Institute of Arthritis and Musculoskeletal and Skin Diseases. (2003). *Scientists identify two key risk factors for hip replacement in women*. Retrieved June 12, 2005, from http://www.niams.nih.gov

National Institute of Neurological Disorders and Stroke. (2005). *NINDS shingles information page*. Retrieved June 12, 2005, from http://www.ninds.nih.gov

National Institute of Neurological Disorders and Stroke. (2008). *Parkinson's disease*. Retrieved June 20, 2008, from http://www.ninds.nih.gov

National Institutes of Health. (2005). *Essential hypertension*. Retrieved October 12, 2005, http://www.nlm.nih.gov/medlineplus/ency/article/000153.htm

National Institutes of Health. (2008). *The seventh report of the Joint National Committee on Prevention, Detection, Evaluation, and Treatment of High Blood Pressure (JNC 7)*. Retrieved June 25, 2008, from http://www.nhlbi.nih.gov/guidelines/hypertension/

National Institutes of Health, Seniors' Health. (2008). *Cancer facts*. Retrieved June 24, 2008, from http://www.nih.gov

National Osteoporosis Foundation. (2008). *Fast facts on osteoporosis*. Retrieved December 28, 2008, from http://www.nof.org/professionals/Fast_Facts_Osteoporosis.pdf

Page, S. J., Levine, P., & Leonard, A. C. (2005). Effects of mental practice on affected limb use and function in chronic stroke. *Archives of Physical Medicine and Rehabilitation, 86*(3), 399–402.

Paun, O., Farran, C. J., Perraud, S., & Loukissa, D. A. (2004). Successful caregiving of persons with Alzheimer's disease: Skill development over time. *Alzheimer's Care Quarterly, 5*(3), 241–251.

Pierce, L. L., Gordon, M., & Steiner, V. (2004). Families dealing with stroke desire information about self-care needs. *Rehabilitation Nursing, 29*(1), 14–17.

Pierce, L. L., Steiner, V., Govoni, A. L., Hicks, B., Cervantez Thompson, T. L., & Friedemann, M. L. (2004). Internet-based support for rural caregivers of persons with stroke shows promise. *Rehabilitation Nursing, 29*(3), 95–99.

Podolsky, M. M. (1998). Exposing glaucoma. *Postgraduate Medicine, 103*(5), 131–152.

Resnick, B. (2005). *Differentiating between and treating delirium, depression, and dementia in older adults*. Retrieved May 25, 2005, from http://www.aanp.org

Reuben, D. B., Herr, K. A., Pacala, J. T., Pollock, B. G., Potter, J. F., & Semla, T. P. (2003). *Geriatrics at your fingertips (6th ed.)*. Malden, MA: American Geriatrics Society.

Reuben, D. B., Herr, K. A., Pacala, J. T., Pollock, B. G., Potter, J. F., & Semla, T. P. (2004). *Geriatrics at your fin-*

gertips (7th ed.). Malden, MA: American Geriatrics Society.

Reuben, D. B., Herr, K. A., Pacala, J. T., Pollock, B. G., Potter, J. F., & Semla, T. P. (2008). *Geriatrics at your fingertips (10th ed.).* Malden, MA: American Geriatrics Society.

Rissner, N., & Murphy, M. (2005). Cervical cancer in older women. *Nurse Practitioner, 30*(3), 61–62.

Rochette, A., Korner-Bitensky, N., & Lavasseur, M. (2006). Optimal participation: A reflective look. *Disability and Rehabilitation, 28*(19), 1231–1235.

Rowan, J., & Tuchman, L. (2003). Management of seizures in the elderly. *Seizure Management, 2*(4), 10–16.

Seftel, D. (2005). *Adult macular degeneration*. Retrieved March 28, 2005, from http://www.eyesight.org

Showalter, A., Burger, S., & Salyer, J. (2000). Patients' and their spouses' needs after total joint arthroplasty: A pilot study. *Orthopaedic Nursing, 19*(1), 49–58.

Smith, R. A., Cokkinides, V., & Eyre, H. J. (2003). *American Cancer Society guidelines for early detection of cancer*. Retrieved April 27, 2005, from http://caonline.amcancersoc.org

Snowden, D. (2004). *Testimony of Dr. David Snowden*. Retrieved October 13, 2005, from http://www.alz.org/advocacy/wherewestand/20040323DS.asp

Spitz, M. (2005). Epilepsy in the elderly. *Epilepsy/Professionals Spotlight, 2*(2), 1–2.

Starr, C. E., Guyer, D. R., & Yannuzzi, L. A. (1998). Age-related macular degeneration. *Postgraduate Medicine, 103*(5), 153–166.

Stefanacci, R. G. (2007, March/April). Let's not lose sight of residents' visual health. *Assisted Living Consult*, 23–26.

Steiner, V., Pierce, L., Drahuschak, S., Nofziger, E., Buchanan, D., & Szirony, T. (2008). Emotional support, physical help and health of caregivers of stroke survivors. *Journal of Neuroscience Nursing, 40*(1), 48–54.

Stotts, N. A., & Deitrich, C. E. (2004). The challenge to come: The care of older adults. *American Journal of Nursing, 104*(8), 40–47.

Trudo, E. W., & Stark, W. J. (1998). Cataracts. *Postgraduate Medicine, 103*(5), 114–130.

Tully, K. C. (2002). Cardiovascular disease in older adults. In V. T. Cotter & N. E. Stumpf (Eds.), *Advanced practice nursing with older adults: Clinical guidelines* (pp. 29–65). New York: McGraw-Hill.

University of Utah. (2008). *Amputation*. Retrieved June 24, 2008, from http://healthcare.utah.edu/healthinfo/adult/Rehab/amput.htm

University of Washington, Department of Ophthalmology. (2008). *Cataract statistics*. Retrieved June 25, 2008, from http://www.universityofwashington/ophthalmology.org

Uthman, B. M. (2004). *Successfully using antiepileptic drugs in the elderly*. Paper presented at the sixth annual U.S. Geriatric and Long Term Care Congress, Orlando, FL.

Velez, I., & Selwa, L. M. (2003). Seizure disorders in the elderly. *American Family Physician, 67*(2), 325–332.

Warlow, C., Sudlow, C., Martin, D., Wardlaw, J., & Sandercock, P. (2003). Stroke. *Lancet, 362*(9391), 1.

Waszynski, C. M. (2001). Confusion assessment method (CAM). *Try This: Best Practices in Nursing Care to Older Adults*, 13.

Watts, S. A., Daly, B., Anthony, M., McDonald, P., Khoury, A., & Dahar, W. (2001). The effect of age, gender, risk level and glycosylated hemoglobin in predicting foot amputation in HMO patients with diabetes. *Journal of the American Academy of Nurse Practitioners, 13*(5), 230–235.

White, N. G., O'Rourke, F., Ong, B. S., Cordato, D. J., & Chan, D. K. Y. (2008). Dysphagia. Causes, assessment, treatment and management. *Geriatrics, 63*(5), 15–18.

Wiesenfeld, L. (2008). Delirium: The ADVISE approach and tips from the frontlines. *Geriatrics, 36*(5), 28–31.

Wiles, R., Ashburn, A., Payne, S., & Murphy, C. (2002). Patients' expectations of recovery following stroke: A qualitative study. *Disability and Rehabilitation, 24*(16), 841–850.

Wiles, R., Ashburn, A., Payne, S., & Murphy, C. (2004). Discharge from physiotherapy following stroke: The management of disappointment. *Social Science & Medicine, 59*(6), 1263–1273.

Williams, K. E., & Bond, M. J. (2002). The roles of self-efficacy, outcome expectancies and social support in the self-care behaviours of diabetics. *Psychology, Health & Medicine, 7*(2), 127–141.

Woolver, D. R., & Beutler, A. I. (2007). Hypothyroidism: A review of the evaluation and management. *Family Practice Recertification, 29*(4), 45–52.

Yurkow, J., & Yudin, J. (2002). Musculoskeletal problems. In V. T. Cotter and N. E. Strumpf (Eds.), *Advanced practice nursing with older adults: Clinical guidelines* (pp. 229–242). New York: McGraw-Hill.

Zann, R. B. (2005). *Joint replacement in normal joints*. Retrieved June 12, 2005, from http://www.orthospine.com

Zucker, D. M. (2002). Chronic heart disease: An approach for intervention. *Rehabilitation Nursing, 27*(5), 187–191.

Zullo, A., Hassan, S., Campo, S. M. A., & Morini, S. (2007). Bleeding peptic ulcer in the elderly: Risk factors and prevention strategies. *Drugs and Aging, 24*(10), 815–828.

CHAPTER 14

Management of Common Problems

Claudia Diebold, RN, MSN, CNE
Frances Fanning-Harding, RN, MSN
Patricia Hanson, PhD, APRN, GNP

LEARNING OBJECTIVES

At the end of this chapter, the reader will be able to:

- Describe the demographics of medication use in the elderly and the possible consequences of polypharmacy in the older adult.
- Identify physiologic changes of aging and their effects on pharmacokinetics (drug absorption, distribution, metabolism, and excretion) and pharmacodynamics.
- Discuss strategies for minimizing adverse consequences of polypharmacy and enhancing medication adherence.
- Develop an understanding of the complex cost issues related to medications for older adults.
- Describe the demographics and identify risk factors for falls in the elderly.
- List components in the evaluation of a fall and identify interventions for fall prevention in the elderly.
- Differentiate between the myths and facts related to restraint use in the elderly.
- Develop a plan to prevent falls and injuries utilizing nonrestraint interventions.
- Explain the effects of and assess and manage problems of depression and anxiety in the older adult.
- Collect the appropriate data related to a patient's urine control and plan nursing care accordingly.
- Initiate behavioral interventions to treat urinary incontinence (UI) and promote continence for those at risk for UI.
- Discuss the effects of and assess and manage sleep disturbances in the older adult.
- Assess and manage pressure ulcers.
- Develop a skin management protocol to prevent pressure ulcers.
- Assess for dysphagia at the bedside.
- Develop a plan to meet the nutritional and hydration needs of a patient with dysphagia.

KEY TERMS

- Adverse drug reaction (ADR)
- Bladder diary
- Bladder training
- Braden Scale for Pressure Ulcer Risk Assessment
- Chemical restraint
- Deglutition
- Delirium
- Dementia
- Dependent continence
- Depression
- Drug-drug interaction
- Dysphagia
- Established incontinence
- Extrinsic risk factors for falls
- Fall

- Functional urinary incontinence
- Generalized anxiety disorder (GAD)
- Independent continence
- Insomnia
- Intrinsic risk factors for falls
- Medication error
- Mixed urinary incontinence
- Nocturia
- Nonadherance
- Nonrapid eye movement (NREM) sleep
- Overflow urinary incontinence
- Panic attacks
- Partial continence
- Pelvic muscle rehabilitation
- Pharmacodynamics
- Pharmacokinetics
- Physical restraint
- Polypharmacy
- Pressure ulcer
- Pressure Ulcer Scale for Healing (PUSH)
- Prompted voiding (PV)
- Rapid eye movement (REM) sleep
- Recurrent falls
- Restless leg syndrome (RLS)
- Sleep apnea
- Social continence
- Stress urinary incontinence
- Total incontinence
- Transient incontinence
- Urge suppression techniques
- Urge urinary incontinence
- Urinary incontinence (UI)

As the aging population grows, so must nursing's ability to provide care that addresses the unique health care needs and characteristics of older adults. Differentiating disease from normal changes that occur with aging and the early recognition of indicators of underlying health problems allow the early initiation of treatment while recovery is still possible (Amella, 2004). The professional nurse's ability to successfully identify, evaluate, and treat the chronic conditions that hallmark impending illness or impair function is essential to promoting the quantity and quality of life. In this chapter, we will present the diagnoses and treatments of multifactorial conditions that may indicate the onset of illness or result in a decline in functioning, including falls, delirium and confusion, anxiety, depression, urinary incontinence, sleep disorders, pressure ulcers, and dysphagia. To start, we will pay special attention to the problem of polypharmacy, a key causative and contributory factor for many common health problems.

POLYPHARMACY

Older adults take considerably more medications than younger people. Despite the fact that older adults constitute only 12.7% of the U.S. population, they consume 34% of all prescription medications and 40% of all nonprescription medications. Persons ages 65 to 69 years old take an average of about 14 prescriptions per year, and those ages 80 to 84 take about 18 prescriptions per year (American Society of Consultant Pharmacists, 2004). The act of taking many medications concurrently is termed **polypharmacy**. The American Nurses Association Position Statement (1990) defines polypharmacy as the "concurrent use of several drugs."

Implications of Polypharmacy

The consequences of polypharmacy in the older adult range from mildly annoying to life threatening. Multiple medication regimens are often perceived as complicated and expensive, resulting in **nonadherence** to the prescribed therapy. Nonadherence is defined as the extent to which patients are not willing to follow the instructions they are given for prescribed treatments. Additionally, other age-related disabilities may hamper adherence, such as visual/hearing impairments, impaired memory or

> **BOX 14-1 Key Point**
>
> "Any symptom in an elderly patient should be considered a drug side effect until proved otherwise."
>
> Source: Gurwitz et al., 1995.

cognition, or arthritis. Polypharmacy and older age are the two most significant predictors of nonadherence (Bedell, Cohen, & Sullivan, 2000).

In addition to nonadherence, polypharmacy may result in a higher incidence of **adverse drug reactions (ADRs)**. An ADR is a detrimental response to a given medication that is undesired, unintended, or unexpected in recommended doses. More than one-third of ADRs involve older persons, and an estimated 95% of those are predictable and preventable (American Society of Consultant Pharmacists, 2004). Once an ADR occurs in an older person, a higher level of care is usually required to treat the adverse event. ADRs have been shown to increase the risk of mortality and nursing home placement in the geriatric population. Clinical manifestations of ADRs may include varying degrees of nausea, constipation, gastrointestinal bleeding, **urinary incontinence (UI)**, muscle aches, sexual dysfunction, insomnia, confusion, dizziness, orthostatic hypotension, and **falls** (Golden, Silverman, & Preston, 2000).

There is an increased incidence of **drug-drug interactions** in a patient experiencing polypharmacy. A drug-drug interaction may occur when two or more drugs are taken concurrently. As the number of medications taken increases, so does the risk for a drug-drug interaction. For example, a patient receiving two different medications has approximately a 6% chance of experiencing an interaction. A patient taking five medications has a 50% chance of an interaction. Finally, this chance rises to nearly 100% if he or she is taking eight medications (Jones, 1997). As with ADRs, more care is usually required to treat these drug-drug interactions in the elderly.

An elderly person experiencing polypharmacy is more susceptible to **medication errors**, defined as taking the wrong medication or the wrong dose at the wrong time or for the wrong purpose. The incidence of errors in medication administration is increasing; deaths attributed to medication errors rose from 198,000 in 1995 to 218,000 in 2000 (Ernst & Grizzle, 2001).

Hospitalization as a consequence of polypharmacy is more prevalent in older adults. Twenty-eight percent of hospitalizations of elderly are a result of ADRs and nonadherence alone. Related complications that result in hospitalization include electrolyte imbalances, gastrointestinal bleeding, and hip fractures associated with falls. The older patient admitted to the hospital and taking three or more medications for chronic conditions has a 33% chance of being readmitted within a month of discharge (American Society of Consultant Pharmacists, 2004).

With the growing concern surrounding identification and prevention of polypharmacy, the nurse also needs to be vigilant regarding the potential underutilization of some drug therapies in the older adult. A number of studies have illustrated the hazards of underprescribing medications, for instance, beta blockers after acute myocardial infarction (Gottlieb, McCarter, & Vogel, 1998), hormone replacement therapy for osteoporosis prevention (Handa, Landerman, & Hanlon, 1996), or antihypertensive drug therapies (Berlowitz, Ash, & Hickey, 1998). Cleeland, Gonin, and Hatfield (1994) demonstrated the amount of opioid analgesia administered to an older person in pain was consistently less than the amount given to younger adults. Withholding therapy based on advanced age may result in increased morbidity and mortality, and reduced quality of life. Unrelieved pain in the elderly can result in decreased cough, decreased gastrointestinal motility, an increase in negative feelings, a preoccupation with the pain, and a longer hospital stay (McCaffery & Pasero, 1999).

Polypharmacy-associated nonadherence, ADRs, drug-drug interactions, and increased incidence of hospitalizations undoubtedly contribute to increased health care costs, both indirectly and directly. Indirect costs are incurred as a result of treating these consequences of polypharmacy. Direct costs stem from the patient literally spending more to obtain the medications. Health care costs in general are rapidly on the rise. In particular, the single leading component of health care expenditure is the cost of prescription drugs. Prescription drugs were projected to account for 18% of total health care spending in 2008 (Ganguli, 2003). The AARP Public Policy Institute (2004) compared prescription drug prices commonly used by the elderly population between 2000 and 2003 and found that the average annual rate of increase in manufacturer list price far exceeded the rate of general inflation during that same time frame.

Even though Medicare covers virtually all adults age 65 and older, its standard benefit package no longer pays for outpatient medications, which is now offered through Medicare Part D (and is discussed in the following sections). A variety of supplementary insurance options is available to the elderly on an individual basis that may provide additional coverage of prescription medicine; however, even with these options, it is estimated that one-third of the beneficiaries have no prescription drug coverage (Klein, Turvey, & Wallace, 2004). This translates into many patients paying hundreds of dollars out-of-pocket per month for medications they literally cannot live without. Despite potentially severe consequences, some older adults are choosing to forgo prescription medications recommended to them. Mojtabai and Olfson (2003) found that in a 2-year period more than 2 million elderly Medicare beneficiaries did not adhere to drug treatment regimens because of cost. Nonadherence with drug therapy tended to be more common among beneficiaries with no or partial medication coverage and was associated with poorer health and higher rates of hospitalization. Clearly, the high cost of medications is taking its toll on the elderly.

Risk Factors for Polypharmacy

There are a number of reasons why the elderly in particular are predisposed to polypharmacy. Older people often have a myriad of chronic comorbidities (chronic illnesses) requiring medications. Cardiovascular disease and diabetes are just two examples of illnesses that may require a multidrug regimen. In addition, many elderly have their care provided by specialty physicians who may be unaware of the medications prescribed by other health care providers. Often there is little or no communication occurring between health care providers, and patients are getting duplicate and unnecessary medications. There are also health care providers who simply write a prescription because that is what the provider thinks the patient wants. It has been estimated that 75% of all visits to a physician result in a written prescription (Larson & Martin, 1999). At other times, a health care provider may unwittingly get caught up in the "prescribing cascade." For example, an elderly patient taking codeine for moderate pain may experience constipation and nausea. If the prescriber adds a phenothiazine (an antiemetic) and a laxative, the patient may become excessively sedated and experience loose stool that may result in fecal incontinence. Consequently, medications may be ordered to treat those symptoms, and so on. Treating adverse drug reactions with more medication will in turn potentiate the possibility of yet more adverse reactions. Tamblyn, McCleod, Abrahamowicz, and Laprise (1996) reported that adverse drug reactions are treated with another drug in 80% of visits to the physician. One study on drug-drug interactions done over a 7-year period included 909 older patients who were hospitalized for drug toxicity. Researchers found that these elderly were prescribed medications known to cause drug-drug interactions, and that many of these hospitalizations could have been avoided (Juurlink, Mamdani, Kopp, Laupacis, & Redelmeier, 2003).

The consequences of polypharmacy in the elderly are complicated by age-related changes in the body that result in altered pharmacokinetics and pharmacodynamics. **Pharmacokinetics** refers to the absorption, distribution, metabolism, and excretion of a given drug, or "what the body does to the drug." **Pharmacodynamics** refers to the biochemical or physiological interactions of drugs, or "what the drug does to the body." The physiological responses to medications are often altered in the older person. The responses to some medications are exaggerated; however, the responses to other medications are often suppressed. See **Table 14-1** for a more detailed description of these age-related changes and their clinical significance.

Recognizing that some medications should be avoided in the elderly because their potential risks outweigh their potential benefits, experts in geriatric medicine and pharmacy have developed explicit criteria for inappropriate drug use in nursing home patients (Beers et al., 1991). These criteria identify medications likely to create problems in the elderly and were developed to predict when the potential for adverse outcomes is greater than the potential for benefit. Beers (1997) updated the original criteria to include elderly patients in all settings (outpatient, inpatient, and nursing homes). Many medications have a high potential for serious adverse outcomes in the elderly; these are described in Chapter 8. The nurse, primary care provider, and pharmacist should refer to the updated list that can be found online (see **Box 14-2**) when considering medication administration in the elderly.

TABLE 14-1 Age-Related Changes Affecting Pharmacokinetics and Pharmacodynamics

Pharmacokinetics	Physiologic Change	Clinical Significance
Absorption	No significant changes in gastric pH; decreased absorptive surface and splanchnic blood flow	Little significance; possibly delayed onset of action and peak effect of medications
Distribution	Increased body fat	Increased volume of distribution of lipid-soluble drugs (e.g., benzodiazepines, barbiturates, phenothiazines, and phenytoin [Dilantin]), resulting in prolonged half-life
	Decreased water compartment	Higher levels of water-soluble drugs (e.g., digoxin and theophylline), increasing risk for toxicity
	Decreased lean body mass	Because creatinine is formed from muscle mass and muscle mass decreases with age, serum creatinine normally decreases with age; therefore, a serum creatinine level of ≤1.2 mg/dl could erroneously be perceived as WNL when in fact renal impairment exists; urine creatinine clearance is a better indicator of renal function in the elderly
	Decreased serum albumin	Risk for toxicity of highly protein-bound drugs due to more free drug circulating
Metabolism	Decreased liver mass and hepatic blood flow	Slowed metabolism, increasing half-life
Excretion	Creatinine clearance reduced	Less efficiently excreted drugs, increasing half-life
Pharmacodynamics	Variable receptor response	Increased response with some drugs (e.g., opiates and benzodiazepines) and decreased response with others (e.g., beta agonists and antagonists)

SOURCE: Dharmarajan & Tota, 2000.

Interventions/Strategies for Care

Nurses play a key role in effective drug therapy. They can implement a number of strategies to enhance medication adherence, minimize adverse consequences of polypharmacy, and in turn improve patient outcomes.

The nurse should be knowledgeable about drug therapy in the elderly and the medications the

BOX 14-2 Web Exploration

An AARP survey (2004) reported that 71% of older adults found paying for prescriptions to be problematic. For more information on medication use in the elderly, see http://www.aarp.org/ppi/.

Review the Web site *Potentially harmful drugs in the elderly: Beers list and more* online at http://www.fmda.org/beers.pdf.

individual patient is taking. Becoming familiar with the medications that have been identified as problematic for the elderly is a good starting point. When medications are being administered that have a high potential for adverse reactions, the nurse should be vigilant about monitoring for adverse effects as well as evaluating the therapeutic effect.

To obtain a comprehensive medication profile when gathering a history, in addition to asking the name, purpose, dose, and administration parameters for each medication taken, also ask the following:

- Do you use over-the-counter (OTC) medications, including vitamins, dietary supplements, or herbal preparations?
- How many alcoholic beverages do you drink a week?
- Do you ever borrow medications?
- How many health care providers are involved in your care?
- Do you request refills without seeing your health care provider?
- Do you have prescription medications from more than one health care provider?
- Do you have prescriptions filled at more than one pharmacy?
- Do you have any vision or hearing problems?

Monitor the patient's serum blood urea nitrogen (BUN) and creatinine because the excretion of most drugs depends on adequately functioning kidneys. However, keep in mind that because lean body mass decreases with advancing age, the serum creatinine level tends to overestimate the older adult's ability to excrete a particular medication. A more accurate measure of renal excretion is the creatinine clearance (CrCl), which measures the glomerular filtration rate (GFR), the number of milliliters of filtrate made by the kidneys per minute. Normal CrCl in males is 107–139 ml/min (or 1.78–2.32 ml/s) and in females is 87–107 ml/min (or 1.45–1.78 ml/s). Values decrease 6.5 ml/min/decade of life because of decreased GFR (Pagana & Pagana, 2005). The Cockroft-Gault (1976) formula should be used to estimate creatinine clearance in older adults. (See **Box 14-3**.)

In comparing and contrasting serum creatinine and CrCl, consider two men with a serum creatinine of 1 mg/dl who both weigh 72 kg (158.7 lb). The first man is 25 years old and the second man is 85 years old. Even though their serum creatinine is the same, their CrCl is significantly different. This difference is especially important with drugs that have a narrow therapeutic index and significant renal excretion.

In addition to monitoring renal function, the nurse should monitor the patient's liver function tests (LFT), aspartate aminotransferase/AST (normal = 0–35 units/l), alanine aminotransferase/ALT (normal = 4–36 units/l), alkaline phosphatase/ALP (normal = 30–120 units/l), and bilirubin (normal = 0.3–1.0 mg/dl). An elevation in LFTs could result in a prolonged half-life of the medication because it is cleared very slowly from the body. As a result, toxicity is a possible outcome of impaired liver metabolism.

Maintain a high index of suspicion. When a patient acquires new symptoms, consider the

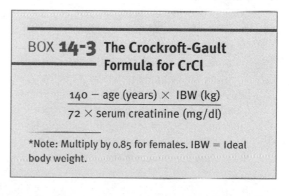

BOX 14-3 The Crockroft-Gault Formula for CrCl

$$\frac{140 - \text{age (years)} \times \text{IBW (kg)}}{72 \times \text{serum creatinine (mg/dl)}}$$

*Note: Multiply by 0.85 for females. IBW = Ideal body weight.

possibility of an ADR until proven otherwise. An alteration in thought processes or behavior (restlessness, irritability, and confusion) may be the first sign of drug toxicity.

Take measures to help simplify and streamline a medication regimen. Use doses with once daily or twice daily dosing, because the less frequent the dosing, the higher the probability of adherence. Avoid alternate day therapy when possible because this can be confusing to the patient. Review regimens regularly and revise as needed, based on patient compliance, satisfaction, and response to the regimen.

Always consider nonpharmacologic approaches (e.g., lifestyle modification) instead of or in addition to drug treatment. For instance, constipation can often be successfully managed with diet and fluid intake rather than laxatives and stool softeners. There is a growing body of evidence identifying effective behavioral interventions to promote continence, safety, relaxation, and sleep. Nonpharmacologic approaches to the treatment of the common health care problems addressed in this chapter are identified and explained in each section.

Ensure that the patient/caregiver is an informed consumer. Encourage the patient and/or caregiver to learn about the medications they are taking. Advise them to ask questions and read package inserts so that they will know the desired therapeutic effects as well as potential ADRs, the correct way to take the medication properly, and potential drug-drug and drug-diet interactions. Suggest that they consider all new medications as trial therapy until the patient and the health care provider determine that they work safely and are effective. Recognize that new symptoms may not be from old age, but from the drugs being taken.

Instruct the patient to obtain all medications (prescription and nonprescription) at one pharmacy so that pharmacists can check for potentially dangerous interactions. The pharmacist can serve as the central figure who maintains a list of medications and screens for drug-drug interactions to avoid harmful situations. Encourage the patient or caregiver to know the pharmacist on a first-name basis. Explain that patients should "brown bag" medications (including prescription and nonprescription medicines, vitamins, and herbal supplements) with every office visit so that the health care provider can review and document medications taken. Suggest the patient invent a system to remember to take medications. Use meals or bedtime as cues for remembering. Drug-taking routines should take into account whether the medicine works better on an empty or a full stomach. Consider using pill boxes, schedules, and/or calendars.

If there are no children or cognitively impaired individuals in the household, the nurse may suggest easy-to-open (nonchildproof) containers. Nonchildproof lids must be requested. Encourage the older person to ask for large type labels or to use a magnifying glass under a bright light to read labels. Large print written instructions should also be requested when needed. Discourage pill sharing and pill hoarding. Medication cabinets should be checked at least annually for outdated medications and medications no longer needed. A home health nurse, family member, or friend may be enlisted to assist the older person with this safety check.

A number of strategies are available to help the patient stretch his or her prescription dollars. When a new prescription is ordered, suggest the patient ask for free drug samples from the physician. If the patient develops undesirable side effects from the medication and has to switch, he or she won't be stuck with a costly bottle of medicine. Encourage the patient to ask for a senior citizen discount at the pharmacy. Generic equivalents and store or discount brand products save money. Be sure the patient understands his or her current drug coverage. Health benefit information can be very confusing.

BOX **14-4** Key Point

Start lower and go slower with new medications.

When initiating pharmacological treatment for chronic or mild disorders in the elderly, the starting dose should be a lower effective dose. If after a predetermined amount of time this dose is not adequate to produce the desired effect, the dose then should be increased slowly until the therapeutic effect is achieved, monitoring closely for ADRs.

Resources

The passage of the Medicare Prescription Drug, Improvement, and Modernization Act of 2003 changed prescription medication accessibility for the elderly. In 2004 and 2005, a prescription discount card was made available to eligible beneficiaries. The card yielded a potential average savings of between 10% and 25% per prescription. In 2006, a full-scale drug benefit replaced the prescription discount card. It allowed beneficiaries to voluntarily sign up with a private plan that offers drug coverage, or sign up for a stand-alone drug benefit. This drug coverage is subject to a monthly premium that varies depending on the type of health insurance in place and the plan chosen. Persons will also pay an annual premium for this benefit as well as a co-pay for the medications, which also varies depending on the plan. Persons with limited financial resources may qualify for additional assistance with obtaining medications through the Medicare prescription drug plan program. Most Medicare drug plans have a coverage gap that occurs when the person has spent a certain amount on medication coverage. In the coverage gap, older adults will have to pay all costs out of pocket until they reach the limit set by their plan. So, for example, if Mrs. Jones has used the amount of drug coverage allowed by her plan and falls within the gap, say hers is between $2,700 and $4,700, she will pay up to the $4,700 out of pocket, after which she will pay a small co-pay and Medicare will pick up the rest after the coverage gap has ended. Medicare Part D especially benefits those with extremely high monthly medication costs. More information can be obtained at http://www.medicare.gov/pdp-basic-information.asp#howmpdc.

Another option for the elderly in financial need is to consider a medication assistance program (MAP). Typically sponsored by pharmaceutical companies, a MAP provides a particular brand of medication at little or no cost to patients who meet certain financial criteria and do not have insurance coverage for prescription drugs. Even though most MAPs require some physician involvement in the application process, nurses can act as advocates to initiate the referral. An Internet site that serves as a directory for these MAPs is http://www.needymeds.com.

In response to the high cost of prescription medications in this country, some people have opted to obtain medications from mail order pharmacies. These pharmacies may be out of state or outside the United States. Depending on the prescription, medications can be bought for a fraction of the cost of purchasing them at the local pharmacy. Critics argue that the lack of regulatory standards puts consumers at risk. Proposals in legislation continue that would legalize the safe importation of prescription drugs, beginning with those from Canada. The AARP states, "though not a final solution to the problem of high drug cost, the safe importation of prescription drugs will help put downward pressure on prices and help individuals secure a degree of savings" (2004, p. 3).

The use of multiple drugs is indicated and appropriate for some medical conditions. However, in the older adult, where it is most prevalent, polypharmacy can cause more harm than good. The nurse plays a key role in making sure the older adult gets the most from his or her drug therapy. It is the nurse's responsibility to be knowledgeable about the medications administered, to astutely assess the patient's response to the drug therapy, and to educate the patient about his or her medication regimen. Nursing intervention can prevent or minimize many of the multiple complications of polypharmacy, such as falls.

FALLS

A fall is defined as "an event which results in a person unintentionally coming to rest on the ground or another lower level; not as a result of a major intrinsic event (such as a stroke) or overwhelming hazard" (Tinetti, Speechley, & Ginter, 1988, p. 1703). For millions of older Americans, falls present a serious health risk. More than one-third of adults ages 65 years and older fall each year (Hausdorff, Rios, & Edelber, 2001). Falls among older adults are not a normal consequence of aging. They are considered a geriatric syndrome most often due to multiple predisposing factors and intrinsic and extrinsic risks (Rubenstein & Josephson, 2006).

Implications of Falls

Falls can result in injury, loss of independence, reduced quality of life, and death in the elderly.

Fractures are the most serious health consequence of falls. Of those who fall, 20–30% suffer moderate to severe injuries such as hip fractures or hip traumas. Eighty-seven percent of all fractures among older adults are due to falls. The most common fractures are of the vertebrae, hip, forearm, leg, ankle, pelvis, upper arm, and hand (Scott, 1990). At least 50% of elderly persons who were ambulatory before fracturing a hip do not recover their prefracture level of mobility (Beers & Berkow, 2005). Falls rank as the eighth leading cause of unintentional injury for older Americans and were responsible for more than 16,000 deaths in 2006 (Centers for Disease Control and Prevention [CDC], 2007).

In addition to fractures, over 50% of falls among elderly persons result in at least some minor injury such as lacerations and bruises (Beers & Berkow, 2005). Quality of life may deteriorate drastically after a fall. If the elderly person remains on the floor for a time after a fall, dehydration, pressure sores, rhabdomyolysis, hypothermia, and pneumonia may result. Elderly persons who fall, particularly those who fall repeatedly, tend to have deficits in activities of daily living and are at high risk of subsequent hospitalization, further disability, institutionalization, and death. Fall-related injuries account for about 5% of hospitalizations in patients 65 years of age or older. About 5% of elderly persons with hip fractures die while hospitalized; overall mortality in the 12 months after a hip fracture ranges from 12% to 67% (Beers & Berkow, 2005). Excess mortality after hip fracture (adjusting for race and age) was 9% in women and 24% in men in the year after fracture, and at 5 years postfracture was 24% in women and 26% in men (Robbins, Biggs, & Cauley, 2006). In 2003 more than 13,700 people age 65 or older died from fall-related injuries. The total cost of all fall injuries for people age 65 or older in 2000 was $19 billion. By 2020, the cost of fall injuries is expected to reach $43.8 billion (CDC, 2007).

Falls that do not result in injury may still have serious consequences. Elderly persons may fear falling again, which can lead to reduced mobility. This reduced mobility can lead to decreased activity, decreased independence, and an increased dependence on others. In addition, decreased activity can increase joint stiffness and weakness, further compromising mobility. Falls are reported to be a contributing factor in 40% of nursing home admissions (Beers & Berkow, 2005).

BOX 14-5 Key Point

In 2001, more than 1.6 million seniors were treated in emergency departments for fall-related injuries and nearly 388,000 were hospitalized.

Source: CDC, 2006.

Risk Factors for Falls

Nurses routinely assess patients and their environment and are instrumental in implementing interventions to prevent falls. In order to accurately assess risk for falls, a comprehensive knowledge of factors that contribute to a fall is essential. Risk factors for falls can be categorized into intrinsic and extrinsic factors. **Intrinsic risk factors** relate to the changes associated with aging and with disorders of physical functions needed to maintain balance. These functions include vestibular, proprioceptive, and visual function, as well as cognition and musculoskeletal function (see **Table 14-2**). Elderly persons who fall in institutions are usually more physically and/or cognitively impaired, and therefore intrinsic factors contribute most to falls and fall-related injuries. **Extrinsic risk factors** are related to environmental hazards and challenges such as poor lighting, stairs, clutter, and throw rugs. Extrinsic factors are implicated in up to 50% of all falls in the elderly in community settings (Beers & Berkow, 2005). In institutionalized patients, the use of restraints and bed rails may increase the risk of falls because patients attempt to free themselves from these constraints.

Among the elderly living in the community, most falls occur during usual activities such as walking. Indoor falls occur most often in the bathroom, bedroom, and kitchen. About 10% of falls occur on stairs, with descent being more hazardous than ascent. The first and last steps are the most dangerous. Common sites of outdoor falls are curbs and steps. In institutions, the most common sites of

TABLE 14-2 Risk Factors for Falls

Intrinsic Factors	Extrinsic Factors
Cognitive impairment	Poor lighting
Medication/alcohol	Poor color distinction
Impaired mobility	Cluttered environment
Fall history	Unfamiliar environment
Acute or chronic illness	Stairs
Elimination problems	Throw rugs
Sensory defects	Unsuitable footwear
Frailty	Restraints
Postural hypotension	Side rails

falls are the bedside (during transfers into or out of bed) and the bathroom (Beers & Berkow, 2005). The use of drugs also is a major risk factor for falls; the risk of falling increases with the number of prescribed drugs. Psychoactive drugs are the drugs most commonly reported as increasing the risk of falls and hip fractures. Other medications that contribute to falls include analgesics, antihypertensives, diuretics, aminoglycosides, and phenothiazines (Beers & Berkow, 2005). The risk of being seriously injured in a fall increases with age. In 2001, the rates for fall injuries for adults 85 or older were four to five times the rates of adults ages 65–74 (Stevens et al., 2005).

Notable Quotes

"Among older adults, falls are the leading cause of injury deaths. They are also the most common cause of nonfatal injuries and hospital admissions for trauma."

CDC, 2006 (from http://www.cdc.gov/ncipc/factsheets/adultfalls.htm paragraph 1)

Fall Assessment

Elderly persons admitted to acute care, rehabilitation, or long-term care settings should have an initial fall risk assessment on admission and at regular intervals throughout their stay (Nicklin, 2006). A number of fall assessment tools are available to assess inpatient risk of falls, but no single tool has been adopted universally. Most tools contain a fall history, an examination of mental and mobility status, a checklist for the presence of sensory deficits, a list of medications the client is receiving, and a list of primary and secondary diagnoses. Two examples are the Tinnetti Performance Oriented Mobility and the Timed Get Up and Go Test. (See http://www.ConsultGeriRN.org for these and other tools.) The Morse Fall Scale is depicted in **Figure 14-1**. To be effective, a fall assessment tool must be short, individualized to the patient, applicable to the setting, readily available to the staff, and have demonstrated validity and reliability. Most important, it must also be followed by individualized interventions to prevent falls specific to the patient. Fall prevention strategies are likely to be more effective if they include a multidisciplinary approach to the process.

In the community setting, elderly patients with known risk for falling should be questioned about falls as part of all their routine screenings. This is necessary because many elderly persons fear being institutionalized and are unlikely to voluntarily admit falling unless they have sustained an injury for which they need medical care. A fall may be an isolated event or recurrent. A **recurrent fall** is defined as more than two falls in a 6-month period (Fuller, 2000). All falls should be carefully evaluated for the underlying cause, but the incidence of recurrent falls is a significant risk factor for serious injury. The person should be asked to describe the circumstances surrounding the fall, such as what activity they were engaged in, the location of the fall, witnesses to the fall, and injuries sustained. The nurse should perform a physical assessment to determine the cause and contributing factors (see **Table 14-3**).

A home visit is important in identifying extrinsic risk factors and planning and implementing appropriate interventions. Home evaluations may be part of discharge planning from an institution or

FIGURE 14-1 **Morse fall scale.**

Criteria:	Circle No/Yes	Score	Patient Score
1. Patient has a history of falling.	No	0	
	Yes	25	
2. Patient has a secondary diagnosis.	No	0	
	Yes	15	
3. Patient uses ambulatory aid:			
None/bedrest/nurse assistant	Yes	0	
Crutch/cane/walker	Yes	15	
Holds on to furniture	Yes	30	
4. Patient is receiving:			
Intravenous therapy/heparin lock	No	0	
	Yes	20	
5. Patient's gait is:			
Normal/bedrest/wheelchair	Yes	0	
Weak	Yes	10	
Impaired	Yes	20	
6. Patient's mental status is:			
Oriented toward own ability	Yes	0	
Overestimates/forgets limitations	Yes	15	
		Total Patient Score:	

Assess the patient for each criterion identified on the scale; circle "No" if the criterion is not present and "Yes" if the criterion is present. Translate the no/yes score into a numerical score and place this number under Patient Score. The score will range from 0 to 125. A patient who scores >25 is at high risk and should have fall prevention strategies in place.

SOURCE: University of Iowa EBP on fall prevention.

conducted during home health visits. A home safety checklist should be used to ensure a thorough evaluation. Important components of a home evaluation are outlined in **Figure 14-2**.

Interventions/Strategies for Fall Prevention

Not all falls can be prevented, but by identifying risk factors and implementing appropriate interventions nurses can play a vital role in preventing falls or minimizing injury. There are a number of strategies for creating a milieu that reduces the risk of falls. Some of the more successful strategies follow.

Modify the Environment

In the inpatient setting, orientation to the environment with an emphasis on safety devices is the first step in preventing falls. Other strategies include non-skid slippers or shoes, hip protectors (Parker, Gillespie, & Gillespie, 2004), removal of obstacles and

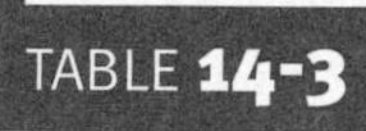

TABLE 14-3 **Components of a Physical Assessment to Identify Intrinsic Risk Factors for Falls**

Physical Assessment	Problem
Pulse	Arrhythmias
Blood pressure	Postural hypotension
Orthostatic blood pressure	
Mental status/LOC/oxygen saturation	Changes in cognition, LOC, hypoxia
Vision screening	Deficits in acuity, depth perception, accommodation, peripheral vision
PERRLA	
Muscle strength	Weakness in one or both sides
ROM in neck, spine, and extremities	Pain, limitation in range of motion
Gait and balance	Deficits in postural control, balance coordination, station, and gait
Gait and movements, Romberg test	

NOTE: LOC: level of consciousness; PERRLA: pupils equal, round, react to light, accommodating; ROM: range of motion

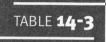

FIGURE 14-2 **Home safety checklist.**

_____ Remove throw rugs.
_____ Secure carpet edges.
_____ Remove low furniture and objects on the floor.
_____ Reduce clutter.
_____ Remove cords and wires on the floor.
_____ Check lighting for adequate illumination at night (especially in the pathway to the bathroom).
_____ Secure carpet or treads on stairs.
_____ Install handrails on staircases.
_____ Eliminate chairs that are too low to sit in and get out of easily.
_____ Avoid floor wax (or use nonskid wax).
_____ Ensure that the telephone can be reached from the floor.

Bathrooms
_____ Install grab bars in the bathtub or shower and by the toilet.
_____ Use rubber mats in the bathtub or shower.
_____ Take up floor mats when the bathtub or shower is not in use.
_____ Install a raised toilet seat.

Outdoors
_____ Repair cracked sidewalks.
_____ Install handrails on stairs and steps.
_____ Trim shrubbery along the pathway to the home.
_____ Install adequate lighting by doorways and along walkways leading to doors.

SOURCE: Ambulatory geriatric care. Rubenstein, L. Z. Falls. In: Yoshikawa, T. T., Cobbs, E. L., & Brummel-Smith, K., eds. 296–304, (1993) with permission from Elsevier.

clutter, having the commode close to the bed, having the call light within easy access, and encouraging use of glasses and hearing aids. The avoidance of physical restraints, such as raised side rails, and maintaining the bed in the lowest position are essential in reducing the severity of falls. Side rails are a common physical restraint that are used to prevent falls but often result in more serious injury because patients attempt to climb over them and may fall from a greater height (O'Keefe, Jack, & Lye, 1996).

Similar interventions applicable to the community setting include removing clutter, throw rugs, and cords and wires; installing handrails on stairs, bathtubs, and showers; using rubber bath mats in the shower and tub; installing a raised toilet; marking stairs and thresholds with fluorescent tape; encouraging the use of eyeglasses and hearing aids; and maintaining adequate lighting throughout the house. Adequate lighting includes installing night-lights throughout the house, using 100-watt nonglare lightbulbs (ceiling lights are best), placing a light switch at the entrance to prevent the elder from entering a dark house or rooms, and ensuring that all stairwells and hallways are well lit to avoid shadows.

Evaluate Gait and Balance

Assess muscle strength and ability frequently and institute appropriate measures for safe mobility and transfer techniques (see Table 14-4). The Tinetti Assessment Tool (Ledford, 1997) provides an objective measure to evaluate gait and balance. Educate patients with gait and balance deficiencies on safety measures such as calling for assistance when getting out of bed. Do not leave patients with gait and balance deficiencies in situations where they can attempt to get up and move without support and assistance; for example, avoid leaving a patient in the bathroom alone.

In the community setting, encourage a regular exercise program to improve balance and coordination, such as tai chi or yoga, based on the individual's abilities. Involve older patients in an exercise program to increase muscle strength, such as low-intensity leg strengthening and weight-bearing exercises. It is important to educate clients on what to do if they fall. Useful techniques include turning from the supine position to the prone position, getting on all fours, crawling to a strong support surface, and pulling up. Having frequent contact with family or friends, a phone that can be reached from the floor, or a remote alarm system can decrease the likelihood of lying on the floor for a long time after a fall (Beers & Berkow, 2005).

If the older person uses an assistive device such as a walker, teach and monitor the proper use of the device. For example, a rolling walker may be safer than a regular walker if the older person is unable to lift the standard walker or attempts to carry the walker. Check the tip end of walkers and canes to be sure they have sufficient smooth tread and replace when necessary. Also make sure all moving parts are clean and any rough edges are smoothed or covered to prevent damage to the skin. Providing hip protectors for patients in institutions with a high incidence of hip fractures appears to reduce the incidence of such fractures (Gillespie, Gillespie, Cummings, Lamb, & Rowe, 2000). However, because they are heavy, are made of polypropylene, and must be worn 24 hours a day, compliance in their use is only between 30% and 50%.

Review Medications

During an inpatient admission is a good time to thoroughly review all the medications the patient is on for desired effect, adverse effect, interactions, and the older person's knowledge base of the medications they are taking. This would include identifying the patient's knowledge of the drug, dosage, administration, and adverse effects, as well as compliance. It is also essential to ask about over-the-counter medications he or she is taking. Patients on four or more medications are at a higher risk for falls (Capezuti, 1996). Special attention should be given to drugs that affect mobility such as sedatives, hypnotics, psychotropics, and antihypertensives. Patients should be taught about interventions to prevent postural hypotension such as changing positions slowly to prevent syncope. When beginning a new medication, elders should be monitored closely, especially if the medication has the potential to affect mobility, balance, and/or cognition. Additional strategies for helping older persons to manage their medications are discussed in the "Polypharmacy" section earlier in the chapter.

Develop a Fall Prevention Plan

Tinniti et al. (1988) found that risk of falling increased with the number of disabilities, but that

TABLE 14-4 Performance-Oriented Assessment of Gait

Components	Observation: Normal = 0	Abnormal = 1	Number
Initiation of gait (patient asked to begin walking down hallway)	Begins walking immediately without observable hesitation; initiation of gait is single, smooth motion	Hesitates; multiple attempts; initiation of gait not a smooth motion	
Step height (begin observing after first few steps: observe one foot, then the other; observe from side)	Swings foot, completely clears floor but by no more than 1–2 inches	Swings foot, not completely raised off floor (may hear scraping) or is raised too high (>1–2 inches)	
Step length (observe distance between toe stance, foot, and heel of swing foot; observe from side; do not judge first few or last few steps; observe one side at a time)	At least the length of individual's foot between the stance toe and swing heel (step length usually longer but foot length provides basis for observation)	Step length less than described under normal conditions	
Step symmetry (observe the middle part of the patch, not the first or last steps; observe from side; observe distance between heel of each swing foot and toe of each stance foot)	Step length same or nearly same on both sides for most step cycles	Step length varies between sides or patient advances with same foot with every step	
Step continuity	Begins raising heel of one foot (toes off) as heel of other foot touches the floor (heel strike); no breaks or stops in stride; step lengths equal over most cycles	Places entire foot (heel and toe) on floor before beginning to raise other foot; or stops completely between steps or step length varies over cycles	
Path deviation, observe from behind; observe one foot over several strides; observe in	Foot follows close to straight line as patient advances	Foot deviates from side to side or toward one direction	

(continues)

TABLE 14-4 (continued)

	Observation		
Components	Normal = 0	Abnormal = 1	Number
relation to line on floor (e.g., tiles) if possible (difficult to assess if patient uses a walker)			
Trunk stability (observe from behind; side to side motion of trunk may be a normal gait pattern; need to differentiate this from instability)	Trunk does not sway; knees or back is not flexed; arms is not abducted in effort to maintain stability	Any of preceding features present	
Walk stance (observe from behind)	Feet should almost touch as one passes other	Feet apart with stepping	
Turning while walking	No staggering; turning is continuous with walking, and steps are continuous while turning	Staggers; stops before initiating turn; or steps are discontinuous	

*Add up numbers in **Number** column to get **TOTAL SCORE:***
A higher score reflects greater risk for falls.

SOURCE: University of Iowa EBP on fall prevention.

modifying just a few factors may reduce the risk. Vassallo et al. (2004) describe a multidisciplinary, proactive approach to fall prevention in a rehabilitation hospital that led to a 15.3% reduction in the number of falls and a 51.1% reduction in patients sustaining an injury. A fall-risk assessment was conducted by the health care team on admission and repeated weekly. At-risk patients were identified with a red armband. Other essential components of a fall prevention program include close routine monitoring, anticipation of needs, offering frequent toileting, bedside commodes, call lights, bed alarms, proper transfer techniques, hip protectors, a regular exercise program, and patient and family education. Treatment of osteoporosis with calcium and vitamin D has resulted in a reduction of fractures and less serious injuries from falls (Gallager, 1994; Gillespie et al., 2004).

The Centers for Disease Control and Prevention (CDC) has funded a number of research studies related to the prevention of falls in the elderly. A description of these studies with related fact sheets and publications can be found at http://cdc.gov/ncipc/duip/FallsPreventionActivity.htm.

Restraint Use

Agitation or confusion caused by delirium is a particularly significant risk for falls (Hayes, 2004). Harrison, Booth, and Algase (2001) reported that patients who experience multiple falls typically have lower cognitive scores. Restrictive procedures were designed to reduce or eliminate maladaptive or unsafe behaviors (e.g., falls, the removal of medical devices, wandering away). However, Tinetti et al. (1988) found that the use of physical restraints failed to prevent falls and was associated with continued fall-related accidents as well as an increase in serious injuries from a fall. Restrictive procedures involve the use of physical restraints and chemical restraints. A **physical restraint** is any physical or mechanical device (e.g., waist restraint, wrist restraint, geriatric chair) that involuntarily restrains a patient as a means of controlling physical activity. A **chemical restraint** refers to the use of a psychopharmacological drug for the purpose of discipline or convenience, and not to treat medical symptoms (Ledford & Mentes, 1997). The deconditioning effect of immobility resulting from the use of a restraint compounded by impaired judgment secondary to dementia were implicated as underlying factors in these findings (Tinetti et al., 1988). Ledford and Mentes (1997) reported 13–47% of older patients who fall in institutional settings are physically restrained.

There are six common myths associated with the use of restraints in the elderly (Evans & Strumph, 1990):

Myth: Elderly clients should be restrained to protect them from falls.
Fact: The risk of falls and injury increases when restraints are used.
Myth: It is a moral duty to protect the elderly from harm by use of restraints.
Fact: Restraints put the elderly at higher risk for problems associated with immobility such as **pressure ulcers**, contractures, and confusion.
Myth: Failure to restrain puts individuals at risk for legal liability.
Fact: U.S. courts are reluctant to hold that there exists a duty to restrain, stating that restraint use is undesirable and decreases the patient's quality of life.
Myth: It doesn't bother the elderly to be restrained.
Fact: Many elderly experience feelings of anger, fear, humiliation, discomfort, demoralization, and punishment when they are restrained (Strumph & Evans, 1988).
Myth: We have to restrain because of inadequate staffing.
Fact: In facilities where restraint-free policies exist, alternatives to restraints appear to consume less staff time than that required by using restraints.
Myth: Alternatives to physical restraints are unavailable.
Fact: Many alternatives exist including companionship or supervision, changing or eliminating bothersome treatment, environmental manipulations, reality orientation, psychosocial interventions, and diversionary and physical activities.

BOX 14-6 Types of Physical Restraints

Wrist and leg restraints
Wheelchair safety bars
Vest restraints
Mitts
Chairs with lapboards
Beds with side rails
Bedsheets
Lap belts

Despite standards aimed at minimal or no restraint use, approximately 15% of nursing home residents spend a portion of the day in restraints or confined inappropriately by side rails. Instead of preventing harm, the use of physical and/or chemical restraints can have an adverse impact on functioning. The use of physical restraints increases the risk for falls, confusion, death by strangulation, and complications of immobility (e.g., contractures, pressure ulcers, pneumonia, UI, and learned helplessness) (Ledford & Mentes, 1997). Falls, hypotension, sedation, tardive dyskinesia, and extrapyramidal and anticholinergic side effects are associated with the use of chemical restraints (Ledford & Mentes, 1997).

A restraint-free environment is the ideal. Nursing care should focus on reducing, and hopefully eliminating, the need for restraints. A variety of interventions have been identified as alternatives to restraints. Providing companionship and supervision from staff, family, friends, or volunteers prevents the patient from being alone. This is most important during the night when patients often become disoriented and wander. Bothersome treatments such as IVs, NG tubes, catheters, and drains need to be assessed for the possibility of being changed or removed. Environments should be designed to decrease confusion, overstimulation, and safety concerns. Examples of this would be lighting that eliminates shadows, low noise levels, beds in low positions with side rails down, accessible call lights, and a quick response to the call light. Reality orientation, therapeutic touch, reality links such as radios and televisions, and active listening are all appropriate interventions to reduce and/or prevent anxiety and confusion. Diversional and physical activities are also helpful in preventing the use of restraints. Other successful interventions include the use of music therapy, pressure-sensitive bed alarms, toileting regimens per the patient's own schedule, placing a sponge ball in the hand to prevent pulling on tubes, giving the patient a picture of a family member to hold, or giving them a small pillow or stuffed animal to hug.

Falls present a serious health problem for millions of elders, often resulting in injury, loss of independence, and a reduction in quality of life. Although all falls are not preventable, identifying an individual's risk factors for falls and implementing appropriate interventions in response to the identified risks can play a vital role in preventing falls and minimizing injuries from a fall. The negative outcomes of physically and/or chemically restraining an elder to prevent injuries are well documented. The ability to minimize injuries and avoid restraints is dependent on the creativity and vigilance of the nursing staff and administrative support. Nurses must strive for a restraint-free environment to prevent physical and psychological harm in the older patient.

ANXIETY

Prevalence

Treatment of mental disorders, including **depression** and anxiety, among older Americans has become a major health need. By 2030, the number of people over the age of 65 with psychiatric disorders is projected to be 15 million. At least 1 in 5 older adults currently suffers from mental disorders, and this number is expected to exceed other age groups within the next 20 years (Jeste et al., 1999). Anxiety is one of the most common mental health problems in older adults and is more common among those with medical conditions and those who live in senior housing (Ayers, Wetherell, Lenze, & Stanley, 2006). The U.S. Surgeon General reported that 11.4% of adults over the age of 55 met criteria for anxiety disorders, with phobic anxiety disorders being the most prevalent in older adults. Nonspecific anxiety rates are reported to be up to 17% in older men and 21% in older women (U.S. Department of Health and Human Services, 1999).

Implications/Relevance of Anxiety

Anxiety is a normal adaptive reaction to new situations or perceived threats and can manifest as tachycardia and palpitations, gastrointestinal disorders, insomnia, and tachypnea. A student may experience this during a class final examination or while performing a skill on a patient for the first time. This physiologic reaction, during which the sympathetic nervous system is dominant, serves to motivate and energize. However, recurring and chronic anxiety can complicate many illnesses, including hypertension, heart disease, chronic obstructive pulmonary disease, and diabetes, and can interfere with activities of daily living. Anxiety in patients with chronic medical conditions significantly increases their duration of disability. The presence of anxiety in the older adult correlates with and predicts cognitive decline and impairment (Sinoff & Werner, 2003). Feeney (2004) measured the relationship between anxiety and pain perception in a population over the age of 65 and found that anxiety significantly elevated acute pain perception. During the relaxation response, the parasympathetic nervous system is dominant.

Warning Signs/Risk Factors for Anxiety

Anxiety disorders include generalized anxiety disorder and panic disorder. **Generalized anxiety disorder (GAD)** is characterized by persistent, excessive worry with fluctuating severity of symptoms that include restlessness, irritability, sleep disturbance, fatigue, and impaired concentration. This disorder typically manifests early in life, but is a chronic condition that continues into the later adult years. Many individuals with GAD also have significant depression.

Panic attacks are characterized by an autonomic arousal that includes tachycardia, difficulty breathing, diaphoresis, light-headedness, trembling, and severe weakness. Between attacks, the individual spends a great deal of time and energy worrying about the next exacerbation. Genetics appear to play a significant role, with a 20% risk among relatives of individuals with panic disorder. The older adult may experience a decreased autonomic response to emotional states and symptoms may be masked (Mohlman et al., 2004); therefore, cues to anxiety problems may be subtle and easily overlooked. Nonspecific complaints such as weakness, feeling light-headed, or a slight increase in heart and respiratory rates may signal anxiety.

Older adults with chronic medical conditions are at a much higher risk for the development of anxiety disorders when compared to those without chronic illnesses (Beekman et al., 1998; Mehta et al., 2003). Psychosocial stressors and negative life events, such as the death of a spouse, significantly increase the incidence of anxiety in older adults. Catastrophic events in early life, poor subjective health, lack of an adequate support network, loneliness, and perceived vulnerability all contribute to the risk of developing anxiety disorders in later life (Beekman et al., 1998).

Assessment

Instruments available to assess anxiety include the State-Trait Anxiety Inventory (STAI) and the Hospital-Anxiety Inventory. An important concept in using assessment instruments is to determine each one's appropriateness in the specific population. An instrument that has been researched only in the critical care setting may not prove as useful in the community-dwelling population. Nursing assessment should include risk identification, medical evaluation, and careful attention to the client's verbalization of thoughts and feelings. Anxiety and depression are often undetected in the older population, and nurses are in key positions to identify both risks and symptoms of these problems. Anxiety can be the most prominent presenting symptom in depression, and this comorbid psychosis is very common in the elderly (Lapid & Rummans, 2003; Lyness, 2008). Successful treatment increases the quality of life in the older adult; a goal of care should be early identification and intervention.

Interventions/Strategies for Care

Nursing interventions in the acute care setting include instructions prior to painful procedures and in self-management of pain. Many interventions for pain, such as relaxation, breathing techniques, distraction, and cognitive restructuring, can simultaneously decrease anxiety (Feeney, 2004). If patients perceive higher levels of control in any situation, anxiety is reduced. Community and social resources should be identified and made available to those

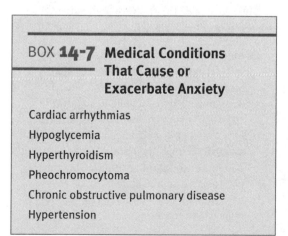

BOX 14-7 Medical Conditions That Cause or Exacerbate Anxiety

- Cardiac arrhythmias
- Hypoglycemia
- Hyperthyroidism
- Pheochromocytoma
- Chronic obstructive pulmonary disease
- Hypertension

BOX 14-8 Drugs That Can Cause or Worsen Anxiety

- Caffeine
- Theophylline
- Pseudoephedrine
- Baclofen

with chronic anxiety disorders. It does not benefit a patient to have a health care practitioner referral if they are unable to arrange transportation or financial support to initiate or continue their care.

BOX 14-9 Nursing Care for the Patient Experiencing Acute Anxiety

Decrease environmental stimuli.

Stay with the patient.

Make no demands and do not ask the patient to make decisions.

Support current coping mechanisms (crying, talking, etc.).

Don't confront or argue with the patient.

Speak slowly in a soft, calm voice.

Avoid reciprocal anxiety. (Emotions can be contagious, and sensing anxiety in the nurse can worsen the patient's anxiety.)

Reassure the patient that the problem can be solved.

Reorient the patient to reality.

Respect the patient's personal space.

BOX 14-10 Deep Breathing Exercises

Have the patient sit in a comfortable chair, with hands on the abdomen. Ask the patient to inhale slowly and deeply, feeling the abdomen rise. Hold the breath for a few seconds. Ask the patient to exhale slowly, allowing the abdomen to deflate. Repeat several times, always speaking in a soft, calm manner.

BOX 14-11 Progressive Muscle Relaxation

The patient should lie down in a comfortable position. Ask the patient to tighten the muscles in his or her hand for a few seconds, and then completely release the tension to relax the muscle. Focusing on a specific muscle by tightening and releasing tension provides a greater relaxation response to the area. Progressively concentrate on the muscles of the arms, shoulders, face, chest, back, abdomen, legs, and feet. Again, use a soft, calm voice to assist the patient through the process.

Medications to treat anxiety include benzodiazepines, selective serotonin reuptake inhibitors (SSRIs), and serotonin-norepinephrine reuptake inhibitors (SNRIs). Adverse reactions with benzodiazepines include drowsiness, fatigue, cognitive and psychomotor problems, confusion, and depression. SSRIs may result in side effects of headache, nausea, sedation, and insomnia. The first line treatment

BOX 14-12 Cognitive-Behavioral Therapy

Cognitive-behavioral therapy assists patients with recognizing cues to anxiety. Once they have identified factors that cause their anxiety, they are able to cognitively "practice" experiencing those situations. Effective coping mechanisms are identified and used during the therapy. When patients encounter the situation in real life, they are able to cope because they have had the opportunity to cognitively review their reactions.

for anxiety disorders is SSRIs, and they have fewer side effects in older adults than the benzodiazepines (which can be potentially harmful and should be avoided).

Individuals of any age often experience anxiety and depression simultaneously. Rates of anxiety in older adults with depression have been reported as high as 47% (Mehta et al., 2003).

DEPRESSION

Prevalence

Although depression is the most common mental health disorder in older adults, it is not a normal consequence of aging. Role changes, major life events, and comorbid illnesses all contribute to an increased rate of depression in the geriatric population. Up to 20% of U.S. adults over the age of 55 experience mental disorders, with depression and anxiety occurring most frequently. In older adults with comorbid illnesses, the rate of depression is as high as 37% (U.S. Department of Health and Human Services, 1999).

Implications/Relevance of Depression

Depression is a significant risk for suicide, and older adults have the highest rates of suicide in the United States. People over the age of 65 comprised only 12% of the U.S. population in 2004, but accounted for 16% of suicide deaths (CDC, 2005). Many geriatric individuals who commit suicide have primary care visits within one month of the suicide, yet symptoms of depression are often undetected or inadequately treated by the medical practitioner. Depression is linked to a decreased quality of life in the older adult, through loss of interest, motivation, creativity, and ability to plan (Fassino et al., 2002). Depressed individuals perceive medical illnesses as having a greater impact on everyday life and have twice the health care costs of nondepressed adults with similar illnesses (Badger & Collins-Joyce, 2000). Older adults with depression have higher mortality rates from coexisting conditions, such as cardiovascular disease and cancer. In an epidemiological study, depression of more than 4 years raised the risk of cancer in older adults by 88% (Pennix et al., 1998). Surgical patients who are depressed have poorer outcomes and lengthier recoveries (Alexopoulous et al., 2002). Therefore, early identification and treatment of depression are of key importance in improving the quality and, possibly, the quantity of life for older adults.

BOX 14-13 Medical Conditions That Increase Risk of Depression

Hypothyroidism	Cancer
Heart disease	Hypertension
Multiple sclerosis	Parkinson's disease
Arthritis	Huntington's disease
Diabetes	Stroke/brain attack

Depression, Dementia, and Delirium

Depression in the older adult can often be difficult to recognize. **Dementia**, **delirium**, medication side effects, and situational grief response can complicate the diagnosis of depression. The American Psychiatric Association (2008) has standard diagnostic criteria for delirium, depression, and dementia. The essential features for delirium include 1) disturbance of consciousness; 2) change in cognition such as memory deficit, language disturbance, or the development of disorientation; and 3) that these changes are of recent onset and fluctuate during the course of the day. Delirium usually arises due to a physiological consequence of a medical condition or medication (Wiesenfeld, 2008). Delirium can often be resolved by altering external or internal factors.

According to Wiesenfeld (2008), delirium can look like many other disorders including sleep pattern disturbances, psychomotor changes, mood and affect disorders, rapid shifts from one psychomotor state to another, delusions (often paranoia), neurologic abnormalities, and personality changes. Delirium may be hyperactive or hypoactive.

Medical conditions that are known to cause delirium may be intercranial or caused by endocrine dysfunction, infections, nutritional deficiencies, electrolyte imbalances, organic encephalopathies, or medication reactions. These disorders can be remembered using Wiesenfeld's IN/OUT approach. Consider causes IN the brain (e.g., stroke, trauma, meningitis, vascular disorder) or OUT of the brain (e.g., endocrine dysfunction, organ failure, infections, metabolic disorders, shock, burns, dehydration, nutritional deficiencies) or consider drugs going IN the body (e.g., opiates, anticholinergic medications, steroids, psychoactive drugs, OTC cold preparations) and drugs going OUT (e.g., alcohol withdrawal, sedative withdrawal, steroid withdrawal, SSRI withdrawal). In detecting and managing delirium he suggests following the mnemonic ADVISE:

A = Advocacy (In this state patients cannot speak for themselves and misdiagnoses are often made unless those closest to the patients advocate for them.)
V = Vigilance (Once the treatment for the delirium begins, the practitioner needs to be very watchful of the patient, monitoring response to treatment.)
I = Integration (Use all resources available to care for the patient. This means using the appropriate pharmacology but also guiding and supporting the patient as the delirium subsides. It won't happen all at once, and this can be very disturbing to the patient and his or her family.)
S = Support (This is a very frightening experience for patients. They know something is not right. They feel the disorientation and may be embarrassed or baffled by what is happening.)
E = Education (Throughout the process, help the family know what is happening; once the delirium resolves, carefully educate both the patient and the family as to the probable cause and how to avoid it in the future—especially if the cause is medication related. Consulting the physician rather than treating a problem with OTC medications needs to be encouraged, as do proper hydration and nutrition.)

Forty-five percent to 59% of hospitalized older adults experience delirium, and in 25% of those cases, irreversible neurological damage or death occurs (Martin & Haynes, 2000). Rapid intervention is of the utmost importance.

Dementia, a group of symptoms accompanying disease, manifests as memory loss; disorientation; changes in mood or personality; and difficulties in abstract thinking, task performance, and language use. Dementia is a gradual, but continuous, cognitive decline. The most common form of dementia is Alzheimer's disease. Other disorders associated with the development of dementia include brain attacks, Huntington's disease, AIDS, and Parkinson's disease (Martin & Haynes, 2000). Antidepressant medications do not improve symptoms of dementia in patients with primary dementia disorders (Raj, 2004).

The American Psychiatric Association (2000) defines depression as a disorder that includes changes in feelings or mood, described as feeling sad, hopeless, pessimistic, or "blue" lasting most of the day, with loss of interest in pleasurable activities. These symptoms represent a change from the person's previous level of functioning. Depression manifests as a loss of interest in life and usual activities, fatigue, decreased concentration and short-term memory, changes in appetite, fluctuations in weight and sleep habits, and irritability and anxiety. Depression, dementia, and delirium can also occur simultaneously, further complicating diagnosis and treatment (Martin & Haynes, 2000).

Assessment

Screening instruments for depression in the geriatric primary care population include the Geriatric Depression Scale (GDS), the Center for Epidemiologic Studies Depression Scale (CES-D), and Self-CARE (D). The Cornell Scale for Depression in Dementia (CSDD) is a reliable and valid instrument

BOX 14-14 Drugs That Can Precipitate Depression

Indomethacin	Digitalis
Diuretics	Cimetidine
Hydralazine	Procainamide
Propanolol	Corticosteroids
Reserpine	Amantadine
Levodopa	Estrogen
Melatonin	

for assessing depression in older adults who also have dementia (Watson & Pignon, 2003). Proper diagnosis and treatment of depression rely on the practitioner's ability to determine underlying medical conditions or medication side effects contributing to or causing the depression. Nursing observations and communication with clients, families, and caregivers are important in identifying older adults with depression and those at risk of developing depression. Many older adults may avoid complaining of sadness or depression. This, along with societal expectations that older adults are more fatigued and less interested in activities, can disguise symptoms of depression and deprive patients of treatment (Amella, 2004).

Interventions/Strategies for Care

Treatment of depression in the older adult is aimed toward remission and prevention of recurrence. Early recognition of risk and appropriate therapy can increase both the quality and quantity of life in the depressed older client. Pharmacological therapy, including tricyclic antidepressants (TCAs) and SSRIs, requires close monitoring because of the increased risk of adverse effects in the older individual. SSRIs are the first choice for treatment of depression in the elderly because they are much safer in overdose and side effects are better tolerated than those of TCAs (Raj, 2004). Care must be taken to avoid drug-drug interactions while considering the older adult's physiological changes in absorption, metabolism, distribution, and excretion of drugs. This is discussed further in Chapter 8. Although older adults respond to antidepressants, their response takes longer than younger adults and they have a higher risk of recurrence.

Venlafaxine, which has a high rate of remission, can cause hypertension, headache, sexual dysfunction, and anxiety. SSRIs can cause sexual dysfunction, nausea, diarrhea, headache, anxiety, and tremor. TCAs have anticholinergic effects, including dry mouth, that can result in an inadequate intake of nutrition, arrhythmias that may be exacerbated in coexisting heart disease, and falls related to orthostatic hypotension.

Serotonin syndrome is a potentially life-threatening condition of elevated serotonin levels. SSRIs, TCAs, and serotonin receptor agonists all increase serotonin and the risk of the syndrome. Symptoms include disorientation, irritability, agitation, anxiety, myoclonus, muscle rigidity, hyperreflexia, tremor, ataxia, hyperthermia, diaphoresis, tachycardia, hypertension, and tachypnea. Treatment consists of withdrawing the medication and managing symptoms.

Cognitive-behavioral therapy (CBT) has the greatest research support among psychosocial interventions for depression (Bartels et al., 2002). This therapy focuses on increasing the awareness of the relationship among thoughts, behaviors, and physiological responses. Symptoms of anxiety and depression are mediated by thoughts and maladaptive behaviors (e.g., tingling of the fingers due to hyperventilation during an anxiety-provoking situation is interpreted as having a massive stroke). CBT uses recognition and relaxation strategies to change these thoughts, and therefore alleviates the anxiety and depression. Individuals are taught to recognize physical symptoms that occur in response to erroneous thoughts and to replace their typical response behaviors and thoughts with those that are more pleasurable and provide the individual with a sense of achievement (Kraus, Kunik, & Stanley, 2007). CBT provides individuals with problem-solving skills that allow them to be active in managing their own mental and physical health.

Nursing interventions that can improve depression include exercise, light therapy, alternative medicine, and counseling (Lam & Kennedy, 2004). Life review therapy, a form of reminiscence, significantly decreases minor depression in nursing home residents, who have much higher rates of depression than their community-dwelling cohorts. Depressed individuals reminisce about their life and reframe decisions and choices made throughout their life (Haight & Michel, 1998). Events or decisions that make the individual unhappy are reintegrated in a more acceptable manner. Mild to moderate exercise releases tension and increases the body's production of endorphins, which can be natural mood elevators. Exercises can be as light as stretching maneuvers such as yoga or tai chi or as strenuous as running, aerobics, or swimming.

URINARY INCONTINENCE

Urinary incontinence (UI) is a common problem of the elderly and has tremendous impact on both the morbidity and quality of life of elderly people (Godfrey, 2008). It is often associated with aging, being female, and particularly as a sequela to bearing children. Although urinary incontinence may be a common problem, it should not be considered a normal part of aging and needs to be evaluated. Urinary incontinence, defined as the involuntary leakage of urine, is a common health problem that affects more than 16 million Americans and may exist in a variety of forms including **stress incontinence**, **urge incontinence**, **mixed incontinence**, **overflow incontinence**, **functional incontinence**, and gross **total incontinence** (Godfrey, 2008; Mayo Clinic.com, 2008). However, it has been estimated that about 80% of adults with UI can experience significant improvement or resolution of their symptoms with evaluation and treatment (Urinary Continence Guideline Panel, 1992). The barrier to realization of this improvement is often a failure in health care to identify those with continence problems, to conduct a comprehensive assessment, and to initiate targeted interventions to address causes and contributing factors. Professional nursing has the knowledge, skills, opportunity, and responsibility to provide beginning continence care: screening patients, performing a basic evaluation, and initiating treatment or referring patients to a specialist if specialized care is indicated (Jirovec, Wyman, & Wells, 1998).

Prevalence

UI affects men and women of all ages, at all levels of health, in all settings. Prevalence estimates vary widely, primarily due to differences in the definition of incontinence, the population studied, sampling approaches, and data collection methods (Godfrey, 2008). It is estimated that about 10% of the total population may experience UI, with the overall prevalence rising to between 30% and 60% of the long-term care population (Royal College of Physicians, 1995). A review of the literature indicates a median range between 30% and 40% among middle-aged women that increases to 30–50% in older women living in the community (Hunskaar et al., 2002). Prevalence rates in men have a similar pattern, although the rates are lower. Prevalence rates range from 1–5% in middle-aged men, with rates increasing to 9–28% in older men living in the community (Hunskaar et al., 2002).

Incontinence may affect up to 43% of acute care patients (Lincoln & Roberts, 1989); prevalence rates in institutions rise to 50% or higher (Hunskaar et al., 2002). Although UI is not a normal consequence of aging, certain physiological changes that accompany aging increase the risk for development of voiding problems, and certain conditions that predispose to continence problems are more likely to occur in older persons. Normal aging changes in the urinary system and their significance in the older adult were discussed in Chapter 6.

Implications of UI

The adverse impact of UI on physical and psychosocial functioning has been frequently discussed in lay and professional literature. Depression and anxiety have long been recognized as potential causes and consequences of incontinence (Dugan et al., 2000; Hajjar, 2004; Heidrich & Wells, 2004; Wells, 1984). Relationships, activities of daily living, socialization, and self-concept are affected by urinary incontinence (Godfrey & Hogg, 2007; Macauly, Stern, Holmes, & Stanton, 1987; Wyman, Harkins, Choi, Taylor, & Fantl, 1987). UI increases the risk of hospitalization and substantially increases the risk of admission to nursing homes in persons over 65 years of age (Thom, Haan, & Van Den Eeden, 1997). Urge incontinence occurring weekly or more frequently is associated with an increased risk of falls and nonspine, nontraumatic fractures in community-dwelling women age 65 years or older (Brown et al., 2000). Incontinence is one of the major risk factors for the development of skin breakdown (U.S. Department of Health and Human Services, 1994).

The economic impact of UI also is significant (Wilson, Brown, Shin, Luc, & Subak, 2001). The cost for management is often an out-of-pocket expense (not covered by insurance) and may interfere with the ability of a person on a fixed income to purchase medications or supplies to manage other health problems.

The nature and degree to which negative consequences result from incontinence are somewhat controversial (Thomas & Morse, 1991). The vast majority of incontinent persons in the community do not seek help for their incontinence because they consider it a normal part of aging (Urinary Continence Guideline Panel, 1992). This raises questions about how people with this problem perceive UI and what determines the significance attributed to the problem. Many noninstitutionalized individuals do not consider incontinence a major problem (Goldstein, Hawthorne, Engeberg, McDowell, & Burgio, 1992; Jeter & Wagner, 1990). However, it is clear that as the degree of incontinence increases the negative impact on lifestyle, and social isolation also increases. It is likely that the total picture of the impact of UI is unknown, because community-dwelling people with UI simply stay home.

Relatively little is known about factors that influence one's perception of incontinence. Women with urge incontinence and mixed incontinence reported more emotional disturbance than an age-matched control group without incontinence, and women with all types of incontinence were more socially isolated than the control group (Grimby, Milson, Molander, Wiklund, & Ekelund, 1993). Other studies support that sensory or irritative symptoms are the most problematic (Wyman, 1994b). The influence of the severity of incontinence on the effects attributed to incontinence is not clear. Interviews with women 31–50 years old suggest the length of time a person has been incontinent influences the impact of the incontinence (Skoner, 1994). Women who had been incontinent longer were more relaxed and spoke more objectively about their incontinence in comparison to those with recent onset of incontinence (Skoner, 1994).

Assessment

An understanding of the types of incontinence and the factors associated with incontinence is necessary to guide evaluation and the development of appropriate targeted interventions. Urinary incontinence is categorized as **transient** (acute) or **established** (chronic) based on onset and etiology. Transient incontinence is caused by the onset of an acute problem that once successfully treated will result in the resolution of incontinence. Multiple causative and contributory factors have been associated with the development or exacerbation of voiding problems, in particular UI. **Table 14-5** lists common transient causes and potentially reversible factors; a brief explanation of the basis for their impact on continence is provided. If transient causes are ruled out or treated and incontinence continues, the problem is considered established and becomes chronic.

> **BOX 14-15 Key Point**
>
> The majority of people with urinary incontinence have not sought help. Health care providers must take the initiative and screen persons at risk.

Chronic incontinence encompasses four basic disorders: stress, urge, overflow, and functional incontinence. Stress incontinence refers to the involuntary loss of urine during activities that increase intra-abdominal pressure (e.g., lifting, coughing, sneezing, and laughing). Stress incontinence is distinguished from urge leakage or overflow incontinence by the absence of bladder contraction or overdistention, respectively. The most common causes of stress incontinence are hypermobility of the bladder neck and urethral sphincter defects. Weakness of the pelvic floor muscles leads to loss of support for the bladder neck and disrupts the normal pressure gradient between the bladder and urethra, resulting in leakage of urine (MayoClinic.com, 2008). Urge incontinence is associated with a strong, abrupt desire to void and the inability to inhibit leakage in time to reach a toilet. Uninhibited bladder contractions usually, but not always, are a precipitating factor. Central nervous system disorders, such as stroke or multiple sclerosis, and local irritations such as infection or ingestion of bladder irritants (e.g., caffeine) are potential causes. Reflex incontinence, a variation of urge incontinence, results from uninhibited bladder contractions with no sensation of needing to void or urgency (MayoClinic.com, 2008). This condition is seen most often in spinal lesions transecting the cord above T10–11. Overflow incontinence refers to overdistention of the bladder due to abnormal emptying. The leakage may be continual or resemble the symptoms of stress or urge incontinence. Overflow incontinence results from a weak or areflexic bladder, neurologic conditions such as diabetes, spinal cord injury below T10–11, or obstruction of the

TABLE 14-5 Transient Causes of Urinary Incontinence

The mnemonic DIAPPERS has been established to list common causes of transient incontinence.

Common Causes	Rationale
Delirium/dementia	Altered cognitive functioning interferes with the ability to recognize the need for toileting or respond in a timely manner.
Infection	The urinary frequency and urgency associated with symptomatic UTI may lead to urinary incontinence.
Atrophic vaginitis/ urethritis	Decreased estrogen in women results in thin, dry, friable vaginal and urethra mucosa.
Psychological	Depression may interfere with an individual's motivation and desire to perform activities of daily living or attend to continence. Anxiety or fear that leakage will occur may contribute to frequency difficulties controlling urge.
Pharmacological agents	Inadequate management of acute or chronic pain can interfere with the ability to attend to toileting needs. Narcotics, a component of many pain management regimens, can lead to constipation and fecal impaction that obstructs the bladder neck, leading to urine retention, overflow incontinence, and urgency. Narcotics can also decrease bladder muscle contraction resulting in urine retention, incomplete bladder emptying, increased risk for UTI, and overflow incontinence. Many medications have adverse or unintended side effects that may directly impact bladder function, bladder relaxation, urinary sphincter relaxation or obstruction, cognitive status (awareness of an effective response to need to void), or urine production. Polypharmacy increases the risk for adverse drug effects and drug interactions.
Endocrine disease	Metabolic conditions (hyperglycemia, hypercalcemia, low albumin states, diabetes insipidus) associated with polyuria increase fluid load on the bladder and increase the risk for urge and stress incontinence.
Restricted mobility	Limited ability to move about interferes with the ability to reach a toilet in time to prevent leakage.
Stool impaction	Overdistention of the rectum or anal canal can obstruct the bladder neck, leading to urine retention, overflow incontinence, and urgency.

bladder outlet or urethra (Urinary Continence Guideline Panel, *Clinical Practice Guidelines*; 1992). Functional incontinence refers to problems from factors external to the lower urinary tract such as cognitive impairments, physical disabilities, and environmental barriers (Urinary Continence Guideline Panel, *Clinical Practice Guidelines*; 1992). Although separate disorders, clinically, patients may exhibit symptoms of more than one type of incontinence. Pure stress and pure urge incontinence were uncommon in a urodynamic evaluation of 263 women and men age 65 years or older (Ouslander, Hepps, Raz, & Su,

1986). The term *mixed incontinence* refers to the existence of the symptoms of urge and stress incontinence at the same time. Diagnosis of the type(s) of UI experienced is essential to the development of interventions that must be designed according to or modified to address varying levels of cognitive and physical functioning.

Variability in the types of voiding problems that may be experienced and the diverse nature of causative and contributing factors necessitate a comprehensive evaluation of urologic functioning. The evaluation recommended by the *Clinical Practice Guidelines on Urinary Incontinence for Adults* outlines the components that should be included in an initial evaluation (Urinary Continence Guideline Panel, 1992). The elements of a basic evaluation are outlined in **Table 14-6** and discussed in greater detail in the following text with respect to the older patient.

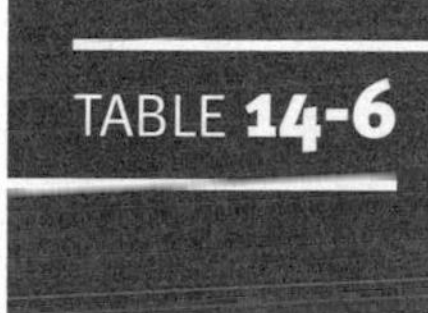

TABLE **14-6** **Components of a Basic Evaluation for Urinary Incontinence**

History
- Focused medical, neurologic, and genitourinary history
- Assessment of risk factors
- Review of medications
- Detailed exploration of the symptoms of incontinence

Physical examination
- General examination
- Abdominal examination
- Rectal examination
- Pelvic examination in women
- Genital examination in men

Postvoided residual volume

Urinalysis

SOURCE: Fantl, J. A., Newman, D. K., Colling J., et al. (1996, March). *Managing Acute and Chronic Incontinence in Adults.* Clinical Practice Guideline, No. 2, 1996 Update. Rockville, MD: U.S. Department of Health and Human Services, Public Health Service, Agency for Health Care Policy and Research. AHCPR Pub No. 96-0686.

History

The first step in the evaluation is a discussion of voiding patterns and problems. Initiating this line of questioning by focusing on usual number of voids during the day and through the night and the presence of other symptoms of voiding problems such as burning, hesitancy, pain, or low pelvic pressure provides a less threatening opening to this topic while securing useful information. It may be necessary to reword questions about the presence of incontinence to determine the occurrence of wetting accidents, their frequency, and volume of urine lost. Asking about the use of padding or protective garments may also provide important clues to the presence of incontinence or the fear of an accident. The onset and duration of voiding problems and activities that precipitate or are associated with their occurrence should be ascertained as well. Of particular relevance is determining the status of bowel functioning and usual bowel habits.

A recall of daily food and fluid intake also provides important information in the evaluation of urological functioning and development of a treatment plan. It is not uncommon for patients with urgency and urge incontinence to report a fluid intake that consists primarily of bladder irritants (e.g., diet drinks, carbonated caffeinated beverages) and minimal to no water. Dietary modifications alone have often significantly reduced urgency and problems precipitated by urge.

The initial interview should help identify potentially reversible causative factors and contributing risk factors for UI. The history should provide clues to the type(s) of incontinence involved. It may be necessary for the patient to complete a detailed **bladder diary** (discussed in the next section) over a period of 3–4 days, noting the information listed previously, in order to obtain a complete picture of factors related to the urinary incontinence.

An awareness of the specific symptoms experienced and the degree of discomfort associated with each can be useful in determining the priority for intervening. Individual responses to incontinence vary greatly (Wyman, 1994b). Identifying those aspects of daily life that incontinence or the fear of incontinence disrupt will help specify outcomes to evaluate the success of treatment. For example, if UI interferes with exercise, then participation in an exercise regimen three times a week might be the goal set with the patient. A specific plan would then need to be established to help the person achieve that goal through management of the urinary incontinence.

Interviews and conversations with persons experiencing incontinence have revealed the difficulty many experience thinking about and discussing this very personal and usually private matter. The use of a tool that provides words and choices for responses frequently facilitates the exchange of information. Short form versions of the Urogenital Distress Inventory/Incontinence Impact Questionnaire (UDI/IIQ) provide objective measurement of the life impact and symptom distress, respectively, of urinary incontinence and related conditions for women. With minor modifications in the wording of some items, the tool can be used with men and can be used from hospitalization through reintegration into the community. A copy of this tool and modifications used with men and hospitalized patients can be found in **Table 14-7**. If the patient has communication or cognitive deficits, information may have to be obtained from or corroborated by family when possible. Previous medical records or observation of current behaviors may be the only source of data available.

Bladder Diary

The bladder diary or bladder record is a critical component of a basic evaluation, regardless of

TABLE 14-7 Urogenital Distress Inventory Short Form (UDI-6) and Incontinence Impact Questionnaire Short Form (IIQ-6)

Do you experience and, if so, how much are you bothered by:

1. Frequent urination
2. Urine leakage related to feeling of urgency
3. Urine leakage related to activity, coughing, or sneezing
4. Small amounts of urine leakage (drops)
5. Difficulty emptying your bladder
6. Pain or discomfort in lower abdominal or genital area

Has urine leakage affected your:

1. Ability to do household chores (cooking, housekeeping, laundry) (daily activities)
2. Physical recreation such as walking, swimming, or other exercise (therapy sessions)
3. Entertainment activities (movies, concerts, etc.)
4. Ability to travel more than 30 minutes from your room or unit
5. Participating in social activities outside your home
6. Emotional health (nervousness, depression, anger)
7. Feeling frustrated

Key to scoring

0 = Not at all
1 = Slightly
2 = Moderately
3 = Greatly

(Information in parentheses are modifications to reflect inpatient activities.)

SOURCE: Uebersax, J. S., Wyaman, J. F., Schumaker, S. A., Fantl, J. A. Continence Program for Woman Research Group. (1995). Short forms to assess life quality and symptom distress for urinary incontinence in women: The incontinence impact questionnaire and the urogenital distress inventory. *Neurourology and Urodynamics*, *14*, 131, 139.

FIGURE 14-3 **A Sample Voiding Diary.**

Your Daily Bladder Diary

This diary will help you and your health care team. Bladder diaries show the causes of bladder control trouble. The "sample" line (below) will show you how to use the diary.

Your name: ____________________

Date: ____________________

Time	Drinks		Urine How much?		ACCIDENTS: Accidental Leaks			ACCIDENTS: Did you feel a strong urge to go?		ACCIDENTS: What were you doing at the time?
	What kind?	How much?	How many times?	Use measuring cups (ml's or oz's)	How much? (check one)			Circle one		Sneezing, exercising, having sex, lifting, etc.
Sample	**Coffee**	**2 cups**		**2 oz or 2 ml**	**sm**	**med**	**lg**	**Yes**	**No**	**Running**
6–7 a.m.								Yes	No	
7–8 a.m.								Yes	No	
8–9 a.m.								Yes	No	
9–10 a.m.								Yes	No	
10–11 a.m.								Yes	No	
11–12 noon								Yes	No	
12–1 p.m.								Yes	No	
1–2 p.m.								Yes	No	
2–3 p.m.								Yes	No	
3–4 p.m.								Yes	No	
4–5 p.m.								Yes	No	
5–6 p.m.								Yes	No	
6–7 p.m.								Yes	No	
7–8 p.m.								Yes	No	
8–9 p.m.								Yes	No	
9–10 p.m.								Yes	No	
10–11 p.m.								Yes	No	
11–12 mid								Yes	No	
12–1 a.m.								Yes	No	
1–2 a.m.								Yes	No	
2–3 a.m.								Yes	No	
3–4 a.m.								Yes	No	
4–5 a.m.								Yes	No	
5–6 a.m.								Yes	No	

the setting (MayoClinic.com, 2008). By outlining the timing, amount, and type of fluid intake with the timing, amount, and continence status for each void, key data are collected to document the severity of incontinence, list any irritating or associated symptoms that are present, identify precipitating events, and detect any patterns to voiding problems (Wyman, 1994a). Bladder record data may be self-reported or completed by caregivers. A bladder diary has been found to be a reliable method for assessing the frequency of voluntary voiding and involuntary incidents of urine loss (Wyman, Choi, Harkins, Wilson, & Fantl, 1988). A 3-day diary provides sufficient data to classify frequency and number of incontinent episodes (Doughty, 2000). See **Figure 14-3** for a sample voiding diary. In the clinical setting, the 3-day diary facilitates the collection of information while allowing patients the opportunity to adjust to the transfer. Patients' and caregivers' participation in the record keeping is advantageous. Many times patients or caregivers completing these records pick up patterns to the occurrence of incontinence and can begin to make positive changes.

The bladder diary is a particularly important source for data to help differentiate factors in nighttime voiding. **Nocturia**, the awakening from sleep to urinate, is a frustrating and common problem for many older persons. Nocturia may result from alterations in normal circadian rhythm of urine output, physiological changes in the lower urinary tract that interfere with storage, or may be an indication of sleep apnea (Donahue & Lowenthal, 1997; Umlauf, Burgoi, Shettar, & Pillion, 1997). Sleep apnea commonly occurs in individuals with cardiovascular disease, and is the root cause of nocturia in this population. Comorbidities of diabetes mellitus and hypertension greatly increase the risk of sleep apnea (Umlauf & Chasens, 2003). Symptoms of the disorder and treatment options are discussed later in the chapter.

Measurement of volume of urine voided throughout a 72-hour period considered with the results of the physical examination and history will help determine factors contributing to nocturia, identify possible strategies for management, and indicate the need for further workup The serious nature of sleep apnea necessitates a careful evaluation of the etiology of nocturia (Pressman, Figueroa, Kendrick-Mohamed, Greenspan, & Peterson, 1996).

Cognitive Status

A client's insight into their voiding status, recall of pertinent health information, and ability to participate in an interview are the first clues to cognitive status. Objective cognitive evaluation may be conducted with the Mini Mental State Examination (MMSE) (Folstein, Folstein, & McHugh, 1973). A more focused assessment of cognitive functioning as it relates to toileting may be accomplished in the 3-day assessment and trial for responsiveness to prompted voiding, discussed under "Interventions/Strategies for Care." The level of severity of cognitive impairment alerts health care professionals to the client's increased risk for persistent incontinence. It also guides selection of options for the first line of intervention.

It is tempting to base the diagnosis of the type of incontinence on the clinical signs and symptoms from the history; however, clinical symptoms alone are not sufficient to determine the pathophysiology of voiding problems (Rich & Pannill, 1999). Focused physical examination of the genitourinary system, rectal area, and neurologic system is a necessary component of the basic evaluation.

Physical Examination

Aspects of a general physical examination with implications for voiding include a focused abdominal assessment, genitourinary assessment, rectal examination, and general examination to detect conditions that may contribute to incontinence such as peripheral edema or neurologic abnormalities that might suggest stroke, Parkinson's, or other neurologic disorders. Gross motor skills (e.g., locomotion, transfer skills, sitting balance), dexterity (e.g., managing buttons, zippers, and toilet paper), and the ability to communicate the need for assistance or reliably respond to verbal or written words must be assessed. Functional deficits and capabilities should be evaluated as barriers and/or assets in continence promotion. Calculating the average time it takes a patient to access a toilet and get on a commode in conjunction with a patient's ability to suppress the urge or delay voiding will help identify therapeutic interventions needed to facilitate continence, goals for the interventions, and the type of continence possible.

An initial and ongoing evaluation of hydration is essential to diagnosing dehydration and minimizing its complications, which range from the local effects on voiding from concentrated, irritative urine to more systemic problems resulting from increased confusion and lethargy that can interfere with all aspects of daily life. Physical parameters of hydration status (e.g., oral mucous membranes, sublingual saliva pool, weight changes, confusion, muscle weakness) may be masked by the deficits of stroke or treatment of concurrent health problems. Monitoring the balance between fluid intake and urine output, urine color, and the specific gravity (SG) for the second void of the day are useful indicators of fluid status. Urine tests are better predictors of a risk for or impending dehydration (Mentes & Iowa Veterans Affairs Nursing Research Consortium, 1998). Urine SG of greater than 1.020 and a dark yellow or brownish-green urine indicate the need for increased fluid intake (Armstrong, 2000). Blood tests such as BUN/creatinine ratio, serum osmolality, and serum sodium are predictors of actual dehydration (Mentes & Iowa Veterans Affairs, 1998). Using height and weight to determine body mass index (BMI) can also assist in identifying persons at risk for hydration problems (BMI <21 or >27) (Mentes & Iowa Veterans Affairs, 1998). In addition, the BMI will provide an indication of the extent of obesity, which contributes to voiding problems.

In women, the pelvic examination should include assessment of the integrity of the perineal skin for lesions, irritation, or inflammation. Evidence of atrophic vaginal changes including pale, thin, dry, friable mucosa and complaints of vaginal itching, dryness, a burning sensation, and dyspareunia should be noted. Vaginal pH levels >5 in women without evidence of a vaginal infection are also indicative of poorly estrogenized tissues (Shull et al., 1999). A urethral carbuncle, a cherry-red lesion at the meatus, is another indicator of estrogen deficiency. Atrophic urethritis and vaginitis contribute to urgency and stress leakage and may be treated with topical estrogen therapy. Women should also be checked for pelvic organ prolapse; prolapse beyond the introitus or that is symptomatic should be referred for further evaluation and treatment. Multiple types and sizes of pessaries are available for correction of prolapse. In men, examination of the external genitalia should include inspection of the skin, location of the urethral meatus, and retractability of the foreskin, if present.

An evaluation of the strength of the pelvic floor muscles is an important component of the examination. However, consideration must be given to the appropriateness of performing an invasive, potentially uncomfortable and embarrassing digital examination, particularly in frail older women or moderately to severely cognitively impaired elders. Lekan-Ruteledge (2004) explains this decision as distinguishing the "nice to know" and "should know" information versus the "must know" information by determining whether the data are essential to developing the treatment plan. If the individual is capable of learning pelvic muscle exercises, adhering to an exercise regimen, and using the pelvic muscles to inhibit an urge or suppress urine flow, a digital examination may not be needed to evaluate pelvic muscle control.

In the pelvic exam, a gloved, lubricated finger is inserted into the vagina and the patient is instructed to contract her pelvic floor muscles against the examiner's finger. One or two fingers are placed in an anterior-posterior plane. The Digital Rating Scale has been found to be a reliable and valid tool to evaluate pelvic muscle strength in women (Brink, Sampselle, Wells, Diokno, & Gillis, 1989). This evaluation also provides key information on the patient's ability to isolate and identify the correct muscles. The strength and duration of contraction of the muscles also may be evaluated rectally in women with vaginal stenosis and in men. If the vaginal exam is not indicated, proceed to the rectal examination.

The rectal examination provides information about the integrity of sacral innervation, pelvic muscle strength, and the presence of a fecal impaction. Resting and active anal sphincter tone is assessed. The ability to voluntarily contract the anal sphincter indicates a functional pelvic floor and intact innervation to the pelvic floor. The presence of sensation of the perineum indicates intact sacral nerve roots for the external urethral and anal sphincters (Schull et al., 1999). This is a particularly important evaluation in diabetics who may experience neuropathy that interferes with normal sensory input, which can result in overdistention and urinary retention.

The digital rectal examination (DRE) is an essential component of the incontinence assessment. In men, the prostate may be palpated proximal to the internal anal sphincter through the anterior rectal wall, noting size, consistency, and tenderness. It must be remembered, however, that prostate size does not correlate well with bladder neck obstruction. During the DRE, strength of the pelvic floor muscles is evaluated and the rectal vault is assessed for the presence of large caliber, hardened stools that suggest constipation or impaction. An impaction must be treated prior to initiating a bladder program.

The abdomen is palpated for tenderness, fullness, or masses that may be indicative of fecal impaction. Bowel sounds are auscultated to evaluate bowel motility. The suprapubic area should also be palpated to detect bladder tenderness or distention.

Difficulties starting the urine stream, intermittent flow, strength of the urine stream, and the presence of postvoid dribbling may be determined in the interview but also may be evaluated directly. The measurement of postvoid residual (PVR) urine volume is recommended in the basic evaluation. PVRs are measured by catheterization or noninvasively with a bladder scanner within a few minutes of voiding. A portable bladder ultrasound is a useful indicator to determine the ability to empty the bladder. The bladder scan's reliability and validity are supported in evaluations in the frail elderly with PVR volumes ≥150 cc (Borrie et al., 2001). PVRs <50 cc are considered normal, whereas volumes >200 cc indicate incomplete emptying. Adding the volume voided and the PVR volume will provide an indication of total bladder capacity.

Urinalysis by dipstick or laboratory testing is a component of the initial evaluation of incontinence. Urine is checked for white blood cells, nitrites, glucose, and blood. Hydration status can also be evaluated with some chemical strips. A UTI should be treated prior to initiation of other treatment for UI. Treatment of a UTI may result in an improvement or resolution of urine leakage, frequency, and/or urgency.

Environmental Resources

The environment must be evaluated as a factor in the development and treatment of urinary incontinence. Structural characteristics; the number, location, and accessibility of toileting facilities; the availability of physical assistance; and adaptive equipment/supplies for toileting are major considerations (Godfrey, 2008). Environmental characteristics of the hospital and potential discharge destinations must be evaluated and compared in the assessment phase. The results should be integrated into the treatment plan to guide the selection and implementation of interventions in order to achieve the optimal level of continence at home.

Goals for Treatment of UI

The goals of treatment for incontinence and the outcomes for evaluation must be addressed and clarified to assist in determining the types of interventions that should be implemented. Understanding the patient's expectations for treatment outcomes and physical abilities provides direction for intervention. The goals of those seeking treatment for incontinence and the conditions for satisfaction with outcomes are multidimensional and do not necessarily require total continence (Sale & Wyman, 1994).

Continence takes several forms, depending upon the conditions or external resources involved in achieving control (Fonda, 1990). Control of voiding occurs on various levels, extending from the loss of control (incontinence) to **independent**

BOX 14-16 Preventing UI Through Healthy Bladder Habits

Encourage all clients to practice healthy bladder habits to minimize their risk for developing UI by reviewing the following strategies:

1. Maintain hydration.
2. Avoid bladder irritants.
3. Empty the bladder on a regular schedule.
4. Avoid constipation.
5. Strengthen and tone the pelvic floor muscles.

continence (control based on the competence of the individual and not requiring the assistance of others). **Dependent continence** requires the physical assistance of and/or reminders from others to maintain continence. **Social continence** refers to situations in which continence cannot be achieved, but urine leakage is contained to maintain dignity and comfort. A category of **partial continence** denotes those situations in which a caregiver's assistance is helpful in achieving continence but is not required all of the time (Palmer, 1996). The effectiveness of interventions can be evaluated more accurately by specifying the level of continence achieved through these categories as opposed to the traditional designation of continent and incontinent. Determination of the effectiveness of the urinary continence promotion intervention must include the degree to which the incontinent individual's personal goals for treatment were met as well as objective measures of changes in the severity of incontinence and occurrence of complications associated with incontinence. The type of continence achieved also must be specified.

Interventions/Strategies for Care

Guidelines for the treatment of different types of UI in specific populations have been developed by national and international panels based on extensive reviews of the literature (Abrams, Khoury, & Wein, 1999; Fantl et al., 1996). The three primary categories of treatment for urinary incontinence are behavioral therapy, pharmacological intervention, and surgery, but treatment also may include lifestyle modification, medication review, and occupational therapy (Godfrey, 2008).

Behavioral management refers to interventions that modify the patient's behavior or environment. Strategies included in a behavioral approach are scheduling regimens, relaxation exercises, **urge suppression techniques**, and pelvic muscle exercises (PME), with and without the addition of biofeedback, vaginal cones, and electrical stimulation as adjuncts to the exercises. Pharmacological treatment involves medications that alter detrusor muscle activity or bladder outlet resistance. Surgical interventions primarily are used to increase bladder outlet resistance and relieve UI and intrinsic sphincteric deficiency or remove a bladder outlet obstruction, relieving overflow incontinence (Fantl et al., 1996).

Behavioral Approaches

Behavioral approaches are recommended as the first line of treatment for urinary incontinence. The clinical practice guidelines identify dietary modifications (hydration and avoidance of bladder irritants), scheduled voiding, **prompted voiding (PV)**, **bladder training**, **pelvic muscle rehabilitation**, and urge suppression techniques as first line approaches in a comprehensive treatment regimen for UI (Abrams et al., 1999; Fantl et al., 1996; Godfrey, 2008).

Behavioral strategies differ in their mechanisms of action, the level of patient participation required, and the technology involved. The interventions are selected for an individual based on the type of incontinence, the mental and physical abilities and limitations of the individual patient, and the environmental resources available (Burgio & Burgio, 1986). The versatility of behavioral therapy enables the care providers to adapt and individualize a treatment plan according to the patient's level of functioning. It also allows changes in treatment approaches that reflect and are congruent with changes in a patient's functional status resulting from recovery and rehabilitation. If successful, behavioral approaches eliminate the added expense and potential risk to health and well-being of an adverse drug reaction from pharmacological intervention and the complications associated with surgery.

Eliminating reversible factors is a first step in treatment in order to optimize urological functioning and the patient's ability to respond favorably to interventions. The results of the evaluation will identify actual or potential risk problems that must be addressed to minimize, prevent, or resolve their occurrence. Of particular concern initially is maintaining hydration, promoting regular bowel function, and removing an indwelling urinary catheter while ensuring the bladder empties completely on a regular basis.

Managing Hydration. Hydration management focuses on maintaining fluid balance. Ensuring an adequate, timely, appropriate fluid intake has long been recognized as essential to a successful continence program. An individualized fluid goal must first be determined. The standard suggested by Skipper (1993) has been suggested as preferable (Mentes & Iowa Veterans Affairs, 1998). To calculate fluid intake according to this standard, take 100 ml/kg for the first 10 kg of weight, 50 ml/kg for the next 10 kg, and 15 ml for the remaining kgs (Skipper, 1993). Because this includes fluid from all sources, to determine the goal for fluid intake alone, 70% of the total volume is used (Mentes & Iowa Veterans Affairs, 1998).

Providing fluids throughout the day will help ensure the fluid goal is met and minimize frequency and urgency that may result from a rapid filling of the bladder from the ingestion of a large volume of intake over a short period. The University of Iowa evidence-based protocol for hydration management suggests delivering 75–80% of fluid at meals and 20–25% during nonmeal times, such as with medications and planned nourishment (Mentes & Iowa Veterans Affairs, 1998). This schedule offers the additional advantage of ensuring supervision is available (if necessary) for patients with swallowing problems. Fluid rounds mid-morning and mid-afternoon, in conjunction with offers of assistance with toileting, have been effective in reducing incontinence and decreasing dehydration in bedfast elderly nursing home residents (Spangler, Risley, & Bilyew, 1984). Fluid breaks can be incorporated into the daily routine. Planned refreshment breaks in a residential program or facility that provide socialization, fluids, and nourishment could be useful and enjoyable opportunities to meet physical and social needs. Fluids should be limited after supper, especially if nocturia is present.

A final consideration in fluid intake concerns the type of fluids consumed, which should be limited to those without a diuretic or irritant effect that provide the appropriate consistency to prevent choking or aspiration. Many common beverages may be irritating to the bladder, causing or contributing to urgency. Carbonated and caffeinated beverages, citrus juices, and aspartame are among the products commonly considered to be bladder irritants. A review of the bladder diary is especially useful in detecting possible agents that precipitate urgency or incontinence. Reducing the intake of caffeinated beverages to two or fewer servings a day is generally recommended for individuals experiencing urgency or urge incontinence (Arya, Myers, & Jackson, 2000). Postum and sun teas are potential alternatives for coffee and tea, respectively. However, water is the better choice of a liquid. Water is not an irritant or a diuretic and will not interfere with diabetic control. If swallowing problems exist, nectars and thick liquids such as buttermilk and V8 juice are acceptable if a mild thickened liquid is needed, according to Cardinal Hill Rehabilitation Hospital. Any liquid may be thickened with commercial products or by mixing it with natural thickeners such as baby food, mashed bananas, or wheat germ (Kain, 2001).

Hydration status should be evaluated on an ongoing basis. A color chart may be particularly helpful in teaching patients and/or caregivers a simple way to self-monitor adequacy of fluid intake. (The color chart is available in the Armstrong [2000] text, *Performing in Extreme Environments*, or may be obtained with the Evidence-Based Hydration Management Protocol from the University of Iowa.)

Maintaining bowel regularity prevents the potential interference with bladder emptying that may result from constipation and promotes fecal continence. Irregular bowel habits, immobility, dehydration, decreased fiber intake, and emotional factors contribute to the development of constipation. Many hospitalized patients identify the lack of privacy and change in daily routines as major factors in their constipation. Planning a set time for defecation consistent with a patient's usual routine had the greatest efficiency and effectiveness for bowel training after stroke when compared in an evaluation of bowel programs differing in the time of day scheduled for bowel training and use of suppositories (Venn, Taft, Carpenter, & Applebaugh, 1992). Maintaining hydration is critical in promoting bowel function as well as bladder activity and has been discussed. The addition of fiber with adequate fluids should be considered if stools are hard. A mild stimulant such as prunes or prune juice 6–8 hours prior to planned defecation may be indicated for hard stool that is difficult to pass. A mixture of applesauce, prune juice, and bran has been effective in decreasing constipation and for laxative use in nursing home patients (Smith & Newman, 1989) and has application in the treatment and prevention of constipation in at-risk patients (see **Table**

14-8). Its thick texture may facilitate administration to patients with swallowing problems. The use of regular grocery store items to prepare the mixture should decrease the overall cost of the bowel program when compared to prescription or over-the-counter products.

Prompted Voiding. Prompted voiding (PV), an intervention to treat a patient's inability to recognize and act on the sensation of the need to void and exert neuromuscular control over initiation of voiding, has been successful in decreasing the frequency of UI in clinical trials with physically and cognitively impaired nursing home residents (Colling, Auslander, Hadley, Eisch, & Campbell, 1992; Fantl et al., 1996; McCormick, Cella, Scheve, & Engel, 1990; Schnelle, 1990). It also has been shown to be effective in home settings (Adkins & Matthews, 1997). Persons with urge, stress, and mixed UI have responded positively to this intervention (Ouslander et al., 1995; Schnelle, 1990). Prompted voiding also has strong support for reducing UI in individuals with cognitive and physical deficits (Abrams et al., 1999; Fantl et al., 1996; Heavner, 1998).

Prompted voiding is a scheduling regimen that initially focuses on the caregiver's behavior in order to change the incontinent person's voiding behavior. PV involves the consistent use of three caregiver behaviors: monitoring, prompting, and praising. The caregiver adheres to a schedule of regular monitoring, asking the incontinent individual if he or she needs to use the toilet, and checking to see if he or she is dry or wet. Prompting involves reminding them to use the toilet and to wait until the caregiver returns to void. Praise is the positive response or feedback for appropriate toileting or dryness. See **Table 14-9** for the steps of the prompted voiding technique and associated caregiver behaviors.

Research evaluating the effectiveness of PV provides clues about the predictors of success and factors in responsiveness. The best predictor of an individual's likelihood to benefit is her or his success during a therapeutic trial (usually lasting 3 days) (Lyons & Specht, 1999; Ouslander et al., 1995). A prompted voiding trial involves assessing the patient's ability to recognize the need to void and to respond to the need appropriately, either by asking to toilet or agreeing to toilet when the bladder is full. If the patient's percentage of appropriate toileting (number of voids in receptacle divided by total number of voids) meets the proportion specified, PV is continued. Although patients are usually checked every 2 hours initially, the pattern and volume of voids recorded guide the interval between voids and determine when the interval is changed. The reader is referred to Schnelle's (1991) text, *Managing Urinary Incontinence in the Elderly*, and the University of Iowa's research-based protocol, *Prompted Voiding for Persons with Urinary Incontinence* (Lyons & Specht, 1999) for an in-depth description of the PV protocol, suggestions for implementation, and forms for documentation. Factors possibly related to lack of success with PV include increased age, high residual urine volumes, low maximum voided volume, and a high frequency of incidents in which the person indicates the need to void and does not void (Lyons & Specht, 1999).

TABLE 14-8 Bran Mixture Recipe for Treating or Preventing Constipation

1 c. applesauce
1 c. unprocessed coarse wheat bran
$^{1}/_{2}$ c. unsweetened prune juice

Mix together. Give 2 T a day with a glass of water or juice. May increase to 3 T twice a day gradually (weekly) until good bowel function is achieved. May be given in hot cereal or added to mashed bananas. Refrigerate the recipe.

Bladder Training. Bladder training focuses on the ability to delay urination and suppress urgency, and is an important component for continence. Bladder training refers to a program of education, scheduled voiding, and reinforcement to provide patients with the skills to improve the ability to control urgency, decrease frequency and incontinent episodes, and prolong the interval between voiding (Wyman, 1994b).

TABLE 14-9 Steps in the Prompted Voiding Protocol

1. Greet the patient by name. Remember to always knock for resident privacy. Close the door and/or privacy curtain.
2. Ask the patient if she or he is wet or dry. Ask a second time if the patient doesn't respond.
3. Check clothes, bedding, or body to determine if he or she is wet or dry. Tell the patient if he or she is correct.
4. If the patient asks for help in toileting:
   a. Praise the resident.
   b. Assist him or her to the toilet.
5. If the patient does not ask for help toileting, you ask the patient if he or she wants to toilet.
   a. Ask a second time if he or she doesn't say yes the first time.
   b. Ask a third time if his or her response is other than yes or no.
6. Assist to toilet only if he or she says yes to your offer.
   a. Praise for appropriate toileting.
   b. Record outcome.
7. Ask if he or she wants something to drink and provide appropriate liquids.
8. Tell the resident when he or she can expect you to be back.

SOURCE: Schnelle, J. F. (1991). *Managing Urinary Incontinence in the Elderly*. New York: Springer Publication.

The steps in a bladder training program include setting a voiding schedule, teaching strategies for controlling urgency, monitoring voiding, and positive reinforcement. The initial voiding schedule is determined from baseline voiding data and prescribed according to the guidelines presented in **Table 14-10**. A 5- to 10-minute window on either side of the scheduled voiding time is allowed for flexibility. The training regimen is followed during waking hours, and the time between voiding is gradually increased by 15–30 minutes until the goal interval between voiding is reached (Sampselle et al., 1997). Although a 3- to 4-hour voiding interval is considered a maximal goal, Wyman and Fantl (1991) report most patients best tolerate an interval of 2–2½ hours. Strategies to suppress urge include relaxation and distraction techniques such as slow deep breathing, concentrating on a task such as talking to someone, and pelvic muscle contractions.

Bladder training has been evaluated and implemented primarily with independent, community-dwelling elderly women. Persons with physical and cognitive impairment have been considered unlikely candidates for bladder training techniques. However, the potential benefit to voiding supports an effort to try this approach. An exercise program to improve walking in cognitively impaired nursing home residents reduced daytime incontinence (Jivorec, 1991). Providing patients the skills to delay voiding until mobility improves or until assistance for toileting can be obtained is a missing element that may decrease incontinence regardless of the level of recovery of mobility.

Pelvic Muscle Relaxation. Another technique is pelvic muscle rehabilitation, which concentrates on increasing the strength, tone, and control of the pelvic floor muscles to facilitate a person's ability to voluntarily control the flow of urine and suppress urgency. The pelvic floor muscles support the pelvic organs. Pelvic muscle rehabilitation refers to an exercise regimen to improve the integrity and function of the pelvic floor. The proposed mechanism of action for pelvic muscle training is that strong and fast pelvic muscle contractions close the urethra and increase urethral pressure to prevent leakage.

TABLE 14-10 Steps in Bladder Training

1. Complete a 72-hour voiding diary.
2. Review the voiding diary. Calculate the number of voids and bladder accidents in a 24-hour period. Determine fluid intake.
3. Examine data for patterns. Does UI occur only during certain times of day? Are accidents associated with certain events (activities, intake of specific type of fluids, medications)? What is the average time between voids and what is the longest interval? Are behaviors different for weekdays or weekends, or workdays vs. nonworkdays, or time when you are at home or out of the home?
4. Establish an initial voiding interval and consider the optimal interval to be achieved. The typical interval for adults is every 4 hours during the day; however, data suggest for older persons every 2 hours may be optimum (Wyman, Choi, Harkins, Wilson, & Fantl, 1988). The objective is to start the voiding routine at the interval that is comfortable to separate urgency from voiding; then, as you develop urge suppression skills, to increase the time between voiding until the goal is reached.
5. Urinate when you wake, after meals, before bedtime, and at the prescribed intervals.
6. If you get the urge to void and it is too soon to void, use the relaxation technique to make the urge go away. Remember, this involves taking very slow deep breaths until the urge goes away. Relax and concentrate when doing this. Contract the pelvic floor muscles quickly 3–5 times. Relax. Contract again.
7. Void at the prescribed time even if you don't feel the need.
8. If after a week it is very easy to wait the assigned time interval, lengthen the time by 15–30 minutes.
9. Begin by only practicing this technique at home, when you are relaxed and the bathroom is nearby.
10. Fluid intake should be kept at six 8-ounce glasses per day. If you awaken frequently during the night to void, drink the majority of your 8 ounces before 6 at night.

    Hints to remember:

    - Do not go to the bathroom before you have the urge to void.
    - Never rush or run to the bathroom—walk slowly.
    - Use the relaxation technique in situations that cause you to have the urge to void before the assigned time interval. For example, if you get the urge to void whenever you start to unlock your front door, stop, relax, and take three slow deep breaths to let the urge pass. Then unlock the door and walk slowly to the bathroom.
    - When you walk slowly to the bathroom, do some pelvic muscle exercises to prevent an accident.
11. Do not despair and get discouraged. In time, this will all fall into place and you will be voiding at the set time interval.

Pelvic muscle contractions may inhibit bladder contractions, helping to suppress urgency.

To teach the individual to identify and isolate the correct muscles, instruct him or her to "draw in" and "lift up" the rectal/anal sphincter muscles. Patients should be instructed to lift up the perivaginal muscles and avoid contracting the abdominal, gluteal, and thigh muscles. To help the patient avoid a bearing down motion, have him or her practice pushing down to feel what not to do. Start with contracting for 2 seconds, and then gradually increase the length of the contraction until a maximum 10-second hold is achieved. A repetition includes relaxing or resting the pelvic floor muscles between contractions for the same amount of time the muscle is being contracted. A typical training regimen involves 10 repetitions two to three times a day.

Once the correct technique has been learned, instruct the patient to use pelvic muscle contraction to prevent urine flow. If leakage occurs with activities that increase intra-abdominal pressure, then a muscle contraction should precede the activity. If urgency is the primary problem, the pelvic floor muscles are used to suppress the urge. The urge suppression technique is outlined in **Table 14-11**.

Biofeedback. Biofeedback is an adjunct to pelvic muscle rehabilitation and bladder contraction inhibition that has strong scientific support for effectiveness with stress and urge urinary incontinence (Abrams et al., 1999; Fantl et al., 1996). In a summary paper on the use of biofeedback-assisted bladder training for urge and stress incontinence, Burgio, Locher, Goode et al. (1998) concluded that this option has particular advantages in that it is very low risk and has had no documented side effects; however, because it relies on learning new behaviors, it may have limited application in patients with cognitive impairment. Much of the initial research evaluated the effectiveness o interventions with cognitively intact, community-dwelling elderly. However, there is compelling evidence supporting the extension of research to a more cognitively impaired population.

Recent studies targeting a more vulnerable population, the homebound frail elderly, report behavioral approaches were effective in reducing UI (Bear, Dwyer, Benveneste, Jeff, & Dougherty, 1997; Engeberg, McDowell, Donovan, Brodak, & Weber, 1997). A pilot study regarding the effect of pelvic muscle exercise and prompted voiding on the frequency of UI in elderly cognitively impaired nursing home residents revealed subjects showed significant reduction in incontinence with the addition of pelvic muscle exercise (PME) to a prompted voiding regimen (Scheve, Engel, McCormick, & Leahy, 1991).

TABLE 14-11 Urge Suppression Techniques

- Stop what you are doing and stay put. Sit down when possible, or stand quietly. Remain very still. When you are still, it is easier to control your urge.
- Squeeze your pelvic floor muscles quickly several times. Do not relax fully in between.
- Relax the rest of your body. Take a few deep breaths to help you relax and let go of your tension.
- Concentrate on suppressing the urge feeling.
- Wait until the urge subsides.
- Walk to the bathroom at a normal pace. Do not rush. Continue squeezing your pelvic floor muscles quickly while you walk.

SOURCE: Fantl, J. A., Newman, D. K., Colling, J., et al. (1996, March). *Managing Acute and Chronic Incontinence in Adults.* Clinical Practice Guideline, No. 2, 1996 Update. Rockville, MD: U.S. Dept. of Health and Human Services, Public Health Service, Agency for Health Care Policy and Research. AHCPR Pub-No. 96-0686.

The importance of ensuring patients can appropriately and adequately perform PME cannot be overemphasized. Bump, Hurt, Fantl, and Wyman (1991) found that verbal instructions were often not sufficient for incontinent women seen in an outpatient program to perform PME. Biofeedback, either through surface electrodes or vaginal or rectal probes, provides visual and/or auditory cues to facilitate incontinent patients' ability to isolate and identify pelvic floor muscles. It also helps decrease patients' tendency to use abdominal or gluteal muscles. In the absence of biofeedback equipment, digital checks can be used to teach and monitor ongoing performance.

The Health Care Financing Administration (HCFA) analyzed scientific data related to the use of biofeedback for treatment of stress, urge, and post-prostatectomy incontinence in a review of the Medicare coverage policy. A decision memorandum summarizing its findings and the recommendations of numerous professional organizations amended HCFA's policy to allow coverage for biofeedback with patients who had failed documented trials of pelvic muscle exercises or who are unable to perform PME (Tunis, Norris, & Simon, 2000). A failed trial is defined as no significant improvement after completing a 4-week period of structured, ordered pelvic muscle reeducation to increase pelvic floor strength (Norris, 2001).

Pelvic Floor Electrical Stimulus. Pelvic floor electrical stimulation (PFES) is another adjunct to PME. PFES refers to the application of electric current to sacral and pudendal afferent fibers via nonimplantable vaginal or anal probes (Fantl et al., 1996). Variable rates of current are used to improve urethral closure by activating pelvic floor muscles, thus exercising and strengthening the pelvic floor (Tunis, Whyte, & Bridger, 2000). PFES also can facilitate an individual's ability to identify and isolate pelvic floor musculature. The Agency for Health Care Policy and Research (AHCPR) guidelines (Fantl et al., 1996) concludes that fair research-based evidence exists that PFES decreases stress urinary incontinence in women and it may be useful for urge and mixed incontinence. The HCFA review panel concluded that PFES is effective for patients with stress and/or urge incontinence, and considers its use as necessary and reasonable if PMEs have been unsuccessful (Tunis et al., 2000). However, the ability to passively exercise the pelvic floor makes this a potentially valuable treatment for individuals unable to perform the exercises.

Pharmacological Management

Medications are available to help treat stress and urge incontinence. Because many older persons have multiple chronic health problems, medications for incontinence should be considered primarily as an adjunct to other behavioral interventions. Pharmacological management of urge urinary incontinence was found to add to the effectiveness of behavioral strategies in frail older persons (Fonda et al., 2002). However, the potential for adverse reactions and added cost must be considered carefully with the patient when a pharmacological intervention is being considered.

Medications prescribed for stress urinary incontinence target the internal urinary sphincter or the urethral/vaginal tissues. The alpha agonist pseudoephedrine acts at the bladder neck, increasing urethral tone, and it may decrease leakage. It is often prescribed for mild cases of stress urinary incontinence; however, its side effects of insomnia, restlessness, nervousness, headache, and potential to increase blood pressure and heart rate limit its usefulness in the older population. Duloxetine, a serotonin and norepinephrine reuptake inhibitor, increases external urethral sphincter tone and is currently under review by the Food and Drug Administration for treating stress urinary incontinence. Estrogen, prescribed to treat urogenital atrophy, increases stimulation of urogenital estrogen receptors and may increase urethral resistance. Evidence of its usefulness in stress UI is inconclusive (Fantl et al., 1996); however, estrogen's effectiveness in treating atrophic tissues can help alleviate irritative symptoms of urgency, which may decrease urge UI.

Drug therapy for urge incontinence has grown over the last few years with new products on the horizon. The primary agents for uninhibited bladder contractions are anticholinergics or antispasmotics that decrease contraction of the detrusor muscle. **Table 14-12** presents

TABLE 14-12 Medications Commonly Used to Treat Urinary Incontinence*

Medication	Dosage	Evidence	Comments
Hyoscyamine	0.375 mg twice daily orally	2/D	Also available in sublingual and elixir forms; it has prominent anticholinergic side effects
Oxbutynin	2.5–5.0 mg thrice daily orally (short-acting) 5–30 mg daily orally (long-acting) 3.9 mg over a 96-hr period (transdermal)	1/A	Long-acting and transdermal preparations have fewer side effects than short-acting preparations The transdermal patch can cause local skin irritation in some patients
Propantheline	15–30 mg 4 times daily orally	2/B	Prominent anticholinergic side effects
Propiverine	15 mg thrice daily orally	1/A	Complex pharmacokinetics with several active metabolites; not currently available in the United States
Tolterodine	1–2 mg twice daily orally (short-acting) 4 mg daily orally (long-acting)	1/A	The long-acting and short-acting preparations have similar efficacy
Trospium	20 mg twice daily orally	1/A	Quaternary ammonium compound, which does not cross the blood–brain barrier and may have fewer cognitive side effects than other anticholinergic agents; not currently available in the United States
Estrogen (for women)			
Vaginal estrogen preparations	Approximately 0.5 g cream applied topically nightly for 2 wk, then twice per week Estradiol ring, replaced every 90 days Estradiol, 1 tablet daily for 2 wk, then 1 tablet twice a week	4/D	Local vaginal preparations are probably more effective than oral estrogen; definitive data on effectiveness lacking

TABLE 14-12 continued

Medication	Dosage	Evidence	Comments
Alpha-Adrenergic Antagonists (for men)			
Alfuzosin	2.5 mg thrice daily orally	4/D*	Useful in men with benign prostatic enlargement
Doxazosin	1–16 mg daily orally		Postural hypotension can be a serious side effect
Prazosin	1–10 mg twice daily orally		
Tamsulosin	0.4–0.8 mg daily orally		
Terazosin	1–10 mg orally each day at bedtime		Doses must be increased gradually to facilitate tolerance
Other drugs			
Imipramine	10–25 mg thrice daily orally	2/C	May be useful for mixed urge-stress incontinence; can cause postural hypotension and bundle-branch block
Desmopressin	20–40 pg of intranasal spray daily at bedtime 0 1–0.4 mg orally 2 hr before bedtime	1/B	Intranasal spray used for primary nocturnal enuresis in children; hyponatremia occurs commonly in older adults, and serum sodium levels must be monitored closely

*Not all drugs listed in this table have proven efficacy specifically for symptoms of overactive bladder.

†Levels of evidence are based on the Oxford System: A score of 1 indicates evidence from randomized, controlled trials; a score of 2, evidence from good-quality prospective cohort studies; a score of 3, evidence from good-quality retrospective case-control studies; and a score of 4, evidence from good-quality case series. The grade of recommendations is based on the definitions used by the International Consultation on Urological Diseases: A indicates consistent level 1 evidence; B, consistent level 2 or 3 evidence or major evidence from randomized, controlled trials; C, level 4 evidence or major evidence from level 2 or 3 studies or expert opinion based on the Delphi method; and D, inconclusive, inconsistent, or nonexistent evidence or evidence based on expert opinion only.

‡The rating is for symptoms of overactive bladder, not for overall symptoms of benign prostatic hyperplasia.

SOURCE: Ouslander, J. G. (2004). Management of the overactive bladder. *NEJM, 350*, 786–799.

(continues)

an overview of the medications used for urge urinary incontinence.

Overflow incontinence in men that is the result of bladder neck obstruction from benign prostatic hypertrophy (BPH) may resolve with treatment of the prostate. Alpha antagonists (doxazosin, tamsulosin, and terazosin) relax the urinary sphincters, improving urine flow and decreasing urine retention and overflow incontinence. However, dizziness and orthostatic hypotension are potential side effects that must be addressed. Other options for BPH treatment are the 5-α reductase inhibitors finesteride and dutasteride. This class of medications blocks the conversion of testosterone to dihydrotestosterone, the form needed for prostate growth. The 5-α reductase inhibitors take about 3 to 6 months to take effect. An important consideration in the prescription and administration of these drugs is their teratogenic effects.

When considering medications it is important to review all medications being taken to determine if any of the medications are actually contributing to the problem of UI. Such medications include hypnotics, antianxiety drugs, and anticholinergics (including antimuscarinics and antinicotinics) (Godfrey, 2008).

Devices and Products

One of the first decisions made in the management of UI is the choice of protective undergarments. A variety of absorbent products is now available to contain urine. It is important that patients use products designed for urine; menstrual pads, a popular choice, are not specifically designed to absorb and contain urine. The absorbent inner core of continence garments wicks the urine away from the skin and allows urine to spread throughout the entire pad, increasing the volume of urine absorbed (Newman, 2002). The volume of urine that needs to be contained and the need for help toileting are important considerations in product selection. The use of pad and pant sets developed for men and for women offers several advantages to the traditional adult diaper. These garments are easier to manipulate to prepare for toileting and for repositioning clothing afterward. They also are more in line with usual or "normal" underclothes, facilitating the expectation of a return to continence and promoting comfort. The introduction of products to accommodate moderate to heavy levels of incontinence has broadened the possibilities for successful containment. Many patients and family have been relieved (especially from an economic perspective) to learn of the availability of nondisposable garments that can be washed and reused.

New and improved products are in the planning and production stages (Mueller, 2004) and will increase the options for management and decrease the control that incontinence and the fear of incontinence exert over an individual's life. Toileting equipment and collection devices are available for men and women to promote self-toileting, including female urinals, wheelchair urinals, and male reusable urinal/pant garments. The National Association for Continence (2004) *Resource Guide* is an excellent resource for all products and their manufacturers and is available for a nominal fee (National Association for Continence at http://www.nafc.org).

Meticulous skin care is essential in the care of persons with incontinence. Moisture barriers and no-rinse incontinence cleansers have been shown to be more effective than soap and water alone in preventing skin breakdown (Byers, Ryan, Regan, Shields, & Carta, 1995). It is important to gently dry the skin after cleaning and to apply moisturizers. Petroleum-based products may be incompatible with some adult briefs, causing skin irritation (Newman, 2002).

Occupational health evaluations of the home may be helpful in modifying the environment to facilitate rapid access to the toilet. Although this may be only one component of urinary incontinence, it may facilitate urination, thus decreasing urinary incontinence.

Indwelling urinary catheters, once the primary means for managing urinary incontinence, are no longer accepted as the first step in an incontinence treatment regimen. However, there are situations that may require catheter use. The Agency for Health Care Policy and Research (now the Agency for Healthcare Research and Quality) identified guidelines for long-term indwelling catheter use (see **Table 14-13**). With long-term use, care must be taken to monitor for common complications of polymicrobial bacteruria (universal by 30 days), fever (1 event per 100 patient days), nephrolithiasis, bladder stones, epididymitis, and chronic renal

TABLE 14-13 AHCPR Guidelines for Long-Term Indwelling Catheter Use

- For patients whose incontinence is caused by obstruction and no other intervention is feasible
- For terminally ill, incontinent patients
- Short-term treatment for patients with pressure ulcers
- For severely impaired individuals in whom alternative interventions are not an option
- For patients who live alone and do not have a caregiver to provide other supportive measures

SOURCE: Fantl, J. A., Newman, D. K., Colling, J., et al. (1996, March). *Managing Acute and Chronic Incontinence In Adults.* Clinical Practice Guideline, No. 2, 1996 Update. Rockville, MD: U.S. Dept. of Health and Human Services, Public Health Service, Agency for Health Care Policy and Research. AHCPR Pub-No. 96-0686.

inflammation and pyelonephritis (Fonda et al., 2002). Maintaining hydration, urine flow, and cleanliness of the system are important components of care. Minimizing urethral trauma by using small-caliber catheters, a 5-cc retention balloon filled with 10 cc of sterile water, and securing the catheter with a thigh strap will promote comfort and may help decrease complications. Emptying the catheter every 4–6 hours to avoid migration of bacteria up the lumen, cleaning the insertion site gently with soap and water daily, and avoiding irrigations may help decrease symptomatic urinary tract infection. Whenever a patient's status changes, such as when pressure ulcers heal or caregivers are available, then a trial without the indwelling catheter should be considered.

Intermittent urinary catheterization is another supportive measure to manage urinary retention (Fantl et al., 1996). In and out catheterization allows regular bladder emptying. Regular emptying reduces pressure within the bladder and improves circulation to the bladder wall, making the mucosa more resistant to infection (Newman, 2002). Sterile technique (ISC) is used in institutions, and clean technique (ICC) is used for catheterizations at home. No studies have been conducted comparing the use of intermittent urinary catheterization and long-term indwelling urinary catheterization in the frail elderly (Fonda et al., 2002). Dexterity and mobility problems may interfere with self-catheterizations. Comfort with intermittent catheterizations is a factor in ISC and ICC performed by caregivers.

Urinary incontinence is a serious, potentially disabling, complication. Incontinence is a common condition in the older population. The introduction of early targeted behavioral interventions should improve urological functioning and limit the impact of uncontrolled incontinence on quality of life. Older patients and their caregivers must be provided the skills—both technical and intellectual—to prevent the development and persistence of elimination problems. These skills are important components in the treatment of sleep problems precipitated by voiding problems.

SLEEP DISORDERS

Sleep is considered a time of restoration for our bodies and minds. Sleep is necessary to heal wounds, maintain normal hormonal function, and provide sound emotional health. Disruptions in sleep of the older adult can worsen chronic illnesses and exacerbate depression. It is necessary for the nurse to understand the normal changes of sleep patterns in the older adult and recognize sleep abnormalities that can negatively impact health.

Sleep Changes Associated with Aging

A sleep cycle consists of two distinct components, **nonrapid eye movement (NREM) sleep** and **rapid eye movement (REM) sleep**. NREM is composed of four stages, beginning with stage I, which is a transitional period of very light sleep. The individual is easily aroused during this stage and may deny having been asleep. Stage I usually lasts less than 7 minutes. This is followed by stage II, a period of deeper relaxation and light sleep. Stage II is the most predominant NREM stage in older adults. Stages III and IV are deeper, more restorative periods of sleep. During these stages, there is a decrease in pulse, blood pressure, and metabolism. Stage IV restores the individual physically, and tissue healing occurs during this time. However, stage IV is the most sensitive to advancing age and begins to decrease during the third decade of life (Honkus, 2003).

REM sleep follows the four stages of NREM, and during REM the body is in the deepest state of relaxation. Large muscles become immobile and the individual is unable to move. However, the autonomic nervous system is very active, and respiratory rate, blood pressure, and heart rate become erratic and frequently elevated. Brain wave activity patterns are similar to those of wakefulness (Hoffman, 2003). REM sleep is the stage of sleep in which dreams occur. It is thought that REM is a time of mental and emotional restoration.

The sleep cycle, usually about 90 minutes long, begins with NREM I, then progresses through NREM II–IV. The individual may return to NREM III and II, and then begin REM sleep. After REM sleep, the sleep pattern returns to stage II. The smallest amount of REM occurs during early cycles and increases with each subsequent cycle through the night. This cycle repeats throughout the night, and the time spent in each stage varies, depending on the individual's age and other factors. When a person is awakened, the sleep cycle always returns to stage I, and the process begins all over again. Therefore, individuals who awaken frequently spend much less time in the restorative phases of sleep.

The older adult spends more time in stage II, takes longer to fall asleep, and is awakened more easily. Sleep can be significantly disrupted in individuals with cardiovascular disease, stroke, endocrine disorders, depression, and Alzheimer's and Parkinson's diseases. Prolonged sleep deprivation can lead to cardiovascular, neuroendocrine, and immune system disorders.

The circadian rhythm that regulates sleep is governed by the suprachiasmatic nucleus (SCN) in the hypothalamus. The SCN responds to transmissions from photoreceptors in the retina that travel along the optic nerve. Most individuals' biological clocks are on an innate 25-hour cycle. Sunlight or other bright light resets the SCN and our circadian rhythm follows the 24-hour cycle of the sun instead of the innate cycle (Medical College of Wisconsin, 1999).

Melatonin is a hormone produced by the pineal gland at night. It is released in response to darkness and inhibits neurotransmitters involved in arousal. Individuals who are exposed to bright lights 24 hours a day can experience a total cessation of melatonin release and subsequent disruption of the sleep cycle. This lack of sleep can lead to delirium in the older adult. It is important that nurses pay close attention to the client's nighttime environment and turn off the lights.

Prevalence of Sleep Disturbances

Sleep difficulties become more prevalent with age. According to the National Sleep Foundation's 2008 *Sleep in America* poll, 32% of adults reported a good night's sleep only a few nights each month. Common sleep complaints in the older adult include frequent awakenings during the night, early morning awakenings, and difficulties falling asleep at night (**Table 14-14**). Those with chronic illnesses tend to have a greater propensity for sleep disturbances. Nearly 80% of men and women over the age of 70 have at least one chronic disease, and those with four or more comorbid conditions are considerably more likely to have sleep disturbances. Individuals with multiple illnesses rate their sleep as being of poorer quality. They sleep less hours, awaken more frequently, report difficulty falling asleep, awaken earlier, and report more significant daytime sleepiness than those with three or fewer medical conditions. The conditions that negatively impact sleep include hypertension, cardiovascular disease, arthritis, diabetes, cancer, stroke, depression, osteoporosis, and respiratory diseases (National Sleep Foundation, 2008).

Types of Sleep Disturbances

Insomnia

Insomnia, or difficulty falling and staying asleep, is more prominent in women. Genetic and environmental factors contribute to insomnia. First-degree relatives of insomniacs have an increased frequency of the disorder. Noise and unfavorable

TABLE 14-14 **Sleep Problems in the Older Adult**

Condition	Description/Significance	Incidence
Sleep disorders—combined	Insomnia, snoring, breathing pauses, or restless legs	55–64 years old: 71% 65–74 years old: 65% 75–84 years old: 64%
Insomnia	Difficulties falling asleep or staying asleep, waking up early or unrefreshed	55–84 years old: 48%
Snoring	Symptom of sleep apnea	55–84 years old: 32%
Breathing pauses	Symptom of sleep apnea; observed or experienced	55–84 years old: 7%
Tingling and discomfort in legs	Symptom of restless leg syndrome	55–84 years old: 17%

SOURCE: Adapted from *Sleep in American Poll* 2003, National Sleep Foundation.

room temperature can contribute to insomnia (Asplund, 1999). Treatment may include benzodiazepines, hypnotics, or antidepressants.

Sleep Apnea

Periods of breathing cessation are the hallmark of **sleep apnea**, and snoring may be present in the individual with this disorder. Sleep apnea can be caused by a central nervous system control-mechanism disturbance (central sleep apnea, CSA) or by the narrowing or loss of tone in the pharyngeal airway (obstructive sleep apnea, OSA). During these episodes of apnea, the soft structures of the throat relax and the airway is closed off. Oxygen levels decrease, carbon dioxide increases, and the blood pH becomes more acidic. The heart rate drops and the brain erroneously interprets the changes as a fluid overload. Hormones are released that awaken the individual and signal the body to get rid of fluid and sodium, resulting in nocturia. Other symptoms usually present with apnea include snoring, restless sleep, and morning head aches. Both forms can result in severe sleep fragmentation, significant daytime sleepiness that interferes with daily life, and an increase in the incidence of several diseases (Asplund, 1999).

Consequences of sleep apnea include hypertension, coronary artery disease, myocardial infarction, pulmonary hypertension, CHF, stroke, neuropsychiatric problems, cognitive impairment, sexual dysfunction, and injury due to accidents (National Commission on Sleep Disorders Research, 1993). Even among healthy adults, a higher risk of death exists in those with longer sleep latencies and poorer sleep quality (Ryff, Singer, & Love, 2004). Nearly 60% of individuals with cardiac disease also have sleep apnea (Anderson, 2004). Patients with sleep apnea have twice the risk of hypertension, three times the risk of coronary artery disease, and a four-fold risk of stroke when compared to national disease prevalence (Chasens, Weaver, & Umlauf, 2003). There is evidence that chronic partial sleep loss, such as delayed onset or frequent awakenings, is more detrimental than short-term total sleep deprivation (Bryant, Trinder, & Curtis, 2004). Poor sleep has been linked to poor memory and work performance, compromised interpersonal relationships, and a diminished quality of life (Cheek, Shaver, & Lentz, 2004). Patients with CHF and untreated sleep apnea consume twice the health care resources as patients with CHF who seek treatment for sleep apnea (Anderson, 2004). Sleep loss has been shown to have a significantly negative impact on memory retention of new skills, such as those learned in the occupational therapy sessions during rehabilitation (DeGroot, Eskes, & Phillips, 2003; Ficca & Salzarulo,

2004). Individuals who exhibit symptoms of sleep apnea should be referred to a sleep center for polysomnography, an overnight evaluation of sleep events. Continuous positive airway pressure (CPAP) devices consistently improve the symptoms of sleep apnea and decrease the individual's risk of developing somatic disease.

Restless Leg Syndrome

Restless leg syndrome (RLS) is a neurological disorder characterized by an uncontrollable urge to move to relieve paraesthesias (abnormal sensations) or dysesthesias (unpleasant abnormal sensations) in the legs. The condition is triggered by lying down to relax. RLS affects up to 12 million Americans, with the highest incidence in middle to older aged individuals. The severity of the disorder also increases with age, with more frequent and longer periods of symptoms.

For mild to moderate cases of RLS, certain lifestyle changes, such as reducing caffeine, alcohol, and tobacco use, may provide some relief. Maintaining a regular sleep pattern can also reduce symptoms. Massage, taking a hot bath, or using heat or ice can relieve symptoms in some individuals (National Institute of Neurological Disorders and Stroke, 2001). Pharmacological treatment of the syndrome includes dopaminergic drugs, dopamine agonists, and benzodiazepines (Asplund, 1999). Ropinirole was approved for the treatment of moderate to severe RLS in 2005. Previously approved for treatment of Parkinson's disease, ropinirole's side effects include somnolence, nausea, vomiting, and headache. Hypotension or syncope can occur during initial dosing of ropinirole (U.S. Food and Drug Administration, 2005).

Sleep Assessment

Daytime sleepiness is a direct result of sleep quality. However, many sleep problems can be a result of poor sleep hygiene, which is the measures an individual takes to promote sleep. Therefore, it is important to also measure the client's sleep habits, such as time of going to bed, rituals prior to bedtime, and established sleep environment. Sleep hygiene should be assessed as well as daytime sleepiness, depression, and anxiety, and a thorough physical examination and medication history should be completed. Many medications can interfere with sleep, and drug-drug interactions can be a contributing factor to sleep disruption.

A cartoon-face sleepiness scale measures sleepiness uncontaminated by emotional state or pain (Maldonado, Bentley, & Mitchell, 2004). The scale requires the client to point to a picture that most represents their perceived level of sleepiness. The pictorial scale has shown validity and reliability in assessing level of sleepiness in sleep-disordered adults, young school-aged children, and adults with low literacy levels.

The Epworth scale is a self-completion report of the likelihood of the patient falling asleep during several daytime activities (Johns, 1991). Ratings are made on a 0–3 scale (0 = never, 3 = a high chance), with an overall score range of 0–24. The Epworth scale can be used to determine whether sleep interferences and frequent awakenings have an impact on daytime sleepiness, which can negatively impact performance and recall of newly learned skills (Ersser et al., 1999).

The Epworth and pictorial scales are valid in differentiating sleepiness and sleep quality without influence of pain or mood state. The pictorial scale is appropriate for clients who are unable to read, including children and clients with decreased cognition. This sleep hygiene assessment measures difficulty falling and staying asleep, daytime somnolence, and individual satisfaction with sleep.

Interventions/Strategies for Care

Nursing therapeutics for sleep promotion include enhanced sleep hygiene (Cheek, Shaver, & Lentz, 2004; Hoffman, 2003), music therapy (Arand & Bonnet, 2000; Fletcher, 1986; Gagner-Tjellesen, Yurkovich, & Gragert, 2001; Johnson, 2003; Mornhinweg & Voignier, 1995), environmental restructuring to enhance sleep (Fontaine, Briggs, & Pope-Smith, 2001), aromatherapy and herbs (Buckle, 2001; Oliff, 2004; Taibi, Bourguignon, & Taylor, 2004), and massage (Field, 1998; Richards, Nagel, Markie, Elwell, & Barone, 2003). Individuals who have delayed sleep onset tend to respond better to nursing interventions than those with sleep maintenance problems. Sleep maintenance disorders, or frequent disruptions after falling asleep due to somatic abnormalities, usually respond better to medical therapy, including CPAP and treatment of underlying causes.

Sleep Hygiene

Clients admitted to the hospital have illness and environment-related disruptions to their sleep. Nursing interventions, including medication administration, taking vital signs, and completing assessments, should be timed to allow long periods of uninterrupted sleep whenever possible. If a client must be awakened, observe for rapid eye movements. If the client is in a state of REM sleep, wait until he or she is experiencing an NREM cycle of sleep to awaken (Honkus, 2003).

Caffeine avoidance is an important measure to enhance sleep. The stimulant increases physiological arousal and prevents the onset of sleep. Caffeine has a half-life of 3–7 hours, and late afternoon to evening abstinence is recommended to avoid its invigorating effect. Alcohol can expedite sleep onset, but interrupts REM and non-REM sleep throughout the night. After alcohol metabolizes, a rebound arousal occurs that can precipitate early morning awakening. The effect can last for several nights based on the individual's metabolism. Smoking also increases awake time and causes a delayed sleep onset (Cheek et al., 2004).

A consistent retiring and awakening time strengthens the circadian rhythm through a homeostatic mechanism and a habitual light-dark cycle exposure. Getting up at the same time each day is more important in establishing synchronization with the light-dark cycle than going to bed at the same time (Cheek et al., 2004; Hoffman, 2003).

Environmental Restructuring

Florence Nightingale was one of the first to address environmental restructuring for improved patient outcomes. She considered lighting, noise, and sensory stimulation as care aspects that could enhance or hinder recovery. Lights should be on during the day and off at night to trigger the normal sleep pattern. Fluorescent light tends to be harsh and can cause visual fatigue and headaches. Natural light through a window can help maintain the circadian rhythm. During a 1975 study of a windowless intensive care unit in Great Britain, the incidence of patient delirium was twice as high as in a unit with windows. Artificial light exposure during the night causes a drop in melatonin levels after 20 minutes, and constant, high-intensity light can lead to a total cessation of melatonin production. Nightingale also incorporated color as a therapeutic tool by using flowers. The colors used in the environment play a role in the sleep cycle. Room colors that promote sleep are soft mixed tones of blue, green, and violet without sharp contrasts. Artwork of nature scenes can decrease use of pain medication, lower blood pressure, and increase the perception of relaxation (Fontaine et al., 2001).

Environmental noise can activate the sympathetic nervous system during sleep. Sleep occurs best at noise levels below 35 decibels (db), and levels above 80 db are related to sleep arousals. Television and talking were the two most frequent disruptive sounds reported in a questionnaire of 203 ICU patients (Fontaine et al., 2001). Environmental "white noise" such as ocean or rain sounds or repetitive tones at 800 Hz tend to enhance sleep (Richards, 1996). Patients with sleep-onset difficulties respond better to relaxation techniques and stimulus control than do those with sleep-maintenance problems (Mantle, 1996).

Relaxation

Music therapy promotes relaxation, deceases anxiety and pain perception, improves sleep quality, and decreases heart rate and systolic pressure (Fontaine et al., 2001; Richards, 1996). Johnson (2003) studied the impact of music therapy on the sleep quality of 52 female participants. Subjects selected their own preference of music, with 64% selecting soothing classical music, 19% selecting sacred music, and 10% selecting new age music.

Each morning, subjects recorded the length of time it took to fall asleep, the number of awakenings, the time they awoke in the morning, and their satisfaction with the night's sleep. Subjects took less time to fall asleep, awoke less often, and reported a quicker return to sleep after awakening. Satisfaction with sleep scores significantly increased. The music therapy became more effective with each consecutive night's use, and a peak effect was reached on the fifth day and was maintained thereafter for the study's 10-night course (Johnson, 2003). Music therapy is the most common independent nursing intervention used for sleep. It elicits the relaxation response, decreases central nervous system arousal, stimulates alpha waves, and triggers endorphin release (Gagner-Tjellesen et al., 2001).

In a systematic review of 22 research articles, Richards, Gibson, and Overton-McCoy (2000) found positive results of massage in sessions as short as 1–2 minutes. Physiologic responses to massage include decreases in heart rate, blood pressure, catecholamine and cortisol production, and muscle activity. Patients with fibromyalgia reported lower anxiety and depression, less pain and stiffness, and fewer difficulties falling asleep (Richards et al., 2000). Field (1998) reported similar results in patients with rheumatoid arthritis. Patients in the massage group slept an average of 1 hour longer than those in the control group. A 3-minute effleurage massage can decrease autonomic arousal and cardiac load in clients with cardiovascular disorders (Gauthier, 1999).

Aromatherapy

Aromatherapy oils such as lavender, chamomile, lemon, peppermint, thyme, geranium, and eucalyptus have been reported to enhance immunity and promote relaxation. Poor industry control and lack of standardization are safety concerns, however. The potential for allergic reactions also exists in patients who are taking multiple medications. Therefore, caution should be used when recommending aromatherapy in the older patient population (Fontaine et al., 2001; Richards et al., 2003).

Lavender oil has a calming effect and decreases insomnia. In a study of elderly individuals with sleep disturbance, lavender was as effective as tranquilizers (Oliff, 2004). True lavender (*Lavandula angustifolia*) produces a sedative effect that is similar to benzodiazepines. It is considered the safest of all essential oils with no irritation or sensitivity reported at dilutions as high as 16%, and no toxicity ever reported (Buckle, 2001). When lavender is inhaled (one to five drops on a tissue inhaled for 10 minutes), the molecules travel to the olfactory bulb and then to the limbic system, where GABA is increased in a response similar to that of diazepam ingestion (Buckle, 2001).

Herbal Therapy

Consumers of herbal products are advised to check with the American Herbal Products Association to ascertain the credibility of manufacturers and safety of compounds. This information is available at http://www.ahpa.org (Taibi et al., 2004). Herbal preparations containing valerian have shown promising results in patients with autoimmune and cardiovascular conditions (Bourguignon et al., 2003; Taibi et al., 2004). Valerian is a root extract that enhances sleep by influencing activity at GABA, adenosine, and serotonin receptors, which regulate normal sleep (Taibi et al., 2004). Some findings suggest that valerian promotes relaxation and increases the depth and quality of sleep. Valerian reduced objective and subjective sleep latency, improved sleep efficiency, and decreased awakenings in patients with rheumatoid arthritis when compared to placebo. Valerian may also have analgesic and spasmolytic properties that reduce pain (Bourguignon, 2003). Valerian does not produce the "hangover" effect similar to that of benzodiazepines. In a review of 28 clinical trials, there were no reported adverse effects of valerian (Taibi et al., 2004). However, drug-drug interactions including hepatotoxicity can occur with valerian, and the herb should be used with caution in older adults.

Medications

When all other means to promote sleep have been unsuccessful, some older adults may require use of medications for sleep. Although medications such as benzodiazepines were once commonly used, these are no longer recommended in the elderly. In fact, triazolam (Halcion) and temazepam (Restoril) have long half-lives that may cause exaggerated side effects in older persons. Flurazepam (Dalmane) also has a long half-life and accumulates over time in the body. Dalmane has been associated with falls and confusion in older adults (Therapeutic Research Center, 2007). Although a low dose of diphenhydramine (Benadryl) used to be commonly prescribed to aid sleep in older adults, it is no longer recommended because of the increased anticholinergic side effects, including hangover effects, often seen in the elderly. The preferred medications for insomnia are the BZD 1 receptor–specific nonbenzodiazepines such as zolpidem (Ambien), zaleplon (Sonata), and eszopiclone (Lunesta). These medications have fewer side effects and a lower abuse potential than the benzodiazepines. For those being treated for major depression and insomnia, a sedating antidepressant may be the drug of choice.

PRESSURE ULCERS

Prevalence

A **pressure ulcer** is a lesion caused by unrelieved pressure with damage to the underlying tissue. Pressure ulcers have significant prevalence in older adults in the acute care setting (3–11%), long-term facilities (24%), and the community (17%). When a stage I ulcer develops, the older adult has a tenfold risk of developing further ulcers (Dhamarajan & Ahmed, 2003). The normal skin changes associated with aging, combined with the effects of illness, contribute to the higher risk of ulcer development in the older population. Skin becomes thinner, has less collagen and moisture, and can lose the ability to protect itself against invading organisms. Blood flow to the dermis is reduced, which results in fewer nutrients reaching the skin and less waste removal. Because of this, the skin takes much longer to heal. The older adult's skin is also more susceptible to friction and shear injuries.

Implications/Relevance of Pressure Ulcers

The most significant contributor to pressure ulcer formation is the ischemia caused by unrelieved pressure. During this time of interrupted blood flow, the skin becomes pale, then hyperemic and blanchable. Nonblanchable erythema is the result of plasma and erythrocytes leaking into the skin tissues. Early identification and pressure-relieving interventions can reverse the effects of ischemia at this point. Once the skin integrity has been compromised, however, the patient is at risk for bacteremia, sepsis, osteomyelitis, and cellulitis.

"In 2007, CMS reported 257,412 cases of preventable pressure ulcers as secondary diagnoses. The average cost for these cases was $43,180 per hospital stay. The incidence of new pressure ulcers in acute-care patients is around 7 percent, with wide variation among institutions" (Beaver, 2008, p. 1). To promote better prevention measures, Medicare will no longer pay for the costs of treatment for pressure ulcers acquired in acute care settings.

> **BOX 14-17 Healthy People 2010**
>
> The Healthy People 2010 target, objective 1–16, is to "reduce the proportion of nursing home residents with current diagnosis of pressure ulcers to no more than 8/1,000 residents." The 1997 baseline data were 16/1,000 residents.

Warning Signs/Risk Factors for Pressure Ulcers

Risk factors for pressure ulcer development include advanced age, immobility, malnutrition, BMI <24, fecal incontinence, diminished level of consciousness, and impaired sensation. External factors that promote pressure ulcer development are pressure, friction, shearing, and moisture. Individuals with intact sensation and ability to move will shift their weight or change positions when pressure or friction is concentrated in an area of the body. However, if a person is immobile or has decreased sensation, the ischemia persists and pressure ulcers can develop in a very short period of time.

Assessment

Risk assessments should be completed on all patients; the **Braden Scale for Pressure Ulcer Risk Assessment** (**Table 14-16**) is the most widely used instrument that determines risk of pressure ulcer development. The scale assesses sensory perception, skin moisture, activity, mobility, nutrition, and friction/shear. Each area is scored on a scale of 1 to 3 or 4, with a possible score of 23 points. The lower the Braden score, the higher the risk of pressure ulcer development (Braden & Bergstrom, 1987). A Braden score of 16 or less indicates a high risk of pressure ulcer development in the general population; a score of 18 or less is indicative of high risk in the older adult or persons with darkly pigmented skin.

Baseline Braden scores should be determined upon admission to the health care facility and at

TABLE 14-15 Braden Scale for Pressure Ulcer Risk Assessment

Sensory Perception Ability to respond meaningfully to pressure-related discomfort	1. *Completely Limited:* Unresponsive (does not moan, flinch, or gasp) to painful stimuli, due to diminished level of consciousness or sedation. OR Limited ability to feel pain over most of body surface.	2. *Very Limited:* Responds only to painful stimuli. Cannot communicate discomfort except by moaning or restlessness. OR Has a sensory impairment, which limits the ability to feel pain or discomfort over half of body.	3. *Slightly Limited:* Responds to verbal commands but cannot always communicate discomfort or need to be turned. OR Has some sensory impairment, which limits ability to feel pain or discomfort in one or two extremities.	4. *No Impairment:* Responds to verbal commands. Has no sensory deficit that would limit ability to feel or voice pain or discomfort.
Moisture Degree to which skin is exposed to moisture	1. *Constantly Moist:* Perspiration, urine, etc. keep skin moist almost constantly. Dampness is detected every time patient is moved or turned.	2. *Moist:* Skin is often but not always moist. Linen must be changed at least once a shift.	3. *Occasionally Moist:* Skin is occasionally moist, requiring an extra linen change approximately once a day.	4. *Rarely Moist:* Skin is usually dry; linen requires changing only at routine intervals.
Activity Degree of physical activity	1. *Bedfast:* Confined to bed.	2. *Chairfast:* Ability to walk is severely limited or nonexistent. Cannot bear own weight and/or must be assisted into chair or wheelchair.	3. *Walks Occasionally:* Walks occasionally during day but for very short distances, with or without assistance. Spends majority of each shift in bed or chair.	4. *Walks Frequently:* Walks outside the room at least twice a day and inside room at least once every 2 hours during waking hours.

Mobility Ability to change and control body position	1. *Completely Immobile:* Does not make even slight changes in body or extremity position without assistance.	2. *Very Limited:* Makes occasional slight changes in body or extremity position but unable to make frequent or significant changes independently.	3. *Slightly Limited:* Makes frequent though slight changes in body or extremity position independently.	4. *No Limitations:* Makes major and frequent changes in position without assistance.
Nutrition Usual food intake pattern	1. *Very Poor:* Never eats a complete meal. Rarely eats more than one-third of any food offered. Eats two servings or less of protein (meat or dairy products) per day. Takes fluids poorly. Does not take a liquid dietary supplement. OR Is NPO and/or maintained on clear liquids or IV for more than 5 days.	2. *Probably Inadequate:* Rarely eats a complete meal and generally eats only about half of any food offered. Protein intake includes only three servings of meat or dairy products per day. Occasionally will take a dietary supplement. OR Receives less than optimum amount of liquid diet or tube feeding.	3. *Adequate:* Eats over half of most meals. Eats a total of four servings of protein (meat, dairy products) each day. Occasionally will refuse a meal, but will usually take a supplement if offered. OR Is on a tube feeding or TPN regimen, which probably meets most of nutritional needs.	4. *Excellent:* Eats most of every meal. Never refuses a meal. Usually eats a total of four or more servings of meat and diary products. Occasionally eats between meals. Does not require supplementation.
Friction and Shear	1. *Problem:* Requires moderate to maximum assistance in moving. Complete lifting without sliding against sheets is impossible. Frequently slides down in bed or chair, requiring frequent repositioning with maximum assistance. Spasticity, contractures, or agitation leads to almost constant friction.	2. *Potential Problem:* Moves feebly or requires minimum assistance. During a move, skin probably slides to some extent against sheets, chair, restraints, or other devices. Maintains relatively good position in chair or bed most of the time but occasionally slides down.	3. *No Apparent Problem:* Moves in bed and in chair independently and has sufficient muscle strength to lift up completely during move. Maintains good position in bed or chair at all times.	
			TOTAL SCORE:	

SOURCE: Copyright Barbara Braden and Nancy Bergstrom, 1988. Reprinted with permission.

regular intervals or when the patient's condition changes. Hospitals and long-term care facilities should implement nursing care policies that determine the frequency of assessment.

Nursing assessment and documentation of pressure ulcers should include staging, measurement, exudate description, wound bed characteristics, pain, condition of surrounding tissue, and any undermining factors. The National Pressure Ulcer Advisory Panel (NPUAP) has defined the stages of pressure ulcers (**Figure 14-4**). Ulcers are staged once and do not heal in a reverse fashion (for example, a stage IV ulcer that heals is not considered a stage I but is referred to as a healed stage IV ulcer). The healing process is described by the Pressure Ulcer Scale for Healing (PUSH) tool, which is discussed later in the chapter.

If an eschar is present, it must be debrided before staging can occur. Prior to debridement (**Table 14-16**), the ulcer should be documented as an eschar-covered pressure ulcer. Structures beneath the epidermis and dermis, including muscle, are more susceptible to the effects of ischemia. Therefore, pressure ulcers are usually much worse

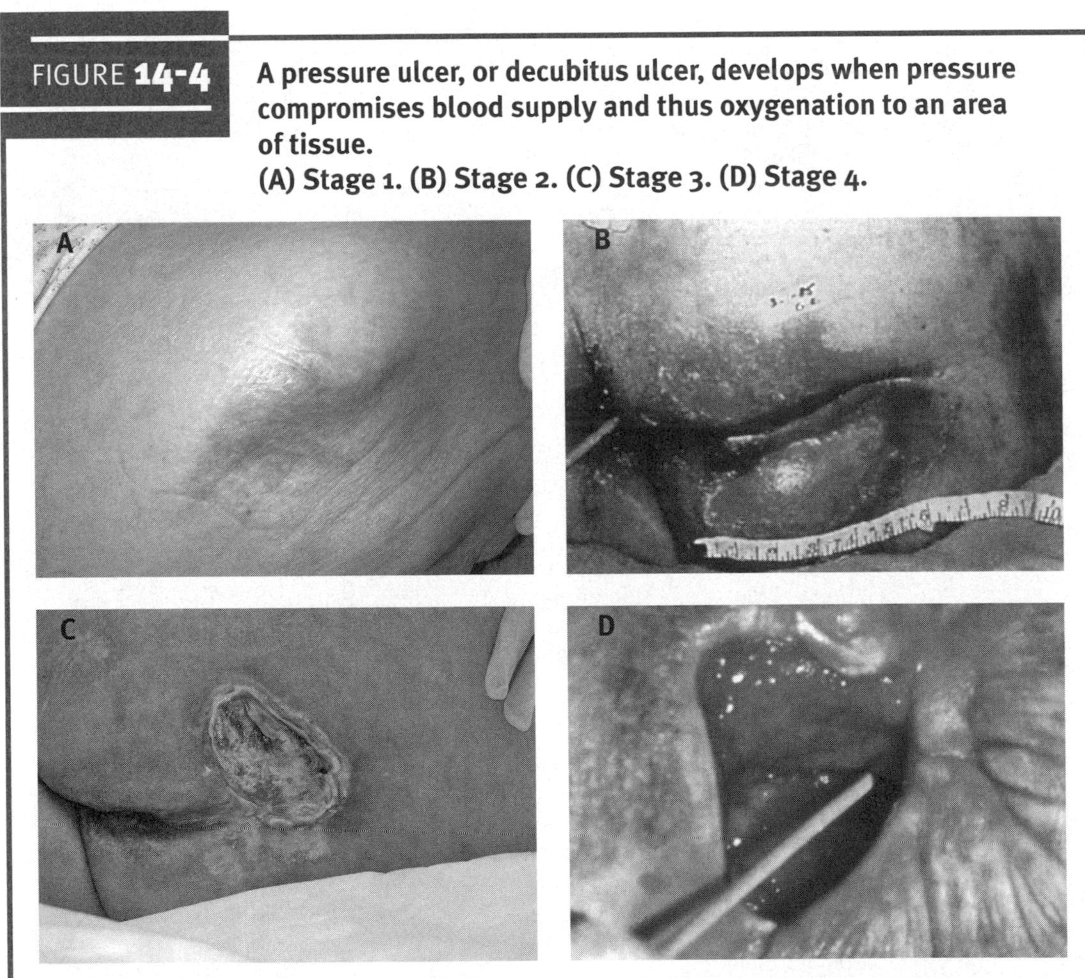

FIGURE **14-4** **A pressure ulcer, or decubitus ulcer, develops when pressure compromises blood supply and thus oxygenation to an area of tissue. (A) Stage 1. (B) Stage 2. (C) Stage 3. (D) Stage 4.**

SOURCE: (A & C) © Chuck Stewart. (B & D) Courtesy of National Pressure Ulcer Advisory Board.

TABLE 14-16 Methods of Pressure Ulcer Debridement

Extrinsic	Factors
Sharp	Devitalized tissue is removed with a scalpel, scissors, or other sharp instrument. The most rapid form of debridement, and can be used for removing areas of thick eschar.
Enzymatic	Topical debriding agents are applied to devitalized tissue areas.
Autolytic	Appropriate for noninfected ulcers only. Synthetic dressings that aid self-digestion of devitalized tissue.
Mechanical	Wet-to-dry dressings, hydrotherapy, and irrigation.

BOX 14-18 Preventing Pressure Ulcers

1. Assess all clients for risk of pressure ulcer development.
2. Identify all factors of risk to determine specific interventions.
3. Inspect the skin at least daily and document results.
4. Use mild cleansing agents for bathing, avoiding hot water, harsh soaps, and friction.
5. Moisturize after bathing and minimize environmental factors that lead to dry skin.
6. Avoid massaging bony prominences.
7. Assess for incontinence. Use skin barriers after cleansing, absorbent underpads or briefs, and monitor frequently for episodes of incontinence.
8. Use dry lubricants, such as cornstarch, on transfer surfaces (linens) to prevent friction.
9. Assess for compromised nutrition, particularly protein and caloric intake. Consider nutritional supplements and support for clients at risk.
10. Maintain or improve client's mobility and activity levels.
11. Reposition bed-bound clients at least every 2 hours and chair-bound clients every hour. Patients should be instructed or assisted to shift their positions more frequently (i.e., every 15 minutes for chair-bound patients and at least every hour for bed-bound).
12. Place at-risk clients on pressure-reducing devices. (Donut devices should not be used—they simply displace the pressure and friction to the periphery of the area that is meant to be protected.)
13. Use lifting devices to transfer clients.
14. Pillows or foam wedges should be used to keep bony prominences from direct contact with each other (e.g., knees, ankles).
15. Avoid positioning the client on the trochanter when lying on his or her side. (Use a 30-degree lateral inclined position.)
16. Elevate the head of the bed at 30 degrees or less. (Shearing injuries can occur at elevations higher than 30 degrees.)
17. Evaluate and document the effectiveness of interventions, and modify the plan of care according to client response.
18. Provide education to clients, family, and caregivers for the prevention of pressure ulcers.

than they appear on the surface, and staging should be to the maximum anatomical depth after necrotic tissue debridement is performed. The structural layers damaged by the ischemia are lost, and the defect is filled with granulation tissue.

The length, width, and depth of pressure ulcers should be measured and documented, with distinction made between healed and nonhealed areas of the ulcer. Photographs are often used to document the occurrence and healing of pressure ulcers. The quantity and characteristics of any exudates and the types of wound bed tissue (necrotic, slough, granulation) are also documented. Pain related to the pressure ulcer should be assessed using an appropriate pain scale. It is also important to identify and document effective pain relief measures and provide analgesia prior to dressing changes or other interventions.

The surrounding skin should be assessed for any maceration or injury (including tape abra-

BOX 14-19 Laboratory Studies Associated with Poor Nutrition

Serum albumin	<3.5 g/dl	
Serum transferrin	<200	
Prealbumin	<11 mg/dl	
Cholesterol	>160	
Lymphocytopenia	<1,500	(<100 indicates severe malnutrition)

Source: Adapted from Best Practices for Care of Older Adults (Clark & Baldwin, 2004).

BOX 14-20 Snacks for Pressure Ulcer Prevention and Management

Protein sources (promote cell production and growth and tissue healing):
- Peanut butter (also a source of zinc)
- Yogurt
- High-protein shakes
- Egg custard

Zinc sources (promote cell production and tissue healing):
- Whole milk
- Wheat bread
- Cheese
- Cereal
- Cocoa

Arginine sources (for the formation of collagen and elastin):
- Walnuts
- Peanuts

Vitamin C sources (for the formation of strong blood vessels):
- Oranges
- Cantaloupe
- Strawberries

Vitamin A sources (promote tissue healing and resistance to infections):
- Carrots
- Pink grapefruit
- Apricots

Vitamin B sources (required for protein synthesis):
- Egg salad
- Chicken

BOX 14-21 Guidelines for Pressure Ulcer Treatments

1. Cleanse the wound with a noncytotoxic cleanser (saline) during each dressing change.
2. If necrotic tissue or slough is present, consider the use of high-pressure irrigation.
3. Debride necrotic tissue.
4. Do not debride dry, black eschar on heels.
5. Perform wound care using topical dressings determined by wound and availability.
6. Choose dressings that provide a moist wound environment, keep the skin surrounding the ulcer dry, control exudates, and eliminate dead space.
7. Reassess the wound with each dressing change to determine whether treatment plan modifications are needed.
8. Identify and manage wound infections.
9. Clients with stage III and IV ulcers that do not respond to conservative therapy may require surgical intervention.

Source: Adapted from National Guideline Clearinghouse *Guideline for Prevention and Management of Pressure Ulcers* (http://www.guideline.gov).

sions). The pressure ulcer may have undermining or sinus tracts, and the presence of these complications should be documented. Pressure ulcers with undermining or tracts often lead to further skin breakdown.

Nutrition

Nutrition is important for the client at risk and for those with pressure ulcers. Nutrients involved in wound healing include protein, arginine, zinc, and vitamins A, B, and C (Mathus-Vliegen, 2004; Singer, 2002). If dietary intake is inadequate, nutritional support (tube feeding) should be used to provide approximately 35 calories/kg/day and 1.5 grams of protein/kg/day (Mathus-Vliegen, 2004). Other identified or suspected nutritional deficiencies should be corrected if possible.

Tissue Load Management

Tissue load is the distribution of friction, pressure, and shear on the tissue. Clients who develop pressure ulcers require a decreased load to the ulcerated area and provision of moisture levels and temperature that enhance healing. Avoid positioning the client on the pressure ulcer and use positioning devices to raise the area off the support surface. Pressure-reducing and pressure-relieving mattresses are available and should be used when positioning techniques are not adequate to reduce the risk of pressure ulcer development or progression.

It is important to measure and document the healing of ulcers that are being treated by nursing and medical interventions. The **Pressure Ulcer Scale for Healing (PUSH)** tool (see **Table 14-17**) provides a consistent method of recording the effectiveness of treatment. The scale has three subscales with a possible score of 17. The score will trend downward when treatment is effective, and a score of 0 indicates complete healing of the pressure ulcer.

Prevention of pressure ulcers is dependent upon nursing assessment and early intervention. The cost of ulcers, both in medical expense and human suffering, is astronomical and is best prevented through aggressive pressure relief methods and nutritional support.

TABLE 14-17 PUSH (Pressure Ulcer Scale for Healing)

Length × Width	**0** 0 cm^2	**1** <0.3 cm^2	**2** 0.3–0.6 cm^2	**3** 0.7–1.0 cm^2	**4** 1.1–2.0 cm^2	**5** 2.1–3.0 cm^2	**Sub-score**
		6 3.1–4.0 cm^2	**7** 4.1–8.0 cm^2	**8** 8.1–12.0 cm^2	**9** 12.1–24.0 cm^2	**10** >24.0 cm^2	
Exudate Amount	**0** None	**1** Light	**2** Moderate	**3** Heavy			**Sub-score**
Tissue Type	**0** Closed	**1** Epithelial tissue	**2** Granulation tissue	**3** Slough	**4** Necrotic tissue		**Sub-score**

Length × Width: Measure the greatest length (head to toe) and the greatest width (side to side) using a centimeter ruler. Multiply these two measurements (length × width) to obtain an estimate of surface area in square centimeters (cm^2). Caveat: Do not guess! Always use a centimeter ruler, and always use the same method each time the ulcer is measured.
Exudate Amount: Estimate the amount of exudate (drainage) present after removal of the dressing and before applying any topical agent to the ulcer. Estimate the exudate (drainage) as none, light, moderate, or heavy.
Tissue Type: This refers to the types of tissue that are present in the wound (ulcer) bed. Score as a 4 if there is any necrotic tissue present. Score as a 3 if there is any amount of slough present and necrotic tissue is absent. Score as a 2 if the wound is clean and contains granulation tissue. A superficial wound that is reepithelializing is scored as a 1. When the wound is closed, score as a 0.
4—Necrotic tissue (eschar): Black, brown, or tan tissue that adheres firmly to the wound bed or ulcer edges and may be either firmer or softer than surrounding skin.
3—Slough: Yellow or white tissue that adheres to the ulcer bed in strings or thick clumps, or is mucinous.
2—Granulation tissue: Pink or beefy red tissue with a shiny, moist, granular appearance.
1—Epithelial tissue: For superficial ulcers, new pink or shiny tissue (skin) that grows in from the edges or as islands on the ulcer surface.
0—Closed/resurfaced: The wound is completely covered with epithelium (new skin).

BOX 14-22 Key Point

Cytotoxic cleansers that should not be used for pressure ulcer management include betadine, peroxide, sodium hypochlorite (Dakin's), iodophor, and acetic acid.

DYSPHAGIA

Prevalence

Dysphagia, or problems with swallowing, is "an underrecognized, poorly diagnosed and poorly managed health problem" that negatively impacts the quality and potentially quantity of life (Ekberg, Hamby, Woisard, Wuttge-Hanning, & Ortega, 2004, p. 143). Although dysphagia may occur at any age, it is more prevalent in the elderly (Morris, 2004; Roy, Stemple, Merrill, & Thomas, 2007; White, O'Rourke, Ong, Cordato, & Chan, 2008). Prevalence data suggest that 13–35% of elderly persons living in the community report dysphagia symptoms (Kawashima, Motohashi, & Fujishima, 2004; Lindgren & Janzon, 1991a; Roy et al., 2007). Between 25% and 30 of hospitalized patients, and approximately 30%–40% of persons in nursing homes, experience dysphagia (Brin & Younger, 1988; Layne, Losinski, Zenner, & Ament, 1989; Stevenson, 2002; Wright, 2007). It was estimated that by 2010, 16.5 million persons would require care for dysphagia (U.S. Census Bureau, 2000).

Implications/Prevalence of Dysphagia

The physiological sequelae of dysphagia have traditionally received the greatest attention. Untreated dysphagia places a person at greater risk for nutritional deficiencies and respiratory problems. Dehydration and malnutrition from inadequate intake predispose persons to the development of many medical problems. Dehydration thickens secretions, increasing the risk for respiratory problems, and aspiration may lead to pneumonia and death. The ability and motivation to be active and involved in daily activities may also be adversely impacted. The development of these complications is dependent on the nature and severity of the dysphagia and the overall health status of the individual.

The social and psychological consequences of dysphagia must also be considered in the treatment and evaluation of care. The effects of dysphagia on quality of life were evaluated in 360 adults with subjective dysphagia complaints living in nursing homes or clinics in four European countries (Ekberg et al., 2004). The findings confirm the serious physiological impact of dysphagia. Fifty-five percent reported their eating habits were affected by their swallowing problems; over 50% ate less, 44% experienced weight loss, and over 30% were still hungry or thirsty after a meal. From a psychosocial perspective, 45% no longer found eating to be enjoyable. More than half indicated dysphagia made life less enjoyable. Loss of self-esteem and an increasing sense of isolation also were reported. Over one-third (36%) avoided eating with others, and 41% experienced anxiety or panic during meals. Of the individuals interviewed, 40% had a confirmed diagnosis, only 32% had received treatment, and just 39% believed dysphagia could be treated (Ekberg et al., 2004). An individual's ability to be nourished physically, emotionally, and socially is threatened by dysphagia. The findings from this study are supported by other literature (Morris, 2004; Roy et al., 2007).

Warning Signs/Risk Factors for Dysphagia

Deglutition is the act of swallowing in which a food or liquid bolus is transported from the mouth through the pharynx and esophagus into the stomach. Swallowing is a complex neuromuscular process that occurs in stages. Dysphagia is usually identified as being either oropharyngeal or esophageal, designating the phase in which dysfunction occurs. In the oropharyngeal phase, food is prepared for swallowing by mastication and mixing with saliva, and then is moved posteriorly, triggering the pharyngeal swallow reflex, which moves the bolus down the pharynx (Logemann, 1998; Morris, 2004). During the pharyngeal swallow, the larynx closes and the epiglottis redirects the bolus around the airway, protecting the respiratory tract (Logemann, 1998; Morris, 2004). The esophageal phase begins when the bolus enters the esophagus at the cricopharyngeal juncture or upper esophageal sphincter (UES). Peristaltic waves propel the bolus through the esophagus to the lower esophageal sphincter, which opens into the stomach (Logemann). Because swallowing is a complex, coordinated event, causes of dysphagia are multiple and diverse. Each type of dysphagia is characterized by specific symptoms and associated with specific disorders.

Oropharyngeal dysphagia is usually related to neuromuscular impairments affecting the tongue, pharynx, and upper esophageal sphincter (Kennedy-Malone, Fletcher, & Plank, 2004). Stroke is the leading cause of oropharyngeal dysfunction (Agency for

Health Care Policy and Research, 1999). Persons experiencing oropharyngeal dysphagia often complain of difficulty initiating a swallow. A cough early in the swallow and nasal regurgitation are symptoms associated with oropharyngeal dysphagia (Kennedy-Malone et al., 2004). The oropharyngeal phase of dysphagia is voluntary and utilizes the motor and sensory pathways to move food posteriorly to the oropharaynx, which then triggers the reflexive/involuntary phase in which the larynx and epiglottis are elevated and lowered, respectively, to prevent aspiration into the trachea (White et al., 2008). Dysphonia and dysarthria indicate motor dysfunction in the structures involved in the oral and pharyngeal phases and may be accompanied by dysphagia (Glenn-Molali, 2002). Inadequate saliva production can also interfere with the formation and movement of the food bolus. Candidiasis, or thrush, a fungal infection identified by white plaques on the mucous membranes of the oral cavity, can cause pain and discomfort when swallowing.

Esophageal dysphagia results from motility problems, neuromuscular problems, or obstruction that interferes with the movement of the food bolus through the esophagus into the stomach (Logemann, 1998; White et al., 2008). Common symptoms of esophageal dysphagia include complaints of food sticking after a swallow and coughing late in the swallow (Kennedy-Malone et al., 2004). Muscular dystrophy, myasthenia gravis, scleroderma, achalasia, and esophageal spasms may cause motility problems. Inflammation of the esophagus, secondary to GERD or a retained pill, is another etiology for esophageal dysphagia. Medications associated with pill-induced irritation or injury include tetracycline, potassium chloride, quinidine, iron, nonsteroidal anti-inflammatory drugs, alendronate sodium, and vitamin C (Amella, 1996). Common medical conditions associated with dysphagia are outlined in **Table 14-18**.

Assessment

Clinical evaluation of swallowing skills in patients with conditions that predispose to dysphagia or who voice complaints that suggest a swallowing disorder should be a priority for nursing. Evaluation, as it relates to dysphagia, can refer to screening or diagnostic testing. Screening involves determining if the patient has signs or symptoms of dysphagia for the purpose of referring for diagnostic evaluation to identify physiological components of swallowing (Smith & Connolly, 2003). Nursing plays a pivotal role in the early detection of swallowing problems and intervening to prevent complications from dysphagia. The findings from a screening evaluation allow prompt referral for diagnostic workup and implementation of interventions to promote safe eating/feeding practices.

TABLE 14-18 Common Medical Conditions Associated with Dysphagia

Classification of Dysphagia	Neuromuscular Causes	Mechanical Causes
Oropharyngeal dysphagia	Cerebrovascular accident Parkinson's disease Multiple sclerosis Zenker's diverticulum	Tumors Inflammatory masses
Esophageal dysphagia	Parkinson's disease Achalasia Scleroderma	Tumors Strictures Foreign bodies Medication irritation Gastroesophageal reflux disease (GERD)

Castell (1996) suggests that 80% of dysphagia can be diagnosed through a history. A careful history of the dysphagia should be obtained during the nursing assessment. Open-ended questions that the nurse can ask of the patient or the caregiver might include: How often do you cough after eating or drinking? How often do you feel that food is caught in your throat or chest? Show me where it sticks. How long does it take for you to eat a meal? Is this a change for you? (Morris, 2004). The patient or caregiver should be asked about the presence of predisposing conditions or warning signs and symptoms. Additional questions might include: What type of food causes the symptoms? Is the swallowing problem intermittent or progressive? Is heartburn present?

The physical examination involves a cognitive, neuromuscular, and respiratory assessment. Important cognitive factors include interest in eating, ability to focus on and complete a meal, and the ability to remember and follow directions for safe eating. Neurological assessment involves testing sensory and motor components of the cranial nerves, in particular cranial nerves V, VII, IX, X, XI, and XII. Breath sounds, the strength of the person's cough, and his or her ability to clear the throat are clues to the integrity of the respiratory structures and the presence of protective mechanisms. Although commonly considered to be protective, the gag reflex is not an indication of the patient's ability to swallow (Logemann, 1998). However, detection of laryngeal elevation during a swallow maneuver grossly suggests airway closure (Amella, 1996). Medications should be reviewed for those that can decrease saliva production (antihistamines, anticholinergics, antihypertensives, cold medications), decrease cognition (sedatives, hypnotics), and/or decrease the strength of the muscles involved in swallowing (antispasticity drugs).

A standard procedure for bedside evaluation has not been formulated (Smith & Connolly, 2003); however, screening protocols have been developed and evaluated. Screening generally involves a checklist for warning signs and symptoms (Logemann, 1998). See **Table 14-19** for warning signs of dysphagia.

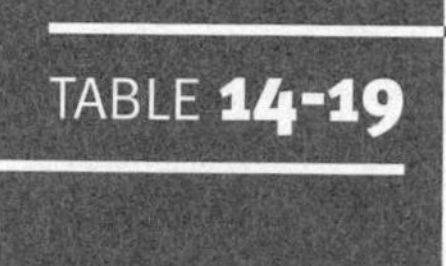

Signs of Swallowing Difficulties or Dysphagia

Inability to recognize foods
Difficulty placing food in the mouth
Inability to control food or saliva
Coughing before, during, or after a swallow
Frequent coughing toward the end of or immediately following a meal
Recurrent pneumonia
Wet, gurgly voice
Weight loss without explanation*
Complaints of swallowing problems

*Weight gain may occur if a large quantity of high calorie beverages such as milkshakes are consumed.

SOURCE: Information taken from Logeman (1998).

The effectiveness of trained nurses to screen for dysphagia after stroke was evaluated in the Collaborative Dysphagia Audit (CODA) Study. Nurses on a stroke unit received training in a simple water screening test and screened acute stroke patients. The findings demonstrated a decrease in the number of patients who kept nothing by mouth (NPO), a decrease in the number of patients with inappropriate feeding orders, and improved referrals (Davies, 2002; Stroke Research Unit, n.d.). The Gatehead Dysphagia Management Model (GDMM), developed from the results of the CODA, provides a decision tree to guide assessment and management of dysphagia (see **Case Study 14-1**).

A careful assessment of the individual eating a meal also is an essential component of an evaluation, even if the initial screening does not suggest a swallowing problem (Davies, 2002). Observations of a prolonged time required to complete a meal, "picking" at food, and active attempts to avoid eating (pushing the food away, turning away from offered food, refusing to open the mouth) may indicate a swallowing problem. Environmental factors that influence intake and eating behaviors, such as distractibility, fatigue, or even compatibility with dining companions or assistants, will not be apparent in a bedside evaluation. Amella (1999) emphasizes the importance of contextual issues in an evaluation, pointing out that fatigue, pain, and anxiety may mask an older person's true abilities.

Case Study 14-1

Mr. C., an 81-year-old widower, is admitted for stroke rehabilitation. He underwent a cystoscopy and transurethral resection of the prostate (TURP) for benign prostatic hypertrophy (BPH) a week ago. After the procedure he experienced a hypotensive episode and mental status changes. A workup revealed a large left middle-cerebral artery stroke. His stroke deficits include expressive aphasia, left neglect, dysphagia, and left hemiplegia. Concurrent health problems include coronary artery disease, hypertension, and hyperlipidemia under good control prior to surgery. Prior to transfer, Mr. C. had a low HCT and hemoccult-positive stool and received a blood transfusion. He was also suspected to have pneumonia and was started on an antibiotic.

On examination, Mr. C. is noted to be thin, pale, and lethargic. He has a weak cough, facial weakness, and a mild case of thrush. An indwelling urinary catheter is draining amber urine. Nonpitting edema is noted in his right hand; his arms have multiple bruises and dry, flaky skin. The transfer report indicates he requires minimal assistance with bed mobility and moderate assistance with transfers including toilet transfers; his sitting balance is fair; and he can self-propel his wheelchair 150 ft. with standby assistance. His son and daughter live out of town and have had to return home. They were not able to accompany him at transfer and will not be able to visit until the weekend (4 days from now).

Orders on admission include a pureed texture diet with moderate thick liquids; Isosource 1.5 cans at 0800 and 1600 and 1 can at 1200 and 2000 with 325 cc free water flush every shift via PEG tube. One scoop of Benefiber is added to tube feeding three times a day. His medication orders include Tenormin, 25 mg once a day; Lipitor, 20 mg at bedtime; Prevacid, 30 mg once a day; ASA, 81 mg once a day; Plavix, 75 mg once a day; amiodarone, 200 mg once a day; and clindamycin, 600 mg three times a day.

Questions:

1. Mr. C. presents multiple challenges. Which of the common health problems discussed in this chapter are relevant to his nursing care?
2. What are the priorities for Mr. C.'s care plan during his first week of rehabilitation?
3. What are key interventions to promote recovery and prevent complications?

After 3 days the physician orders to discontinue his indwelling catheter. He experiences frequency, urgency, and incontinence. He has developed symptoms of an allergy—he is suffering from runny nose and dry cough. His tube feeding is being decreased as his dietary intake increases. When his family arrives, they ask about putting him on that medicine advertised on TV for overactive bladder and bring his OTC allergy medicine (Sudafed) for his cold. They also bring him his favorite soda.

Questions:

4. How would you respond to the family?
5. What actions would you take to address the problems and concerns raised?
6. How would your goals for care evolve over the next weeks of his stay?
7. What interventions would you institute to prevent the development of common health problems during his hospitalization and upon return to the community?

Assessment for aspiration is also important. Aspiration occurs when material passes into the larynx below the true vocal cords; silent aspiration refers to situations in which aspiration does not produce the typical cough or change in voice quality (Smith & Connolly, 2003). Pulse oximetry has been found to be an effective, efficient tool to detect aspiration while eating. In a review of trends in the evaluation and treatment of dysphagia after stroke, Smith and Connolly report that a 2% drop in oxygen saturation levels from baseline detects 86% of penetration/aspiration. When followed by a 10 ml water swallow test at the bedside, the ability to detect aspiration increases to 95%.

Persons at risk should be assessed upon admission to a facility or community caseload; if deterioration occurs after admission, the individual should be reassessed at that time. Persons with degenerative conditions should be reassessed on a regular basis and when the condition progresses. (Monitoring lung sounds, respiration rate and quality, and other vital signs remains an important component of ongoing assessment and evaluation of care.) If screening suggests dysphagia, a referral for diagnostic evaluation should be ordered. A more focused examination may be conducted by a speech-language therapist (SLT). Occupational therapists (OTs) also may be prepared to complete an extensive examination. Further testing to confirm the diagnosis and determine the presence of and conditions surrounding aspiration are conducted by radiology or gastroenterology subspecialists.

Interventions/Strategies for Care

Actual treatment of the dysphagia depends on the specific diagnosis and the level of dysfunction. Restoration of swallowing has been attempted using a variety of strategies ranging from electrical stimulation to thermal stimulation, muscle exercises, and even black pepper oil—all with varying success at restoring muscular function and normal swallowing. Forthcoming should be the results of trials of Shaker exercises (which provide another way to open the upper esophageal sphincter through postural maneuvering) vs. standard treatment and muscle exercises vs. sensory postural therapy. Those studies may shed new light on the problem of restoration of normal swallowing function (White et al., 2008). Nursing interventions to manage dysphagia in order to minimize the risk of aspiration and promote nutrition and hydration involve compensatory eating techniques, diet modification, and oral care, and may require adaptive equipment.

Compensatory Eating Techniques

Specific interventions are developed for persons with dysphagia based on the swallowing problems identified. The results of a diagnostic workup or referral to an SLT or OT should provide specific recommendations for eating techniques. However, appropriate positioning is critical for safe eating and swallowing for all individuals. An upright position with the arms and feet supported, the head midline in a neutral position, and the chin slightly tucked is recommended to minimize the possibility of aspiration. The upright position should be maintained for at least 30 to 60 minutes after eating (the longer interval is necessary for esophageal dysphagia) (Avery-Smith, 1992). The location of food placement in the mouth as well as the size, consistency, and temperature of food items are important sensory cues to promote safe swallowing. If the individual has a sensory loss or oral muscular weakness, placing food on the unaffected or least affected side may help improve control over the bolus and its movement to the back of the mouth. If movement of the food to the back of the mouth is the problem, then placement of the bolus at the back of the tongue may be necessary to trigger the swallow (Martin-Harris & Cherney, 1996). The bolus size also influences swallow. A small bolus will not enter the pharynx as quickly as a large bolus, decreasing the risk of aspiration. However, a large bolus improves movement through the oral cavity in persons with delayed oral transit and also prolongs laryngeal elevation and closure (Martin-Harris & Cherney, 1996). For persons with decreased oral sensation or the impaired oral movement of food, cold items may improve posterior tongue movements and laryngeal swallow; for other persons a warm bolus facilitates swallowing (Glenn-Molali, 2002). Careful questioning and observation of the conditions that result in optimal intake without evidence of swallowing problems and those associated with apparent problems will help guide eating techniques and feeding strategies. Having said this, a recent study looking at dysphagia among Parkinson's and dementia patients found that honey-thick foods were more effective than nectar-thick foods in preventing aspiration; the chin-down swallowing posture was least effective (Loggmann et al., 2008).

Characteristics of the environment, including assistive personnel and dining partners, are factors that can facilitate or interfere with a safe, efficient swallow and adequate intake. For the first meal or eating/feeding session (and subsequent meals in some cases) a quiet room is preferable to decrease distractions and allow greater concentration on eating. The health care provider should sit down to assist with eating, positioning herself or himself and the food tray directly across from the patient in order to maintain the proper posture for the patient and ensure that she or he can see and reach food items and utensils (Avery-Smith, 1992). An unhurried, calm demeanor is important. Conversation should be limited to after a swallow is completed and before the next bite is taken. However, interaction that requires a response from the person eating is necessary to provide information about changes in voice quality as well as to promote a more pleasant social experience.

Diet Modifications

Modifying the texture of the food and fluids consumed is a common response to suspected swallowing problems. Alterations in diet consistency should be tailored to the type of swallowing disorder. An example of levels for food consistency is provided in **Table 14-20**. Foods can be prepared in blenders or food processors to the approved consistency or purchased in the infant–child food section. Attention to seasoning may improve flavor and therefore adherence to and intake of a modified diet.

Thickened fluids frequently present a challenge to adequate hydration. Complaints about the texture, taste, and ability to quench thirst are common. The Dysphagia Diet Task Force has standardized food and fluid textures (see Table 14-22). Certain fluids have a thicker consistency naturally, whereas others will require thickening to the appropriate consistency with commercial or natural thickeners. Instant potato flakes, instant baby rice cereal, and mashed bananas are natural thickeners, but may not meet special diet requirements and may change the taste of the thickened items. Commercial thickening agents differ with respect to the directions for preparation and the effect of time on consistency. The type and temperature of the fluid to be thickened also affect mixing directions, so it is important to be familiar with the product used by the facility or individual at home.

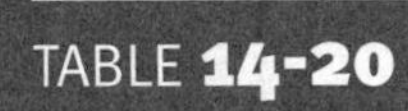

The National Dysphagia Diet (NDD)

The National Dysphagia Diet (NDD) provides guidelines for progressive diets to be used nationally in the treatment of dysphagia. The following are some examples:

- **Dysphagia Pureed (NDD 1):** "Pudding-like" consistencies; pureed, no chunks or small pieces; avoid scrambled eggs, cereals with lumps.
- **Dysphagia Mechanically Altered (NDD 2):** Moist, soft foods; easily formed into a bolus; ground meats; soft, tender vegetables; soft fruit; slightly moistened dry cereal with little texture. No bread or foods such as peas and corn.
  Avoid skins and seeds.
  Mechanical Soft: Same as the mechanically altered, but allows bread, cakes, and rice.
- **Dysphagia Advanced (NDD 3):** Regular textured foods except those that are very hard, sticky, or crunchy. Avoid hard fruit and vegetables, corn, skins, nuts, and seeds.
  LIQUID CONSISTENCIES:
  Spoon thick
  Honey-like
  Nectar-like
  Thin: All beverages such as water, ice, milk, milkshakes, juices, coffee, tea, sodas

SOURCE: Adapted from *Journal of the American Dietetic Association*, *103*(3), McCallum S. L. © 2003 American Dietetic Association.

Encouraging fluid intake with thickened liquids often requires creativity and persistence. Some facilities allow dysphagia patients to drink plain water between meals while requiring thickened liquids with meals. There are contradictory beliefs about the likelihood that allowing plain water will lead to aspiration pneumonia (Garon, Engle, & Ormison, 1997; Panther, 2005). Oral care appears to be a crucial link in the aspiration to pneumonia process (Langmore et al., 1998; White et al., 2008). Frequent oral care to ensure the oral cavity is clear of food particles and to prevent the growth of bacteria is a critical component of liberalized fluid programs and an essential strategy to minimize the risk for pneumonia.

> **BOX 14-23 Key Point**
>
> **Providing adequate fluid before and after administering medications will help maintain moisture and decrease the likelihood of impaired transport and esophageal irritation.**

Oral Hygiene

Examination of the relative risk of multiple factors (medical/health status, functional status, dysphagia/gastroesophageal reflux, feeding/mode of nutritional intake, and oral/dental status) in the development of pneumonia in older persons suggests that colonization and host resistance are key contributors (Langmore et al., 1998). Oropharyngeal colonization from inadequate oral care, decayed teeth, or periodontal disease is the initial process that can lead to the development of pneumonia. Aspiration of these organisms in liquids, food, or saliva combined with decreased immunity increases the risk for development of pneumonia.

Regular cleaning of the teeth or dentures, gums, and tongue and maintaining moisture in the mouth are essential components of an oral hygiene protocol. (See Johnson and Chalmers [2002] for tools and strategies to address various problems in providing oral care.) A soft toothbrush, gauze-covered swabs, or foam toothettes may be used to scrub the surfaces of the oral cavity after meals. Electric toothbrushes may also be useful tools and, depending on the person's physical and cognitive abilities, may enable the older person with limited hand grasp and movement to more adequately and independently clean the mouth's surfaces. Individuals who receive non-oral feedings also need to have regular oral care to remove debris. The teeth and mouth should be cleaned upon awakening, after meals (or snacks for persons with dysphagia), and before bed. Dentures should be taken out and scrubbed at least daily with a brush; chemical denture cleaner tablets may be used in addition to brushing with soap or toothpaste (Johnson & Chalmers, 2002). Soaking dentures in a solution of white wine vinegar and cold water (a 50:50 solution) will help remove built-up calculus. Denture cups must also be cleaned or replaced regularly. A weekly cleaning and soaking of the denture cup in a diluted hypochlorite solution for an hour followed by thorough washing with soap and water will help sterilize the container (Johnson & Chalmers, 2002) if frequent replacement is not feasible.

Maintaining moist mucous membranes is essential to the health and integrity of the oral cavity. Dry membranes contribute to an increased rate of plaque accumulation (Almstahl & Wikstrom, 1999), and dental and denture plaque serves as a major reservoir for pathogenic organisms in the elderly (Aiden et al., 2004). Many of the medications prescribed for chronic conditions result in a dry mouth. Limited fluid intake and infrequent oral care, especially for persons who are ordered nothing by mouth, contribute to dryness. Meticulous oral care as outlined previously is crucial; however, additional measures may be needed. Saliva substitutes, toothpaste and mouth rinses without alcohol or excessive additives such as in the Biotene range, water or mouthwash in spray bottles to spritz inside the mouth, water-soluble lubricants applied to the tongue and cheeks, and Vaseline or lanolin applied frequently to the lips are among the strategies recommended for combating dry mouth in the physically dependent or cognitively impaired older adult (Johnson & Chalmers, 2002).

Adaptive Equipment

The modification of utensils or use of adaptive equipment is frequently necessary to promote independence in eating and to facilitate safe swallowing. However, careful evaluation of eating is needed for each person to ensure safe and effective tools are used. Using a straw to drink moves a fluid bolus quickly through the mouth and can exacerbate problems with swallowing. Drinking from a cup requires the head to be tilted to empty the glass; this maneuver (hyperextension) can increase the risk of aspiration. Specially designed cups with a cutout for the nose can be purchased or made to prevent the need to tilt the head back. Similarly, shallow bowls on spoons may be helpful in preventing hypertension when eating with a spoon (Glenn-Molali, 2002). An ongoing assessment of abilities and problems at meal time will help ensure that necessary changes to the plan of care are made in a timely manner. Rehabilitation nurses and texts and continuing education programs focusing on swallowing evaluation and feeding techniques are resources for new tools and techniques. Physical, occupational, and speech-language therapists can recommend specific techniques and equipment for safe intake and can help modify available tools. Their expertise and assistance should be sought.

Non-Oral Feedings

The initiation of tube feedings is a complicated decision made by the patient, health care provider, and family or health care surrogate. Often prescribed to maintain adequate nutrition and hydration levels and prevent aspiration, persons receiving non-oral feedings are still at risk for aspiration (Logemann, 1998; White et al., 2008) and inadequate nutritional intake. Attention to positioning during and after a feeding and meticulous oral hygiene are very important in preventing or minimizing the risk for aspiration in persons receiving enteral nutrition. In a literature review on GI motility, feeding tube site, and aspiration, Metheny, Schallom, and Edwards (2004) reported that the "aspiration risk exists to some extent in all tube-fed patients, depending on GI dysmotility patterns and individual patient characteristics. However, regardless of the feeding site, it is ultimately regurgitated gastric contents that are aspirated into the lungs. For this reason, the assessment of greatest interest for tube-fed patients is the evaluation of gastric emptying" (p. 131). Although the need for additional research is indicated, Edwards and Metheny (2000) suggest McClave et al.'s (1999) recommendation that a residual volume (RV) greater than or equal to 200 cc for nasogastric tubes and greater than or equal to 100 cc for gastrostomy tubes should raise concern about intolerance. Although these volumes were associated with dysmotility, McClave et al. emphasize the importance of giving consideration to other symptoms of intolerance before holding feedings. Interruptions and incomplete feedings interfere with the nutritional adequacy of non-oral diets. Nausea/vomiting, absent bowel sounds, abdominal distention, and stool pattern are clues to intolerance that should be evaluated and factored into the decision.

> **BOX 14-24 Key Point**
>
> **Monitor abdominal distention by measuring the abdominal circumference from iliac crest to iliac crest. An increase in measurement of 8–10 cm beyond baseline is considered distention.**

The administration of medications to patients with dysphagia remains a challenge for nurses. If a patient is eating but needs changes in food consistency to promote swallowing, the problem then arises—should medications be crushed? The answer is simple and has been identified as being the best practice in delivering medications to patients with dysphagia: Only medications that have been specifically designed to be crushed or opened (in the case of capsules) may be administered in that way. To crush or open capsules not designed for that purpose alters the pharmacodynamics and pharmacokinetics of the drug and must not be done. If the patient cannot take the medications, the nurse's responsibility is to contact the prescribing practitioner and seek a different medication. To not do so is negligence on the part of the nurse and potentially life threatening for the patient (Griffith, 2008).

Managing GERD

The relationship between gastroesophageal reflux disease (GERD) and enteral nutrition remains unclear; however, interventions to prevent the development of reflux or esophageal irritation and treat GERD are supported by data implicating reflux in the development of aspiration. An individual's diet pattern, in particular food or fluids associated with heartburn or discomfort, should be evaluated. Coffee, spicy foods, fatty foods, citrus fruits, alcohol, and smoking may weaken the lower esophageal sphincter and contribute to the development of the symptoms of reflux (Kennedy-Malone et al., 2004). Diet modification can be a simple, effective strategy. Sitting up for at least an hour after eating and/or raising the head of the bed 4 to 6 inches with blocks may help control the onset of symptoms, too. An oral proton pump inhibitor taken 60 minutes before a meal may be indicated (Kennedy-Malone et al., 2004). Be sure an adequate amount of fluid is consumed before and after oral medications are administered to avoid esophageal irritation.

SUMMARY

The prevention and early recognition and management of common health problems in the elderly require knowledge of the person and his or her lifestyle, an understanding of risk factors and warning signs of health problems, an awareness of options for treatment, and the ability to work with the older person and/or caregiver to establish goals and implement a plan of care. Intellectual, technical, and interpersonal skills must be interwoven to support and maintain health. "Nurses weave a tapestry of care, knowledge, relationship, and trust that is critical to a patient's survival" (Gordon, 1997, p. 12). This tapestry is also essential to maintaining the dignity, unique identity, and quality of life in the elderly by preventing the development of conditions that limit function and fulfillment.

BOX 14-25 Research Highlight

Aim: This study evaluated the relationship between urge urinary incontinence and the risk of falls and fractures in older women.

Methods: Community-dwelling women age 65 years or older, participating in the Study of Osteoporotic Fractures (SOF), were recruited. Of 7,847 subjects in the SOF, 6,049 met criteria and completed data collection. Participants completed a self-administered questionnaire on demographic data, personal habits, medical conditions, and medications. Cognitive and functional examinations were conducted. The women were asked to call the study staff as soon as possible if a fracture occurred. Every 4 months participants were sent a postcard to return reporting any falls or fractures. Radiographic verifications of fractures were obtained.

Findings: The sample was composed of white women with an average age of 78.5 years; the majority (80%) was considered in good health and only 5% had poor cognitive function. Fifty-five percent reported at least one fall over a mean follow-up period of 3.0 years (range 90 days to 4.2 years). About 20% reported one fall per year, with 5% reporting an average of one fall a year; 8.5% experienced a fracture. Almost half (46.6%) reported at least one episode of UI per month over the past year. One-quarter of the participants ($n = 1{,}493$) had urge incontinence at least weekly, and 18.8% ($n = 1{,}137$) reported at least weekly stress incontinence. Seven hundred eight women (11.7%) had both stress and urge incontinence. Weekly or more frequent urge incontinence was independently

BOX 14-25 continued

associated with falling (odds ratio [OR] 1.26; $P < .001$), whereas weekly or more frequent stress incontinence was not associated with falls (OR 1.06, $P = .3$). Weekly or more frequent urge incontinence was also independently associated with the risk of fractures (relative hazard [RH] 1.34; $P = .02$). Weekly or more frequent urge urinary incontinence independently increased the risk of falls 26% and the risk of fractures 34%.

Application to practice: Identification and treatment of urge urinary incontinence may be an effective intervention to decrease falls and fractures in community-dwelling women.

Source: Brown, J. S., et al. (2000). Urinary incontinence: Does it increase risk for falls and fractures? *Journal of the American Geriatrics Society, 48*, 721–725.

BOX 14-26 Recommended Resources

ConsultGeriRN. Provides free resources, including assessment instruments and specialty nursing Web links (http://www.consultgerirn.org).

Morse, J. (1997). *Preventing patient falls*. Thousand Oaks, CA: Sage.

National Association for Continence (NAFC). Advocate and informational resource for the public and professionals on continence, its management, and resources (http://www.nafc.org).

Simon Foundation. Advocate and educational resource for the public and professionals on urinary continence (http://www.simonfoundation.org).

Try This: Best Practices in Nursing Care to Older Adults from the Hartford Institute for Geriatric Nursing, Division of Nursing, New York University. Addresses topics such as preventing aspiration, avoiding restraint use in patients with dementia, and oral assessment. Material may be downloaded and/or distributed in electronic format (http://www.hartfordign.org).

University of Iowa Gerontological Nursing Interventions Research Center. Research-based protocols on a variety of common health problems including prompted voiding, restraint use, prevention of falls, oral care, and depression (http://www.nursing.uiowa.edu/excellence/nursing_interventions/ index.htm).

Critical Thinking Exercises

1. Mrs. Jones, an 80-year-old widow living alone in the community, was recently diagnosed with congestive heart failure. Concurrent health problems include osteoarthritis and osteoporosis. During the initial home health visit, the nurse notices the faint odor of urine. Upon questioning, Mrs. Jones reports she often is up several times a night to urinate. She says she has done this for years and has adjusted. Should this be considered a problem? What additional information is needed for decision making? What evidence can the nurse provide to Mrs. Jones to support a need for further evaluation and treatment of this problem?
2. Your grandfather has been admitted to the hospital with pneumonia. He lives independently and is cognitively alert. When you go to the hospital to stay with him, you find him confused and disoriented. He is in bilateral arm restraints. Upon questioning the nursing staff about the restraints, they report that he has been trying to pull his IV out and gets out of bed without calling for assistance. His nurse states that they do not have time to stay with him. What interventions would you discuss implementing with his nursing staff?
3. A 60-year-old African American woman has been admitted to the rehabilitation hospital for exacerbation of rheumatoid arthritis. Her past medical history includes congestive heart failure, type 2 diabetes mellitus, and hypertension. While obtaining her history, you note that she was diagnosed with obstructive sleep apnea a year ago and has been using a CPAP appliance for the past 11 months. She states that she "sleeps much better" since beginning the CPAP, but still takes a couple of hours to fall asleep at night. She drinks a small glass of brandy each night at around 10:00 p.m. and listens to the television while trying to fall asleep. She goes to bed at 11:00 p.m., but gets up at different times each morning. Why is she at risk for sleep problems? How would you assess the effect of her delayed sleep onset? What nursing interventions may help improve her sleep habits?

Personal Reflections

1. The nursing staff in a long-term care facility insist that checking residents every 3 hours for incontinence and changing undergarments when needed is more cost-effective and labor-saving than bladder training. They point out that no one has developed skin breakdown. Develop a plan to promote continence and a rationale to support implementation. Consider your philosophy of nursing and conception of care for elderly in the rationale.
2. You have been involved in a motor vehicle accident and wake up in the ICU with both arms restrained. Discuss the emotions you would experience. What would you want the nursing staff to say or do?
3. Wear a protective undergarment for 24 hours and follow a 2-hour toileting schedule during the day. How do the experiences influence your activity and your mood?
4. Have someone feed you an entire meal. What was your interaction like (who talked, what were the topics of conversation)? How did it feel to be fed? Did your pattern for eating or the amount of food and fluid consumed differ from normal?

References

AARP. (2004, May 20). *Press center: Congressional testimony. Statement for the Senate Committee on Health, Education, Labor, and Pensions on prescription drug importation*. Retrieved October 5, 2005, from http://www.aarp.org/research/press-center/testmony/a2004-05-20-medicare.html

Abrams, P., Khoury, S., & Wein, A. (Eds.). (1999). *Incontinence.* Plymouth, UK: Health Publication.

Adkins, V. K., & Matthews, R. M. (1997). Prompted voiding to reduce incontinence in community-dwelling older adults. *Journal of Applied Behavioral Analysis, 30*, 153–156.

Agency for Health Care Policy and Research. (1999). *Diagnosis and treatment of swallowing disorders (dysphagia) in acute care stroke patients: Evidence report/technology assessment, 8*. AHCPR 99-EO23. Rockville, MD: Author.

Aiden, E., Feldman, P. A., Madeb, R., Steinberg, J., Merlin, S., Sabo, E., et al. (2004). *Candida albicans* colonization of dental plaque in elderly dysphagia patients. *IMAGE, 6*, 342–345.

Alexopoulos, G., Buckwater, K., Olin, J., Martinez, R., Wainscott, C., & Krishnan, K. (2002). Comorbidity of late life depression: An opportunity for research on mechanisms and treatment. *Biological Psychiatry, 52*(6), 543–558.

Amella, E. J. (1996). Choking—Aspiration in the elderly. In C. W. Bradway (Ed.), *Nursing care of geriatric emergencies* (pp. 154–169). New York: Springer.

Amella, E. J. (1999). Dysphagia—The differential diagnosis in long-term care. *Primary Care Practice, 3*(2), 135–149.

Amella, E. J. (2004). Presentation of illness in older adults. *American Journal of Nursing, 104*(10), 40–51.

American Dietetic Association. (2003). National Dysphagia Diet. *Journal of the American Dietetic Association, 103*(3).

American Nurses Association. (1990). *Position statement: Polypharmacy and the older adult*. Retrieved December 27, 2004, from http://www.ana.org/readroom/position/drug/drpoly.htm

American Psychiatric Association. (2000). *The diagnostic and statistical manual of mental disorders* (4th ed.). Washington, DC: Author.

American Society of Consultant Pharmacists. (2004). *Seniors at risk: Designing the system to protect America's most vulnerable citizens from medication-related problems*. Retrieved July 27, 2008, from http://www.ascp.com/publications/seniorsatrisk/upload/AtRisk.pdf

Anderson, J. (2004, Winter). Sleep apnea and heart failure. *Focus*, p. 30.

Arand, D., & Bonnet, M. (2000). The impact of music upon sleep tendency as measured by the multiple sleep latency test and maintenance of wakefulness test. *Physiology and Behavior, 71*(5), 485–492.

Armstrong, L. E. (2000). *Performing in extreme environments*. Champaign, IL: Human Kinetics.

Arya, L. A., Myers, D. L., & Jackson, N. D. (2000). Dietary caffeine intake and the risk of detrusor instability: A case-control study. *Obstetrics and Gynecology, 96*(1), 85–89.

Asplund, R. (1999). Sleep disorders in the elderly. *Drugs and Aging, 14*(2), 91–103.

Avery-Smith, W. (1992). Management of neurologic disorders: The first feeding session. In M. E. Groher (Ed.), *Dysphagia: Diagnosis and management* (2nd ed., pp. 219–236). Boston: Butterworth-Heinemann.

Ayers, C., Wetherell, J. L., Lenze, E. J., & Stanley, M. A. (2006). Treating late-life anxiety. *Psychiatric Times, 23*(3), 1–2.

Badger, T., & Collins-Joyce, P. (2000). Depression, psychosocial resources, and functional ability in older adults. *Clinical Nursing Research, 9*(3), 238–255.

Bartels, S. J., Dums, A. R., Oxman, T. E., Schneider, L. S., Arean, P. A., Alexopoulos, G. S., et al. (2002). Evidence-based practices in geriatric mental health care. *Psychiatric Services, 53*, 1419–1431.

Bear, M., Dwyer, J. W., Benveneste, D., Jett, K., & Dougherty, M. (1997). Home-based management of urinary incontinence: A pilot study with both frail and independent elders. *Journal of Wounds, Ostomy, and Continence Nurses, 24*, 163–171.

Beaver, M. (2008). *CMS to Put Pressure on Providers for Decubitus Ulcer Prevention*. Retrieved on December 30, 2008, from http://www.infectioncontroltoday.com/articles/decubitus-ulcer-prevention.html

Bedell, J. R., Cohen, N. L., & Sullivan, A. (2000). Case management: The best current practices and the next generation of innovation. *Community Mental Health Journal, 36*(2), 179–194.

Beekman, A. T., Bremmer, M. A., Deeg, D. J., Van Balkom, A. J., Smith, J. H., De Beurs, E., et al. (1998). Anxiety disorders in later life: A report from the longitudinal aging study Amsterdam. *International Journal of Geriatric Psychiatry, 13*, 717–726.

Beers, M. (1997). Explicit criteria for determining potentially inappropriate medication use by the elderly: An update. *Archives of Internal Medicine, 157*, 1531–1536.

Beers, M., & Berkow, R. (2005). *The Merck manual of geriatrics* (5th ed.). Whitehouse Station, NJ: Merck.

Beers, M., Ouslander, J. G., Rolinger, I., Reuben, D. B., Brooks, J., & Beck, J. C. (1991). Explicit criteria for determining inappropriate medication use in nursing home residents. *Archives of Internal Medicine, 151*, 1825–1832.

Berlowitz, D. R., Ash, A. S., & Hickey, E. C. (1998). Inadequate management of blood pressure in a hypertensive population. *New England Journal of Medicine, 339*, 1957–1963.

Borrie, M. J., Campbell, K., Arcese, Z. A., Bray, J., Labate, T., & Hesch, P. (2001). Urinary retention in patients in a geriatric rehabilitation unit: Prevalence, risk factors, and validity of bladder scan evaluation. *Rehabilitation Nursing, 26*(5), 187–191.

Bourguignon, C., Labyak, S., & Taibi, D. (2003). Investigating sleep disturbances in adults with rheumatoid arthritis. *Holistic Nursing Practice, 17*(5), 241–249.

Braden, B., & Bergstrom, N. (1987). A conceptual schema for the study of the etiology of pressure sores. *Rehabilitation Nursing, 12*, 8–12, 16.

Brin, M. F., & Younger, D. (1988). Neurologic disorders and aspiration. *Otolaryngeal Clinics of North America, 21*, 691–699.

Brink, C. A., Sampselle, C. M., Wells, T. J., Diokno, A. C., & Gillis, G. L. (1989). A digital test for pelvic muscle strength in older women with urinary incontinence. *Nursing Research, 38*(4), 196–199.

Brown, J. S., Vittinghoff, E., Wyman, J. F., Stone, K. L., Nevitt, M. C., Ensrud, K. E., et al. (2000). Urinary incontinence: Does it increase risk for falls and fractures? *Journal of the American Geriatrics Society, 48*, 721–725.

Bryant, P., Trinder, J., & Curtis, N. (2004). Sick and tired: Does sleep have a vital role in the immune system? *Nature Reviews Immunology, 4*, 457–467.

Buckle, J. (2001). The role of aromatherapy in nursing care. *Nursing Clinics of North America, 36*(1), 57–67.

Bump, R., Hurt, W., Fantl, J., & Wyman, J. (1991). Assessment of Kegel exercise training for stress urinary incontinence. *American Journal of Obstetrics and Gynecology, 165*, 322–329.

Burgio, K. L., & Burgio, L. D. (1986). Behavioral therapies for urinary incontinence in the elderly. *Clinics in Geriatric Medicine, 2*(4), 809–827.

Burgio, K. L., Locher, J. L., Goode, P. S., Hardin, J. M., McDowell, B. J., Dombrowski, M., et al., (1998). Behavioral vs drug treatment for urge urinary incontinence in older women: A randomized controlled trial. *Journal of the American Medical Association, 280*, 1995–2000.

Byers, P. H., Ryan, P. A., Regan, M. D., Shields, A., & Carta, S. G. (1995). Effects of skin care cleansing regimens on skin integrity. *Journal of Wound, Ostomy, and Continence Nursing, 22*(4), 187–192.

Capezuti, E. (1996). Falls. In R. J. Lavizzo-Mourey & M. A. Forciea (Eds.), *Geriatric secrets* (pp. 110–115). Philadelphia: Hanley & Belfus.

Carlson, E. V., Kemp, M. G., & Shott, S. (1999). Predicting the risk of ulcers in critically ill patients. *American Journal of Critical Care, 8*(4), 262–269.

Castell, D. O. (1996). The efficient dysphagia work-up. *Emergency Medicine, 58*(2), 73–77.

Centers for Disease Control and Prevention. (2006). *What you can do to prevent falls*. Retrieved December 29, 2008, from http://www.cdc.gov/ncipc/pub-res/toolkit/WhatYouCanDoToPreventFalls.htm

Centers for Disease Control and Prevention, National Center for Injury Prevention and Control. (2005). *Web-based injury statistics query and reporting system (WISQARS)*. Retrieved November 11, 2007, from http://www.cdc.gov/ncipc/wisqars

Chasens, E., Weaver, T., & Umlauf, M. (2003). Insulin resistance and obstructive sleep apnea: Is increased sympathetic stimulation the link? *Biological Research for Nursing, 5*(2), 87–96.

Cheek, R., Shaver, J. L., & Lentz, M. J. (2004). Variations of sleep hygiene practices of women with and without insomnia. *Research in Nursing and Health, 27*(4), 225–236.

Clark, A. P., & Baldwin, K. (2004). Best practices for care of older adults: Highlights and summary from the preconference. *Clinical Nurse Specialist, 18*(6), 289–301.

Cleeland, C. S., Gonin, R., & Hatfield, A. K. (1994). Pain and its treatment in outpatients with metastatic cancer. *New England Journal of Medicine, 330*, 592–596.

Cockroft, D. W., & Gault, M. H. (1976). Prediction of creatinine clearance from serum creatinine. *Nephron, 16*, 31–41.

Colling, J. C., Auslander, J. G., Hadley, B. J., Eisch, T., & Campbell, E. (1992). The effects of patterned urge-response toileting on urinary incontinence among nursing home residents. *Journal of the American Gerontological Society, 40*, 135–141.

Consensus Conference, Urinary Continence Guideline Panel. (1992). *Urinary incontinence in adults*. AHCPR Pub No. 92-0038. Rockville, MD: U.S. Department of Health and Human Services.

Davies, S. (2002). An interdisciplinary approach to the management of dysphagia. *Professional Nurse, 18*(1), 22–25.

DeGroot, M., Eskes, G., & Phillips, S. J. (2003). Fatigue associated with stroke and other neurologic conditions: Implications for stroke rehabilitation. *Archives of Physical Medicine and Rehabilitation, 84*(11), 1714–1720.

Dharmarajan, T., & Ahmed, S. (2003). The growing problem of pressure ulcers. *Postgraduate Medicine, 113*(5), 77–84.

Donahue, J. L., & Lowenthal, D. T. (1997). Nocturnal polyuria in the elderly person. *American Journal of Medical Sciences, 314*, 232–237.

Doughty, D. (2000). *Urinary and fecal incontinence: Nursing management*. St. Louis: Mosby.

Dugan, E., Cohen, S. J., Bland, S. R., Priesser, J. S., Davis, C. C., Suggs, P. K., et al. (2000). The association of depressive symptoms and urinary incontinence among older adults. *Journal of the American Geriatrics Association, 48*(4), 413–416.

Edwards, S. J., & Metheny, N. A. (2000). Measurement of gastric residual volume: State of the science. *MEDSURG Nursing, 9*(3), 125–128.

Ekberg, O., Hamby, S., Woisard, V., Wuttge-Hanning, A., & Ortega, P. (2004). Social and psychological burden of dysphagia: Its impact on diagnosis and treatment. *Dysphagia, 17*, 139–146.

Engeberg, S., McDowell, J., Donovan, N., Brodak, I., & Weber, E. (1997). Treatment of urinary incontinence in homebound older adults: Interface between research and practice. *Ostomy/Wound Management, 43*(10), 18–25.

Ernst, F., & Grizzle, A. (2001, March/April). Drug-related morbidity and mortality. *Journal of the American Pharmaceutical Association, 1*(2), 41.

Ersser, S., Wiles, A., Taylor, H., Wade, S., Walsh, R., & Bentley, T. (1999). The sleep of older people in hospital and nursing homes. *Journal of Clinical Nursing, 8*(4), 360–373.

Evans, L. R., & Strumph, N. E. (1990). Myths about elder restraint. *Image, 22*(2), 122–128.

Fantl, J. A., Newman, D. K., Colling, J., DeLancey, J. O. L., Keeys, C., Loughery, R., et al. (1996). *Urinary incontinence in adults: Acute and chronic management. Clinical practice guideline, 2*. AHCPR Pub No. 96-0682. Rockville, MD: U.S. Department of Health Care Policy and Research.

Fassino, S., Leombruni, P., Daga, G., Brustolin, A., Rovera, G., & Fabris, F. (2002). Quality of life in dependent older adults living at home. *Archives of Gerontology and Geriatrics, 35*(1), 9–20.

Feeney, S. L. (2004). The relationship between pain and negative affect in older adults: Anxiety as a predictor of pain. *Journal of Anxiety Disorders, 18*, 733–744.

Ficca, G., & Salzarulo, P. (2004). What in sleep is for memory? *Sleep Medicine, 5*(3), 225–230.

Field, T. (1998). Massage therapy effects. *American Psychology, 53*, 1270–1281.

Fletcher, D. (1986). Coping with insomnia: Helping patients manage sleeplessness without drugs. *Postgraduate Medicine, 79*(2), 265–274.

Folstein, M. F., Folstein, S. E., & McHugh, P. R. (1975). "Mini-mental state." A practical method for grading the cognitive state of patients for the clinician. *Journal of Psychiatric Research, 12*, 189–198.

Fonda, A. (1990). Improving management of urinary incontinence in geriatric centers and nursing homes. *Australian Clinical Review, 10*, 536–540.

Fonda, D., Benvenuti, F., Cottenden, A., DuBeau, C., Kirshner-Hermanns, R., Miller, K., et al. (2002). Urinary incontinence and bladder dysfunction in older persons. In P. Abrams, L. Cardozo, S. Khoury, & A. Wein (Eds.), *Incontinence, proceedings from the Second International Consulta-tion on Incontinence*. Plymouth, UK: Health Publication.

Fontaine, D., Briggs, L., & Pope-Smith, B. (2001). Designing humanistic critical care environments. *Critical Care Nursing Quarterly, 24*(3), 21–34.

Fuller, G. F. (2000). Falls in the elderly. *American Family Physician, 61*(7), 1969–1972, 2159–2168, 2173–2174.

Gagner-Tjellesen, D., Yurkovich, E., & Gragert, M. (2001). Use of music therapy and other ITNIs in acute care. *Journal of Psychosocial Nursing and Mental Health Services, 39*(10), 26–37.

Gallagher, E. M. (1994). *Falls and the elderly*. Victoria, BC: School of Nursing, University of Victoria.

Ganguli, G. (2003). Consumers devise drug cost-cutting measures: Medical and legal issues to consider. *Health Care Manager, 22*(3), 275–281.

Garon, B. R., Engle, M., & Ormison, C. (1997). A randomized control study to determine the effects of unlimited oral intake of water. *Journal of Neurological Rehabilitation, 11*, 139–148.

Gauthier, D. M. (1999). The healing potential of back massage. *Online Journal of Knowledge Synthesis for Nursing, 6*(5).

Gillespie, L. D., Gillespie, W. J., Cummings, R., Lamb, S. E., & Rowe, B. H. (2000). Interventions for preventing falls in the elderly. *The Cochrane Library*, 2.

Glenn-Molali, N. H. (2002). Nourishment and swallowing. In S. P. Hoeman (Ed.), *Rehabilitation nursing* (3rd ed., pp. 322–346). St. Louis: Mosby.

Godfrey, H. (2008). Older people, continence and catheters: Dilemmas and resolutions. *British Journal of Nursing, 17*(9), S4–S11.

Godfrey, H., & Hogg, A. (2007). Links between social isolation and incontinence. *British Journal of Nursing, 1*(3), S1–S8.

Golden, A. D., Silverman, M. A., & Preston, R. A. (2000). Prescribing medications for geriatric patients in managed care setting. *American Journal of Managed Care, 6*(5), 610–621.

Goldstein, M., Hawthorne, M. E., Engeberg, S., McDowell, B. J., & Burgio, K. (1992). Urinary incontinence—Why people do not seek help. *Journal of Gerontological Nursing, 18*(4), 15–20.

Gordon, S. (1997). *Life support. Three nurses on the front lines*. New York: Little, Brown.

Gottlieb, S. S., McCarter, R. J., & Vogel, R. A. (1998). Effect of beta-blockade on mortality among high-risk and low-risk patients after myocardial infarction. *New England Journal of Medicine, 339*, 489–497.

Grimby, A., Milson, J., Molander, U., Wiklund, I., & Ekelund, P. (1993). The influence of urinary incontinence on the quality of life in the elderly woman. *Age and Aging, 22*(2), 82–89.

Haight, B. K., & Michel, Y. (1998). Life review: Preventing despair in nursing home residents: Short and long-term effects. *International Journal of Aging and Human Development, 47*(2), 119–143.

Hajjar, P. R. (2004). Psychosocial impact of urinary incontinence in the elderly population. *Clinical Geriatric Medicine, 20*(3), 553–564.

Handa, V. L., Landerman, R., & Hanlon, J. T. (1996). Do older women use estrogen replacement? *Journal of the American Geriatric Society, 44*, 1–6.

Harrison, B., Booth, D., & Algase, D. (2001). Studying fall risk factors among nursing home residents who fell. *Journal of Gerontological Nursing, 27*(10), 26–34.

Hausdorff, J. M., Rios, D. A., & Edelber, H. K. (2001). Gait variability and fall risk in community-living older adults: A 1-year prospective study. *Archives of Physical Medicine and Rehabilitation, 82*(8), 1050–1056.

Hayes, N. (2004). Prevention of falls among older patients in the hospital environment. *British Journal of Nursing, 13*(15), 896–898, 899–901.

Heavner, K. (1998). Urinary incontinence in extended care facilities: A literature review and proposal for continuous quality improvement. *Ostomy/Wound Management, 44*(12), 46–53.

Heidrich, S., & Wells, T. J. (2004). Effects of urinary incontinence: Psychosocial well-being and distress in older community dwelling women. *Journal of Gerontological Nursing, 39*(5), 47–54.

Hoffman, S. (2003). Sleep in the older adult: Implications for nurses. *Geriatric Nursing, 24*(4), 210–216.

Honkus, V. L. (2003). Sleep deprivation in critical care units. *Critical Care Nursing Quarterly, 26*(3), 179–189.

Hunskaar, S., Burgio, K., Diokno, A. C., Herzog, A. R., Hjalmas, K., & Lapitan, M. C. (2002). Epidemiology and natural history of urinary incontinence (UI). In P. Abrams, L. Cardozo, S. Khoury, & A. Wein (Eds.), *Incontinence, proceedings from the Second International Consultation on Incontinence* (pp. 165–201). Plymouth, UK: Health Publication.

Jeste, D. V., Alexopoulous, G. S., Bartels, S. J., Cummings, J. L., Gallo, J. J., Gottlieb, G. L., et al. (1999). Consensus statement on the upcoming crisis in geriatric mental health: Research agenda for the next 2 decades. *Archives of General Psychiatry, 56*(9), 848–853.

Jeter, K. F., & Wagner, B. A. (1990). Incontinence in the American home. *Journal of the American Geriatrics Society, 38*, 379–383.

Jivorec, M. M. (1991). The impact of daily exercise on the mobility, balance, and urine control of cognitively impaired nursing home residents. *International Journal of Nursing Studies, 28*(2), 145–151.

Jirovec, M. M., Wyman, J. F., & Wells, T. J. (1998). Addressing urinary incontinence with educational continence care competencies. *Image: Journal of Nursing Scholarship, 30*(4), 375–378.

Johns, M. W. (1991). A new method for measuring daytime sleepiness: The Epworth Sleepiness Scale. *SLEEP, 14*, 540–545.

Johnson, J. E. (2003). The use of music to promote sleep in older women. *Journal of Community Health Nursing, 20*(1), 27–35.

Johnson, V., & Chalmers, J. (2002). *Oral hygiene care for functionally dependent and cognitively impaired older adults—Evidence-based protocol.* Iowa City: University of Iowa Gerontological Nursing Intervention Research Center, Research Dissemination Core.

Jones, B. (1997). Decreasing polypharmacy in clients most at risk. *AACN Clinical Issues, 8*, 627.

Juurlink, D. N., Mamdani, M., Kopp, A., Laupacis, A., & Redelmeier, D. A. (2003). Drug-drug interactions among elderly patients hospitalized for drug toxicity. *Journal of the American Medical Association, 289*(13), 1652–1658.

Kain, M. (2001, September 6). Personal communication.

Kawashima, K., Motohashi, Y., & Fujishima, I. (2004). Prevalence of dysphagia among community-dwelling elderly individuals as estimated using a questionnaire for dysphagia screening. *Dysphagia, 19*, 266–271.

Kennedy-Malone, L., Fletcher, K. R., & Plank, L. M. (2004). *Management guidelines for nurse practitioners working with older adults* (2nd ed.). Philadelphia: F. A. Davis.

Klein, D., Turvey, C., & Wallace, R. (2004). Elders who delay medication because of cost: Health insurance, demographic, health, and financial correlates. *The Gerontologist, 44*(6), 779–787.

Kraus, C. A., Kunik, M. E., & Stanley, M. A. (2007). Use of cognitive behavioral therapy in late-life psychiatric disorders. *Geriatrics, 62*(6), 21–26.

Lam, R. W., & Kennedy, S. H. (2004). Evidence-based strategies for achieving and sustaining full remission in depression: Focus on meta-analyses. *Canadian Journal of Psychiatry, 49*(1), 17S–26S.

Langmore, S. E., Terpenning, M. S., Schork, A., Chen, Y., Murray, J. T., Lopatin, D., et al. (1998). Predictors of aspiration pneumonia: How important is dysphagia? *Dysphagia, 13*, 69–81.

Lapid, M. I., & Rummans, T. A. (2003). Evaluation and management of geriatric depression in primary care. *Mayo Clinic Proceedings, 78*, 1423–1429.

Larson, D., & Martin, J. H. (1999). Polypharmacy and elderly patients. *AORN Journal, 69*(3), 619–628.

Layne, K. A., Losinki, D. S., Zenner, P. M., & Ament, J. A. (1989). Using the Flemish index of dysphagia to establish prevalence. *Dysphagia, 4*, 39–42.

Ledford, L. (1997). *Research-based protocol: Prevention of falls.* Iowa City: University of Iowa Gerontological Nursing Intervention Research Center, Research Dissemination Core.

Ledford, L., & Mentes, J. (1997). *Research-based protocol: Restraints.* Iowa City: University of Iowa Gerontological Nursing Intervention Research Center, Research Dissemination Core.

Lekan-Rutledge, D. (2004). Urinary incontinence strategies for frail elderly women. *Urologic Nursing, 24*(4), 281–283, 287–302.

Lincoln, R., & Roberts, R. (1989). Continence issues in acute care. *Nursing Clinics of North America, 24*(3), 741–754.

Lindgren, S., & Janzon, L. (1991a). Evaluating dysphagia. *American Family Physician, 61*(12), 147–152.

Lindgren, S., & Janzon, L. (1991b). Prevalence of swallowing complaints and clinical findings among 50–79 year old men and women in an urban population. *Dysphagia, 6*(4), 187–192.

Logemann, J. A. (1998). *Evaluation and treatment of swallowing disorders* (2nd ed.). Austin, TX: Pro-ed.

Logemann, J. A., Gesler, G., Robbins, J., et al. (2008). A randomized study of three interventions for aspiration of thin liquids in patients with dementia or Parkinson's disease. *Journal of Speech, Language and Hearing Research, 5*(1), 173–183.

Lyness, J. M. (2008). Depression and comorbidity: Objects in the mirror are more complex than they appear. *American Journal for Geriatric Psychiatry, 16*(3), 181–185.

Lyons, S. S., & Specht, J. K. P. (1999). *Prompted voiding for persons with urinary incontinence.* Iowa City: University of Iowa Gerontological Nursing Intervention Research Center, Research Dissemination Core.

Macauly, A. J., Stern, R. S., Holmes, D. M., & Stanton, S. L. (1987). Micturition and the mind: Psychological factors in the treatment of urinary symptoms. *British Medical Journal, 294*, 540–543.

Maldonado, C. C., Bentley, A. J., & Mitchell, D. (2004). A pictorial sleepiness scale based on cartoon face. *Sleep, 27*(3), 541–546.

Mantle, F. (1996). Complementary therapies: Sleepless and unsettled. *Nursing Times, 92*(23), 46–47.

Martin, J., & Haynes, L. (2000). Depression, delirium, and dementia in the elderly patient. *Journal of the Association of Perioperative Registered Nurses, 72*(2), 209–217.

Martin-Harris, B., & Cherney, L. R. (1996). Treating swallowing disorders following stroke. In L. R. Cherney

& A. S. Halper (Eds.), *Topics in stroke rehabilitation* (3rd ed., pp. 27–40). Frederick, MD: Aspen.

Mathus-Vliegen, E. (2004). Old age, malnutrition, and pressure sores: An ill-fated alliance. *Journal of Gerontology, 59A*(4), 355–360.

MayoClinic.com. (2008). *Urinary incontinence*. Retrieved July 27, 2008, from http://www.mayoclinic.com/health/urinary-incontinence/DS00404/DSECTION=symptoms

McCaffery, M., & Pasero, C. (1999). *Pain: Clinical manual* (2nd ed.). St. Louis: Mosby.

McCormick, K. A., Cella, M., Scheve, A., & Engel, B. T. (1990). Cost effectiveness of treating incontinence in severely mobility-impaired long-term care residents. *Quality Review Bulletin, 16*, 439–443.

Medical College of Wisconsin. (1999). *Sleep and circadian rhythms*. Retrieved January 1, 2005, from http://healthlink.mcw.edu/article/922567322.html

Mehta, K. M., Simonsick, E. M., Penninx, B. W., Schulz, R. X., Rubin, S. M., Satterfield, S., et al. (2003). Prevalence and correlates of anxiety symptoms in well-functioning older adults: Findings from the Health Aging and Body Composition Study. *Journal of the American Geriatrics Society, 51*(4), 499–504.

Mentes, J. C., & Iowa Veterans Affairs Nursing Research Consortium. (1998). *Hydration management*. Iowa City: University of Iowa Gerontological Nursing Intervention Research Center.

Metheny, N. A., Schallom, M. E., & Edwards, S. J. (2004). Effect of gastrointestinal motility and feeding tube site on aspiration risk in critically ill patients: A review. *Heart and Lung, 33*(3), 131–145.

Miller, C. (2002). Helping older adults reduce the cost of the drugs they need. *Geriatric Nursing, 23*(4), 230–232.

Mohlman, J., De Jesus, M., Gorenstein, E. E., Kleber, M., Gorman, J. M., & Papp, L. A. (2004). Distinguishing generalized anxiety disorder, panic disorder, and mixed anxiety states in older treatment-seeking adults. *Journal of Anxiety Disorders, 18*(3), 275–290.

Mojtabai, R., & Olfson, M. (2003). Medication costs, adherence, and health outcomes among Medicare beneficiaries. *Health Affairs, 22*(4), 220–229.

Mornhinweg, G., & Voignier, R. (1995). Music for sleep disturbance in the elderly. *Journal of Holistic Medicine, 13*(3), 248–254.

Morris, H. (2004). Dysphagia in the elderly: A management challenge for nurses. *British Journal of Nursing, 15*(10), 558–562.

Mueller, N. (2004). What the future holds for incontinence care. *Urologic Nurse, 24*(3), 181–186.

National Association for Continence. (2004). *Resource guide—Products and services for incontinence*. Charleston, SC: Author.

National Commission on Sleep Disorders Research. (1993). *Wake up America: A national sleep alert, executive summary and report*. Retrieved October 21, 2004, from http://www.medhelp.org/lib/breadiso.htm

National Guideline Clearinghouse. (2003). *Guideline for prevention and management of pressure ulcers*. Retrieved January 19, 2005, from http://www.guideline.gov

National Institute of Neurological Disorders and Stroke. (2001). *Restless leg syndrome fact sheet*. NIH Pub No. 01-4847. Bethesda, MD: National Institutes of Health.

National Pressure Ulcer Advisory Panel. (2003). *NPUAP staging report*. Retrieved July 28, 2007, from http://www.npuap.org

National Sleep Foundation. (2008). *Sleep in America poll 2008*. American Academy of Sleep Medicine. Retrieved June 1, 2008, from http://www.sleepfoundation.org

Newman, D. K. (2002). *Managing and treating urinary incontinence*. Baltimore, MD: Health Professions Press.

Nicklin, D. (2006). Physical assessment. In J. J. Gallo, H. K. Bogner, T. Fulmer, & G. H. Paveza (Eds.), *Handbook of geriatric assessment* (4th ed., pp. 273–317). Sudbury, MA: Jones and Bartlett.

Norris, A. (2001, January 1). HCFA correspondence.

O'Keeffe, S., Jack, C. I., & Lye, M. (1996). Use of restraints and bedrails in a British hospital. *Journal of the American Geriatric Society, 44*(9), 1086–1088.

Oliff, H. S. (2004). *Herbal supplements to treat sleeplessness*. SkyLine Medical Center. Retrieved October 5, 2005, from http://www.skylinemedicalcenter.com

Ouslander, J. G., Hepps, K., Raz, S., & Su, H. L. (1986). Genitourinary dysfunction in a geriatric population. *Journal of the American Geriatrics Society, 34*(7), 507–514.

Ouslander, J. G., Schnelle, J. F., Uman, G., Fingold, S., Nigam, J. G., Tulco, E., et al. (1995). Does oxybutynin add to the effectiveness of prompted voiding for urinary incontinence among nursing home residents? *Journal of the American Geriatrics Society, 43*(6), 610–617.

Pagana, K. D., & Pagana, T. J. (2005). *Mosby's diagnostic and laboratory test reference* (7th ed.). Williamsport, PA: Elsevier/Mosby.

Palmer, M. H. (1996). A new framework for urinary continence outcomes in long-term care. *Urologic Nursing, 16*(4), 146–150

Panther, K. (2005). The Frazier free water protocol. *Perspectives on Swallowing and Swallowing Disorders (Dysphagia), 14*(1), 4–9.

Parker, M., Gillespie, L., & Gillespie, W. (2004). Hip protectors for preventing hip fractures in the elderly. (Cochrane Review). *Cochrane Library, 1*. Chichester: John Wiley & Sons.

Pennix, B., Guralnik, J., Pahor, M., Ferrucci, L., Cerhan, J., Wallace, R., et al. (1998). Chronically depressed mood and cancer risk in older persons. *Journal of the National Cancer Institute, 90*, 1888–1893.

Pressman, M. R., Figueroa, W. G., Kendrick-Mohamed, J., Greenspan, L. W., & Peterson, D. D. (1996). Nocturia: A seldom recognized symptom of sleep apnea and other occult sleep disorders. *Archives of Internal Medicine, 156*, 545–555.

Raj, A. (2004). Depression in the elderly. *Postgraduate Medicine, 115*(6), 26–35.

Rich, S. A., & Panill, F. C. (1999). Urinary incontinence. In E. R. Black, D. R. Bordley, T. G. Tape, & R. J. Panzer (Eds.), *Diagnostic strategies for common medical problems* (2nd ed.). Philadelphia: American College of Physicians.

Richards, K. (1996). Sleep promotion. *Critical Care Nursing Clinics of North America, 8*(1), 39–50.

Richards, K., Gibson, R., & Overton-McCoy, A. (2000). Effects of massage in acute and critical care. *AACN Clinical Issues, 11*(1), 77–96.

Richards, K., Nagel, C., Markie, M., Elwell, J., & Barone, C. (2003). Use of complementary and alternative therapies to promote sleep in critically ill patients. *Critical Care Nursing Clinicians of North America, 15*(3), 329–340.

Robbins, J. A., Biggs, M. L., & Cauley, J. (2006). Adjusted mortality after hip fracture: From the cardiovascular health study. *Journal of the American Geriatrics Society, 54*(12), 1885–1891.

Roy, N., Stemple, J., Merrill, R. M., & Thomas, L. (2007). Dysphagia in the elderly: Preliminary evidence of prevalence, risk factors and socioemotional effects. *Annals of Otology, Rhinology and Laryngology, 111*(11), 858–865.

Royal College of Physicians. (1995). *Incontinence: Causes, management and provision of services*. London: Author.

Rubenstein, L. Z. (2003). Falls. In T. T. Yoshikawa, E. L. Cobbs, & K. Brummel-Smith (Eds.), *Ambulatory geriatric care* (pp. 296–304). Philadelphia: Elsevier.

Rubenstein, L. Z., & Josephson, K. R. (2006). Falls and their prevention in the elderly: What does the evidence show? *Medical Clinics of North America, 90*(5), 807–824.

Ryff, C. D., Singer, B. H., & Love, G. D. (2004). Positive health: Connecting well-being with biology. *Philosophical Transactions, Royal Society of London, 359*, 1383–1394.

Sale, P. G., & Wyman, J. (1994). Achievement of goals associated with bladder training by older incontinent women. *Applied Nursing Research, 7*(2), 93–96.

Sampselle, C. M., Burns, P. A., Dougherty, M. C., Newman, D. K., Thomas, K. K., & Wyman, J. F. (1997). Continence for women: Evidence-based practice. *Journal of Obstetrical, Gynecological and Neonatal Nurses, 26*, 375-385.

Scheve, A. A., Engel, B. T., McCormick, K. A., & Leahy, E. G. (1991). Exercise in continence. *Geriatric Nursing, 12*(3), 124.

Schnelle, J. F. (1990). Treatment of urinary incontinence in nursing home patients by prompted voiding. *Journal of the American Geriatrics Society, 38*, 356–360.

Schnelle, J. F. (1991). *Managing urinary incontinence in the elderly*. New York: Springer.

Scott, J. C. (1990). Osteoporosis and hip fractures. *Rheumatic Disease Clinics of North America, 16*(3), 717–740.

Shull, B. L., Halaska, M., Hurst, G., Laycock, J., Palmtag, H., Reilly, N., et al. (1999). Physical examination. In P. Abrams, S. Khoury, & A. Wein (Eds.), *Incontinence*. Plymouth, UK: Health Publication.

Singer, P. (2002). Nutritional care to prevent and heal pressure ulcers. *Israel Medical Association Journal, 4*, 713–716.

Sinoff, G., & Werner, P. (2003). Anxiety disorder and accompanying subjective memory loss in the elderly as a predictor of future cognitive decline. *International Journal of Geriatric Psychiatry, 18*, 951–959.

Skipper, A. (1993). *Dietician's handbook of enteral and parenteral nutrition*. Rockville, MD: Aspen.

Skoner, M. M. (1994). Self-management of urinary incontinence among women 31 to 50 years. *Rehabilitation Nursing, 19*(6), 339–343.

Smith, D., & Newman, D. (1989, September). Beating the cycle of constipation, laxative abuse, and fecal incontinence. *Today's Nursing Home*, 12–13.

Smith, H. A., & Connolly, M. J. (2003). Evaluation and treatment of dysphagia following stroke. *Topics in Geriatric Rehabilitation, 19*(1), 43–59.

Spangler, P., Risley, T., & Bilyew, D. (1984). The management of dehydration and incontinence in nonambulatory geriatric patients. *Journal of Applied Behavior Analysis, 17*, 397–401.

Spieker, M. R. (2000). Evaluating dysphagia. *American Family Physician, 61*(12), 3639–3648, 3547–3550, 3749.

Stevens, J. A. (2005). Falls among older adults—Risk factors and prevention strategies. *NCOA Falls Free: Promoting a National Falls Prevention Action Plan.* Research Review Papers. Washington, DC: National Council on Aging.

Stevenson, J. (2002) Meeting the challenge of dysphagia. *Nurse2Nurse, 3*, 2–3.

Stroke Research Unit, Queen Elizabeth Hospital, Gateshead. *Collaborative Dysphagia Audit (CODA) Study*. Retrieved April 10, 2005, from http://www.ncl.ac.uk/stroke-research-unit/coda/cointro.htm

Strumpf, N. E. & Evans, L. K. (1988). Physical restraints of the hospitalized elderly: Perceptions of patients and nurses. *Nursing Research, 37*, 132–137.

Taibi, D., Bourguignon, C., & Taylor, A. (2004). Valerian use for sleep disturbances related to rheumatoid arthritis. *Holistic Nursing Practice, 18*(3), 120–126.

Tamblyn, R. M., McLeod, P. J., Abrahamowicz, M., & Laprise, R. (1996). Do too many cooks spoil the broth? Multiple physician involvement in medical management of elderly patients and potentially inappropriate drug combinations. *Canadian Medical Association Journal, 154*(8), 1177–1184.

Therapeutic Research Center. (2007). Potentially harmful drugs in the elderly: Beers list and more. *Pharmacist's Letter/Prescriber's Letter, 23*(230907).

Thom, D. H., Haan, M. N., & Van Den Eeden, S. K. (1997). Medically recognized urinary incontinence and the risks of hospitalization, nursing home admission and mortality. *Age and Ageing, 26*, 367–374.

Thomas, A. M., & Morse, J. M. (1991). Managing urinary incontinence with self-care practices. *Journal of Gerontological Nursing, 17*(6), 9–14.

Tinetti, M. E., Speechley, M., & Ginter, S. F. (1988). Risk factors for falls among elderly persons living in the community. *New England Journal of Medicine, 319*, 1701 1707.

Tunis, S. R., Norris, A., & Simon, K. (2000). *Medicare coverage policy decisions. Biofeedback for treatment of urinary incontinence.* #CAG-00020. Washington, DC: Health Care Financing Administration.

Tunis, S. R., Whyte, J. J., & Bridger, P. (2000). *Medicare coverage policy decisions. Pelvic floor electrical stimulation for treatment of urinary incontinence.* #CAG-00021. Washington, DC: Health Care Financing Administration.

Uebersax, J. S., Wyaman, J. F., Schumaker, S. A., & Fantl, J. A., Continence Program for Woman Research Group. (1995). Short forms to assess life quality and symptom distress for urinary incontinence in women: The incontinence impact questionnaire and the urogenital distress inventory. *Neurourology and Urodynamics, 14*, 131, 139.

Umlauf, M., & Chasens, E. (2003). Sleep disordered breathing and nocturnal polyuria: Nocturia and enuresis. *Sleep, 7*(5), 373–376.

Umlauf, M. G., Burgio, K. L., Shetter, S., & Pillion, D. (1997). Nocturia and nocturnal urine production in obstructive sleep apnea. *Applied Nursing Research, 10*(4), 198–201.

University of Iowa Clinical Guidelines. (2004). *Fall prevention for older adults*. Retrieved on December 29, 2008, from http://www.guideline.gov/summary/summary.aspx?doc_id=4833

Urinary Continence Guideline Panel. (1992). *Urinary incontinence in adults.* AHCPR Pub. No. 92-0038. Rockville, MD: U.S. Department of Health and Human Services.

U.S. Department of Health and Human Services. (1994). *Treatment of pressure ulcers*. AHCPR Pub. No. 95-0652. Rockville, MD: Agency for Public Health Policy and Research.

U.S. Department of Health and Human Services. (1999). *Mental health: A report of the surgeon general—executive summary*. Rockville, MD: U.S. Department of Health and Human Services, Substance Abuse and Mental Health Services Administration, Center for Mental Health Services, National Institutes of Health, National Institute of Mental Health.

U.S. Food and Drug Administration. (2005). *FDA approves Requip for restless leg syndrome*. FDA Talk Paper. Washington, DC: Author.

Vassallo, M., Vignaraja, R., Sharma, J., Hallam, H., Binns, K., Briggs, R., et al. (2004). The effects of changing practice on fall prevention in a rehabilitation: The hospital injury prevention study. *Journal of the American Geriatrics Society, 52*, 335–339.

Venn, M. R., Taft, L., Carpenter, B., & Applebaugh, G. (1992). The influence of timing and suppository use on efficiency and effectiveness of bowel training after a stroke. *Rehabilitation Nursing, 17*, 116–120.

Watson, L., & Pignon, M. (2003). Screening accuracy for late-life depression in primary care: A systematic review. *Journal of Family Practice, 52*(12), 956–964.

Wells, T. (1984). Social and psychological implications of incontinence. In J. C. Brocklehurst (Ed.), *Urology in the elderly* (pp. 107–126). New York: Churchill Livingston.

Wiesenfeld, L. (2008). Delirium: The ADVISE approach and tips from the frontline. *Geriatrics, 63*(5), 28–31.

White, G., O'Rourke, F., Ong, B. S., Cordato, D. J., & Chan, D. Y. K. (2008). Dysphagia: Causes, assessment, treatment and management. *Geriatrics, 63*(5), 15–20.

Wilson, L., Brown, J. S., Shin, G. P., Luc, K., & Subak, L. L. (2001). Annual direct cost of incontinence. *Obstetrics and Gynecology, 98*, 398–406.

Wyman, J., Harkins, S. W., Choi, S. C., Taylor, J. R., & Fantl, A. (1987). Psychosocial impact of urinary incontinence in women. *Obstetrics and Gynecology, 70*(1), 378–381.

Wyman, J. F. (1994a). Level 3: Comprehensive assessment and management of urinary incontinence by continence nurse specialists. *Nurse Practitioner Forum, 5*(3), 177–185.

Wyman, J. F. (1994b). The psychiatric and emotional impact of female pelvic floor dysfunction. *Current Opinion in Obstetrics and Gynecology, 6*, 336–339.

Wyman, J. F., Choi, S. C., Harkins, S. W., Wilson, M. S., & Fantl, J. A. (1988). The urinary diary in evaluation of incontinent women: A test-retest analysis. *Obstetrics and Gynecology, 71*(6), 812–817.

CHAPTER 15

Nursing Management of Dementia

Christine E. Schwartzkopf, MSN, RN, CRRN
Prudence Twigg, PhD, RN, ANP-BC, GNP-BC

LEARNING OBJECTIVES

At the end of this chapter, the reader will be able to:

- Differentiate among dementia, depression, and delirium.
- Identify the stages and clinical features of dementia.
- Describe procedures for diagnosing dementia.
- Recognize and address the common causes of delirium.
- Discuss the theoretical foundations of nursing care for persons with dementia.
- Contrast pharmacological and nonpharmacological interventions for dementia, delirium, and depression.
- Apply basic principles to provide safe and effective care for persons with dementia.
- List specific nursing interventions for behavioral and psychological symptoms of dementia.
- Recognize the role of adult day services in the care of persons with dementia.

KEY TERMS

- Acetylcholine
- Agnosia
- Alzheimer's disease (AD)
- Anticholinergic
- Aphasia
- Apolipoprotein E-e4
- Apraxia
- Beta-amyloid plaques
- Cholinesterase
- Cholinesterase inhibitor (CEI)
- Delirium
- Dementia
- Depression
- Executive function
- Hallucinations
- Neurofibrillary tangles
- Neurotransmitter
- Paranoia

The purpose of this chapter is to present basic information about dementia, delirium, and depression. These conditions are sometimes referred to as the "3Ds" of geriatrics because they are fairly common in older adults and their signs and symptoms often overlap. Additionally, this chapter includes information on pharmacological and nonpharmacological treatments and care approaches to improve care for older adults with dementia.

DEMENTIA

Dementia is a general term that refers to progressive, degenerative brain dysfunction, including deterioration in memory, concentration, language skills, visuospatial skills, and reasoning, that interferes with a person's daily functioning. Although

BOX 15-1 Web Exploration

Review the following resources about dementia, delirium, and depression:

Alzheimer's Association: http://www.alz.org

American Association for Geriatric Psychiatry: http://www.aagpgpa.org

National Institute of Mental Health: http://www.nimh.nih.gov

National Institute of Neurological Disorders and Stroke: http://www.ninds.nih.gov

National Institute on Aging: http://www.nia. nih.gov

dementia is much more common in older adults than in younger persons, dementia is not considered a normal part of aging. The most common type of dementia is **Alzheimer's disease (AD)**, named after Dr. Alois Alzheimer, who first described the condition about 100 years ago. AD did not begin to be commonly diagnosed and systemically studied until the 1970s (National Institute on Aging, 2007).

Currently, about 4 million people in the United States have Alzheimer's disease. With the changing demographics of the U.S. population leading to a higher percentage of older adults, the number of Americans with AD is expected to rise to about 14 million by the year 2050. As will be discussed throughout this chapter, the needs of persons with dementia are complex and costly, both financially and psychologically, with families providing most of the care. There are no specific interventions for the prevention of AD, and the current treatments offer only modest benefits (National Institute on Aging, 2007).

Although the aging brain undergoes many developmental changes, these changes do not significantly interfere with the daily functioning of most older adults. Persons with AD, however, have numerous pathological brain changes that contribute to their symptoms. The pathological hallmarks of AD are **beta-amyloid plaques** and **neurofibrillary tangles**. The plaques are dense deposits around neurons. The tangles build up inside nerve cells. Together, the plaques and tangles interfere with normal nerve cell function and lead to neuronal death (National Institute on Aging, 2007). See the section on the nervous system in Chapter 6 for more specific information about brain changes with aging and Alzheimer's disease.

Alzheimer's dementia is the most common type of dementia, accounting for approximately 50–70% of all cases, although several other types of dementia are also commonly seen in older adults. Vascular dementia is the second most common type of dementia, and combinations of Alzheimer's and vascular dementia are also quite common (called "mixed dementia"). Vascular dementia may occur rather acutely after a cerebrovascular accident (CVA, or stroke) or more insidiously due to chronic atherosclerosis of cerebral arteries. Much like the coronary arteries, cerebral arteries are negatively affected by factors such as hyperlipidemia, smoking, and hypertension, causing decreased blood flow to the brain and neuronal death (Alzheimer's Association, 2008). The clinical signs and symptoms of dementia due to Alzheimer's and vascular causes are similar, and generally, the assessment of and interventions for these dementias are similar.

Parkinson's disease (PD) is a chronic neurodegenerative disease characterized by motor symptoms in the early stages, but cognitive symptoms and dementia may develop in the later stages of PD. Dementia with Lewy bodies, or Lewy body dementia (LBD), is a variant of dementia with a specific pathological finding in the brain (abnormal deposits of a protein, alpha-synuclein). Clinically, LBD can be distinguished from AD by:

- Motor symptoms in the early stage of LBD (which occur in the late stage of AD)
- Visual hallucinations in early LBD (which occur in the middle stage of AD, if at all)
- Fluctuating mental status as a feature of LDD (which usually occurs only due to delirium in AD)

It is not uncommon for persons with LBD to initially be suspected of having PD, due to their motor symptoms (e.g., decreased range of motion and gait instability), although their motor symptoms do not respond to dopaminergic agents given for PD.

Frontotemporal dementia or frontal lobe dementia (FLD) affects the frontal and temporal lobes of the brain and is often characterized by early deficiencies in executive functioning (e.g., planning and making decisions), while memory may initially remain fairly intact. Persons with FLD often experience personality changes and disinhibition (saying and doing inappropriate things) much earlier than persons with AD (Alzheimer's Association, 2008).

Normal pressure hydrocephalus (NPH) is a relatively rare type of dementia, but an important subtype, primarily because, if identified early, it may be partially reversible with surgical intervention. The symptoms of NPH are related to an abnormal accumulation of cerebrospinal fluid and are clinically distinguishable from other dementias by a triad of symptoms: slowed cognitive processes, gait disturbances, and urinary incontinence with a relatively acute onset (Alzheimer's Association, 2008).

Other, less common dementias include Huntington's disease (hereditary), Wernicke-Korsakoff's syndrome (most commonly caused by chronic alcoholism), and Creutzfeldt-Jakob disease (a very rare, rapidly progressing dementia related to "mad cow disease"). Down's syndrome is also associated with the eventual development of dementia. About 65% of persons with Down's syndrome who are over 60 years old will have dementia. Although there are many types of dementia, the majority of cases are attributable to Alzheimer's and/or vascular dementia (Alzheimer's Association, 2008).

BOX 15-2 Most Common Types of Dementia in Older Adults

Alzheimer's disease

Vascular dementia

Mixed Alzheimer's/vascular dementia

Parkinson's dementia

Lewy body dementia

Frontotemporal lobe dementia

Risk Factors for Dementia

The main risk factor for developing Alzheimer's-type dementia is age. The risk for AD doubles every 5 years after age 65 years. By age 85, about one-half of people will have symptoms of Alzheimer's. Family history also plays a role in the risk for developing dementia. Having a first-degree relative (parent, sibling, or child) with Alzheimer's increases the risk, and the risk increases even more if more than one first-degree relative has had the disease. Some of the increased risk is genetic, but environmental factors may also play a role in the increased risk within families (Alzheimer's Association, 2008).

One gene that increases the risk for Alzheimer's in the general population is the presence of **apolipoprotein E-e4** (APOE-e4). The other common forms of the APOE gene (e2 and e3) are not associated with Alzheimer's. Each person inherits two APOE genes, so some people will have no APOE-e4, some may have one APOE-e4 (higher risk for AD), and a few may have two copies of APOE-e4 (highest risk for AD). The APOE-e4 gene has varying penetrance, however, so even persons at the highest risk may never develop the disease. The APOE gene codes for proteins associated with cholesterol transport in the body. There are rarer genes that are associated with the risk for Alzheimer's, but these genes tend to be concentrated within a few hundred well-identified families (Alzheimer's Association, 2008). Although many people worry about having the APOE-e4 gene, routine genetic screening is not recommended. The value of having such knowledge is questionable because of the varying predictive ability and lack of treatment for the presence of the gene.

On the other hand, there are several modifiable risk factors that can lower one's risk for developing Alzheimer's and/or vascular dementia. Persons with a history of head injury have a higher risk for developing dementia later in life. Protecting the head from injury by using seatbelts and bicycle/motorcycle helmets throughout the life span is one way to lower the risk for dementia. Vascular disease contributes to the risk for dementia, so taking care of one's brain, in much the same way that one can prevent heart disease, is another good way to lower the risk for dementia. Maintenance of ideal body weight, exercising, avoiding smoking, and

BOX 15-3 Risk Factors for Dementia

Age

Family history

Genetic factors

History of head trauma

Vascular disease

Certain types of infections

controlling hyperlipidemia and hypertension may all help to lower the risk of dementia. Finally, exercising the brain with lifelong cognitive activity may help lower the risk of dementia (Alzheimer's Association, 2008).

Medical Diagnosis of Alzheimer's Disease/Dementia

When an older adult and/or their family members suspect memory problems and possibly dementia, the first step is a visit to the primary care provider (PCP). It is not uncommon for family members and friends to notice changes and request an evaluation even though the older adult him- or herself may not think there are any problems. Conversely, some older adults without significant cognitive problems may be overly concerned about mild memory lapses and request evaluations. Whenever the cognitive function of an older adult is in question, the best course of action is to seek a medical evaluation. More and more PCPs are routinely screening for cognitive impairment in older adults using short questionnaires at office visits for other medical problems. The goal of this practice is to identify and treat dementia in the early stage, before the symptoms are more apparent and when interventions tend to be more successful.

Alzheimer's disease has several clinical features including, but not limited to, memory impairment (see **Box 15-5**). Memory impairment alone does not indicate AD; rather, the cognitive deficits and memory impairment must significantly interfere with functioning. Additionally, the diagnostic criteria require that one of the following features also be present: impaired executive function, aphasia, apraxia, or agnosia. **Executive function** refers to higher level functions such as the ability to think abstractly, plan, organize, complete sequences of action, and make decisions. Impaired executive function significantly affects a person's ability to complete day-to-day tasks. Even an activity as simple as getting dressed in the morning requires planning, decision making, and sequencing. **Aphasia** refers to language deficits, typically a lack of complex language (e.g., less vocabulary) and word finding difficulties (e.g., can't think of the right word to speak) early in AD. **Apraxia** is the inability to carry out motor activities, even though there are no motor deficits (e.g., unable to comb one's hair even though the arms have full range of motion). **Agnosia** refers to the failure to recognize sensory stimuli (e.g., cannot look at a wristwatch and name what it is). In AD, the history of the cognitive deficits is that they have occurred gradually over a relatively long period of time (months to a few years).

In addition to having the preceding deficits, to make a diagnosis of AD, the clinician must ensure that nothing else but AD accounts for the deficits observed. Therefore, a significant part of diagnosing AD is ruling out other possible causes of cognitive deficits such as **delirium**, **depression**, other

BOX 15-4 Possible Warning Signs of Dementia

Frequent forgetfulness, especially of recent events

Difficulty with common tasks (e.g., cooking)

Forgetting common words

Becoming lost in familiar areas

Poor judgment, especially with finances

Misplacing objects in unusual places (e.g., puts clothes in bathtub, puts purse in oven)

Changes in mood, behavior, or personality

Lack of interest/involvement in life activities

BOX 15-5 Diagnostic Criteria for Alzheimer's Disease

- Multiple cognitive deficits/impairment
  1. Impaired short- or long-term memory AND
  2. At least one of the following:
     - Impaired executive function (abstraction, planning, organizing, sequencing)
     - Aphasia (language disturbance)
     - Apraxia (impaired purposeful movements)
     - Agnosia (inability to recognize sensory stimuli)
- The changes significantly interfere with social and/or occupational function and represent a decline from previous level of function.
- The course has been a gradual onset and continuing decline.
- The changes do not occur exclusively during delirium.
- The changes are not better accounted for by another condition (systemic disorders, central nervous system disorders, substances, other psychiatric conditions).

central nervous system disorders, medication side effects, and numerous medical conditions that impact cognitive function.

The primary care provider (PCP) evaluating cognitive problems in an older adult will conduct a history and physical examination. The medical history, particularly the onset, type, and duration of symptoms, may help distinguish chronic from acute cognitive changes. A thorough physical examination, including laboratory tests, may help identify possible reversible causes of the cognitive changes. Several medical disorders that can be identified with laboratory tests can contribute to cognitive problems in older adults including severe liver disease, hypothyroidism, vitamin B_{12} deficiency, hypercalcemia, and latent syphilis. The patient's medication list should be carefully reviewed to determine any current medications that may be causing or worsening cognitive impairment. (A pharmacist may be enlisted to help with this review.) Box 15-10 lists common medications that may cause or worsen cognitive impairment. Many of these medications appear on a list that is famous, or perhaps infamous, in the world of geriatrics: Beers's criteria for potentially inappropriate drugs in older adults (Fick et al., 2003). Medication issues will be discussed in more detail later in this chapter.

Usually, imaging of the head/brain will be conducted. Although Alzheimer's disease cannot be directly diagnosed by a computed tomography (CT) scan of the head or magnetic resonance imaging (MRI) of the brain, these studies may identify or rule out other possible causes of cognitive decline and may confirm previous strokes or the presence of vascular disease. The American Association for Geriatric Psychiatry (AAGP) has recommended that a CT or MRI be conducted as part of a dementia workup and that positron emission tomography (PET) scans not be used routinely to diagnose dementia (AAGP, 2004b). PET scans of the brain are more commonly used in dementia research than in clinical practice.

Any possible medical problems contributing to cognitive changes will usually be treated before concluding that the older adult has dementia. Notably, delirium should be excluded and depression should be excluded or diagnosed and treated before a diagnosis of dementia can be firmly established.

The PCP may do simple "paper and pencil" screening tests to determine the presence and degree of cognitive impairment. If the screening tests are suspicious for cognitive impairment, the PCP may refer the older adult to a psychologist and/or psychiatrist for further testing, although many PCPs are comfortable making the diagnosis of dementia without referral to a specialist. The AAGP, however, recommends that the diagnosis of dementia be made by physicians with experience in geriatrics: geriatric internists, geriatric psychiatrists, neurologists with training in the area of cognitive disorders, or family practitioners with expertise in geriatrics (AAGP, 2004b).

There are several common neuropsychological screening tests that can be administered to older adults. In the past, the most popular screening test was the Mini Mental State Examination (MMSE), which is scored from 0–30; 30 is considered normal (Folstein, Folstein, & McHugh, 1975). The MMSE, however, is no longer available in the public domain and so is not as commonly used, though you may still hear clinicians refer to it. Alternatives to the MMSE include the Mini Cog (Borson, Scanlan, Brush, Vitallano, & Dokmak, 2000) and the St. Louis University Mental Status (SLUMS) examination (Tariq, Tumosa, Chibnall, Perry, & Morley, 2006). (See Box 15-31 at the end of this chapter to access these and other assessment tests referred to in this chapter.) Psychologists and/or psychiatrists administering neuropsychological tests for cognitive impairment may administer much more complicated and time-intensive tests to determine the exact nature of the cognitive deficits.

Many persons with a new diagnosis of dementia and/or their families may believe that the diagnosis is incorrect. Receiving a diagnosis of dementia is almost uniformly devastating to the client and/or family, and initially, denial is a common psychological coping mechanism. When the previously mentioned diagnostic steps are completed, however, the diagnostic certainty for the diagnosis of "probable dementia" is quite high (about 90%), higher than for many other medical illnesses (National Institute on Aging, 2007). Clients and families who remain uncertain about the diagnosis should be counseled to seek a second opinion from a physician specializing in the diagnosis and treatment of dementia. From a medical, psychosocial, and financial planning perspective, acceptance of the diagnosis by the client and family and subsequent steps to act on the knowledge can positively influence care outcomes. Prolonged denial of the diagnosis tends to worsen the situation for both the client and family and delay necessary treatment. Older adults with dementia and their families should be referred to the Alzheimer's Association (http://www.alz.org), a national organization with local chapters, for support services.

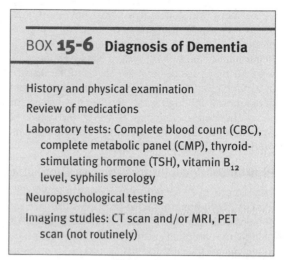

BOX 15-6 Diagnosis of Dementia

History and physical examination

Review of medications

Laboratory tests: Complete blood count (CBC), complete metabolic panel (CMP), thyroid-stimulating hormone (TSH), vitamin B_{12} level, syphilis serology

Neuropsychological testing

Imaging studies: CT scan and/or MRI, PET scan (not routinely)

Stages of Alzheimer's Disease

Alzheimer's disease (AD) is commonly divided into three stages for the purpose of clinical management: mild, moderate, and severe (National Institute on Aging, 2007). (See **Box 15-7**.) During the mild stage of AD, symptoms are often subtle and may go unnoticed by the person and his or her family and friends or may be attributed to "just getting older," resulting in a delay in diagnosis and appropriate treatment. Behavioral and psychological symptoms of dementia (BPSD) are most commonly exhibited during the moderate stage and often lead to institutionalization due to the need for 24-hour supervision. BPSD will be discussed in more detail later in this chapter. The person with severe AD requires total care for all needs and will most often die of complications (aspiration pneumonia) related to dysphagia, unless another medical condition causes death sooner.

Reisberg and colleagues (2002) have identified seven stages of AD (ranging from Stage 1: "no impairment" to Stage 7: "very severe cognitive decline"). Regardless of the staging system employed, persons with AD may pass through the stages of the disease at varying rates, but generally die within 4 to 6 years of diagnosis, although most have had the disease for some time before diagnosis. However, the course of AD is quite variable and can range from 3 to 20 years (Alzheimer's Association, 2008).

Pharmacological Intervention for Dementia

The American Association for Geriatric Psychiatry (AAGP, 2006) has published principles for care for persons with Alzheimer's disease, including principles of pharmacological management. Ideally, pharmacological therapy for AD would prevent beta-amyloid plaques and/or ameliorate the neuronal damage caused by the plaques and neurofibrillary tangles. Unfortunately, currently no medications are available that have this mechanism of action, although many new promising agents are being studied. Two classes of medications currently are approved for the treatment of Alzheimer's dementia: **cholinesterase inhibitors (CEIs)** and N-methyl-D-aspartate (NMDA) receptor antagonists. Both classes have their therapeutic effect by acting on **neurotransmitters**. Several neurotransmitters in the brain are affected by the pathological changes associated with Alzheimer's disease.

Notable Quotes

"The intuitive mind is a sacred gift, and the rational mind its faithful servant. We have created a society that honors the servant and has forgotten the gift."

—Albert Einstein

Acetylcholine is a neurotransmitter in the brain, known to be important for memory. Medications or diseases that inhibit acetylcholine interfere with memory. Early in the course of AD, neuronal loss causes a decrease in the acetylcholine available for normal neurotransmission. Direct supplementation with acetylcholine is not currently feasible. Acetylcholine is naturally degraded in the brain by an enzyme, acetylcholinesterase. Cholinesterase inhibitors (CEIs) exert their therapeutic effect by blocking the enzyme, resulting in a net increase in acetylcholine.

The first CEI developed was tacrine (Cognex); however, this agent is no longer commonly used due to its dosing schedule (four times a day) and potential liver complications. Three CEIs commonly are prescribed for AD: donepezil (Aricept), rivastigmine (Exelon), and galantamine (Razadyne). The CEIs are generally started as early as possible in AD and continued throughout the disease course until no longer effective based on clinical judgment, although only donepezil is approved by the FDA for use in severe AD. The CEIs are generally well tolerated, although, when initiated, clients may complain of gastrointestinal (GI) side effects (nausea, diarrhea), due to the cholinergic effects of the medication on the GI tract. For this reason, the CEIs are usually started at low doses and then gradually titrated up (usually over a period of about 6 weeks) to the target dose in order to lessen side effects. Rivastigmine is also approved for use in mild to moderate Parkinson's dementia. All of the CEIs, however, are often prescribed off-label for dementias other than AD.

Glutamate is the main excitatory neurotransmitter in the brain. Glutamate excitotoxicity (due to excess glutamate) has been implicated in the pathogenesis of AD. When neurons die due to plaques and tangles, glutamate is released in large amounts into the extracellular fluid, increasing N-methyl-D-aspartate (NMDA) receptor activation and intracellular calcium influx into adjacent neurons. Excess intracellular calcium kills the remaining healthy neurons. Although excess glutamate is not the cause of AD per se, the cascading effect of neuronal death, excess glutamate, and further neuronal loss is believed to play a role in the progression of the disease.

Memantine (Namenda) is an NMDA noncompetitive receptor antagonist, currently the only medication in this class, and helps to protect neurons from glutamate excitotoxicity without completely eliminating the glutamate necessary for normal neurological function. Memantine is generally well tolerated, can be safely administered with donepezil or other **cholinesterase** inhibitors, and the combination has been found to be more effective than cholinesterase inhibitors alone. Memantine is currently approved for moderate to severe stage AD, although some clinicians may prescribe the medication for early stage AD or other dementias (off-label use). Memantine, like the CEIs, is generally started at a low dose and gradually titrated up to the target dose (usually over a period of about 4–6 weeks) to lessen side effects.

The cholinesterase inhibitors and memantine slow the progression of dementia, but do not stop the decline. After several months or years of treatment, however, the person receiving treatment may have significantly higher function than if he or she had not been treated at all. For this reason, once the medications are started, they are usually not discontinued unless significant side effects develop (rare after

BOX 15-7 Characteristics of Alzheimer's Disease by Stage

Mild Stage

- Memory loss
- Getting lost in familiar places
- Having more difficulty doing normal daily tasks
- Difficulty with managing finances
- Making bad decisions
- Not being as talkative or verbally fluent
- Being more moody or anxious

Moderate Stage

- Increased memory loss and confusion
- Short attention span
- Difficulty with language, numbers
- Difficulty with reasoning
- Inability to learn new things or to adapt to new situations
- Restlessness, agitation, anxiety, tearfulness, wandering—especially in the late afternoon or at night ("sundowner syndrome")
- Repetitive statements, questions, or movements
- Hallucinations, delusions, paranoia, irritability
- Impulsivity (saying or doing things he or she normally would not)
- Perceptual-motor problems (interfering with activities of daily living)

Severe Stage

- Weight loss
- Seizures in some patients
- Dysphagia (difficulty swallowing)
- Vocalizations, but speech usually unintelligible
- Increased time spent sleeping
- Bowel and bladder incontinence
- Loss of recognition of family
- Pressure ulcers
- Neuromuscular symptoms (contractures)

continuous use). Suddenly discontinuing the medications may result in a significant observable decline that may not be reversed by restarting the medications. If the medications are stopped for some reason for a period of days or weeks, and then restarted, the lowest dose is restarted and then titration proceeds back up to the target dose. Eventually, when the client is in the most advanced stage of AD and is clearly no longer benefiting from the medications (nonambulatory, mute, unable to recognize family members), the medications are usually weaned off.

Indirectly, good treatment for other medical conditions, particularly the management of vascular disease and associated conditions such as hypertension, hyperlipidemia, hyperglycemia, and elevated homocysteine levels, may help slow the progression of dementia. Vitamin E supplementation, as an antioxidant, is available over the counter and may be recommended for AD by some clinicians, although the daily dose should not exceed 400 IU due to concerns about toxicity and cardiovascular side effects. Medications *not* currently recommended for the treatment of Alzheimer's disease include estrogen replacement, anti-inflammatory agents (e.g., ibuprofen), and gingko biloba, although estrogen and ibuprofen may be appropriate for other uses (AAGP, 2006).

Numerous new medications for Alzheimer's disease are being investigated in drug trials. The next generation of drugs is designed to prevent and/or destroy deposits of beta-amyloid plaque that kill the brain's nerve cells, which leads to the devastating loss of cognition and function that characterizes Alzheimer's. Some trials are exploring the strong correlation between heart disease and diabetes as Alzheimer's risk factors. Cholesterol-lowering drugs (statins) and the diabetes drug rosiglitazone (Avandia) are being trialed for Alzheimer's disease.

Medications That Can Cause or Worsen Confusion

With an understanding of some of the neurotransmitters affected by Alzheimer's disease and the medications used to treat dementia, one can imagine that some medications could worsen confusion in persons with dementia. This is, indeed, the case. Particularly problematic are agents that block acetylcholine. Medications classified as **anticholinergic** or medications otherwise classified but with significant anticholinergic effects can be expected to worsen cognitive function in persons with dementia (see **Box 15-10**). Additionally, any medications that have central nervous system effects have the potential to negatively affect cognitive functioning.

DELIRIUM

Delirium is a syndrome (group of symptoms) that occurs relatively acutely and is often called *acute confusion*, unlike dementia, which is characterized as chronic confusion. Delirium typically develops over a period of hours or days and is caused by

BOX 15-8 Medication Treatment for Alzheimer's Disease

Medication	Target Dose
Cholinesterase inhibitors (CEIs)	
Donepezil (Aricept)	10 mg po q. daily
Galantamine (Razadyne ER)	24 mg po q. daily
Rivastigmine (Exelon)	6 mg po bid or 9.5 mg patch q. daily
N-methyl-D-aspartate (NMDA) receptor antagonists	
Memantine (Namenda)	10 mg po bid

Refer to a pharmacology text for more specific information about medications for dementia.

BOX 15-9 Research Highlight

Aim: This review study evaluated the evidence for the effectiveness of cholinesterase inhibitors and memantine in achieving clinically relevant outcomes for patients with Alzheimer's disease.

Methods: A literature search for all published English-language randomized controlled clinical trials that evaluated the pharmacologic agents for adults with AD yielded 96 publications of 59 unique studies eligible for review.

Findings: Both cholinesterase inhibitors and memantine demonstrated consistent clinical effects in the areas of cognition and global assessment; however, the effect sizes were small. Most of the studies were short (6 months), limiting the ability to make conclusions about the effects of the medications on the progression of dementia. Other limitations included inclusion of only patients with mild or moderate AD, poor reporting of adverse effects of the medications, and limited evaluation of behavior and quality of life as possible outcome indicators.

Application to practice: Cholinesterase inhibitors and memantine for the treatment of AD show statistically significant results but only marginal clinical improvement in cognition and global (overall) assessment measures. Nurses should use this knowledge when teaching patients and families about the benefits of medication therapy in AD.

Source: Raina, P., Santaguida, P., Ismaila, A., Patterson, C., Cowan, D., Levine, M., Booker, L., & Oremus, M. (2008). Effectiveness of cholinesterase inhibitors and memantine for treating dementia: Evidence review for a clinical practice guideline. *Annals of Internal Medicine, 148*, 379–397.

some other underlying medical problem. A person of any age, when acutely ill, may experience delirium or acute confusion; however, older adults are at higher risk than younger adults, and older adults with pre-existing dementia are at highest risk for developing delirium when acutely ill or injured. Not surprisingly, there is a high incidence of delirium among older adults in acute care hospitals, estimated to be as high as 80% (Foreman, Wakefield, Culp, & Milisen, 2001).

Inouye and colleagues (1990) developed an instrument, the Confusion Assessment Method (CAM), to assist nurses and others to identify delirium quickly and accurately using the four basic features of delirium: 1) acute onset or fluctuating course, 2) inattention, 3) disorganized thinking, and 4) altered level of consciousness. A diagnosis of delirium is made if both features 1 and 2 are present along with either of features 3 or 4. The CAM can be accessed online (see Box 15-31 at the end of this chapter).

The nurse plays a critical role in identifying whether an older adult has experienced an acute change in mental status that could be delirium, assessing for delirium (using an instrument like the CAM), reporting the change to the physician or nurse practitioner, implementing appropriate interventions, and continuing to evaluate the client for signs and symptoms of further decline or improvement.

The primary treatment for delirium is to discover and treat the etiology or cause. The typical medical workup for the possible causes of delirium includes physical examination, laboratory tests (complete blood count, basic metabolic panel, and urinalysis), and imaging of the head/brain if trauma is suspected (e.g., delirium occurring after a recent fall). The medication list should be scrutinized for agents that are known to cause or worsen confusion (see Box 15-10). Particular attention should be paid to medications that have recently been started or increased. A pharmacist may be enlisted to assist with the review of medications.

BOX 15-10 Common Medications That Can Cause or Worsen Confusion

Any anticholinergic agents or those with significant anticholinergic effects

Analgesics

- Propoxyphene (found in Darvon and Darvocet)
- Meperidine (Demerol)
- Opiates in excessive doses

Antiemetics

- Promethazine (Phenergan)—anticholinergic

Antihistamines

- Diphenhydramine (Benadryl)—anticholinergic

Antihypertensives

- Clonodine (Catapres)

Antipruritics

- Hydroxyzine (Atarax)—anticholinergic

Antiseizure medications (most, to some degree)

- Phenobarbital

Anxiolytics

- Meprobamate (Equanil)
- Benzodiazepines (Ativan, Xanax, Valium)

Bladder relaxants

- Oxybutynin (Ditropan)—anticholinergic

Gastrointestinal antispasmodics

- Dicyclomine (Bentyl)—anticholinergic
- Hyoscyamine (Levsin)—anticholinergic

H2 antagonists

- Cimetidine (Tagamet)—anticholinergic

Muscle relaxants

- Cyclobenzaprine (Flexeril)—anticholinergic

Tricyclic antidepressants

- Amitriptyline (Elavil)—anticholinergic

Secondary interventions for delirium include keeping the patient comfortable, treating symptoms (e.g., with pain medication, oxygen, or intravenous fluids), and ensuring the safety of the client. Some persons with delirium may be quite lethargic (hypoactive delirium) whereas others may be very agitated (hyperactive delirium). Either situation presents a nursing challenge. For the lethargic client, oral intake may be compromised and the client is at risk for dehydration and aspiration pneumonia; impaired mobility increases the risk for pressure ulcers. The client with agitated delirium may be at risk for harming self and/or others and may require the judicious use of medications (e.g., benzodiazepines, antipsychotics). Physical restraints should be avoided if at all possible because they tend to cause more panic and agitation in older adults with delirium and can result in serious injury.

Other nursing interventions include moving the older adult to a room nearer the nursing station (for closer observation), implementing risk for falls protocols, providing one-to-one care and supervision, eliminating "tethers" when medically feasible (e.g., indwelling catheters, oxygen tubing), and

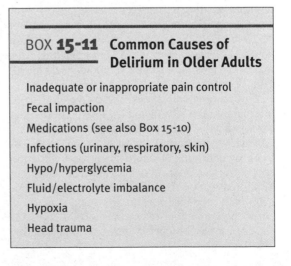

BOX 15-11 Common Causes of Delirium in Older Adults

- Inadequate or inappropriate pain control
- Fecal impaction
- Medications (see also Box 15-10)
- Infections (urinary, respiratory, skin)
- Hypo/hyperglycemia
- Fluid/electrolyte imbalance
- Hypoxia
- Head trauma

eliminating confusing external stimuli (e.g., television). Generally, a calm, quiet environment is the most beneficial for a client with delirium. With appropriate medical care, delirium will eventually clear. One of the main goals of nursing care for delirium is to prevent further complications from developing during this acute syndrome.

DEPRESSION

The risk for depression increases in older adults with chronic illnesses, including dementia. Content in Chapters 13 and 14 also discussed delirium and depression. Depression in the older adult is often not as obvious or as easily diagnosed as in young or middle-aged adults. Older adults may deny depression due to the stigma that this cohort often attaches to mental illness. Older adults, their families, and/or health care providers may incorrectly attribute depressive symptoms to normal aging. Many older adults do not meet the strict criteria for a diagnosis of major depression (see **Box 15-12**), and yet have significant depressive symptoms. Although the prevalence of major depression in older adults is actually lower than that of younger and middle-aged adults, about 8–20% of older adults living in the community and 25–40% of older adult nursing home residents have significant depressive symptoms (American Association for Geriatric Psychiatry, 2004a).

The nurse can play an important role in recognizing possible symptoms of depression and reporting them to the primary care provider, screening for depression, and educating older adult clients and their families about depression. The most commonly used screening tool for depression in older adults is the Geriatric Depression Scale (GDS), a 30-item yes-no questionnaire developed by Yesavage and colleagues (1983), and subsequently shortened to a 15-item scale (Sheikh & Yesavage, 1986). See Box 15-31 at the end of this chapter to access the GDS online. The GDS and other screening tools, however, do not replace the need for a clinical examination to diagnose the condition. Many clinicians are qualified to diagnose and treat geriatric depression including primary

BOX 15-12 Diagnostic Criteria for Major Depression

At least five of the following symptoms for at least 2 weeks:

- Depressed mood*
- Diminished interest or pleasure*
- Significant involuntary weight loss/gain or appetite change
- Insomnia/hypersomnia
- Psychomotor agitation/retardation
- Fatigue/loss of energy
- Feelings of worthlessness/guilt
- Impaired concentration
- Recurrent thoughts of death or suicide

*Must have one of these symptoms

The symptoms cause significant distress or impaired function.

The symptoms are not better accounted for by other medical conditions, substances, or bereavement.

Source: Modified from American Psychiatric Association (2000). *Diagnostic and statistical manual of mental disorders* (4th ed., text revision). Washington, DC: Author.

care providers, psychiatrists, and psychiatric clinical nurse specialists.

Symptoms of depression may overlap with symptoms of dementia. For example, persons with depression frequently have poor concentration that may worsen performance on cognitive tests. Ordinarily, older adults with cognitive symptoms will be evaluated for both dementia and depression. If depressive symptoms are present, treatment with antidepressants and/or psychotherapy will be initiated. Mild cognitive symptoms in older adults often improve with the treatment of depression; however, some older adults will eventually be diagnosed with both dementia and depression.

Depression in older adults (with or without dementia) often includes symptoms of anxiety (see Chapter 14), agitation, and insomnia. Therefore, an important step in evaluating these symptoms in older adults is to screen for depression. Unfortunately, some older adults with depression are inappropriately treated for months or years with sedating medications to control these symptoms without ever being treated for the primary cause of their symptoms, depression. A complete discussion of geriatric depression is beyond the scope of this text; the reader is referred to mental health nursing texts for more information on the evaluation for and treatment of depression. The symptoms of dementia, delirium, and depression often overlap. See **Table 15-1** for a summary of some of the key similarities and differences.

BOX 15-13 Important Points About Depression in Older Adults

Prevalent condition

Often underrecognized

Often undertreated

May not meet strict diagnostic criteria

May present with anxiety, agitation, or insomnia

Symptoms may overlap with dementia

Common cause of excess disability

Potentially life-threatening

Treatable

CARING FOR THE PERSON WITH DEMENTIA

Theories of Dementia Care

Several theories of dementia care have been developed and tested. The Progressively Lowered Stress Threshold (PLST) model of Hall and Buckwalter (1987) focuses on the relationship between environmental stimuli and the lowered stress threshold of the person with dementia, identifying common stressors that may lead to behavioral and psychological symptoms; for example, misleading or inappropriate stimuli, excessive external demands, physical stressors, and changes in the environment, routine, or caregiver (Hall, 1994). Using this model, nurses focus on supporting the personal resources of the person with dementia (e.g., providing rest periods) and controlling that person's environment (e.g., assigning the same nursing assistant to care for the person when possible).

The Enablement Model of dementia care (Dawson, Wells, & Kline, 1993) focuses on supporting the remaining abilities of the person with dementia in order to avoid excess disability (i.e., functional impairment above and beyond what should be expected based on degree of dementia). Using this model, when abilities are still present (e.g., self-feeding), nurses focus on promoting the use of the retained abilities (e.g., setting up the meal tray for the client). When abilities have been lost due to progressive dementia (e.g., drinking from a glass without spilling), nurses focus on assisting the client and manipulating the environment to support the client (e.g., providing a "sippy" cup with a lid).

The Need-Driven Dementia-Compromised Behavior (NDB) model has conceptualized behavioral and psychological symptoms of dementia as resulting from background and proximal factors (Algase et al., 1996; Kolanowski, 1999). Background factors are person-related and more enduring; these include neurological factors, cognitive abilities, health status, and psychosocial history. Proximal factors are more amenable to change and include

TABLE 15-1 Comparison of Signs and Symptoms of Dementia, Depression, and Delirium

	Dementia	Depression	Delirium
Onset	Gradual over months to years.	Usually gradual.	Acute over hours to days.
Course	Slowly progressive, irreversible, minimally treatable.	Chronic but sometimes abrupt with psychosocial stressors. Treatable.	Fluctuating. Reversible with identification and treatment of cause.
Level of Consciousness	Alert.	Alert.	Altered, clouded, fluctuating.
Memory	Impaired. Initially short-term memory loss, eventually long-term memory loss.	Intact, but may exhibit poor effort on memory tests.	Short-term memory loss.
Orientation	Impaired to time, then place, and eventually person, including self.	Intact.	Impaired. Fluctuating.
Psychomotor speed	Normal. Slowed in advanced stages.	May be normal, hypoactive, or hyperactive.	Hypoactive, hyperactive, or mixed.
Language	Word-finding difficulties. Impairment increases with disease progression.	Normal. May not initiate much conversation.	Often incoherent.
Hallucinations	Usually visual if present. Most common in middle stage.	None unless psychotic depression.	Common, tend to be visual and tactile.

physiological and psychological need states, and the physical and social environment. The background and proximal factors interact to produce need-driven behaviors. The nurse considers the background factors in providing care and intervenes to change proximal factors that may be contributing to behavioral symptoms.

The antecedent-behavior-consequence (ABC) model can be used to analyze and understand the behavioral symptoms of persons with dementia (Smith, Buckwalter, & Mitchell, 1993). Using the ABC model, the nurse would first observe and describe the behavior. Next, the nurse would identify the antecedents or "triggers" that occurred before the behavior. Common triggers for behavioral symptoms in persons with dementia include, but are not limited to, personal care discomfort or embarrassment (e.g., bathing, toileting), the person with dementia misinterpreting environmental cues (e.g., a misplaced personal item must have been stolen), and caregiver approaches (e.g., rushing tasks). Finally, the nurse considers the consequences or reactions that may have worsened the behavior (e.g., yelling at the person with dementia who is resisting a bath). After analyzing the behavior using the ABC model, the nurse can plan changes to the antecedents and consequences to help prevent the behavioral symptom from recurring.

Retrogenesis theory, sometimes referred to as "reverse Piaget theory," describes the decline in cognition and function of persons with dementia in terms of reverse development (Reisberg et al., 2002). Retrogenesis theory posits that persons with dementia tend to lose cognition and function in the reverse order of acquisition. Using this theory, the nurse would understand why a person with severe dementia may put nonfood items in the mouth (analogous to Piaget's sensorimotor stage of infant development). The nurse would focus on providing an environment and activities consistent with the client's cognitive developmental stage. An important caveat to the use of this theory is that we do not want to fall into the habit of treating persons with dementia like children or referring to them as "babies." Persons with dementia should always be treated as adults, but knowledge of their cognitive stage of development can enhance understanding and promote more appropriate interventions.

Lawton's person-environment (P-E) fit theory (1982) can be used as a theoretical basis for providing care to persons with dementia. (See the discussion of this theory in Chapter 3.) The environmental docility hypothesis, formulated by Lawton, posits that persons with disability, including dementia, will be more dependent upon the physical and social environment. An appropriate environment will support higher functioning. "Environmental press" is the degree to which the environment challenges the individual. If the environment is too complex, a person with dementia may become frustrated and withdraw from activity. Conversely, if the environment is too trivial, the person with dementia will not be challenged to maintain cognitive and functional abilities. Using the P-E fit theory, the nurse can formulate plans of care that adjust the environmental conditions to challenge, without frustrating, the person with dementia.

Person-centered care, based on the work of Kitwood (1997), is not a true theory, but an approach to dementia care that incorporates several principles: 1) learning about the history and preferences of the person with dementia, 2) developing genuine relationships between persons with dementia and caregivers, 3) promoting physical and emotional comfort, and 4) respecting the choices of persons with dementia and their families (Talerico, O'Brien, & Swafford, 2003).

Behavioral and Psychological Symptoms of Dementia (BPSD)

In the past, persons with Alzheimer's disease and other dementias were often labeled as having "problem behaviors" or "behavioral disturbances." You may still hear some clinicians using these terms. A consensus group of the International Psychogeriatric Association (IPA, 2002), however, has recommended that the term *behavioral and psychological symptoms of dementia* or *BPSD* be used instead, emphasizing the understanding that such symptoms are disease-related. BPSD includes symptoms of disturbed perception, thought content, mood, or behavior. Behavioral symptoms can typically be assessed objectively by observing the person with dementia. Psychological symptoms are usually assessed by talking to the person with dementia and/or their families and caregivers.

BOX 15-14 Behavioral and Psychological Symptoms of Dementia (BPSD)

Behavioral Symptoms

Physical aggression (hitting, kicking, biting)
Verbal agitation (screaming, meaningless vocalizations)
Physical agitation (restlessness, purposeless movements)
Wandering (continuous walking around aimlessly)
Sexual disinhibition (exposing genitals, masturbating in public)
Hoarding (keeping/hiding unusually large amounts of what are often useless items)
Verbal aggression (swearing at, threatening others)
Shadowing (following another person around closely for long periods of time)

Psychological Symptoms

Anxiety
Depressive symptoms (feeling sad, poor sleep and/or appetite, lack of interest in life)
Hallucinations (seeing or hearing things that others do not)
Delusions (holding false beliefs)
Paranoia (having unreasonable fears)

The estimated frequency of BPSD varies considerably. Anywhere from 20–73% of persons with dementia may experience delusions, 15–29% have **hallucinations**, up to 20% show aggression and hostility, and as many as 80% have depressive symptoms (Finkel, 1998). If left untreated, BPSD contributes to premature institutionalization, increased financial costs, increased caregiver stress, excess disability for the person with dementia, and decreased quality of life for the person with dementia and their caregivers (IPA, 2002). The frequency of BPSD tends to peak in the middle stages of dementia and wane in the later stages.

Some types of BPSD are more common in certain types of dementia. For example, visual hallucinations and sexual disinhibition are more common in Lewy body dementia and frontotemporal lobe dementia, respectively. Common delusions in dementia include the belief that others are stealing things, that one's spouse is having an affair, that one's spouse or other loved one is an imposter, or that one has been abandoned. One of the more difficult situations nurses employed in nursing homes often encounter is trying to find out if a particular item really was stolen from an older adult (a crime) or if the belief is falsely held by the older adult (a delusion). Visual hallucinations are more common than auditory hallucinations in persons with dementia and are more common in persons with visual deficits, who are presumably misinterpreting visual stimuli. Close attention to lighting, eliminating confusing visual stimuli, and providing visual aids may decrease visual hallucinations. When a person with dementia has ongoing disturbing hallucinations, delusions, and/or **paranoia**, a diagnosis of "psychosis of Alzheimer's disease" may be made, and the condition may be treated with antipsychotic medication.

Agitation is a nonspecific term often applied to the behavior of persons with dementia. Cohen-Mansfield (1996) studied agitation extensively and identified four subtypes of agitation: physically nonaggressive behaviors (e.g., restlessness, pacing), verbally nonaggressive behaviors (e.g., complaining, interrupting), verbally aggressive behaviors (e.g., screaming, swearing), and physically aggressive behaviors (e.g., hitting, kicking, biting). When a person with dementia becomes agitated, the possibility of delirium should be considered.

Pharmacological Treatment for Behavioral and Psychological Symptoms of Dementia (BPSD)

Generally, nonpharmacological treatments for BPSD are initiated first and preferred due to potential medication side effects in older adults. When symptoms are uncomfortable for the person with dementia or the behaviors endanger self or others, and have not responded to nonpharmacological treatments, then medications are prescribed. See **Box 15-15** for a list of medications commonly prescribed for BPSD.

Older antidepressants, such as amitriptyline (Elavil), are generally avoided in older adults with dementia due to their adverse side effect profiles (anticholinergic). Generally, the selective serotonin reuptake inhibitors (SSRIs) and serotonin norepinephrine reuptake inhibitors (SNRIs) are safe and effective with minimal side effects. The most common side effect of these classes is gastrointestinal upset when the medications are started, so starting doses are usually low and gradually titrated upward. Paroxetine (Paxil) is often avoided because this agent has the most anticholinergic side effects in its class. Although gradual dose reductions, unless contraindicated, of all psychotropic medications are mandated in the nursing home setting, many clinicians continue antidepressants indefinitely due to the high rate of recurrence of geriatric depressive symptoms when medications are withdrawn (AAGP, 2004b).

Antipsychotics are generally reserved for psychotic or serious behaviors endangering self or others. Antipsychotics are not considered effective for dementia per se. The atypical antipsychotics carry a "black box warning" concerning the increased risk for adverse cardiovascular events (AAGP, 2004b). Generally, the atypical antipsychotics are preferred over the conventional antipsychotics due to the side effect profiles, although haloperidol (Haldol) is commonly used in acute care for delirium. Benzodiazepines are used cautiously in older adults due to their side effect profile, particularly increased risk for falls. Psychotropic drug use in the nursing home setting is highly regulated. Regular review of the risks and benefits along with trials of periodic gradual dose reductions are mandated unless clinically contraindicated.

A more complete discussion of pharmacological therapy for persons with dementia is beyond the scope of this chapter. For more information, please consult psychiatric nursing and pharmacology texts.

Nonpharmacological Treatment for Dementia

Nurses, as an interdependent intervention, administer medications prescribed for persons with dementia. The largest role for nurses in dementia care, however, is applying the nursing process to promote comfort, function, and dignity for persons with dementia. The nurse uses theories about dementia care to guide assessment, nursing diagnosis, planning, intervention, and ongoing evaluation. The role of the nurse is particularly important in assessing and treating behavioral and psychological symptoms of dementia (BPSD). When evaluating any acute changes in the cognition, behavior, and mood of persons with dementia, recall that delirium is a common cause of these changes.

General Interventions

Reality orientation is a technique that presents information to persons with dementia about themselves and their orientation in time and place. Nurses using reality orientation frequently remind the person with words and other cues (e.g., clocks, calendars). A systematic review of studies of reality orientation found that the technique could improve both cognitive and behavioral outcomes (Spector, Orrell, Davies, & Woods, 2008). Reality orientation, however, may actually increase distress in some persons with dementia, who may be convinced of some other reality and resent being "corrected."

Validation therapy (VT), which was developed by Naomi Feil (1993), is a systematic method for communicating with and caring for persons with dementia in an empathic and individualized manner. Validation therapy recognizes that older adults with dementia are unique, valuable individuals who should be accepted nonjudgmentally. Within the VT framework, the behavior of persons with dementia is viewed as having meaning and is not just caused by physical and functional changes in the brain (the medical model of dementia). Furthermore, VT posits that older adults with impaired memory are often trying to resolve uncompleted developmental tasks from earlier in life, thus accounting for their tendency to dwell more on remote rather than recent memories. Feil developed

BOX 15-15 Common Medications Prescribed for BPSD

Class/Medications	Common Uses
Selective serotonin reuptake inhibitors	Depression, agitation, and/or anxiety attributed to depression
Fluoxetine (Prozac)	
Sertraline (Zoloft)	
Paroxetine (Paxil)	
Citalopram (Celexa)	
Serotonin norepinephrine reuptake inhibitors	Depression, agitation, and/or anxiety attributed to depression
Venlafaxine (Effexor)	
Duloxetine (Cymbalta)	
Other antidepressants	
Mirtazapine (Remeron)	Depression, used at lower doses for insomnia and appetite stimulation
Trazadone (Desyrel)	
Mood stabilizers	Low doses for insomnia
Divalproex (Depakote)	Bipolar-type depression, agitation
Benzodiazepines*	Anxiety, agitation
Antipsychotics	Psychotic symptoms, mania, adjunct therapy for depression, violent behavior
Risperidone (Risperdal)	
Olanzapine (Zyprexa)	
Quetiapine (Seroquel)	
Aripiprazole (Abilify)	
Ziprasidone (Geodon)	
Conventional/typical antipsychotics	Delirium, violent behavior
Haloperidol (Haldol)	

*Check the Beers list for cautions in older adults.

her own classification of chronic confusion in older adults called the four stages of resolution: malorientation, time confusion, repetitive motion, and vegetation. Communication and care are based on the stage of resolution. The goals of VT are to reduce anxiety, restore a sense of self-worth, and improve function for the person with dementia. A systematic review of VT for persons with dementia concluded that there were too few good studies and relatively small numbers of subjects to draw

BOX 15-16 General Approaches to Managing Behavioral and Psychological Symptoms of Dementia (BPSD)

Try nonpharmacological before pharmacological interventions.

Maintain a calm, familiar environment and routine.

For specific BPSD:

- Identify and describe the behavior in as much detail as possible.
- Identify the antecedents (triggers) and consequences of the behavior (per the ABC model).
- Identify the desired behavioral outcome.
- Implement interventions.
- Evaluate the effectiveness of interventions.

any conclusions about the effectiveness of VT (Neal & Barton Wright, 2008).

Validation and reminiscence therapy (RT) share several principles and approaches, though validation therapy relies less on cognitive ability and thus can theoretically be used into much later stages of dementia. Reminiscence therapy was developed for use with older adults by Norris (1986), based on Butler's work on life review (1963). The purpose of RT is to promote adjustment and integrity for older adults through structured remembering and reflecting on the past. RT may be conducted individually, but is frequently a group activity for persons with dementia living in institutions, often incorporating refreshments. A systematic review of RT for persons with dementia concluded that there were too few good studies and too many variations in treatment protocols to evaluate the effectiveness of RT (Woods, Spector, Jones, Orrell, & Davies, 2008).

Environmental Interventions

Managing the environment of the person with dementia is a component of most theories of dementia care. The acute care environment, with its multiple and competing stimuli, can be very stressful for persons with dementia, who have decreased ability to adapt to change. Nurses should assess and modify the environment to control the information the patient is receiving.

The impact the environment has on patient behavior may fluctuate, depending on the degree of activity occurring at any given time. Behavioral symptoms are more likely to occur during periods of high activity: 7 to 10 a.m., noon to 2 p.m., and 4 to 7 p.m. In an acute care environment, these times represent periods of high activity: shift changes, meal times, sending and receiving patients from operating rooms, doctor rounds, and visiting hours. Carefully planning activities to minimize additional procedures and demands during peak periods may prevent unnecessary stress and behavioral outbursts (Gitlin, Liebman, & Winter, 2003).

Physical Comfort Interventions

Interventions to promote elimination, comfort, sensory function, and adequate sleep and nutrition

BOX 15-17 Examples of Environmental Interventions

Physical Environment

- Areas for safe wandering.
- Alarms on exits and/or the person to detect elopement.
- Adequate, but not harsh, lighting during the day.
- Low lighting at night.
- Soft background music.
- Appropriate, nonconfusing sensory stimuli.
- Comfortable room temperature.

Temporal Environment

- Establish a meaningful routine.
- Alternate activity and rest periods.

(discussed in other areas of this text) will contribute to overall well-being for persons with dementia and reduce the risk for BPSD.

Pain Management and Alzheimer's Disease

Many people with Alzheimer's disease are unable to report their pain. In such cases, nurses must rely on observation to assess for pain behaviors. Each person might have a "pain signature," which means that one person's pain may cause him or her to become agitated and combative, whereas another may withdraw. Failure to recognize and treat pain can lead to sleep disturbances, malnutrition, depression, decreased mobility, needless suffering, and inappropriate psychotropic medication use (American Geriatrics Society [AGS], 2002).

One of the most important steps in evaluating any patient, especially for those with Alzheimer's disease, is to obtain a baseline pain assessment. Changes in baseline are then used to determine the need for adjustments in the treatment plan, such as the addition of an analgesic or dose adjustment. Because self-report is the single most reliable indicator of pain, those who are able to communicate verbally should be asked about their pain level. A pain assessment, such as a 0–10 scale or a faces pain rating scale, should be used to determine pain intensity. For more impaired clients, the nurse should assess for crying, moaning, groaning, and other verbalizations that may be indicative of pain, along with possible nonverbal expressions of pain (see **Box 15-18**). It is important to assess pain at rest and during activity. Pain behaviors are often more obvious during activities such as repositioning and bathing. See Box 15-31 at the end of this chapter for more information on how to assess for pain in persons with dementia.

The principles of good pain management for adults with Alzheimer's apply universally to those with the disease. Nonpharmacological interventions (see **Box 15-19**) should be tried first for mild pain and used along with pharmacological interventions in moderate to severe pain. Nonopioid analgesics should be considered for mild to moderate pain. Opioid analgesics are added to the treatment plan for more severe pain. If neuropathic pain is suspected, adjuvant analgesics such as local anesthetics, anticonvulsants, and antidepressants may be indicated. Opioid analgesics are generally started at very low doses and titrated upward based on continuing evaluation. When opioids are administered, it is particularly important to assess bowel function, because the person with dementia may not be able to report constipation (AGS, 2002).

BOX 15-18 Possible Nonverbal Expressions of Pain

Agitation

Increased confusion

Decreased mobility

Combativeness

Resistance to care

Guarding

Grimacing

Restlessness

Changes in eating and sleeping habits

Withdrawal

Aggression

Rubbing/holding a particular area of the body

Rapid breathing

BOX 15-19 Nonpharmacological Interventions for Pain

Distraction

Massage

Heat/cold application

Gentle movement/repositioning

Participation in normal activities as able

Activity Interventions

Persons with dementia need a balance between stimulating and calming activities. Too much or too

BOX 15-20 Key Points for Pain Control

Persons with dementia may not be as able to report pain.

Always consider pain as a possible cause of behavioral symptoms.

Assess for possible objective indicators of pain.

Administer analgesics routinely for painful conditions when the person cannot ask.

little activity may lead to behavioral and psychological symptoms (BPSD). When evaluating behavioral symptoms, note the time of day and the level of activity at the time the symptoms occurred.

Interdisciplinary teamwork between nursing and the activities service is needed to assess the person's normal schedule of activities, looking for prolonged periods of activity or inactivity. Adjustments can be made to increase or decrease activity. In addition to the quantity of activity, the quality of activity is important. Generally, persons with dementia respond most positively to meaningful activities that are connected to their personal history and preferences. Lifelong personality characteristics may also be used to help choose appropriate activities (Kolanowski & Buettner, 2008). More extroverted individuals may prefer small group activities; more introverted individuals may prefer one-on-one or individual activities. Group physical activity can help meet both exercise and socialization needs (Netz, Axelrad, & Argov, 2007).

Communication Interventions

Language and speech become progressively impaired in dementia, but maintaining communication is critical to effective care for persons with dementia. Keep in mind that behavior is a form of communication, and as dementia progresses it becomes more and more important for the nurse to analyze and interpret the behavior of a person with dementia in that context. For example, a person with dementia who is exhibiting a behavioral symptom may just need food, fluids, or to be toileted, but be unable to express that need. Nurses who routinely care for persons with dementia in long-term care become experts at interpreting the meaning of particular behaviors. See **Box 15-21** for suggested communication techniques.

Interventions for Particular Behaviors

Nurses caring for persons with dementia are often challenged to address particular behaviors. Keeping in mind that these behaviors are most often symptoms of the disease process, the nurse can analyze the behaviors using the ABC model. An important step in this process is examining the possible

BOX 15-21 Suggested Communication Techniques

Speak to the person distinctly and in simple phrases/sentences.

Speak as one adult to another.

Smile.

Avoid "elderspeak" (sing-song baby talk).

Keep the pace of the conversation slow.

Listen.

Allow sufficient time for responses.

Be calm, remain patient, and speak softly.

Maintain eye contact.

Use nonverbal cues: Point or demonstrate what you want done.

Repeat instructions as often as necessary.

Lower voice to accommodate age-related hearing changes.

For persons with limited speech, try using yes-no questions.

Observe carefully for a person's nonverbal cues.

antecedents, causes, or triggers for the behavior (see **Box 15-22**). When the antecedents of the behavior have been identified, the nurse can plan care to help prevent that behavior in the future. For example, if a person with dementia becomes agitated every time he or she has to void, scheduled toileting could be implemented to avoid this behavior. Nursing care for the behavioral symptoms of dementia is quite individualized because the cause of and approach to the behavior are very much dependent on the personal and contextual factors. There are, however, some general approaches to particular behaviors (see **Boxes 15-23** to **15-27**).

Notable Quotes

"The journey into dementia has its disappointments to be endured as well as its triumphs to be cherished. In all of the ambiguities and confusion there may also be signs of hope, for this is a journey with intersecting signposts; reminders of the past and pointers to the future. There are always fresh opportunities for a new walk on a new day."

—Rosalie Hudson. (2006). Spirited walking. In M. Marshall & K. Allan (Eds.), *Dementia: Walking not wandering* (p. 113). London: Hawker.

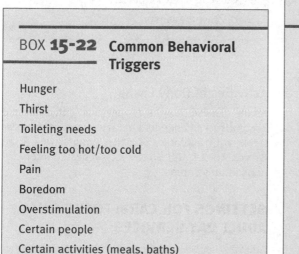

BOX 15-22 Common Behavioral Triggers

Hunger

Thirst

Toileting needs

Feeling too hot/too cold

Pain

Boredom

Overstimulation

Certain people

Certain activities (meals, baths)

BOX 15-23 Suggested Interventions for Agitation/Aggression

Avoid provoking situations.

Intervene early, before the behavior escalates.

Remain calm; speak in a soft voice.

Approach slowly from the front.

Avoid startling the person.

Stay at the eye level of the person.

Avoid touching initially; wait until the person is calmer.

Distract the person.

Avoid rational arguments.

Avoid physical restraint if at all possible.

Identify and address unmet needs (food, fluid, toileting).

BOX 15-24 Suggested Interventions for Resistance to Bathing

Remain calm.

Use a soft voice.

Choose a time when the person is most rested and least confused.

Consider the person's lifelong preferences:

- Shower vs. bath
- Morning vs. evening

Maintain a leisurely pace. Avoid rushing the person.

(continues)

BOX 15-24 Continued

Premedicate with analgesics if pain with movement is an issue.

Allow the person to wear underwear or a patient gown, if desired.

Avoid spraying water directly on the head or face.

Pantomime the desired hygiene activities.

Use distraction: conversation, snacks, or music.

When complete, give praise for clean appearance.

BOX 15-25 Suggested Interventions for Wandering

Assess for unmet needs.

Reassure the person that he or she is in the right place.

Use identification bracelets (in case he or she gets lost).

Place alarms on the person and/or doors to detect elopement.

Provide a safe wandering "path."

Provide alternative activities.

Minimize medication use (to reduce risk for falls).

Visually disguise exits.

Provide daily exercise.

Provide simple snack foods to be eaten "on the run."

BOX 15-26 Suggested Interventions for Delusions/Paranoia

Assist the person to keep track of personal items.

Avoid defensiveness if accused.

Do not argue with the person.

Maintain a simple, noncluttered environment.

Avoid whispering in front of the person.

Note: Antipsychotic medications are often required.

BOX 15-27 Suggested Interventions for Inappropriate Sexual Behavior

If disrobed, offer clothing.

If masturbating:

- Avoid laughing, scolding, or confrontation.
- Guide to a private place.
- Distract the person.

Activities of Daily Living

As the disease progresses, persons with dementia become more dependent upon caregivers for assistance with activities of daily living (ADLs). See **Boxes 15-28** and **15-29** for suggested interventions in these areas.

SETTINGS FOR CARE: FOCUS ON ADULT DAY SERVICES

Adult day services are the cornerstone of community-based, long-term care alternatives. These services

BOX 15-28 Suggested Interventions for Eating/Feeding Issues

Thoroughly prepare meal trays (open cartons, cut food).

Offer small, frequent meals and snacks.

At meals, provide one food and one utensil at a time.

Provide nutritious finger foods.

Provide nutritional supplements, if indicated.

Offer fluids in containers that can be self-managed ("sippy" cups, sports bottles).

Request speech therapy (ST) and occupational therapy (OT) services, if needed.

Provide adaptive utensils, if indicated. (OT will order.)

Assist the client to feed self, rather than feeding, whenever possible.

Use "hand-over-hand" feeding (your hand guides theirs).

Gently cue the person to continue eating, chewing, and swallowing.

Avoid making comments about manners or messiness.

Provide the person with dignified protection for clothing.

If agitation develops during feeding, stop and retry a little later.

Avoid force feeding.

Reassure the person that his or her food has been paid for (a common concern).

Monitor body weight to detect gains or losses.

BOX 15-29 Suggested Interventions to Promote Continence/Toileting

Ensure that toilets are visible.

- Keep bathroom doors open.
- Place signs/pictures as visual cues.

Keep paths to the bathroom clear.

Systematically assess voiding and bowel patterns.

Offer toileting frequently.

Use incontinence pads/briefs, as needed.

For persons who can still toilet, use "pull-up" type protective products.

Provide adequate fluids during the day.

Limit fluids at bedtime.

Avoid beverages with caffeine.

Ensure adequate fiber in diet.

BOX 15-30 Typical Adult Day Services

Recreational therapy/activities

Meals

Social services

Transportation

Personal care: bathing, hair and nail care

Nursing services

Rehabilitation services (less commonly offered)

Medical services (less commonly offered)

are designed to meet the needs of cognitively and functionally impaired adults through individualized plans of care (National Adult Day Services Association [NADSA], n.d.). Most frequently referred to as adult day care (ADC), these services offer consumers the opportunity to continue living at home while receiving needed services in a safe, structured environment. They offer a comprehensive program that provides a variety of health, social, and related services in a protective setting during the daytime hours: mid-day meals, structured recreational activities, socialization opportunities, and appropriate cognitive stimulation (see **Box 15-30**). Over the past 10 years, the number of adult day services has increased to about 3,400 nationwide, serving about 150,000 older adults each day (NADSA, n.d.). Consumers of adult day care increasingly have more health care and functional needs. Over 50% of ADC consumers have dementia.

As the older adult population increases, adult day services will undoubtedly become more appealing to consumers. Caregivers using ADC for older adults with dementia have more time to rest, run errands, and do other business. Adult day services assist persons with dementia to function at their highest level, strengthen caregivers' abilities and coping skills, and delay institutionalization.

SUMMARY

In conclusion, there are many challenges that face the gerontological nurse who is working with patients with dementia. As the population continues to age, the number of persons with dementia will also grow, so nurses need to be well informed about dementia care. There are reliable assessment tools to assist nurses in recognizing dementia in earlier stages. The content of this chapter presented many suggestions of interventions for the common behaviors encountered among persons with dementia.

BOX 15-31 Resources for Assessment Available on the Internet

Assessing and Managing Delirium in Older Adults with Dementia:

http://consultgerirn.org/uploads/File/trythis/AssesMangeDeleriumWDementia.pdf

Assessing Pain in Persons with Dementia:

http://consultgerirn.org/uploads/File/trythis/assessingPain.pdf

Avoiding restraints in patients with dementia:

http://www.nursingcenter.com/prodev/ce_article.asp?tid=776342

(continues)

Beers Criteria for Potentially Inappropriate Medication Use in Older Adults: Parts I and II:
http://consultgerirn.org/uploads/File/trythis/issue16_1.pdf
http://consultgerirn.org/uploads/File/trythis/issue16_2.pdf

Brief Evaluation of Executive Dysfunction:
http://consultgerirn.org/uploads/File/trythis/issue_d3.pdf

Communication Difficulties: Assessment and Interventions in Hospitalized Older Adults with Dementia:
http://www.nursingcenter.com/prodev/ce_article.asp?tid=776481

Confusion Assessment Method (CAM):
http://www.nursingcenter.com/prodev/ce_article.asp?tid=756744

Decision Making and Dementia:
http://consultgerirn.org/uploads/File/trythis/issue_d9.pdf

Eating and Feeding Issues in Older Adults with Dementia: Parts I and II:
http://consultgerirn.org/uploads/File/trythis/issue11_1.pdf
http://consultgerirn.org/uploads/File/trythis/issue11_2.pdf

Geriatric Depression Scale (GDS):
http://www.nursingcenter.com/prodev/ce_article.asp?tid=743421

Mental Status Assessment of Older Adults: The Mini-Cog:
http://www.nursingcenter.com/prodev/ce_article.asp?tid=743421

Nursing Standard of Practice Protocol: Recognition and Management of Dementia:
http://consultgerirn.org/topics/dementia/want_to_know_more

St. Louis University Mental Status Examination (SLUMS):
http://medschool.slu.edu/agingsuccessfully/pdfsurveys/slumsexam_05.pdf

Critical Thinking *Exercises*

1. Delirium may present as hypoactive or hyperactive. Which type of delirium do you think is more likely to be identified by nurses in the clinical setting, and why?
2. Evaluate the medication list of one of your clinical clients with dementia or delirium in relation to the Beers criteria for potentially inappropriate medications for older adults.
3. Given the modest benefits of cholinesterase inhibitors and memantine in the treatment of dementia, debate the pros and cons of administering these medications for persons with dementia.
4. Choose a client in your clinical setting who has dementia. Practice communication strategies.

Personal **Reflections**

1. Have you ever cared for a patient or family member with dementia? How did you feel about this experience? What did you find most frustrating? How did you handle specific symptoms that caused changes in behavior?
2. What risk factors do you personally have for AD? Are there any activities that you can do to decrease your personal risk?
3. This chapter focused on the nurse's role, but what challenges do you think family members face in caring for loved ones with AD?

References

Algase, D. L., Beck, C., Kolanowski, A., Whall, A., Berent, S., Richards, K., et al. (1996). Need-driven dementia-compromised behavior: An alternative view of disruptive behavior. *American Journal of Alzheimer's Disease, 11*(6), 10–19.

Alzheimer's Association. (2008). *Alzheimer's disease.* Retrieved July 27, 2008, from http://www.alz.org/alzheimers_disease_alzheimers_disease.asp

American Association for Geriatric Psychiatry. (2004a). *Geriatrics and mental health: The facts.* Retrieved July 30, 2008, from http://www.aagponline.org/prof/facts_mh.asp

American Association for Geriatric Psychiatry. (2004b). *PET scans for the diagnosis of Alzheimer's disease.* Retrieved July 27, 2008, from http://www.aagpgpa.org/prof/facts_PETscans2004.asp

American Association for Geriatric Psychiatry. (2006). *Position statement: Principles of care for patients with dementia resulting from Alzheimer disease.* Retrieved July 27, 2008, from http://www.aagpgpa.org/prof/position_caredmnalz.asp

American Geriatrics Society, Panel on Persistent Pain in Older Persons. (2002). The management of persistent pain in older persons. *Journal of the American Geriatrics Society, 50*(6 Suppl.), S205–S224. Retrieved July 28, 2008, from http://www.americangeriatrics.org/products/positionpapers/JGS5071.pdf

American Psychiatric Association. (2000). *Diagnostic and statistical manual of mental disorders* (4th ed., text rev.). Washington, DC: Author.

Borson, S., Scanlan, J. M., Brush, M., Vitallano, P., & Dokmak, A. (2000). The Mini-Cog: A cognitive "vital signs" measure for dementia screening in multilingual elderly. *International Journal of Geriatric Psychiatry, 15*(11), 1021–1027.

Butler, R. N. (1963). The life review: An interpretation of reminiscence in the aged. *Psychiatry, 26*, 65–68.

Cohen-Mansfield, J. (1996). Conceptualization of agitation results based on the Cohen-Mansfield Agitation Inventory and the Agitation Behavior Mapping Instrument. *International Psychogeriatrics, 8*(3 Suppl.), 309–315.

Dawson, P., Wells, D. L., & Kline, K. (1993). *Enhancing the abilities of persons with Alzheimer's and related dementias: A nursing perspective.* New York: Springer.

Feil, N. (1993). *The validation breakthrough: Simple techniques for communicating with people with Alzheimer's-type dementia.* Baltimore: Health Professions Press.

Fick, D. M., Cooper, J. W., Wade, W. E., Waller, J. L., Maclean, J. R., & Beers, M. H. (2003). Updating the Beers criteria for potentially inappropriate medication use in older adults. *Archives of Internal Medicine, 163*, 2716–2725.

Finkel, S. I. (1998). The signs of the behavioural and psychological symptoms of dementia. *Clinician, 16*(1), 33–42.

Folstein, M., Folstein, S. E., & McHugh, P. R. (1975). "Mini-Mental State": A practical method for grading the cognitive state of patients for the clinician. *Journal of Psychiatric Research, 12*(3), 189–198.

Foreman, M. D., Wakefield, B., Culp, K., & Milisen, K. (2001). Delirium in elderly patients: An overview of the state of the science. *Journal of Gerontological Nursing, 27*(4), 12–20.

Gitlin, L. N., Liebman, J., & Winter, L. (2003). Are environmental interventions effective in the management of Alzheimer's disease and related disorders?: A synthesis of the evidence. *Alzheimer's Care Quarterly, 4*(2), 85–107.

Hall, G. R. (1994). Caring for people with Alzheimer's disease using the conceptual model of Progressively Lowered Stress Threshold in the clinical setting. *Nursing Clinics of North America, 29*(1), 129–141.

Hall, G. R., & Buckwalter, K. C. (1987). Progressively lowered stress threshold: A conceptual model for the care of adults with Alzheimer's disease. *Archives of Psychiatric Nursing, 1*, 399–406.

Inouye, S., van Dyck, C., Alessi, C., Balkin, S., Siegal, A., & Horwitz, R. (1990). Clarifying confusion: The confusion assessment method. *Annals of Internal Medicine, 113*(12), 941–948.

International Psychogeriatric Association. (2002). *Behavioral and psychological symptoms of dementia (BPSD)*. Retrieved July 27, 2008, from http://www.ipaonline.org/ipaonlinev3/ipaprograms/bpsdarchives/bpsdrev/1BPSDfinal.pdf

Kitwood, T. (1997). *Dementia reconsidered: The person comes first*. Buckingham: Open University Press.

Kolanowski, A., & Buettner, L. (2008). Prescribing activities that engage passive residents: An innovative method. *Journal of Gerontological Nursing, 34*(1), 13–18.

Kolanowski, A. M. (1999). An overview of the need-driven, dementia-compromised behavior model. *Journal of Gerontological Nursing, 25*(9), 7–9.

Lawton, M. P. (1982). Competence, environmental press, and the adaptation of older people. In M. P. Lawton, P. G. Windley, & T. O. Byerts (Eds.), *Aging and the environment: Theoretical approaches* (pp. 33–59). New York: Springer.

National Adult Day Services Association. (n.d.). *Adult day services: The facts*. Retrieved July 31, 2008, from http://www.nadsa.org

National Institute on Aging. (2007). *Alzheimer's disease: Unraveling the mystery*. Retrieved July 27, 2008, from http://www.nia.nih.gov/Alzheimers/Publications/Unravelingthemystery

Neal, M., & Barton Wright, P. (2008). Validation therapy for dementia. [Systematic Review]. *Cochrane Dementia and Cognitive Improvement Group Cochrane Database of Systematic Reviews, 2*.

Netz, Y., Axelrad, S., & Argov, E. (2007). Group physical activity for demented older adults: Feasibility and effectiveness. *Clinical Rehabilitation, 21*(11), 977–986.

Norris, A. D. (1986). *Reminiscence with elderly people*. London: Winslow.

Raina, P., Pasqualina, S., Ismaila, A., Patterson, C., Cowan, D., Levine, M., et al. (2008). Effectiveness of cholinesterase inhibitors and memantine for treating dementia: Evidence review for a clinical practice guideline. *Annals of Internal Medicine, 148*, 379–397.

Reisberg, B., Franssen, E. H., Souren, L. E. M., Auer, S. R., Akram, I., & Kenowsky, S. (2002). Evidence and mechanisms of retrogenesis in Alzheimer's and other dementias. *American Journal of Alzheimer's Disease and Other Dementias, 17*(4), 202–212.

Sheikh, J. I., & Yesavage, J. A. (1986). Geriatric Depression Scale (GDS). Recent evidence and development of a shorter version. In T. L. Brink (Ed.), *Clinical gerontology: A guide to assessment and intervention* (pp. 165–173). New York: Haworth Press.

Smith, M., Buckwalter, K., & Mitchell, S. (1993). Acting up and acting out: Assessment and management of aggressive and acting out behaviors. In M. Smith, K. Buckwalter, & C. M. Mitchell (Eds.), *The geriatric mental health training series*. New York: Springer.

Spector, A., Orrell, M., Davies, S., & Woods, B. (2008). Reality orientation for dementia. [Systematic Review]. *Cochrane Dementia and Cognitive Improvement Group Cochrane Database of Systematic Reviews, 2*.

Talerico, K. A., O'Brien, J. A., & Swafford, K. L. (2003). Person-centered care: An important approach for 21st century health care. *Journal of Psychosocial Nursing and Mental Health Services, 41*(11), 12–16.

Tariq, S. H., Tumosa, N., Chibnall, J. T., Perry, M. H., & Morley, J. E. (2006). Comparison of the Saint Louis University Mental Status Examination and the Mini-Mental State Examination for detecting dementia and mild neurocognitive disorder: A pilot study. *American Journal of Geriatric Psychiatry, 14*, 900–910.

Woods, B., Spector, A., Jones, C., Orrell,, M., & Davies, S. (2008). Reminiscence therapy for dementia. [Systematic Review]. *Cochrane Dementia and Cognitive Improvement Group Cochrane Database of Systematic Reviews, 2*.

Yesavage, J. A., Brink, T. L., Rose, T. L., Lum, O., Huang, V., Adey, M. B., et al. (1983). Development and validation of a geriatric depression screening scale: A preliminary report. *Journal of Psychiatric Research, 17*, 37–49.

SECTION

6

Information and Health Care Technologies

(Competencies 16–17)

CHAPTER 16

Using Assistive Technology to Promote Quality of Life for Older Adults

Linda L. Pierce, PhD, RN, CNS, CRRN, FAHA

Victoria Steiner, PhD

LEARNING OBJECTIVES

At the end of this chapter, the reader will be able to:

- Identify assistive technology and methods for teaching older adults about its use.
- Recognize common applications of assistive technology to enhance older adults' functioning, independence, and safety.
- Describe Internet and Web approaches for assistive technology, including learning activities, health information, and health care services that can be used in caring for older adults and their families, along with teaching strategies for its access.
- Discuss new assistive technologies on the horizon.

KEY TERMS

- Assistive device
- Assistive technology
- Augmentative and alternative communication (AAC)
- Emergency response system (ERS)
- Environmental controls
- Internet
- Nursing informatics
- World Wide Web

This century reflects a time of change for nursing and the way nurses deliver health care to the population over the age of 65 years. Americans are living longer, and this age cohort will increase from about 30 million in the 1990s to more than 70 million by the year 2030 (U.S. Census Bureau, 2004). Most of these individuals expect to have an active life in the community well into their seventh decade. Each decade of life past age 65 often brings with it acute illnesses and chronic conditions accompanied by increased disability (Centers for Disease Control and Prevention [CDC], 2007). Nurses caring for older adults must advocate for and use new ways to provide care to these adults that promotes their quality of life. The purpose of this chapter is to provide information about the integration of nursing care with the latest **assistive technologies** that support the care of older adults, as well as to describe the technologies on the horizon.

INTRODUCTION TO ASSISTIVE TECHNOLOGY

The growing population of older adults will change many aspects of health care. One change will be an increase in the number of people who experience a disabling condition. As individuals age or become disabled, mental and physical changes may influence their ability to live as independently and productively as they would wish. A lessening or loss of strength, balance, visual and auditory acuity, cognitive processing, and/or memory may affect the way they are able to function at home.

Assistive technology devices are mechanical aids that substitute for or enhance the function of some physical or mental ability that is impaired (Kelker, 1997; Spillman, 2004). The term *assistive technology* encompasses a broad range of devices from "low tech" (e.g., pencil grips, splints, paper stabilizers) to "high tech" (e.g., computers, voice synthesizers, Braille readers). These devices include the entire range of supportive tools and equipment, from adapted spoons to wheelchairs and computer systems for environment control.

As a tool for living, the primary purpose of assistive technology is to bridge the gap between an older person's declining capabilities and the unchanging environmental demands of home and community (Gitlin, 1998; Spillman, 2004). The use of **assistive devices** may enable independent performance, increase safety, reduce risk of injury, improve balance and mobility, improve communication, and limit complications of an illness or disability. These devices are not just for those who are disabled or have functional limitations. Assistive devices can also help individuals who are aging and who may benefit from using them to promote safety and reduce the risk of injury. Individuals experiencing age-related changes or functional decline may also benefit from equipment and devices that enable independent performance and prevent disability.

Norburn and colleagues (1995) found that a large number of older adults practice some form of self-care, even in the absence of reported disability. Their study determined the "extent to which self-care coping strategies, defined as modifying the environment, changing behavior, and/or using special equipment and devices, are employed by older adults at all levels of functioning in order to maintain a viable and independent social life without the need for institutional care" (p. S101). More than 75% of the subjects made behavioral changes in their daily routines (e.g., doing things more slowly) during the year before the survey. About 42% of the subjects reported using assistive devices, and almost one-third had modified their built environment.

Assistive Device Use

Living at home can be made easier with the use of assistive devices. The increased independence afforded individuals who use these devices may ultimately result in their being able to remain in their homes for longer periods of time with reduced concerns for safety. Many of these devices are inexpensive and easy to obtain, but the general population's knowledge of them is poor. Consequently, individuals who are aging or disabled may not be living their lives to their fullest potential.

There is no evidence to suggest that older adults use assistive technology and devices less than young adults, but it is not known whether there is greater reluctance among the elderly to use high-technology vs. low technology solutions. A number of research and service programs are currently evaluating the willingness of older adults to use high technology, such as computer-based systems to increase communication, and social integration and smart house arrangements to increase safety and function (Gitlin, Schemm, Landsberg, & Burgh, 1996; Johnson, Davenport, & Mann, 2007; Mann, Belchior, Tomita, & Kemp, 2007; Tomita, Mann, Stanton, Tomita, & Sundar, 2007). A smart home is an environment constructed with various technological applications and devices that are directed by a central control unit to assist the residents in performing daily activities.

Johnson, Davenport, and Mann (2007) gathered input from potential smart home users in an effort to develop more beneficial and usable applications. Many older adults felt that these technologies were for others or that they could use them in the future. Individuals also expressed concern that if they relied on technology to do tasks for them that they would lose abilities, but were willing to use technology for things they were unable to do themselves. Users were most favorable regarding applications that were related to their type of impairment. For example, individuals with mobility impairments liked smart door applications, which allowed them to answer the door and enter the house hands-free. Older adults were also willing to receive assistance from smart technology if it enabled them to remain independent and stay in their home.

The probability of engaging in self-care practices and the type of strategy employed vary with levels of impairment. Older adults with moderate levels of impairment rely more on special equipment and assistive devices, whereas those with slight functional impairments tend to change their behavior (Norburn et al., 1995). "Of importance is the consistent finding that device use has a dual outcome: At the same time that a device promotes independence, it appears to also raise concerns about social stigma, feelings of embarrassment, and issues related to personal identity and self-definition" (Gitlin, 1998, p. 154). There is no stigma involved in the use of developmentally appropriate equipment or tools for children (e.g., jumbo crayons), so why should equipment and device use in older adults be seen as a response to disability (e.g., wide Dr. Grip pens)?

Mann, Hurren, and Tomita (1993) studied assistive device use by interviewing 157 noninstitutionalized older persons in their homes. Study participants were not selected randomly, however, but were individuals who were recently or currently receiving services from a human service agency, hospital, or nursing home. The researchers used the definition of an assistive device provided in the Technology-Related Assistance for Individuals with Disabilities Act of 1988: "Any item, piece of equipment, or product system, whether acquired commercially off the shelf, modified, or customized that is used to increase, maintain, or improve functional capabilities of individuals with disabilities" (U.S. Congress, 1988). They found that subjects owned a mean of 13.7 devices and used 10.8 of the devices. Older persons with multiple impairments that included physical impairments used the greatest number of devices. Subjects also expressed a need for additional equipment and devices.

Another study by Mann, Hurren, and Tomita (1995) examined the need for and current use of assistive devices by home-based older adults with arthritis. Subjects were assigned to a moderate or a severe arthritis group according to the impact of arthritis on their activities. Subjects in the severe arthritis group had more chronic diseases, a higher level of pain, and a lower level of independence in self-care activities than subjects in the moderate group. Both groups reported using a high number of assistive devices (about 10 per person) and expressed the need for additional devices, such as reachers, magnifiers, jar openers, grab bars, and hearing aids. Generally, there was a high rate of satisfaction with the equipment and devices used.

More recently, Kraskowsky and Finlayson (2001) reported usage rates from 47% to 82% of equipment and devices prescribed. Mann, Goodall, Justiss, and Tomita (2002) found that study participants owned a mean of 14.2 assistive devices, used 84.8% of the devices, and were satisfied with 84.2% of the devices they owned. Mann, Llanes, Justiss, and Tomita (2004) looked at the value older individuals themselves place on their equipment and devices by interviewing 1,016 home-based frail older adults in western New York and northern Florida, specifically asking them what they considered their "most important" assistive device and why. Although "importance" is a general construct, it embodies the perception of "usefulness" and impact on ability to do tasks and participate in activities. Not considering the number of users, the top five most important equipment and devices were eyeglasses, canes, wheelchairs, walkers, and telephones. Controlling for the number of people using the device, the top five most important devices were oxygen tanks, dentures, 3-in-1 commodes, computers, and wheelchairs.

Mann, Ottenbacher, Frass, Tomita, and Granger (1999) studied the effectiveness of assistive devices and environmental modifications in maintaining independence and reducing home care costs. Researchers assigned 104 frail older adults recently referred to home health care to either a treatment group or a control group. Individuals in the treatment group received a functional assessment, a home assessment, and any necessary equipment and/or assistive devices and environmental interventions. The control group received usual care services. The frail older adults in the study experienced functional decline over time, but the control group declined significantly more. Costs related to hospitalization and nursing home stays were more than three times higher for the control group. This randomized controlled trial provided strong evidence that appropriate and necessary equipment or devices can slow the rate of functional decline and reduce health-related costs.

Based on the literature, a number of conclusions can be drawn. Although studies have shown varied results, a consistent finding is that older adults are willing to use assistive devices. Studies have also concluded that some individuals, particularly those who are less impaired, might be more likely to modify their behaviors than use equipment or devices for assistance. Unfortunately, the definition of assistive devices varies across studies, as do the characteristics of the individuals studied; for example, Mann and colleagues tended to seek older adult subjects who were impaired or at risk for needing assistive devices. Regardless of the study, however, researchers have stated that older adults are lacking adequate information about assistive technology that could improve quality of life.

Evaluating the Use of Assistive Technology

Use of assistive technology is a type of health behavior among older adults to maintain their independence and enable them to live at home. This type of technology offers the potential of increasing independence and quality of life for older individuals, as well as reducing health-related costs. From the viewpoints of the national health economy and the quality of life of older adults and caregivers, it is important to understand who does not use devices and why they do not.

A study by Mann, Goodall, Justiss, and Tomita (2002) sought to identify those types of equipment and devices with a higher frequency of nonuse and the reasons given by older adults for not using them. Based on the Rehabilitation Engineering Research Center on Aging Consumer Assessments Study, 1,056 subjects reported use or nonuse of assistive devices. Of these subjects, 873 identified reasons for not using or being dissatisfied with certain equipment and devices. These were grouped into categories based on the type of impairment they addressed (hearing, vision, cognition, and musculoskeletal/neuromotor). Study participants owned the largest number of equipment and devices in the musculoskeletal/neuromotor category, such as canes. Equipment and devices in the hearing impairment category were rated lowest by participants in terms of satisfaction. Almost half of all reasons listed for not using certain assistive devices related to perceived lack of need.

The purpose of a study by Tomita, Mann, Frass, and Stanton (2004) was to identify predictors of the use of assistive devices that address physical impairments among cognitively intact, physically frail older adults living at home. Interviewers who visited their homes identified equipment and devices in use. White elders who live alone in the south, are physically disabled, take more medications, and are less depressed tend to use more equipment and devices to address physical impairments than nonwhite elders who are living with someone in the northern United States and who have less severity of physical disability, take fewer medications, and are more depressed. Among all the variables, physical disability was the most significant predictor of use. Consistent with findings from previous studies, income, education, and marital status were not associated with their use. In addition, age and gender were not significant.

Kraskowsky and Finlayson (2001) compared 14 studies of factors influencing use of assistive devices by older adults. They found that use of them decreased over time. The primary reason for nonuse was lack of fit between the device, the person, and the person's environment. They suggested a range of factors to consider when prescribing assistive technology to older adults, including personal (client) factors, the equipment and device's fit with the client's environment, and intervention-related factors. Creating a positive expectation for the use of the equipment and/or device, when it is introduced, can influence the client factor. Knowing what to expect in the client's environment when prescribing an assistive device can influence its fit within the environment. Increasing the frequency and duration of education on the assistive device can positively influence use.

A careful evaluation of older adults is an important step in determining their need for assistive devices and equipment to enhance and maintain independence and quality of life (Kraskowsky & Finlayson, 2001). The evaluation may occur during acute care, inpatient rehabilitation, home care, or outpatient visits (Roelands, Van Oost, Depoorter, & Buysse, 2002) by any interdisciplinary team member (i.e., nurse, physician, therapist, dietitian, or social worker). Typically, an occupational therapist determines whether the equipment is appropriate for older adults and their environment and educates them and their caregivers on use and care of assistive devices. However, all team members have a responsibility for evaluation and follow-up, as needed. Appropriate fit between the person's ability, the demands of the environment, and each piece of equipment or device is essential to successful task performance.

Assistive devices and equipment are typically first introduced in the hospital, outpatient, or home care setting, primarily to enhance independence in self-care. During inpatient rehabilitation, an older adult will receive an average of eight pieces of equipment and/or devices to use in the home for mobility, dressing, seating, bathing, grooming, and feeding. Those living in the community with a functional impairment report having an average of 14 pieces of equipment and/or devices in the home, including those for hearing and vision (Gitlin et al., 1996). With shortened hospital stays and briefer exposure to occupational and physical therapy, the need for efficient and effective instruction in assistive device use becomes that much more important for nurses. Teaching an elderly person to use technology should not be limited to the person alone, but should include caregivers and other family members. Education must be sensitive to any physical, cognitive, psychological, and environmental factors that affect the elderly person. When introducing technology to the elderly and teaching them to use it, there are several guidelines that can be employed (see **Box 16-1**).

COMMON APPLICATIONS OF ASSISTIVE TECHNOLOGY

The following are common applications for assistive technology (Kelker, 1997): 1) position and mobility, 2) environmental access and control, 3) self-care, 4) sensory impairment, 5) social interaction and recreation, and 6) computer-related technology.

Position and Mobility

Older adults may need assistance with their positions for seating so that they can effectively participate in activities and interact with others. Generally, nurses or therapists try to achieve an upright, forward-facing position for the individual by using padding, structured chairs, straps, supports, or restraints to hold the body in a stable and comfortable manner (Kelker, 1997). Examples of equipment used for different types of positioning are walkers, floor sitters, chair inserts, wheelchairs, straps, traps, and standing aids. Conversely, older adults whose physical impairments limit their

BOX 16-1 Guidelines for Introducing Technology and Teaching the Elderly About Its Use

- The use of technology must be perceived as needed and meaningful, and must be linked to the lifestyle of the person.
- Cautions and disbelief in one's capability may be an obstacle in accepting new technology and must be considered when creating the learning environment.
- A generous amount of time as well as repeated short training sessions should be allowed.
- More stress should be placed on the practical application of the device than on its technical features.
- Only selective, central facts should be presented.
- Mnemonics and cues will favorably affect self-efficacy in handling new products.
- Training sessions should be held in the home or natural meeting places of the elderly.
- The instructor should be well known by the elderly or introduced well in advance of the training.
- The attitudes of the instructors toward the aged must be positive and realistic.

Source: Idaho Assistive Technology Project. (1995). *Assistive technology and older adults.* Information Sheet #25. Retrieved January 5, 2009, from http://www.idahoat.org/files/factsheets/25%20OlderPersonsAT.pdf

mobility may need a device to help them get around or participate in activities. Mobility devices include self-propelled walkers, manual or powered wheelchairs, and powered recreational vehicles like bikes and scooters.

Environmental Access and Control

Access to shopping centers, places of business, schools, recreation, and transportation is possible because of assistive technology modifications. This kind of assistive technology includes modifications to buildings, rooms, or other facilities that allow people with physical impairments to use ramps and door openers to enter, allow people with visual disabilities to follow Braille directions and move more freely within a facility, and allow people of short stature or people who use wheelchairs to reach pay phones or operate elevators (Kelker, 1997).

Once inside a building, various types of **environmental controls**, including remote control switches and special adaptations of on/off switches to make them accessible (e.g., Velcro attachments, pointer sticks), can promote independent use of equipment by an older adult. Robotic arms and other environmental control systems turn lights on and off, open doors, and operate appliances. For example, X-10 is an electronic environmental control that allows individuals to control lights, heating, and cooling, as well as just about any electrical piece of equipment, such as curtains, garage doors, and gates. Basic installation is very easy for lamps and plug-in items. The minimum requirements are one control unit and one control module. No wiring is required. First, the control unit is plugged in, then the lamp to be controlled is plugged into a module, and finally the module is plugged into an outlet. There are also several types of modules and switches available to replace existing wall switches (X-10, 2005).

Self-Care

Assistive devices for self-care include such items as robotics, electric feeders, adapted utensils, specially designed toilet seats, and aids for tooth brushing, washing, dressing, and grooming. An **emergency response system (ERS)** can increase the safety of an individual who requires assistance with self-care activities. The most common ERS is the telephone-based personal emergency response system (PERS), which consists of the subscriber wearing a small help button as a necklace or wristband, with a home communicator that is connected to a residential phone line (Mihailidis & Lee, 2007). In the event of an emergency, the subscriber presses the help button and is connected to a live emergency response center, which arranges for appropriate help, such as calling paramedics or the person's family.

Remote health monitoring devices also have been developed that measure and track various physiological parameters, such as pulse, skin temperature, and blood pressure (Mihailidis & Lee, 2007). These systems are less commonly found in the home, but are growing in demand despite their restrictions. They require the user to wear the device at all times and/or to manually take the required measurements and enter the data into the system, which then automatically transmits to an evaluation and emergency service station.

Many of the PERS and physiological-based monitoring systems are inappropriate, obtrusive, and difficult for an older adult to operate. These systems require effort from the person, sometimes long training times in order for the person to learn how to use the required features, and they become ineffective during more serious emergency situations, such as if the person has a stroke (Mihailidis & Lee, 2007). As a result, new systems are being developed that do not require manual interaction from the user and that use nonphysiological measures to determine health parameters.

Studies have shown that a decline in an older adult's ability to complete activities of daily living (ADLs) is a strong indicator of declining health and may increase the likelihood of an emergency situation occurring (Mihailidis & Lee, 2007). Several researchers are developing systems that can monitor ADLs in the home. These systems use simple switches, sensors, and transducers located at various places in the user's environment and attached to various objects to detect which tasks are being completed.

Sensory Impairment

Older adults may experience impairment in their speech, hearing, or sight. From 2 to 2.5 million Americans have communication disorders too severe to permit them to meet their daily communication needs using only natural speech and handwriting (National Institutes of Health [NIH], 2000). The term **augmentative and alternative communication (AAC)** refers to all forms of communication that enhance or supplement speech and writing, either temporarily or permanently. AAC can both enhance (augmentative) and replace (alternative) conventional forms of expression for people who cannot communicate through speech, writing, or gestures. Augmentative and alternative communication devices offer dynamic displays (i.e., electronic displays that change with user input) and synthesized (computer-generated) and digitalized (recorded) speech, and are accessible through many input modalities, including touchscreen, keyboard, and infrared headpointers (Dickerson, Stone, Panchura, & Usiak, 2002). Chapter 5 provides further discussion of AAC.

The goal of AAC is to encourage and support the development of communicative competence so that people can participate as fully as possible in home and community environments, and to improve the efficiency and use of communication aids. Selecting the communication methods that are best for an individual is not as simple as getting a prescription for eyeglasses (American Speech-Language-Hearing Association [ASHA], 2002). Language is complex, and individuals learn to use it every day. Indeed, developing the best communication system for a person with a severe speech and language problem requires evaluation by many specialists (ASHA), all of whom may not have offices in the same building or even in the same city. Communication boards, which use pictures as symbols for words, may need to be made. Vocabulary to meet the needs of a wide range of communication disorder situations must be selected. Equipment may need to be ordered and paid for. Health plans or other third-party payers may need to be contacted.

Once all the parts of the communication plan are in place, the user must learn to operate each part of the system effectively and efficiently. Professionals (e.g., nurses, therapists) need to help the user and his or her communication partners learn a variety of skills and strategies, which might include the meaning of certain hand shapes and how to make them, starting and stopping a piece of electronic equipment at a desired word or picture, ways to get a person's attention, ways to help a communication partner understand a message, and increasing the rate of communication (ASHA, 2002). Without effort by the user, professional help, ongoing practice, and support from friends, family, and colleagues, the promises of augmentative communication may not be realized.

Much of the time, individuals are expected to learn through listening. Hearing impairments can interfere with an older adult's speaking, reading, and ability to follow directions. Assistive devices to help with hearing and auditory processing problems include hearing aids, personal FM units, Phonic Ear, or closed caption TV.

Vision is also a major learning mode. General methods for assisting with vision problems include increasing contrast, enlarging stimuli, and making use of tactile and auditory assistive devices. Devices that assist with vision include screen readers, screen enlargers, magnifiers, large-type books, taped books, Braillers, light boxes, high contrast materials, and scanners.

Social Interaction and Recreation

Older adults still want to have fun and interact socially with others. Assistive technology can help them to participate in all sorts of interactive recreational activities with friends (Kelker, 1997). Some adapted recreational activities include drawing software, computer games, computer simulations, painting with a head or mouth wand, adapted puzzles, or online computer games.

Computer-Based Assistive Technology

Some older adults may require special devices that provide access to computers. Controllable anatomical movements like eye blinks, head or neck movements, or mouth movements may be used to operate equipment that provides access to the computer. Once a controllable anatomical site has been determined, decisions can be made about input devices including switches, alternative keyboards, mouse, trackball, touch window, speech recognition, and head pointers (Kelker, 1997).

Computers are an important type of assistive technology because they open up so many exciting possibilities for writing, speaking, finding information, or controlling an individual's environment. Software can provide the tools for written expression, calculation, reading, basic reasoning, and higher level thinking skills. The computer can also be used to access a wide variety of databases.

Many examples of the assistive devices mentioned earlier can be found on the ABLEDATA Web site (http://www.abledata.com). It is a federally funded project whose primary mission is to provide information on assistive technology, including all types of adaptive equipment and assistive devices, available from domestic and international sources to consumers, organizations, professionals, and caregivers within the United States. The ABLEDATA database contains information on more than 30,000 assistive technology products (over 20,000 of which are currently available), from white canes to voice output programs. The database contains detailed descriptions of each product, including price and company information. The database also contains information on noncommercial prototypes, customized and one-of-a-kind products, and do-it-yourself designs.

THE INTERNET AND THE WORLD WIDE WEB

The **Internet** is not just about data; it is an international community of people who share information, interact, and communicate. From the point of view of its users, the Internet as an assistive technology is a vast collection of resources that includes people, information, and multimedia. The Internet is best characterized as the biggest labyrinth of computer networks on earth (Encarta World English Dictionary, 2007). A computer network is a data communications system made up of hardware and software that transmits data from one computer to another. In part, a computer network includes a physical infrastructure of hardware, like wires, cables, fiber-optic lines, undersea cables, and satellites. The other part of a network is the software to keep it running. Computer networks can connect to other computer networks to produce an even bigger computer network. Thus, the Internet is a set of connected computer networks. In contrast, the **World Wide Web** (WWW or Web) is not a network. The Web is not the Internet itself, nor is it a proprietary system like America Online. Instead, the Web is a system of clients (Web browsers) and servers that use the Internet to exchange data (Encarta World English Dictionary, 2007).

The Internet and the World Wide Web are evolving into an environment for collaboration, content exchange, mentorship, and creative endeavors (see **Box 16-2**). This virtual environment is becoming an accessible place for the building of intellectual assets, where knowledge can be effectively identified, distributed, and shared. Nursing professionals are joining this growing evolution in a number of different ways. Many nurses work hard to shape at least some of the Internet and World Wide Web into a milieu for active participation that serves to inform, educate, and advocate for older adults. Some nurses may specialize in nursing informatics.

Nursing Informatics

Nursing informatics is a 21st-century science with great potential for improving the quality,

BOX 16-2 Common Applications of Assistive Technology: Resource List

AARP: http://www.aarp.org

Adaptive and Assistive Technology: http://www.rehabtool.com

BrainBashers Games and Puzzles: http://brainbashers.com

CataList, the official catalog of LISTSERV lists: http://www.lsoft.com/lists/listref.html

ElderWeb: http://www.elderweb.com/home/

Free Greeting Cards: http://www.123greetings.com

Healthfinder: http://www.healthfinder.gov

Learn the Net: http://www.learnthenet.com/english/index.html

National Library of Medicine: http://www.nlm.nih.gov

SeniorNet: http://www.seniornet.org

safety, and efficiency of health care. About 20 years ago, Kathryn Hannah proposed a simple definition for nursing informatics. She said that nursing informatics encompasses the use of information technologies in relation to any functions that are within the sphere of nursing and that are carried out by nurses in the performance of their practice (Ball & Hannah, 1988).

Graves and Corcoran (1989) presented a more complex definition of nursing informatics. They argued that "nursing informatics is a combination of computer science, information science and nursing science, designed to assist in the management and processing of nursing data, information and knowledge to support the practice of nursing and the delivery of nursing care" (p. 227). The American Nurses Association (ANA) modified the Graves and Corcoran definition when it developed the *Scope and Practice for Nursing Informatics* and distinguished between practice and theory (ANA, 1994) (see **Box 16-3**). The ANA more recently defined nursing informatics as "a specialty that integrates nursing science, computer science, and information science to manage and communicate data, information, and knowledge in nursing practice . . . to support patients, nurses, and other providers in their decision-making . . . using information structures, information processes and information technology" (2001, p. 46).

The *Scope and Standards of Nursing Informatics Practice* (now known as *Nursing Informatics: Scope and Standards of Practice*) is a professional guideline and an essential reference for nurses that emphasizes competencies and functional areas (ANA, 2001, 2008). It articulates the essentials of nursing informatics, including the who, what, when, where, and how of its practice for both specialists and generalists. This booklet, revised by the American Nursing Informatics Association (http://www.ania.org) in 2008, builds upon historical knowledge and includes new, state-of-the-science material for the specialty. Although nursing informatics is a growing area of

BOX 16-3 Recommended Readings

American Nurses Association. (2001). *The scope and standards of nursing informatics practice*. Washington, DC: American Nurses Publishing.

American Nurses Association. (2008). *Nursing informatics: Scope and standards of practice*. Washington, DC: American Nurses Publishing.

Burdick, D. C., & Kwon, S. (Eds.). (2004). *Gerotechnology: Research and practice in technology and aging: A textbook and reference for multiple disciplines*. New York: Springer.

Charness, N., & Schaie, K. W. (Eds.). (2003). *Impact of technology on successful aging*. New York: Springer.

Hart, T. (2004). Evaluation of Websites for older adults: How "senior-friendly" are they? *Usability News, 6*(1). Retrieved September 20, 2007, from http://psychology.wichita.edu/surl/usability_news.html

Miller, J. (2006). *The savvy senior: Computers made simple and easy: Step by step*. New York: Golden Savvy Communications.

Nicoll, L. (2001). *Nurses' guide to the Internet*. Philadelphia: Lippincott Williams & Wilkins.

Richmond, C. (2006). *Computers for klutzes: Basics, email, and Internet: A familiarization course for older adults*. Bloomington, IN: AuthorHouse.

Thede, L. (2003). *Informatics and nursing: Opportunities and challenges*. Philadelphia: Lippincott Williams & Wilkins.

specialization, all nurses can employ basic information technology in their practice.

Using the Web

The Pew Internet and American Life Project (2006) found that in January 2006, 34% of Americans age 65 or older go online, up from 29% in January 2005. In the year 2000, about 60% of older adult Web users were men and about 40% were women (Pew Internet and American Life Project, 2004). The gender ratio among these users has now shifted to 50% men and 50% women (Pew Internet and American Life Project, 2005). Computer ownership also has increased among older adults; 40% of these adults currently report having a personal computer at home, compared to 29% in 1995. Additionally, 1 in 10 older adults without access to the Internet from home or from work say that they sometimes access the Internet from another place such as a friend's, neighbor's, or relative's home or the public library (Center for Medicare Education, 2002). Approximately one-third of the users logged on several times a day (Pew Internet and American Life Project, 2005). Older adults spend more than 8 hours online each week, using Web-based materials or electronic documents in various formats and media (**Figure 16–1**).

Researchers have found that Web use by older adults enhances self-esteem and increases a sense of productivity and accomplishment (Purnell & Sullivan-Schroyer, 1997) as well as increasing their social interaction (Kautzmann, 1990; Post, 1996). Web use also meets older adults' needs for personal control (McConatha, McConatha, & Dermigny, 1994), mental stimulation, and fun (Weisman, 1983). They are passive and active participants who primarily use e-mail, send pictures, and search for health care information (Interest Survey, 2004). And once the baby boomer generation, most of whom are already computer-literate, becomes the Medicare generation, older adult Web use will soar. Therefore, gearing access to and design of Web sites toward this older population becomes an important task.

FIGURE **16-1** **Older adults obtain many benefits from computer use including social interactions, mental stimulation, and exploring health information.**

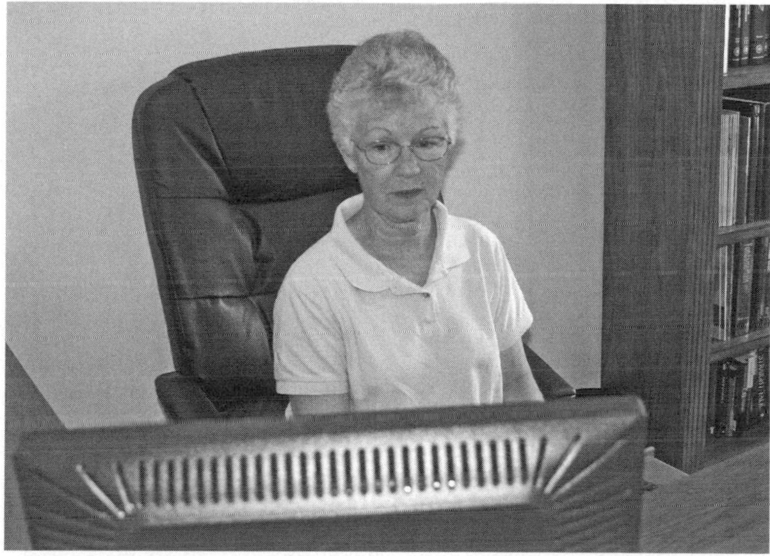

Web Site Design

Designers for Web sites sometimes fail to recognize older adults as a potential user group for their technology. Industry has only recently begun adapting access to hardware and designing software that make accommodations for the needs of older adults. This age group has specific abilities and performance attributes that need to be addressed to coincide with several life changes. Functional limitations related to visual, hearing, and mobility changes are common among older adults as a result of bodily changes secondary to the aging process. These changes may deter their ability to use the Web. After age 65, a large proportion of this population begins to demonstrate significant visual acuity deficits. In addition, beyond age 65, one in four older adults is affected by hearing loss and some of them may develop essential benign tremor that may impair their fine motor skills (Reuben et al., 2004). Increasing font size to at least 18 points or using computer magnification screens compensates for decreased visual acuity, using the Tab key or a touch screen attached to a monitor eliminates the necessity to have fine motor skills to move the cursor, and using external speakers or headphones for increased amplification can compensate for sensory and mobility impairments.

In general, older adults are slower in using the computer (Czaja & Sharit, 1998), travel to fewer Web pages (Liao, Groff, Chaparro, Chaparro, & Stumpfhauser, 2000), and spend more time selecting targets for tasks than younger users (Chaparro, Bohan, Fernandez, Choi, & Kattel, 1999). Many groups and researchers have developed comprehensive sets of guidelines to improve Web design, and thus accessibility for older adults (e.g., Web Content Accessibility Guidelines and Web Accessibility Initiative from the World Wide Web Consortium [W3C, 2004] and the government-instituted U.S. Section 508 Guidelines [GSA, 2002] (**Case Study 16-1**)). The National Institute on Aging (NIA) and the National Library of Medicine (NLM) advanced the preceding guidelines one step further by developing specifications that are even more geared to the older adult Web user. They published *Making Your Web Site Senior Friendly: A Checklist,* consisting of 25 empirically based guidelines for Web sites targeting these users (NIA & NLM, 2002). Research in aging, cognition, human factors, and print materials led to the development of these guidelines that cover three areas of design: 1) designing readable text, 2) increasing memory and

Case Study 16-1

Roscoe Brown is a 73-year-old man who recently had a stroke that resulted in left hemiparesis. He was admitted to an acute care hospital where he was diagnosed with a right middle cerebral artery thrombosis. After a course of medication, the thrombosis dissolved and Mr. Brown demonstrated neurological gains. He has been transferred to the rehabilitation unit and has been assigned to your team. He can walk 50 feet with some assistance, his speech is slow and his words are slurred, but his short-term memory is intact. He owns his home and has $75,000 in a savings account that he is saving for a "rainy day." Just prior to his stroke, your team learned that Mr. Brown was the primary caregiver for his wife, Verna, who has senile dementia. The Browns have no children. Mr. Brown expressed a desire to get home as soon as possible so that he can once again care for his wife.

Assuming that Mr. Brown is able to be discharged home and care for his wife:

1. What Web sites would you use to help in identifying community resources for Mr. and Mrs. Brown?
2. Discuss the community resources suggested to Mr. Brown.
3. What Web sites might be helpful for Mr. Brown in terms of education and social support for a) stroke and b) dementia?
4. What assistive devices might you suggest for Mr. Brown? Where did you find information about this equipment and/or devices, and, if appropriate, how would you teach Mr. Brown about their use?

Assuming Mr. Brown is unable to return home and care for his wife:

1. Discuss home care and/or placement options for both Mr. and Mrs. Brown, including Web-based information about these options.

comprehension of Web content, and 3) increasing the ease of navigation. These guidelines for Web site design may result in greater accessibility to Web-based information for older adults, leading to a future willingness to explore the Web and increased enthusiasm toward technology (see **Box 16-4**).

BOX 16-4 The Internet and the World Wide Web "Senior-Friendly" Guidelines for Web Page Construction Recommended by the National Institute on Aging

1. *Phrasing:* Use the active voice.
2. *Scrolling:* Avoid automatically scrolling text and provide a scrolling icon.
3. *Mouse:* Use single clicks to access information.
4. *Lettering:* Use upper- and lowercase for body text and reserve all capitals for headlines.
5. *Justification:* Use left-justified text.
6. *Style:* Use positive phrasing and present information in a clear manner without need for inferences.
7. *Menus:* Use pull-down and cascading menus sparingly.
8. *Simplicity:* Use simple language for text; provide a glossary for technical terms.
9. *Typeface:* Use a san serif typeface that is not condensed.
10. *Color:* Avoid using yellow, blue, and green in proximity to each other.
11. *Backgrounds:* Use light text on dark backgrounds or vice versa; avoid patterns.
12. *Consistent layout:* Use a standard page design, and provide the same navigation on each page.
13. *Organization:* Use a standard format; break lengthy documents into short sections.
14. *Navigation:* Use explicit step-by-step navigation procedures; simple and straightforward.
15. *Help and information:* Offer a tutorial on the Web site or offer contact information.
16. *Icons and buttons:* Use large buttons; incorporate text with an icon when possible.
17. *Text alternatives:* Provide text alternatives for all other media types.
18. *Illustrations and photos:* Use text-relevant images only.
19. *Type weight:* Use medium or boldface type.
20. *Type size:* Use 12- or 14-point type for body text.
21. *Site maps:* Use a site map to show how the site is organized.
22. *Hyperlinks:* Use icons with text as hyperlinks.
23. *Animation, video, and audio:* Use short segments to reduce download time.
24. *Backward/forward navigation:* Use buttons such as "previous" and "next" for reviewing text.
25. *Physical spacing:* Use double spacing in body text.

Source: National Institute on Aging & National Library of Medicine. (2002). *Making your Web site senior friendly.* Retrieved September 18, 2007, from http://www.nlm.nih.gov/pubs/checklist.pdf

Teaching about Accessing Web Sites

To begin teaching older adults how to access Web sites, the nurse needs to be knowledgeable about the capacity of the learner. The older adult must: 1) be oriented; 2) have an attention span and be capable of short-term memory; 3) not be agitated, combative, or destructive; and 4) be able to respond to one-step commands and make choices. For those individuals with severe motor disability, they must be able to raise an eyebrow, puff with the mouth, tap with a finger or foot, or talk to make selections. Adaptive or assistive devices can be used to expedite the learning process. In 1991, McNeely (1991) identified eight factors affecting teaching-learning outcomes for Web-based instruction and older adults that are useful. Each factor is described and expanded upon in the following list:

1. The rate of presentation of information needs to be individualized. Older adults need training that is self-paced and includes ways to ask questions. Enough time needs to be given to perform the task.
2. All new information needs to be presented in a highly organized manner. Initially, the task and end goals need to be introduced. Then, parts should be identified and each related to the preceding step(s) and to the whole. Visual displays should be simple and demonstrate only important information. Relevant information is presented and social chatter is avoided to help prevent the older adult from getting distracted.
3. Older adults need to feel that they can practice as much as they like without slowing the pace of the instruction. Thus, older and younger adults need separate training sessions. This will also prevent a situation in which older adults would hesitate to ask questions around younger people for fear of embarrassment.
4. There needs to be an opportunity for practice because it not only improves learning and mastery, but also has a direct influence on older adults' attitude. Unlimited trials need to be given. Cognitive support through use of software is important, because it offers nonthreatening and repetitive tutoring that does not judge a person's mistakes.
5. Web use that is interesting and personally meaningful to the older adult has been related to a positive attitude change. Older adults should dictate what they need and want from the Web. People perform best when the task is relevant to their lives.
6. Teaching older adults about Web usage needs to be done in a comfortable environment. A calm, patient, unhurried, sensitive, interested, and knowledgeable instructor can decrease situational stress and promote a climate of acceptance and reassurance.
7. Step-by-step graphic instructions or even video demonstration rather than relying on manuals provided by vendors are helpful in teaching older adults. Use concrete language as often as possible, because it is absorbed more readily and efficiently than abstract information. Printing a hard copy of their work is beneficial. Seeing work in print may increase enthusiasm and a sense of productivity and provide stimulus for further participation.
8. Supportive verbal feedback may improve the older adult's performance. This should be done right after an activity. Interactive feedback via Web-based instruction may stimulate learning (McNeely, 1991).

Learning Activities

Many adults participate in Web-based learning activities that lead to increased interaction and shared learning. They use the Web to create their own letters and use e-mail, greeting cards, and posters in addition to playing word and board games and participating in music and art activities. In fact, Malcolm and associates (2001) found that most physically frail older adults primarily used e-mail, and that they also played games. E-mail letters provide an opportunity to reconnect with old friends and distant family. E-mail also can be used to resolve a billing question with a cable company, find out about services at a local volunteer organization, track down old classmates, or request information from a national organization. And it would be impossible to overstate the satisfaction older adults can feel when they are called "the coolest grandparent in the world" because they have sent an e-mail or e-greeting card or poster to a grandchild.

Online games and activities can be a fun way to engage the older person's mind when no one else is around. For example, Garfield (http://www.garfield.com) is an interactive Web site that can be used by all ages to play games, create electronic cards, or build their own comic strip. Jigzone (http://www.jigzone.com) is a jigsaw puzzle site containing hundreds of picture puzzle shapes with a controlled level of difficulty. There are also several joke Web sites (see **Box 16-5**) that are fun and easy to use. At the Web site http://www.fiftiesweb.com, older adults can find the words to some of those common songs that they knew as young adults. The Web fulfills older adults' needs for fun and mental stimulation.

Health Information

The emphasis on early discharge and the movement of care from inpatient settings to the home mandates the development of electronic information systems to augment and extend services. The use of information searching on the Web is a promising tool for older adults. Information provided on the Web can help to inform and educate about acute illnesses, chronic conditions, and health promotion as well as resource availability. The following are just some of the resources available:

- As previously mentioned, the ABLEDATA Web site can be used to locate companies that sell particular assistive devices.
- The National Institutes of Health and the U.S. National Library of Medicine currently maintain several Web sites designed to provide accurate health information to consumers. MEDLINEplus (http://medlineplus.gov) has sections in English and Spanish on health topics, medications, physicians, and medical terminology that are easy to use and understand. Information on this site can be accessed through alphabetical menus and through buttons and the search window. There is also a site from the National Institutes of Health (http://nihseniorhealth.gov) just for older adults that contains information on age-related health topics, remedies, and help for caregivers.
- The Department of Health and Human Services (http://www.dhhs.gov) is a comprehensive source on health information, diseases, and aging, and contains a resource locator.
- A nationwide locator service, Eldercare Locator (http://www.eldercare.gov/Eldercare/Public/Home.asp), helps people find local services that are provided to older adults. Users simply enter their state and ZIP code, and the Eldercare Locator will link to information, referral services, and their state and area agencies on aging.

These programs all help consumers identify appropriate services in the area where they reside.

> **BOX 16-5 Web Exploration**
>
> Visit these Web sites to find some humor for the day:
>
> - http://www.comedycentral.com/jokes/index.jhtml
> - http://www.joke-of-the-day.com
> - http://www.cleanjokes4u.com
> - http://www.jokesclean.com
>
> Check out this interesting 2008 report about technology and aging from the Center for Aging Services Technologies:
>
> http://www.agingtech.org/documents/bscf_state_technoloy_summary.pdf

Health Care Services

Beyond information searches, the Internet has other applications. For many years, traditional face-to-face support groups facilitated by nurses and other professionals have been used extensively with positive outcomes for persons and their family members dealing with chronic diseases and long-term illnesses (Broadhead & Kaplan, 1991) (see **Box 16-6**). Web-based support groups managed by professional providers, including nurses, are gaining credibility, as positive outcomes are obtained (Larkin, 2000). Emotional and social support are gained by the participants in these Internet-based groups, in addition to information about best treatments, doctors, medical centers, and more (Veggeberg, 1996). According to White and Dorman (2000) and Northhouse and Peters-Golden (1993), members of Internet support groups share experiences and opinions that often

BOX 16-6 Research Highlight

Aim: This descriptive study examined problems and successes that a sample of 73 adult caregivers new to the role expressed in the first year of caring for stroke survivors. Data were collected from May 2002 to December 2005.

Method: Bi-monthly, trained telephone interviewers asked the participants open-ended questions to elicit their experience in caregiving. Guided by Friedemann's framework of systemic organization, the data were analyzed, using Colaizzi's method of content analysis.

Results: There were 2,455 problems and 2,687 successes reported. Three themes emerged from the problems: being frustrated in day-to-day situations (*system maintenance* in Friedemann's terms), feeling inadequate and turning to others for help (*coherence*), and struggling and looking for "normal" in caring (*system maintenance* versus *change*). Three themes were attributed to the successes: making it through and striving for independence (*system maintenance*), doing things together and seeing accomplishments in the other (*coherence*), and reaching a new sense of normal and finding balance in life (*individuation* and *system maintenance*).

Application to practice: These findings provided an in-depth, theory-based description of the experience of being a new caregiver and helped increase understanding of how caring can be a difficult yet rewarding experience. Knowledge of the changes over time allows health care professionals to tailor their interventions, understanding, and support. Nurses should be aware that caregivers of stroke survivors may experience common frustrations and challenges in the caring role and that the successes reported in this study may be enhanced by nursing interventions to promote positive family adjustment to the poststroke experience.

Source: Pierce, L., Steiner, V., Govoni, A., Thompson, T., & Friedemann, M. (2007). Two sides to the caregiving story. *Topics in Stroke Rehabilitation, 14*(2), 13–20.

include helping persons cope with body changes or providing encouragement to other group members, such as helping persons work through health care problems. For instance, international, national, and local organizations and medical centers offer group discussion. The Wellness Community (TWC) is a nonprofit organization dedicated to providing support to individuals dealing with cancer (Wellness Community, 2007). In 2002, in collaboration with the University of California at San Francisco and Stanford University, TWC established an online support group at http://www.thewellnesscommunity.org for those individuals. Researchers at the University of Toledo in Ohio tested Caring~Web, a restricted Web site geared toward providing education and support services for caregivers of persons with stroke (see **Box 16-7**).

Some other Web sites are interactive and include monitoring devices that enable the person to send temperature, blood pressure, glucose levels, and other health data to health care providers electronically. Televisual Web sites allow health care providers to conduct virtual house calls with older adults (Spry Foundation, 2005). For example, Brennan and associates (2001) demonstrated the effectiveness of computer-mediated information and support services for patients recovering from coronary artery bypass graft surgery, and McKay, Glasgow, Feil, Boles, and Barrera (2002) suggested that Web-based information and support interventions exert a positive impact on health-promoting behaviors of patients with type 2 diabetes.

BOX 16-7 Research Highlight

Aim: The primary aim was to test the feasibility of providing Caring~Web, a Web-based education and support intervention, to caregivers living in rural settings, including caregivers' satisfaction with the intervention. A secondary aim was to examine their experience of caring.

Introduction: After initial hospitalization and stroke rehabilitation, 80% of persons with stroke return to the community, relying on their family members' emotional, informational, and instrumental support for daily living.

Methods: Nine adult caregivers of persons with stroke were enrolled during 2002–2003 in this descriptive study. They were chosen from rehabilitation centers in northwestern Ohio and southeastern Michigan. Participants were given access to the Caring~Web site from their home via MSN/WebTV or a computer for 3 months. Each participant completed a bi-monthly telephone survey regarding use of Caring~Web and the experience of caring, guided by Friedemann's framework of systemic organization. Data were collected from the interviews and the e-mail communications. Caring~Web provides education and support through: 1) an opportunity to ask a nurse specialist any questions, 2) a nonstructured e-mail discussion for caregivers, 3) Web sites about stroke, and 4) customized educational information. Procedures were tested for use in a larger study and data were collected on the use of the intervention and the experience of caring.

Results: All participants agreed they were adequately trained and satisfied, in general, with Caring~Web. Seventy-eight percent of participants used the intervention 1–2 hours/week. Procedures were found valid for use in a larger study. Using Friedemann's framework, a coding system was developed for the qualitative e-mail data on the experience of caring. Five main themes emerged: changing roles and solving problems (system change and maintenance in Friedemann's terms), seeing others' success or failure as own (individuation), pulling together (coherence), being spiritual (spirituality), and balancing successes/problems (congruence).

Application to practice: These findings helped expand knowledge about caregivers of persons with stroke and laid the groundwork for a larger, comprehensive examination of outcomes from Caring~Web and further exploration of the experience of caring. The Caring~Web intervention and those like it may help caregivers understand the myriad of educational information available and have the potential to offer emotional and social support to persons affected by stroke. Nurses should be alert to the possibility of Web-based support for patients in their geographic location, particularly for those who live in rural communities who may be isolated from more traditional educational and support activities.

Source: Pierce, L., Steiner, V., Govoni, A., Hicks, B., Thompson, T., & Friedemann, M. (2004). Caring~Web: Internet-based support for rural caregivers of persons with stroke shows promise. *Rehabilitation Nursing, 29*(3), 95–99, 103.

TECHNOLOGIES ON THE HORIZON

A number of organizations are testing computer-based technologies that have the potential to provide help for people dealing with chronic illness and disability. The practical application of these technologies may be especially important for older adults and their caregivers living in community settings.

Robotic Assistance

Two factors suggest that now is the time to establish mobile robots in the home-care arena. First, technology is available to develop robots that exhibit the necessary power, reliability, and level of competence. Second, now more than ever, there is a need for cost-effective solutions to maintain older adults in home settings. Researchers from the University of Pittsburgh, University of Michigan, and Carnegie Mellon University (2005) are collaborating to produce a personal robotic assistant for older adults, called Nursebot. The goal of this project is to develop mobile personal service robots that assist older adults suffering from chronic disorders in their everyday life. An autonomous mobile robot "lives" in the private home of a chronically ill person. The robot provides a research platform on which to test out a range of ideas for assisting these adults, such as:

- *Intelligent reminding:* Many older adults have to give up independent living because of memory loss. They forget to visit the restroom, to take medicine, to drink, or to see the doctor. One project explores the effectiveness of a robotic reminder, which follows people around, so they cannot become lost.
- *Tele-presence:* Professional caregivers can use the robot to establish a "tele-presence" and interact directly with remote care recipients. This makes many doctor visits unnecessary.
- *Data collection and surveillance:* Robots can be used for a wide range of emergency conditions that can be avoided with systematic data collection (e.g., certain types of heart failures).
- *Mobile manipulation:* A semi-intelligent mobile manipulator integrates robotic strength with a person's senses and intellect. This mobile manipulation can overcome barriers in handling objects (e.g., refrigerator, laundry, and microwave) that currently force older adults to move into assisted-living facilities. This technology could be used for any person dealing with function problems, such as arthritis, as the main reason for giving up independent living.
- *Social interaction deprivation:* This affects a huge number of elderly people who are forced to live alone. This project seeks to explore whether robots can take over certain social functions for these older adults (University of Pittsburgh et al., 2005).

Testing is under way at a retirement community with a Nursebot named Pearl. If this project is successful, it could change the way health care is delivered to an ever-growing contingent of older adults, while significantly advancing the state of the art for mobile service robotics and human–robot interaction (Jajeh, 2005; University of Pittsburgh et al., 2005).

Sensor-Based Monitoring

The Medical Automation Research Center (MARC), at the University of Virginia, has developed and is testing technological solutions for in-home distance monitoring of the functional abilities of older adults. The goal of this system is to enable older adults with disabilities to remain in their own homes for as long as possible. The system is composed of unobtrusive and low-cost sensors (no cameras or microphones) that detect movement and pressure. There is a data logging and communications module, in addition to an integrated data management system, linked to the Internet. Using the appropriate data analysis tools, important observations about activities of daily living can be made from the data generated by the monitored person. These observations may yield early indicators of the onset of a disease or a sudden change of activity (or inactivity) that can indicate an accident. Although the system is not meant as an emergency prompt system, the caregiver may receive alerts over the Internet or urgent notifications over the phone in case of such sudden accident-indicating changes. Additionally, there is a potential for information about sickness or accidents to be transmitted immediately to a service provider (MARC, 2005).

In a 4-month pilot project, MARC's health status monitoring system was evaluated in regard to the functional independence and quality of life of 13 older adult caregivers in a home care setting (Alwan et al., 2007). Strain and burden of the informal caregivers and workloads of 16 professional caregivers were also examined. As expected there was no change in their pre- and postmonitoring functional independence assessment scores, due to the short period of the project. Results showed that there was an increase in quality of life of these monitored older adults that could be attributed to improved quality of care and/or to increased sense of security, due to the use of the monitoring technology. For these monitored adults, their caregivers had reduced levels of strain, but there was no change in their level of burden. The professional caregivers experienced no change in their workload assessment score after monitoring, indicating that the technology did not add to their workloads. Based on these results, the researchers suggested further testing with larger sample sizes and over longer periods of time (Alwan et al., 2007).

Notable Quotes

"Imagine homes of the future as places equipped with a variety of technological devices that work together to support their older occupants. Such homes would feature health and wellness technologies that allow caregivers and health care providers to monitor the occupants' ability to carry out activities of daily living. These technologies would also facilitate the collection of important health information that could help older people take proactive steps to maintain their own health and control their care; give informal caregivers an objective assessment of an older relative's ability to live independently; help professional caregivers coordinate, dispatch and track the delivery of needed care and services; and allow health care providers to identify early onset of disease, prescribe appropriate interventions and monitor the efficacy of those interventions."

—Marj Alwan, PhD, and Jeremy Noble, MD, MPH, in a 2008 report for the Center for Aging Services Technologies (p. 2)

Intel's Assistance Program

The Alzheimer's Association and Intel Corporation have formed a consortium to spur development of technologies for the home to help support the care of older adults. This group grew out of several separate and ongoing efforts. In 2001, the Alzheimer's Association convened a group of caregivers as well as experts from diverse disciplines including bioengineering, robotics, artificial intelligence, communications, systems design, software engineering, medicine, nursing, biology, economics, finance, and business. Around the same time, Intel funded and conducted research on the ways in which computing and communications technologies could support the daily health and wellness needs of people of all ages in their homes and everyday lives. An example of Intel's technology is a wireless "sensor network" made up of thousands of small sensing devices that could someday be embedded throughout the home to monitor important behavioral tendencies, such as sleep and eating patterns. It could also send prompts to a person, such as reminders to take medication (Assisted Living, 2003).

Continuing this work, the Alzheimer's Association and Intel Corporation in partnership with Agilent Technologies worked with university professors at Florida Tech to develop a portable caregiver support system called PocketBuddy (Rhine, 2005). This system would issue audio and text messages to caregivers that could include medication information, appointment reminders, and automated checklists for daily support. Imbedded information could contain the location of important documents and emergency contact names. The creators project that family and friends might access information about the person with Alzheimer's disease and their caregivers via a Web log, a "Buddy Blog," linked to a PocketPC. This technology could bridge time and space barriers that separate these individuals. A study is under way to test and validate the use and acceptance of this technology (Rhine, 2005).

Another example is the COACH (Cognitive Orthosis for Activities in the Home) prototype of an intelligent supportive environment (Mihailidis, 2007). The COACH is being developed by the Alzheimer's Disease Association of Canada and Intel Corporation, in collaboration with researchers at the University of Toronto and several other universities, to assist people with dementia to complete activities of daily living with less dependence on a caregiver. The COACH represents one of the first clinically tested supportive devices to use artificial intelligence techniques. Using a personal (desktop) computer and a single video camera to unobtrusively track a user during an ADL, this device provides prerecorded (visual or video) prompts when necessary (Mihailidis, 2007). In pilot studies, two successive prototypes of the COACH system have been trialed with subjects who had moderate to severe dementia based around the ADL of handwashing (Mihailidis, Barbenel, & Fernie, 2004; Mihailidis, Boger, Canido, & Hoey, 2007). These trials showed that the number of steps in handwashing that the subjects were able to complete without assistance from the caregiver increased noticeably when the device was present (Mihailidis et al., 2004; Mihailidis et al., 2007). Planned future studies will examine, for example, 1) a new color tracking system that is able to track the position of both hands of the person with dementia, the position of task objects (e.g., soap and towel), and the interaction between them; and 2) a new system that implements algorithms, which allow for good decision making under conditions of uncertainty (Mihailidis, 2007).

SUMMARY

Today's technologies provide many opportunities for older adults to maintain their independence and stay connected to the world even when functional limitations are present. Nurses should be aware of the latest trends in technology, the use of computers among the older adult population, and how assistive devices help promote autonomy for this cohort. In addition, nurses can use the strategies suggested in this chapter to enhance learning and teaching with older adults by incorporating technology into the care of both well and ill elderly.

Critical Thinking Exercises

1. If someone stopped you on the street and demanded to know your definition of the Internet and World Wide Web, what would you say? Define the Internet in your own words. How is the Web different from the Internet? Discuss your findings with another student nurse in one of your clinical groups.
2. Explore the Web sites of the American Stroke Association (http://www.americanstroke.org) and the National Stroke Association (http://www.stroke.org). What are differences and similarities between these Web sites? Discuss your findings with another student nurse in one of your clinical groups.
3. Discuss with students in your clinical group at least two factors affecting teaching–learning outcomes for Web-based instruction and older adults.
4. Describe an assistive device to students in your clinical group, and tell how you would teach the patient and/or caregiver about its use when discharging a patient to a home setting.
5. How can information be located about the assistive technology and assistive devices currently available for consumers' use?

Personal Reflections

1. Do you know an older adult who is a novice computer user? Interview this person: Ask how his or her life has changed (what is better and/or worse) since becoming a user. Think about how these changes may affect his or her quality of life.
2. How do you feel about older adults becoming part of the technology revolution? Do you feel that they are using the computer and World Wide Web more often? Do you know any older adults who use iPods, iPhones, mp3 players, PDAs, Flash drives, or other gadgets used by the younger population today? How is their use the same as or different from your generation?

References

Alwan, M., Kell, S., Dalal, S., Turner, B., Mack, D., Wolfe, M., et al. (2007). *Impact of passive in-home health status monitoring on older adults, informal caregivers, and professional caregivers in home care settings*. Retrieved September 20, 2007, from http://www.agingtech.org

American Nurses Association. (1994). *The scope and practice for nursing informatics*. Washington, DC: American Nurses Publishing.

American Nurses Association. (2001). *Scope and standards of nursing informatics practice*. Washington, DC: Author.

American Nurses Association. (2008). *Nursing informatics: Scope and standards of practice*. Washington, DC: American Nurses Publishing.

American Speech-Language-Hearing Association. (2002). *Augmentative and alternative communication: Knowledge and skills for service delivery*. Retrieved October 11, 2007, from http://www.asha.org/policy

Assisted Living. (2003). *The Alzheimer's Association, Intel team up to expand home care technology research*. Retrieved September 20, 2007, from http://www.alsuccess.com/hotnews/37h25103519.html

Ball, M., & Hannah, K. (1988). What is informatics and what does it mean to nursing? In M. Ball, K. Hannah, U. Gerdin Jelger, & H. Peterson (Eds.), *Nursing informatics: Where caring and technology meet* (pp. 81–87). New York: Springer Verlag.

Brennan, P. F., Moore, S. M., Bjornsdottir, G., Jones, J., Visovsky, C., & Rogers, M. (2001). HeartCare: An Internet-based information and support system for patient home recovery after coronary artery bypass graft (CABG) surgery. *Journal of Advanced Nursing, 35*(5), 699–708.

Broadhead, W., & Kaplan, W. (1991). Social support and the cancer patient: Implications for future research and clinical care. *Cancer, 67*(3), 794–799.

Center for Medicare Education. (2002). *Creating senior-friendly Web sites*. Retrieved September 20, 2007, from http://www.futureofaging.org/PublicationFiles/V1N4.pdf

Centers for Disease Control and Prevention. (2007). *Health-related quality of life*. Retrieved September 20, 2007, from http://www.cdc.gov

Chaparro, A., Bohan, M., Fernandez, J., Choi, S., & Kattel, B. (1999). The impact of age on computer input device use: Psychophysical and physiological measures. *International Journal of Industrial Ergonomics, 24*, 503–513.

Czaja, S., & Sharit, J. (1998). Age differences in attitudes toward computers. *Journal of Gerontology, 53B*(5), 329–340.

Dickerson, S. S., Stone, V. I., Panchura, C., & Usiak, D. J. (2002). The meaning of communication: Experiences with augmentative communication devices. *Rehabilitation Nursing, 27*(6), 215–221.

Encarta World English Dictionary. (2007). *Assistive technology*. Retrieved September 19, 2007, from http://encarta.msn.com/encnet/features/dictionary/

General Service Administration. (2002). *U.S. section 508 guidelines*. Retrieved September 20, 2007, from http://www.section508.gov

Gitlin, L. (1998). The role of social science research in understanding technology use among older adults. In M. G. Ory & G. H. DeFriese (Eds.), *Self-care in later life* (pp. 142–169). New York: Springer.

Gitlin, L., Schemm, R., Landsberg, L., & Burgh, D. (1996). Factors predicting assistive device use in the home by older people following rehabilitation. *Journal of Aging and Health, 8*(4), 554–575.

Graves, J., & Corcoran, S. (1989). The study of nursing informatics. *Image: Journal of Nursing Scholarship, 21*(4), 227–231.

Idaho Assistive Technology Project. (1995). *Assistive technology and older adults*. Information Sheet #25. Retrieved January 5, 2009, from http://www.idahoat.org/files/factsheets/25%20OlderPersonsAT.pdf

Interest Survey 2004. (2004). Retrieved September 20, 2007, from http://www.seniornet.org

Jajeh, D. (2005). *Robot nurse escorts and schmoozes the elderly*. Retrieved September 19, 2007, from http://www.globalaging.org/elderrights/us/2005/escorts.htm

Johnson, J. L., Davenport, R., & Mann, W. C. (2007). Consumer feedback on smart home applications. *Topics in Geriatric Rehabilitation, 23*(1), 60–72.

Kautzmann, L. (1990). Introducing computers to the elderly. *Physical and Occupational Therapy in Geriatrics, 9*, 27–36.

Kelker, K. (Ed.). (1997). *Family guide to assistive technology*. Retrieved September 20, 2007, from http://www.pluk.org/AT1.html

Kraskowsky, L. H., & Finlayson, M. (2001). Factors affecting older adults' use of adaptive equipment: Review of the literature. *American Journal of Occupational Therapy*, *55*(3), 303–310.

Larkin, M. (2000). Online support groups gaining credibility. *Lancet*, *355*(9217), 1834.

Liao, C., Groff, L., Chaparro, A., Chaparro, B., & Stumpfhauser, L. (2000). A comparison of Web site usage between young adults and the elderly. *Proceedings of the IEA 2000/HGES 2000 Congress*. San Diego, CA: Human Factors and Ergonomics Society.

Malcolm, M., Mann, W., Tomita, M., Fraas, L., Stanton, K., & Gitlin, L. (2001). Computer and Internet use in physically frail elders. *Physical and Occupational Therapy in Geriatrics*, *19*(3), 15–32.

Mann, W., Belchior, P., Tomita, M. R., & Kemp, B. J. (2007). Older adults' perception and use of PDAs, home automation system, and home health monitoring system. *Topics in Geriatric Rehabilitation, 23*(1), 35–46.

Mann, W., Goodall, S., Justiss, M., & Tomita, M. (2002). Dissatisfaction and nonuse of assistive devices among frail elders. *Assistive Technology*, *14*(2), 130–139.

Mann, W., Hurren, D., & Tomita, M. (1993). Comparison of assistive device use and needs of home-based older persons, with different impairments. *American Journal of Occupational Therapy*, *47*(11), 980–987.

Mann, W., Hurren, D., & Tomita, M. (1995). Assistive devices used by home-based elderly persons with arthritis. *American Journal of Occupational Therapy*, *49*(8), 810–820.

Mann, W., Llanes, C., Justiss, M. D., & Tomita, M. (2004). Frail older adults' self-report of their most important assistive devices. *OTJR: Occupation, Participation, and Health*, *24*(1), 4–12.

Mann, W., Ottenbacher, K. J., Fraas, L., Tomita, M., & Granger, C. V. (1999). Effectiveness of assistive technology and environmental interventions in maintaining independence and reducing home care costs for the frail elderly. *Archives of Family Medicine*, *8*, 210–217.

McConatha, D., McConatha, J., & Dermigny, R. (1994). The use of interactive computer services to enhance the quality of life for long-term care residents. *The Gerontologist*, *34*, 553–556.

McKay, H. G., Glasgow, R. E., Feil, E. G., Boles, S. M., & Barrera, M. M. (2002). Internet-based diabetes self-management and support: Initial outcomes from the Diabetes Network Project. *Rehabilitation Psychology*, *47*, 31–48.

McNeely, E. (1991). Computer-assisted instruction and the older-adult learner. *Educational Gerontology*, *17*, 229–237.

Medical Automation Research Center. (2005). *Smart in-home monitoring system*. Retrieved September 20, 2007, from http://marc.med.virginia.edu/projects_smarthomemonitor.html

Mihailidis, A. (2007). *Intelligent supportive environments for older adults (COACH project)*. Retrieved September 20, 2007, from http://www.ot.utoronto.ca

Mihailidis, A., Barbenel, J., & Fernie, G. (2004). The efficacy of an intelligent cognitive orthosis to facilitate handwashing by persons with moderate-to-severe dementia. *Neuropsychological Rehabilitation*, *14*(1/2), 135–171.

Mihailidis, A., Boger, J., Canido, M., & Hoey, J. (2007). The use of an intelligent prompting system for people with dementia: A case study. *ACM Interactions*, *14*(4), 34–37.

Mihailidis, A., & Lee, T. (2007). *Intelligent emergency response and fall detection system*. Retrieved September 20, 2007, from http://www.ot.utoronto.ca/iatsl/projects/ers.htm

National Institute on Aging & National Library of Medicine. (2002). *Making your Web site senior friendly*. Retrieved September 20, 2007, from http://www.nlm.nih.gov/pubs/staffpubs/od/ocpl/agingchecklist.html

National Institutes of Health. (2000). *Communicative competence of users of augmentative and alternative communication (AAC) systems*. Retrieved September 20, 2007, from http://grants.nih.gov/grants/guide/pa-files/PA-96-032.htm

Norburn, J., Bernard, S. L., Konrad, T. R., Woomert, A., DeFriese, G. H., Kalsbeek, W. D., et al. (1995). Self-care and assistance from others in coping with functional status limitations among a national sample of older adults. *Journals of Gerontology: Series B, Psychological Sciences and Social Sciences*, *50*(2), S101–S109.

Northouse, L., & Peters-Golden, H. (1993). Cancer and the family: Strategies to assist spouses. *Seminars in Oncology Nursing*, *9*(2), 74–82.

Pew Internet and American Life Project. (2004). *Demographics: Older Americans and the Internet*. Retrieved September 20, 2007, from http://www.pewinternet.org/PPF/r/117/report_display.asp

Pew Internet and American Life Project. (2005). *How men and women use the Internet*. Retrieved September 19, 2007, from http://www.pewinternet.org

Pew Internet and American Life Project. (2006). *Are "wired seniors" sitting ducks?* Retrieved October 15, 2007, from http://www.pewinternet.org/PPF/r/180/report_display.asp

Pierce, L., Steiner, V., Govoni, A., Hicks, B., Thompson, T., & Friedemann, M. (2004). Caring~Web: Internet-based support for rural caregivers of persons with stroke shows promise. *Rehabilitation Nursing, 29*(3), 95–99, 103.

Pierce, L., Steiner, V., Govoni, A., Thompson, T., & Friedemann, M. (2007). Two sides to the caregiving story. *Topics in Stroke Rehabilitation, 14*(2), 13–20.

Post, J. (1996). Internet resources on aging: Seniors on the Net. *The Gerontologist, 36*, 565–569.

Purnell, M., & Sullivan-Schroyer, P. (1997). Nursing home residents using computers: The Winchester houses experience. *Generations, 21*(3), 61–62.

Reuben, D., Herr, K., Pacala, J., Pollock, B., Potter, J., & Semla, T. (2004). *Geriatrics at your fingertips*. Malden, MA: Blackwell.

Rhine, K. (2005). *A pocketful of help for Alzheimer's sufferers and caregivers*. Retrieved September 20, 2007, from http://www.eurekalert.org

Roelands, M., Van Oost, P., Depoorter, A., & Buysse, A. (2002). A social-cognitive model to predict the use of assistive devices for mobility and self-care in elderly people. *The Gerontologist, 42*(10), 39–50.

Spillman, B. C. (2004). Changes in elderly disability rates and the implications for health care utilization and cost. *Milbank Quarterly, 82*(1), 157–194.

Spry Foundation. (2005). *Computer-based technology and caregiving of older adults*. Retrieved September 20, 2007, from http://www.spry.org

Tomita, M., Mann, W. C., Fraas, L. F., & Stanton, K. M. (2004). Predictors of the use of assistive devices that address physical impairments among community-based frail elders. *Journal of Applied Gerontology, 23*(2), 141–155.

Tomita, M. R., Mann, W. C., Stanton, K., Tomita, A. D., & Sundar, V. (2007). Use of currently available smart home technology by frail elders: Process and outcomes. *Topics in Geriatric Rehabilitation, 23*(1), 24–34.

University of Pittsburgh, University of Michigan, & Carnegie Mellon University. (2005). *Nursebot project*. Retrieved September 19, 2007, from http://www.cs.cmu.edu/~nursebot/

U.S. Census Bureau. (2004). *Interim projections consistent with Census 2000*. Retrieved September 20, 2007, from http://www.census.gov

U.S. Congress. (1988). *Technology-Related Assistance for Individuals with Disabilities Act of 1988*. Retrieved September 20, 2007, from http://www.resna.org/taproject/library/laws/techact88.htm

Veggeberg, S. (1996). Online health and healing. *Molecular Medicine Today, 2*(8), 315.

Weisman, S. (1983). Computer games for the frail elderly. *The Gerontologist, 23*, 361–363.

Wellness Community. (2007). *Cancer support, education and hope*. Retrieved September 19, 2007, from http://www.thewellnesscommunity.org

White, M., & Dorman, S. (2000). Online support for caregivers: Analysis of an Internet Alzheimer mailgroup. *Computers in Nursing, 18*(4), 168–176.

World Wide Web Consortium. (2004). *Web content accessibility guidelines*. Retrieved November 17, 2004, from http://www.w3.org/TR/

X-10. (2005). *Affordable solutions for everyday life*. Retrieved September 20, 2007, from www.x10.com

SECTION

7

Ethics

(Competencies 18–19)

CHAPTER 17

Ethical/Legal Principles and Issues

Pamela A. Masters-Farrell, MSN, RN, CRRN

LEARNING OBJECTIVES

At the end of this chapter, the reader will be able to:

- Define key ethical constructs as they relate to the care of geriatric patients.
- Discuss concepts of ethics and the implications in the care of geriatric patients.
- Recognize the influence of personal values, attitudes, and expectations about aging on care of older adults and their families.
- Analyze the impact of fiscal, sociocultural, and medico-legal factors on decision making in the care of geriatric patients.
- Identify strategies for facilitating appropriate levels of autonomy and decision making in the care of geriatric patients.

KEY TERMS

- Advance directives
- Advocacy
- Autonomy
- Beneficence
- Codes of ethics
- Competence
- Confidentiality
- Conflict
- Conflict of interest
- Cost-benefit analysis
- Dilemma
- Ethics of care
- Failure to rescue
- Fidelity
- Fiduciary responsibility
- Informed consent
- Justice
- Moral dilemma
- Moral distress
- Moral principles
- Moral uncertainty
- Nonmaleficence
- Paternalism
- Patient rights
- Quality of life
- Reciprocity
- Sanctity of life
- Values
- Veracity

The **ethics of care** in the geriatric population, as in others, include compassion, equity, fairness, dignity, confidentiality, and mindfulness of a person's autonomy within the realm of the person's abilities and mental capacity. It is not possible to care for this population without being faced with difficult choices surrounding issues relating to the ability to live independently. Independence in the community requires some level of self-sufficiency in the management of medications, health care, driving, and maintaining and running a home (self-care, pet care, meals, housekeeping, shopping, banking, etc.). Self-sufficiency, issues of finance, and personal choices directly impact adherence to a plan of care.

These basic issues of autonomy are further challenged by the effects of aging and chronic disease on cognitive functioning and decision making. Advance directives, informed consent, and refusal of treatment are dependent on clarity of mind. Difficult choices call for judgments and serious consideration of what is right or best for patients, their families, and their communities. These personal choices are further compounded by social pressures associated with technological developments, options for end-of-life care, genetic research, and resource allocation. Technology and science have moved forward at their own paces without concern for consequences, asking not if something is needed, only whether or not it can be done (Coverston & Rogers, 2000).

Notable Quotes

"Everyone has the right to a standard of living adequate for the health and well-being of himself and of his family, including food, clothing, housing and medical care and necessary social services, and the right to security in the event of unemployment, sickness, disability, widowhood, old age or other lack of livelihood in circumstances beyond his control."

—Article 25 from the Universal Declaration of Human Rights (General Assembly, res. 217a (III), December 10, 1948)

Ethical concepts are principles that facilitate decision making and guide our professional behavior. They evolve from our beliefs and **values**, and therefore have their foundations in religion, culture, and family expectations. Ethical decision making is driven by moral reasoning—our determination of what is right and wrong. Ethical concepts and personal values define our character and are expressed in our conduct and actions. Professional codes or standards within the profession of nursing help to define ethical actions. Changes in our social networks, including global awareness, cultural diversity, and advances in science, medicine, and technology, have created increasingly complex conflicts and dilemmas. Therefore, nurses must have a clear understanding of their own values and a strategy for decision making because a nurse's personal beliefs may be quite different from the patient's, from the organization's values and expectations, or from the community's public rules.

CONFLICT AND DILEMMA

Conflict occurs when a choice must be made between two equal possibilities. Three types of moral conflict are described by Redman and Fry (1998). **Moral distress** occurs when someone wants to do the right thing but is limited by the constraints of the organization or society. **Moral uncertainty** defines the confusion surrounding situations in which a person is uncertain what the moral problem is or which moral principles or values apply to it. A **moral dilemma** arises when two or more moral principles apply that support mutually inconsistent actions. A true **dilemma** occurs when it appears there are no acceptable choices. To qualify as a dilemma, there must be active engagement in the situation that forces an evaluation of and need for choices. Actions are uncertain because alternatives are equally unattractive (Sletteboe, 1997). **Case Study 17-1** provides an example of a dilemma.

Case Study 17-1

Mr. Bowen is 64 years old. He has been very healthy by report and very active working as a dairy farmer. He had a stroke affecting his right side 2 weeks ago and currently has a moderate leg weakness with a more significant arm weakness, slurred speech, and mild dysphagia (swallowing difficulty). He is predicted to be ambulatory with a cane, though prognosis of arm function returning is more guarded. It is likely he will improve speech function and swallowing ability but will require some specialization of diet to prevent aspiration.

Mr. Bowen has chosen to stop eating, stating that he does not want to live as an invalid. His family is very distressed and wants him to be forced to eat. They cannot imagine why he has made this choice when his prognosis is so good compared to others they have seen in the rehabilitation setting with much more severe deficits. He has been evaluated for depression and an antidepressant has been recommended, which he refuses to take along with all other medications recommended for his newly diagnosed cardiovascular disease. Mr. Bowen is oriented and has not had competence questioned prior to taking this stand.

Some of the staff supports his decision and others do not. Discussion with the family reveals that Mr. Bowen has frequently made deriding remarks about persons with disability, including remarks like "If I ever end up that way, just take me out behind the barn and shoot me." The psychologist comments that Mr. Bowen is frankly depressed and that part of this depression is related to the location of his stroke. He also points out that he feels strongly that should the depression be resolved, Mr. Bowen would likely change his opinion.

Questions:

1. How is this situation best handled?
2. Does Mr. Bowen have the right to refuse to eat and take medications when he is clearly not in an end-of-life situation?
3. How does the team resolve the situation when the depression is so prevalent and he refuses treatment for it?
4. Will you be able to care for Mr. Bowen if his wishes are granted?

Dilemmas are inherent in the health care of the geriatric population, creating ethical problems for those providing care. Differences in values and opinions can lead to conflicts between caregivers and health care providers and are more common in diverse communities where cultural values may be quite different (Ellis & Hartley, 2004). There are seldom perfect solutions to ethical dilemmas. Those forced to make them are often required to justify their decisions and actions. Some conflicts are resolved through dialogue, others are legislated, and others are defined by agreements regarding basic rights. Many health care organizations utilize ethics committees to resolve such dilemmas in real time.

MORAL PRINCIPLES

Moral principles are incorporated into professional **codes of ethics**, organizational value statements, and position statements published by professional groups such as the American Nurses Association (ANA). The ANA posts the *Code of Ethics for Nurses* on its Web site at http://www.nursingworld.org/MainMenuCategories/ThePracticeofProfessionalNursing/EthicsStandards/CodeofEthics.aspx. This code forms the cornerstone of nursing practice. The purpose of this code is to provide nurses with tools for identifying ethical responsibilities and to guide decision making within the primary goals, values, and obligations of the profession (Hook & White, 2003). The ANA has issued many position statements speaking to ethics and human rights and is currently active in addressing issues of genetic research, confidentiality, privacy, managed care, health services for undocumented persons, and the health care system's impact on the profession of nursing using moral principles and *Nursing's Agenda for Health Care Reform* as a guide for action (ANA, 2005b). A nurse's understanding of moral principles facilitates ethical decision making in daily practice.

Advocacy

Advocacy refers to loyalty and a championing of the needs and interests of others, requiring the nurse to educate patients and their families so that they know their rights, are fully informed, and are able to access all the benefits they are entitled to (Hoeman & Duchene, 2002). Advocacy is implicit in the social contract between the profession of nursing and society and is based on other ethical concepts such as justice and autonomy (Falk Rafael, 1995). Our increasingly complex health care system often calls for advocacy efforts to help patients and families negotiate it and receive appropriate services. Nurses also advocate for patients by supporting them in their efforts to retain as much autonomy as their abilities allow. At times, nurses advocate for the expressed desires of the patient within the context of team and family discussions in which the patient is not present, ensuring true

BOX 17-1 Ethical/Moral Principles

Advocacy
Autonomy
Beneficence/nonmaleficence
Confidentiality
Fidelity
Fiduciary responsibility
Justice
Quality of life
Reciprocity
Sanctity of life
Veracity

representation of the patient's desires when known. Other situations require advocacy efforts to prevent abuse, neglect, and exploitation.

Advocacy also refers to maintaining the status of safe care. The nurse is committed to the well-being of the patient and thus must take appropriate action in the event that incompetent, illegal, unethical, or impaired practice puts a patient at risk. Nurses are obligated to address the issue with the person involved and, if necessary, with higher authorities so that patients are not placed in jeopardy (ANA, 2005a). Most health care organizations have processes in place for reporting and managing such behaviors. Utilization of official channels reduces the risk of reprisal against the reporting nurse (ANA, 2005a).

Autonomy

Autonomy is the concept that each person has a right to make independent choices and decisions. It is reflected in guidelines and laws regarding patient rights and self-determination. Inherent in the concept of autonomy is respect for another and their decisions and that each person should be treated with dignity as a unique individual with inherent worth. Evidence of respect for autonomy is found in care that considers the patient's lifestyle, value system, and religious beliefs. Such respect does not mean that the nurse condones those beliefs or choices, but rather that the nurse respects the patient as a person with autonomy and rights (ANA, 2005a). Autonomy may be limited by cognitive deficits that impair clarity of thought and the ability of the patient to make decisions.

Autonomous choices are based on values and experiences. In order for patients and their families to make sound choices, they must have appropriate resources and information available. Thus, autonomy is supported by informed consent and patient and family education. **Informed consent** means making sure that consent has been granted, not assumed, following an educational process that facilitates the weighing of benefits, risks, and available options (Aveyard, 2005). Informed consent is not compliance, but ensuring that voluntariness is honored.

Although consent is not required for routine activities for which the risks are commonly understood, patients often comply with actions and activities during nursing care procedures because they

BOX 17-2 Informed Consent

Elements to include in discussion:

- The specific condition requiring treatment
- The purpose and distinct nature of the procedure or treatment
- Potential complications or risks associated with the procedure or treatment
- Reasonable alternatives with a discussion of their relative risks and benefits
- Discussion of the option of taking no action
- The probability of success of the recommended treatment or procedure

Source: Adapted from Quallich, S. A. (2004). The practice of informed consent. *Urologic Nursing, 24*(6), 513–515.

believe that is what is expected of them (Quallich, 2004). This does not mean they have provided informed consent for those activities not considered routine by the patient. All too often nurses discover that patients do not really understand why they are doing something that was prescribed by a health care provider. We often err by assuming they understood and provided consent because they were participating (Aveyard, 2005).

Unmistakably, autonomy also means that nurses and other health professionals can educate, provide support, and provide resources, but they cannot force compliance with recommended treatment. Thus, it is important to recognize that informed consent also means that consent can be denied, can be withdrawn after it has been given, and that such requests should be respectfully honored. Refusal of treatment is a patient right. Care should be taken that health care providers do not abuse their power in the relationship by persuading patients to comply with recommended treatment. Patients and their families have been badgered into agreeing to an intervention that they did not want to pursue (Aveyard, 2005). It is important to recognize the impact of previous experiences on choices made by patients and to actively address barriers through support and education.

Conflicts around autonomy can occur with issues of chronic or life-threatening illness, when patients and family members fail to conform to expected behavior patterns, or when they disagree with the recommendations of professionals. Patients are labeled noncompliant and families are labeled dysfunctional. **Paternalism** has been prevalent in the medical field, and health care providers, including nurses, are at risk for paternalistic behavior when patients are perceived as difficult to work with. Paternalism is easily supported by the distribution of power in relationships with patients and families in many health care settings. Paternalism fails to support autonomy and limits the development of trusting partnerships. The best outcomes are achieved when autonomy is supported through a shared responsibility for decision making that allows the patient and family to be vested in the plan.

The burden of health care has been steadily shifting to the community. Nurses and other health care providers are wise to invest in the development of strong relationships and partnerships with family caregivers. This ethic of negotiation and accommodation means providing information in a timely manner in a way that is easily understood. It means taking the time to prepare and train the patient and caregiver for both the technical and emotional aspects of their changing roles. And it means being compassionate about their anxiety, suffering, and hard work. Caregivers need direction, guidance, and support in defining their roles and responsibilities in patient care and decision making. They also need support and permission to set fair limits on their sacrifices, supporting their autonomy and conditions of choice (Levine, 2000).

As models of health care change and resource allotment shifts or diminishes, autonomy can be lost by the directives or requirements of those who control the flow of money. Elderly patients are often overwhelmed by the choices they must make regarding insurance offerings and health care access. Decisions regarding living arrangements, transportation, and support services also stress resources and potentially limit autonomy.

Elder patients may need support from health care professionals to be assertive regarding their needs and expectations. Health care professionals across the continuum of care should actively include elders in decision making and care planning as long as they are able to participate. Some elders may have the resources to work around the system and its regulations, but many will not. But that does not need to result in allowing those with fewer resources to simply be victims of the system. Health care professionals are in a unique position of being able to direct elders to community resources and to educate and support them should they appeal the system. Feedback to regulatory bodies regarding patient needs by patients and health care professionals alike provides opportunities for changing regulations. The Older Americans Act of 1965 was updated in 2006 due to efforts of providers and recipients alike. This act provides resources to the elderly and preserves advocacy and coordination of the national aging network of services as its primary mission. The act directs the actions of the Administration on Aging, which coordinates a large number of services that support autonomy and independence for aging Americans. These services include information and referral services, nutrition support services, transportation, community-based long-term care, legal services, nursing home ombudsman programs, identification and prevention of elder abuse, senior community service jobs, mental health screening and treatment, and funding for the National Family Caregiver Support Program and the Native American Caregiver Program. This act directs support to those with the greatest social or economic need (Administration on Aging, 2007).

Nurses may face ethical dilemmas when they advocate for autonomy in the face of being forced to comply with regulatory guidelines (Hoeman, Duchene, & Vierling, 2007). Nurses can facilitate autonomy in elder patients by:

- Encouraging completion of **advance directives**, living wills, powers of attorney, or other documents that can ensure that personal preferences are met should cognitive capacity decline
- Providing patient-centered care
- Providing appropriate education and training
- Ensuring that consents are truly *informed*
- Actively supporting and educating patients about their rights
- Staying informed of regulatory guidelines and appeal processes and knowing how to help patients access resources to navigate insurance and health care systems
- Staying politically informed and active in providing feedback to those developing laws and allotting patient access and resources
- Creatively devising care strategies that support autonomy while complying with regulations
- Referring patients to ombudsmen, community care managers, or other resources to help them navigate issues of insurance, living arrangements, transportation, and health care access

Beneficence/Nonmaleficence

These concepts of do good (**beneficence**) and do no harm (**nonmaleficence**) are integral to health care. Nurses intend to do good for their patients. Nurses are also concerned about situations that can result in harm to patients, such as understaffing. Consider the situation on a busy medical unit where a nurse does a cursory assessment due to workload demands and the apparent comfort of the patient on rounds. The patient is a very social and talkative elderly woman who has had a recent crisis with heart failure and is having her medications adjusted. She has become significantly deconditioned and has spent much of the last couple of weeks in her recliner prior to admission. Near the end of the shift the patient complains of severe chest pain and anxiety. An emergent work-up determines that she has a deep vein thrombosis with pulmonary embolism. Is this an example of maleficence (doing harm)? Obviously, purposeful behavior such as administering a lethal dose of medication is an example of maleficence, but where does failure to rescue fall on the ethical scale?

Failure to rescue refers to effectiveness in rescuing a patient from a complication vs. preventing a complication (National Quality Measures Clearinghouse, 2005). Failure to rescue data are collected by measuring the number of deaths occurring out of those discharges with potential complications of care listed in the failure to rescue definitions (pneumonia, deep vein thrombosis/pulmonary embolism, sepsis, acute renal failure, shock/cardiac arrest, or gastrointestinal hemorrhage/acute ulcer). It is a patient safety quality monitor for the National Institutes of Health and Agency for Healthcare Research and Quality. Failure to rescue has many causes, from situations as simple as educational background, inexperience, and lack of knowledge to more complex issues such as attitudes toward work, staffing patterns, and resource allocation (see **Case Study 17-2**). It can be an issue of omission as much as an issue of commission. It behooves all nurses to think carefully about the issue of failure to rescue and to investigate practice situations so that such circumstances are not issues of maleficence.

Confidentiality

The ANA Code of Ethics (2001) emphasizes respect for human dignity that is demonstrated in daily work. This includes respect for privacy and maintaining **confidentiality**. So much value is placed on the concept of confidentiality that it is considered a right—the right to privacy. The right to privacy has been inferred from the U.S. Constitution but has been legislated more directly in recent years by the Health Insurance Portability and Accountability Act (HIPAA).

Driving forces for these laws relate to the spread of socially stigmatized diseases such as AIDS and concerns over the large volumes of information transmitted electronically containing sensitive material, detailed descriptions of interactions with health care workers, and genetic data that can result in potential invasions of privacy or be utilized for discrimination in the workplace or denial of insurance coverage (Ellis & Hartley, 2004). HIPAA requires that providers educate their patients regarding their rights under HIPAA and that they release only information the patient specifically designates as sharable with others. HIPAA regulations protect privacy so strongly that even admitting the patient is in your care is a violation unless the patient has expressly agreed that such information can be shared. This has changed many practices related to confidentiality in health care settings.

HIPAA has legislated the concept of confidentiality inherent in practice by requiring that only persons with a need to know access the patient's record or receive information about the patient. Nurses are entrusted with personal information in the course of providing care that should be shared only as necessary to facilitate that patient's care. In addition to the personal responsibility for protecting privacy, legal ramifications for failure to comply with this law are steep; the nurse should be well informed of organizational guidelines for compliance with this regulation. Health care providers can be held liable for harm that results from sharing information without permission. Nurses should be able to easily access appropriate administrative personnel in the event that a request for patient information is questionable.

Fidelity

Fidelity refers to keeping promises or being true to another; being faithful to commitments and responsibilities (Ellis & Hartley, 2004). Fidelity is particularly important in the care of geriatric patients because of the amount of trust they put into the health care system. Fidelity is also important in relationships with team members and the organization at which the nurse works. The team and the organization need to be able to trust the nurse to keep promises and honor relationships with them.

BOX 17-3 Web Exploration

Agency for Healthcare Research and Quality: http://www.ahrq.gov. An excellent site for tracking and learning about quality of care initiatives that support autonomy, safety, and appropriate access to care.

American Hospital Association: http://www.aha.org. A site emphasizing better health care for persons and communities; contains multiple links related to health policy, research, and advocacy.

American Nurses Association: http://www. nursingworld.org. Contains multiple sections on ethics in nursing.

Berman Institute of Bioethics at Johns Hopkins University: http://www.bioethicsinstitute.org. A wealth of information on bioethics, including discussions on genetic research.

National Quality Measures Clearinghouse: http://www.qualitymeasures.ahrq.gov. Learn about the quality measures that reflect data on failure to rescue and many other topics.

The Patient Care Partnership: Understanding Expectations, Rights and Responsibilities: http://www.aha.org/aha/ptcommunication/partnership/index.html. An excellent resource for involving patients in their care.

Trust is earned, and fidelity is demonstrated in daily work and the relationships therein.

Fiduciary Responsibility

In this age of diminishing health care resources it is important that all nurses have an understanding of the costs and benefits of care that is given. Health care professionals have an ethical obligation to good stewardship of both the patient's and the organization's funds—**fiduciary responsibility**. This refers to using both fiscal reserves and care-giving resources wisely, potentially requiring a **cost-benefit analysis** to facilitate decision making. It becomes more difficult to deal with persons who are noncompliant or who have conditions that could have been prevented through healthier lifestyles as resources and manpower decline (Hoeman & Duchene, 2002). For many, rehabilitation and other special health care programs are not a right, they are a privilege that is rationed and controlled by those who control funding.

Justice

Fiduciary responsibility and fidelity are some of the moral principles that help to determine what is just. **Justice** refers to the fairness of an act or situation. Health care is replete with issues of justice. Is it just for one patient to receive rehabilitation following a stroke and another to be sent to a nursing home without acute rehabilitation? Is it just for a person who has attempted suicide and severely damaged his liver to receive a transplant before another who has been patiently waiting for the same liver? Who decides what is just and right? Does age make a difference? Why should one person receive more resources than another? Is the government responsible for providing resources to those unable to provide for themselves?

Many geriatric patients depend on Medicare and Medicaid for insurance, so nurses in the field of geriatrics should conscientiously follow the government's efforts to determine just distribution of its dollars. The Medicare Prospective Payment System has been mandated by the Balanced Budget Act of 1997 and requires strict accounting for where its dollars go in postacute care. This has led to a redistribution of services and limiting of access to home health, outpatient, and rehabilitation services for the geriatric population.

This situation quickly reinforces the issue of access, of whether we all deserve the same sort of care and who should decide what that care should be. Care of geriatric patients is burdened with age-related biases regarding resource allocation and rationales for resource allotment. Resources are limited. Elderly persons are usually on fixed incomes with restricted benefits and strict criteria for access to services, especially supportive assistance in the home. This increases the burden on caregivers, creating a difficult, isolated, and often unsupported role (Hoeman & Duchene, 2002). Success in this role is further hampered by the complexities of the system and limitations on time spent with patients and caregivers.

Levine (2000) comments that caregivers lamented the incomplete information they received regarding basic information about diagnosis and prognosis, key elements of the treatment plan, side effects of medication, symptoms to watch for at home, and whom to call for assistance or problems. Others have reported difficulties with compliance and learning about their loved one's care needs due to conflicting information from health care

Case Study 17-2

Mr. Jacobs, a young-acting 72-year-old who is rather obese, was admitted for trauma following a motorcycle accident in which he broke his femur. He is 24 hours post op and has requested pain meds at 0400. The medications were given, and the nurse glanced in the room 2 hours later and noted he appeared to be sleeping. At 0700, the nurse on the next shift enters the room and turns on the light to see the patient is cyanotic and difficult to arouse. Aggressive stimulation and oxygen revived him. Discussion with the patient noted a history of sleep apnea that appeared to be worsened by the effects of the pain medication.

Questions:

1. Was this a near miss or failure to rescue?
2. Did the night shift nurse adhere to principles of beneficence and nonmaleficence?
3. What should the nurse have done differently?

providers. One also has to question the justice in a system that impairs the caregiver's ability to learn because professionals share information in such hurried and technical manners that anxious and stressed caregivers can hardly be expected to absorb it (Levine, 2000). These failures in communication hardly support a fair or just health care system; rather, they contribute to serious problems that can increase both morbidity and mortality.

Quality and Sanctity of Life

The issues of justice and access to care remind us that many decisions regarding self-determination and autonomy are related to **quality of life**, or one's personal perception of the conditions of life, and **sanctity of life**, referring to the value of life and the right to live. Quality of life is a perception based on personal values and beliefs. Views on quality of life are widely variable and likely to change when circumstances differ. They are influenced by emotional, physical, economic, and social needs. Quality of life is enhanced by prevention and management of chronic disease through preventive care, support for healthy lifestyle choices, education, and home evaluations to reduce risk of injury. However, even the best nurse cannot prevent injury or reduce risk of complications in those who continue to make unhealthy choices or fail to heed health or safety recommendations (Hoeman & Duchene, 2002). Some quality-of-life decisions are made in direct relation to the burden being placed on others. Sometimes it is not the big things such as limitations in mobility that cause the greatest burden on quality of life, but rather the indignity and emotional burden associated with problems such as incontinence and dependency.

Sanctity of life supports the belief that all life is of value and that this value is not based on how functional or effective a person's life is, simply that we all have a right to life. The meeting of personal perspectives on quality and sanctity of life can thus be expressed in an individual's advance directives. Conflicts in health care are rife with issues related to values surrounding sanctity of life and end-of-life care issues. The ANA (2005a) has addressed this directly in the *Code of Ethics for Nurses*, stating that nurses may not act with the intent to end life but may support and act on well-thought-out decisions regarding resuscitation status, withholding and withdrawing of life-sustaining care including nutrition and hydration, and aggressively managing pain and other symptoms at the end of life even if such care hastens death.

Reciprocity

Reciprocity is a feature of integrity concerned with the ability to be true to one's self while respecting and supporting the values and views of another. Living according to this principle is particularly important when values and views are different. Nurses need to be impartial once a plan of care is agreed on, actively facilitating achievement of intended goals and outcomes. Passive resistance does not support reciprocity or trust. If a nurse or other health care provider cannot demonstrate reciprocity, another should take his or her place in the care of the patient.

Veracity

Veracity means truthfulness and refers to telling the truth, or, at the very least, not misleading or deceiving patients or their families. Veracity forms the basis of informed consent—without truthfulness and an explanation of options, the patient cannot possibly make the best choice. Failure to be truthful impairs trust and reliability (Ellis & Hartley, 2004). But issues of truthfulness create conflict as well. Do you tell the truth when you know it will cause harm or distress? How do you maintain hope while sharing a poor prognosis? It is possible to support hopefulness and decrease stress with truthfulness through careful choices of words. It is as simple as the difference between stating, "You will not likely walk again considering the severity of this stroke" and compassionately saying, "It will take considerable work and fortunate healing of your brain in order for you to walk again, but we will work with you and see what happens."

PATIENT RIGHTS

Patient rights direct actions on ethical issues in the care of geriatric populations. The concept of rights forms the basis of many of our laws and is indeed the basis for the foundation of the U.S. Constitution. Rights are considered basic to human life, and each person is entitled to them on a legal, moral, or ethical basis (Ellis & Hartley, 2004). Over the last several decades considerable effort has been put into defining patients' rights. These rights are defined by organizational values, accreditation standards, professional codes, and legislative guidelines. The American Hospital Association has published a document addressing patient rights and hospital responsibility, entitled *The Patient Care Partnership: Understanding Expectations, Rights and Responsibilities*, in an effort to define these rights and to hold hospitals and patients accountable to them. This document is available at http://www.aha.org/aha/ptcommunication/partnership/index.html.

Rights also evolve as values within a cultural or social group change. The right to decide what can and cannot be done to a person evolved as a legal definition due to a malpractice lawsuit in 1957 (Quallich, 2004). The right to effective pain management has evolved due to changes in perception and studies assessing the impact of poor pain management on outcomes. This development was supported by the Joint Commission when it added accreditation standards related to effective pain management and by rulings of the courts related to failure to manage terminal pain (Furrow, 2001).

Advance Directives and Living Wills

The most fundamental patient right is the right to decide. The Patient Self-Determination Act of 1990 was enacted to reduce the risk that life would be shortened or prolonged against the wishes of the individual. Following the belief that each person has a fundamental right to decide (autonomy), this law requires that patients are provided the opportunity to express their preferences regarding life-saving or life-sustaining care on entering any health care service, including hospitals, long-term care centers, and home care agencies. The law also requires that adequate information be supplied to the patient so that he or she can make informed decisions regarding self-determination.

Decisions regarding life-saving or life-sustaining care are recorded in legal documents known as advance directives. Advance directives describe actions to be taken in a situation where the patient is no longer able to provide informed consent. Living wills are alternative documents that direct preferences for end-of-life care issues, providing an "if . . . then . . ." plan. They often include what type of care to provide and whether resuscitation measures should be taken. The "if" condition (e.g., If I am terminally ill and not expected to recover) must be confirmed by a physician (Ellis & Hartley, 2004). Laws vary from state to state regarding living wills, and some require two physicians to agree to the status of the patient before enacting directives. In states where living wills have been enacted into law, health care providers who do not agree with a patient's directives must remove themselves from the case (Ellis & Hartley, 2004). Remember that living wills are equally as likely to indicate that resuscitation efforts be limited as they are that all possible efforts be taken.

Durable Power of Attorney

A living will may include a durable power of attorney, a legal document designating an alternative decision maker in the event the person is incapacitated. This document supersedes all other general legal designations for decision makers. In other words, a patient may designate a close friend with durable power of attorney, superseding the designation of immediate family members in decision making in a situation where the patient is incapacitated. The living will in this situation provides direction to the decision maker. The use of a durable power of attorney can decrease conflicts between family members and allows the designated decision maker to perform in roles negotiated in advance with the patient (Ellis & Hartley, 2004).

The absence of a living will or "do not resuscitate" order requires that all possible efforts at resuscitation should be initiated. Care of the incapacitated person is greatly simplified by an advance directive or living will. However, the issues of paternalism and boundary violations can cause ethical conflicts in the pursuit of such directives if not handled empathetically. It is imperative that information be supplied in an ethically appropriate manner for each patient because the manner in which alternatives are discussed greatly influences choices made (Elliot & Hartley, 2004). Cultural values influence decisions made as well as the way in which decisions are made. Whereas one family may see the decision as solely up to the individual involved, others may feel it is a family decision because of duty, compassion, or the concern of those ultimately assuming the burden of care. The nurse supports the preferences of the patient in resolving self-determination issues.

Competence

Competence refers to one's clarity and appropriateness in decision making. Competence must be present for persons to exercise autonomy and their right to decide. Inherent in autonomy is the right to choose, the right to be informed, and the right to refuse treatment, including whether to participate in research. Loss of competence due to impaired memory or sensory function significantly impacts one's ability to make such informed decisions. There is a difference between being declared legally incompetent and situations of evidence of impaired competence that may be transient due to health problems or side effects of medications. Legal competence is determined by the courts, and if a person is deemed legally incompetent, a legal guardian is appointed.

Informed consent means that the person clearly understands the choices offered. Problems develop when one no longer has the capacity to make health care decisions. Nurses should involve patients in the planning of their own health care to the extent that they are able to participate. But what do we do when the patient is confused and refusing care that is necessary for both comfort and health? Do we perform that care against the person's will, documenting that clarity of thought was limited? We do. Under our ethical standards, we are equally obligated to provide the best care under the circumstances (ANA, 2005a). This default condition becomes uncomfortable for many nurses when the patient is combative or agitated with the care being delivered (Aveyard, 2005). Discomfort can be reduced and confidence in proceeding enhanced by discussing such care with designated decision makers. Each state has laws indicating who is designated as a decision maker in the event a person becomes confused, unconscious, or considered incompetent to make informed decisions. Organizational guidelines are established in line with these laws to guide staff in management of such situations. If a physician determines a person is no longer competent for such decision making, it should be noted in writing with an explanation of the probable cause and its likely duration. This allows the nurse to follow legal and institutional guidelines for using an advance directive or alternative decision maker (Butler, 2004).

Assisted Suicide

Another ethical issue of self-determination and autonomy is that of assisted suicide. As Hoeman and Duchene (2002) comment, if "social values dictate beliefs about self-determination and life satisfaction, persons with chronic, disabling disorders are at risk for promoted suicide even if they are not terminally ill. Hospice and palliative care are rejected in favor of aids to rapid death" (p. 53). Refusal of treatment is considered a right and protected under self-determination directives. The recent movement toward legislation regarding assisted suicide forces the judgment of when suicide should be used on the basis of health status, age, or other attributes and counters the ethical principle on which self-determination is based (Hoeman & Duchene, 2002). Does this create the potential of targeting those with severe disabilities, whether the condition is terminal or not? Does it create a double standard for treatment and survival? Is it a plan of managing devalued persons (Hoeman & Duchene, 2002)? The ANA published a statement on assisted suicide in 1994 and does not support it in any form, stating that it is a violation of the *Code of Ethics for Nurses*. Instead, it suggests that nurses focus on providing competent, comprehensive, and compassionate end-of-life care (ANA, 1994). Chapter 24 of this text focuses on such care of elders at end of life.

Oregon enacted the Death with Dignity Act in 1997 to allow terminally ill residents of Oregon to use voluntary self-administration of lethal medications to end their lives. These medications are expressly prescribed by physicians for this purpose. The law applies only to mentally competent adults who must:

- Provide written documentation of their intentions
- Be diagnosed as terminally ill
- Participate in a prescribed waiting period
- Take the prescribed medication themselves—medications must be taken orally

The Death with Dignity Act specifically disallows lethal injection, mercy killing, or active euthanasia and protects those who participate in the process

BOX 17-4 Recommended Reading

American Nurses Association. (2008). *Some nurses still need end-of-life education*. Retrieved April 26, 2008, from http://nursingworld.org/MainMenuCategories/ThePracticeofProfessionalNursing/EthicsStandards/CEHR/IssuesUpdate/UpdateArchive/IssuesUpdateSpring2001/EndofLifeEducation.aspx

Anthony, J. S. (2007). Self-advocacy in health care: Decision-making among elderly African Americans. *Journal of Cultural Diversity, 17*(2), 88–97.

Butler, K. A. (2004). Ethics paramount when patient lacks capacity. *Nursing Management, 35*(11), 18, 20, 52.

Mathes, M. (2004). Ethical decision making and nursing. *MEDSURG Nursing, 13*(6), 429–431.

Joint Commission. (2007). *"What did the doctor say?": Improving health literacy to protect patient safety.* Oakbrook Terrace, IL: Author.

Slettebo, A., & Bunch, E. H. (2004). Solving ethically difficult care situations in nursing homes. *Nursing Ethics, 11*(6), 543–552.

from liability and criminal prosecution (Oregon Department of Human Services, 1997). There were many concerns that outsiders would flock to Oregon to take advantage of the law, but that has not happened. As of 2006, only 292 persons had died under the terms of the law since its inception, and numbers have not exceeded 50 in any given year (Oregon Department of Human Services, 2007).

ETHICS IN PRACTICE

Ethical dilemmas and conflicts surround us in real life, and ethical principles alone are not likely to address many of the quandaries and dilemmas occurring in the care of geriatric patients. Living by these principles requires reflection and consideration of one's own beliefs and how they interface with the professional code of ethics, organizational statements, and beliefs of patients in the community in which the nurse practices. Nurses must prepare for such dilemmas by considering the influence of their own personal values, attitudes, and expectations about aging on the care of older adults and their families. Without such reflections, the patient may lose autonomy, the right to self-determination, and justice.

Nurses must learn how to assess competency as related to specific features of care in the geriatric population. Developing skills in probing the expressed wishes of patients and advocating for those wishes to be followed facilitates respect and the honoring of self-determination. Nurses also need to recognize that clarity of thought is fluid, and lucid moments can return or appear. These moments should be recognized and viewed as opportunities for discussion. Nurses, as patient advocates, also bear responsibility for effective communication of a patient's preferences through documentation and reporting processes. They are also responsible for creatively thinking about and problem-solving situations that limit functional status and safety to support quality of life and independent living.

Mistakes

Mistakes happen, and happened more often than the public was aware of prior to the 2000 report by the Institute of Medicine that stated such errors are common and often life threatening (Kohn, Corrigan, & Donaldson, 2001). Since that time, considerable effort has been put into reducing mistakes and improving patient safety. However, even the most conscientious nurse will make a mistake or two. Responding to mistakes is intimidating, embarrassing, and risky for most. Ethical responses to mistakes include:

- Honestly admitting the error occurred in a neutral and objective manner
- Taking proper steps to correct the situation
- Apologizing for the mistake
- Making amends as possible
- Evaluating how to prevent such mistakes in the future

Disclosure of mistakes in an honest and willing manner reduces the threat of the situation and also reduces the threat of liability (**Case Study 17-3**). Honesty and humility decrease the mental anguish of those who make errors in practice (Crigger, 2004). Compassionate and caring relationships with team members create support systems in which health care providers can help each other weather such storms.

Conflict of Interest

Conflict of interest situations arise from competing loyalties and opportunities. These may include conflicts of values between the nurse's value system and choices made by the patients, their families, other health care team members, the organization, or the insurance company. This is particularly evident in discussions related to resource allocation and end-of-life care. Other conflicts occur when incentive systems or other financial gains create conflict between professional integrity and self-interest. Nurses should facilitate resolution of conflicts by disclosing potential or actual conflicts of interest or withdraw from participation in care or processes that are causing the conflict (ANA, 2005a).

SUMMARY

Nurses must respect the worth, dignity, and rights of the elderly and must provide care that meets

BOX 17-5 Research Highlight

Aim: The purpose of this study was to characterize patient-related errors that contribute to adverse drug events (ADEs) and to determine which patients are at high risk for these errors.

Methods: Thirty thousand Medicare enrollees of a large multispecialty group practice were followed for 12 months. Data were collected and analyzed for ADEs and potential ADEs, and the subset of data related to patient errors was identified.

Findings: Most errors (32%) were related to administering a medication, modifying a medication regimen (42%), or not following clinical advice regarding the use of medications (22%). The medications most often involved in patient-related errors were hypoglycemic medications (29%), cardiovascular medications (22%), anticoagulants (19%), and diuretics (10%). The patients at the highest risk for errors were those taking more regularly scheduled medications, regardless of age or sex.

Application to practice: The authors concluded that the medication regimens of older adults create a range of difficulties with the potential for harm. Strategies are needed that specifically address the management of complex drug regimens in this population. Nurses may be able to decrease the likelihood of patient-related medication errors through careful patient teaching and follow-up, especially for those noted in this study to be at higher risk.

Source: Field, T. S., Mazor, K. M., Briesacher, B., DeBellis, K. R., & Gurwitz, J. H. (2007). Adverse drug events resulting from patient errors in older adults. *Journal of the American Geriatrics Society, 55*(2), 271–276.

Case Study 17-3

Jane is a junior-level baccalaureate nursing student who is doing her clinical rotation in a long-term care facility. She is assigned to care for a resident who occupies a double room, 111-2. The resident assigned to Jane is named Iva Wittacker, and Iva's roommate is Ida Wallace. Both residents are elderly women and have the same initials. While passing out medications, Jane asks the nursing assistant to identify Ms. Wittacker, because the residents do not wear armbands, Ms. Wittacker's picture is missing from the medication book, and Jane has not cared for this resident in the past. The CNA points to a white-haired woman in room 111. Jane administers the medications to the resident, and then her roommate enters the room and asks where her pills are. Jane asks the woman's name and she states she is Iva Wittacker. Jane realizes that she has administered medications to the wrong resident.

Questions:

1. What should Jane do immediately in this situation?
2. What could and should have been done to prevent such an error from occurring?
3. Who is responsible for Jane's mistake? What about accountability of the facility, the CNA, and/or the clinical instructor?
4. What are the ethical and legal implications in this situation?
5. Discuss what might happen if this mistake occurred in the facility where you are practicing.

their comprehensive needs across the continuum. Their fundamental commitment to the uniqueness of the patient creates opportunities for participation in planning and directing care. Their vigilance in advocating for dignified, just, and humane care establishes a standard that can be appreciated, and potentially needed, by all of us. It is not the rules and regulations that create ethical care delivery; it is the little actions done by each and every nurse in every day of practice.

As nurses, each of us is held to the ethical standards of practice of our profession (Esterhuizen, 1996). Providing respectful care that puts the patient's safety and welfare first helps us to avoid situations that can result in failure to rescue, abuse of power, exploitation, and over-involvement (Ellis & Hartley, 2004). Developing a framework for ethical decision making provides a foundation for discussion when dilemmas present themselves, smoothing the way for integrity-saving compromise. The nurse's conscientious effort to follow ethical standards in daily practices supports the quality of care we all want to experience.

Critical Thinking Exercises

1. Are your patients truly informed about their care? Ask five patients why they are taking the medications they are prescribed, and evaluate their responses.
2. Mrs. Gomez is confused and at times combative. Her family regularly visits and is actively involved in her care. She has been agitated and wandering the unit for the last several days and has not had a bowel movement for 6 days. She is constantly complaining of stomach pain and refuses all oral or rectal medications to facilitate bowel emptying. Her bowel sounds are diminished, and a hard mass

continues

Critical Thinking (continued)

suspected to be stool can be felt in the descending colon. Will you restrain her and give her an enema to prevent further complications?

3. You see a good friend while you are shopping at the mall. She inquires, "Hey, is my aunt on your unit? Can you tell me how she is doing? I just haven't had the time to get over and see her." How do you respond?
4. You answer the phone and a woman, indicating she is the daughter of your patient, asks you about her status. How will you respond considering confidentiality and privacy issues?
5. You observe a fellow nurse undressing an elderly woman and restraining her hands. The woman has been crying and yelling out for much of the night and is obviously confused. She leaves the woman naked on the stripped bed and walks out of the room, closing the door behind her and commenting as she passes you, "There, let her wet herself all night, I am done with her." What should you do?

Personal **Reflections**

1. As you prepare to care for older adults, what values, conflicts, or ethical dilemmas do you anticipate you will face?
2. Assess your feelings about the right to die and assisted suicide. Do you agree with the ANA's stand on this issue? How would you respond in the event that an elderly patient asks "please help me die" when death is not near?
3. An elderly person is becoming unsafe living alone and has been identified as at risk for serious injury. During admission to an alternative living setting, the person appears oriented and appropriate. Furthermore, the person expresses disagreement with the recommendations for this admission. How would you respond in this situation?

References

Administration on Aging. (2007). *The Administration on Aging gateway to the Older Americans Act Amendments of 2006*. Retrieved October 30, 2007, from http://www.aoa.gov/OAA2006/Main_Site/

American Nurses Association. (1994). *Position statement on assisted suicide*. Washington, DC: Author.

American Nurses Association. (2001). *Code of ethics for nurses with interpretive statements*. Washington, DC: Author.

American Nurses Association. (2005a). *ANA code of ethics—2001 updates*. Washington, DC: Author. Retrieved April 26, 2008, from http://www.nursingworld.org/MainMenuCategories/ThePracticeofProfessionalNursing/EthicsStandards/CodeofEthics.aspx

American Nurses Association. (2005b). *Center for ethics and human rights*. Retrieved April 26, 2008, from http://nursingworld.org/MainMenuCategories/ThePracticeofProfessionalNursing/EthicsStandards/CEHR.aspx

Aveyard, H. (2005). Informed consent prior to nursing care procedures. *Nursing Ethics, 12*(1), 19–29.

Coverston, D., & Rogers, S. (2000). Winding roads and faded signs: Ethical decision-making in a postmodern world. *Journal of Perinatal and Neonatal Nursing, 17*(2), 1–11. Retrieved January 24, 2005, from EBSCO.

Crigger, N. J. (2004). Always having to say you're sorry: An ethical response to making mistakes in professional practice. *Nursing Ethics, 11*(6), 568–576.

Ellis, J. R., & Hartley, C. L. (2004). *Nursing in today's world: Trends, issues and management* (8th ed.). Philadelphia: Lippincott Williams & Wilkins.

Esterhuizen, P. (1996). Is the professional code still the cornerstone of clinical nursing practice? *Journal of Advanced Nursing, 23*(1), 25–31.

Falk Rafael, A. R. (1995). Advocacy and empowerment: Dichotomous or synchronous concepts? *Advances in Nursing Science, 18*(2), 25–32. Retrieved January 24, 2005, from EBSCO.

Field, T. S., Mazor, K. M., Briesacher, B., DeBellis, K. R., & Gurwitz, J. H. (2007). Adverse drug events resulting from patient errors in older adults. *Journal of the American Geriatrics Society, 55*(2), 271–276.

Furrow, B. R. (2001). Pain management and provider liability: No more excuses. *Journal of Law, Medicine, and Ethics, 29*, 28–51. Retrieved January 31, 2005, from http://www.painandthelaw.org/mayday/jlme_29.1.php

Hoeman, S. P., & Duchene, P. M. (2002). Ethical matters in rehabilitation. In S. P. Hoeman (Ed.), *Rehabilitation nursing process, application, and outcomes* (3rd ed., pp.28-35). St. Louis: Mosby.

Hoeman, S. P., Duchene, P. M., & Vierlin, J. D. (2007). Ethical and legal issues in rehabilitation nursing. In S. P. Hoeman (Ed.), *Rehabilitation nursing process, application, and outcomes* (4th ed., pp.30-44). St. Louis: Mosby Elsevier.

Hook, K. G., & White, G. B. (2003). *Code for nurses with interpretive statements: An independent study module.* Washington, DC: American Nurses Association. Retrieved January 7, 2009, from http://nursingworld.org/mods/mod580/cecdevers.htm

Kohn, L. T., Corrigan, J., & Donaldson, M. S. (Eds.). (2001). *To err is human: Building a safer healthcare system*. Washington, DC: National Academy Press.

Levine, C. (Ed.). (2000). *Always on call: When illness turns families into caregivers*. New York: United Hospital Fund of New York.

National Quality Measures Clearinghouse. (2005). *Failure to rescue*. Rockville, MD: Agency for Healthcare Research and Quality, U.S. Department of Health and Human Services. Retrieved February 11, 2005, from http://www.qualitymeasures.ahrq.gov/resources/summaryarchive.aspx#611

Oregon Department of Human Services. (1997). *Death with Dignity Act*. Retrieved October 30, 2007, from http://www.oregon.gov/DHS/ph/pas/ors.shtml

Oregon Department of Human Services. (2007). *Summary of Oregon's Death with Dignity Act—2006*. Retrieved October 30, 2007, from http://egov.oregon.gov/DHS/ph/pas/docs/year9.pdf

Quallich, S. A. (2004). The practice of informed consent. *Urologic Nursing, 24*(6), 513–515.

Redman, B., & Fry, S. (1998). Ethical conflicts reported by certified registered rehabilitation nurses. *Rehabilitation Nursing, 23*(4), 179–184.

Sletteboe, A. (1997). Dilemma: A concept analysis. *Journal of Advanced Nursing, 26*(3), 449–454.

SECTION

8

HUMAN DIVERSITY
(Competency 20)

CHAPTER 18

Appreciating Diversity and Enhancing Intimacy

Donald D. Kautz, PhD, RN, CNRN, CRRN-A
Ramesh C. Upadhyaya, PhD, RN, CRRN, MBA

LEARNING OBJECTIVES

At the end of this chapter, the reader will be able to:

- Contrast the meanings of heritage, ethnicity, and nationality.
- Appreciate the diversity of older adults.
- Describe basic health and religious beliefs and health disparities of major ethnic groups in the United States.
- Identify strategies to enhance the care of a diverse elder population.
- Implement strategies to prevent and overcome racism in patients and the health care team.
- Discuss the sexual development of older adults and changes in the sexual response due to aging and chronic illness.
- Identify strategies to overcome vaginal dryness and erectile dysfunction.
- Implement appropriate policies that promote intimacy in community and long-term care settings.
- List strategies to extinguish sexually inappropriate behavior.

KEY TERMS

- Acculturation
- Culture
- Diversity
- Dyspareunia
- Erectile dysfunction (ED)
- Ethnicity
- Heritage
- Human sexual response
- Nationality
- Race
- Racism
- Religion
- Sexuality
- Spirituality

This chapter addresses **diversity** issues in providing holistic nursing care for older adults. Sexual expression and romantic intimacy are viewed as a part of holistic care and also are a major part of this chapter.

DIVERSITY AND HOLISTIC NURSING CARE

Does taking a person's **culture** into consideration matter when providing nursing care? Well, think about it. Do you perform better when you've had enough sleep, or when you're sleep deprived? What does sleep have to do with culture? Do you have certain "bedtime rituals" that you do to prepare for sleep? Do you like to shower before you go to bed? Brush your teeth? Read a book? Watch television? Do you sleep on a certain side of the bed? What happens when something happens to change your routine? Do you have a harder time falling asleep?

Consider what may happen when nurses and other health care providers impose their values and beliefs onto someone from another culture. A growing body of research shows that patients whose culture is taken into consideration have better outcomes than those whose culture is not considered.

What makes one person different from another? Is it physical characteristics, personality, or some combination of the two? It turns out the answer is not as easy as it would seem. Many times it has to do with the definitions we use. The physical differences between people may be a result of normal age-related changes, pathophysiology, gender, or biological variations within a race. But this is only the outward appearance; it represents a small part of the overall picture when it comes to treating the whole person—mind, body, and spirit. What lies underneath the surface is often more complex and requires more assessment and observation than what can be ascertained by a person's outward appearance.

Notable Quotes

"In times of grief and sorrow I will hold you and rock you, and take your grief and make it my own. When you cry, I cry, and when you hurt, I hurt. And together we will try to hold back the floods of tears and despair and make it through the potholed streets of life."

—From a character in *The Notebook* by Nicholas Sparks

One characteristic that must be considered is **heritage**. Heritage encompasses a person's ethnic origin (or ethnicity), nationality, religion, and culture (Spector, 2004). **Ethnicity** (or ethnic origin) refers to what some have called **race**. Ethnically, a person may be, for example, African, European, Asian, or Native American. **Nationality** refers to the geographic location of the person's birth (or the country with which he or she identifies); for example, a person could be born and raised in Italy, but be of Egyptian descent. **Religion** refers to a belief system based on a higher power. This higher power may be monotheistic, as in Islam, where Allah is god, or polytheistic, as in Hinduism, where dozens of gods and goddesses are worshipped. Culture refers to the group to which the person belongs and which influences the person's values and beliefs. Culture may cut across nationality, religion, and ethnicity because culture represents shared beliefs. For example, the elderly represent a culture within the United States, as they do in other countries. People with disabilities are another example of a culture that cuts across other descriptors. Often there is more variation within a particular culture than there is between cultures.

Diversity of Elders

Adults over 65 years old are much more diverse than any other age group, because of the wide range of their life experiences, lifestyles, and health status, and the variations in their socioeconomic status. Although the majority of elders in the United States are presently white and female, this is changing (see Chapter 2). The increasing number of elders of color, and differences in diets, leisure, and health care beliefs present tremendous challenges to nurses. Food is one example. What people eat differs widely: Some elders have tried many different foods throughout their lives, whereas others have limited their diet to a few foods, even though great variety may be readily available. To illustrate, some elders have eaten pork their whole lives, others have avoided it for religious reasons, and still others have avoided pork products with the belief that they are too high in fat. Elders are not alone in these behaviors. The authors recently conducted a diversity exercise with nurses. They were given a list of 20 foods from the menus of restaurants within a one-mile radius of their hospital, but only a few had eaten more than 5–10 items on the list.

Providing food that is consistent with cultural, ethnic, religious, and personal preferences in hospitals and long-term care settings is a tremendous challenge. ElGindy (2004) actually suggests that patients who are in a hospital or nursing home may need to check out, even against medical advice, if the facility is unable to meet their dietary needs. ElGindy makes these recommendations for cultural dietary assessments: Remember that each individual is unique, and that adherence to dietary traditions and guidelines varies. Personal food habits are a part of cultural norms, yet the nurse can recommend subtle changes that can have profound effects on health. For example, switching from regular soy sauce to a low sodium brand is culturally sensitive but cuts salt intake by half. The nurse may need to use pictures of foods to get a clear idea of what a patient likes to eat. To determine how flexible the individual may be in making dietary changes, ask if the patient's special dietary need is a cultural norm, a personal preference, or a religious mandate. The wording a nurse uses may help. For example, Seventh-Day Adventists believe that eating between meals is an undesirable habit; thus, persons with diabetes can be taught to divide their intake among five or six small meals, rather than being told to include a snack. Finally, encouraging patients to perform special customs or religious practices before or after meals may increase the likelihood that they will adhere to treatment-related dietary restrictions.

A key strategy for achieving cultural competence is to learn about different cultural and religious preferences, customs, and restrictions, and then use this knowledge in planning and providing care. In the journal *Minority Nurse*, ElGindy (2004) has written guides to meeting the special dietary needs of those of several faiths, including Jewish, Muslim, Hindu, and Buddhist. When an elder is in the hospital or extended care facility, encourage the family to bring in favorite foods from home, unless there are dietary restrictions that prevent this. Encourage the family to eat together. Hostler (1999) found that bringing in food promoted both family integrity and recovery in families of hospitalized children, and it is likely bringing in food for elders will also promote recovery. Again, remember that food preferences within a cultural group, even within families, vary greatly.

Economic diversity is also great among elders. Some are barely getting by whereas others are among the wealthiest in society (see **Case Study 18-1**). Ensuring that all have adequate food, shelter, and health care has always been a societal problem. The effects of age also differ. Some 60-year-olds who have lived with chronic illness may be frail and disabled, though the majority of persons at this age are active, productive, and independent. Many 80-year-olds are frail, yet a growing number are still active, productive, and independent. The key for nurses is to assess each individual's level of activity, health status, and heritage, and plan care accordingly, rather than relying on age in planning care.

Case Study 18-1

A nurse is in charge of an intercity clinic that serves the uninsured, underinsured, and the "working poor" in a location where the majority of older persons are from minority groups. Getting medications prescribed by the clinic's doctor for those who cannot even afford to put food on their tables is a constant challenge that the nurse in charge wishes to address.

Questions:

1. What resources are available at the local, county, state, and federal levels for such a clinic?
2. How would the nurse begin finding funding sources to help those at the clinic?
3. What is the role of drug representatives and drug companies in clinics such as these regarding providing samples of or free medications?
4. To whom could the nurse go for assistance in addressing the issues in this community?
5. What would the nurse likely see as typical medical problems among this group of older adults?

Another aspect of diversity is religion and faith practices. Again, the elderly are a very diverse group. Some have practiced only one faith for their entire lives, whereas others may have made many changes in a lifelong spiritual quest. Faith communities provide a great deal of support for some elderly. These communities are active in promoting health for elders and in overcoming health disparities.

Health care for elders is also diverse. Those who are wealthy, well educated, and used to having power have access to the best care. Those who are poor, poorly educated, and used to living on the margins of society suffer from health disparities and often have poor access to care.

Health Care Disparities

The second goal of the Healthy People 2010 project is to eliminate race- and ethnicity-based health disparities. In an article examining the 10 largest racial and ethnic disparities for each of five ethnic groups in the United States, Keppel (2007) noted that about half of the 900 objectives of Healthy People 2010 are based on characteristics of persons in the population. The top five for each group are included later in this chapter.

The challenge for nurses is to develop reliable, evidence-based, culturally competent nursing interventions for minority elders. The differences between healthy aging and aging impeded by the clinical manifestations of chronic illnesses and disability are largely due to the adoption of health promotion behaviors and the ability to obtain appropriate medications and treatments. Assisting elders to make healthy decisions and adhere to medication and treatment regimens is addressed in more detail elsewhere in this text; however, the key is to adapt our nursing interventions to make them appropriate for elders of different races and ethnic groups. The American Academy of Nursing (Giger et al., 2007) has developed recommendations to increase the diversity of nurses, assist nurses in providing culturally competent care, and eliminate health disparities in vulnerable populations. Harrison and Falco (2005) advocate that nurses reach out to alleviate human suffering, which is the most significant consequence of racial disparity, by recognizing and studying **racism** and cultivating advocacy based on respect for each client's life choices.

It is likely that as we pay closer attention to the causes of disparities and strategies to eliminate them, we will reframe some of our thinking, as recommended by Dr. Kathleen Fuller, a cultural anthropologist. Fuller, director of AnthroHealth (http://www.AnthroHealth.net), recommends reframing the problem of health disparities from a racial issue to one of a phenotype/environmental mismatch that cuts across current racial groups. Fuller (2007) points out that cultural behaviors and biological variations are rarely based on race, and there really are no biological races. U.S. Census data from 2000 confirm this: 7 million people checked more than one box for race. Focusing on racial disparities ignores the diversity within racial groups and leads us away from the true issue, the higher incidence of diseases in certain individuals. One example Fuller cites is the high incidence of hypertension in people of color in the United States. Fuller points to research suggesting that a significant factor contributing to hypertension is low serum vitamin D levels. In order to activate vitamin D, those with darker pigmented skin, regardless of racial background, need more exposure to ultraviolet B (UVB) radiation than those with lighter skin pigment. Thus, people of color in the United States may need more exposure to UVB radiation or prophylactic doses of vitamin D in order to reduce hypertension and the incidence of myocardial infarctions (MI). Fuller recommends determining the degree of pigmentation in all patients using the Minolta 508d spectrophotometer, which is noninvasive and takes about 3 seconds, rather than asking about racial designation on health care forms. Appropriate treatment would be based on an individual's skin color, the latitude at which they live, their current serum vitamin D level, and their risk for disease. Fuller also makes convincing arguments for reframing the incidence disparities of prostate cancer, low-birth-weight infants, infant mortality, rickets, and melanoma as interactions among degree of skin pigmentation, amount of exposure to UVB radiation, and levels of serum vitamin D.

Characteristics of Five Major Ethnic Groups in the United States

This section of the chapter will briefly explore five major ethnic groups in the United States: European Americans, African Americans, Hispanic Americans, Asian Americans, and Native Americans. Some basic health and religious beliefs of each group will be explored, followed by the top five health disparities for each group. Disparities, according to Keppel (2007), "were measured as the percent difference between each of the other group rates and the rate for the best group" (p. 98), with "all indicators being expressed as adverse events" (p. 97). So, to simplify the discussion, one might consider the disparities discussed here as the most significant health-related differences found among ethnic groups, based on Keppel's research. Brief summaries of culturally sensitive nursing research to promote health in each ethnic group are also discussed in this section.

European Americans

Currently, European Americans constitute the majority of the population in the United States. This demographic is changing, however, and by the year 2050, European Americans will no longer be the prevalent cultural group (Supple & Small, 2006). The majority of European Americans describe themselves as Christian (Nelson-Becker, 2005). Within this sect, European Americans include the two major Christian denominations: Catholics and Protestants. Protestant denominations further fracture into, among others, Lutherans (Scandinavian Americans), Presbyterians (German Americans), Methodists (Scottish Americans), and Episcopalians (Anglo Americans). Of note is that these sects are not hard-and-fast rules; many Irish and Italian Americans are not Catholics, but Protestants; likewise many German and Anglo Americans are Catholic. Furthermore, many of these churches, upon movement to the United States, split off from their parent churches and evolved into nondenominational Christian churches (Kelley, Small, & Tripp-Reimer, 2004). European Americans are less likely to turn to religion or **spirituality** as coping or problem-solving mechanisms. European Americans tend to rely on science to explain health and illness, rather than one's communion with God. European Americans also are more likely to turn to government as the responsible caretaker for the infirm and/or elderly (Walker, Lester, & Joe, 2006).

European Americans generally do not have as close ties to their extended families as other cultural groups within the United States. European Americans tend to be individualistic when it comes to health care, often presenting a stoic attitude about illness, so as not to "be a burden" on others. This is represented by the value system of European Americans as "doers." Upon reaching retirement, European Americans can lose their sense of self-worth (Giger & Davidhizar, 2004). European Americans are more accepting of the paternalistic nature of the health care system, are generally more trusting of authority, and therefore tend to follow the advice of health care providers to engage in more physical and mental activity than other cultural groups within the United States (Njoku, Jason, & Torres-Harding, 2005).

The top five health disparities for European Americans (white non-Hispanic) are 1) smoking by pregnant women, 2) drug-induced deaths, 3) deaths from poisoning, 4) deaths from melanoma, and 5) deaths from chronic lower respiratory disease before age 45 (Keppel, 2007). Notice that only one of these, deaths from melanoma, is a specific concern for older adults. The U.S. health care system is primarily designed to meet the needs of European Americans.

Crespo and Arbesman's (2003) analysis of the differences in factors associated with obesity in different cultural and ethnic groups is an excellent way to emphasize the importance of cultural assessments when providing nursing care. The prevalence of obesity is higher among African American (35%) and Hispanic (33%) women than among European American women (22%). In African Americans and Hispanics, obesity is associated with poverty. It may not be safe to walk or run for exercise in poorer neighborhoods, and there may not be affordable gyms nearby. Poverty is associated with higher fat diets; higher fat foods are less expensive. In African Americans and Hispanics with higher education and higher income levels, obesity levels are similar to European Americans. On the other hand, obesity in European Americans is associated with higher income and less education, or is truly a disease of excess living. In all groups, increased time watching television is associated with obesity. Thus, when intervening with older adults who are obese, it is important to identify specific factors that are contributing to obesity, and make culturally sensitive recommendations to exercise more, reduce fat and calorie intake, and watch television less.

African Americans

As seen in Chapter 2, African Americans make up the second largest minority population in the United States, only recently being overtaken by Hispanics. The majority of African Americans live in the South (54.8%); in the remaining regions of the country, the majority of African Americans live in large metropolitan areas such as New York City, Chicago, Detroit, Philadelphia, and Baltimore (Cherry & Giger, 2004). African Americans' religions vary as much as European Americans, but most African Americans are Protestant (Baptist, Pentecostal, and others). A fair number of African Americans are Muslim, or followers of Islam. It is therefore of vital importance not to generalize about any particular culture, but to inquire about religious beliefs and practices, instead of making assumptions (Nelson-Becker, 2005).

The role of religion and spirituality plays an important part in the African American health and wellness belief system. Often African Americans equate good luck, good fortune, and good health with "being right with God." Therefore, disease and illness can be thought of as being in disfavor with God and incurring His wrath. Likewise, African Americans believe they have less control over their health and well-being than God, and illness and disease are part of "God's plan" (Walker et al., 2006). This is, however, an oversimplification of a much more complex locus of control discussion that is beyond the scope of this chapter.

Despite the systematic destruction of the family unit by 200 years of slavery in the United States, African Americans have much closer ties to their extended families as compared to other cultural groups within the United States. African Americans tend to rely on their close family ties or close neighbors when in need of support rather than turning inward, as with other cultural groups. Along with slavery, other historical injustices, such as segregation and economic disparity, have influenced African Americans' distrust of authority. African Americans are particularly distrustful of health care personnel because of discrimination in medical care and because most authority figures in health care are not African Americans. Wallace et al. (2007) found that the "Tuskegee Syphilis Study continues to influence the relationship of the African American patient and the biomedical community" (p. 722). A study of older, community-dwelling African Americans identified the following categories of coping strategies for chronic health conditions: dealing with it, engaging in life, exercising, seeking information, relying on God, changing dietary patterns, medicating, self-monitoring, and self-advocacy (Loeb, 2006).

Notice the dramatic difference in health disparities for African Americans when compared to those noted earlier for European Americans. The top five for African Americans are 1 and 2) new cases of gonorrhea, 3) congenital syphilis, 4) new cases of AIDS, and 5) deaths due to HIV infection. None of these are even in the top 10 for European Americans. Obviously, as a nation, we are much better at identifying and treating sexually transmitted diseases in European Americans than African Americans. The authors worked with a community housing project that had an outbreak of syphilis and gonorrhea among elderly residents who did not think they were at risk, and thus engaged in unprotected sex. Culturally sensitive educational efforts by African American staff and volunteers quickly controlled the outbreak, which has not reoccurred.

The impact of racism toward African Americans has long been considered one of the factors that contribute to decreased longevity and increases in chronic illnesses. Moody-Ayers, Stewart, Covinsky, and Inouye (2005) studied the prevalence and correlates of perceived societal racism in African American adults age 50 or older with type 2 diabetes mellitus. The investigators found that 92% of the sample experienced social racism, which correlated with fair or poor health. The investigators caution health care providers that day-to-day societal racism may affect patients' trust in health care providers, adherence with medical advice, and self-management of chronic health problems.

Hispanic Americans

Hispanic Americans have recently become the second largest population demographic in the United States, and as a result of immigration and higher than average birth rates, the number of Hispanic Americans (people of Latin descent) is projected to comprise 29% of the U.S. population by the year 2050 (Passel & Cohn, 2008; Supple & Small, 2006). It is for these reasons, and others, that it is important for health care providers to understand the needs of this population and find ways to meet those needs.

Most Hispanic Americans place a high value on family, religion, and community. Hispanic cultures emphasize family interdependence over independence. For this population, self-care is not as important as receiving care in recovery from illness. An individual who becomes ill will turn to the family first before seeking outside health care. The Hispanic culture, especially the elderly, will seek the use of homeopathic remedies in conjunction with religious artifacts before engaging a health care professional. Additionally, direct disagreement with a health care provider is uncommon; the usual response to a decision that the patient or the family disagrees with is silence and noncompliance. Other Hispanic Americans may choose not to seek health care because they, like members of other cultures and religions, feel that their affliction is a punishment for sins. However, a growing number of Hispanic Americans do not seek health care because they do not have access to health care. This could be because they lack health insurance, have communication difficulties, or fear legal ramifications for residing in the country illegally (Gonzalez & Kuipers, 2004; Padilla & Villalobos, 2007).

Most Hispanic Americans are Catholic, but as with most cultures, the role that religion plays in health practices varies greatly from person to person. Those Hispanic Americans who have been **acculturated** to the United States generally accept the scientific theory of health and illness, although many subscribe to a more naturalistic approach. This approach in the Hispanic American culture strives to achieve a balance between "hot" and "cold" within the body. Illnesses are categorized as either hot or cold, and treated with the reciprocal type of substance, found in either medicine or food (Gonzalez & Kuipers, 2004).

The top five health disparities for Hispanic Americans are 1) congenital syphilis, 2) new cases of tuberculosis, 3) new cases of AIDS, 4) exposure to particulate matter, and 5) cirrhosis deaths (Keppel, 2007). Note that all except congenital syphilis affect older adults, and exposure to infectious disease, particulate matter, and liver disease all have increased consequences the longer one's body is exposed and/or not treated.

Diabetes and heart disease are two health problems that have an increased prevalence and mortality in Hispanic Americans. Whittemore (2007) conducted a systematic review of the literature to identify culturally competent interventions for Hispanic adults with type 2 diabetes. In reviewing 11 studies, Whittemore found that providing educational sessions and written materials, in both English and Spanish; employing bilingual Hispanic staff; including family members in an informal atmosphere in health care encounters; incorporating cultural traditions in interventions; developing culturally relevant program literature; and providing fact sheets about risk and potential poor outcomes of chronic conditions such as diabetes will increase the effectiveness of interventions.

Asian Americans

Often immigrants from China, India, the Philippines, Vietnam, Korea, and the Middle East are grouped together as Asian Americans. But to do so not only is a gross oversimplification, but also does an injustice to the ancient histories of these cultures, with recorded history going back 10,000 years (Spector, 2004). The majority of Asian Americans in the United States are Chinese Americans, and this section will briefly cover health and religious practices of the Chinese culture.

Most Asian Americans' health beliefs and practices follow the same trajectory as other cultures within the United States; that is, the more acculturated to Western traditions, the more they move toward the scientific theory of health and illness. Hsiung and Ferrans (2007) identified four Chinese American groups in the acculturation continuum: the most traditional and least acculturated elderly immigrants; less acculturated elderly immigrants of working class, bi-acculturated professionals; and Chinese Americans born and raised in the United States. The most traditional and least acculturated elderly Asian Americans may still practice holistic (naturalistic) medicine and may incorporate this as an adjunct to allopathic (Western) medicine. Some of these herbal supplements may have undesired effects when combined with prescribed medications; therefore, it is vital that all complementary medicine and treatment be taken into consideration in directing care for individuals (Giger & Davidhizar, 2004).

Chinese cultural beliefs are influenced by forms of Buddhism, Confucianism, and Taoism; however, the majority of the influence comes from Confucianism. Confucianism stresses accommodation and avoids confrontation, and heavily influences health beliefs and practices. Confucianism follows a naturalistic perspective, defining health and illness as a balance between the individual and the world around the individual. Individuals are a component of the universe, and it is believed that the individual should strive to be in harmony with the universe in which he or she lives. The basic concept of Chinese medicine is that all things, including the body, are composed of opposing forces called yin and yang. Health is said to depend on the balance of these forces. Chinese medicine focuses on maintaining the yin–yang balance to maintain health and prevent illness. If the balance between yin and yang is broken, it is essential to restore this balance to bring about health. To regain balance, the belief is that the balance between the internal body organs and the external elements of earth, fire, water, wood, and metal must be adjusted.

Treatment to regain balance may involve:

- Acupuncture
- Moxibustion (the burning of herbal leaves on or near the body)
- Cupping (the use of warmed glass jars to create suction on certain points of the body)
- Massage
- Herbal remedies
- Movement and concentration exercises (such as tai chi) (Xu & Chang, 2004)

Some elderly Chinese patients may forgo life-sustaining treatment because of the principle of *ren*. Ren is considered the golden rule of Chinese decision making and is embodied in Confucius's axiom, "Do not do to others what you do not want done to yourself" (Hsiung & Ferrans, 2007, p. 135).

Keppel (2007) lists the top five health disparities for Asian Americans as 1) new cases of tuberculosis, 2) congenital syphilis, 3) no Papanicolaou (Pap) test among females older than 18, 4) exposure to particulate matter, and 5) carbon monoxide exposure. All of these problems except congenital syphilis have an increased impact on adults as they age. Of note is that the lack of Papanicolaou test does not rank in the top 10 for any other racial or ethnic group in the United States. This is an excellent example of the need for culturally sensitive approaches for health promotion measures in Asian Americans, most likely individualized for different subgroups of Asian Americans, as is illustrated by the following studies.

Two recent nursing studies of health promotion interventions to prevent breast and cervical cancer among Asian Americans confirm that nurses need to modify interventions for subgroups of Asian Americans, because the strongest correlations were within the specific subgroups of Chinese, Filipino, Korean, Japanese, or Vietnamese descent; however, there were no correlations with Asian Americans when lumped together in a single group (Kim, Ashing-Giwa, Singer, & Tejero, 2006; Lee-Lin & Menon, 2005). These studies show how important it is to not lump people who may look alike to the European American, when the differences among diverse Asian cultures may be even greater than the differences between European American culture and all Asian cultures.

One example of a nursing study that focused specifically on the needs of a subgroup, Taiwanese Americans, is Suen and Morris's (2006) study of depression. The investigators found depression was underdiagnosed in Taiwanese American older adults, and they recommended the establishment of support groups and health promotion activities at local Taiwan Centers, because many elders go to these centers every day to talk to friends, sing, and participate in leisure activities. The investigators believe that the resulting discussion and sharing will promote mental health and assist in both preventing and treating depression, which often accompanies chronic illness in this population.

Native Americans

There are about 500 different Native American tribes within the United States. Nearly half of these 2.4 million people reside in the western part of the country due to forced migration. The two predominant tribes are the Cherokee and the Navajo, each with more than a quarter million people (Spector, 2004). American Indians did not immigrate to the United States; therefore, the process of acculturation does not apply. In fact, many American Indians' culture is insulated from the rest of the country, either literally (by way of land reservation) or in other ways such as linguistically. For example, the majority of Navajo people speak both English and Navajo, but many speak Navajo alone and require an interpreter when interacting with someone who does not speak Navajo (Hanley, 2004).

Like other cultures throughout the world, Native Americans follow a naturalistic approach to health and illness, believing that health is a balance of the mind, body, and spirit, and illness occurs when there is an imbalance or disharmony with nature (Spector, 2004). Native American religion is centered on legends of sacred spirits that take many forms, some human and some animal. Native American health beliefs and practices are blended with religion, thus carrying a magic facet as well as holistic and naturalistic approaches (Hanley, 2004).

The top five health disparities for Native Americans and Alaska Natives are 1) fetal alcohol syndrome, 2) smoking by pregnant women, 3) alcohol-related motor vehicle deaths, 4) cirrhosis deaths, and 5) new cases of gonorrhea (Keppel, 2007). All of these disparities point to the lack of effective programs to reduce alcohol consumption among those Native American individuals who are at high risk of alcoholism. There continues to be a pressing need for culturally sensitive interventions to address major health problems in Native Americans. The authors are aware of a project in a tribe in Wisconsin to promote walking and a return to a traditional diet, which includes wild rice, venison, trout, and salmon, all harvested locally. The concept is to promote weight maintenance and glycemic control in order to reduce the incidence of diabetes, heart disease, and alcoholism. The prevention of high and low blood sugar in those who are at risk of alcoholism may be an effective prevention strategy. Poor glycemic control is also considered a risk factor for diabetes and heart disease. In a review of cardiovascular research in Native Americans, Eschiti (2005) found only one study, conducted by nurses, that the existing research of other disciplines relies on only a few tribes of the more than 500 tribes in the United States, and very little intervention research. Eschiti recommends that studies focus on the establishment of trust with providers as well as those working in governmental agencies by involving tribal members in all aspects of program design, implementation, and evaluation. Miller and Clements (2006) also call for active partnerships between health care providers and tribal communities to identify the extent of elder abuse and effective treatment measures that are sensitive and responsive to tribal cultures and conditions in order to assist Native Americans in their desire to care for and honor their elders.

Implications for Nursing

A 2002 issue of *Generations* contained an interview with E. Percil Stanford and Fernando Torres-Gil, two leaders in the field of aging who have long focused on diversity. This interview (Kaufman, 2002) contains several points crucial to consider when caring for diverse older adults. The first is that diversity has been mainstream for over a decade in the field of aging, and elders with diverse points of view have long been in leadership positions in the American Society on Aging, the Gerontological Society of America, and AARP. Some minority elders who were once overlooked now have a well-heard voice. The first lesson for nurses here is that to ensure culturally competent care, elders who are being cared for need to have a voice in their care and give regular input into how care is delivered, for themselves and their loved ones. The second point is the need to use well elders as volunteers and as paid staff when providing care and to ensure that they have educational and training opportunities, as well as the support to remain active members of their communities and their health care organizations. Virtually all elders will eventually require some level of assistance or health care. Helping them stay healthy as long as possible and then helping them plan for their own care is key to the financial survival of our health care system. We need to help elders make sound health care decisions early on, before a crisis occurs, and to ensure that all family members are in agreement with the decision. A third point is the need to seek out individuals who are not being served, who are still marginalized, and who lack resources, and to target care to those who really need the care. Not all elders need all resources; the focus needs to be on those who are in the greatest need.

Diversity in the Health Care Team

Traditionally, nurses have been primarily white and female; however, the diversity of the health care teams who care for elders is increasing dramatically, especially in race and ethnicity. These changes will have a profound impact on elder care. In order to ensure quality of care, we must promote diversity while preventing stereotyping, become culturally competent, cope with and overcome racism, overcome language barriers, and learn effective health promotion strategies for those with varying lifestyles. In 1998, the American Nurses Association published a position statement titled *Discrimination and Racism in Health Care*, which is still available at http://www.nursingworld.org. Diversity education for nursing staff should be included as a part of routine educational programs in all schools of nursing and all health care facilities. Harrison and Falco (2005) recommend we understand the importance of folk idiom, kinship bonds, ancestry, and cultural wisdom when teaching nursing and when providing care. They also recommend putting a face on the human suffering of health disparity through imaginative literature and by studying discrimination as clients experience it in health care encounters. Smith and colleagues' (2007) recommendations for teaching physicians about racial and ethnic disparities is an excellent source for nursing educators and students who wish to adapt their ideas to nursing curriculum. Smith and colleagues point out that a first step is to assist health care providers to examine and understand the attitudes, such as mistrust, subconscious bias, and stereotyping, that both patients and practitioners may bring to a clinical encounter.

In 2006 and 2007, much of the nursing literature that outlined ways for nursing staff to promote both morale and quality care when working with a diverse staff came from authors from the United Kingdom, as the British deal with racism in their health care system. Several U.S. authors have also outlined several strategies to include in programs that train nursing staff to be culturally competent. Carol (2007), a regular contributing author in the journal *Minority Nurse*, recommended that all programs include content to address the linguistic needs of patients who speak limited English, as outlined in the National Standards on Culturally and Linguistically Appropriate Services (CLAS) in health care developed by the Office of Minority Health in 2000, as well as a frank discussion of how bias, prejudice, and stereotyping by health care providers may be contributing to lower quality care for some patients. Eshleman and Davidhizar (2006) outlined strategies to encourage cultural competency in an RN to BSN program, and Jacobson, Chu, Pascucci, and Gaskins (2005) provided recommendations for conducting culturally competent research. Shattell (2007) shared a strategy that has been successful in engaging students and faculty through the use of diverse first-person narratives in small interpretive research groups in a psychiatric mental health nursing course. Shattell developed the first-person narratives from previous or current studies. Small groups of 8 to 10 students and 1 to 2 faculty members are given copies of patient interview transcripts stripped of all identifying characteristics, and these are read aloud by volunteers in the group. Reading the conversation aloud is a powerful method of bringing the patient to life over a 2- to 3-hour session in which the faculty members and students share the personal and collective experiences of others.

Williamson (2007) discussed how to provide leadership in a culturally diverse workplace and provides several resources for diverse staff to work together, drawing on individual strengths. Unfortunately, prejudice, poor teamwork, conflict, and low job satisfaction may also occur. In a discussion on communicating with individuals from other cultures, Williamson pointed out that two key issues to keep in mind, especially when working with those who speak English as a second language, is to be sure yes really means yes, and to ensure that communication is still occurring when someone uses a nonconfrontational communication style. When people whose English is poor are asked whether they understand or whether they will do something, they may say "yes" even though they really mean "no," because they want to be polite, or not offend, or not call attention to themselves. They may use nonconfrontational communication, believing it is better to say yes and go along, than to say no. Staff working together can ask each other to repeat what is expected or being taught, and ensure that additional, nonthreatening opportunities are made available to raise concerns or objections at a later time.

Covert Racism in the Health Care Team

The ANA's statement on discrimination and racism notes that "Discrimination and racism continue to be a part of the fabric and tradition of American society and have adversely affected minority populations, the health care system in general, and the profession of nursing" (ANA, 1998). Although more covert than in earlier decades, racism still occurs in health care settings, resulting in health care disparities for minority patients and a difficult working environment for minority health care staff. Policies to prevent racism will diminish the overt expression of racist comments and actions among staff, but they do not address the underlying need to appreciate and increase diversity in the health care team. In the authors' view, policies alone will not prevent or overcome racism, and even in those trying to become more aware, racist attitudes emerge.

The journal *Minority Nurse* regularly addresses the subject of racism among staff. In one article, Carol (2005) recommended that when a coworker makes a culturally insensitive remark and a heated exchange takes place, managers need to be informed. Later, when those involved have cooled down, the situation can be discussed with the manager present. A sincere apology may be all that is needed, and this may prevent further insensitive behaviors. If culturally insensitive remarks continue, counseling needs to occur.

Nursing staff working on a diverse team need to regularly explore ways to maximize each other's strengths. One-on-one efforts may be the only way we can prevent or overcome covert racism and stereotyping and become culturally competent.

Racist Comments from Patients

There are few mentions in the nursing literature about elderly patients who make racist comments toward staff from different ethnic groups. However, anecdotal reports by staff reveal that some patients appear to lose their inhibitions as they age, and those with dementia may be especially prone to making racist comments. Redirecting patients and telling them that the comments are inappropriate may be helpful in modifying the behavior. One group of personal care aides used the strategy of "giving themselves a time out," and coming back later to provide care. Minority nurses who have "been there" also suggest trying to understand the patient's intent. Racist remarks may occur because the patient is confused, frustrated, and feeling vulnerable, and is unable to think of anything else to say (Carol, 2005).

Effective strategies for preventing racist comments have not been tested through research, and as noted previously, the problems are rarely mentioned in the literature, nor are they brought up by staff. The first step for a staff member who experiences a racist comment is to report the comment to the nurse manager, who can later discuss the inappropriateness of the comments with the patient (Carol, 2005). Just as effective strategies have been identified to reduce residents' behavioral manifestations of dementia, including fighting and resisting taking a bath, strategies can be developed to extinguish racist comments.

Providing Culturally Competent Care for Culturally Diverse Patients

Walsh (2004) has developed a plan of care, based on NANDA nursing diagnoses, that is culturally competent. The care plan focuses on communication, health maintenance, health education, nutrition, and family coping. Strategies are briefly summarized in this section and supplemented with additional ideas. All of these strategies need to be studied further by nurses working with the elderly (**Figure 18-1**).

If a client speaks a foreign language, or is unable to speak, assess for the need for and provide an interpreter to ensure that the patient and family will be able to communicate their needs and understand instructions, and use resources that are printed in the patient's and family's dominant language. Also use alternative communication methods, such as sign language and printed pictures of basic needs. Additionally, laminate one or two pages of common questions and appropriate responses in both English and the patient's dominant language that nursing staff and patients can refer to. Electronic hand-held English and foreign language dictionaries that actu-

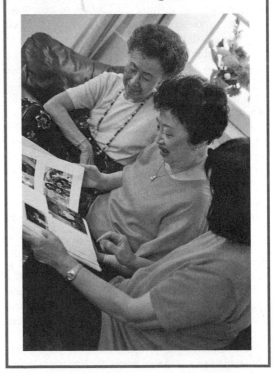

FIGURE **18-1** **Nurses should be sensitive to ethnic and cultural differences among families.**

ally speak the words may be helpful. Language classes could be made a requirement both in nursing schools and in practice settings for all staff. The Joint Commission Web site (http://www.jointcommission.org) contains several recommended strategies that 60 hospitals across the country have implemented to provide quality health care to culturally and linguistically diverse patient populations (Wilson-Stronks & Galvez, 2007).

Health maintenance and health education efforts by staff, especially efforts to change dietary habits, may be hindered by cultural patterns of dominant and minority populations. For example, the practice of encouraging children of all cultures to "eat everything on the plate" has contributed to obesity in Americans. Nursing staff can assess for unhealthy patterns and religious or cultural beliefs that support unhealthy patterns, then assist patients to adopt new behaviors consistent with their cultural and religious beliefs. For example, encourage clients to replace traditional foods that are high in calories and fat with other foods that are also traditional but lower in fat. A traditional food of Southern whites and blacks is "greens" (collard greens, mustard greens, turnip greens, and kale) cooked in bacon grease or pork fatback. Substituting a low-salt chicken broth or ham bouillon and a few pieces of low-fat meat will create a similar flavor but significantly cut the calories, fat, and salt. Greens are a great source of both vitamins and antioxidants, and cooked in this manner, they are a healthy dietary choice.

Family coping may be compromised in any health care setting if the family feels a lack of privacy, feels that staff members do not respect their spiritual beliefs, or feels unwelcome. Nurses can assess the effects of a patient's illness on the family and encourage families to participate in care. Religious and cultural requests should be honored whenever possible. By being sensitive to a family's typical patterns and providing support, as well as referring the family to other appropriate support services, the nurse can aid the family in providing care to the patient while in the hospital or long-term care setting, and in caring for the patient at home after discharge.

BOX 18-1 Research Highlight

Aim: To test the effectiveness of an intervention to reduce the uncertainty of diabetes management.

Methods: Researchers conducted a randomized controlled trial with 68 African Americans over 50 with diabetes. The experimental group received weekly phone calls for 4 weeks, lasting from 10 minutes to an hour, in which an African American nurse practitioner answered their concerns. The control group received the usual care of regular visits for primary and specialty care, but no telephone interventions.

Findings: Those in the treatment group showed an increase in cognitive reframing of their diabetes, increased problem-solving skills regarding their diabetes, and increased diabetes knowledge. However, only the increase in problem-solving skills was correlated with a reduction in uncertainty.

Application to practice: Teaching problem-solving skills and assisting patients to apply these skills may be the most useful tools health care providers can give their patients, especially older African American women, to reduce the burden of managing a chronic illness.

Source: Amoako, E., & Skelly, A. H. (2007). Managing uncertainty in diabetes: An intervention for older African-American women. *Ethnicity and Disease, 17*, 515–521.

Providing Spiritually Competent Care for Spiritually Diverse Patients

Providing spiritually competent care goes hand in hand with providing culturally competent care. Spirituality is an important and essential component of culture, and it bears special mention here. Religion and spirituality are commonly used interchangeably, but they are not the same. Religion is an organized worship or specific faith to which a person subscribes, whereas spirituality is a broad term referring to feelings of being connected with something higher than oneself, often without wishing to be called "religious."

For many older adults, spirituality is an important part of their lives and family. Schmidt (2004), summarizing research findings on spirituality in health, concluded several factors are related to spirituality in older adults. First, "Spirituality is related to a sense of well-being in older adults" (p. 308). Patients may believe that an illness or disability is a punishment from God, or that God has deserted them (Gaskamp, Sutter, Meraviglia, Adams, & Titler, 2006; Vitek, Rosenzwig, & Stollings, 2007). Further, a positive relationship exists between emotional wellbeing and self-transcendence (Schmidt, 2004).

Nurses are responsible for finding out each patient's spiritual practices and preferences as part of a holistic plan of care. Meraviglia, Adams, and Titler (2006) have developed an evidence-based guideline for promoting spirituality in the older adult.

The patient and family members may be excellent sources of information. Older persons should always be asked if they wish their spiritual leader or adviser to be included in the interdisciplinary team or notified of hospitalization. Local churches, parishes, or synagogues can be helpful in locating resources and spiritual support for those with spiritual beliefs different from the nurse's own. Books and Web sites can provide additional insights, although the patient, if able, will provide the most accurate insights into what is needed to provide competent spiritual care. Spiritual care takes on particular significance at the end of life and is discussed further in Chapter 24.

Taking Lifestyle into Account When Promoting Health

A final component of promoting healthy lifestyle practices to diverse groups is taking into account lifestyles that are very diverse. (The topic of health promotion is addressed in detail in other chapters.) Considering the diversity of lifestyles is key in planning care. Some older adults have always exercised and will continue to do so if they can find a way to continue, despite the effects of aging and changes due to chronic illness. For example, those who have always been active but now have severe arthritis pain or mobility limitations may attend a water aerobics class if the class is reasonably priced and conducted at a convenient time, and transportation is provided. Chair aerobics may be another option. However, motivating someone who has never or only sporadically exercised will require intensive efforts, possibly on a daily basis, for many weeks, with continued monitoring and motivating for months until the change becomes a habit and the older person can see a real difference in how he or she feels.

The importance of patient adherence to medications and diet in order to prevent or slow down the complications of chronic illnesses is well documented. The key is for nursing staff to individualize the plan of care, periodically check to be sure the plan is working, and make adjustments as needed. Continued support, either by other elders making the same change or by health care workers, may be necessary until the changes become established in the elder's routine.

ENHANCING SEXUAL INTIMACY

A basic human need of people of all ages is intimacy with others. Loneliness, loss, and lack of meaningful social relationships have been addressed in other chapters in this text. This chapter is designed to assist the nurse in enhancing romantic intimacy and sexual function in older adults. Those over 50 are a very diverse group, and when it comes to romantic intimacy and sexual expression, they are probably more diverse than any other age group.

Despite decades of research showing that older adults want to discuss intimacy and sexual concerns (Bauer, McAuliffe, & Nay, 2007; Higgins, Barker, & Begley, 2006; Magnan, Reynolds, & Galvin, 2006), these needs continue to be ignored by health care professionals, for several reasons. Sex is not seen as a priority for either the patient or the provider, and sexual concerns have not traditionally been addressed in health care encounters. As nurses, we do not see any consequences to not addressing sexual concerns. **Sexuality** is seen as separate from health care concerns, rather than integral to quality of life. Anxiety and fear of embarrassment prevent both patients and nurses from bringing up sexual concerns. Further, we fear that we may not have the resources to assist patients to overcome sexual problems.

Most sexual concerns that result from aging or chronic health problems are within the realm of nursing practice (Kautz, 2007; McAuliffe, Bauer, & Nay, 2007; Mick, 2007). Yet instead of helping, we may contribute to sexual dysfunction by ignoring the underlying health problems that lead to sexual problems. For example, urge or stress incontinence in women may lead to vaginal infections and **dyspareunia** or painful intercourse; in addition, the woman or her partner may be turned off by the smell. Yet hospital nurses rarely ask about this type of incontinence when a patient is admitted. Acute respiratory infections, abdominal surgery, and mobility limitations following surgery may all lead to temporary urge or stress incontinence, but nurses do not routinely warn patients about this possibility, or treat or refer those with problems. Sending a patient home with an indwelling Foley catheter will certainly interfere with sexual intercourse. Teaching a woman to tape the catheter up on her abdomen and wear some type of t-shirt to prevent the catheter from rubbing during intercourse, or to wear a crotchless teddy or crotchless panties, will keep the catheter out of the way. Men can fold the catheter back over an erect penis, and then put on a condom. Partners report not being able to feel the catheter during intercourse, and ejaculation will occur unimpeded around the catheter. Both of these techniques have been recommended for decades, and they are not thought to increase the chances of urinary tract infection (Cournan, Kautz, & Conrad, 2007). Yet again, nurses regularly fail to teach clients who are discharged with catheters these effective and safe techniques.

We also miss many opportunities to assist our clients in overcoming problems. Most health promotion strategies have the potential to make a positive impact on sexual relationships and sexual function. Quitting smoking, limiting fat in the diet, losing weight, and exercising all may reverse the sexual changes that occur due to aging. If our patients realize that heightened intimacy and regained sexual function may result from these lifestyle changes, they may be more motivated to make the changes.

Sexuality and Quality of Life

In 2004, AARP conducted a survey with 1,682 respondents, whose average age was 61 years. The majority of participants were non-Hispanic whites. AARP (2005) found that sexuality was an essential part of the life of those 45 or older. Approximately two-thirds of the participants were married or living with a partner, and most had been with their partner for over 10 years. Approximately one-third reported sexual intercourse once a week or more often. Robinson and Molzahn (2007) found that satisfaction with personal relationships, health status, and sexual activity strongly contributed to quality of life in a sample of 426 older adults, regardless of gender, marital status, and education. These studies add to the evidence that intimacy and sexuality are important regardless of age.

Romantic Relationships in the Elderly

Elders differ greatly in their romantic relationships. Some older adults have been in the same romantic relationship for 50 years and have developed a profoundly deep relationship. (See **Box 18-2** in which Tim, an 81-year-old man, and Teresa, a 79-year-old woman, discuss how they feel about their 50-year relationship.)

Some people become involved in a romantic relationship for the first time after retiring. Indeed, Aleman's (2003) ethnographic study shows romance may be a key part of older adults' identities as men and women. Some older adults have been married many times; others not at all. Some have had literally hundreds of partners over their lifetime; others only a few, others one, and still others none. Some were nuns and priests or celibate for other reasons, and then gave up being celibate in order to be in a romantic relationship. Others became nuns or priests or otherwise became celibate after being married when younger. May–September relationships also occur, and an elder may have a partner who is 30 or even 40 years younger. Some elders have been gay or straight for their whole

BOX 18-2 Tim and Teresa

Tim (81)

"I think she feels about me just about the same way I feel about her. I'm sure I come first in her life and I'm sure she's first in my life. It's always been that way. She was the girl that I wanted. I got her and I still want her. Both of us try to please each other. One of the most important things in a marriage is a connection. That if you do [have a connection] show your relationship in love and with expressions of love. We say it every day, two or three times. I love you."

Teresa (79)

"I couldn't live without him. I like to know where he is every minute. I like to touch him, I like him by me in bed. I like him. I just like him. Tim married for keeps and so did I. We're always together, and most of the time either holding hands or he has his arm around me or I have my hand on his knee. And there's not just one, it's not just Teresa, and it's not just Tim, it's Teresa and Tim."

Source: Kautz, D. D. (1995). The maturing of sexual intimacy in chronically ill, older adult couples. (Doctoral dissertation, University of Kentucky). *Dissertation Abstracts International* (UMI Order #PUZ9527436), 55.

lives; others are bisexual and were in gay or lesbian relationships when younger, then later got married and had children. The opposite is true as well. The 2004 movie *De-Lovely* about Cole Porter portrayed the passion of his homosexual relationships during his long-lasting and loving heterosexual marriage.

Gender identity may be an issue that a man or woman struggles with all his or her life, and then acts on the desire to become the opposite gender when older. A poignant example is a man who had transsexual surgery at 74 (Docter, 1985). When asked why he had not pursued the change earlier, he said that he was married to the love of his life for decades, and if she had known that he wanted to be a woman, it would have crushed her. Several years after her death, he had the surgery and lived out his last 3 years as a woman.

As a society, we continually try to come to terms with the diversity of romantic relationships. As nurses, remaining nonjudgmental will ensure that our care includes and is respectful of those who are most important to our patients, regardless of whether we believe their romantic relationships to be healthy or morally or politically correct. Indeed, excluding the love or loves of a patient's life when the person is ill or dying may potentiate complications or hasten death, while including the love may speed recovery. We need to ask, "Who should I call?" rather than asking about marital status. Unfortunately, those who are most important to our patients may stay away out of fear or unease when their partner is admitted to a health care facility. Nurses have a unique opportunity to be welcoming to those our patients love.

The loss of one's romantic partner is common for older adults through divorce and death. However, the sexual loss is overlooked by most of society. Research on grieving completely ignores how people who lose a lifelong romantic partner adjust to the loss of sex and what we as health professionals can do to assist them in coping with and overcoming their loss. Of course, not all experience grief; the last years of a long-term relationship may have been sexless and filled with anger and pain. Nevertheless, nurses need to assess for the loss of intimacy and sex, acknowledge the loss, and listen to our patients as they express grief and anger.

Sexual Development in Older Adults

Contrary to what some think, adults continue to develop sexually throughout their lives. Chronic illnesses have the potential to affect sexual function, and those who are older who continue to have sex have to adapt to many changes. Most adults who are now over 65 were raised not to talk about sex, and they may not talk with their partners about their sexual desires or preferences. They may see this silence as a way of protecting their partner, even though the silence results in loss of intimacy. The oldest among us have lived through several sexual revolutions. The first was in the roaring twenties, when women gained the right to vote and gained a great deal of sexual freedom. The second came shortly after World War II, when Kinsey published *Sexuality in the Human Male* in 1948 and *Sexuality in the Human Female* in 1952. The third was in the 1960s and early 1970s, with the advent of the birth control pill and legalization of abortion. A fourth revolution occurred with the discovery of HIV, which led to the promotion of safe sex and the use of condoms (**Box 18-3**). Some might argue that another sexual revolution is occurring now due to the advent of better treatments for **erectile dysfunction (ED)** and vaginal dryness.

Triphasic Human Response and Changes with Aging

Kaplan (1990), building on early work by Masters and Johnson, identified a triphasic model of **human sexual response**. The three phases are desire, excitement, and orgasm. The desire phase includes the sensations that move one to seek sexual pleasure. Sexual desire is probably stimulated by endorphins; pleasure centers are stimulated by sex, whereas pain inhibits sexual desire. Love is a powerful stimulus to sexual desire. The excitement phase primarily occurs due to myotonia, or increased muscle tone and vasodilation of the genital blood vessels. In men the penis becomes erect. In women the vagina becomes lubricated, the clitoris and vagina become longer and wider, and the labia minora extend outward. Sexual excitement is

BOX 18-3 Research on Older Adults with HIV

- People over 50 comprise over 30% of the people living with HIV, largely due to the success of anti-HIV drugs (HAART), which increase the quality of life and life expectancy of those with HIV.
- Heterosexual sex is the dominant mode of HIV transmission in older adults.
- African American and Hispanic women report higher levels of risk-taking behaviors.
- The poor make up a disproportionate number of those with HIV.
- Elders may not reveal risky behaviors that are socially unacceptable.
- Depression is undertreated in older adults with HIV infection.
- Comorbid conditions (heart disease, arthritis, hypertension, diabetes), normal aging, and age-related changes in drug absorption and distribution may increase adverse drug reactions, drug interactions, and mortality among those with HIV.

Nursing strategies:

- Identify those at risk and provide referrals, social support, and educational materials.
- Target HIV prevention efforts to older adults.
- Increase public education to reduce HIV stigma, homophobia, and ageism in health care.
- Promote more qualitative and quantitative research on elders and HIV.

controlled by the sympathetic nervous system, and fear will inhibit sexual excitement. The orgasm phase is a climactic release of the genital vasodilation and myotonia of the excitement phase. Orgasm is an automatic spinal reflex response. Typically sexual problems can be classified as either desire, excitement, or orgasm phase disorders, or combinations of the three.

Changes in sexual response have for decades been considered normal consequences of aging. Desire may or may not change with aging; levels of desire may remain the same throughout life. However, both men and women experience changes in excitement with age. Achieving an erection may require more direct stimulation and take longer, and the erection may be softer. Ejaculation may not be as forceful, and it may not occur with every sexual encounter. Vaginal lubrication is often decreased, and women find the need for more direct stimulation. Orgasms for women include uterine contractions, and changes in the uterus may change the way an orgasm feels.

Elders differ greatly in their response to these changes. Some couples adapt by increased genital fondling and caressing, taking more time, and paying more attention to each other's needs. Sex may be better than when they were younger. Other couples may welcome an end to sex. Still others may transcend the need for sex and actually become closer (Kautz, 1995). If an elder abstains from sex for months to years when in a sexless relationship or due to loss of a sexual partner, desire will eventually decrease. This loss of sexual desire has been thought to be permanent; however, there are anecdotal reports that when a person who has not been involved in a sexual relationship for many years meets a new partner, desire will return. When those who have stopped having sex for many years start with a new partner, some regain erectile function and vaginal lubrication after several weeks of manual or oral genital stimulation. Still others may seek help from their health care provider, which has led to what some call the Viagra revolution, or what MacDougall (2006) described as a remaking of the "real-man."

Vaginal Dryness and Erectile Dysfunction (ED)

The decreased ability of a man to achieve and maintain an erection and the decreased ability for a woman to achieve vaginal lubrication have, for decades, been considered normal consequences of aging (Ebersole, Hess, Touhy, Jett, & Luggen, 2007). As with most changes associated with aging, changes in sexual function may begin as early as age 40, and they occur in almost every adult by age 80. In a recent study (Lindau et al., 2007) with a diverse sample of 3,005 adults ages 57 to 85, several problems were identified. Among women, 43% complained of low desire, 39% complained of vaginal dryness, and 34% had problems with orgasm. Erectile dysfunction (ED) was the most common problem among men (37%). Yet some have estimated that less than 50% of men (Steggall, 2007) and women seek treatment (Malatesta, 2007), either because of embarrassment or because they are not bothered by the problems. Some may not discuss the issue with their partners.

ED and vaginal dryness are also associated with diabetes, heart disease, hypertension, and arthritis (Malatesta, 2007; Steggall, 2007). Current recommendations for the therapeutic management of ED and vaginal dryness include stopping smoking, drinking only a moderate amount of alcohol, exercising more, and reducing obesity, especially belly fat. The physiologic rationale for this is that smoking, obesity, and a sedentary lifestyle increase atherosclerosis in genital blood vessels, and there is excellent evidence that stopping smoking, losing weight, and doing aerobic exercises reverse this process. Vaginal dryness in women is the physiologic correlate of ED in men, and thus it is possible that the same illnesses and lifestyle habits are correlated with vaginal dryness in women.

The introduction of sildenafil (Viagra) in 1998, and more recently vardenafil (Levitra) and tadalafil (Cialis) have changed the norms for sexual dysfunction. The constant barrage of ads in print media and junk mail, on television, and through Internet providers such as AOL and MSN imply that ED is common, almost expected, and the norm is to seek treatment. Twenty years ago, ED and vaginal dryness may have been a private matter for a couple; however, it is now literally impossible for couples to escape these ads. Ads put pressure on men and women to seek treatment who otherwise might not have considered treatment or not thought the problem was important. In addition, a woman may not want sex anymore, but she may go along when the man seeks treatment because she believes that whether or not they have sex is the man's decision (Kautz, 1995).

Traditionally, vaginal dryness has been treated with lubricants or the oral or cream form of estrogen. Although there are no medications for women that are direct corollaries of Viagra, Levitra, and Cialis, women are bombarded with ads to relieve vaginal dryness and increase sexual desire with hormonal medications and nutritional/natural supplements. There are also constant ads for nutritional supplements and natural remedies for erectile dysfunction.

Clinical literature has long recommended that maintaining a healthy lifestyle will lead to more satisfying sexual relationships. Many reputable Web sites, maintained by health care organizations including the Mayo Clinic and Dr. Dean Ornish, and self-help groups such as the Diabetes and Heart Associations, advocate healthy behaviors as a first step in overcoming problems with erections and vaginal dryness. Books such as *A Lifetime of Sex* (George & Caine, 1998), *Sex over 50* (Block & Bakos, 1999), and *The Good Mood Diet: Feel Great While You Lose Weight* (Kleiner, 2007) recommend aerobic exercise, a low fat diet, and stopping smoking as ways to improve sexual performance for both men and women. Nurses can focus patient education on the adoption of healthy behaviors as one step in overcoming sexual dysfunction. Because both erectile dysfunction and vaginal dryness may be early signs of hypertension, heart disease, dementia, or diabetes (Lewis, Rosen, Goldstein, & Consensus Panel of Health Care Clinician Management of Erectile Dysfunction, 2003), all patients should be told to see their physician for problems with erectile dysfunction or vaginal dryness to ensure that there are no underlying problems and to explore all treatment options.

One approach to adopting healthy behaviors to prevent or alleviate sexual dysfunction is the popular *South Beach Diet* by Agatston (2003). One of the diet's claims to fame is the loss of belly fat first. Belly fat, especially a waist of over 40 inches in either men or women, has been associated with both erectile dysfunction and vaginal dryness. Loss of belly fat, when combined with exercise, is an effective treatment for erectile dysfunction (McCoid, 2007) in men and vaginal dryness in women (Malatesta, 2007). Loss of belly fat is recommended in the clinical literature, on reputable Web sites, and in books such as *In Bed with the Food Doctor, Eat Your Way to Better Sex and Better Sleep* (Edgson & Marber, 2001) and *The Better Sex Diet Book* (Fischer, 2002) as a way to increase erectile ability in men and vaginal lubrication in women. Similarly, adopting a Mediterranean diet, which also decreases belly fat, has been shown to increase erectile ability (Giugliano, Giugliano, & Espositio, 2006).

Although studies have examined the effectiveness of Viagra in improving both erectile function and quality of life in men, little is known about couples' experiences with these medications. Men receive the prescription for Viagra, but it is possible that women may be the ones taking the medication. Researchers are now beginning to study the effectiveness of Viagra in women (Basson, McInnes, Smith, Hodgson, & Koppiker, 2002). And, Dr. Irwin Goldstein, director of the Institute of Sexual Medicine at Boston University School of Medicine, recently suggested that women use Viagra for vaginal dryness. It is also unclear whether couples use lubricants during intercourse to help the man achieve an erection through stimulation or to assist the woman to overcome vaginal dryness. Finally, the differences in views and experiences of men and women are unknown. Most studies of Viagra have only examined the men taking it, not their partners. One study (Potts, Gavey, Grace, & Vares, 2003) noted a dearth of information on the perspectives and experiences of women whose partners take Viagra and found that there were several detrimental effects for women when their partners took Viagra.

Promoting Sexual Function in Community-Dwelling Elders

Nurses can have a tremendous impact in assisting elders who reside in the community and wish to maintain sexual function in spite of a myriad of health problems and physical limitations due to aging. Those who wish to maintain an active sex life will need to learn to overcome and compensate for the changes. Articles have been written by nurses to assist clients to overcome sexual problems due to stroke (Kautz, 2007), heart and lung disease (Steinke, 2005), and the sexual problems of psychotropic medications taken to treat depression

(Higgins, 2007). Whatever the underlying cause(s), the three major obstacles to sexual intimacy that elders need to overcome are fatigue, pain, and finding comfortable positions for giving and receiving of pleasure. These obstacles may occur for either men or women, and for either one partner or both. However, there are practical ways to help overcome these problems.

Overcoming Fatigue and Pain

Overcoming fatigue and pain is essential to feeling desire and having the stamina to give and receive pleasure. Fatigue and pain are addressed in detail elsewhere in this text. Common ways to overcome fatigue are to plan for sex when rested, which is often in the morning. Kautz (1995) and others have found that elders who continue to have sex tend to have sex in the morning. Another key factor is to plan one's activities to save some time and energy for pleasure.

Pain is a hallmark of aging. Arthritis and other chronic illnesses have a chronic pain component that lasts until one dies. Most pain management strategies leave some residual pain, which may interfere with sexual desire and sexual excitement. The irritability, fatigue, and depression that accompany chronic pain can also have an impact on a couple's sexual relationship. Recommendations include planning for sex at a time when the pain is at its lowest level, often mid-morning for those with rheumatoid arthritis, or when pain medications have their peak action. Incorporating massage, a hot bath for chronic arthritic pain, or cold packs for acute inflammation, or using an electric massager or vibrator may relax sore muscles, relieve stiffened joints, and, when done with a partner, stimulate sexual excitement. Women may focus the water jets from a hot tub on their clitoris, and both men and women may use the vibrator for sexual stimulation. Anecdotal reports from those with arthritis suggest that the relaxing effects of these pain relief strategies and orgasm actually relieve chronic pain for many hours. This effect is thought to be due to endorphin release during the relaxing treatment and sexual stimulation.

Adopting New Positions and Learning New Techniques for Lovemaking

Because of limitations from disease and disability, some elders need to adopt new positions for lovemaking. **Table 18-1** lists resources that give suggestions for comfortable positions as well as additional information about sex and intimacy with specific chronic illnesses. The illustrations in **Figure 18-2** provide examples of positions for intercourse when adapting to chronic illness or disability. **Table 18-2** lists resources where couples can obtain educational materials and products through reputable sex education Web sites. Two books written to assist older couples with specific chronic illnesses in overcoming clinical manifestations interfering with intimacy and sexual function are:

- Silverburg, C., Kautfman, M., & Odette, F. (2003). *The Ultimate Guide to Sex and Disability: For All of Us Who Live with Disabilities, Chronic Pain and Illness*, published by Cleis Press.
- Corn, L. (2001). *The Great American Sex Diet: Where the Only Thing You Nibble on Is Your Partner*, published by William Morrow.

BOX 18-4 Sexuality and Alzheimer's Disease: Can the Two Go Together?

In an article in *Nursing Forum*, Tabak and Shemesh-Kigli (2006) examine the ethical issue of sexual relations in nursing homes among those who are demented. The authors demonstrated that staff is often untrained and may be confused about patient/resident rights related to sexual relations within a nursing home. Two case studies are used to illustrate the dilemmas confronting nurses. Recommendations are given for nurses, the nursing profession, owners of nursing homes, and those making policy.

TABLE 18-1 Resources for Information and Comfortable Positions for Intercourse

- *Being Close. COPD and Intimacy*. Available from: http://lungline.njc.org
- *Chronic Low Back Pain and How It May Affect Sexuality*. Available from: http://ukhealthcare.uky.edu/patiented/booklets.htm
- *Sex and Arthritis*. Available from: http://www.orthop.washington.edu
- Sex and cancer (several Web articles by American Cancer Society). Available from: http://www.cancer.org
- *Sex After Stroke*. Available from: http://www.strokeassociation.org
- *Intimacy and Diabetes*. Available from: http://www.netdoctor.co.uk

FIGURE 18-2 These positions may be used by men and women when either or both have limited endurance, COPD, hip or knee replacement, stroke. Those with GERD may find sitting in the chair will not exacerbate their symptoms.

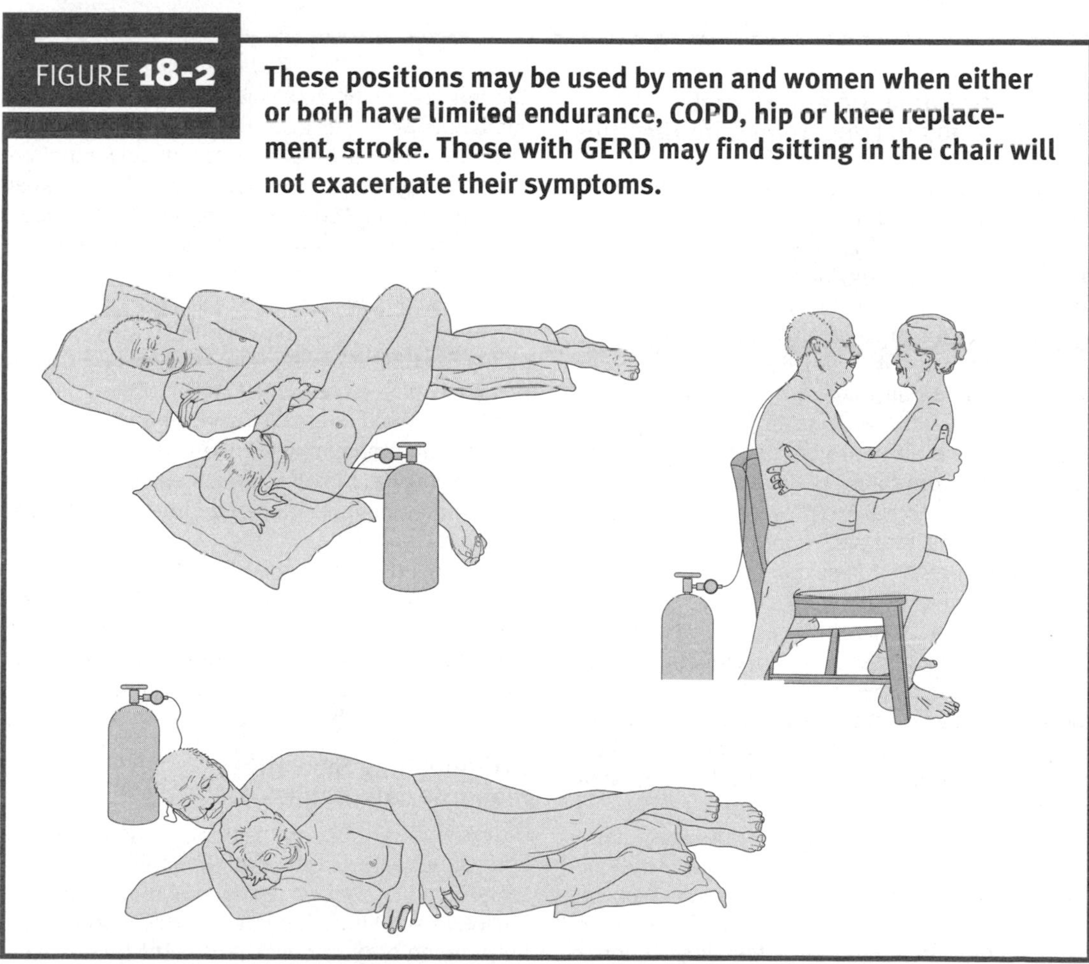

TABLE 18-2 Web Links: Sex Education Web Sites

The following are a few professional Web sites that are highly recommended by the authors for older people to obtain sex education materials. Reassure older adults these are legitimate sex education Web sites and are not "porno sites."

- http://www.hivwisdom.org (HIV Wisdom for Older Women)
- http://www.womenshealth.org (Estronaut: A Forum for Women's Health)
- http://www.erectile-dysfunction-impotence.org
- http://marriage.about.com (About.com: Marriage)
- http://www.sexualhealth.com (Sexual Health Network)
- http://www.4woman.gov (National Women's Health Information Center, contains information on sexuality and disability for women)

Promoting Romantic and Sexual Relationships in Long-Term Care Facilities

Another issue that is rarely addressed in the literature is intimacy and sex among elders residing in long-term care facilities. Barriers exist in virtually all facilities, including lack of privacy and door locks, lack of queen size beds, and literally lack of opportunities for romance. Inability to leave a facility overnight without "losing the bed" prevents couples who have had long-term relationships from getting away for even one night. Although it is important for staff to protect patients from sexual abuse and ensure safety, policies and environmental design go overboard to prevent intimacy. Recent studies confirm that staff continue to be uncomfortable with residents' sexual behavior (Bouman, Arcelus, & Benbow, 2006; Roach, 2004). A timeless story of love in a nursing home, *The Notebook* by Nicholas Sparks (1999), shows us what is possible if nursing staff respect the rights and privacy of those who have entrusted us with the last years of their lives. Some staff may actually promote romance and sex in long-term care, but they do not reveal these efforts for fear of reprisal.

The American Medical Directors Association (AMDA) of long-term care facilities has developed policies that are available on the AMDA Web site, *Caring for the Ages*, at http://www.amda.com/caring/february2002/sex.htm. Messinger-Rapport, Sandhu, and Hujer (2003) provide guidelines for sex in the nursing home, taking into account the issues of what to do if a resident is cognitively impaired, the health needs of the residents, and how to keep the staff informed so that the privacy of the couple can be maintained. The authors recommend the video *Freedom of Sexual Expression: Dementia and Resident Rights in Long Term Care Facilities*, developed by the Hebrew Home for the Aged, a facility that is nationally known for its policies promoting intimacy between residents. (Their current policies can be obtained at http://www.hebrewhome.org.) This film and many others on a wide range of topics on aging, including intimacy and sexuality, are available through Terra Nova Films, http://www.terranova.org.

Evidence-based practice guidelines that balance safety with the lifelong need for intimacy are needed. The need to be touched and held by someone who loves us, and the need to feel loved, not just cared for, does not diminish with age, or with physical or cognitive impairment (Edwards, 2004).

Extinguishing Sexually Inappropriate Behavior

Unfortunately, nursing staff may sometimes be confronted with an older adult, either a man or a woman, who displays sexually inappropriate behavior. Most of the incidents reported involve men, but women may display these behaviors as well.

Sexually inappropriate behaviors include inappropriate language ("Won't you get in the bed with me?"), inappropriate requests for personal care ("Make sure and wash my penis really good"), inappropriate gestures (such as sticking the tongue out and wiggling it at staff), exposing one's self or masturbating in public places, and inappropriate touching (grabbing a breast or buttock when in close proximity). All of these behaviors constitute sexual harassment and are not to be tolerated. These behaviors may reflect a power issue, a loss of inhibition due to cognitive impairment, or a combination of these. The behaviors make it difficult or impossible to care for the patient exhibiting them.

The goal is to extinguish the behavior while maintaining the dignity of the patient. Nursing staff need to confront the patient calmly and firmly, saying, "This behavior is inappropriate, interferes with me doing my job, and will not be tolerated." Laughing it off, reacting violently, or showing anger all are likely to encourage the behavior. Saying, "Oh, Mr. Smith, you wouldn't know what to do even if you could," although meant lightheartedly, is demeaning and may encourage the patient to try the behavior with someone else. Ask other staff if the behavior is a pattern and be sure to inform others so that they will not be caught off guard. One quadriplegic client told the authors he had rubbed the breasts of every nursing staff member on the unit with his upper arm when they were leaning over him to assist in dressing. He had gotten away with this behavior for weeks because the staff had not talked with each other about this behavior. We informed the staff, and two nursing staff firmly and compassionately confronted him together, and the behavior ended. Confronting him led several staff to talk with him about his fears of dating and being seen as attractive, which was the underlying need behind this behavior.

Although extinguishing sexually inappropriate behavior is necessary to care for older adults, there is some "good news" about this behavior. It is an indicator of recovery in a client who has been too ill to think or worry about his or her sexuality. It may be an expression of power or anger, both of which are expressions of independence. Interest in sexuality can aid in the rehabilitation process. After confronting a patient and ensuring that the client is not going to act out again, the nurse can initiate discussions about recovery and how to take an active role in that process.

Confronting cognitively impaired clients who act out may be effective in extinguishing the behavior. If this strategy does not work, other strategies may extinguish the behavior. If a client has a habit of inappropriately touching staff during a bath or bed-to-chair transfer, put a washrag in the client's hand during the bath, or place the patient's hand on the armrest to assist in the transfer. Approach a client from the weaker side, which will both protect the staff member and discourage the client from acting out. Another strategy is to encourage appropriate behaviors and ignore inappropriate behaviors. In rehabilitative settings, rewarding appropriate behaviors can be included as a part of a behavioral modification program. If possible, get family involved in extinguishing the behavior. Do not assume that the behavior is a premorbid or lifelong behavior, and try not to feed into perceptions of the client as a "dirty old man." Another strategy is to avoid using language the client may misinterpret as sexual. Nurses typically say, "I am your nurse today," or "I am going to take care of you," both of which may be misinterpreted as flirting. Instead say, "I am going to work with you" or "I am going to assist you," which sound much more businesslike. Lesser, Hughes, Jemelka, and Griffith (2005) outline pharmacologic therapies that may be necessary when sexually inappropriate behaviors continue despite the interventions outlined previously.

Dealing with Masturbation in Public Places in Hospitals or Long-Term Care

Masturbation is self-limiting and has no known harmful effects. It does not spread sexually transmitted diseases, and it can be performed with minimal cognitive and hand function. The comedian Phyllis Diller has been quoted as saying that another advantage is "You don't have to get dressed up." However, masturbation is only appropriate in private. Public masturbation is best extinguished using the strategies described previously for sexually inappropriate behaviors. The goal is to allow privacy, yet not draw undue attention. If "privacy" signs are necessary, keep them inconspicuous. Try to provide privacy even if clients' rooms are only semi-private, by giving the client some private time. Schover and Jenson (1988), who worked extensively with head injury survivors, noted that some clients benefited from an inflatable doll to have intercourse with. Clients using sex toys or explicit materials should do so in private and store them in their own private space, away from public view.

Patients Displaying Sexually Explicit Materials on the Unit or in the Home

Display of sexually explicit materials is a problem that is ignored in the nursing literature. Nursing staff may need to set some ground rules with patients in regard to posters, jokes, magazines, or cards on display on the patient's room wall or on dressers or over-bed tables. Staff need to recognize that although having these materials is the patient's choice, openly displaying them is a form of sexual harassment. A good rule is that materials with a PG-13 rating, such as the *Sports Illustrated* swimsuit issue, are acceptable, but those with naked bodies are not. Rules apply equally to men and women and apply regardless of the patient's sexual orientation. Rules also apply to staff areas; the inside of a staff member's locker may be his or her private space, but when the door is open in a public lounge and others have to view the pictures, that is a form of sexual harassment. Pictures are not the only problem; get-well cards that overtly encourage sexual relationships with patients and nursing staff are also inappropriate. If a patient has displayed these materials, calmly tell the patient why they are inappropriate and encourage the patient or family to remove them. Use respect when approaching a patient about offensive material. It is the patient's home too, especially in a long-term care setting. Try a compassionate approach first, focusing on your feelings. Keep the confrontation one on one if possible.

Occasionally, nursing staff who visit patients in their homes may encounter sexually explicit materials on display. Tell patients you cannot work with them in the rooms in which the materials are displayed. Negotiate with the patient for one room of the house where treatment can occur where there are no explicit materials.

This section of the chapter has addressed a wide variety of areas related to sexuality and intimacy. The goal is to promote intimacy when appropriate by assisting older adults to overcome the effects of age and chronic illness.

Critical Thinking *Exercises*

1. Mr. Song is an older patient of Chinese descent. He wishes to observe a specific diet while in the hospital, but the menus he receives do not include the foods he eats. What is the nurse's best response in this situation? How does the nurse advocate for Mr. Song? What are some alternative solutions if the hospital cannot prepare food that Mr. Song can eat on his diet?
2. Rabbi Steinberg is an Orthodox Jewish rabbi. He observes strict practices related to his religion, including kosher diet restrictions. If the nurse is unfamiliar with these traditions, what information does she need to provide spiritually and culturally sensitive care for Rabbi Steinberg? To whom could the nurse look as a resource for information?
3. Mrs. Smith is an African American widow who is 89 years old. She has been admitted with complaints of severe chest pain. She confides to the nurse that she has no insurance and does not know how she will pay for the tests they wish to run to diagnose her problem. What is the nurse's responsibility in this situation? How can he advocate for this patient and ensure that proper medical and nursing care is provided? What resources are available to help with these medical costs?

Personal **Reflections**

1. Have you ever cared for an older person from a culture or ethnic group different from your own? How did you feel about that experience? What did you learn?
2. Have you ever cared for an older person from a religion different from your own? How did you feel about that experience? What did you learn?
3. If an older patient was having problems dealing with sexuality after a life-changing event, how could you assist him or her? What is your comfort level with discussing sexual information with patients? How could you become more comfortable with this important aspect of nursing?
4. What resources are available in your area for older persons or those with disabilities who may need additional information and counseling about sexuality after an event such as a stroke or heart attack?

References

AARP. (2005). *Sexuality at midlife and beyond.* Retrieved December 11, 2007, from http://www.aarp.org

Agatston, A. (2003). *The south beach diet*. Emmaus, PA: Rodale Press.

Aleman, M. W. (2003). "You should get yourself a boyfriend" but "Let's not get serious": Communicating a code of romance in a retirement community. *Qualitative Research Reports in Communication, 4,* 31–37.

American Nurses Association. (1998, March 26). *Ethics and human rights position statements: Discrimination and racism in health care*. Retrieved March 29, 2005, from http://www.nursingworld.org/readroom/position/ethics/etdisrac.htm

Basson, R., McInnes, R., Smith, M. D., Hodgson, G., & Koppiker, N. (2002). Efficacy and safety of sildenafil citrate in women with sexual dysfunction associated with female sexual arousal disorder. *Journal of Women's Health and Gender Based Medicine, 11*, 367–377.

Bauer, M., McAuliffe, L., & Nay, R. (2007). Sexuality, health care and the older person: An overview of the literature. *International Journal of Older People Nursing, 2,* 63–68.

Block, J. D., & Bakos, S. C. (1999). *Sex over 50.* Paramus, NJ: Reward Books.

Bouman, W. P., Arcelus, J., & Benbow, S. M. (2006). Nottingham Study of sexuality and ageing (NoSSA I). Attitudes regarding sexuality and older people: A review of the literature. *Sexuality and Relationship Therapy, 21,* 149–161.

Carol, R. (2005, Winter). Overcoming bias in the workplace. *Minority Nurse,* 38–32.

Carol, R. (2007, Winter). Providing cultural competency training for your nursing staff. *Minority Nurse,* 32–37.

Cherry, B., & Giger, J. N. (2004). African-Americans. In J. N. Giger & R. E. Davidhizar (Eds.), *Transcultural nursing assessment and intervention* (4th ed., pp. 177–219). St. Louis: Mosby.

Crespo, C. J., & Arbesman, J. (2007). Obesity in the United States: A worrisome epidemic. *Physician and Sportsmedicine, 31*(11), 23–28.

Docter, R. F. (1985). Transsexual surgery at 74: A case report. *Archives of Sexual Behavior, 14*, 271–277.

Ebersole, P., Hess, P., Touhy, T., Jett, K., & Luggen, A. S. (2007). *Towards healthy aging: Human needs and nursing response* (7th ed.). Philadelphia: Elsevier.

Edgson, V., & Marber, I. (2001). *In bed with the food doctor.* New York: Collins & Brown.

Edwards, D. J. (2004). Sex and intimacy in the nursing home. *Nursing Homes, 52*(2), 18–23.

ElGindy, G. (2004, Fall). We are what we eat: Cultural competence and dietary needs. *Minority Nurse,* 54–55.

Eshleman, J., & Davidhizar, R. E. (2006). Strategies for developing cultural competency in an RN-BSN program. *Journal of Transcultural Nursing, 17,* 179–183.

Fischer, L. (2002). *The better sex diet book*. New York: St. Martin's Press.

Fuller, K. E. (2007). Your skin color and your health. *AnthroHealth News, 6*(4), 1–7. Retrieved January 7, 2008, from http://www.anthrohealth.net/AHV6N4.htm

Gaskamp, C., Sutter, R., Meraviglia, M., Adams, S., & Titler, M. G. (2006). Evidence-based guideline: Promoting spirituality in the older adult. *Journal of Gerontological Nursing, 32*(11), 8–13.

George, S. C., Caine, K. W., & Editors of Men's Health Books. (1998). *A lifetime of sex*. Emmaus, PA: Rodale Press.

Giger, J., Davidhizar, R. E., Purnell, L., Harden, J. T., Phillips, J., & Strickland, O. (2007). American Academy of Nursing expert panel report: Developing cultural competence to eliminate disparities in ethnic minorities and other vulnerable populations. *Journal of Transcultural Nursing, 17,* 95–102.

Giger, J. N., & Davidhizar, R. E. (2004). *Transcultural nursing assessment and intervention* (4th ed.). St. Louis: Mosby.

Giugliano, D., Giugliano, F., & Esposito, K. (2006). Sexual dysfunction and the Mediterranean diet. *Public Health Nutrition, 9,* 1118–1120.

Gonzalez, T., & Kuipers, J. (2004). Hispanic-Americans. In J. N. Giger & R. E. Davidhizar (Eds.), *Transcultural nursing assessment and intervention* (4th ed., pp. 221–253). St. Louis: Mosby.

Hanley, C. (2004). Navajos. In J. N. Giger & R. E. Davidhizar (Eds.), *Transcultural nursing assessment and intervention* (4th ed., pp. 255–277). St. Louis: Mosby.

Harrison, E., & Falco, S. M. (2005). Health disparity and the nurse advocate: Reaching out to alleviate suffering. *Advances in Nursing Science, 28,* 252–264.

Higgins, A. (2007). Impact of psychotropic medication on sexuality: Literature review. *British Journal of Nursing, 16,* 545–549.

Higgins, A., Barker, P., & Begley, C. M. (2006). Sexuality: The challenge to espoused holistic care. *International Journal of Nursing Practice, 12,* 345–351.

Hostler, S. L. (1999). Pediatric family-centered rehabilitation. *Journal of Head Trauma Rehabilitation, 14,* 384–393.

Jacobson, S. F., Chu, N. L-L., Pascucci, M. A., & Gaskins, S. W. (2005). Culturally competent scholarship in nursing research. *Journal of Transcultural Nursing, 16,* 202–209.

Kaplan, H. S. (1990). Sex, intimacy, and the aging process. *Journal of the American Academy of Psychoanalysis, 18,* 185–205.

Karpiak, S. E., Shippy, R. A., & Cantor, M. H. (2006). *Research on older adults with HIV.* New York: AIDS Community Research Initiative of America.

Kaufman, J. (2002). Looking at the past and the future of diversity and aging: An interview with E. Percil Stanford and Fernando Torres-Gil. *Generations, 26*(3), 74–78.

Kautz, D. D. (1995). The maturing of sexual intimacy in chronically ill, older adult couples. (Doctoral dissertation, University of Kentucky). *Dissertation Abstracts International* (UMI Order #PUZ9527436).

Kautz, D. D. (2007). Hope for love: Practical advice for intimacy and sex after stroke. *Rehabilitation Nursing, 32,* 95–103.

Kelley, L. S., Small, C. C., & Tripp-Reimer, T. (2004). Appalachians. In J. N. Giger & R. E. Davidhizar (Eds.), *Transcultural nursing assessment and intervention* (4th ed., pp. 279–299). St. Louis: Mosby.

Keppel, K. G. (2007). Ten largest racial and ethnic health disparities in the United States based on Healthy People 2010 objectives. *American Journal of Epidemiology, 166,* 97–103.

Kim, J., Ashing-Giwa, K. T., Singer, M. K., & Tejero, J. S. (2006). Breast cancer among Asian-Americans: Is acculturation related to health-related quality of life? *Oncology Nursing Forum, 33,* 1071.

Kleiner, S. (2007). *The good mood diet: Feel great while you lose weight.* New York: Warner Books.

Lee-Lin, F., & Menon, U. (2005). Breast and cervical cancer screening practices and interventions among Chinese, Japanese, and Vietnamese Americans. *Oncology Nursing Forum, 32,* 995–1003.

Lesser, J. M., Hughes, S. V., Jemelka, J. R., & Griffith, J. (2005). Sexually inappropriate behaviors: Assessment necessitates careful medical and psychological evaluation and sensitivity. *Geriatrics, 60,* 34–37.

Lewis, J. H., Rosen, R., Goldstein, I., & Consensus Panel of Health Care Clinician Management of Erectile Dysfunction. (2003). Erectile dysfunction: A panel's recommendations for management. *American Journal of Nursing, 103*(10), 48–57.

Lindau, S. T., Schumm, L. P., Laumann, E. O., Levinson, W., O'Muircheataigh, C. A., & Waite, L. J. (2007). A study of sexuality and health among older adults in the United States. *New England Journal of Medicine, 357,* 762–774.

Loeb, S. J. (2006). African-American older adults coping with chronic health conditions. *Journal of Transcultural Nursing, 17,* 139–147.

MacDougall, R. (2006). Remaking the real man: Erectile dysfunction palliatives and the social re-construction of the male heterosexual life cycle. *Sexuality and Culture, 10*(3), 59–90.

Magnan, M. A., Reynolds, K. E., & Galvin, E. A. (2006). Barriers to addressing patient sexuality in nursing practice. *Dermatology Nursing, 18,* 448–454.

Malatesta, V. J. (2007). Sexual problems, women and aging: An overview. *Mental Health Issues of Older Women:*

A Comprehensive Review for Health Care Professionals, 19, 139–154.

McAuliffe, L., Bauer, M., & Nay, R. (2007). Barriers to the expression of sexuality in the older person. *International Journal of Older People Nursing, 2,* 69–75.

McCoid, J. D. (2007). Therapeutic management of erectile dysfunction. *Nurse Prescribing, 5,* 143–147.

Messinger-Rapport, B. J., Sandhu, S. K., & Hujer, M. E. (2003). Sex and sexuality: Is it over after 60? *Clinical Geriatrics, 11*(10), 45–53.

Mick, J. M. (2007). Sexuality assessment: 10 strategies for improvement. *Clinical Journal of Oncology Nursing, 11,* 671–675.

Miller, R. I., & Clements, P. T. (2006). Fresh tears over old griefs: Expanding the forensic nursing research agenda with Native American elders. *Journal of Forensic Nursing, 2,* 147–153.

Moody-Ayers, S. Y., Stewart, A. L., Covinsky, K. E., & Inouye, S. K. (2005). Prevalence and correlates of perceived societal racism in older African-American adults with type 2 diabetes mellitus. *Journal of the American Geriatrics Society, 53,* 2202–2208.

Nelson-Becker, H. (2005). Religion and coping in older adults: A social work perspective. *Journal of Gerontological Social Work, 45*(1/2), 51–67.

Njoku, M. G. C., Jason, L. A., & Torres-Harding, S. R. (2005). The relationships among coping styles and fatigue in an ethnically diverse sample. *Ethnicity and Health, 10*(4), 263–278.

Padilla, Y. C., & Villalobos, G. (2007). Cultural responses to health among Hispanic American women and their families. *Family and Community Health, 30*(18), S24–S33.

Passel, J. S., & Cohn, D. (2008). *U.S. population projections 2005–2050*. Pew Research Center. Retrieved July 2, 2008, from http://pewhispanic.org/files/reports/85.pdf

Potts, A., Gavey, N., Grace, V. M., & Vares, T. (2003). The downside of Viagra, women's experiences and concerns. *Sociology of Health and Illness, 25,* 697–719.

Roach, S. M. (2004). Sexual behaviour of nursing home residents: Staff perceptions and responses. *Journal of Advanced Nursing, 48,* 317–379.

Robinson, J. G., & Molzahn, A. E. (2007). Sexuality and quality of life. *Journal of Gerontological Nursing, 33*(3), 19–27.

Schmidt, N. A. (2004). Nursing research about spirituality and health. In K. L. Mauk & N. A. Schmidt (Eds.), *Spiritual care in nursing practice* (pp. 303–326). Philadelphia: Lippincott.

Schover, I. R., & Jenson, S. B. (1988). *Sexuality and chronic illness: A comprehensive approach*. New York: Guilford Press.

Shattell, M. M. (2007). Engaging students and faculty with diverse first-person experiences: Use of an interpretive research group. *Journal of Nursing Education, 46,* 572–575.

Smith, W. R., Betancourt, J. R., Wynia, M. K., Bussey-Jones, J., Stone, V. E., & Phillips, C. O., et al. (2007). Recommendations for teaching about racial and ethnic disparities in health and health care. *Annals of Internal Medicine, 147,* 654–665.

Sparks, N. (1999). *The notebook*. New York: Warner Books.

Spector, R. E. (2004). *Cultural diversity in health and illness* (6th ed.). Upper Saddle River, NJ: Prentice Hall.

Steggall, M. J. (2007). Erectile dysfunction: Physiology, causes and patient management. *Nursing Standard, 21*(43), 49–56.

Steinke, E. E. (2005). Intimacy needs and chronic illness: Strategies for sexual-counseling and self-management. *Journal of Gerontological Nursing, 31*(5), 40–50.

Suen, L.-J. W., & Morris, D. L. (2006). Depression and gender differences: Focus on Taiwanese-American older adults. *Journal of Gerontological Nursing, 34*(4), 28–36.

Supple, A. J., & Small, S. A. (2006). The influence of parental support, knowledge, and authoritative parenting on Hmong and European American adolescent development. *Journal of Family Issues, 27*(9), 1214–1232.

Tabak, N., & Shemesh-Kigli, R. (2006). Sexuality and Alzheimer's disease: Can the two go together? *Nursing Forum, 41,* 158–166.

Walker, R. L., Lester, D., & Joe, S. (2006). Lay theories of suicide: An examination of culturally relevant suicide beliefs and attributions among African Americans and European Americans. *Journal of Black Psychology, 32*(3), 320–334.

Walsh, S. (2004). Formulation of a plan of care for culturally diverse patients. *International Journal of Nursing Terminologies and Classifications, 15*(1), 17–26.

Whittemore, R. (2007). Culturally competent interventions for Hispanic adults with type 2 diabetes: A systematic review. *Journal of Transcultural Nursing, 18,* 157–166.

Williamson, G. (2007). Providing leadership in a culturally diverse workplace. *AAOHN Journal, 55,* 329–335.

Wilson-Stronks, A., & Galvez, E. (2007). *Hospitals, language, and culture: A snapshot of the nation*. Retrieved January 9, 2008, from http://www.jointcommission.org

Xu, Y., & Chang, K. (2004). Chinese Americans. In J. N. Giger & R. E. Davidhizar (Eds.), *Transcultural nursing assessment and intervention* (4th ed., pp. 407–427). St. Louis: Mosby.

SECTION

9

Global Health Care, Health Care Systems, and Policy

(Competencies 21–24)

CHAPTER 19

Global Models of Health Care

Carole A. Pepa, PhD, RN

LEARNING OBJECTIVES

At the end of this chapter, the reader will be able to:

- Compare the aging policies of Japan, Germany, England, and Canada with those of the United States.
- Describe the effects of an aging population on health policy.
- Explain how morbidity and mortality can influence policies for the elderly.
- Analyze the benefits of social security.
- Contrast the Medicare and Medicaid programs.
- List the benefits and barriers to long-term care insurance.
- Assess the long-term care continuum.

KEY TERMS

- Acute care
- Assisted living
- Copayment
- Deductible
- Delayed retirement credit (DRC)
- Home care
- Life expectancy
- Long-term care
- Medicaid
- Medicare
- Minimum Data Set (MDS)
- Mortality
- Nursing home
- Outcome and Assessment Information Set (OASIS)
- Prospective payment system
- Social Security

Meeting the needs of a rapidly growing older adult population is a challenge worldwide (Flesner, 2004). Comparing models of health care around the world may provide greater insights into how best to meet the challenges the growth in the aging population will create. Some countries, like Japan and the United States, have separate care models for the elderly. Other countries, like Canada and England, have health care delivery models that include all citizens.

INTERNATIONAL MODELS OF HEALTH CARE

Japan

Japan has a universal health care system. Insurance is provided through the National Health Insurance or through Employees' Health Insurance. A citizen must be covered under one of these two plans.

Employee Health Insurance covers those individuals working for medium to large companies, national or local governments, or private schools.

Provisions are also available for small business employees. Premiums are based on monthly salary; half of the premium is paid by the employer and half is paid by the employee. The average cost is 4% of a person's salary (National Coalition on Health Care, n.d.). **Copayments** are required for hospital and outpatient care, and may be required for prescriptions. Copayments are between 20% and 30% of the bill. After an out-of-pocket payment ceiling is reached, patients are no longer required to pay copayments, and they receive full coverage. Patients who suffer from long-term illnesses receive an allowance based on salary; in case of death, a funeral allowance is paid.

The National Health Insurance covers workers in agriculture, forestry, or fisheries; the self-employed; and those not employed, including students. Copayments are required for both inpatient and outpatient services and for prescriptions. Premiums are based on resources, including salary and property, and on the number of dependents; they amount to about 4% of a salary. Coverage includes sickness, injury, necessary dental work, childbirth, and death of the insured or their dependents (National Coalition on Health Care, n.d.).

There is also a health plan for people over the age of 70 years. Aging in Japan is occurring at a rapid pace. In 2000, persons age 65 or over comprised 17% of the population. It is estimated that by 2020, the 65 or older population will comprise 27% of the total population (Houde, Gautam, & Kai, 2007). In comparison, the elderly are expected to make up 16.6% of the total population in the United States, and just over 24% of the population in Italy in 2020 (Elderly workers, 2001). Currently, the elderly in Japan enjoy the longest **life expectancy** in the world.

Since World War II, policies related to the elderly in Japan have undergone several changes. In 1954, the Pension Reform Act covered about 20% of the labor workforce; payments into the program were contributed by both the employee and the employer (Usui & Palley, 1997). Beginning in 1961, the National Pension Law provided coverage for the entire population. In the 1970s, benefits for the elderly were expanded to include free medical care; pension benefits were also significantly increased (Usui & Palley, 1997). However, policies in place encouraged an overuse of acute care hospitals, and during the 1980s, Japan experienced a large increase in health care expenses (Usui & Palley, 1997). The Health Care for the Aged Law of 1982 terminated free medical care to the elderly; with this initiative, the elderly had to pay a small **deductible** for outpatient and hospital care. By 1985, coinsurance and copayments were also required. In addition to coinsurance and copayments, the 1985 act also discouraged the use of acute hospitals for **long-term care**. The law called for an increased use of intermediate nursing care, rehabilitation, and other lower cost strategies to support discharged elderly patients (Usui & Palley, 1997). The Gold Plan of 1989 (formally called the Ten-Year Strategy to Promise Health and Welfare for the Aged) was a 10-year plan that targeted health promotion and welfare for the elderly while trying to control future cost escalation. The Gold Plan promoted three services: home help, short-stay institutions, and day services (Usui & Palley, 1997). It also included education regarding normal aging to prevent misuse of health resources by persons acting as they thought elderly persons should act. For instance, many elderly were bedridden because they believed elderly people were supposed to be bedridden (Usui & Palley, 1997). The Gold Plan was modified in 1994 to place even more emphasis on community-based care, such as respite care for caregivers, daycare centers, short-stay nursing homes, and in-home care. Although in-home care appeared to be a solution to the overuse of hospital facilities, each year 100,000 people had to leave their jobs to care for elderly family members (Watts, 2000). In addition, the system was becoming more expensive, and the administrative structure for determining eligibility was becoming too cumbersome (Ikegami, Yamauchi, & Yamada, 2003).

On April 1, 2000, the Long-Term Care Insurance (LTCI) program was introduced. The purpose of the LTCI system was to "support the independence and quality of life for frail and impaired elderly persons by providing them with adequate health and welfare services" (Asahara, Momose, & Murashima, 2003, p. 770). Under this program, all those age 65 or older were entitled to receive long-term care according to their eligibility levels. The six levels of care were determined by physical and mental status; availability of family support was not considered when determining the level of care required (Ikegami et al., 2003). With the allotted benefit, people could choose among agencies providing services. To fund the program, a 0.9% premium on monthly income was levied on those ages 40–64; an average of $23 (U.S. dollars) is deducted from the pensions of those 65 years or older (Ikegami et al., 2003). People over the age of 64 pay 10% of their nursing costs and also are charged a monthly premium. Payments from those 40 years of age and older provide 50% of the revenue for the LTCI. The remaining 50% is financed through national and local taxes, with 25% from the national government, 12.5% from the prefecture, and 12.5% from the local municipality (Asahara et al., 2003). The LTCI program is administered by the municipalities with support from one of the 47 prefectures and follows national government guidelines (Tsutsui & Muramastu, 2007).

Notable Quotes

"The secret of health for both mind and body is not to mourn for the past, nor to worry about the future, but to live the present moment wisely and earnestly."

—Buddha

With the emphasis on in-home caregivers for the Japanese elderly, elder abuse has received additional attention. The Japan Federation of Bar Associations submitted a report to the Health, Labor and Welfare Ministry at the end of 2004 that included recommendations to assist both the victims and abusers (Roundup, 2005a). According to the report, the elderly were reluctant to report abuse because they felt responsible when their children were the perpetrators because they raised them (Roundup, 2005a). The report also revealed that the nursing care insurance program was too complicated for some people to understand. Consequently, not everyone was receiving the assistance that could help with caregiving (Roundup, 2005b). The attorney group also discovered that families caring for their elderly relatives were experiencing mental, physical, and economic hardships (Roundup, 2005a) (**Box 19-1**). In addition, current law creates a barrier to professionals wanting to report suspected elder abuse. Although citizens are encouraged to report child abuse and domestic violence, those who report suspected elder abuse could be charged with violating confidentiality (Roundup, 2005b).

A 5-year review of LTCI revealed that both the number of certified users and home care users increased more than 100%; institutional users increased by 56% (Tsutsui & Muramatsu, 2007). Several reasons were posited for the increase in use as well as cost of the program. First, elders no longer had to meet a means test to be eligible for service, so elders who were not eligible in the past were able to secure services. Second, under the 2000 LTCI plan, it was less expensive for seniors to pay the copayment for a nursing home with food and around-the-clock care than to pay for rent and utilities for most apartments or copayment for community-based settings, such as a group home. However, institutional care costs the LTCI program more than three times the cost of community-based settings (Tsutsui & Muramatsu, 2007). Last, municipalities had little control over the type and quality of services provided. Originally, public health nurses were scheduled to act as care managers to create care plans based on a senior's certified need, but the shortage of public health nurses led to other health professionals with at least 5 years' experience being able to assume this role.

These weaknesses were addressed with the 2005 reforms to the LTCI. One reform increased the standard copayment for a nursing resident approximately 50%, effective in May 2005. Lower income seniors are exempt from this increase. The goal of this increase is to lessen the gap in cost between institutional and community-based care.

Germany

Germany was the first country to establish a national health care program. Social insurance in Germany is a mandatory transfer system whereby employees and employers make equal contributions for long-term care (LTC), social health insurance, pension funds, unemployment, and worker's compensation. Only employers contribute to the accident fund (Geraedts, Heller, & Harrington, 2000). The Federal Employment Agency makes contributions to the insurance funds for those who are unemployed. Those on pensions pay 50% of their premiums for health and LTC insurance; the other 50% is paid by their pension insurance fund (Geraedts et al., 2000). If family members of an employee are not employed, they are covered by the employee's health and LTC insurance at no additional cost. Families with only

BOX 19-1 Criteria for Medicare Reimbursement of Home Care Visits

Aim: The purpose of this study was to examine whether the use of care services reduces the feelings of burden among family caregivers in Japan. Three hypotheses were tested: 1) severity of impairment among the disabled elderly increases feelings of burden among family caregivers, and support from family members decreases burden; 2) the amount of services used among the elderly and caregivers is affected by the severity of impairment among the disabled elderly and the amount of support from family caregivers; and 3) once severity is taken into account, the use of care services under the LTCI program is associated with lower feelings of burden among family caregivers.

Methods: This descriptive study used a cross-sectional observational design. Participants were recruited from community-dwelling "registered disabled elderly" who had applied for services under LTCI in a town in northern Japan. Eighty-two elderly and their caregivers returned completed questionnaires out of 88 eligible participants. Each caregiver competed a self-report questionnaire that included the Japanese version of the Zarit Burden Interview, demographic information, questions about the type and severity of the elder's disability, and identification of the public care services used. Data were analyzed using measures of central tendency, correlational analysis to determine possible covariates to include in the model, and structural equation modeling.

Results: The model supported the hypotheses. First, caregivers of people with greater deficits had higher burden, but those caregivers receiving more support from family members identified a lower burden. Second, caregivers assisting people with greater deficits used more care services, whereas those who received more support from family members used fewer services. Finally, utilization of care services had a negative relation to caregiver burden, indicating that the more services were used, the less the caregiver burden.

Application to practice: Nurses should consider the effects of caregiver burden to be an influential one for families providing long-term care. The model tested in this study suggests that the support of family members can decrease caregiver burden as well as potentially decrease the use of care services. Social support continues to be an important factor in relation to caregiver burden. In addition, encouraging caregivers to use available home care services may lessen the perceived burden of family members caring for disabled older relatives.

Source: Kumamoto, K., Arai, Y., & Zarit, S. H. (2006). Use of home care services effectively reduces feelings of burden among family caregivers of disabled elderly in Japan: Preliminary results. *International Journal of Geriatric Psychiatry, 21*, 163–170.

one employed member pay the same amount for insurance as a single person in the same income bracket (Geraedts et al., 2000). German social insurance is based on the "solidarity principle," which states that "members of society are responsible for providing adequately for another's well-being through collective action" (Geraedts et al., 2000, p. 378). Insurers are known as sickness funds, and citizens are free to choose a fund; they can change sickness funds once a year without penalty (Green & Irvine, 2001). German citizens also have access to private insurance, and premiums are based on risk. In addition, under private insurance, coverage for family dependents increases premiums. Private insurance enables a beneficiary to access amenities such as a private room (Green & Irvine, 2001).

In Germany, primary care physicians act as gatekeepers to hospital access, but German citizens can access specialists without a primary care referral. In turn, some of these specialists have direct hospital access, so it is possible to circumvent the primary care physician gatekeeping (Green & Irvine, 2001). Unlike some other countries' health care systems, there is little or no waiting for physician or care access in Germany.

Like other countries, Germany faces a growth in its elderly population. In 1995, those age 60 or older comprised 21% of the German population; by 2030, 36% of the population will be 60 years of age or older (Geraedts et al., 2000). Aware of the projected need, the German government integrated long-term-care (LTC) coverage into the social security system.

The goal of the LTC insurance law was to provide relief from the financial burden of long-term disability and illness (Geraedts et al., 2000). Before LTC insurance, 80% of the elderly in nursing homes depended on public assistance, funded by local communities (Geraedts et al., 2000). This situation created a financial strain for the local communities. In addition, more family members were fulfilling the role of informal caregivers. Mental strain, lack of support, and financial hardships created when the caregiver was no longer employed outside the home made family members reluctant to assume caregiving responsibilities. To fund the LTC insurance program, one paid holiday was eliminated in all states but Saxony; this equaled 75% of the employers' contributions to the plan. (Geraedts et al., 2000). German citizens can also purchase private LTC in place of the LTC purchased with statutory health insurance. This private insurance is closely monitored because as citizens age, the premiums of private insurance increase as risk increases, and LTC premiums may become unaffordable (Busse, 2002).

Although most aging Germans are still cared for by relatives, the LTC insurance provides incentives to establish additional home health care agencies, short-term institutional care facilities, and assisted living facilities (Geraedts et al., 2000). LTC insurance also provides cash to family caregivers and makes contributions to the pension fund if the caregiver provides more than 14 hours of caregiving a week (Geraedts et al., 2000).

More research is encouraged to evaluate the quality of care provided under LTC insurance. Costs of the program have remained within the budget, but adjustments may be required in the future as the aging population increases.

England

The National Health Service (NHS) in England (Great Britain) was established in 1948. It is a universal system of health care based on clinical need rather than employment status; care is free at point of care. The NHS is divided into two basic sections: primary and secondary care. Primary care is usually the patient's first contact with a health care provider. Primary care providers are independent contractors with the NHS and may be general practitioners, dentists, pharmacists, or optometrists.

Over 75% of the funding for the health care comes from taxes, with a little over 10% coming from user charges. Nearly 100% of the population of Great Britain has access to health services. To better meet the needs of their population, the NHS has undergone some changes within the past few years.

Primary Care Trusts (PCTs) control about 75% of the health care budget. These trusts are responsible for addressing the local needs of a community. It is the responsibility of the PCT to ensure that services are accessible and that collaboration occurs among services, and to commission services that best match the community's needs (Holtz, 2008). PCTs also manage nurse-led walk-in centers. These centers are open past regular business hours and provide initial services available to anyone, without an appointment (Holtz, 2008). General practitioners belong to PCTs and serve as the gatekeepers of the health care system. Although the general practitioners maintain ownership of their practices, they must belong to a PCT, and they can belong to only one. Physicians are paid by capitation, although there is some fee-for-service present. A patient in England can choose to see the general practitioner of choice as long as the physician has an opening for patients; the resident can also change physicians. The PCT Web site enables a resident to evaluate physicians based on outcomes, waits, and other criteria. If additional care is needed, the patient is referred to secondary care: specialists, the local hospital, or a regional or national hospital. Except in emergencies, general practitioners do not provide hospital services, but rather they must refer to the specialists. Specialists are also employees of the National Heath Service.

Private health services are available in England, although they are much smaller than the National Health Service. The private sector provides services similar to those offered by the National Health Service, but those in the private sector do not have to follow the national treatment guidelines nor do they have a focus on the health of the community (BBC, 2008).

When the NHS was established in 1948, it was a leader in the provision of health care. By 2000, however, there was dissatisfaction with the system, as reflected by anecdotal evidence and public opinion polls. One of the leading reasons for dissatisfaction was the long waiting times (Monitor, 2005). These concerns were investigated, and changes were made in the system. First, additional financial resources were allocated to the NHS. In addition, Patient Choice was introduced. Under this system, the patients have a choice regarding which hospital they want to go to (Monitor, 2005). In a review of survey data conducted on sicker adults in five countries to determine their concerns, British adults reported the most satisfaction with their health care system, even though they reported problems with waiting times (Blendon, Schoen, DesRoches, Osborn, & Zapert, 2003).

Canada

The Canadian health care system, known as medicare, provides universal coverage at no cost at the point of case access. Each of the 10 provinces is responsible for establishing, maintaining, and evaluating the provision of health care services within the province following national guidelines: universal, portable, ability to access, and publicly administered (Irvine, Ferguson, & Cackett, 2005). In addition, the services must be based on need rather than ability to pay, sharing of best practices, accountability, and flexibility among provinces (Storch, 2005). Therefore, even though each province has a slightly different coverage plan, a resident could receive covered care in another province if it were necessary.

The health care system in Canada is funded primarily through tax monies. Although the federal government provides some money to the provinces, most of the costs are covered by the provinces, which in turn, levy taxes to pay for health care. Most physicians are in private practice, and they charge on a fee-for-service basis. They cannot charge, however, more than the negotiated fee. Hospitals are pri marily private, not-for-profit institutions.

One criticism of the Canadian system is the long waiting periods. Reforms are aimed at controlling escalating costs (Irvine et al., 2005; Schoen et al., 2005). The Canadian Institute for Health Information (2007) stated that in 2005, about 13% of people reported they had to wait more than 3 months to see a specialist for a new medical problem. A scarcity of diagnostic equipment can also create increased wait times. For example, in January 2006, there were about 6 MRI and 12 CT scanners for every 1 million Canadians (Canadian Institute for Health Information, 2007). In an attempt to provide quality care to all Canadians, each territory and province was required to specify its intention to implement a plan to reduce wait times (Health Council of Canada, 2007).

In addition to medical services, most provinces and territories cover the cost of regular vision and dental care for children, seniors, and social assistance recipients. Also, most public drug plans cover seniors as well as those in low income groups. Persons with diseases that require potentially high drug costs such as cancer, diabetes, and HIV/AIDS are also covered under many drug plans. For others, drug coverage varies among provinces (Canadian Institute for Health Information, 2007).

U.S. HEALTH CARE SYSTEM AND POLICIES

Effects of an Aging Society

The elderly population of the United States also is expected to increase, consistent with the increase in the elderly population worldwide. By the year 2050, projections indicate that 30% of the population will be over the age of 65 years; the population over the age of 85 is expected to double, and the population under the age of 35 years will decline by 10% (Sultz & Young, 2004). This increase in the elderly population is expected to bring challenges to policymakers. The future population of the elderly is expected to be better educated, more active, and more culturally diverse than the current population (Sultz & Young, 2004). This increase in the elderly population will create economic challenges such as how to finance long-term care. The shift in the demographic makeup of the population will create disequilibrium in the ratio between the working middle age population and the traditionally retired elderly population. Currently, there are 3.3 workers for every Social Security beneficiary; by the year 2030, there will be 2.2 workers for every beneficiary (Triest, 1997). More financial support will be needed. In response to these needs, creative health care delivery models will be required.

Effects of Mortality

The population age 65 years or older is increasing rapidly. From 1950 to 2005, the total population of the United States sustained an average growth rate of 1.2%; the population 65 years of age or older grew an average of 2% (Health Center for Health Statistics, 2007). By 2029, all the baby boomers (those born between 1946 and 1964) will be 65 or older. Consequently, the population ages 65–74 will increase from 6% to 10% of the total population between 2005 and 2030 (Health Center for Health Statistics, 2007). With an increase in the aging population, a concomitant increase in chronic diseases is expected (Anderson & Knickman, 2005; Flesner, 2004; Sultz & Young, 2004). Interdisciplinary teams of health care providers with expertise in geriatrics will be needed to meet the physical and psychosocial consequences of these illnesses (Sultz & Young, 2004).

Life expectancy, as a summary measure of **mortality**, is often used as an indicator of the health of a country (Health Center for Health Statistics, 2007). For a child born in 2008, life expectancy in the United States is 78.14 years; however, the United States is behind the countries of Andorra (the highest at 83.53 years), Japan (82.07 years), Canada (81.16 years), France (80.87 years), Germany (79.10 years), and the United Kingdom (78.85). According to the Central Intelligence Agency (2008), the United States ranks 47th in life expectancy at birth out of the 223 countries listed.

Health practices in childhood and young adulthood influence the health of individuals as they age (Rowland, 2007). People are living longer, so measures that support health promotion and illness prevention in childhood and through young and middle adulthood may produce a healthier older adult population. An emphasis on preventing some chronic illnesses or decreasing their debilitating effects will help to decrease the cost of health care for the elderly. Currently, health expenditures by and for the elderly are disproportionate to the distribution of the elderly in the general population (Joyce, Keeler, Shang, & Goldman, 2005; Kramarow, Lubitz, Lentzner, & Gorina, 2007).

Social Security

During the Great Depression, unemployment affected nearly 25% of the elderly (Kart & Kinney, 2001). Many middle and upper income individuals were affected as estate values and financial resources plummeted. It was during this time of financial stress that interest in an old-age pension was sparked. With the passing of the **Social Security** Act of 1935, the United States became one of the last industrial nations to establish a federal old-age pension program. However, the original Social Security Act did not provide benefits comparable to those provided by other industrial nations. The Social Security Act was strengthened, however, with the addition of survivors' and dependents' benefits (1939), disability insurance (1956), Medicare (1965), and automatic adjustment of benefits for inflation and supplemental income (1972). The Social Security Act provided a safety net of income in return for a lifetime of employment; it never was intended to be the sole source of retirement income. It also provided a standard age by which retirement could be defined (Kart & Kinney, 2001). Participation in the Social Security system is mandatory through payroll taxes called "contributions" (Kart & Kinney, 2001). No means test is required to receive benefits; rather, it is an earnings-related program. Benefits are financed by payroll taxes paid by employees and employers on income up to a certain level.

Basic benefits, available at full retirement age, are based on a worker's average indexed monthly earnings in covered employment (Kart & Kinney, 2001). For those individuals born before 1938, the full retirement age is 65 years; this is the age when one traditionally thinks of retirement. However, since 2003, the full retirement age has been rising. For example, a person born in 1955 will reach full retirement age at 66 years and 2 months; an individual born in 1960 will not reach full retirement age until 67 years (Social Security Administration, 2008). If retiring before the age of full retirement, individuals may receive reduced Social Security benefits beginning at age 62; benefits are reduced by 1/180 for each month before full retirement age that an individual begins to collect benefits. Conversely, an eligible worker can increase full Social Security benefits through **delayed retirement credit (DRC)**. If a worker postpones retirement past full retirement age and up to age 70, the worker will receive more than the earned full benefit for which he or she was eligible for at age 65 (Social Security Administration, 2008). The Social Security Administration uses a retirement test to determine whether a person is actually retired and eligible for Social Security benefits. Until age 70, benefits are reduced to those individuals who earn a certain amount of money while "retired" (Kart & Kinney, 2001). A criticism of the retirement test is that it is a disincentive to those who continue to work at another job while officially retired.

Social Security has decreased poverty rates of the elderly, particularly for female elderly. Half of the older women in the United States would live in poverty without their Social Security income (Meier, 2000). Approximately 75% of the poor elderly are women who largely depend on Social Security as the major source of their income; many have no other source of income (Meier, 2000). Women represent 60% of all Social Security recipients at age 65; at age 85, women represent 71% of all Social Security recipients (Meier, 2001).

Medicare

Medicare is Title XVIII of the Social Security Act; it was passed in 1965, after years of trying to provide some kind of universal health insurance. It is an insurance program for those 65 or over who have paid into the Social Security system, the railroad fund, or are diagnosed with end stage renal disease. Those collecting Social Security Disability Insurance (SSDI) are eligible for Medicare after a 24-month waiting period. When Medicare was enacted, nearly one in three elderly were poor, and about half of America's elderly did not have hospital insurance (De Lew, 2000).

The Original Medicare Plan, managed by the federal government, provides Part A and Part B. Medicare Part A helps to cover inpatient hospital care, inpatient care in a skilled nursing facility (for transitional, but *not* custodial care), hospice care, and home health care services (Centers for Medicare and Medicaid Services [CMS], 2008). Financed by payroll taxes paid by the employer and employee, Medicare Part A is available without charge for those who are eligible to receive Social Security or Railroad Retirement benefits. If an individual is 65 years of age and has not worked 10 years (40 quarters) in a job that has paid Medicare taxes, he or she can still receive Medicare Part A by paying a premium. In 2008, this premium was $423/month (CMS, 2008). Part B, previously referred to as Supplemental Medical Insurance (SMI), is considered medical insurance. It covers some of the cost for laboratory services, home health care services, doctor services, some outpatient therapies, mental health services, and outpatient hospital services. Participation in Medicare Part B is not mandatory and is not funded by the Medicare trust fund. Participants may pay for Part B out of their Social Security checks. In 2008, premiums for Medicare Part B were based on income; for example, if an individual reported yearly income of $82,000 or below ($164,000 for a joint return) on his or her income tax return, the monthly premium was $96.40. This premium increases incrementally as income increases, to a high of $238.40 for individuals with a yearly reported income above $205,000 (above $410,000 for a couple). In addition to monthly premiums, beneficiaries must pay a yearly deductible ($135 for 2008); this was up from $110 in 2005. In addition to the deductible, beneficiaries are required to pay 20% of the usual and customary charges (CMS, 2008). If a physician accepts Medicare assignment, then the physician must accept whatever Medicare provides as reimbursement. If the physician does not accept Medicare assignment, then the patient is responsible for any additional cost Medicare does not reimburse the physician. This is a question that all older adults should ask of their physicians prior to a visit.

For reimbursement purposes under Part A, Medicare establishes benefit periods, which consist of 90 days of inpatient hospital care. When a patient is admitted to a hospital for inpatient care, the benefit period begins. In 2008, for each benefit period, the beneficiary was required to pay a deductible of $1,024. If a patient were in the hospital for more than 60 days, a further charge of $256/day was incurred.

If a patient were in the hospital for more than 90 days, then the beneficiary begins to use his or her lifetime reserve of 60 days. The cost of using lifetime reserve days was $512/day. All figures are amounts due in 2008; these charges have increased every year (CMS, 2008). If an individual requires additional skilled care in the transition from hospital to home, Medicare Part A will cover the first 20 days of each benefit period in a skilled nursing facility for no out-of-pocket expense. However, for days 21–100, the 2008 out-of-pocket cost was $128/day. After 100 days in a skilled nursing facility, the individual is responsible for all costs in the benefit period (CMS, 2008).

In addition to the Traditional Medicare Plan with Parts A and B, Medicare also offers a plan called Medicare Advantage, also referred to as Medicare Part C. This option offers managed care plans like health maintenance organizations (HMOs) and preferred provider organizations (PPOs). Medicare Advantage plans provide all of the benefits of the hospital and medical insurance plans under original Medicare, but can charge different copayments and deductibles.

With the passing of the Medicare Prescription Drug Improvement and Modernization Act of 2003, Medicare Part D was added. This is the Medicare prescription option, and it offers multiple plans from which the beneficiary can choose. Each plan identifies the prescription medication it covers as well as the pharmacy, premium, deductible, and copayment. Consequently, the beneficiary must determine the plan that covers most of the medications prescribed as well as determine whether to choose a higher premium or higher deductible. A beneficiary may change plans for the next year during the open enrollment period of November and December of the current year. Once enrolled, the beneficiary must remain on the chosen plan until the next open enrollment period. One criticism of Medicare Part D is the coverage gap, or what some call the doughnut hole. Once a beneficiary has spent a certain amount of money during a year, all medication costs are out of pocket until the beneficiary is eligible for catastrophic coverage. In 2008, for most plans, once beneficiaries paid $4,050 for covered medications, they would only have to pay a coinsurance of 5% of the drug cost or a copayment of less than $6 (CMS, 2008). Choosing a prescription plan is very complex, and plans vary among states. In the booklet *Medicare & You*, plans and options are outlined so beneficiaries can determine which plans to contact for additional information (**Box 19-2**). Even though this prescription option has saved the elderly money, medication costs can still be very expensive.

When Medicare was proposed, private sector insurance plans were used as the models for coverage, administration, and payment methods (De Lew, 2000). Initially, Medicare did not cover dental care, routine eye care and glasses, hearing aids, preventive services, prescriptions, or long-term care. Today, in addition to covering prescriptions with Part D, Medicare does reimburse for some screenings on a regular basis and a physical exam when the beneficiary first becomes eligible for Medicare services after the deductible has been met. Medicare also covers hospice care for those patients who have been certified by the physician as having 6 months or less to live. Medicare covers care provided by a Medicare-certified hospice agency. Medicare also covers home care provided by a Medicare-certified agency (**Box 19-3**). All of these services have criteria that must be met for reimbursement (CMS, 2008).

The Balanced Budget Act (1997) included extensive changes to the Medicare system. Some of the changes included: 1) payments to providers were reduced; 2) preventive benefits were expanded; 3) Medicare + Choice, a managed care option, and other health plan choices with a coordinated open enrollment process were added; and 4) new home health, skilled nursing facility, inpatient rehabilitation, and outpatient hospital prospective payment guidelines for Medicare services were included to help decrease spending growth (De Lew, 2000). The Balanced Budget Refinement Act (1999) restored some of the Medicare payments that had been reduced in the 1997 Balanced Budget Act. In 2005, the managed

BOX 19-2 Web Link

Browse the free online version of *Medicare & You*, available at http://www.medicare.gov/publications/pubs/pdf/10050.pdf.

BOX 19-3 Criteria for Medicare Reimbursement of Home Care Visits

1. Care must be provided by a Medicare-certified agency.
2. The plan of care must be certified by a physician every 60 days.
3. The client must be homebound.
4. The client must require intermittent skilled nursing care or physical, occupational, or speech therapy.

care options for Medicare were changed from Medicare + Choice to Medicare Advantage.

Medicaid

Medicaid is Title XIX of the Social Security Act. It is an assistance program that is jointly financed by the state and federal governments, but is administered by the state; therefore, coverage and eligibility differ from state to state. To qualify for Medicaid, an individual must fit into a category of eligibility and meet certain financial and resource standards. Medicaid provides three types of health protection: 1) health insurance for low-income families and people with disabilities, 2) long-term care (LTC) for older Americans and persons with disabilities, and 3) supplemental coverage for low-income Medicare beneficiaries for services not covered by Medicare (e.g., eyeglasses, hearing aids, prescription drugs) as well as Medicare Part B premiums and Medicare Parts A and B deductibles and copayments (Provost & Hughes, 2000).

Federal funding for Medicaid comes from the general revenues; there is no trust fund set up for Medicaid as there is for Medicare. The state Medicaid office directly pays the doctor, hospital, nursing home, or other health care provider. Not all physicians will accept Medicaid patients because physicians must accept as payment whatever Medicaid reimburses. In some instances, this reimbursement may be less than the cost to provide the service.

The elderly account for a disproportionate share of Medicaid costs. For example, in 1998, although only about 11% of Medicaid recipients were elderly, they accounted for approximately 31% of Medicaid reimbursement (Provost & Hughes, 2000). The fact that Medicaid is the primary reimbursement mechanism for long-term care explains this phenomenon (Provost & Hughes, 2000). In an attempt to decrease high-cost nursing home care, Medicaid instituted a waiver program to facilitate home and community-based care delivery (Provost & Hughes, 2000). Many states have instituted programs that support low-income elderly in their homes to prevent or delay nursing home placement. In another attempt to curtail Medicaid spending, many states have initiated a managed care model for Medicaid services.

Although eligibility for Medicaid is different in each state, each state does require an individual and family to use their own resources (spend down) before they can become eligible to receive Medicaid reimbursement for LTC. Usually, an unmarried individual is allowed a small amount of personal property (in Indiana, for example, this is $1,500). If the recipient of nursing home care is married, and the spouse is remaining in the couple's home, the spouse is allowed to keep one half of the total nonexempt resources jointly owned when the individual entered the nursing home. There are upper as well as lower limits to the amount the spouse can keep. Rules also cover property given away as a gift, so family members cannot give away as gifts resources that could be used to pay for care.

Long-Term Care Insurance

Long-term care insurance is designed to cover those expenses of long-term care that are not covered by traditional health insurance or Medicare (U.S. Department of Health and Human Services [HHS], 2008). Although it has increased in popularity, long-term care insurance plays a relatively minor role in financing long-term care (Bodenheimer & Grumbach, 2005). One barrier to long term care insurance is the cost. For the elderly, because they are a population at high risk to use the benefits, the cost is high when compared with income. For instance, according to HHS (2008), the average cost of a comprehensive policy for an eligible person ages 65–69 would be $2,003 per year. Ideally, healthy middle-aged adults would be buying long-term care insurance against future need, but this is not happening to a large degree. Many employers are now offering long-term care insurance as an employee benefit. As a rule, companies offering long-term care insurance as a benefit do not contribute to offset the cost, but they do provide group rates for their employees (Sultz & Young, 2004).

Long-term care insurance can provide a wide spectrum of benefits; home care, assisted living, adult daycare centers, respite services, and nursing home care are among the care options that may be covered. Examples of services not included under these policies are care provided by a family member who is not an employee of a contracted service, care or services for which there would be no charge if insurance were not present, care for alcoholism and drug addiction, services usually covered by Medicare, and services or care for self-inflicted injury.

Long-term care insurance policies can be complex, and it is important to understand how these policies work. Long-term care insurances refer to benefit amounts, and these range from $90/day to $500/day, with most individuals choosing $150–200/day (Shore, 2007). Benefits can be paid on either a daily basis or a monthly basis. If daily benefits are chosen, then if costs exceed the daily amount, the difference would be paid out of pocket. For example, if a $90/day benefit were chosen, and the expenses for one day are $180, the $90 difference would be paid out of pocket. However, if a $360/month benefit were chosen, then expenses up to the monthly limit would be covered, regardless of when they were incurred during the month. Benefit periods refer to how long an individual wants the benefits to continue after they begin, usually a period of 5 years. If the total amount of coverage is not used during the benefit period, then the benefit period may be extended until the entire benefit amount is used. Long-term care insurance policies also have waiting periods, or elimination periods. This is the time a beneficiary must pay out of pocket before the policy begins to cover expenses; the shorter the waiting period, the more expensive the policy premiums will be. Policies may also include an escalator to help cover the increase in care costs over time.

Depending on benefit amount, waiting or elimination period, and age of the purchaser, even with long-term care insurance, out-of-pocket expenses for long-term care services could be considerable. In addition, not everyone who would like to purchase long-term care insurance is eligible to do so. Anyone who is currently using long-term care services or who has a progressive health condition may be precluded from purchasing long-term care insurance.

Residents in five states, California, Connecticut, Indiana, Iowa, and New York, have the opportunity to participate in private/public programs that link long-term care insurance with Medicaid. Although the specifics of these partnerships vary with the state, all enable the beneficiary to retain more of their assets should they need to apply for Medicaid to assist in paying for long-term care services (HHS, 2008). According to HHS, this is a program that is growing and may be an incentive for more people to purchase long-term care insurance.

SETTINGS FOR CARE IN THE UNITED STATES

Acute Care

The elderly use **acute care** hospitals at a rate greater than any other age group. The rate of hospitalization for the elderly increased by 23% over the past 30 years in spite of a decline in hospitalizations in the 1980s; hospitalizations for other age groups declined overall (Hall & Owings, 2002). From 1990–2000, the discharge rate among the elderly increased 8% whereas the rate among 15–44 year olds decreased by 18%, and by 16% among 45–64 year olds. The discharge rate for children 15 and under did not change (Hall & Owings, 2002). The elderly comprised 20% of all hospital discharges and used one-third of the hospital days in 1970. In 2000, the elderly compiled nearly 40% of the discharges and used almost one-half of the hospital days (Hall & Owings, 2002). Overall, average lengths of stay for those 65 or older were longer than for any other age group (Hall & Owings, 2002; Shi & Singh, 2005).

Medicare may reimburse for acute care of the elderly after deductibles and copayments are paid. Under the diagnosis-related groupings (DRG) system, hospitals have an incentive to discharge a patient as soon as medically possible. The combination of high use and incentive for discharge as quickly as medically possible creates a need for discharge planning and a continuum of services and nurses with expertise in geriatric physical assessment.

Long-Term Care

Long-term care "refers to health, mental health, social, and residential services provided to a temporality or chronically disabled person over an extended period of time with a goal of enabling the person to function as independently as possible" (Evashwick, 2002, p. 236). Most long-term care is community and institutionally based.

Home Care

Home care is part of the continuum of long-term care. It includes skilled nursing care and therapies, personal care services, homemaker/handyman services, durable medical equipment, high-technology home services, and hospice (Evashwick, 2002). These services may be provided by one agency or by a group of agencies. Home care agencies may be freestanding or facility based. Freestanding agencies include visiting nurses associations, which are voluntary, not-for-profit organizations governed by a board of directors. Now sometimes a generic term for all home care agencies, originally visiting nurses associations were discrete agencies with a common history of being part of the Visiting Nurses movement (Evashwick, 2002). Public or official agencies are government agencies supported by tax dollars and operated by a local, county, or state government. Public agencies may provide home care services, but their primary purpose is public health. Proprietary home care agencies are free-standing for-profit agencies. Private not-for-profit agencies are privately owned and operated. Facility-based agencies may be hospital-based, which are an integral part of the hospital organization; skilled nursing facilities; agencies based in skilled nursing facilities; or rehabilitation, which are agencies based in rehabilitation hospitals or clinics. Home care agencies are further divided as Medicare certified and non-Medicare certified.

Home visits to the elderly who are eligible for Medicare are reimbursed if certain conditions are met. Agency evaluation of the home visit process is achieved through agency outcomes-based quality improvement projects and through the **Outcome and Assessment Information Set (OASIS)**. OASIS information must be obtained at the beginning and end of service and every 60 days, coinciding with the certification period. Data are submitted to a national database, and results are compared with other similar agencies. The agencies receive both the results and the comparisons (Stanhope & Lancaster, 2008). Consumers as well as health care providers can use the OASIS data to compare agencies through the Medicare Web site at http://www.medicare.gov.

Assisted Living

Assisted living is another component of the long-term care continuum. Although there is no common definition for assisted living, policies in many states include the philosophies of resident independence, autonomy, and dignity (Beel-Bates, Ziemba, & Algase, 2007). In an assisted living environment, residents can determine which services they receive as well as when and how these services will be delivered (National Center for Assisted Living, 2007). Services generally included in an assisted living facility are congregate meals (although residents can choose to eat some meals in their rooms to decrease costs), 24-hour monitoring for emergencies, medication supervision, recreational activities, and security (HHS, 2005; Sultz & Young, 2004). If residents require intermittent skilled nursing care for a dressing change, that care often will be provided through a home care agency.

Aging in place has been an integral philosophy of assisted living facilities. Key to this philosophy is that a facility must adjust its service provision and level of care to meet the residents' changing needs (Chapin & Dobbs-Kepper, 2001). Most residents seek assisted living facilities because they need help with activities of daily living, but they do not require constant care (**Case Study 19-1**). Assisted living facilities are not substitutes for **nursing home** care; instead, they bridge the care need between living independently at home and nursing home care. About 36% of assisted living residents eventually go to a nursing home because their needs can no longer be met at the assisted living facility. Another 2% go to nursing homes because they can no longer afford their care (Is assisted living, 2001). One concern of assisted living is its affordability. "Affordability is critical in trying to make independent, autonomous, and dignified living available for all seniors, no matter their financial resources" (Piotrowski, 2003, p. 26). Currently, the cost of care at an assisted living facility can exceed $4,000 a month, depending on the size of the unit and the services required (Is assisted living, 2001), although the average monthly cost is estimated at $1,800 (Sultz & Young, 2004). Most costs for assisted living are paid for out of pocket, but long-term care insurance, Social Security Supplemental Income, and, in 37 states, Medicaid may assist with the cost (Sultz & Young, 2004). Facilities may charge fees for additional services such as meal choices and additional personal care (Is assisted living, 2001).

LONG-TERM CARE FACILITY (NURSING HOME)

According to Nursing Home Info (2003), a nursing home "provides skilled nursing care and rehabilitation services to people with illnesses, injuries, or functional disabilities." Nursing homes may provide both skilled nursing and intermediate care. Nursing homes with skilled nursing facilities (SNF) can provide nursing care to individuals who require a higher level of care for a short amount of time. Skilled nursing units often bridge the care needs between hospital and home care. When patients are medically stable, have used hospital days allotted to them under the **prospective payment system**, and yet are not ready to be cared for at home, Medicare will reimburse for skilled nursing care in

Case Study 19-1

Anna Broom is a 76-year-old widow who recently had bilateral knee replacements. She is completing her inpatient rehabilitation, and the nurses are exploring with her the need for referral to postdischarge care. Anna's husband of 52 years died 2 years ago from renal failure subsequent to sepsis, and she lived alone in a tri-level home before her surgery. Two of her children live in the same city. Both work and they are concerned about their mother's safety upon discharge because she must go up eight stairs to get to the bedroom and bathroom in her own home. Before surgery, Anna was taking atenolol and a baby aspirin; she was also getting a little forgetful. Upon discharge, Anna will be on warfarin (Coumadin) for at least 2 weeks, so she will need a protime and INR drawn weekly to determine dosage. She will resume her atenolol, but not the baby aspirin.

Questions:

1. What are Anna's options for care after discharge?
2. What assessments should the nurse make to help determine an appropriate postdischarge referral?
3. What decision should be made about postdischarge care?

BOX 19-4 Resource List

Aging and Policy

American Association for Long-Term Care Insurance: http://www.aaltci.org

Centers for Medicare and Medicaid Services: http://cms.hhs.gov

Department of Health and Human Services: http://www.hhs.gov

Medicare National Nursing Home Database and Surveys: http://www.medicare.gov/NHcompare/home.asp

U.S. Administration on Aging: http://www.aoa.dhhs.gov

Settings for Care

Assisted Living Federation of America: http://www.alfa.org

National Association for Home Care and Hospice: http://www.nahc.org

National Center for Assisted Living: http://www.ncal.org

Nursing Home Info: http://www.nursinghomeinfo.com

a Medicare-certified agency for 100 days each benefit period. After 20 days in a skilled nursing facility, the beneficiary must pay a copayment (CMS, 2008). A benefit begins the day of admission to an SNF and ends when skilled nursing care has not been received for 60 days in a row (CMS, 2008).

Individuals who require constant nursing care for stable, chronic conditions are not eligible for Medicare reimbursement. For these patients, care in a nursing home as part of the continuum of long-term care is an option. Each state defines what constitutes a nursing home; no federal guidelines define a nursing home. Nursing homes may be owned by private, for-profit corporations; not-for-profit organizations; religious-affiliated organizations; or government entities. All nursing homes that want to provide beds for residents who qualify for Medicaid must be Medicaid certified, indicating that they have met defined standards of care and services. Nursing homes may have beds certified as Medicaid, Medicare (SNF), or private pay.

BOX 19-5 Recommended Readings

Adeniran, R. (2004). The United Kingdom and United States health care systems: A comparison. *Home Health Care Management & Practice, 16,* 109–116.

Ball, M. M., Perkins, M. M., Whittington, F. J., Connell, B. R., Hollingsworth, C., King, C. V., & Elrod, C. L., et al. (2004). Managing decline in assisted living: The key to aging in place. *Journals of Gerontology: Series B: Psychological Sciences and Social Sciences, 59B,* S202–S212.

Benjamin-Coleman, R., & Alexy, B. (1999). Use of the SF-36 to identify community dwelling rural elderly at risk for hospitalization. *Public Health Nursing, 16,* 223–227.

Grabowski, D. C., Angelelli, A., & Mor, V. (2004). Medicaid payment and risk-adjusted nursing home quality measures. *Health Affairs, 23,* 243–252.

Harrington, C. (2005). Nurse staffing in nursing homes in the United States Part II. *Journal of Gerontological Nursing, 31*(3), 9–15.

Li, H. (2004). Post-acute home care and hospital readmission of elderly patients with congestive heart failure. *Health and Social Work, 29,* 275–285.

Light, D. W. (2003). Universal health care: Lessons from the British experience. *American Journal of Public Health, 93,* 25–30.

Mackenzie, A. E., Lee, D. T. F., & Ross, F. M. (2004). The context, measures, and outcomes of psychosocial care interventions in long-term health care for older people. *International Journal of Nursing Practice, 10,* 39–44.

Naylor, M. D., Brooten, D. A., Campbell, R. L., Maislin, G., McCauley, K. M., & Schwartz, J. S. (2004). Transitional care of older adults hospitalized with heart failure: A randomized controlled trial. *Journal of the American Geriatrics Society, 52,* 675–684.

Stone, R. I., & Reinhard, S. C. (2007). The place of assisted living in long-term care and related service systems. *Gerontologist, Special Issue 3,* 23–32.

Tsutsui, T., & Muramatsu, N. (2007). Japan's universal long-term care system reform of 2005: Containing costs and realizing a vision. *Journal of the American Geriatrics Society, 55,* 1458–1463.

Two major concerns face nursing homes today. One is the overall quality of care, and the second is the decline in Medicaid reimbursement. As the cost of care increases, and Medicaid reimbursement remains flat, in effect, reimbursement has declined because the percentage of actual cost covered by the reimbursement is less. Hicks, Rantz, Petroski, and Mukamel (2004) investigated the relationship between variable nursing home costs and outcome of care measures. Outcome measures used were 1) decline in ADLs, 2) development of pressure ulcers, 3) weight loss, and 4) psychotropic drug use. Results indicated that, collectively, these quality outcome measures can substantially impact the cost of nursing home care. The balance of cost and quality can place nursing homes in a precarious position because they are under constant pressure to improve performance and keep costs down (Scott, Vojir, Jones, & Moore, 2005). Nursing homes must compile data on resident health and outcomes on a regular basis; data are collected in a **Minimum Data Set (MDS)**. These data are used to compare performances of nursing homes nationwide. The Medicare Nursing Home Report Card comparing nursing homes is available on the Medicare Web site at http://www.medicare.gov.

Maas (2004) proposed the need for a new paradigm for long-term care. According to Maas, in today's nursing home environment, medical care is assumed most important, with the accompanying custodial care considered satisfactory. She posited a new paradigm that would abandon the medical-custodial model in favor of one that emphasized holistic, interdisciplinary care with multiple strategies to meet the needs of the older adult. In this paradigm, the roles of gerontological nurses and gerontological nursing best practices would be emphasized. Maas also proposed extending Medicare and Medicaid reimbursement to advanced practice nurses and nurses with specific gerontological training for nurse case management and interventions.

SUMMARY

The international policies on aging within models of health care vary between countries. This chapter presented information on Japan, Germany, England, Canada, and the United States to provide comparisons and contrasts between care delivery systems. Gerontological nursing care may be provided in a variety of settings from home care to long-term care. Each setting presents various challenges for payment. Gerontological nurses can assist patients and families to navigate the health care system by understanding reimbursement issues related to particular benefits.

Critical Thinking *Exercises*

1. Access the Medicare Web site at http://www.medicare.gov and compare the long-term care facilities in your area. What are the comparison indicators? How do the facilities compare? Explain how the nurse would use this information when discussing care options with an older adult.
2. In a small group, create a model for health care delivery for the year 2030. Identify which features would be present, why these features would be necessary, and how it would be financed. Explain the role of the professional nurse and the advanced practice nurse as well as other health care providers.
3. In a small group, compare health care policies for the elderly in Japan, England, Canada, Germany, and the United States. Identify the strengths and weaknesses of each model.
4. Box 19-5 lists some recommended readings. Choose one reference of interest to read, and share the information with a classmate.

Personal Reflections

1. Access the Medicare Web site at http://www.medicare.gov and review the home health agency comparison data. Explain how the care you provided an elderly client and family through a home care agency is reflected in these comparison data.
2. Visit an assisted living facility and a nursing home in your area. What was your impression of the two settings for care?
3. Interview someone who has come from another country. Explore with this person how the elderly were cared for in his or her country. Would that health policy be a viable model for the United States?

References

Anderson, G., & Knickman, J. R. (2005). Chronic care. In A. R. Kovner & J. R. Knickman (Eds.), *Jonas & Kovner's health care delivery in the United States* (8th ed., pp. 248–273). New York: Springer.

Asahara, K., Momose, Y., & Murashima, S. (2003). Long-term care insurance in Japan. Its frameworks, issues, and roles. *Disease Management & Health Outcomes, 11,* 769–777.

Beel-Bates, C. A., Ziemba, R., & Algase, D. L. (2007). Families' perceptions of services in assisted living residences: Role of RNs and implications for policy. *Gerontological Nursing, 33*(12), 5–12.

Blendon, R. J., Schoen, C., DesRoches, C., Osborn, R., & Zapert, K. (2003). Common concerns amid diverse systems: Health care experiences in five countries. *Health Affairs, 22,* 106–121.

Bodenheimer, T. S., & Grumbach, K. (2005). *Understanding health policy: A clinical approach.* New York: McGraw-Hill.

British Broadcasting Corporation. (2008). *How the health-care system works in England.* Retrieved April 27, 2008, from http://www.bbc.co.uk/dna/h2g2/A2454978

Busse, R. (2002). Germany. In A. Dixon & E. Mossialos (Eds.), *Health care systems in eight countries: Trends and challenges* (pp. 48–60). Retrieved September 14, 2006, from http://www.who.dk/document/OBS/hcs8countries.pdf

Canadian Institute for Health Information. (2007). *Health care in Canada 2007.* Retrieved May 23, 2008, from http://secure.cihi.ca/cihiweb/dispPage.jsp?cw_page=media_20sep2007_e

Centers for Medicare and Medicaid Services. (2008). *Medicare & you 2008.* Baltimore, MD: Author.

Central Intelligence Agency. (2008). *The world factbook. Rank order: Life expectancy at birth.* Retrieved May 24, 2008, from https://www.cia.gov/library/publications/the-world-factbook/rankorder/2102rank.html

Chapin, R., & Dobbs-Kepper, D. (2001). Aging in place in assisted living: Philosophy versus policy. *The Gerontologist, 41,* 43–50.

De Lew, N. (2000). Medicare: 35 years of service. *Health Care Financing Review, 22*(1). Retrieved June 9, 2005, from Expanded Academic ASAP Plus database.

Elderly workers solution for Japan. (2001). *Business Asia, 9*(18), 46. Retrieved June 5, 2005, from Expanded Academic ASAP Plus database.

Evashwick, C. J. (2002). The continuum of long-term care. In S. J. Williams & P. R. Torrens (Eds.), *Introduction to health services* (6th ed., pp. 234–279). Albany, NY: Delmar.

Flesner, M. K. (2004). Care of the elderly as a global nursing issue. *Nursing Administration Quarterly, 28*(1), 67–72.

Geraedts, M., Heller, G. V., & Harrington, C. A. (2000). Germany's long-term-care insurance: Putting a social insurance model into practice. *The Milbank Quarterly, 78*(3), 375–401.

Green, D. G., & Irvine, B. (2001). *Health care in France and Germany: Lessons for the UK.* London: Civitas.

Hall, M. J., & Owings, M. F. (2002). *2000 national hospital discharge survey. Advance data from vital and health statistics*. Hyattsville, MD: Department of Health and Human Services.

Health Center for Health Statistics. (2007). *Health, United States, 2007 with chartbook on trends in the health of Americans*. Hyattsville, MD: Author. Retrieved May 22, 2008, from http://www.cdc.gov/nchs/data/hus/hus07.pdf

Health Council of Canada. (2007). *Wading though wait times: What do meaningful reductions and guarantees mean?* Retrieved May 23, 2008, from http://healthcouncilcanada.ca/en/index.php?option=com_content&task=view&id+202 &itemid=10

Hicks, L. L., Rantz, M. J., Petroski, G. F., & Mukamel, D. B. (2004). Nursing home costs and quality of care outcomes. *Nursing Economics, 22,* 178–192.

Holtz, C. (2008). Global health in developed societies: Examples in the United States, United Kingdom, Sweden, and Israel. In C. Holtz (Ed.), *Global health care: Issues and policies* (pp. 1–37). Sudbury, MA: Jones and Bartlett.

Houde, S. C., Gautam, R., & Kai, I. (2007). Long-term care insurance in Japan. *Journal of Gerontological Nursing, 33*(1), 7–13.

Ikegami, N., Yamauchi, K., & Yamada, Y. (2003). The long term care insurance law in Japan: Impact on institutional care facilities. *International Journal of Geriatric Psychiatry, 14,* 217–221.

Irvine, B., Ferguson, S., & Cackett, B. (2005). *Background briefing: The Canadian health care system.* Retrieved May 24, 2008, from http://www.civitas.org.uk/pdf/Canada.pdf

Is assisted living the right choice? (2001). *Consumer Reports, 66*(1), 26–31.

Joyce, G. F., Keeler, E. B., Shang, B., & Goldman, D. P. (2005). The lifetime burden of chronic disease among the elderly. *Health Affairs, 5,* R18–R29.

Kart, C. S., & Kinney, J. M. (2001). *The realities of aging: An introduction to gerontology.* Boston: Allyn & Bacon.

Kramarow, E., Lubitz, J., Lentzner, H., & Gorina, Y. (2007). Trends in the health of older Americans, 1970–2005. *Health Affairs, 26,* 1417–1425.

Kumamoto, K., Arai, Y., & Zarit, S. H. (2006). Use of home care services effectively reduces feelings of burden among family caregivers of disabled elderly in Japan: Preliminary results. *International Journal of Geriatric Psychiatry, 21,* 163–170.

Maas, M. (2004). Long-term care for older adults. *Journal of Gerontological Nursing, 30*(10), 3–4.

Meier, E. (2000). Medicare, Social Security, and competitive benefits are neglected nursing issues. *Nursing Economics, 18*(3), 168–170.

Monitor. (2005). *Securing an effective healthcare system for England.* Retrieved April 27, 2008, from http://www.monitor-nhsft.gov.uk/publications.php?id=906

National Center for Assisted Living. (2007). *Consumer information.* Retrieved May 26, 2008, from http://www.ncal.org/consumer/index.cfm

National Coalition on Health Care. (n.d.). *Health care in Japan.* Retrieved August 26, 2007, from http://www.nchc.org/facts/Japan.pdf

Nursing Home Info. (2003). *What is a nursing home?* Retrieved March 17, 2005, from http://www.nursinghomeinfo.com/nhserve.html

Piotrowski, J. (2003). Weighing in on assisted living. *Modern Healthcare, 23*(20), 26.

Provost, C., & Hughes, P. (2000). Medicaid: 35 years of service. *Health Care Financing Review, 22*(1). Retrieved June 9, 2005, from Expanded Academic ASAP Plus database.

Roundup: Japan seeks efforts to stem abuse of elderly (part one). (2005a, January 10). *Xinhua News Agency.* Retrieved June 5, 2005, from Expanded Academic ASAP Plus database.

Roundup: Japan seeks efforts to stem abuse of elderly (part two). (2005b, January 10). *Xinhua News Agency.* Retrieved June 5, 2005, from Expanded Academic ASAP Plus database.

Rowland, T. W. (2007). Promoting physical activity for children's health: Rationale and strategies. *Sports Medicine, 37,* 929–936.

Schoen, C., Osburn, R., Huynh, P. T., Doty, M., Zapert, K., Peugh, J., et al. (2005). Taking the pulse of health care systems: Experiences of patients with health problems in six countries. *Health Affairs-Web Exclusive, 24,* W5-509–W5-525.

Scott, J., Vojir, C., Jones, K., & Moore, L. (2005). Assessing nursing home capacity to create and sustain improvement. *Journal of Nursing Care Quality, 20,* 36–42.

Shi, L., & Singh, D. (2005). *Essentials of the U.S. health care system.* Sudbury, MA: Jones and Bartlett.

Shore, R. M. (2007). Buying long-term care insurance? *The Maryland Nurse, 8*(3), 24.

Social Security Administration. (2008). *Understanding the benefits.* Retrieved May 22, 2008, from http://www.ssa.gov/pubs/10024.html

Stanhope, M., & Lancaster, J. (2008). *Public health nursing: Population-centered health care in the community* (7th ed.). St. Louis, MO: Mosby.

Storch, J. L. (2005). Country profile: Canada's health care system. *Nursing Ethics, 12,* 414–418.

Sultz, H. A., & Young, K. M. (2004). *Health care USA: Understanding its organization and delivery* (4th ed.). Sudbury, MA: Jones and Bartlett.

Triest, R. K. (1997). Social security reform: An overview. *New England Economic Review.* Retrieved June 9, 2005, from Expanded Academic ASAP Plus database.

Tsutsui, T., & Muramatsu, N. (2007). Japan's universal long-term care system reform of 2005: Containing costs and realizing a vision. *Journal of the American Geriatrics Society, 55,* 1458–1463.

U.S. Department of Health and Human Services. (2005). *Eldercare locator fact sheet.* Retrieved May 26, 2008, from http://www.eldercare.gov/eldercare/Public/resources/fact_sheets/assisted_living.asp

U.S. Department of Health and Human Services. (2008). *National clearinghouse for long-term care information.* Retrieved May 24, 2008, from http://www.longtermcare.gov/LTC/Main_Site/Paying_LTC/Private_Programs/LTC_Insurance/index.aspx

Usui, C., & Palley, H. A. (1997). The development of social policy for the elderly in Japan. *Social Services Review, 71*(3), 360–388. Retrieved June 5, 2005, from Expanded Academic ASAP Plus database.

Watts, J. (2000). Japan launches nursing insurance scheme for the elderly. *Bulletin of the World Health Organization, 78*(5), 710. Retrieved June 5, 2005, from Expanded Academic ASAP Plus database.

Unit Two

Role Development

SECTION

10

PROVIDER OF CARE

(Competencies 25–26)

CHAPTER 20

The Interdisciplinary Team

Teresa Cervantez Thompson, PhD, RN, CRRN-A
Deborah Dunn, EdD (c), MSN, GNP-BC, ACNS-BC

LEARNING OBJECTIVES

At the end of this chapter, the reader will be able to:

- Distinguish among multidisciplinary, interdisciplinary, and intradisciplinary teams.
- Describe the roles and educational background of each team member.
- Discuss the challenges and benefits of interdisciplinary geriatric teams.
- Appreciate the unique contributions that the interdisciplinary geriatric team can make toward helping older adults achieve their maximal levels of independence.

KEY TERMS

- Acute care for elders (ACE)
- Geriatric assessment interdisciplinary team (GAIT)
- Geriatric assessment team (GAT)
- Geriatric evaluation and management (GEM)
- Geriatric interdisciplinary team training (GITT)
- Interdisciplinary team
- Intradisciplinary team
- Multidisciplinary team
- Palliative care and hospice team

The elderly deal with normal age changes, the impact of chronic illness, and the realities of real or potential changes in function or cognition. Their needs for health care are best served through a comprehensive collaborative approach to assessment and care (Reuben et al., 2004). This collaboration is most frequently referred to as an **interdisciplinary team**. The elderly also may be facing end-of-life and palliative care issues that may bring another set of professionals into their care. Working together within or between teams or with professionals outside the team is required to provide the most comprehensive care for the individual.

The concept of interdisciplinary teams has been discussed in the health care literature since early in the twentieth century. The underlying "assumption [is] that an interdisciplinary team will bring together diverse skills and expertise to provide more effective, better coordinated, [and] better quality services for clients" (Ducanis & Golin, 1979, p. 1). Formal efforts made by the Department of Veterans Affairs (Reuben et al., 2004), along with grants that supported the development of geriatric assessment centers and **geriatric interdisciplinary team training (GITT)** (Siegler, Hyer, Fulmer, & Mezey, 1998), have increased the understanding of, awareness of, and interest in collaboration.

This chapter begins with an overview of the concept of teams. A discussion of geriatric teams and their potential members along with educational efforts to prepare health professionals for collaborative roles is presented. The realities and issues that surround other teams, new team members, or temporary team members coming into the mix of care will then be shared. The chapter concludes with a discussion of common challenges and benefits found in the geriatric team experience.

TEAMS

Teams have been defined in terms of why they exist; for example, they may be client centered or task centered (Ducanis & Golin, 1979). They also are defined in terms of how the team is seen to function, for example, as multidisciplinary or interdisciplinary.

There is no one consistent definition of *team* in health care. The idea of teams conjures up sports analogies as one thinks of groups of individuals with various skills and roles working together for a common end: *winning a game*. A batter alone does not win a baseball game and neither does a quarterback win the football game. Instead, all the team's players bring different perspectives and skills and work together to complement or build on one another's efforts to achieve the common goal of winning. This analogy fits well when one considers a variety of health professionals, each with different perspectives, knowledge, and skills, all wanting to provide effective care for the same individual. Where the analogy fails is the lack of a common vision of what the process and end products are and how professionals can effectively work together. Various disciplines have different views of teams and teamwork. Some may see teams as collaborative and egalitarian whereas others see teams as groups of individuals having a top-down perspective with one person in charge. With no common language among health professionals or expectation of interdependence, health care teams continue to be a work in progress.

Notable Quotes

"Alone we can do so little; together we can do so much."

—Helen Keller

Early literature related to health care teams is found in psychiatric and rehabilitation arenas (Ducanis & Golin, 1979). In these specialties, a number of different disciplines consistently work in the same settings with the same patients. Efforts to come together in assessing needs and developing treatment plans became part of their practice due to this proximity along with an appreciation of or frustration with each other's roles. Over the past 50 years, discussions of teams and team approaches have evolved, working to define the roles and responsibilities of different team efforts.

Multidisciplinary teams function as a group (multiple) of professionals who work loosely in the same area or with the same client. **Interdisciplinary teams** are an interconnected group of professionals who have common and collective goals. Another way to describe multidisciplinary and interdisciplinary is to see multidisciplinary as sequential, with each discipline applying its assessment and intervention within its own silo (Siegler et al., 1998), whereas interdisciplinary teams have an interactive approach to care. Two other terms have arisen related to teams: transdisciplinary and intradisciplinary. The use of the term *transdisciplinary* began in the rehabilitation arena in an effort to describe the circumstance of rising above the discipline to a team of professionals that worked more as rehabilitationists who then worked across the team. Lessard, Morin, and Sylvain (2008) see the transdisciplinary team as one in which the group has "accepted that decisions, roles and professional responsibilities will be shared (p. 13). The term **intradisciplinary team** is used to indicate that the work and relationship are within a discipline but members may be at different levels of preparation (Pierce, 2005). This may also be call unidisciplinary. Today the terms *multidisciplinary*, *transdisciplinary*, *intradisciplinary*, and *interdisciplinary* are often used interchangeably, which further confuses the issue. The concepts of an evolving and interconnected team are the target of the terminology. To limit any confusion, this chapter acknowledges the variety of terms but will focus on the term *interdisciplinary* as the most common and will assume the inclusion of the other terms.

Interdisciplinary teams include members from different disciplines who together undertake specified activities as a group with the client. Although each of the health professionals brings his or her own expertise (Greiner & Knebel, 2003), collectively they assume the basic roles of sharing information and have a common objective of coordinating care to provide a coherent and cohesive service to the client (Bokhour, 2006; Lessard et al., 2008). On a more advanced level, the members of an interdisciplinary team tackle complex problem solving, are interdependent in their work, and as one share accountability for outcomes. Rowe (1998) notes, "an interdisciplinary approach recognizes that many clinical problems outstrip the tools of individual disciplines and entails several health care providers simultaneously and cooperatively evaluating the patient and developing a joint plan of action" (p. vii). In the most effective teams the client (and/or caregiver) is an active team member and is expected to participate in goal setting and care planning. Most would say the client is always part of an interdisciplinary team or it is not a true team. (The use of the term *client*, *patient*, or *resident* is often used based on the setting in which the care is provided. In this chapter the terms should be considered interchangeable.) Interdisciplinary teamwork is an evolving process requiring communication and negotiation in a mutually respectful environment by all involved (Lindeke & Sieckert, 2005).

In geriatrics, teams are seen in all aspects of care, but the most common areas are in geriatric assessment and geriatric treatment. The needs for a team are based on the complex issues presented by the elderly; the benefits include coordination and integration of care assessment and planning (Bokhour, 2006; Howe, Sherman, Amato, & Banc, 2002; Tsukuda, 1998; Vazirani, Hays, Shapiro, & Cowan, 2005). The American Geriatric Society adopted a position statement entitled *Interdisciplinary Care for Older Adults with Complex Needs* (Geriatric Interdisciplinary Advisory Group, 2006). This position statement postulates that interdisciplinary care addresses the "complex needs of older adults," improves care and outcomes, and benefits the health care system and caregivers (p. 849). It further supports the positive impact of interdisciplinary training. In all, an interdisciplinary approach provides more holistic and comprehensive care and is valued by the professionals in the field.

Table 20-1 provides a summary of the common disciplines involved in geriatric teams. Adapted from a geriatrics interdisciplinary curriculum (Howe et al., 2002), this table shares professional titles, a description of education, and roles/skills important to the elderly, and also includes links to the professional organizations and/or specific gerontology resources for the profession. The most common reason for the member to be on the team is the unique body of knowledge that person brings to the assessment or treatment aspect of the services offered and of course the client's need(s) (**Box 20-1**).

As can be seen in Table 20-1, the "who" in a team can include any number of health care professionals along with the client and family or caregiver. If, instead of a series of appointments, a geriatric team provided assessments, this might be accomplished in a consultative assessment visit with the team (**Case Study 20-1**). The deciding factor for team membership is the aim of the assessment or treatment. Beyond the client, teams may include any combination of geriatricians, registered nurses, nurse practitioners, clinical nurse

Case Study 20-1

Mr. J., an 84-year-old man, has type 2 diabetes and hypertension. He notices some decrease in his activities of daily living due to unsteadiness on his feet. He is mourning the loss of his wife, who died 6 months ago. His daughter-in-law is concerned about the number of medications he is on and if he is taking them correctly. Mr. J. has been eating frozen dinners and spends most of his days sitting in the front room watching television.

Questions:

1. Who is the correct person for him to see: the physician, the social worker, the registered nurse or nurse practitioner, the pharmacist, the dietician, the physical therapist, or the occupational therapist?
2. Should the physician be an internist, an endocrinologist, a psychiatrist, or a gerontologist?
3. Should Mr. J. see all of these individuals and have multiple evaluations, treatment plans, and follow-up appointments? If so, which professional should he see first?
4. Is it possible for the different treatment plans to be duplicative or counterproductive to each other?

TABLE 20-1 Disciplines, Education, Roles in Gerontology and Web Resources

Discipline	Education/Certification Certification Licensure	Role(s) in Gerontology	Web Resource
Audiologist	Master's degree Certificate of clinical competence National exam	Hearing assessment including audiometric studies, evoked potentials, and other diagnostic procedures, and treatment of hearing loss	The Role of Speech-Language Pathologists and Audiologists in Working with Older Persons: American Speech-Language-Hearing Association (ASHA) http://www.asha.org/docs/html/PS1988-00231.html
Caregiver		Varying degrees of expertise	National Family Caregivers Association http://www.nfcacares.org/index.cfm Empowering Caregivers http://www.care-givers.com/pages/elderly.html
Title based on religion; some include Chaplain Priest Rabbi Minister	Education varies depending on requirements of religion and requirements of institution	Provide support to the client/patient, family, and others as it relates to spiritual needs. May assist in identifying resources from within congregation for support, visitation, or respite	Center for Aging and Spirituality http://www.spirituality4aging.org/about.htm American Society on Aging: Forum on Religion, Spirituality and Aging http://www.asaging.org/networks/index.cfm?cg=FORSA
Client/patient	Life experience	Expert in their experience	
Dietician	Bachelor's degree Internship National exam	Assess nutritional status and implementation of a nutritional plan	Gerontological Nutritionists http://www.gndpg.org
Geriatrician	Licensed medical physician with fellowship (2 years) in gerontology post medical internship and residency Board certification	Use knowledge of normal aging as part of assessment Specialize in the diagnosis and treatment of the elderly	Geriatric Medical Education and Training in the United States http://homepage.vghtpe.gov.tw/~jcma/68/12/547.pdf The American Geriatric Society http://www.americangeriatrics.org

(continues)

TABLE **20-1** Continued

Discipline	Education/Certification Certification Licensure	Role(s) in Gerontology	Web Resource
Advanced practice gerontological nurse practitioner (GNP)	Master's degree as a gerontological nurse practitioner National certification State licensure May also be prepared at the Doctor of Nursing Practice level with same certification and licensure requirements	Provide primary care including history and physical, chronic disease management Note: Adult nurse practitioners, family nurse practitioners, and palliative nursing practitioners may also have a role in geriatrics.	National Conference of Gerontological Nurse Practitioners http://www.ncgnp.org
Advanced practice gerontological clinical nurse specialist (GCNS)	Master's degree as a gerontological clinical nurse specialist National certification State licensure May also be prepared at the Doctor of Nursing Practice level with same certification and licensure	Provide advanced care for older adults, their families, and significant others in a variety of settings Note: Adult health, public, and community CNSs may have a role in geriatric care.	National Association of Clinical Nurse Specialists http://www.nacns.org National Gerontological Nursing Association https://www.ngna.org
Occupational therapist	Master's degree as an occupational therapist National certification State licensure Specialty certification in gerontology May also be prepared as a Doctor of Occupational Therapy	Assess and treat functional, sensory, and perceptual deficits that impact on ADLs Assess need for assistive devices Assess and treat cognitive deficits Rehabilitative services in geropsychiatrics	Aging Blueprint http://www.agingblueprint.org American Occupational Therapy Association http://www.aota.org
Physical therapist	DPT (Doctor of Physical Therapy) transitioning from MPT Licensure exam Specialty certification in gerontology is available State licensure	Assess mobility and functional capacity of the elderly Treatment includes rehabilitation, strengthening, mobility, and use of assistive devices	American Physical Therapy Association: Section on Geriatrics http://geriatricspt.org
Pharmacist	PharmD, 4 years beyond prerequisite 2 years National exam NABPLEX State licensure required Certification available as geriatric pharmacist	Prepare and dispense medication Clinical consultation and education for patient and geriatric team	American Society of Consultant Pharmacists http://www.ascp.com/about/ Commission for Certification in Geriatric Pharmacy http://www.ccgp.org/

Discipline	Education/Certification Certification Licensure	Role(s) in Gerontology	Web Resource
Physician	Professional doctorate with a degree in allopathic or osteopathic medicine	Dependent on the area of residency, specialty focus is on the area/disease process as it relate to aging	
Physician assistant	Two-year education, usually postbachelor's degree State licensure required	Midlevel practitioner	American Academy of Physician Assistants http://www.aapa.org
Psychiatrist	Medical degree with residency and board certification in psychiatry State licensure	Geropsychiatry evaluation, treatment, and management of mental health issues faced by the elderly Includes pharmacotherapy, evaluation of cognition, and psychotherapy	American Association for Geriatric Psychiatry http://www.aagponline.org
Psychologist	Graduate education, usually at the PhD or PsyD level State licensure required	Geropsychology assessment, consultation, intervention, and management of conditions related to adaptation, bereavement, counseling, and treatment for clinical cognitive and behavioral needs	American Psychological Association Committee on Aging http://www.apa.org/pi/aging/cona01.html Clinical Geropsychology http://www.geropsych.org Psychology of Adult Development and Aging Division 20 (APA) http://apadiv20.phhp.ufl.edu
Registered nurse	Associate degree, diploma, or bachelor's degree National Board exam NCLEX Optional certification in gerontology State licensure required	Assessment, planning, providing, coordinating, and evaluating care, which focuses on health, optimal wellness, disease prevention, and advocacy	Hartford Geriatric Nursing Initiative http://www.hgni.org National Gerontological Nursing Association https://www.ngna.org
Social worker	Bachelor's degree in social work (LSW) Master's degree in social work (MSW) State licensure	Assist with coping and problem solving as individuals and families adjust and face changes with aging and chronic illness Provide counseling and psychotherapy	Geriatric Social Work Initiative: http://www.jhartfound.org/pro gram/social_workers.htm National Association of Social Workers http://www.naswdc.org

(continues)

TABLE **20-1** Continued

Discipline	Education/Certification Certification Licensure	Role(s) in Gerontology	Web Resource
Speech-language pathologist	Master's degree and clinical fellowship (CFY) State licensure	Assess and treat communication disorders, which include speech, language, hearing, swallowing, and cognitive deficits	The Roles of Speech-Language Pathologists and Audiologists in Working with Older Persons: American Speech-Language-Hearing Association (ASHA) http://www.asha.org/docs/html/PS1988-00231.html

BOX **20-1** Reflections on the Case Study

The assessment team for Mr. J. in Case Study 20-1 may include a geriatrician, gerontological nurse practitioner, social worker, dietician, physical and occupational therapist, pharmacist, and psychologist or psychiatrist. Together they could assess Mr. J. for diabetes control and the presence of peripheral neuropathy, which may be affecting his mobility, and rule out a minor stroke given his history of hypertension and diabetes. From that point they could assess his need for physical or occupational therapy for functional mobility. The dietician could analyze his diet and, based on Mr. J.'s diabetes, recommend dietary needs. Depending on the assessment for grieving or depression, recommendations for counseling, medication, or socialization might be needed. Referrals could be made as needed for Meals on Wheels or for some socialization activities at a senior center.

specialists, physicians, physician assistants, social workers, psychologists, psychiatrists, pharmacists, occupational therapists, physical therapists, speech pathologists, dieticians, discharge planners, and chaplains (Agostini, Baker, Inouye, & Bogardus, 2001; Benedict, Robinson, & Holder, 2006; Howe et al., 2002; John A. Hartford Foundation, 2001b; Siegler et al., 1998). Wieland and Ferruci (2008) describe trials of home visit programs guiding care for chronic conditions as examples of comprehensive geriatric assessment. Going beyond the traditional health care team seen in inpatient and outpatient settings, teams may also be formed by including others outside of health care that are also vital to the focus of the team's work. An example would be a team focused on elder abuse assessment, which may include collaboration with adult protective services (Dyer et al., 1999; Dyer, Goodwin, Pickens-Pace, Burnett, & Kelly, 2007).

Together, the geriatric team can identify needs based on a wide array of assessment parameters. Working together allows the patient to be seen as a whole and treatment to be more effective.

TEAM DEVELOPMENT

Unfortunately, until very recently none of the individual professions required educational coursework or consistent experience in interdisciplinary work. This is just beginning to change as an outgrowth of two Institute of Medicine (IOM) reports. The value of health professionals learning to work in interdisciplinary teams is not limited to gerontology and has become an area of concern and need for all health professionals. In its *Crossing the Quality Chasm* report (2001), the IOM notes, "effective teams have a culture that fosters openness, collaboration, teamwork, and learning from mistakes" (p. 132). The IOM expanded this to a mandate for interdisciplinary education in its publication, *Health Professions Education: A Bridge to Quality* (Greiner & Knebel, 2003). It reports the need to work in interdisciplinary teams for patient safety and quality care. To do this, professionals need to learn to cooperate, collaborate, communicate, and integrate care in teams to ensure that care is continuous and reliable. Developing core competencies of providing patient-centered care based on current evidence, quality improvement strategies, and informatics through work in interdisciplinary teams is key to effective care (p. 46). The initiatives in quality and safety that are evolving from the IOM work are becoming evident in the various disciplines as well as in organizations. An example in nursing is Quality and Safety Education for Nursing (QSEN), in which competencies are identified specifying the knowledge, skills, and attitudes needed for each competency (Cronenwett et al., 2007). Included in these competencies are teamwork and collaboration, which are defined as "[the nurse] functions effectively within nursing and inter-professional teams, fostering open communication, mutual respect, and shared decision-making to achieve quality patient care" (p. 126).

Notable Quotes

"It is amazing what can be accomplished when nobody cares about who gets the credit."

—Robert Yates

In a review of the literature on collaboration, San Martin-Rodriguez, Beaulieu, D'Amour, and Ferrada-Videla (2005) identified the systemic factors of social, cultural, professional, and educational systems as influences in interprofessional collaboration. Organizational determinants are also identified as having the potential to enhance or discourage collaboration through structure, philosophy, and support. They also identify the interactional determinants as major components in collaboration. In all, to develop teams an understanding is needed and, as noted from the IOM reports, a change in the foundational socialization, enculturation, and education of all health care professionals. Organizations need to understand and value collaborative efforts to invest in them. Finally, the individuals need to develop a mutual respect for each other's contribution and develop a trust relationship that is nurtured through effective communication.

In 1994, the John A. Hartford Foundation began its efforts for geriatric interdisciplinary team training (GITT) by establishing an advisory committee to consider the feasibility for a training program (Hyer, 1998). From that advisory committee a plan was implemented that offered grants to initiate training programs. That initial group of grant programs included students from advanced practice nursing, medicine, occupational therapy, physical therapy, ethics, law, social work, audiology, dentistry, nutrition and dietetics, pharmacy, administration, psychology, pastoral counseling, physician assistants, and speech and language pathology. The target was to expose these health professionals to group interaction, group norms, and growth during their educational process. This initial project has gone beyond the education of the participants to the development of a core curriculum in interdisciplinary training (John A. Hartford Foundation, 2001a).

In 2005, Fulmer et al. provided a full description of the GITT evaluation results. This report identified that 1,341 health professionals completed the GITT programs. Outcome data included the valuable education curriculum developed; the impact on the knowledge, attitudes, and skill of the professionals; and the challenges faced in demonstrating patient outcomes. **Box 20-2** provides online resources for GITT along with other Web resources.

Another team education model is the **geriatric assessment interdisciplinary team (GAIT)**, funded in Maryland as part of the Geriatric and Gerontology Education and Research Program (GGEAR). This is an elective for students from Maryland schools of medicine, gerontology, psychology, recreation therapy, social work, nursing, physician assistants, speech and language, dental, law, pharmacy, and occupational and physical therapy that includes a series of 2-day rotations between various geriatric programs. The components of the training include a core curriculum as well as experience in working in a team environment. Content related to the professional roles of the various team members, their education, and scope of practice is foundational to working together. The content includes meanings and definitions found in geriatrics. Additional material deals with team-building exercises and roles played within a team, which may or may not reflect the individual's professional role. Finally, the team's forming, storming, norming, and performing phases are shared as a means of understanding the dynamic of a team's developmental process (Siegler et al., 1998; Smith, 2005).

Teams in geriatrics are usually focused on assessment, consultation, or management. **Geriatric assessment teams (GATs)** or geriatric consultation teams vary with the purpose of the consultation and may occur in an inpatient or outpatient setting. For example, if the team focuses on dementia or Alzheimer's assessment, there may be members who can evaluate other causes of confusion, ascertain cognitive function, or identify stages of the disease process and the potential resources available to the individual. If instead the GAT is focused on functional assessment, the emphasis may be on activities of daily living, home assessment, and the etiology of the functional changes. Geriatric teams are frequently called in to evaluate "functional, social, fall risk, nutrition, medication, depression, cognition, and incontinence" problems (Dellasaga, Salerno, Lacko, & Wasser, 2001, p. 202; Hickman, Newton, Halcomb, Chang, & Davidson, 2007; Robinson, 2007; Wright, Goldman, & Beresin, 2007).

In a meta-analysis of multidisciplinary geriatric consultation, Agostini, Baker, Inouye, and Bogardus (2001) noted that fewer than half of all hospitals offer comprehensive geriatric assessment. These consultation teams can provide services throughout the hospital to the attending physician. Unfortunately, these services are requested for only a small number of the hospitalized elderly. The recommendation from the analysis is that further study is needed to identify the potential effects of geriatric consultation, especially in the area of functional loss due to hospitalization.

There are also treatment and management teams, which may occur in the inpatient or outpatient setting. In the inpatient setting, if there are designated units, these are often referred to as inpatient **geriatric evaluation and management (GEM)** units. Another term used is **acute care for elders (ACE)** units. In GEM and ACE units, patients are admitted to the geriatric service and the unit is staffed with geriatric team members. Spinewine et al. (2007) report on their GEM team's randomized controlled trial on prescribing for geriatric inpatients. In this study, the inclusion of the pharmaceutical care "improved the appropriate use of medicines during hospital stay and after discharge" (p. 658). Studies to date for these types of teams, interventions, and research are still limited in the literature. Agostini, Baker, and Bogardus (2001) do note there were indications of increased likelihood of discharge home in the studies reviewed. Moving to application, Amador, Reed, and Lehman (2007) share that the outcomes an ACE unit can track include "patient satisfaction, medication compliance and a decrease in readmission" (p. 130).

In addition to the "within team" work needed to effectively provide care, there may be concurrent or intersecting teams working with a client. This may occur when the rehabilitation and geriatric teams have similar professionals represented but work as separate teams. At times it may seem confusing that the same disciplines on different teams may or may not understand the roles of their counterparts. This is very understandable, however, when one looks at the subspecialties within disciplines that focus on their own cores of knowledge, skills, and abilities.

Opportunities for optimizing care of the elderly are present when geriatric teams collaborate with palliative care and hospice interdisciplinary teams to provide comprehensive end-of-life care. Today, **palliative care and hospice teams** are active across care settings where geriatric teams are also found, including in hospitals, extended care, and rehabilitation centers. Palliative care and hospice teams are composed of the disciplines seen in geriatric teams: medical specialists, nurse practitioners, registered nurses, dieticians, pharmacists, social workers, psychologists, and additionally include chaplain services and specially trained volunteers. The goal of palliative care is "to prevent and relieve suffering and to provide the best possible quality of life for patients and their families regardless of the stage of their disease or need for other therapies" (National Consensus Project for Quality Palliative Care, 2004). Palliative care and hospice teams provide care that addresses end-of-life physical, psychosocial, and spiritual issues and eases the transition from purely curative care to supportive care. The decision-making style of palliative care and hospice teams is client centered; care goals are determined by the patient and family. Team members work collaboratively toward attainment of these patient-centered care goals. Adding collaboration with the geriatric team, it is possible to use the expertise of both in enhancing the care provided. The elderly often have multiple chronic health care issues that may confound the palliative intervention focus. Together the two teams' knowledge may be able to ensure a relief of suffering while managing the chronic conditions that might negatively impact on the relief efforts if not controlled.

There is little study to date on the intersection of geriatric and palliative care teams in optimizing end-of-life care of the elderly. However, the opportunity exists to structure systems, policies, and processes that can bring geriatric and palliative care teams together to optimize end-of-life care for elders (**Case Study 20-2**).

Each team has specific expertise, goals, approaches to care, and ways in which the team works together. The reality is that without the communication and collaboration between teams, the same issues of fragmented care or competing priorities and values may exist. Working together the two (or more) teams may identify which is best to take some leadership and coordination of the care to limit confusion and improve the patient's outcomes.

CHALLENGES AND BENEFITS

The challenges begin with the reality that each professional discipline has been educated to think in a specific way. That socialization rarely includes the expectation to work within an interdisciplinary team. The move into a team role means a blurring of discipline-specific roles and of some long-held norms. Only nursing and social work are noted to have a history of collaboration (Reuben et al., 2004). Most of the professionals are accustomed to being dependent on physician orders. This experience, as well as the physician's experience of writing orders, may impact the manner in which a team initially works together. A lack of understanding about each other's professional education, roles, and scope of practice can lead to misunderstandings and unrealistic or limited expectations. Hall (2005) expands on the challenges by introducing the concept of professional cultures as one of the barriers to team-

Case Study 20-2

J.B. is an 83-year-old female who was recently discharged home from a long-term care facility after completing a course of rehabilitation following a 5-day hospitalization for congestive heart failure and management of pleural effusion related to metastatic lung carcinoma secondary to breast cancer. Her medical problems include chronic atrial fibrillation, hypertension, coronary artery disease, hypothyroidism, and treatment of metastatic cancer for 8 years. She was discharged with medications for management of her chronic conditions and in-home oxygen for her chronic shortness of breath. Her oncologist has referred her to her primary care provider (a geriatric service) for further management, indicating that further oncologic treatment will not be beneficial. Her functional status is ambulatory with a cane for short distances; she is able to complete her activities of daily living, although she fatigues easily. She relies on her daughter for grocery shopping, making doctor appointments, paying bills, and banking.

Questions:

1. What services would be appropriate for the geriatric team to provide J.B.?
2. Could J.B. benefit from palliative care team consultation?
3. How could the consultation/collaboration with the geriatric service enhance care?
4. How would you approach prioritizing care for J.B.?

BOX 20-2 Reflections on the Case Study

In Case Study 20-2, the geriatric team can act as the coordinator of care, carefully assessing J.B.'s functional status in the most supportive yet least restrictive care setting. The team can help J.B. to establish the goals of care and determine advance directives, including her desire for future hospital care. A treatment plan for management of symptoms related to J.B.'s chronic illnesses, supportive home care services, and possibly in-home medical visits can be explored. Additionally, the team can discuss with J.B. and her family their understanding of the oncologist's prognosis and care recommendations. These discussions can include the exploration of palliative care and completion of advance care directives. If J.B. and her family select a palliative course of care, the geriatric team can explore palliation and hospice care with J.B. and her family and can make a referral to or consult with the palliative care team. The priority of care for J.B. is to assess her and her family's understanding of her health condition, impact on functional status, and need for supportive care and advance directives in order to maintain J.B.'s quality of life. Establishing the goals of care in the face of the unpredictable course of illness J.B. is likely to experience is essential. Geriatric and palliative care teams working together will best be able to meet the complex care needs of J.B.

BOX 20-3 Geriatric Team Resources

American Geriatric Society: http://www.americangeriatrics.org/education/geristudents/interdisciplinary.shtml

The American Geriatric Society GITT site: http://www.americangeriatrics.org/education/gitt/gitt.shtml

National Council on the Aging: http://www.ncoa.org

Discover Nursing links: http://www.discovernursing.com/jnj-specialtyID_238-dsc-specialty_detail.aspx

Interdisciplinary Care of Older Adults: A Web-Based Case Project: http://geri-ed.umaryland.edu/assessTools.asp

work. In essence, each profession incorporates into their education and writings a worldview from that profession's perspective. This can result in a completely different view of the presenting clinical situation and indeed opposing or counterproductive interventions being proposed. Without understanding each other's position and rationale there can be a diminishing or discounting of the value of each other's perspective on the outcome of care. All these issues need to be part of the initial work as a team comes together. Trust and respect are key components in the development of a successful team (San Martin-Rodriguez et al., 2005).

A barrier not found in the literature is that team members are not consistently the same individuals. Most of the discussions on teams have as an assumption that the members have the potential of being and staying a part of the interdisciplinary process. This is ideal, but the reality of service rotations, the coming and going of students and residents, shift differences, and turnover need to be part of the discussion. Another factor is that some of the professional services (e.g., rehabilitation therapies) may be outsourced to an external company for services. This means that team members may not be from the same organization, may be hired and paid by different entities, and may have different organizational expectations for performance. Although interested in interdisciplinary teamwork, they may not be encouraged or expected to participate. How does a team fully reach collaboration when the individuals may be continually changing or if the members have dual memberships or competing priorities? There is no one answer, but there can be no assumptions that a team will form and have the same mutual commitment and understanding of the process unless there is a concerted effort to make this happen. Effective orientations, negotiation for consistency in staffing, and ongoing orientation and education are all key components to addressing this barrier.

Although there have been training programs as well as curricula, the initial educational work has been done with students working in teams. These students may then go into the work setting and find that the ideal taught in the classroom is not practiced in the clinical world. Implementing geriatric teams in the work setting requires an investment in time to develop a team and work through a team-building effort. It is likely that professionals have not had experience or training in working in an interdisciplinary team. The bottom line of cost is also an issue. There is no real funding or reimbursement for team development. This requires institutional as well as professional commitment (Reuben et al., 2003).

There may even be regulatory and accreditation barriers that do not recognize team structures. Administrators or the team itself may continue to look at the silo approach to care. Reimbursement is another issue. Not all disciplines can bill for services, but these disciplines may be key to providing a comprehensive assessment.

Finally, there is the issue of shared power. This is an issue within the team because, as mentioned earlier, professional norms indicate who writes orders and who follows them. This is also an issue when power is shared with the patient. In an interdisciplinary team, the patient and/or caregiver are equal members of the team and are expected to participate in the goal setting and planning for their own care. The role of the patient and/or caregiver as expert is not common in this country and may cause dissonance for some professionals.

The benefits of geriatric teams center on the potential benefit for the elderly as they receive patient-centered assessment and interventions that take into account the whole person, the context in which they find themselves, and their presenting concerns. Because the professionals on a geriatric team have advanced knowledge of aging, chronic illness, and disease as well as functional loss prevention, the elderly they treat receive a more comprehensive approach to their care. Satisfaction is increased through the inclusion of the patient or caregiver in the assessment as well as the planning and goal setting. Care is viewed as more respectful when the patient's values, impressions, and preferences are included in the process (Greiner & Knebel, 2003; Melnyk & Fineout-Overholt, 2006). The quality of care is increased by the inclusion of evidence from a number of different disciplines' perspectives as part of the assessment and treatment process. In general, it is more cost effective to provide care using a geriatric team because there is less redundancy in the services provided and the team has representatives that view the presenting issues from a multitude of perspectives at the same time (Vazirani et al., 2005).

From a professional standpoint, the benefits include shared values, goals, and responsibilities for the care of the elderly. The opportunity to work together and learn from one another has the potential for growth of the team members within the specialty. Another advantage to working in teams is the development of new skills in communication, collaboration, negotiation, conflict resolution, and time management as one gains comfort working within a team.

The potential for time saving and increased productivity is also part of a team effort. The time saving relates not only to the patient, but also to the professional who does not need to wait for consultations, avoids duplication of assessment information, and maintains an understanding of what resources are available within the team. An increase in productivity occurs through team meetings, versus individual contacts, with all involved in the assessment or treatment of a patient.

SUMMARY

In general, once the investment is made in the team concept, there is great opportunity for professional growth. The potential for collaboration in planning, decision making, problem solving, and goal setting has great promise in health care (Gardner, 2005; Greiner & Knebel, 2003; Hall, 2005). Geriatric interdisciplinary teams offer the most effective way to meet the needs of the elderly in all settings.

BOX 20-4 Research Highlight

Aim: The purpose of this study was to identify the effectiveness of using simple screening tools in assessing elderly adults with varying cognitive impairments.

Methods: Demographic, cognitive (using a variety of testing measures), and health data were collected from a sample of 130 older adults living in nursing homes, assisted living facilities, and retirement communities. Analysis by a team of a PhD-prepared nurses and neuropsychologists with nurse practitioners classified the participants' cognitive status using consensus and discriminant function analysis.

Findings: "Discriminant function analysis correctly classified 95.2% of the participants in agreement with classifications of the consensus conference" (p. 44). This supported the usefulness of the screening measures (Dementia Rating Scale-2 and Hopkins Verbal Learning Test) in identifying amnestic mild cognitive impairment. It also found that these tools exceeded the effectiveness of the Mini Mental State Examination (MMSE) in assessing those with mild cognitive impairment (MCI).

Application to practice: The results support the potential of primary care providers such as nurse practitioners using these tools to detect MCI in a variety of settings. Gerontological nurses may consider using the tools mentioned in addition to or in place of the MMSE to assess those with MCI.

Source: Elliot, A. F., Horgas, A. L., & Marsiske, M. (2008). Nurses' role in identifying mild cognitive impairment in older adults. *Geriatric Nursing, 29*(1), 38–47.

BOX 20-5 Web Exploration

Check out this interesting PDF on teamwork in health care from the Canada Health Services Research Foundation (2006) at http://www.chsrf.ca/research_themes/pdf/teamwork-synthesis-report_e.pdf.

Critical Thinking Exercises

1. If an older person is having difficulty with home maintenance skills such as eating or using the laundry facilities, which team member would best address this?
2. For a person having gait problems, which team member could the nurse go to for advice and assistance?

continues

Critical Thinking (continued)

3. If an individual with aphasia wishes to improve his speech, which team member will be working closely with him?
4. A person with a tube feeding who is not tolerating the formula well might benefit from the nurse and which other team member when discussing this problem?
5. As a new member of an interdisciplinary team, how would you help build trust within the team related to your own abilities?

Personal Reflections

1. Have you ever worked with a team in any area? Have you ever worked with an interdisciplinary team in a health care setting? If so, how did you feel about that experience? If not, have you ever observed such a team in action? Which of the team members are you most familiar with? How important to you in your future career is the opportunity to work within a well-functioning team?
2. If you were assigned to work on an ACE unit, what differences would you expect to see compared to a general medical-surgical unit? What types of backgrounds, educational levels, or experiences would team members likely have?
3. Consider the various aspects of effective teamwork. How would you develop trust and respect within a team? How would you develop your negotiation and collaboration skills? Which strategies or interpersonal skills would you need to develop?

References

Agostini, J. V., Baker, D. I., & Bogardus, S. T. (2001). Geriatric evaluation and management units for hospitalized patients. *Agency for Healthcare Research and Quality Evidence Report 43: Making Health Care Safer: A Critical Analysis of Patient Safety Practices.* U.S. Department of Health and Human Services. Retrieved November 28, 2007, from http://www.ncbi.nlm.nih.gov/books/bv.fcgi?rid=hstat1.section.61048

Agostini, J. V., Baker, D. I., Inouye, S. K., & Bogardus, S. T. (2001). Multidisciplinary geriatric consultation services. *Agency for Healthcare Research and Quality Evidence Report 43: Making Health Care Safer: A Critical Analysis of Patient Safety Practices.* U.S. Department of Health and Human Services. Retrieved November 28, 2007, from http://www.ncbi.nlm.nih.gov/books/bv.fcgi?rid=hstat1.section.61010

Amador, L. F., Reed, D., & Lehman, C. A. (2007). The acute care for elder unit: Taking the rehabilitation model into the hospital setting. *Rehabilitation Nursing, 32*(3), 126–132.

Benedict, L., Robinson, K., & Holder, C. (2006). Clinical nurse specialist practice within the Acute Care for Elders interdisciplinary team model. *Clinical Nurse Specialist, 20*(5), 248–251.

Bokhour, B. G. (2006). Communication in interdisciplinary team meeting: What are we talking about. *Journal of Interprofessional Care, 20*(4), 349–363.

Cronenwett, L. Sherwood, G., Barnsteiner, J., Disch, J., Johnson, J., Mitchell, P., et al. (2007). Quality and safety education for nurses. *Nursing Outlook, 55*(3), 122–131.

Dellasaga, C. A., Salerno, F. A., Lacko, L. A., & Wasser, T. E. (2001). The impact of a geriatric assessment team on patient problems and outcomes. *MEDSURG Nursing, 1*, 202–209.

Ducanis, A. J., & Golin, A. K. (1979). *The interdisciplinary health care team: A handbook*. Rockville, MD: Aspen.

Dyer, C. B., Gleason, M. S., Murphy, K. P., Pavlik, V. N., Portal, B., Regev, T., et al. (1999). Treating elder neglect: Collaboration between a geriatrics assessment team and adult protective services. *Southern Medical Journal, 92*(2), 242–244.

Dyer, C. B., Goodwin, J. S., Pickens-Pace, S., Burnett, J., & Kelly, P. A. (2007). Self-neglect among the elderly: A model based on more than 500 patients seen by a geriatric medicine team. *American Journal of Public Health, 97*(9), 1671–1677.

Elliot, A. F., Horgas, A. L., & Marsiske, M. (2008). Nurses' role in identifying mild cognitive impairment in older adults. *Geriatric Nursing, 29*(1), 38–47.

Fulmer, T., Hyer, K., Flaherty, E., Mezey, M., Whitelaw, N., Jacobs, M. O., et al. (2005). Geriatric interdisciplinary team training program evaluation results. *Journal of Aging and Health, 17*(4), 443–470.

Gardner, D. B. (2005). Ten lessons in collaboration. *Online Journal of Issues in Nursing, 10*(1). Retrieved November 28, 2007, from http://nursingworld.org/MainMenuCategories/ANAMarketplace/ANAPeriodicals/OJIN/TableofContents/Volume102005/No1January31/tpc26_116008.aspx

Geriatric Interdisciplinary Advisory Group. (2006). Interdisciplinary care for older adults with complex needs: American Geriatrics Society position paper. *Journal of the American Geriatrics Society, 54*(5), 849–852.

Greiner, A. C., & Knebel, E. (Eds.). (2003). The core competencies needed for healthcare professionals. *Health Professions Education: A Bridge to Quality*. Retrieved November 28, 2007, from http://books.nap.edu/openbook.php?record_id=10681&page=R1

Hall, P. (2005). Interprofessional teamwork: Professional cultures as barriers. *Journal of Interprofessional Care, 19*(Suppl. I), 188–196.

Hickman, L., Newton, P., Halcomb, E. J., Chang, E., & Davidson, P. (2007). Best practice interventions to improve the management of older people in acute settings: A literature review. *Journal of Advanced Nursing, 60*(2), 113.

Howe, J. L., Sherman, D. W., Amato, N. L., & Banc, T. (2002). *Introduction to team work. Geriatrics, palliative care and interprofessional teamwork: An interdisciplinary teamwork*. Bronx, NY: VA Medical Center.

Hyer, K. (1998). The John A. Hartford Foundation geriatric interdisciplinary team training program. In E. L. Siegler, K. Hyer, T. Fulmer, & M. Mezey (Eds.), *Geriatric interdisciplinary team* (pp. 3–12). New York: Springer.

Institute of Medicine. (2001). *Crossing the quality chasm: A new health system for the 21st century*. Washington, DC: National Academy Press.

John A. Hartford Foundation. (2001a). *The John A. Hartford Foundation geriatric interdisciplinary team training (GITT) program*. (Implementation Manual). New York: Author.

John A. Hartford Foundation. (2001b). *Topic 2: Team member roles and responsibilities*. GITT Core Curriculum. Retrieved November 28, 2007, from http://www.americangeriatrics.org/education/gitt/2_topic.pdf

Lessard, L., Morin, D., & Sylvain, H. (2008). Understanding teams and teamwork. *The Canadian Nurse, 104*(3), 12–13.

Lindeke, L. L., & Sieckert, A. M. (2005). Nurse-physician workplace collaboration. *Online Journal of Issues in Nursing, 10*(1). Retrieved November 28, 2007, from http://nursingworld.org/MainMenuCategories/ANAMarketplace/ANAPeriodicals/OJIN/TableofContents/Volume102005/No1January31/tpc26_416011.aspx

Melnyk, B. M., & Fineout-Overholt, E. (2006). Consumer preferences and values as an integral key to evidence-based practice. *Nursing Administrative Quarterly, 30*(2), 123.

National Consensus Project for Quality Palliative Care. (2004). *Clinical practice guidelines for quality palliative care*. Pittsburgh, PA: Author.

Pierce, L. L. (2005). Rehabilitation nurses working as collaborative research teams. *Rehabilitation Nursing, 30*(4), 132–139.

Reuben, D. B., Levy-Storms, L., Yee, M. N., Lee, M., Cole, K., Waite, M., et al. (2004). Disciplinary split: A threat to geriatrics interdisciplinary team training. *Journal of the American Geriatric Society, 53*(6), 1000–1006.

Reuben, D. B., Yee, M. N., Cole, K. D., Waite, M. S., Nichols, L. O., Benjamin, B. A., et al. (2003). Organizational issues in establishing geriatrics interdisciplinary team training. *Gerontology and Geriatrics Education, 24*(2), 13–34.

Robinson, J. G. (2007). Utilizing best practice in dementia care. *Canadian Nursing Home, 18*(1), 21–27.

Rowe. J. W. (1998). Foreword. In E. L. Siegler, K. Hyer, T. Fulmer, & M. Mezey (Eds.), *Geriatric interdisciplinary team* (pp. vii–viii). New York: Springer.

San Martin-Rodriguez, L., Beaulieu, M.-D., D'Amour, D., & Ferrada-Videla, M. (2005). The determinants of successful collaboration: A review of the theoretical and empirical studies. *Journal of Interprofessional Care, 15*(Suppl. 1), 132–147.

Siegler, E. L., Hyer, K., Fulmer, T., & Mezey, M. (Eds.). (1998). *Geriatric interdisciplinary team*. New York: Springer.

Smith, M. K. (2005). Bruce W. Tuckman—forming, storming, norming and performing in groups. *The Encyclopaedia of Informal Education*. Retrieved January 12, 2009, from http://www.infed.org/thinkers/tuckman.htm

Spinewine, A., Swine, C., Dhillon, S., Lambert, P., Nachega, J. B., Wilmotte, L., et al. (2007). Effect of a collaborative approach on the quality of prescribing for geriatric inpatients: A randomized, controlled trial. *Journal of the American Geriatrics Society, 55*(3), 658–665.

Tsukuda, R. A. (1998). A perspective on healthcare teams and team training. In E. L. Siegler, K. Hyer, T. Fulmer, & M. Mezey (Eds.), *Geriatric interdisciplinary team* (pp. 21–37). New York: Springer.

Vazirani, S., Hays, R. D., Shapiro, M. F., & Cowan, M. (2005). Effect of a multidisciplinary intervention on communication and collaboration among physicians and nurses. *American Journal of Critical Care, 14*(1), 71–77.

Wieland, D., & Ferrucci, L. (2008). Multidimensional geriatric assessment: Back to the future. *Journals of Gerontology: Series A: Biological Sciences and Medical Sciences, 63*(3), 272–274.

Wright, S., Goldman, B., & Beresin, N. (2007). Three essentials for successful fall management: Communication, policies and procedures, and teamwork. *Journal of Gerontological Nursing, 33*(8), 42–48.

CHAPTER 21

ALTERNATIVE HEALTH MODALITIES

CAROLE A. PEPA, PHD, RN

LEARNING OBJECTIVES

At the end of this chapter, the reader will be able to:

- Explain what constitutes CAM.
- Explain each classification of CAM.
- Discuss nursing interventions associated with the most popular herbal products.
- Compare the benefits and drawbacks of the diets identified under biologically based therapies.
- Distinguish the differences between veritable and putative energy fields.
- Discuss why older adults may use CAM.
- Contrast Ayurveda and traditional Chinese medicine (TCM) systems.
- Discuss the benefits and supports for mind-body interventions.

KEY TERMS

- Acupuncture
- Ayurveda
- Biofeedback
- Biologically based practices
- Chiropractic practice
- Dosha
- Guided imagery
- Homeopathy
- Massage therapy
- Meditation
- Mind-body medicine
- Music therapy
- Naturopathic medicine
- Pet-assisted therapy
- Prayer
- Putative energy field
- Qi (chi)
- Reiki
- Sound energy therapy
- Therapeutic (healing) touch
- Traditional Chinese medicine
- Veritable energy field
- Yang
- Yin

The use of complementary and alternative medicine (CAM) has been steadily increasing in both the United States and worldwide (Barnes, Powell-Griner, McFann, & Nahin, 2004; Bielory, 2002; Eisenberg et al., 1998; Milden & Stokols, 2004). The widespread use of CAM therapies among those 65 years of age or older was documented by Ness, Cirillo, Weir, Nisly, and Wallace (2005). This widespread use of CAM therapies requires health care providers to be knowledgeable about these modalities and to educate clients and patients about the safety of their use.

WHAT IS COMPLEMENTARY AND ALTERNATIVE MEDICINE?

According to the National Center for Complementary and Alternative Medicine (NCCAM), CAM "is a group of diverse medical and health care systems, practices, and products that are not presently considered part of conventional medicine" in the United States (National Center for Complementary and Alternative Medicine [NCCAM], 2007f). In their classic article on unconventional medicine in the United States, Eisenberg et al. (1993) defined unconventional or alternative therapies as "medical interventions not taught widely at U.S. medical schools or generally available at U.S. hospitals" (p. 246). Although considered alternative or complementary in the United States, many of the modalities under this umbrella term are considered mainstream medicine in other countries (Bielory, 2002). In addition, the definition of what is complementary or alternative today may be considered a mainstream modality in 10 years. According to the White House Commission on Complementary and Alternative Medicine Policy (WHCCAMP) (2002), CAM is used to treat illness and promote health and well-being

CLASSIFICATIONS OF CAM

The NCCAM classifies CAM into five domains: 1) whole medical systems, 2) **mind-body medicine**, 3) **biologically based practices**, 4) manipulative and body-based practices, and 5) energy medicine. Although these classifications are widely recognized in literature and research, there is some overlap in the categories, particularly in mind-body medicine and energy medicine.

Whole Medical Systems

Whole medical systems "involve complete systems of theory and practice that have evolved independently from or parallel to allopathic medicine" (NCCAM, 2007e, para. 1). Examples from the United States are homeopathic medicine and naturopathic medicine.

Homeopathy originated with German physician Dr. Samuel Hahnemann's natural law of "like cures like" or the Principle of Similars (Kuhn, 1999; Rosser, 2004). According to homeopathic theory, when a person's vital force or self-healing response is out of balance, health problems will develop. The goal of homeopathy is to stimulate the body's own healing responses to prevent or treat illnesses (NCCAM, 2003). Homeopathic remedies are prepared by diluting certain substances and then gradually increasing the dilution until no actual measurement of the original substance exists. Although there are no active ingredients in a homeopathic solution, it helps the body to begin to heal itself by using its own defense mechanisms. Homeopathic remedies are recognized and regulated by the Food and Drug Administration (FDA). Remedies are also listed in the *Homoeopathic Pharmacopoeia of the United States.*

According to Kuhn, homeopathic remedies enhance healing without harmful side effects. Homeopathy has been used to treat illnesses such as respiratory infections, headaches, ear infections, neck stiffness, postoperative infections, dental pain, flu, motion sickness, and general aches and pains as well as sprains, bruises, and burns (Kuhn, 1999). The use of homeopathy has been controversial because of how the remedies are created using the dilution process. Research studies designed to support the efficacy of homeopathic remedies have demonstrated mixed results (NCCAM, 2003).

Naturopathic medicine focuses on keeping the person healthy as well as treating diseases. It is practiced in Europe, Australia, New Zealand, Canada, and the United States (NCCAM, 2007e). Principles of naturopathy include "(a) the healing power of nature, (b) identification of the cause and treatment of disease, (c) the concept of 'do no harm,' (d) doctor as teacher, (e) treatment of the whole person, and (f) prevention" (NCCAM, 2007e). It encompasses a variety of healing practices, including diet and nutrition, hydrotherapy, spine and soft tissue manipulation, acupuncture and acupressure, herbs, exercise, counseling, and light therapy (Kuhn, 1999; NCCAM, 2007e). In naturopathy, if the body is supported and barriers to cure are removed, the body will heal itself. There are minimal risks to naturopathic medicine, but natural healing takes longer than traditional allopathic medicine. Therefore, symptoms may last longer before they are eradicated.

Traditional medical systems of non-Western cultures are also included under this category of CAM. **Ayurveda** and **traditional Chinese medicine** are examples of these systems. Ayurveda dates to 4500 B.C. and is rooted in the ancient Hindu medical texts called *Vedas* (Gormley, 2000). Sanskrit for "knowledge or science of life,"

Ayurveda is a comprehensive system that encompasses the body, mind, and consciousness connection and seeks to restore a person's harmony or balance. It emphasizes prevention and encourages maintaining health. Ayurveda includes geriatrics as one of eight medical divisions. Practices in Ayurveda medicine include 1) diet, 2) exercise, 3) meditation, 4) herbs, 5) massage, 6) exposure to sunlight, 7) controlled breathing, and 8) detoxification (Pohl, 2001). According to Ayurveda, five elements make up all things: 1) space or ether, 2) air, 3) fire, 4) water, and 5) earth. These elements are not static, but rather are always in flux. In addition to the five elements, Ayurveda identifies three types of energy, or **doshas**. Vata is the energy of movements and comes from ether and air. Pitta is the energy of digestion and comes from fire and water, and kapha comes from water and earth and is the energy of lubrication and structure, which keeps the cellular body together (Gormley, 2000; Pohl, 2001). In Ayurvedic medicine, each person has a unique energy pattern. Disease is caused by an imbalance in the body, or disorder. Diagnosis is made through symptomatology rather than through traditional laboratory diagnostics. The goal of treatment is to bring the body into balance. Although the Ayurvedic physician has many treatments available, most of the research evaluated by the Agency for Healthcare Research and Quality (AHRQ) focused on herbal remedies (Southern California Evidence-Based Practice Center & RAND, 2001).

Traditional Chinese medicine (TCM) dates back in written form to 200 B.C. Korea, Japan, and Vietnam all have medical systems based on the traditional medical systems in China. TCM includes the therapies of acupuncture, herbal medicine, massage, and meditation. According to TCM, the body is a balance of two opposing forces: **yin** and **yang**. Yin represents the cold, slow, darkness, or passive principle, usually considered the female aspect. Yang, on the other hand, simulates fire and is the hot, excited, active principle, usually considered the male aspect. In this tradition of medicine, health is balance. Disease is seen as an imbalance between yin and yang; this imbalance impedes the flow of vital energy (**qi** or **chi**) and blood along pathways called meridians (NCCAM, 2007e). The system of qi forms the basis for diagnosis and treatment of illness as well as for promoting health and preventing illness (Chen, 2001). Diagnosis of disharmony is made on the basis of a patient's complaints and report of the experience of being sick (Fan, 2003). The evaluation of the quality of the pulse at nine particular points in the body and the appearance of the tongue are also taken into account when diagnosing disharmony.

Acupuncture is an integral part of TCM; it promotes the flow of qi through pathways in the body called meridians. There are 14 major meridians used in acupuncture; each meridian consists of an internal pathway, which often connects with an internal organ, and a corresponding external pathway. A total of 361 regular acupuncture points fall on the external pathways of the 14 meridians. An additional 40 acupuncture points fall outside the meridians (Lee, LaRiccia, & Newberg, 2004). Based on patient history and a physical examination, the acupuncturist determines which points on the external pathway of a meridian to stimulate and for how long (Lee et al., 2004). Very thin, solid, metallic needles are inserted at the appropriate acupuncture point to increase the circulation of qi and to bring the body back into balance. Nothing in allopathic medicine compares to the meridians in TCM.

Although acupuncture originated in China more than 2,000 years ago, it did not become well known in the United States until 1971, when a *New York Times* reporter wrote about how acupuncture eased his pain postoperatively (NCCAM, 2004). Burke, Upchurch, Dye, and Chyu (2006) reported that 4.1% of the adults in a 2002 National Health Interview Survey had used acupuncture at some time, and 1.1% had used acupuncture in the past year. According to the World Health Organization (WHO, 2003), there is support for the use of acupuncture to relieve postoperative pain, chemotherapy-induced nausea and vomiting, nausea associated with pregnancy, and dental pain. In a systematic review completed to determine the effects of acupuncture for individuals with neck pain, Trinh et al. (2006) found that there is moderate evidence that acupuncture relieves pain better than some sham treatments and moderate evidence that those who received acupuncture reported less pain at short-term follow-up than those on a waiting list. It is believed that acupuncture releases endogenous opioids, the same mechanism behind the use of transcutaneous electrical nerve stimulation (TENS) (Gloth, 2001). Promising results have been shown in the treatment of headache, stroke rehabilitation, osteoarthritis, low back pain, carpel tunnel syndrome, and asthma, but more research needs to be done to support the efficacy of acupuncture in treating these problems (National Institutes of Health Consensus Development Panel on Acupuncture, 1998).

Mind-Body Interventions

Mind-body interventions are among the most widely used of the complementary/alternative modalities (Barnes et al., 2004). Among the therapies included in this category are prayer, deep breathing, meditation, yoga, biofeedback, tai chi, and guided imagery (**Table 21-1**). Other modalities that would fit under this category are pet therapy and music therapy. Mind-body interventions acknowledge that emotional, mental, social, spiritual, and behavioral factors can directly affect health (NCCAM, 2007d). The mind-body connection entails two physiological pathways that involve the nervous, immune, and endocrine systems (Maier-Lorentz, 2004). The sympathetic-adrenal-medullary (SAM) pathway activates the autonomic nervous system; neurotransmitters and neuropeptides communicate with the immune cells. The hypothalamic-pituitary-adrenal (HPA) pathway signals the endocrine system to release hormones, particularly thyroid and adrenal, which have a direct effect on the immune system (Maier-Lorentz, 2004). The impact of stressors and hormones on the immune system is discussed in Chapter 6.

Notable Quotes

"For a completely safe and effective form of balance training, I recommend tai chi, the slow-motion, patterned movements sometimes called 'Chinese shadow boxing' or 'swimming in air.' . . . Older people who practice tai chi are less likely to fall and less likely to suffer injury if they do fall."

—Andrew Weil, MD, from his bestselling book *Healthy Aging: A Lifelong Guide to Your Well-Being*, pp. 233–234

TABLE 21-1 CAM Most Identified Mind-Body Therapies Ranked by Reported Use

Prayed for own health	52.1%
Others ever prayed for your health	31.3
Participate in a prayer group	23.0
Deep breathing exercises	14.6
Meditation	10.2
Yoga	7.5
Healing ritual for own health	4.6
Progressive relaxation	4.2
Guided imagery	3.0
Tai chi	2.5
Hypnosis	1.8
Energy healing therapy (Reiki)	1.1
Biofeedback	1.0
Qi gong	0.5

SOURCE: Barnes, P. M., Powell-Griner, E., McFann, K., & Nahin, R. L. (2004). *CDC Advance data report # 343. Complementary and alternative medicine use among adults: United States, 2002*. Bethesda, MD: Author.

Several of the mind-body interventions have their roots in religious traditions. **Prayer** is the most widely used CAM. In a report released by the National Center for Health Statistics, 45% of the adults surveyed in 2002 had used prayer for health or spiritual healing during the past 12 months (Barnes et al., 2004). Belief in God or a higher being is not required for prayer to occur because prayer can be defined as turning one's heart and mind to the sacred (Ameling, 2000). Although prayer is widely used and accepted, research studies as well as a systematic review supporting the value of prayer and healing have led to inconclusive results (Gundersen, 2000; Maier-Lorentz, 2004; Roberts, Ahmed, & Hall, 2007; Sending Prayers, 2002; Sicher, Targ, Moore, & Smith, 1998). Difficulties in standardizing methods, including treating prayer, religion, and spirituality as the same concept, may be responsible for some of the mixed results (Gundersen, 2000; Maier-Lorentz, 2004; Roberts et al., 2007). **Meditation** is closely related to prayer; it is a conscious process that induces the relaxation response (NCCAM, 2007d). There are two types of meditation. In concentrative meditation, the individual focuses on a mantra, sound, or visual image and is able to quiet the mind by concentrating on this focal point. The second type of meditation, mindfulness or vipassana meditation, begins with the individual focusing on breathing and continues until he or she develops a nonjudgmental awareness of the present. Meditation can be practiced by individuals of all ages and has been used to reduce stress, promote relaxation, and remove pain from the main focus of an individual's mind (Ott, 2004; Roberts, 2004).

The practice of yoga, which has its roots in India, integrates physical, mental, and spiritual health so that the individual can be in harmony with the universe. There are different schools of yoga, and each has a different focus, but basically, yoga combines disciplined breathing, defined gestures, and specific postures (*asanas*) to achieve a sense of harmony. Studies have supported the benefits of yoga for a wide variety of medical conditions and a wide variety of ages (Raub, 2002).

Tai chi is an ancient Chinese martial art. Although it can be used as a method of self-defense, it is practiced by many as an exercise to promote mental tranquility, improve physical fitness, and increase circulation (Chen, 1973). It also has been used to decrease the symptoms of arthritis and hypertension, and to improve balance. The mental concentration, deep breathing, and body movements work together to generate a tremendous amount of vital energy (qi) throughout the body system, resulting in the slow, fluid movements of tai chi (Chen, 1973, p. vi).

Imagery is any perception that comes through the senses (Naparstek, 1994). Sights, sounds, smells, or tastes can be used to create mental images to aid in relaxation and manage physical symptoms of stress and anxiety. These created mental images, called **guided imagery**, are considered a powerful self-help technique that is easy to learn and can be used by individuals of all ages (Menzies & Taylor, 2004; Miller, 2003). Guided imagery has been used by chemotherapy patients to decrease the side effects of treatments.

Biofeedback is now used in traditional therapies as well as complementary and alternative therapies. An individual uses machines to receive information about bodily functions such as skin temperature, brain waves (electroencephalography [EEG]), breathing, blood pressure, and heart rate. The individual receives information about the function in the form of audible or visual signals and is trained to focus on controlling the targeted bodily function. Reinforcement is received through feedback from the audible or visual signals. With practice, the individual becomes more skilled at controlling the targeted function. Eventually, the individual can control the function without the use of the machine to provide feedback. Studies have demonstrated that biofeedback has been used successfully to control a variety of symptoms such as headaches, chronic pain, hot flashes, and incontinence (Kuhn, 1999).

Another mind-body therapy not listed in the NCCAM categories is **pet-assisted therapy**, or pet-assisted visitation. Pet-assisted therapy and visitation is gaining in popularity, especially with children and older adults. A variety of animals (dogs, cats, horses, and rabbits) have been used to decrease stress and increase feelings of well-being. Although sometimes the terms are used synonymously, animal-assisted therapy is different from animal-assisted visitation. In animal-assisted visitation, certified therapy animals visit patients and families in a common room or at the bedside. A trained professional, on the other hand, performs animal-assisted therapy (Stanley-Hermanns & Miller, 2002). Research studies tend to support the effectiveness of pet-assisted visitation and therapy (Hooker, Freeman, & Stewart, 2002; Stanley-Hermanns & Miller, 2002). To initiate a pet therapy or visitation program, disease prevention strategies must be undertaken. Animals must be examined by a veterinarian to make sure they are free of any disease or parasites and are up-to-date on vaccinations. Animals should be bathed within the 24 hours before visiting and should be under the handler's control at all times (Stanley-Hermanns & Miller, 2002).

Music therapy is becoming more and more popular as a nonpharmacologic intervention to enhance the physical and psychological well-being of individuals in a variety of settings. Aldridge (1994) described two basic types of music therapy: active and passive. In active music therapy, the individual participates in singing or playing a musical instrument with the therapist. Passive music therapy is most often used in clinical settings in the United States. With passive music therapy, the individual listens to recorded music. This music may be chosen for the individual from selections known to provide a calming effect or the individual may make his or her own selections from music provided by the therapist or nurse. A third option is that the individual provides his or her own musical selections from personal favorites. The effect of music therapy to decrease anxiety or reduce pain has been reported in the literature, and the findings are mixed. Vanderboom (2007) conducted an integrative review to determine if music should be used as an intervention to modify the anxiety-provoking stimuli experienced by patients undergoing interventional radiology procedures. The review identified that the music intervention may be effective in decreasing blood pressure and reducing the need for medication, but the evidence was limited. Richards, Johnson, Sparks, and Emerson (2007) and Daniel, O'Keefe, and Pepa (2002) each conducted reviews of current research related to the effect of music therapy on patients. Both groups of researchers concluded that although music may be helpful in reducing pain and anxiety, the evidence was limited and findings could not be generalized to all patient populations. These findings are consistent with the findings of the systematic review by Cepeda, Carr, Lau, and Alverez (2006), which stated that, although music reduced pain levels and the need for opioids, the magnitude of the benefits was small.

Biologically Based Therapies

In CAM, biologically based practices include botanicals, animal-derived extracts, vitamins, minerals, fatty acids, proteins, prebiotics and probiotics, whole diets, and functional foods (NCCAM, 2007a). Vegetarian, macrobiotic, Atkins, Pritikin, Ornish, and Zone are examples of whole diets included in the biologically based category (**Table 21-2**). Although some whole diet therapies may be used to prevent or treat health conditions, others may not provide all the micronutrients an individual may need. This is especially true of fad diets. Nurses should include questions about whole diet practices in their assessments.

Dietary supplements, which may include vitamins, minerals, herbs or other botanicals, amino acids, and substances such as enzymes, organ tissues, glandulars, and metabolites, are a subset of this category (NCAAM, 2007a). According to Barnes et al. (2004), nearly 19% of adults who used complementary and alternative medicine within the past year used nonvitamin and natural products, 3.5% used diet therapies, and 2.8% used megavitamin therapy. Because this category includes natural products, individuals, particularly the elderly, may have the mistaken belief that there are no side effects or concerns in using these products. However, caution must be taken in using these products with certain prescribed medications. The ingredients listed on the labels of dietary supplements may be long and printed in a font size difficult for the older adult to read easily. Consequently, ingredients with the potential for interactions with medications could be overlooked.

Vitamins are compounds the body needs to maintain health. The concern, however, is that some individuals believe that "if a little is good, more must be better," and they take megadoses of vitamins. A list of potential risks of large doses of vitamins is found in **Table 21-3**. Vitamin deficiencies can also cause problems beyond those related to vitamin action. For example, older adults may have difficulty absorbing vitamin B_{12} from unfortified foods. These adults can absorb the vitamin from fortified foods and supplements, however. A vitamin B_{12} deficiency may mimic signs of dementia, including memory loss, disorientation, hallucinations, and tingling in the arms and legs (Harvard School of Public Health, n.d.). A daily vitamin from a reliable manufacturer that supplies nearly 100% of the daily requirements is a good choice for older adults.

Table 21-4 displays the 10 most commonly used natural products identified by those who used complementary and alternate medicine in the year preceding the 2002 National Health Interview Survey (NHIS). Actions, uses, and contraindications for these products are also included. In addition to those natural products listed in Table 21-4, other medicinal herbs also are popular. Valerian root is used as a sedative and sleep aid. It should not be used in conjunction with alcohol, sedatives, and anti-anxiety medication. Side effects include mild headache or upset stomach; it is not addictive. Kava kava (*Piper methysticum*) has been shown to relax

TABLE 21-2 **Popular Diets Listed Under Biologically Based Therapies**

Diet	Description
Atkins	Emphasizes low carbohydrates (40 g or less) with an increase in fat and protein (Barnes et al., 2004).
Macrobiotic	Low-fat diet emphasizes whole grains and vegetables and a decrease in fluid intake. Meat, dairy products, eggs, alcohol, sugar, sweets, coffee, and caffeinated tea are avoided.
Ornish	High-fiber, low-fat vegetarian diet promotes weight loss by restricting the types of food rather than calories.
Pritikin	Low-fat (10% or less) diet emphasizes consumption of foods with a large volume of fiber and water (low in calorie density). Diet includes many vegetables, fruits, beans, and unprocessed grains.
Zone	Each meal consists of 30% low fat protein, 30% fat, and 40% fiber-rich fruits and vegetables. The goal of this diet is to control key hormone production to alter metabolism.
Vegetarian	Diet excludes meat, fish, fowl, or products containing these foods.
Lacto-ovo-vegetarian	Diet is based on grains, vegetables, fruit, seeds, nuts, legumes, dairy products, and eggs. It excludes meat, fish, and fowl.
Lacto vegetarian	Diet excludes eggs, meat, fish, and fowl, but includes dairy.
Vegan vegetarian	Diet excludes dairy, eggs, meat, fish, fowl, and other animal products.

SOURCE: Mangels, Messina, & Melina, 2003.

skeletal muscles. It is used for anxiety, stress, restlessness, and insomnia. Its use is contraindicated in individuals with liver disease or depression. It should not be used with antidepressives, alcohol, or tranquilizers. Side effects include dizziness, headache, drowsiness, and hepatic toxicity (Deglin & Vallerand, 2007; Ernst, 2002). Saw palmetto has been used for treating benign prostatic hyperplasia (BPH), and studies have supported its efficacy (Ernst, 2002; Gordon & Shaughnessy, 2003; Wilt, Ishani, & MacDonald, 2002). Side effects include mild gastrointestinal upset; there are no reported drug interactions. The biggest concern about the use of saw palmetto is that individuals may self-medicate without verifying the diagnosis of BPH, and, therefore, more serious diseases of the prostate could be missed. Capsaicin cream, derived from hot peppers, is used topically to relieve pain from neuralgias, osteoarthritis, rheumatoid arthritis, back pain, and nerve pain, among other conditions. Capsaicin produces a stinging or burning sensation when initially used. Clients should be instructed to keep capsaicin away from the eyes and other sensitive areas of the body. Randomized control studies supported capsaicin use over the use of placebo (Wong, 2006).

Even though herbs are natural products, some medicinal herbs have side effects that could have adverse effects for the elderly. Yohimbe, for example, is used to treat impotence. Although it has been shown to be effective, it is not recommended by the U.S. Food and Drug Administration (FDA). When combined with tricyclic antidepressants, side effects include hypertension, renal failure,

TABLE 21-3 Potential Side Effects of Large Doses of Vitamins

Vitamin	Side Effects of Large Doses
A (retinol)	Nausea, vomiting, headache, dizziness, blurred vision, possible risk of osteoporosis (U. S. Food and Drug Administration, 2007). Beta carotene (a precursor to vitamin A) is less toxic than preformed A (retinol) at high levels of intake (Vitamins, 2007).
B_3 (niacin)	Flushing, redness of skin, upset stomach (U. S. Food and Drug Administration, 2007).
B_6 (pyridoxine)	Nerve damage to limbs (U.S. Food and Drug Administration, 2007).
C (ascorbic acid)	Upset stomach, kidney stones, increased iron absorption (U.S. Food and Drug Administration, 2007).
D (calciferol)	Nausea, vomiting, poor appetite, constipation, weight loss, confusion (U.S. Food and Drug Administration, 2007).
Folic acid (folate)	Hides signs of vitamin B_{12} deficiency (U.S. Food and Drug Administration, 2007).

seizures, hypotension, tachycardia, and dizziness. Comfrey has been used for gastritis, gastrointestinal ulcers, rheumatism, bronchitis, internal bleeding, diarrhea, and sprains and pulled ligaments. Because of the potential side effect of liver toxicity, however, the FDA has identified comfrey as a possible health hazard. In 2001, the FDA required oral comfrey removed from all dietary supplement products. Although topical products containing comfrey are available, comfrey should not be applied to open wounds or on broken skin (University of Maryland Medical Center, 2007). The FDA also proposed a limit to the amount of ephedrine alkaloids in dietary supplements (ephedra, Ma Huang, Chinese ephedra). The use of ephedrine has been linked with nervousness, dizziness, heart attack, stroke, seizures, and death (FDA, 2004). Consumers must be instructed to read labels because ephedrine may be an ingredient in supplements imported from other countries.

Although most of the herbal medications are safe when used as recommended, the concern is that many older adults do not tell their nurse practitioners, physicians, or other health care providers about the botanicals they are taking. This increases the possibility of drug interactions (Astin, Pelletier, Marie, & Haskell, 2000). Also, many times health care providers do not ask their patients about what natural substances they are taking (Milden & Stokols, 2004). Patients taking prescription drugs such as blood thinners, blood pressure medications, cyclosporine, digoxin, hypoglycemic agents, phenytoin, theophylline, and antidepressants should avoid herbal medications (Kuhn, 2002; Williamson, Fletcher, & Dawson, 2003). In addition, many safety concerns and drug interactions are under-researched in the elderly. Consumers should be cautioned when using herbal remedies to buy only reputable products, because the FDA does not regulate herbal manufacturing (**Case Study 21-1**).

Manipulation and Body-Based Practices

Manipulation and body-based practices primarily focus on the structures and systems of the body These practices are not new; some are rooted in

TABLE 21-4 Ten Most Often Used Natural Products

Name	Actions/Use	Contradications/Side Effects
Echinacea purpurea (Echinacea)	Anti-infective; stimulates immune response Uses: treatment and prevention of coughs, colds, flu, and bronchitis; wounds and burns; fevers	May interfere with immunosuppressant drugs; contraindicated in diseases related to immune response, multiple sclerosis, tuberculosis, AIDS, and autoimmune diseases Should not be used for more than 8-week intervals or immune system may be depressed (Deglin & Vallerand, 2007)
Panax ginseng (Asian ginseng) *Panax quinquefolius* (American ginseng)	Uses: improve physical and mental stamina; treatment of diabetes; sedative; aphrodisiac; increase immune response; increase appetite	May decrease effectiveness of warfarin; may interfere with MAO inhibitors; may have hypoglycemic effects; caffeine may increase herb effect; use with caution with estrogen; may increase risk of bleeding if used with antiplatelet herbs; may prolong QT interval if used with bitter orange; may interfere with immunosuppressant therapy Side effects: agitation, insomnia, tachycardia, depression, hypertension (Deglin & Vallerand, 2007)
Gingko biloba (Gingko) Standardized: 24% flavonoid glycosides 6% terpenelactones	Uses: symptomatic relief of organic brain dysfunction; intermittent claudication; vertigo and tinnitus (vascular origin); sexual dysfunction; improve peripheral circulation	Use with caution if individuals are on anticoagulant or antiplatelet therapy or have diabetes Contraindicated if individuals have bleeding disorders or increased blood sugars Side effects: headache, dizziness, GI disturbances
Garlic supplements	Vasodilator, antiplatelet properties Uses: hypertension, lowering cholesterol	May increase bleeding; not as effective in lowering cholesterol as other medications (Deglin & Vallerand, 2007)

Name	Actions/Use	Contradications/Side Effects
Glucosamine	May stimulate cartilage growth Use: osteoarthritis	Contraindicated if shellfish allergy is present May interfere with glucose regulation in diabetics (Deglin & Vallerand, 2007)
St. John's wort (*Hypericum perforatum*)	Antidepressant; when used topically, may have antiviral, anti-inflammatory, antibacterial activity Uses: mild to moderate depression	Alcohol and other antidepressives may increase CNS side effects Side effects: dizziness, restlessness, sleep disturbance, hypertension, bloating, abdominal pain, flatulence (Deglin & Vallerand, 2007)
Peppermint	Muscle relaxant, particularly in the digestive tract; reduces inflammation in nasal passages Uses: irritable bowel syndrome, nausea and vomiting, congestion related to colds and allergies	May cause choking feeling if applied to chest or nostrils of a child under 5; may intensify symptoms in hiatal hernia; avoid large doses if pregnant because it can relax uterine muscles Side effects: none identified (Supplements: Peppermint, 2005)
Fish oils/omega fatty acids	May decrease risk of coronary artery disease; may protect against irregular heartbeats Uses: protect against heart disease	None
Ginger supplements	Inhibit platelets, prostaglandins; improve digestion, appetite; may be hypoglycemic Uses: nausea and vomiting; joint pain	Use with caution in patients with bleeding tendencies or on anti coagulant therapy or with diabetics Side effects: heartburn
Soy supplements	Lowers total cholesterol and low-density lipoprotein (LDL)	Controversy that isoflavones, a component of soy, are phytoestrogens, a weak estrogen, and may increase cancer risk; other evidence supports that soy may protect against breast cancer (Henkel, 2000)

traditional medical systems and others have been practiced in the United States for over 150 years. Those practitioners of manipulation and body-based practices believe that parts of the body are interdependent and the body has the ability to heal itself. Chiropractic and osteopathic manipulation, massage therapy, reflexology, and rolfing are examples of practices from this category (NCCAM, 2007c). Both chiropractic care and massage were reported to be among the 10 most used CAM therapies (Barnes et al., 2004).

Chiropractic practice is considered a holistic approach to health. It is thought to provide benefit by helping place the body in proper alignment. Many

Case Study 21-1

Mr. Walters, 85, is receiving home care following a hospitalization for an exacerbation of congestive heart failure (CHF). He is diagnosed with atrial fibrillation and peripheral vascular disease. His legs are dry with scales; they are discolored from mid-calf to the foot. Both feet are warm to the touch. He was sent home on oxygen at 3 liters with an oxygen concentrator. He is taking the following medications:

Lanoxin 0.125 mg every day
Enteric coated aspirin 325 mg daily
Enalapril 25 mg twice a day
Furosemide 40 mg each morning
Vitamin E 400 IU every day
Gingko biloba 120 mg leaf extract twice a day
Panax ginseng 200 mg every day
Capsaicin to his back and legs when he has been working in the garden

Questions:

1. What assessments would the home health nurse make during home visits?
2. What instructions should Mr. Walters receive from the nurse?
3. What would be appropriate follow-up for the next visit?

third-party payers for health care provide some reimbursement for chiropractic care. Although satisfaction with chiropractic care is high (Hertzman-Miller, 2002; NCCAM, 2007c), empirical evidence about the long-term efficacy is mixed (Bove & Nilsson, 1998; Cherkin, Sherman, Deyo, & Shekelle, 2003; Ernst & Canter, 2003; NCCAM, 2007c).

Massage therapy includes various techniques that involve the manipulation of soft tissue through pressure and movement. Massage promotes circulation of blood and lymph, stimulates nerve endings, increases nutrients to the tissues, and removes waste products (Mitzel-Wilkinson, 2000). Many individuals use massage therapy to increase relaxation and reduce stress, recover from muscle stress and strain, heal injuries, and relieve pain. Satisfaction with massage treatments is very high (NCCAM, 2007c). In addition, research studies have supported the use of massage in a variety of situations (Billhult, Bergbom, & Stener-Victorin, 2007; Furlan, Brosseau, Imamura, & Irvin, 2002; Gatlin & Schulmeister, 2007). Although massage is considered a low risk intervention, it is contraindicated under several circumstances, including deep vein thrombosis, burns, skin infections, eczema, open wounds, bone fractures, and advanced osteoporosis (Gatlin & Schulmeister, 2007).

Energy Medicine

Energy medicine encompasses two basic types of energy fields: veritable, which can be measured, and putative, which currently cannot be measured. Examples of **veritable energy fields** include mechanical vibration and electromagnetic forces. **Putative energy fields** (biofields) include the vital energy (qi) of TCM, doshas in Ayurvedic medicine, ki in the Japanese Kampo system, and prana, etheric energy, fohat, orgone, odic force, and homeopathic resonance in other systems (NCCAM, 2007b). Therapists claim they work with this energy to improve health by reducing pain, anxiety, and blood pressure; increasing wound healing; and providing a sense of well-being (NCCAM, 2007b). Examples of practices using putative energy fields include Reiki, qi gong, healing (or therapeutic) touch, and prayer for the health of others (intercessory prayer). As a group, these are the most controversial of CAM practices because the energy fields cannot be measured, making traditional scientific research methodology difficult.

Also, there is an overlap between the CAM designations of mind-body medicine and putative energy fields. This can add some confusion to the CAM categories and, consequently, to consumers. It also illustrates that many of the CAM modalities cannot be investigated in isolation, but, rather, must be studied within the larger context. Those modalities that were covered under mind-body medicine, such as acupuncture, Ayurvedic medicine, homeopathy, and music therapy, will not be explained again. *Qi gong* refers to exercises that improve health and increase a sense of harmony by manipulating qi (vital energy) through movement and meditation. Currently, qi gong is considered an umbrella term for all energy exercises, such as yoga, Reiki, and meditation. It is widely practiced in

Chinese hospitals and clinics, but there have been no large clinical trials outside China to support this practice. Studies, however, have demonstrated some evidence to support the influence of qi gong (Chen, Hassett, Hou, Staller, & Lichtbroun, 2006; Sancier & Holman, 2004; Tsang, Fung, Chan, Lee, & Chan, 2006).

Therapeutic (healing) touch and **Reiki** both involve movement of a practitioner's hands over the patient's body to balance energy fields (NCCAM, 2007b). Reiki is a form of healing through the manipulation of ki (Japanese for life energy; similar to Chinese qi). Therapeutic touch may involve either physically touching the body or noncontact touch. When the body is not physically touched, the touch refers to the "touching" or movement of the individual's energy field (Eschiti, 2007). The purpose of therapeutic touch is to transfer life energy through the therapist's hands to the client, who will use the energy to rebalance and restore health. Certification in healing touch can be obtained through Healing Touch International, Inc.; healing touch classes are taught worldwide. Although anecdotal evidence and relatively small research studies tend to support therapeutic touch (NCCAM, 2007b; Eschiti, 2007), no large scale controlled studies have been conducted with these therapies. A systematic review to determine the effects of therapeutic touch on the healing of acute wounds produced no evidence that therapeutic touch promotes the healing of wounds (O'Mathuna & Ashford, 2003).

Several electromagnetic fields, part of veritable energy medicine, have been used in conventional medicine. Magnetic resonance imagery, cardiac pacemakers, transcutaneous electrical nerve stimulators (TENS), and radiation therapy are all examples of the use of these fields. Another veritable energy modality is magnetic therapy, which is the use of static magnets to relieve pain or increase energy levels. Anecdotal reports support the efficacy of static magnets, but more scientific research is needed to support this therapy (NCCAM, 2007b).

Sound energy therapy includes music therapy. The basis of sound energy therapy is that specific sound frequencies can facilitate the body's healing (NCCAM, 2007b). Music therapy is also a mind-body modality, further supporting the overlap of mind-body interventions and energy medicine. Light therapy has been used to treat seasonal affective disorder successfully, but other uses do not have as much empirical support (NCCAM, 2007b). This is an area for further research.

REASONS FOR CAM USE

Older adults use CAM for pain relief, to increase quality of life, and to maintain health and fitness (Astin et al., 2000; Williamson et al., 2003). Some view CAM as a return to a "kinder and gentler medicine" (Barrett et al., 2004); however, most use CAM in combination with conventional medication rather than as a primary source of treatment (Barnes et al., 2004; Bausell, Lee, & Berman, 2001). In addition, most rely on family and friends to provide information about choosing a modality (Najm, Reinsch, Hoehler, & Tobis, 2003). As a rule, elders choose CAM because of the belief system behind the modality, not because of dissatisfaction with conventional care (Smith, 2004). However, the nurse cannot overlook the fact the some elders may use CAM because they have difficulty accessing traditional medical care or medications (Pagan & Pauly, 2005).

NURSING INTERVENTIONS

When performing assessments, nurses must ask clients about their use of CAM, why particular modalities are used, the source of the therapy, and their knowledge of side effects (King, Pettigrew, & Reed, 2000). These questions should be phrased in a nonjudgmental manner and should also be phrased in such a way as to cover the variety of modalities. Clients may not acknowledge they are taking herbal medicines, but may identify that they are taking natural products. This is particularly important when clients are on prescribed medications for blood thinning, blood pressure, depression, anxiety, or insomnia. Also, elders may not consider vitamins or minerals as medications because they are considered dietary supplements; however, if taken in conjunction with some prescribed medications or in large doses, vitamins may interfere with the actions of the medications and produce side effects. Good communication skills are a key to a thorough assessment of CAM use. Integrated care, a combination of allopathy and CAM, may be the best model of care for an older adult. The nurse must be a knowledgeable member of this integrated health care team to be able to provide comprehensive, holistic care (Killinger, Morley, Kettner, & Kauric, 2001). To facilitate cultural competency and to provide holistic care to clients and patients, nursing and medical schools have added content on complementary and alternative medicine to their curricula.

SUMMARY

As CAM becomes more widely used by the elderly as well as by the general population, the nurse has a responsibility to be knowledgeable about the modalities clients may be using. The World Health Organization (WHO) estimates that 80% of the world's population uses some form of CAM (Bielory, 2002; Milden & Stokols, 2004), so knowledge of CAM may be considered part of culturally competent care (Cueller, Cahill, Ford, & Aycock, 2003). Nurses should have basic knowledge of the most commonly used CAM therapies in order to provide holistic care to older adults who may wish to incorporate these modalities into their treatment plan. Remember that the effectiveness of some CAM therapies with the older population has not been well researched. Nurses will need to tailor their care to the needs of each individual.

BOX **21-1** Research Highlight

Aim: This two-group randomized study examined the effects of guided imagery on pain perception, functional status, and self-efficacy in persons with fibromyalgia.

Methods: This longitudinal experimental study randomly assigned volunteer participants with fibromyalgia into two groups. The experimental group ($n = 24$) received usual care as well as three guided imagery audiotapes for a 6-week treatment phase and a 4-week follow-up phase. The control group ($n = 24$) received usual care. Demographic information was collected at baseline. Pain, functional status, and self-efficacy were measured at baseline, at week 6, and week 10. Pain was measured by the Short-Form McGill Pain Questionnaire; functional status was measured by the Fibromyalgia Impact Questionnaire; and self-efficacy was measured by the Arthritis Self-Efficacy Scale. The self-efficacy scale was modified to be specific for persons with fibromyalgia.

Findings: The groups were similar on demographic and outcome variables at baseline. Over time, the group receiving guided imagery showed significant improvements in functional status and self-efficacy for managing pain when compared to the group receiving usual care alone. There were no significant differences between the groups over time in perceived pain.

Application to practice: Although the perception of pain did not change over time for either group, guided imagery made a difference in the functional status and self-efficacy in the ability to manage pain in this population. This has implications for improving quality of life. More research needs to be done to provide a body of evidence to support the efficacy of guided imagery as a nonpharmacological intervention to assist patients living with chronic pain.

Source: Menzies, V., Taylor, A. G., & Bourguignon, C. (2007). Effects of guided imagery on outcomes of pain, functional status, and self-efficacy in persons diagnosed with fibromyalgia. *Journal of Alternative and Complementary Medicine*, *12*, 23–30.

BOX 21-2 Resource List

General

The Cochrane Collaboration for systematic reviews: http://www.cochrane.org

Institute of Medicine Board: Health Promotion and Disease Prevention. (2005). *Use of complementary and alternative medicine (CAM) by the American public.* Washinton, DC: Author.

National Center for Complementary and Alternative Medicine (NCCAM): http://nccam.nih.gov

University of Maryland Medical Center Complementary and Alternative Medicine Index (CAM): http://www.umm.edu/altmed

University of Pittsburgh—The Alternative Medicine Homepage: http://www.pitt.edu/~cbw/altm.html

Diet and Herbs

Alternative Medicine Foundation: http://www.herbmed.org

Blumenthal, M. (Ed.). (1998). *The complete German commission E monographs: Therapeutic guide to herbal medicines.* Austin, TX: American Botanical Council.

Complementary/Integrative Medicine Program at the University of Texas M. D. Anderson Cancer Center: http://www.mdanderson.org/CIMER

Pet Therapy

Delta Society: http://www.deltasociety.org

Therapet Animal Assisted Therapy Foundation: http://www.therapet.com

BOX 21-3 Web Exploration

Explore conferences, products, certifications, and careers in music therapy at American Music Therapy Association (AMTA): http://www.musictherapy.org

Check out Canine Companions for Independence, an association that facilitates the breeding, raising, and training of dogs to be working companions to those with disabilities: http://www.cci.org/site/c.cdKGIRNqEmG/b.3978475/

BOX 21-4 Recommended Readings

Adams, L. L., Gatchel, R. J., & Gentry, C. (2001). Complementary and alternative medicine: Applications and implications for cognitive functioning in elderly populations. *Alternative Therapies in Health and Medicine, 7*(2), 52–61.

Astin, J. A. (1998). Why patients use alternative medicine: Results of a national study. *Journal of the American Medical Association, 279,* 1548–1553.

Barrett, B. (2003). Alternative, complementary, and conventional medicine: Is integration upon us? *Journal of Alternative and Complementary Medicine, 9,* 417–427.

Birch, S., Hesselink, J. K., Jonkman, F. A. M., Hekker, T. A. M., & Bos, A. (2004). Clinical research on acupuncture: Part I. What have reviews of the efficacy and safety of acupuncture told us so far? *Journal of Alternative and Complementary Medicine, 10,* 468–480.

Cartwright, T (2007). "Getting on with life": The experiences of older people using complementary health care. *Social Science and Medicine, 64,* 1692–1703.

Doherty, D., Wright, S., Aveyard, B., & Sykes, M. (2006). Therapeutic touch and dementia: An ongoing journey. *Nursing Older People, 18*(11), 27–30.

Dossey, L. (1993). *Healing words: The power of prayer and the practice of medicine.* San Francisco: Harper.

Gloth, F. M. (2001). Pain management in older adults: Prevention and treatment. *Journal of the American Geriatrics Society, 49,* 188–199.

Jonas, W. B., Kaptchuk, T. J., & Linde, K. (2003). A critical overview of homeopathy. *Annals of Internal Medicine, 138,* 393–399.

Schofield, P., Smith, P., Aveyard, B., & Black, C. (2007). Complementary therapies for pain management in palliative care. *Journal of Community Nursing, 21*(8), 10, 12–14.

Steyer, T. E. (2001). Complementary and alternative medicine: A primer. *Family Practice Management, 8*(3), 37–42, 61–62.

Vangsness, S., Moffitt, R., & Herbold, N. H. (2005). Education and knowledge of dietetic interns regarding herbs and dietary supplements: Preparing for practice. *Topics of Clinical Nutrition, 20,* 269–276.

Critical Thinking *Exercises*

1. Access the National Center for Complementary and Alternative Medicine Web site (http://nccam.nih.gov) and explore one of the CAM therapies listed. Review the information presented from the per-

continues

Critical Thinking (continued)

spective of a consumer with no medical knowledge. What is the reading level? Is the material easy to understand? What would you add and why? What would you delete and why?

2. Interview several older adults and ask them what supplements, vitamins, or herbals they use and why. During the course of conversation, ask them if they inform their health care providers about their practices and why. Discuss your findings with a group of nursing students. As a group, identify nursing interventions appropriate for the adults interviewed.
3. In a group, critique research articles exploring the efficacy of a CAM modality with research reports on clinical trials of allopathic medicines. Compare the levels of evidence of each report.

Personal Reflections

1. Think about what CAM therapies you have used personally. If you have not used any, think about one therapy you think you may want to try. Why did you use CAM or why would you use CAM? Think about patients that you have had who have used CAM. What was your reaction to the information? Have you changed your mind about CAM since reading the chapter? Did the patients use CAM for the same reasons you did or thought you may?
2. Look through your local newspaper for a week. What references to CAM do you find? How many references were directed at the older adult? Were you surprised by what you found?

References

Aldridge, D. (1994). An overview of music therapy research. *Complementary Therapies in Medicine, 2,* 204–216.

Ameling, A. (2000). Prayer: An ancient healing practice becomes new again. *Holistic Nursing Practice, 14*(3), 40–48.

Astin, J. A., Pelletier, K. R., Marie, A., & Haskell, W. L. (2000). Complementary and alternative medicine use among elderly persons: One-year analysis of a Blue Shield Medicare supplement. *Journals of Gerontology, 55A,* M4–M9.

Barnes, P. M., Powell-Griner, E., McFann, K., & Nahin, R. L. (2004, May 27). *CDC advance data report #343. Complementary and alternative medicine use among adults: United States, 2002.* Bethesda, MD: Author.

Barrett, B., Marchand, L., Scheder, J., Applebaum, D., Plane, M. B., Blustein, J., et al. (2004). What complementary and alternative practitioners say about health and health care. *Annals of Family Medicine, 2,* 253–259.

Bausell, R. B., Lee, W. L., & Berman, B. M. (2001). Demographic and health-related correlates of visits to complementary and alternative medical providers. *Medical Care, 39,* 190–196.

Bielory, L. (2002). "Complementary and alternative medicine" population based studies: A growing focus on allergy and asthma. *Allergy, 57,* 655–658.

Billhult, A., Bergbom, I., & Stener-Victorin, E. (2007). Massage relieves nausea in women with breast cancer who are undergoing chemotherapy. *Journal of Alternative and Complementary Medicine, 13,* 53–57.

Bove, G., & Nilsson, N. (1998). Spinal manipulation in the treatment of episodic tension-type headache.

Journal of the American Medical Association, 280, 1576–1579.

Burke, A., Upchurch, D. M., Dye, C., & Chyu, L. (2006). Acupuncture use in the United States: Findings from the National Health Interview Survey. *Journal of Alternative and Complementary Medicine, 12,* 639–648.

Cepeda, M. S., Carr, D. B., Lau, J., & Alvarez, H. (2006). Music for pain relief. *Cochrane Database of Systematic Reviews, 2,* Art. No.: CD004843. DOI:10.1002/14651858.CD004843.pub2.

Chen, K. W., Hassett, A. L., Hou, F., Staller, J., & Lichtbroun, A. S. (2006). A pilot study of external *qigong* therapy for patients with fibromyalgia. *Journal of Alternative and Complementary Medicine, 12,* 851–856.

Chen, W. C. C. (1973). *Body mechanics of tai chi chuan.* New York: William C. C. Chen.

Chen, Y. (2001). Chinese values, health, and nursing. *Journal of Advanced Nursing, 36,* 270–273.

Cherkin, D. C., Sherman, K. J., Deyo, R. A., & Shekelle, P. G. (2003). A review of the evidence for the effectiveness, safety, and cost of acupuncture, massage therapy, and spinal manipulation for back pain. *Annals of Internal Medicine, 138,* 898–906.

Cuellar, N. G., Cahill, B., Ford, J., & Aycock, T. (2003). The development of an educational workshop on complementary and alternative medicine: What every nurse should know. *Journal of Continuing Education in Nursing, 34,* 128–135.

Daniel, C., O'Keefe, P., & Pepa, C. A. (2002, November). *The use of music therapy in selected clinical areas: An integrative review.* Paper presented at the 10th annual Northwest Indiana Nursing Research Consortium conference, Merrillville, IN.

Deglin, J. H., & Vallerand, A. H. (2007). *Davis's drug guide for nurses* (10th ed.). Philadelphia: F. A. Davis.

Eisenberg, D. M., Davis, R. B., Ettner, S. L., Appel, S., Wikey, S., Van Rompay, M., et al. (1998). Trends in alternative medicine use in the United States, 1990–1997. *Journal of the American Medical Association, 280,* 1569–1575.

Eisenberg, D. M., Kessler, R. C., Foster, C., Norlock, F. E., Calkins, D. R., & Delbanco, T. L. (1993). Unconventional medicine in the United States. *New England Journal of Medicine, 328,* 246–252.

Ernst, E. (2002). The risk-benefit profile of community-used herbal therapies: Gingko, St. John's wort, ginseng, echinacea, saw palmetto, and kava. *Annals of Internal Medicine, 136,* 42–53.

Ernst, E., & Canter, P. H. (2003). Chiropractic spinal manipulation treatment for back pain? A systematic review of randomized clinical trials. *Physical Therapy Reviews, 8,* 85–91.

Eschiti, V. S. (2007). Healing touch: A low-tech intervention in high-tech settings. *Dimensions of Critical Care Nursing, 26*(1), 9–14.

Fan, R. (2003). Modern Western science as a standard for traditional Chinese medicine: A critical appraisal. *Journal of Law, Medicine and Ethics, 31,* 213–221.

Furlan, A. D., Brosseau, L., Imamura, M., & Irvin, E. (2002). Massage for low-back pain. *Cochrane Database of Systematic Reviews, 2.* Art. No.: CD001929. DOI: 10:1002/14651858.CD001929.

Gatlin, C. G., & Schulmeister, L. (2007). When medication is not enough: Nonpharmacologic management of pain. *Clinical Journal of Oncology Nursing, 11,* 699–704.

Gloth, F. M. (2001). Pain management in older adults: Prevention and treatment. *Journal of the American Geriatrics Society, 49,* 188–199.

Gordon, A. E., & Shaughnessy, A. F. (2003). Saw palmetto for prostate disorder. *American Family Physician, 67,* 1281–1283.

Gormley, J. J. (2000). Ayurveda: Wisdom, science, and healing for today. *Better Nutrition, 62*(10), 80–82, 84.

Gundersen, L. (2000). Faith and healing. *Annals of Internal Medicine, 132,* 169–172.

Harvard School of Public Health. (n.d.). *Vitamins.* Retrieved January 2, 2008, from http://www.hsph.harvard.edu/nutritionsource/vitamins.html

Henkel, J. (2000). Soy: Health claims for soy protein, questions about other components. *FDA Consumer Magazine.* Retrieved January 3, 2008, from http://www.cfsan.fda.gov/~dms/fdsoypr.html

Hertzman-Miller, R. P. (2002). Comparing the satisfaction of low back pain patients randomized to receive medical or chiropractic care: Results from the UCLA low-back pain study. *American Journal of Public Health, 92,* 1628–1633.

Hooker, S. D., Freeman, L. H., & Steward, P. (2002). Pet therapy research: A historical review. *Holistic Nursing Practice, 17*(1), 17–23.

Killinger, L. Z., Morley, J. E., Kettner, N. W., & Kauric, E. (2001). Integrated care of the older patient. *Topics in Clinical Chiropractic, 8*(2), 46–54.

King, M. O., Pettigrew, A. C., & Reed, F. C. (2000). Complementary, alternative, integrative: Have nurses kept pace with their clients? *Dermatology Nursing, 12,* 41–44, 47–50.

Kuhn, M. (1999). *Complementary therapies for health care providers.* Philadelphia: Lippincott Williams & Wilkins.

Kuhn, M. A. (2002). Herbal remedies: Drug-herb interactions. *Critical Care Nurse, 22*(2), 22–30.

Lee, B. Y., LaRiccia, P. J., & Newberg, A. B. (2004). Acupuncture in theory and practice Part I: Theoretical basis and physiologic effects. *Hospital Physician, 40*(4), 11–18.

Maier-Lorentz, M. M. (2004). The importance of prayer for mind/body healing. *Nursing Forum, 39*(3), 23–32.

Mangels, A. R., Messina, V., & Melina, V. (2003). Position of the American Dietetic Association and Dietitians of Canada: Vegetarian diets. *Journal of the American Dietetic Association, 103*, 748–765.

Menzies, V., & Taylor, A. G. (2004). The idea of imagination: An analysis of "imagery." *Advances in Mind Body Medicine, 20*(2), 4–10.

Menzies, V., Taylor, A. G., & Bourguignon, C. (2007). Effects of guided imagery on outcomes of pain, functional status, and self-efficacy in persons diagnosed with fibromyalgia. *Journal of Alternative and Complementary Medicine, 12,* 23–30.

Milden, S. P., & Stokols, D. (2004). Physicians' attitudes and practices regarding complementary and alternative medicine. *Behavioral Medicine, 30,* 73–82.

Miller, R. (2003). Nurses at community hospital welcome guided imagery tool. *Dimensions of Critical Care Nursing, 22,* 225–226.

Mitzel-Wilkinson, A. (2000). Massage therapy as a nursing practice. *Holistic Nursing Practice, 14*(2), 48–56.

Najm, W., Reinsch, S., Hoehler, F., & Tobis, J. (2003). Use of complementary and alternative medicine among the ethnic elderly. *Alternative Therapies in Health and Medicine, 9*(3), 50–57.

Naparstek, B. (1994). *Staying well with guided imagery.* New York: Werner Books.

National Center for Complementary and Alternative Medicine. (2003). *Research report. Questions and answers about homeopathy.* NCCAM Publication No. D183. Retrieved December 30, 2007, from http://nccam.nih.gov/health/homeopathy

National Center for Complementary and Alternative Medicine. (2004). *Backgrounder. An introduction to acupuncture.* NCCAM Publication No. D003. Retrieved September 27, 2007, from http://nccam.nih.gov/health/acupuncture

National Center for Complementary and Alternative Medicine. (2007a). *Backgrounder. Biologically based practices: An overview.* NCCAM Publication No. D237. Retrieved November 29, 2007, from http://nccam.nih.gov/health/backgrounds/biobasedprac.htm

National Center for Complementary and Alternative Medicine. (2007b). *Backgrounder. Energy medicine: An overview.* NCCAM Publication No. D235. Retrieved November 29, 2007, from http://nccam.nih.gov/health/backgrounds/energymed.htm

National Center for Complementary and Alternative Medicine. (2007c). *Backgrounder. Manipulative and body-based practices: An overview.* NCCAM Publication No. D238. Retrieved November 29, 2007, from http://nccam.nih.gov/health/backgrounds/manipulative.htm

National Center for Complementary and Alternative Medicine. (2007d). *Backgrounder. Mind-body medicine: An overview.* NCCAM Publication No. D239. Retrieved November 29, 2007, from http://nccam.nih.gov/health/backgrounds/mindbody.htm

National Center for Complementary and Alternative Medicine. (2007e). *Backgrounder. Whole medical systems: An overview.* NCCAM Publication No. D236. Retrieved November 29, 2007, from http://nccam.nih.gov/health/backgrounds/wholemed.htm

National Center for Complementary and Alternative Medicine. (2007f). *CAMBasics: What is CAM?* NCCAM Publication No. D347. Retrieved October 25, 2007, from http://nccam.nih.gov/health/whatiscam/

National Institutes of Health Consensus Development Panel on Acupuncture. (1998). Acupuncture. *Journal of the American Medical Association, 280,* 1518–1524.

Ness, J., Cirillo, D. J., Weir, D. R., Nisly, N. L., & Wallace, R. B. (2005). Use of complementary medicine in older Americans: Results from the health and retirement study. *The Gerontologist, 45,* 516–524.

O'Mathuna, D. P., & Ashford, R. L. (2003). Therapeutic touch for healing acute wounds. *Cochrane Database of Systematic Reviews, 4.* Art. No.: CD002766. DOI: 10.1002/14651858.CD002766.

Ott, M. J. (2004). Mindfulness meditation: A path of transformation and healing. *Journal of Psychosocial Nursing and Mental Health Services, 42*(7), 22–29.

Pagan, J. A., & Pauly, M. V. (2005). Access to conventional medical care and the use of complementary and alternative medicine. *Health Affairs, 24,* 255–262.

Pohl, T. (2001). Ayurveda: The science of life. *New Mexico Nurse, 46*(2), 13–14.

Raub, J. A. (2002). Psychophysiologic effects of hatha yoga on musculoskeletal and cardiopulmonary function: A literature review. *Journal of Alternative and Complementary Medicine, 8,* 797–812.

Richards, T., Johnson, J., Sparks, A., & Emerson, H. (2007). The effect of music therapy on patients' perception and manifestation of pain, anxiety, and patient satisfaction. *MEDSURG Nursing, 16,* 7–14.

Roberts, D. (2004). Alternative therapies for arthritis treatment. *Holistic Nursing Practice, 18,* 167–174.

Roberts, L., Ahmed, I., & Hall, S. (2007). Intercessory prayer for the alleviation of ill health. *Cochrane Database of Systematic Reviews, 1.* Article No.: CD000368. DOI: 10.1002/14651858.CD000368.pub2.

Rosser, C. (2004). Homeopathy in cancer care: Part I—An introduction to "like curing like." *Clinical Journal of Oncology Nursing, 8,* 324–326.

Sancier, K. M., & Holman, D. (2004). Commentary: Multifaceted health benefits of medical *qigong. Journal of Alternative and Complementary Medicine, 10,* 163–165.

Sending prayers: Does it help? (2002). *Harvard Health Letter, 27*(7), 7.

Sicher, F., Targ, E., Moore, D., & Smith, D. (1998). A randomized double-blind study of the effect of distant healing in a population with advanced AIDS: Report of a small scale sample. *Western Journal of Medicine, 169,* 356–363.

Smith, S. S. (2004). Who uses complementary therapies? *Holistic Nursing Practice, 18,* 176.

Southern California Evidence-Based Practice Center & RAND. (2001). Ayurvedic interventions for diabetes mellitus: A systematic review. *AHRQ Evidence Reports No. 41.* Retrieved December 29, 2007, from http://www.ncbi.nlm.nih.gov/books/bv.fcgi?rid=hstat1.section.95397

Stanley-Hermanns, M., & Miller, J. (2002). Animal assisted therapy. *American Journal of Nursing, 102*(10), 69–76.

Supplements: Peppermint. (n.d.). Retrieved March 12, 2005, from http://www.wholehealthmd.com

Trinh, K. V., Graham, N., Gross, A. R., Goldsmith, C. H., Wang, E., Cameron, I. D., et al. (2006). Acupuncture for neck disorders. *Cochrane Database of Systematic Reviews, 3.* Art No.: CD004870. DOI: 10.1002/14651858.CD004870.pub3.

Tsang, H. W. H., Fung, K. M. T., Chan, A. S. M., Lee, E., & Chan, F. (2006). Effect of *qigong* exercise programme on elderly with depression. *International Journal of Geriatric Psychiatry, 21,* 890–897.

University of Maryland Medical Center. (2007). *Comfrey.* Retrieved January 2, 2008, from http://www.umm.edu/altmed/articles/comfrey-000234.htm

U.S. Food and Drug Administration. (2004). *An FDA guide to dietary supplements.* Center for Food Safety and Applied Nutrition. Retrieved March 10, 2005, from http://vm.cfsan.fda.gov

U.S. Food and Drug Administration. (2007). *Fortify your knowledge about vitamins.* Retrieved on January 12, 2009, from http://www.fda.gov/CONSUMER/updates/vitamins111907.html

Vanderboom, T. (2007). Does music reduce anxiety during invasive procedures with procedural sedation? An integrative research review. *Journal of Radiology Nursing, 26,* 15–17.

White House Commission on Complementary and Alternative Medicine Policy. (2002). *Final Report March 2002* (NIH Publication 03-5411). Washington, DC: NIH. Retrieved December 29, 2007, from http://www.whccamp.hhs.gov

Williamson, A. T., Fletcher, P. C., & Dawson, K. A. (2003). Complementary and alternative medicine: Use in an older population. *Journal of Gerontological Nursing, 29*(5), 20–29.

Wilt, T., Ishani, A., & MacDonald, R. (2002). *Serenoa repens* for benign prostatic hyperplasia. *Cochrane Database of Systematic Reviews, 2.* Art. No.: CD001423. DOI: 10.1002/14651858.CD001423.

Wong, C. (2006). *What is capsaicin cream?* Retrieved January 2, 2008, from http://altmedicine.about.com/od/completeazindex/a/capsaicin_cream.htm

World Health Organization. (2003). *Traditional medicine.* Retrieved January 1, 2008, from http://www.who.int/mediacentre/factsheets/fs134/en/print.html

SECTION

11

DESIGNER/MANAGER/ COORDINATOR OF CARE

(Competencies 27–29)

CHAPTER 22

Promoting Quality of Life

Sonya R. Hardin, PhD, RN, CCRN, ACNS-BC

LEARNING OBJECTIVES

At the end of this chapter, the reader will be able to:

- Define quality of life for the elderly.
- Describe a theoretical model for promoting quality of life.
- Discuss the active aging framework proposed by the World Health Organization.
- Identify components of each determinant of the active aging framework.
- Utilize select strategies to promote optimal active aging.

KEY TERMS

- Active aging
- Activity
- Autonomy
- Determinants of health
- Food Guide Pyramid for Older Adults
- Health-related quality of life (HRQOL)
- Independence
- Quality of life

Quality of life is a concept that has many definitions; to date there is no consensus regarding the meaning of the term. Given the concept's multidisciplinary nature, it has been defined as a degree of satisfaction or dissatisfaction with life (Abrams, 1973; Campbell, Converse, & Rogers, 1976), a person's sense of well-being (Dalkey & Rourke, 1973; Hanestad, 1990), and as dimensions such as health function, comfort, emotional response, economics, spirituality, and social support (Gough, Furnival, Schilder, & Grove, 1983; Patterson, 1975). Older people talk about quality of life in terms of family relationships, social contacts and activities, general health, and functional status (Farquhar, 1995a). These items are deemed important to the individual.

Quality of life is

> *. . . an individual's perception of his or her position in life in the context of the culture and value system where they live and in relation to their goals, expectations, standards and concerns. It is a broad-ranging concept, incorporating a person's physical health, psychological state, level of independence, social relationships, personal beliefs and relationships to salient features in the environment. (World Health Organization [WHO], 1994, p. 90)*

As people age, their quality of life is dependent upon their ability to maintain autonomy and independence. Besides the WHO, the Centers for Disease Control and Prevention (CDC) has an interest in quality of life for the population. The CDC's focus has been on the concept of **health-related quality of life (HRQOL)**. The CDC measures HRQOL using an instrument that assesses the number of healthy days an individuals has in a given month. **Box 22-1** displays the four questions used to measure population HRQOL. Utilizing this instrument, the CDC reports that in the United States, individuals feel physically or mentally unhealthy about 6 days a month. Almost one-third of the population reports suffering from some mental or emotional problem monthly. Approximately 10% of the population reports experiencing poor mental health at least 14 or more days a month. Native Americans and Alaska Natives have reported the highest levels of unhealthy days among the various U.S. racial/ethnic groups. Adults with the lowest income or education reported more unhealthy days than did those with higher income or education (CDC, 2005).

QUALITY OF LIFE MODELS

Grant, Ferrell, Schmidt, Fonbuena, Niland, and Forman (1992) have proposed a model for understanding the components of quality of life. The Ferrell and Grant quality of life model (**Figure 22-1**) was developed using qualitative methodology and identifies the four concepts of quality of life: physical well-being, psychological well-being, social well-being, and spiritual well-being. **Table 22-1** displays the major concepts of this model. Subsequent cross-cultural work with African Americans and Mexican Americans has provided evidence that the elements of the model appropriately reflect quality of life for these populations.

Quality of life has been linked with successful aging and active aging. Successful aging means that a person has avoided disease and disease-related disability, and has a high level of cognitive and physical functioning that allows the individual to be engaged with life. Numerous studies have focused on successful aging (e.g., Ouwehand, de Ridder, & Bensing, 2007). Several models, such as the Selective Optimization with Compensation model (SOC model) developed by Baltes and Baltes (1990) and Rowe and Kahn's Model of Successful Aging (1998), equate engagement in life, minimal

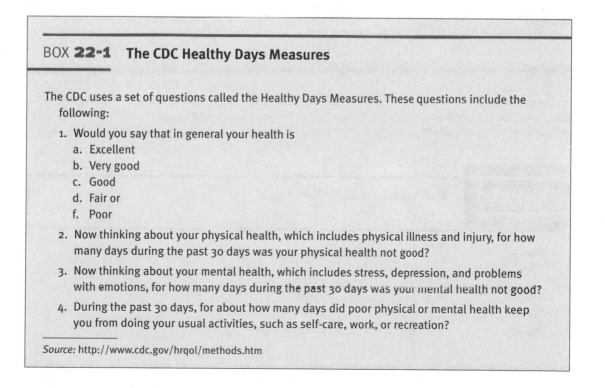

BOX 22-1 The CDC Healthy Days Measures

The CDC uses a set of questions called the Healthy Days Measures. These questions include the following:

1. Would you say that in general your health is
   a. Excellent
   b. Very good
   c. Good
   d. Fair or
   f. Poor
2. Now thinking about your physical health, which includes physical illness and injury, for how many days during the past 30 days was your physical health not good?
3. Now thinking about your mental health, which includes stress, depression, and problems with emotions, for how many days during the past 30 days was your mental health not good?
4. During the past 30 days, for about how many days did poor physical or mental health keep you from doing your usual activities, such as self-care, work, or recreation?

Source: http://www.cdc.gov/hrqol/methods.htm

FIGURE 22-1 Quality of Life Model.

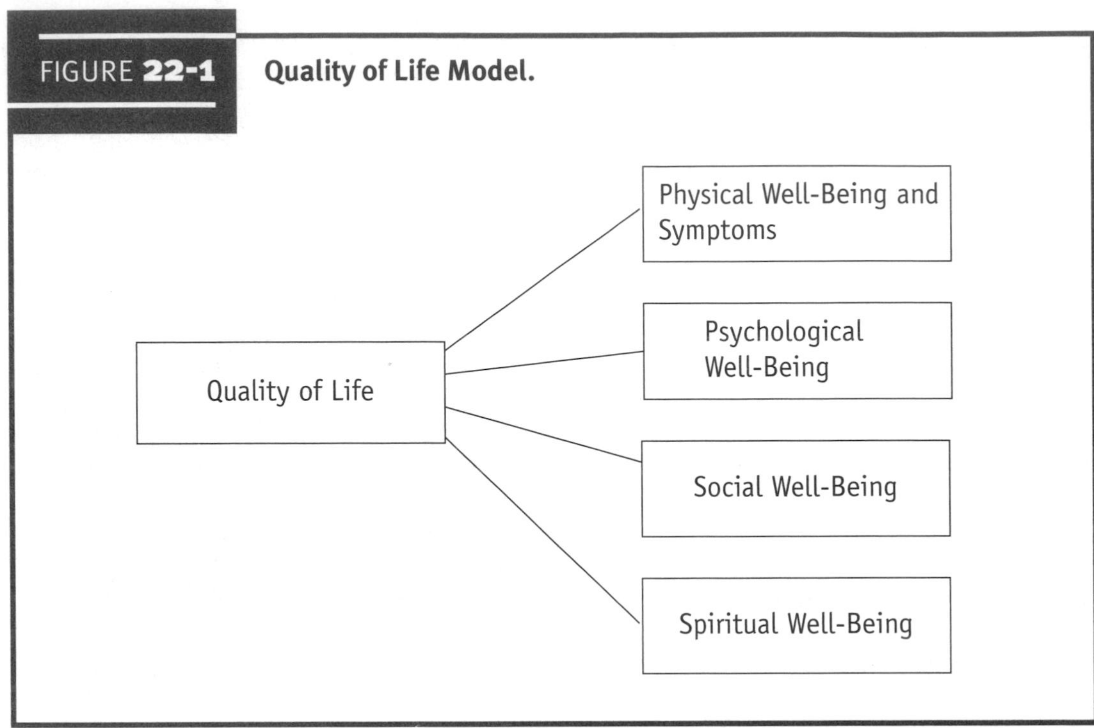

SOURCE: Ferrans, C. E. (1996). Development of a conceptual model of quality of life. *Scholarly Inquiry for Nursing Practice: An International Journal, 10*(3), 293–304. Springer Publishing Company, Inc., New York 10012. Used by permission.

disability, and high levels of physical and mental abilities with successful aging. These same concepts are often utilized in quality of life models. The SOC model identifies the processes that older adults use to cope with the changes of aging, whereas the Rowe and Kahn model stresses that successful aging is maximized when engagement in life and physical and mental abilities are enhanced.

Health services researchers typically identify quality of life as including dimensions of health

TABLE 22-1 **Distinguishers of Well-Being**

Physical Well-Being	Psychological Well-Being	Social Well-Being	Spiritual Well-Being
Functional ability, strength/fatigue, sleep/rest, nausea, appetite, constipation	Anxiety, depression, enjoyment/leisure, pain distress, happiness, fear, cognition/attention	Caregiver burden, roles and relationships, affection/sexual function, appearance	Suffering, meaning of pain, religiosity, transcendence

(physical and psychological) and functional status (Farquhar, 1995b). Much of the conceptual framework for measuring quality of life is derived from the WHO definition of health as a state of complete physical, mental, and social well-being (WHO, 1958). These are all components of quality of life. So is there a distinction between health and quality of life? The WHO has integrated health and quality of life into a program called **active aging**. This program is designed to help people remain independent and active as they age. Active aging encourages older individuals to continue to work according to their capacity and to delay disabilities and chronic diseases (see **Figure 22-2**). Active aging is being promoted by the WHO as a process of optimizing opportunities for health, participation in the community, and safe living in order to enhance quality of life as people age (WHO, 2002, p. 12). Maintaining quality of life is at the center of active aging. This chapter will look at each of the determinants described by the WHO program on active aging.

ACTIVE AGING

The term *active aging* was adopted by the WHO in the late 1990s to allow inclusion of additional factors related to healthy aging. The active aging approach is based on the human rights of older people and the United Nations' principles of **independence**, participation, dignity, care, and self-fulfillment. Such an approach requires thinking to shift from "needs-based" to "rights-based" in treatment as an individual grows older. This supports an individual's right to receive interventions to enhance **autonomy**, independence, and **activity**.

An active aging approach to strategies that promote quality of life has the potential to decrease

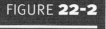

FIGURE **22-2** **Many older adults continue to work into their 70s as this veterinarian is.**

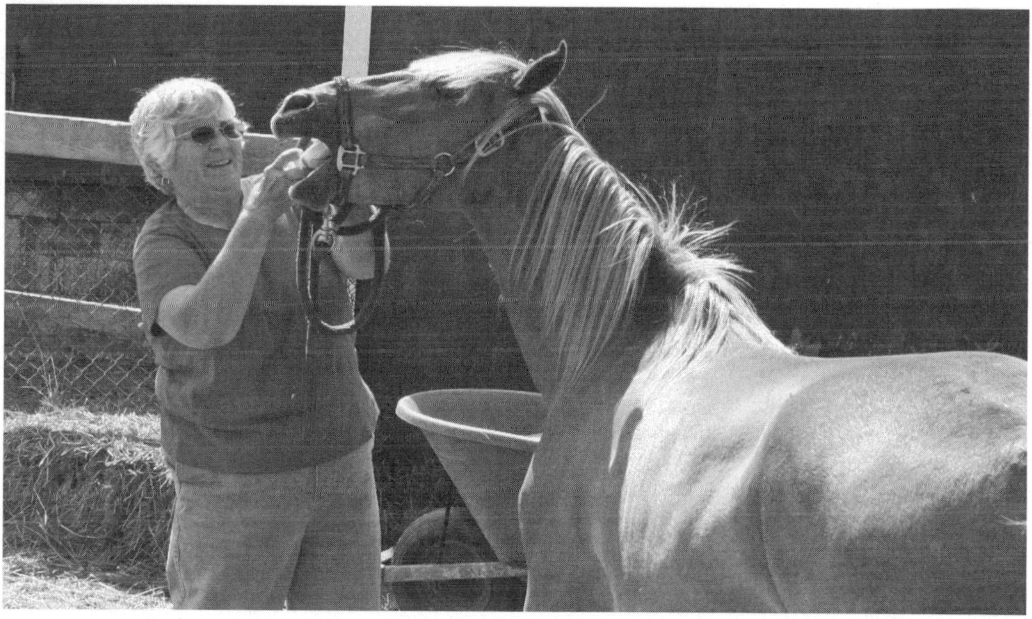

disabilities associated with chronic illness; increase elders' participation in the social, cultural, economic, and political aspects of society; and lower the cost of medical treatment. These interventions recognize the need to encourage individuals to plan and prepare for older age and to choose healthy lifestyles. Active aging can enhance and ensure one's quality of life in later years.

The World Health Organization has identified **determinants of health** that affect aging and the quality of life of individuals, communities, and nations. Healthy aging is influenced by gender and culture in addition to the following determinants: behavioral, social and physical environments, and personal, economic, and social service systems. Behavioral determinants include physical activity, nutrition, smoking, alcohol ingestion, and medication adherence. Determinants related to personal characteristics include genetics and psychological factors. Physical environment determinants include neighborhoods and safe housing. Social support, education and literacy, violence, and abuse make up the social environment determinants. Economic determinants include income and social protection. Determinants related to social services include health promotion and disease prevention.

Gender and culture influence all the determinants of healthy aging. In many countries females have a lower social status and less access to food, education, and health care; however, males are more likely to engage in behaviors such as smoking, alcohol, drug consumption, and strenuous labor. Values and traditions determine how a society views aging. Some societies view aging as a natural period of decline without expectations of a high quality of life, and thus are less likely to provide prevention, early detection, and tailored interventions for the elderly when symptoms are attributed to the aging process. Aging is viewed as a life process, one in which ultimate deterioration is expected and should be accepted. Health-seeking behaviors also are influenced by culture and values. By enhancing individual quality of life, one must respect diverse ethnicities while educating to overcome folk medicine beliefs or prejudice against formal biomedicine.

Behavioral Determinants

Behavioral determinants refer to behaviors that promote healthy lifestyles. Healthy behaviors are just as important to older persons as to the young. Aging should not deter an individual from improving quality of life through engaging in physical activity, healthy eating, social support, and medication compliance as well as avoiding tobacco and limiting alcohol intake.

Physical Activity

The literature is clear that physical activity, even if initiated in later years, contributes to high physical and cognitive functioning, overall health, and engagement with life (Aranceta, Perez-Rodrigo, Gondra, & Orduna, 2001; Fillit et al., 2002; Houde & Melillo, 2002; Mattson, Chan, & Duan, 2002; Oguma, Sesso, Paffenbarger, & Lee, 2002). Specifically, physical activity contributes to muscle strength, flexibility, balance, cardiovascular health, and positive mood, and improves cognition. It also has been found to prevent falls and improve brain function, even after brain injury (Aranceta et al., 2001; Houde & Melillo, 2002; Mattson et al., 2002). Physical activity as well as resistance exercise training have been found to promote muscle functioning in elders by strengthening muscles, improving flexibility and strength, and preventing muscle loss (Schulte & Yarasheski, 2001; Thompson, 2002). Participation in moderate-intensity physical activity is associated with longevity and well-being (Aranceta et al., 2001; Mattson et al., 2002; Oguma et al., 2002). Physical activity also has been found to lower the risk of developing vascular dementia but not of developing Alzheimer's disease (Ravaglia et al., 2008). Seniors who engage in an active lifestyle improve their physical well-being and social activities (Aranceta et al., 2001). Conversely, physical inactivity is associated with muscle atrophy, reduced endurance and muscle strength, increased falls, and increased mortality (Oguma et al., 2002; Thompson, 2002). Physical inactivity leads to a decline in physical function and recreational and social opportunities. Dependence on others for assistance with activities of daily living is a critical outcome resulting from decreased activity and predicts loss of independence and nursing home admission (Oguma et al., 2002; Schulte & Yarasheski, 2001; Thompson, 2002; Wilkins, 2001). Physical activity is essential for optimal physical, cognitive, and emotional functioning. Therefore, increasing physical activity may be the primary factor for promoting optimal aging.

The potential for regular exercise to offset the deleterious effects of aging is well established. In fact, the pronounced health benefits attributed to regular exercise, including improvements in resting blood pressure, cholesterol profile, osteoarthritis, osteoporosis, diabetes mellitus, and cognitive functioning can be achieved even in those individuals who start physical conditioning programs later in life. Yet, despite these impressive data, approximately 70% of elderly Americans are physically inactive (King, 2001). A hypokinetic state not only negatively affects the health status of the elderly, but also significantly influences health care costs as more Americans are attaining octogenarian status. Health care workers should actively encourage elderly individuals to maintain or start an exercise program. Such recommendations may help to decrease comorbid conditions associated with the aging process, increase functional independence, and attenuate skyrocketing health care costs associated with treating the growing elderly population (Dejong & Franklin, 2004).

Notable Quotes

"Beautiful young people are accidents of nature, but beautiful old people are works of art."

—Eleanor Roosevelt (1884–1962)

Many studies have examined the benefits of exercise in frail elders living in skilled nursing facilities, where the effect of group-centered interventions is easy to assess (Fisher, Pendergast, & Calkins, 1991; McMurdo & Rennie, 1993; Sauvage et al., 1992; Schnelle, MacRae, Ouslander, Simmons, & Nitta, 1995). These institutionalized populations, who often have varying degrees of cognitive impairment, can be challenging, both when trying to establish motivation for exercise and when creating opportunities for group reinforcement and participation. Study variables on which exercise interventions have had an impact include those directly related to the exercise itself—changes in mobility or strength. More indirect but perhaps more functionally relevant benefits also accrue from exercise, such as improved sleep, improved mood, and overall well-being of the participants (King, Rejeski, & Buchner, 1998). Older adults may be easily discouraged by a belief that for exercise to be beneficial, one must walk very fast, lift weights at a gym, or exercise every day. Many exercise programs for the elderly that have extended independence and improved activities of daily living include very simple regimens such as lifting cans of vegetables of varying weights, doing leg lifts from a sitting position, or walking lengths of the hall a few times in one's home a couple of times a day. One should set very low goals to guarantee success. Diaries have been shown to be effective in increasing activity. Any movement is better than none, so every little activity should be encouraged (van der Bij, Laurant, & Wensing, 2002).

Physical activity interventions are not always effective because older adults often do not comply with planned exercise for the long term. For older adults, interventions should be tailored to individuals' preferences and should be directed toward home-based intervention. Intense long-term strategies and behavioral strategies will promote adherence (van der Bij et al., 2002).

Individuals living at home must be coached about completing a safety check to ensure a safe pathway through their home. Establishing hand rails along a hall can ensure safety for those individuals with health concerns such as dizziness or for whom conditions may force them to stay inside. Others may benefit from watching and moving with a televised program; for example, a colleague reported that after working with African Americans in a housing development, by having them play Motown records and dance around for 20 minutes a day, they were later able to increase their ability to walk around the building. Health care providers may do well to use neutral words such as *movement* or *activity* rather than *exercise*, which raises self-expectations to an extreme for some.

One major intervention study conducted in a supervised group setting used daytime arm and leg exercises as a means to improve the sleep of nursing home residents. The investigators found that participants' quality and quantity of sleep improved by about 40% during subsequent nighttime observations (Alessi, Yoon, Schnelle, Al-Samarrai, & Cruise, 1999). Another institutionally based study examined the effect of weight training on strength and stair climbing in a selected group of very old (mean age 87 years) nursing home residents

(Fiatarone et al., 1994). Participants assigned to the intervention group receiving a socialization intervention had enhanced overall mobility compared with the control group. This study provides the best evidence that exercise can produce short-term, highly relevant improvements for even the oldest frail elders. In another group of nursing home patients for whom stair climbing was considered well beyond their functional capacity, a structured strength-training program using resistance exercise of upper extremities dramatically improved spontaneous activity (Evans, 1999).

Interventions to promote physical activity in older adults can be organized by level of impact using individual and interpersonal approaches through environmental- and societal-level interventions (Marcus et al., 2007; King, 1991). Interventions that facilitate physical activity among the elderly include goal setting, self-monitoring, feedback, support, stimulus control, and relapse-prevention training (Young & King, 1995). Using both positive self-talk and goal-setting produces greater physical activity adherence (Atkins, Kaplan, Timms, Reinsh, & Lofback, 1984). Also useful is telephone supervision and home-based physical activity programs (King, Haskell, Taylor, Kraemer, & DeBunk, 1991).

The relationship between health-related quality of life and physical activity in the literature was systematically evaluated and found to be correlated in the general population. Higher levels of physical activity were found in individuals with a high HRQOL score (Bize, Johnson, & Plotnikoff, 2007). The CDC conducted a study to assess the percentage of adults who were questioned about physical activity by their health care provider. Over half of the respondents (52%) reported their health care providers had asked about their level of physical activity or exercise. Women, older adults, and those with decreased education were less likely to be asked. The likelihood of being asked increased for individuals who were obese (CDC, 2002).

Nutrition

The literature provides evidence that proper nutrition is a powerful, modifiable lifestyle factor that may delay or prevent chronic diseases in later life and, more importantly, will potentially lead to additional years of health, productivity, and high functioning. For those who are inactive, good nutrition enhances skin integrity and prevents skin breakdown (Shikany & White, 2000). However, older adults may be at risk for inadequate nutrition because of physiological changes related to organ function declines, which can affect digestion, metabolism, and absorption of nutrients (Lueckenotte, 2000). Additionally, older adults' nutritional intake may be compromised because of the development of poor eating habits related to chewing or swallowing difficulties as well as diminished interest in food resulting from sensory loss (e.g., taste and smell) (Swartzberg, Margen, & Editors, 2001). Physically active seniors' diets are relatively higher in dairy products and fruits than are the diets of sedentary older adults (Aranceta et al., 2001). Proper nutrition, with an emphasis on consuming fruits and vegetables, has long-term health benefits and contributes to physical, cognitive, and overall well-being (Lange-Collette, 2002; Pullen & Walker, 2002). However the costs associated with healthier foods on a limited budget are an issue for many elderly.

Evidence suggests that adequate nutrition has great benefits; however, researchers have noted that many older adults are deficient in particular vitamins and minerals, including vitamins B_6, B_{12}, D, and K; folic acid; the antioxidant vitamins A, C, E, and beta carotene; and the minerals selenium, calcium, and iron, which are essential for overall health (Fillit et al., 2002). Cognitive function can be impacted by nutrition; specifically, malnutrition can cause long-term cognitive impairment (Fillit et al., 2002). Research findings also indicate that elders with various vitamin deficiencies, especially of B_{12}, may be at risk for cognitive disorders (including dementia) that were previously considered to be due to normal cognitive aging; other nutrients, such as antioxidants and vitamin C, may protect against cognitive decline (Fillit et al., 2002; Mattson et al., 2002).

Other dietary factors associated with health in advancing age, particularly for women, may be the consumption of significantly lower percentages of calories from fat and a higher percentage of calories from complex carbohydrates (Klein et al., 2004). In relation to dietary fats, future health in both men and women was predicted by higher baseline high-density lipoprotein cholesterol levels, as well as lower low-density lipoprotein cholesterol levels for women. Eating a healthy diet has been found to assist with weight reduction and decrease serum cholesterol, and has been associated with decreasing incidence of coronary artery disease (CAD), diabetes, colon cancer, and osteoporosis, although these require early dietary intervention (Lange-Collette, 2002).

Additional findings suggest that optimal calcium intake is critically related to reducing the risk of bone loss and osteoporosis and decreasing the incidence of fractures in both men and women (Shikany & White, 2002). A diet with high soy protein combined with regular weight-bearing physical activity may protect against osteoporosis (Lange-Collette, 2002). Osteoporosis can prevent optimal physical activity and, in turn, participation in social and community recreational activities, thus denying the benefits of such participation. Dietary intake is often associated with income and living arrangements. It is clear that health care providers must be sensitive to individuals' income levels and ability to apply for public assistance as well as cultural constraints on food selections. Some individuals may benefit from having a high-potency vitamin prescribed so that their insurance or pharmacy plan may cover the costs. Others may be unaware of simple requirements such as the amount of protein recommended on a daily basis. Health care providers should consider the individual's budget and realize that fresh vegetables and fruit may be cost prohibitive. Always ask the person to make out a grocery list or save store receipts so that the health care provider can help the individual review his or her choices.

The **Food Guide Pyramid for Older Adults**, known as MyPyramid, has been updated by Tufts University researchers. The new version continues to emphasize nutrient-dense food choices and foods that meet the unique needs of older adults. Added to the new pyramid is a foundation depicting physical activities characteristic of older adults, such as walking, yard work, and swimming as well as a row of glasses indicating the need for fluids. Also included at the top of the pyramid is a flag that indicates the need for calcium, vitamin D, and vitamin B_{12} (Lichtenstein, 2008).

Smoking

In countries that report deaths that are attributable to smoking, cigarettes were responsible for an estimated 21 million deaths from 1990 to 1999, with more than half of those deaths occurring in people 35 to 69 years of age (Joint Committee on Smoking and Health, 1995). The 1990 report of the Surgeon General differentiates smoking-related deaths in the United States by disease category. Cigarette smoking accounts annually for an estimated 131,503 deaths from heart disease, 125,100 deaths from lung cancer, 35,272 deaths from other cancers, 77,665 deaths from chronic obstructive pulmonary disease (COPD), and 16,492 deaths from strokes. In addition to these extraordinary mortality rates, the annual direct financial burden of smoking is estimated to exceed $167 billion (CDC, 2006). Currently, 23.9% of adult men and 18.0% of adult women in the United States smoke, representing 45.3 million lives (CDC, 2007).

Smoking is the single most important preventable risk factor to human health in developed countries and an important cause of premature death worldwide (Joint Committee on Smoking and Health, 1995). Approximately 70% of individuals that smoke would like to quit smoking (CDC, 2006). A population-based survey (Goldstein et al., 1997) found that less than 15% of smokers who saw a physician in the past year were offered assistance in quitting smoking and only 3% had a follow-up appointment to address tobacco use.

The first step in treating tobacco use and dependence is to identify tobacco users. The effective identification of tobacco use status not only opens the doors for successful interventions, but also guides clinicians to identify appropriate interventions based on a patient's willingness to quit. A guideline that was developed by a private-sector panel of experts convened by a consortium of federal and nonfederal partners recommended the implementation of an office-wide protocol that systematically solicits and documents the tobacco-use status of each patient at every visit. Such a practice can be done effectively by expanding the number of vital signs to include smoking status or by placing an appropriate tobacco-use sticker on all patient charts. In clinical settings where tobacco use has been universally documented, the rate at which physicians then asked their patients about smoking and provided specific advice on quitting approximately doubled (Fiore et al., 1995). The 2000 guideline documents that clinical interventions as brief as 3 minutes can substantially increase cessation success. This finding supports the idea that a personalized clinician message meaningfully enhances the likelihood that a smoker will make a successful attempt to quit smoking. Therefore, it is essential to provide at least a brief intervention for all tobacco users at each clinic visit.

Because effective tobacco dependence treatments are available, every patient who uses tobacco should be offered at least one of the following treatments:

- Patients willing to try to quit using tobacco should be provided with treatments that are identified as effective in the guideline.
- Patients unwilling to try to quit using tobacco should be provided with a brief intervention that is designed to increase their motivation to quit.

For Patients Willing to Quit: The 5 As. The "5 As" were designed as a brief and effective intervention for tobacco users willing to make an attempt to quit smoking (**Table 22-2**). It is important for the clinician to ask patients whether they use tobacco; to advise them to quit in a clear, strong, and personalized manner; and to assess their willingness to make an attempt to quit at that time. If the patient agrees to attempt cessation, the clinician should then assist in making a quit attempt and should arrange for follow-up contacts to prevent a relapse (**Box 22-2**).

For Patients Not Ready to Quit: The 5 Rs. For patients not willing to make an attempt to quit at the time of an assessment or hospital admission, health professionals should provide a brief intervention that is designed to promote the motivation to quit (the "5 Rs"; **Table 22-3**). Patients may be unwilling to make an attempt to quit for a variety of reasons. Many older individuals may view an attempt to quit as too late in their stage of life. They may not realize how side effects of smoking are relevant to their personal health history. These patients may, however, respond to a motivational intervention that provides the health care provider an opportunity to educate and reassure the patient by means of the following 5 Rs: relevance, risks, rewards, roadblocks, and repetition (Colby et al., 1998; Prochaska & Goldstein, 1991).

Pharmacotherapies for Smoking Cessation. Numerous effective pharmacotherapies for smoking cessation now exist. Except in the presence of contraindication(s), these should be used with all patients who are attempting to quit smoking. The treatment of tobacco dependence, like the treatment of other chronic diseases, requires the use of multiple modalities. Pharmacotherapy is an essential element of a multicomponent approach.

The seven first-line medications with an established empirical record of efficacy in smoking cessation are varenicline (Chantix), bupropion SR (Zyban), the nicotine patch, nicotine gum, nicotine lozenge, nicotine inhaler (Nicotrol Inhaler), and nicotine nasal spray (Nicotrol NS). These medications are summarized in **Table 22-4**. Combining the nicotine patch with a self-administered form of nicotine replacement therapy (NRT), such as the gum, the inhaler, or the nasal spray, is more efficacious than a single form of nicotine replacement. Patients should be encouraged to use combined treatments if they are unable to quit using a single method.

Alcohol

Alcohol abuse and alcoholism are underrecognized problems in the elderly population. One-third of older alcoholic persons have developed alcoholism in later life; the other two-thirds of the population will grow older with the medical and psychosocial sequelae of early-onset alcoholism. Sixty-two percent of community-dwelling adults ages 60 to 94 were found to drink alcohol (Mirand & Welte, 1996). In the elderly, the effects of alcohol may be increased because of pharmacologic changes associated with aging. Interactions between alcohol and drugs, prescription and over-the-counter, may also be more serious in elderly persons. Physiologic changes related to aging can alter the presentation of medical complications of alcoholism (Rigler, 2000, p. 171). The National Institute on Alcohol Abuse and Alcoholism considers one drink per day to be the maximum amount for "moderate" alcohol use in individuals over the age of 65 (O'Connor & Schottenfeld, 1998).

Binge drinking is a significant problem even among moderate drinkers and is associated with particularly high social and economic costs. The elderly are also commonly prescribed an average of

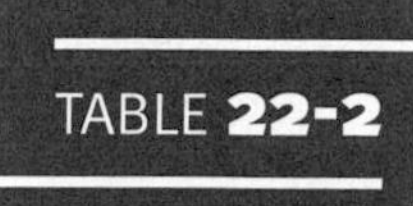

TABLE 22-2 Brief Strategies: Helping the Patient Willing to Quit

Action	Strategies for Implementation
Ask: Systematically identify all tobacco users at every visit.	
Query patient at every office visit.	Expand the vital signs to include tobacco use or use an alternative universal identification system.
Advise: Strongly urge all tobacco users to quit.	
Urge every tobacco user to quit.	Advice should be: "I think it is important for you to quit smoking now and I can help you. Cutting down while you are ill is not enough." **Strong:** "As your clinician, I need you to know that quitting smoking is the most important thing you can do to protect your health now and in the future. The clinic staff and I will help you." **Personalized:** Tie tobacco use to current health/illness, and/or its social and economic costs, motivation level/readiness to quit, and/or the impact of tobacco use on children and others in the household.
Assess: Determine willingness to make a quit attempt.	
Ask if he or she is willing to make an attempt at this time (e.g., within the next 30 days).	Assess patient's willingness to quit: If the patient is willing to make an attempt to quit at this time, provide assistance. If the patient will participate in an intensive treatment, deliver such a treatment or refer him or her to an intensive intervention. If the patient clearly states he or she is unwilling to make an attempt to quit at this time, provide a motivational intervention. If the patient is a member of a special population (e.g., adolescent, pregnant, racial/ethnic minority), consider providing additional information.
Assist: Aid the patient in quitting.	
Help the patient with a plan to quit.	A patient's preparations for quitting (STAR): Set a quit date; ideally, the quit date should be within 2 weeks. Tell family, friends, and coworkers about quitting, and request understanding and support. Anticipate challenges to the planned quit attempt, particularly during the critical first few weeks; these include nicotine withdrawal symptoms. Remove tobacco products from your environment; prior to quitting,

(continues)

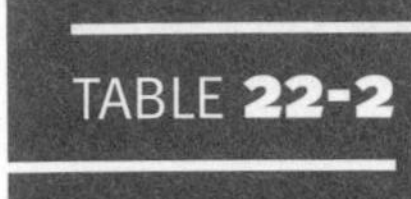

TABLE **22-2** **(continued)**

Action	Strategies for Implementation
	avoid smoking in places where you spend a lot of time (e.g., work, home, car).
Provide practical counseling (problem solving/skills training).	Abstinence: Total abstinence is essential; "not even a single puff after the quit date." Past quitting experience: Review past quit attempts, including identification of what helped during the quit attempt and what factors contributed to relapse. Anticipate triggers or challenges in the upcoming attempt: Discuss challenges/triggers and how the patient will successfully overcome them. Alcohol: Drinking alcohol is highly associated with relapse; the patient should consider limiting/abstaining from alcohol during the quit process. Other smokers in the household: The presence of other smokers in the household, particularly a spouse or partner, is associated with lower abstinence rates. Patients should encourage significant others to quit with them. If others continue to smoke, they should be asked to smoke outdoors and not in the quitter's presence.
Provide intratreatment social support.	Provide a supportive clinical environment while encouraging the patient in his or her quit attempt: "My office staff and I are available to assist you."
Help patient obtain extratreatment social support.	Help the patient develop social support for his or her attempt to quit in his or her environments outside of treatment: "Ask your spouse/partner, friends, and coworkers to support you in your quit attempt."
Recommend pharmacotherapy.	Recommend the use of pharmacotherapies; explain how these medications increase smoking cessation success and reduce withdrawal symptoms. The first-line pharmacotherapy medications include the following: bupropion SR, nicotine gum, nicotine inhaler, nicotine nasal spray, and nicotine patch.
Provide supplementary materials.	Sources: Federal agencies, nonprofit agencies, or local/state departments Type: Culturally/racially/educationally/age-appropriate for the patient Location: Readily available at every clinician's workstation
Arrange: Schedule follow-up contact.	
Schedule follow-up contact, either in person or via telephone.	Timing: Follow-up contact should occur soon after the quit date, preferably during the first week. A second follow-up contact is recommended within the first month; schedule further follow-up contacts as indicated.

Action	Strategies for Implementation
	Actions during follow-up contact: Congratulate success; if tobacco use has occurred, review circumstances and elicit recommitment to total abstinence. Remind the patient that a lapse can be used as a learning experience. Identify problems already encountered and anticipate challenges in the immediate future. Assess pharmacotherapy use and problems. Consider use or referral to more intensive treatment.

SOURCE: Fiore, M. C., et al. (2000). *Treating tobacco use and dependence: Clinical practice guideline*. Rockville, MD: U.S. Department of Health and Human Services, Public Health Service.

BOX 22-2 Research Highlight

Aim: The aim of this study was to describe sleep characteristics with health-related quality of life in old age.

Methods: A cross-sectional, descriptive study of 64 older adults without sleep/wake complaints participated in the study. Diary-based, laboratory-based, and actigraphic measures of sleep, health-related quality of life, mental health, social support, and coping strategies were collected. A 2-week sleep-wake log was maintained by subjects, who also wore a wrist activity monitor. A polysomnography was performed at a university-based sleep lab. Daytime sleepiness was assessed using multiple sleep latency tests; general physical and mental health and health-related quality of life and medical comorbidity were measured with the Outcome Survey (MOS) Short Form (SF)-36, the Depression Cumulative Illness Rating Scale—Geriatric, and the Hamilton Rating Scale for Depression. Psychological symptom burden was measured with the Hamilton Rating Scale for Anxiety. Cognitive functioning was measured by the Logical Memory test, the Letter-Numbering Sequencing test, the test of Nonverbal Intelligence III, and the Folstein Mini Mental Status Exam. Sleep and circadian functioning was measured using the Composite Scale of Morningness. Perceived social support was measured by the Interpersonal Support Evaluation List, and coping strategies were measured by the Brief COPE instrument.

Findings: Women experienced a greater depth and continuity of sleep than men. The sleep diary correlated with physical and mental health–related quality of life.

Application to practice: Sleep quality and daytime alertness can be considered an aspect of successful aging. Good health was associated with satisfactory sleep quality. Nurses should assess the sleep quality of older adults using a reliable and valid tool. Strategies to promote satisfactory sleep quality should be implemented to promote optimal health in older adults.

Source: Driscoll, H. C., Serody, L., Patrick, S., Maurer, J., Bensasi, S., et al. (2008). Sleeping well, aging well: A descriptive and cross-sectional study of sleep in "successful agers" 75 and older. *American Journal of Geriatric Psychiatry, 16*(1), 74–82.

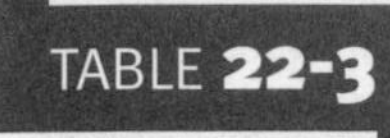

TABLE 22-3 Enhancing Motivation to Quit Tobacco: The 5 Rs

Motivation	Description
Relevance	Encourage the patient to indicate why quitting is personally relevant, being as specific as possible. Motivational information has the greatest impact if it is relevant to a patient's disease status or risk, family or social situation (e.g., having children in the home), health concerns, age, gender, and other important patient characteristics (e.g., prior quitting experience, personal barriers to cessation).
Risks	The clinician should ask the patient to identify potential negative consequences of tobacco use; the clinician may suggest and highlight those that seem to be the most relevant to the patient. The clinician should emphasize that smoking low-tar/low-nicotine cigarettes or use of other forms of tobacco (e.g., smokeless tobacco, cigars, and pipes) will not eliminate these risks. Examples of risks are: **Acute risks:** Shortness of breath, exacerbation of asthma, harm to pregnancy, impotence, infertility, increased serum carbon monoxide **Long-term risks:** Heart attacks and strokes, lung and other cancers (larynx, oral cavity, pharynx, esophagus, pancreas, bladder, cervix), chronic obstructive pulmonary diseases (chronic bronchitis and emphysema), long-term disability and need for extended care **Environmental risks:** Increased risk of lung cancer and heart disease in spouses; higher rates of smoking by children of tobacco users; increased risk for low birth weight, SIDS, asthma, middle ear disease, and respiratory infections in children of smokers
Rewards	The clinician should ask the patient to identify potential benefits of stopping tobacco use. The clinician may suggest and highlight those that seem to be the most relevant to the patient. Examples of rewards include the following: • Improved health • Food will taste better • Improved sense of smell • Save money • Feel better about yourself • Home, car, clothing, breath will smell better • Can stop worrying about quitting • Set a good example for kids • Have healthier babies and children • Not worry about exposing others to smoke • Feel better physically • Perform better in physical activities • Reduced wrinkling/aging of skin

Motivation	Description
Roadblocks	The clinician should ask the patient to identify barriers or impediments to quitting and note elements of treatment (i.e., problem solving, pharmacotherapy) that could address barriers. Typical barriers might include: • Withdrawal symptoms • Fear of failure • Weight gain • Lack of support • Depression • Enjoyment of tobacco
Repetition	The motivational intervention should be repeated every time an unmotivated patient visits the clinic setting; tobacco users who have failed in previous quit attempts should be told that most people make repeated quit attempts before they are successful.

SOURCE: Fiore, M. C., et al. (2000). *Treating tobacco use and dependence: Clinical practice guideline*. Rockville, MD: U.S. Department of Health and Human Services, Public Health Service.

7–8 medications, many of which are negatively affected by alcohol. A cautious approach should be emphasized for those individuals who drink even small amounts of alcohol. Many elderly are taking antianxiety drugs such as Valium and Xanax that can be potentiated by the use of alcohol. Also, the regular use of alcohol should be discouraged in those individuals with depressive illnesses where alcohol taken in combination with other drugs as common as Tylenol may contribute to a suicide attempt.

Benefits of Light to Moderate Alcohol Consumption. Published health benefits of regular light to moderate alcohol consumption include lower myocardial infarction rates, reduced heart failure rates, reduced risk of ischemic stroke, lower risk for dementia, decreased risk of diabetes, and reduced risk of osteoporosis. Numerous complementary biochemical changes have been identified that explain the beneficial effects of moderate alcohol consumption. Heavy alcohol consumption, however, can negatively affect neurologic, cardiac, gastrointestinal, hematologic, immune, psychiatric, and musculoskeletal organ systems (Rigler, 2000).

An American Heart Association (AHA) position statement cautions that if someone chooses to drink alcohol, they should do so in moderation. Moderation is considered an average of one to two drinks per day for men and one drink per day for women. It further cautions people *not* to start drinking, and to consult their doctor on the benefits and risks of consuming alcohol in moderation (AHA, 2008).

The popularity of the topic of the health benefits of moderate alcohol intake in both medical journals and the lay press gives rise to increased discussion of the subject. A recent column by a popular wine journalist reported on medical studies that moderate drinking can help prevent strokes, amputated limbs, and dementia. The cardiac benefits of low-dose alcohol are evident in study after study. He quoted Abigail Zuger's *New York Times* article titled, "The Case for Drinking," which describes the growing body of evidence that people who consume wine in moderation tend to be healthier and live longer (Zuger, 2002). He further decried the political correctness of institutions and authorities that at worst cover up the results of the Framingham study and at best are too timid to go so far as to recommend wine in moderation. He concludes by advising his readers to discuss the topic with their family physicians (Garr, 2003).

Individuals who are currently abstinent and comfortable with that lifestyle should not be encouraged to start drinking solely for the potential health benefits. Although convincing data do not currently exist, the risks of developing abusive drinking patterns and the associated detrimental health effects potentially outweigh the advantage of light to moderate drinking (Cherpitel et al., 1995;

TABLE 22-4 Pharmacotherapy for Smoking Cessation

Factor	Varenicline	Bupropion SR	Patch	Gum	Inhaler	Nasal Spray
Treatment period	3–6 mo.	7–12 wk. Take for 1–2 wk before quitting smoking. May use for maintenance for up to 6 mo.	6–8 wk.	Up to 12 wk. May use for longer time as needed.	3–6 mo. Taper use over last few weeks.	T3–6 mo.Taper use over last few weeks.
Dosage	Start 1 week prior to stop date of smoking at 0.5 mg once daily for 3 days, followed by 0.5 mg twice daily for 4 days, followed by 1 mg twice daily for 3 months.	Days 1–3: 150-mg tablet each morning. Days 4–end: 150-mg tablet in morning and evening.	One patch each day. Taper dose if using: 21 mg for 4 wk, 14 mg for 2 wk, 7 mg for 2 wk. No taper if using 15 mg for 8 wk. Light smokers (10 cigarettes/d) can start with lower dose.	2 mg. 4 mg (heavy smokers). Chew one piece every 1–2 h (10–15 pieces/d). Many people do not use enough gum—chew gum whenever you need it!	6–16 cartridges/d. Need to inhale about 80 times to use up cartridge. Can use part of cartridge and save the rest for later that day.	One dose equals one squirt to each nostril. Dose 1–2 times/h as needed: minimum = 8 doses/d; maximum = 40 doses/d.
Pros	Easy to use. Reduces urges to smoke.	Easy to use. Reduces urges to smoke.	Easy to use. Steady dose of nicotine.	Can control your own dose. Helps with predictable urges (e.g., after meals). Keeps mouth busy.	Can control your own dose. Helps with predictable urges. Keeps hands and mouth busy.	Can control your own dose. Fastest acting for relief of urges.
Cons	In February 2008, the FDA added a warning regarding the use with psy-	May disturb sleep. May cause dry mouth.	May irritate skin. May disturb sleep. Cannot adjust amount of nicotine in	Need to chew correctly—"chew and park." May stick to den-	May irritate mouth and throat (improves with use). Does not	Need to use correctly (do not inhale it). May irritate nose

	chiatric history. A depressed mood, agitation, changes in behavior, and suicidal ideation have been reported.		response to urges.	tures. Should not drink acidic beverages while chewing gum.	work well < 40°. Should not drink acidic beverages while using inhaler.	(improves with use). May cause dependence.
Caution	Psychiatric history in patients.	Do not use if you have a seizure disorder, an eating disorder, or are already taking a monoamine oxidase inhibitor.	Do not use if you have severe uncontrolled eczema or psoriasis.	Caution with dentures.		Do not use if you have severe reactive airway disease (asthma).
Availability	Prescription only.	Prescription only.	Over the counter (regular/mint/orange flavors).	Over the counter.	Prescription only.	Prescription only.

SOURCE: Fiore, M. C., et al. (2000). *Treating tobacco use and dependence: Clinical practice guideline.* Rockville, MD: U.S. Department of Health and Human Services, Public Health Service. AHCPR (2006). AHCPR (2008). Clinical guidelines for prescribing medication for treating tobacco use and dependence accessed at: http://www.ncbi.nlm.nih.gov/books/bv.fcgi?rid=hstat2.table.29458

BOX 22-3 Web Links

Smoking cessation resources for health care professionals available on the Internet include the following:

- Smokefree.gov (http://www.smokefree.gov): Sponsored by the National Cancer Institute, provides smoking-related resources for health professionals; includes Web sites and government reports.
- Treatobacco.net (http://www.treatobacco.net): Sponsored by the Society for Research on Nicotine and Tobacco and the World Health Organization Europe, provides evidence-based information on treating tobacco dependence.
- Smoking and Tobacco Use (http://www.cdc.gov/tobacco): Sponsored by the Centers for Disease Control and Prevention, provides a wealth of information regarding smoking, including reports, statistics, resources, and past Surgeon General reports.
- Tobacco Cessation—You Can Quit Smoking Now! (http://www.surgeongeneral.gov/tobacco/): Sponsored by the Surgeon General, provides smoking cessation materials for both clinicians and consumers.

Exercise resources available on the Internet for health care professionals include the following:

- *Physical Activity and Health: A Report of the Surgeon General* (1996): http://profiles.nlm.nih.gov/NN/B/B/H/B/
- Physical Activity and Older Americans: Benefits and Strategies: http://www.ahrq.gov/ppip/activity.htm
- Growing Stronger—Strength Training for Older Adults: http://www.cdc.gov/nccdphp/dnpa/physical/growing_stronger/

Nutrition resources available on the Internet for health care professionals include the following:

- The Food Guide Pyramid: http://www.mypyramid.gov
- Nutrition for Older Adults: http://www.nal.usda.gov/foodstamp/Topics/elderly_nutrition.html

Alcohol resources available on the Internet for health care professionals include the following:

- Worldwide recommendations on alcohol consumption: http://www.drinkingandyou.com/site/uk/biggy.htm
  Helping patients who drink too much: A clinician's guide: http://pubs.niaaa.nih.gov/publications/Practitioner/CliniciansGuide2005/guide.pdf

Dawson, 2001). Exceptions to this conservative stance may be considered for the patient who 1) is well known to the physician, 2) has no apparent abuse liability, and 3) has cardiovascular risks that demand aggressive intervention and is on no medications that prohibit alcohol use. For those choosing to initiate alcohol consumption, a conservative prescription-like recommendation of a precise amount at a given time (e.g., one glass of red wine with the evening meal) would seem indicated. Careful monitoring for escalating usage and/or adverse health consequences is appropriate.

For individuals who have established an adaptive and enjoyable pattern of appropriate alcohol use, and have no identified health problems that could be adversely affected by alcohol use, there appears to be no compelling reason to encourage them to abstain (Rehm, Greenfield, & Rogers, 2001), although continued monitoring is indicated. After assessing for contraindications, individuals who do not have a history of alcohol abuse can be counseled regarding the health benefits of light to moderate consumption (Ellison, 2002). Although some studies show no difference in the beneficial effects of different forms of alcohol (Gaziano et al., 1999), others have found red wine to be most beneficial (GrønbÊk et al., 2000).

Recommendations regarding alcohol intake should be individualized based on age and gender as well as physical and mental health status (Drory, 2001). Individuals with medical, psychiatric, or pharmacologic contraindications, and those with personal and/or family histories of substance abuse should be encouraged not to drink at all; however, lower limits may be appropriate for those with hypertension or diabetes (Meister, Whelan, & Kava, 2000). Everyone should be cautioned regarding the effect of even moderate drinking on motor skill activities such as driving (Drory, 2001).

Alcoholism in the Elderly. The following are four steps for treating alcoholism in the elderly:

1. Identify individuals requiring treatment.
2. Determine individuals' readiness to discuss treatment.
3. Assess individuals requiring detoxification.
4. Plan for postdetoxification treatment in coordination with other professionals.

When assessing the elderly for alcohol use, health care providers should assess for cognitive decline, nonadherence with appointments, psychiatric history, insomnia, poorly controlled hypertension, frequent falls, gastrointestinal problems, nutritional deficiencies, delirium during hospitalization, elevated corpuscular volume on CBC, and family problems. Cancers of the head, neck, and esophagus are associated with chronic alcohol abuse. Also, liver cancer is associated with cirrhosis as a side effect of chronic alcohol abuse.

Hospitalization is recommended for detoxification of those elderly who are dependent on alcohol. Older individuals with multiple medical conditions have a decreased reserve and are at risk for delirium and seizure during withdrawal. Treatment typically consists of benzodiazepines, specifically shorter-acting benzodiazepines, as well as thiamine and other vitamin supplements. Following detoxification, older patients should be directed into elder-specific outpatient therapy for long-term adherence (Rigler, 2000).

Medication Adherence

In the past few decades, hundreds of research articles have been published on nonadherence. Dozens of devices and programs have been developed to assess and resolve adherence-related problems. Yet, despite the tremendous efforts of pharmacists and other health care providers, medication nonadherence remains a major public health problem, particularly for aging persons. Indeed, the National Council on Patient Information and Education (NCPIE) has aptly termed nonadherence "America's other drug problem" (NCPIE, 2007). NCPIE has noted that nonadherence can take a variety of forms, including not having a prescription filled; taking an incorrect dose; taking a medication at the wrong time; forgetting to take doses; or stopping therapy too soon due to the costs, a logical decision, or side effects unknown to the physician. Medication adherence can be influenced by herb use and over-the-counter medications as first choices prior to utilizing prescription drugs.

Medication nonadherence is a major public health problem that has been called an "invisible epidemic" (Fincham & Wertheimer, 1985; Smith, 1996). Nonadherence to pharmacotherapy has been reported to range from 13% to 93%, with an average rate of 40% (Bond & Hussar, 1991). The problem encompasses all ages and ethnic groups, but is even more prevalent in the elderly; it has been estimated that 55% of the elderly are nonadherent (Bruce, Berger, Krueger, & Felkey, 2004). A host of individual characteristics may also influence adherence, such as the patient's religion, health beliefs, social support system, and ethnicity. Although a plethora of attributes and variables has been evaluated as predictors of adherence, the frequency of dose has been identified by multiple studies as contributing to nonadherence.

Rates of nonadherence vary with different disease states. For example, the nonadherence rate for hypertension is reported to be 40%, whereas that for arthritis has been found to range between 55% and 70% (Task Force for Compliance, 1994). Nonadherence rates are especially high among patients with chronic diseases (Blandford et al., 1999). These patients, who typically require long-term, if not lifelong, medications to control symptoms and prevent complications, often must make significant behavioral changes to adhere with pharmacotherapy. Such changes can be difficult to integrate into everyday life.

Direct and indirect methods of assessing medication adherence can be utilized to identify elderly people having difficulty in adhering to prescribed regimens. Health care professionals can monitor blood levels and/or urine assays for drug metabolites or marker compounds. Indirect methods of assessing adherence include patient interviews, pill counts, refill records, medication organizers, and measurement of health outcomes. The interview method is inexpensive and allows the health care professional to show concern for the patient and provide immediate feedback. A drawback of this method is that it can overestimate adherence, and its accuracy depends on the patient's cognitive abilities and the honesty of his or her replies, as well as the interviewer's correct interpretation of responses. Pill counts provide an objective measure of the quantity of drug taken over a given time period; however, this method is time-consuming and assumes that medication not in the container was consumed. The refill record provides an objective measure of quantities obtained at given intervals, but assumes that the patient obtained the medication only from the recorded source and assumes the individual actually takes the pills.

Strategies to improve adherence should target the specific risk factors and causes identified during the patient assessment (**Case Study 22-1**). Adherence aids, such as medication organizers, may be used alone or in combination, but should be tailored to the individual patient. For example, a forgetful patient may benefit from a special package or container that provides a visual reminder that a medication was taken (for example, blister packaging or a computer-aided compliance package). Patients should be advised to take dosages in conjunction with other routine daily activities that are highly habituated and not likely to be skipped, such as at mealtimes or before tooth brushing. Refill reminders or automatic delivery to the home also can be valuable for the forgetful patient, as can simplification of the dosage schedule, such as changing to a once-daily prescription. Cues or prompts, including phone calls, medication diaries, and medication organizers, are reported to be helpful across multiple age groups. It is crucial that the individual's perception of the environment and his or her view of the feasibility of the support system or aid, such as a medication organizer, be considered. Health care providers should plan with the individual, given they know their adaptive strategies the best as well as what aids they are willing to use. Individuals should be encouraged to monitor "outcome" variables and maintain a medication diary instead of taking medication based on "perceived symptoms," which leads to poor adherence.

Once the initial adherence plan is implemented, follow-up is important to gauge how well the plan

Case Study 22-1

Mr. Lopez is an 82-year-old man with a history of hypertension, coronary artery disease (stent × 2), type 2 diabetes, and gout. His BMI is 30. He comes to the medical clinic today complaining of headaches, tiredness, and fatigue. Upon taking his vital signs, the nurse notes a regular heart rate of 98, blood pressure of 189/92, and normal temperature. In taking his history, the nurse asks about the medications he is taking. He states that he has pills for his blood pressure. The nurse asks him if he takes his medicine every day. He states that he takes part of his medicine every day. When the nurse asks how he does this, he replies that he cuts his medicine into quarters so that the medicine will last longer.

Questions:

1. As the nurse, what would be your plan of care for this patient?
2. How would you address his medication adherence problem?
3. What resources could help you in providing his care?
4. What underlying causes may be present that explain this patient's behavior?

is working and whether changes are needed. Therefore, the pharmaceutical care plan must include periodic reinforcement strategies for long-term success. The plan should also be reevaluated from time to time to assess its effectiveness and determine how well it meets patient expectations.

Although care plans should be individualized, some adherence-promoting strategies tend to be helpful for the majority of patients. Whenever possible, health care providers should strive to:

Promote self-efficacy: Encourage patients to assume an active role in their own treatment plans. In general, the more confident people feel about their ability to manage a problem, the more likely they will be to take positive action to solve that problem. Involving patients in decisions about their care is important for promoting self-efficacy.

Empower patients to become informed medication consumers: A medication care plan to enhance adherence should first focus on educating the patient and family members or caregivers about the patient's disease and medications. Nurses should provide both written and oral information to address such basic questions as: What is the disease? Which treatments have been prescribed or recommended and why? What is the patient's role in managing the disease? Which adverse effects may occur?

Avoid strategies that could intimidate: Scaring patients or giving them dire warnings about the consequences of less-than-perfect adherence can backfire and may actually worsen adherence. A more constructive approach is to help the patient focus on ways to integrate medication-taking into his or her daily routine. Investigate the individual's belief about his or her medications and their perceived values.

Help the patient to develop a list of short-term and long-term goals: These goals should be realistic, achievable, and individualized. The health care provider can also make "contractual" agreements with the patient to encourage development of constructive behaviors, such as getting more exercise or beginning a smoking cessation program.

Plan for regular follow-up: The health care provider should plan to interact with the patient at regular, usually brief intervals to reinforce the adherence plan. For example, brief appointments can be scheduled prior to when patients need to visit the pharmacy for prescription refills. The plan should be adapted to the patient's lifestyle and be reevaluated from time to time to adjust for life changes, such as aging or a change in work or school schedules. If possible, the time for counseling on adherence should be separated from the dispensing and pick-up functions.

Implement a reward system: Giving prescription coupons or specific product discounts for successfully reaching a goal in the treatment plan can help to increase adherence, particularly in patients with low motivation.

Although older Americans (age 65 or older) account for less than 15% of the population, they consume about 33% of all prescription medications and 40% of nonprescription drugs (NCPIE, 2007). Poor adherence in the elderly often leads to additional physician or emergency department visits, hospitalization, and uncontrolled chronic diseases. One study estimated that about 17% of elderly hospitalizations are due to adverse medication reactions—nearly six times the rate in the nonelderly population (Nanada, Fanale, & Kronholm, 1990).

A variety of interacting risk factors increase the risk of nonadherence among the elderly. Risk factors in this population include:

- *Polypharmacy:* Elderly patients are more likely to take multiple medications, including both prescription and nonprescription products. Whenever possible, the medication regimen should be simplified. Health care providers also should consider the extent to which the mode of drug delivery (e.g., pill, patch, or inhaler) may influence adherence.
- *Physical impairments:* Age-related physical disabilities, such as difficulty getting out of bed or a chair, may limit an elderly person's ability to take medication consistently. Traditional packaging of medication also may be an impediment to some elderly patients; for example, individuals with arthritis in their hands may have trouble opening containers. For these patients, consider options such as unit-of-use packaging, unit-dose packing, or blister packaging.
- *Cognitive limitations:* Memory loss and other cognitive problems may interfere with adher-

ence by causing patients to fail to understand or remember medication instructions (Mallet, 1992). For these patients, health care providers may need to provide medication instructions several times and in different formats, such as both verbal and written information.

- *Limited access to or affordability of health care services:* Many elderly patients are on fixed incomes. Elderly patients who are unable to afford certain medications may be eligible for various forms of state or federal aid, or special discounts from pharmaceutical manufacturers.
- *Low-literacy patients:* Patients who read poorly or not at all are at high risk for poor adherence. According to the U.S. Department of Education Health Literacy Survey (Kirsch et al., 1993), 40 million people in the United States are functionally illiterate and another 55 million are only marginally literate. Patients with low literacy skills are less likely to be adherent to their medication regimens and appointments, or to present for care early in the course of their disease (Malveaux et al., 1996). Patients with low literacy can be taught to color code their bottles with colored tape or to use an organizer that separates daily doses into morning, noon, evening, and night.

Personal Determinants

Determinants related to personal factors refer to the biological and genetic impact of the aging process. The rate of aging and maximum life span vary among species, and therefore must be at least partly under genetic control (Hekimi & Guarente, 2003; Miller, 2002). Up to 25% of the variation in human life span is inheritable (Mitchell et al., 2001); the rest is due to environmental exposures, accidents and injuries, and chance. Very long life, to beyond age 90 years, appears to have an even stronger genetic basis (Perls et al., 2002), which explains why centenarians and near-centenarians tend to cluster in families. At the other extreme, the progeroid syndromes of accelerated aging and death at an early age have known genetic causes (Martin, Oshima, Gray, & Poot, 1999).

However, many genes that are associated with human life span are not "longevity genes" per se; for example, mutations in the tumor suppressor genes BRCA-1 and BRCA-2 are associated with breast and/or ovarian cancer (King, Marks, & Mandell, 2003). However, these genes are rare among long-living women, accounting for only 5–10% of breast and ovarian cancer cases. Conversely, genes that reduce the risk of atherosclerosis may be more common in centenarians; two such genes may have been identified. The first involves a mutation in the cholesteryl ester transfer protein (CETP) gene that leads to larger-sized lipoproteins and a reduced prevalence of cardiovascular disease (Barzilai et al., 2003). The second involves variations in the gene for microsomal transfer protein (MTP)—the rate-limiting step in lipoprotein synthesis (Geesaman et al., 2003). Although such genes may have substantial effects on longevity, they do not appear to modulate the aging process.

In contrast, longevity genes should delay the onset and/or reduce the rate of aging (Pletcher, Khazaeli, & Curtsinger, 2000), perhaps by slowing cellular senescence, improving repair mechanisms, increasing resistance to stresses such as infection and injury, or lowering metabolic rate. These requirements are consistent with the observation that children of centenarians have much lower rates of diabetes and ischemic heart disease, and better self-rated health, than do age-matched controls (Terry, Wilcox, McCormick, Lawler, & Perls, 2003). Therefore, these persons inherited from their long-lived parent a longevity gene, or a set of genes, that protects against these infirmities.

There is evolutionary pressure to select genetic mutations that are beneficial throughout life and that manifest as extreme longevity. But why should evolution select mutations that just increase survival beyond the reproductive years? Indeed, the opposite might be true, because evolution should select mutations that increase reproductive success even if they have adverse consequences later in life. A recent study (Lahdenpera, Lummaa, Helle, Tremblay, & Russell, 2004) has found evidence for the so-called grandmother effect (Hawkes, 2003), in which longer survival after menopause increases reproductive fitness among a woman's descendants, because she is available to assist in childrearing.

Psychological Determinants

Psychological factors such as intelligence and cognitive capacity are strong predictors of active aging and longevity (Smits, Deeg, Kriegsman, & Schmand, 1999). During normal aging, some cognitive capacities (including learning speed and memory) naturally decline with age; however, these losses can be compensated for by gains in wisdom, knowledge, and experience. Often, declines in cognitive functioning are triggered by disuse (lack of practice), illness (such as depression), behavioral factors (such as the use of alcohol and medications), psychological factors (such as lack of motivation, low expectations, and lack of confidence), and social factors (such as loneliness and isolation), rather than aging per se. Other psychological factors such as self-efficacy are linked to personal behavior choices as one ages and in preparation for retirement. Coping styles determine how well people adapt to the transitions of aging. A further discussion of such factors appears in Chapter 9.

Physical Environment Determinants

Physical environments that are safe can make the difference between independence and dependence for all individuals, but are of particular importance for older adults. Hazards in the physical environment can lead to debilitating and painful injuries among older people. Injuries from falls, fires, and traffic collisions are the most common. Chapters 9 and 12 provide additional discussions about these issues.

Safe Housing

Safe, adequate housing and neighborhoods are essential to the well-being of young and old. For older people, location, including proximity to family members, services, and transportation, can mean the difference between positive social interaction and isolation. Building codes need to take the health and safety needs of older people into account. Household hazards that increase the risk of falling need to be remedied or removed. Strategies for extending independence in the home include the use of handrails in the shower, monitoring devices, elevated commode seats, and an environmental survey for risks.

There is an increasing trend for older people to live alone—especially unattached older women who are mainly widows and are often poor, even in developed countries. Others may be forced to live in arrangements that are not of their choice, such as with relatives in already crowded households. The solution to social isolation may be through social programs developed at the local level for the elderly. Programs on aging have developed alliances with senior centers for facilitating social interaction.

Social Environment Determinants

Social environment determinants include social support, violence and abuse, and education and literacy. These determinants impact quality of life in the elderly by influencing their environment positively or negatively.

Social Support

Social support is an important factor in the promotion and maintenance of overall long-term health by contributing to physical and cognitive functioning and supporting engagement with life (Lange-Collette, 2002). Social support is very influential not only in relation to health behavior, both prevention and treatment, but also in the way individuals with serious medical problems react to and recuperate from various diseases (Hurdle, 2001). For example, one study found that minority women who had stronger social networks and support made greater use of cancer screening methods, mammography, and occult blood examinations than did women with fewer relationships and less social support (Hurdle, 2001). Epidemiologic data confirm that social support (i.e., strong social networks and high social contact) is related to longevity and mortality (Frisby & Hoeber, 2002); both are related to quality of life.

Another study found that older adults who were socially engaged with others and with their communities and who used additional information resources in solving daily problems demonstrated greater cognitive vitality (Fillit et al., 2002). Conversely, social disengagement in cognitively intact elders was found to be an independent risk factor for cognitive decline. Multiple satisfying social engagement patterns, avoidance of social isolation, and engagement in continuing complex nonoccupational activities appear to support cognitive vitality and be protective against dementia in late life (Fillit et al., 2002). Moreover, these findings suggest that volunteerism and continued participation in the workforce after retirement may play a role in maintaining cognitive reserve and vitality (Fillit et al., 2002).

Seniors who engage in an active lifestyle report an improvement in their social relations (Aranceta et al., 2001). One study found that social function was promoted and maintained when older women on low incomes had access to community recreation. A program conducted to address this issue focused on improving the health of women living below the poverty line, fostered personal and social changes, and involved the collaborative efforts of a municipal recreation department, several community partners, a research team, and these women. Several positive outcomes were achieved, the most notable being self-reported improvements in physical and mental health, increased participation rates, the formation of new community partnerships, and municipal recreation policy changes (Frisby & Hoeber, 2002). Social interactions, proper nutrition, and physical activity have been found to help maintain healthy behaviors and thus promote optimal aging.

Violence and Abuse

Older people who are frail or live alone may feel particularly vulnerable to crimes such as theft and assault. A common form of violence against older people is elder abuse committed by family members and institutionalized caregivers who are well known to the victims. Elder abuse occurs in families at all economic levels. It is likely to escalate in societies experiencing economic upheaval and social disorganization when overall crime and exploitation tend to increase. Elder abuse includes physical, sexual, psychological, and financial abuse as well as neglect. Older people themselves perceive abuse as including the following societal factors: neglect, violation, and deprivation (WHO/International Network for the Prevention of Elder Abuse, 2002). Elder abuse is a violation of human rights and a significant cause of injury, illness, lost productivity, isolation, and despair. Assessment of elder abuse should be conducted with each home visit, physician visit, and emergency room visit.

Families and health care providers should be taught to not disregard any reports by an elderly individual that sound abusive or harmful. Comments such as "I put on the lights and no one comes" or "I called and then finally went to the bathroom by myself" indicate that neglect is occurring. Caregivers also need to have respite care so that they are less likely to become overwhelmed. Also, low levels of neglect, such as inadequate staffing to offer foods and fluids by hand, are common in many licensed facilities. Neglect may also be noted by observing the individual's body and skin for open areas or bruises.

Education and Literacy

Low levels of education and illiteracy are associated with increased risks for disability and death among people as they age, as well as higher rates of unemployment. Education in early life combined with opportunities for lifelong learning can help people develop the skills and confidence they need to adapt and stay independent as they grow older.

Studies have shown that employment problems of older workers are often rooted in their relatively low literacy skills, not in aging per se. If people are to remain engaged in meaningful and productive activities as they grow older, there is a need for continuous training in the workplace and lifelong learning opportunities in the community (Organisation for Economic Co-operation and Development, 1998). Also, patient education material is needed for illiterate elders.

Economic Determinants

Income and Social Protection

Active aging policies need to intersect with broader schemes to reduce poverty at all ages. Although poor people of all ages face an increased risk of ill health and disabilities, older people are particularly vulnerable.

In developed countries, older people who need assistance tend to rely on family support, informal service transfers, and personal savings. Social insurance programs in Germany and Japan, discussed in Chapter 19, may provide protection to all citizens.

Social Services Determinants

Social services determinants refer to integrated, coordinated, and cost-effective efforts organized to provide health care. Services should include respect and dignity for older persons. To promote quality of life for older persons, health systems need to focus on health promotion, disease prevention, and equitable access to care. Health promotion and preventive strategies need to be designed to reduce the risk of disabilities. Health promotion is the process of enabling individuals to improve their overall health and ultimately their quality of life through behavior management. Prevention is focused on strategies to delay or prevent diseases. The availability of these services influences quality of life.

As individuals age, their risk for disease increases as does the demand for medication used to treat disease. The affordability of medications influences older adults' ability to adhere to treatment interventions and to delay the progression of a disease. Services within communities, such as mental health programs, long-term care, aging programs, and senior-focused organizations, can provide resources that promote the quality of life among older persons.

SUMMARY

The challenges of the population aging are global, national, and local. Meeting the challenges of improving the quality of life of the elderly will require substantive policy reforms in developed countries and innovative interventions. Promoting quality of life is a multidimensional endeavor. Health care professionals must continuously evaluate programs that can enhance successful active aging. A higher quality of life and active aging are more likely to be achieved by the following behaviors: daily weight-bearing or resistance exercise, appropriate nutritional intake, social support and involvement, participation in medication adherence plans, securing safe environments, and activities that strengthen mental cognitive acuity such as conversations, playing cards, and working on puzzles. By focusing on active aging determinants and strategies to increase healthy living, health care providers will aid elders in achieving optimal quality of life.

Critical Thinking Exercises

1. Which determinant of active aging is most influential in healthy aging, and why?
2. What approach should be utilized in counseling patients regarding smoking cessation options?
3. If a patient asks you if he or she should start drinking wine every day, how would you respond?
4. What does the active aging agenda support? How can it be used in the care of older adults?

Personal Reflections

1. Keep a diary for one week identifying all personal choices that indicate you are promoting your quality of life.
2. How do you feel about being involved in smoking cessation for older adults? Are there any groups in your area or at the local university in which you could become involved?
3. What is your opinion about the active aging information presented in this chapter? How could it be useful to you personally? Professionally?
4. How does your culture impact your decisions regarding quality of life?

References

Abrams, M. A. (1973). Subjective social indications. *Social Trends, 4*, 35–56.

Agency for Health Care Policy and Research. (2006). *Clinical guidelines for prescribing medication for treating tobacco use and dependence.* Retrieved June 25, 2008, from http://www.ncbi.nlm.nih.gov/books/bv.fcgi?rid=hstat2.table.29458

Alessi, C. A., Yoon, E. J, Schnelle, J. F., Al-Samarrai, N. R., & Cruise, P. A. (1999). A randomized trial of a combined physical activity and environmental intervention in nursing home residents: Do sleep and agitation improve? *Journal of the American Geriatrics Society, 47*, 784–791.

American Heart Association. (2008). *Alcohol, wine and cardiovascular disease.* Retrieved June 28, 2008, from http://www.americanheart.org/presenter.jhtml?identifier=4422

Aranceta, J., Perez-Rodrigo, C., Gondra, J., & Orduna, J. (2001). Community-based programme to promote physical activity among elderly people: The Gerobilbo study. *Journal of Nutrition, Health, and Aging, 5*, 238–242.

Atkins, C. J., Kaplan, R. M., Timms, R. M., Reinsh, S., & Lofback, K. (1984). Behavioral exercise programs in the management of chronic obstructive pulmonary disease. *Journal of Consulting and Clinical Psychology, 52*, 591–603.

Baltes, P. B., & Baltes, M. M. (1990). Psychological perspectives on successful aging: The model of selective optimization with compensation. In P. B. Baltes & M. M. Baltes (Eds.), *Successful aging: Perspectives from the behavioral sciences* (pp. 1–34). New York: Cambridge University Press.

Barzilai, N., Atzmon, G., Schechter, C., Schaefer, E. J., Cupples, A. L., Lipton, R., et al. (2003). Unique lipoprotein phenotype and genotype associated with exceptional longevity. *Journal of the American Medical Association, 290*, 2030–2040.

Bize, R., Johnson, J. A., & Plotnikoff, R. C. (2007). Physical activity level and health-related quality of life in the general adult population: A systematic review. *Preventive Medicine*, 45(6), 401–415.

Blandford, L., Dans, P. E., Ober, J. D., & Wheelock, C. (1999). Analyzing variations in medication compliance related to individual drug, drug class, and prescribing physician. *Journal of Managed Care Pharmacy, 5*(1), 47–51.

Bond, W. S., & Hussar, D. A. (1991). Detection methods and strategies for improving medication compliance. *American Journal of Hospital Pharmacy, 48*, 1978–1988.

Browner, W. S., Kahn, A. J., Ziv, E., Reiner, A. P., Oshima, J., Cawthon, R. M., et al. (2004). The genetics of human longevity. *American Journal of Medicine, 117*(11), 851–860.

Bruce, A., Berger, B. A., Krueger, K. P., & Felkey, B. G. (2004). The pharmacist's role in treatment adherence part 1: Extent of the problem. *U.S. Pharmacist, 29*(11), 50–54.

Campbell, A., Converse, P. E., & Rogers, W. L. (1976). *The quality of American life.* New York: Russell Sage Foundation.

Centers for Disease Control and Prevention. (2002). Prevalence of health care providers asking older adults about their physical activity levels—United States, 1998. *Morbidity and Mortality Weekly Report, 51*(19), 412–414. Retrieved June 25, 2006, from http://www.cdc.gov/mmwr/preview/mmwrhtml/mm5119a2.htm

Centers for Disease Control and Prevention. (2005). *Health-related quality of life: Methods and measures.* Retrieved January 12, 2009, from http://www.cdc.gov/hrqol/methods.htm

Centers for Disease Control and Prevention. (2007). Cigarette smoking among adults—United States, 2006. *Morbidity and Mortality Weekly Report, 56*(44), 1157–1161. Retrieved January 12, 2009, from http://www.cdc.gov/mmwr/preview/mmwrhtml/mm5644a2.htm

Cherpitel, C. J., Tam, T., Midanik, L., Caetano, R., & Greenfield, T. (1995). Alcohol and non-fatal injury in the U.S. general population: A risk function analysis. *Accident, Analysis and Prevention, 27*, 651–661.

Colby, S. M., Barnett, N. P., Monti, P. M., Rohsenow, D. J., Weissman, K., Spirito, A., et al. (1998). Brief motivational interviewing in a hospital setting for adolescent smoking: A preliminary study. *Journal of Consulting and Clinical Psychology, 66*, 574–578.

Dalkey, N., & Rourke, D. (1973). The Delphi procedure and rating quality of life factors. In N. Dalkey & D. Rourke (Eds.), *Quality of life concept* (pp. 209–221). Washington, DC: Environmental Protection Agency.

Dawson, D. A. (2001). Alcohol and mortality from external causes. *Journal of Studies on Alcohol, 62*, 790–797.

Dejong, A. A., & Franklin, B. A. (2004). Prescribing exercise for the elderly: Current research and recommendations. *Current Sports Medicine Report, 3*(6), 337–343.

Driscoll, H. C., Serody, L., Patrick, S., Maurer, J., Bensasi, S., Houck, S., et al. (2008). Sleeping well, aging well: A descriptive and cross-sectional study of sleep in "successful agers" 75 and older. *American Journal of Geriatric Psychiatry, 16*(1), 74–82.

Drory, Y. (2001). Is drinking alcohol good for your health? [in Hebrew]. *Harefuah, 140*, 1032–1037, 1117.

Ellison, R. C. (2002). Balancing the risks and benefits of moderate drinking. *Annals of the New York Academy of Science, 957*, 1–6.

Evans, W. J. (1999). Exercise training guidelines for the elderly. *Medicine and Science in Sports and Exercise, 31*, 12–17.

Farquhar, M. (1995a). Definitions of quality of life: A taxonomy. *Journal of Advanced Nursing, 22*, 502–508.

Farquhar, M. (1995b). Elderly people's definitions of quality of life. *Social Science and Medicine, 41*(10), 1439–1446.

Ferrans, C. E. (1996). Development of a conceptual model of quality of life. *Scholarly Inquiry for Nursing Practice, 10*(3), 293–304.

Fiatarone, M. A., O'Neill, E. F., Ryan, N. D., Clements, K. M., Solares, G. R., Nelson, M. E., et al. (1994). Exercise training and nutritional supplementation for physical frailty in very elderly people. *New England Journal of Medicine, 330*, 1769–1775.

Fillit, H. M., Butler, R. N., O'Connell, A. W., Albert, M.S., Birren, J. E., Cotman, C. W., et al. (2002). Achieving and maintaining cognitive vitality with aging. *Mayo Clinic Proceedings, 77*, 681–696.

Fincham, J. E., & Wertheimer, A. I. (1985). Using the health belief model to predict initial drug therapy defaulting. *Social Science and Medicine, 20*(1), 101–105.

Fiore, M. C., Bailey, W. C., Cohen, S. J., Dorfman, S. F., Goldstein, M. G., Gritz, E. R., et al. (2000). *Treating tobacco use and dependence: Clinical practice guideline*. Rockville, MD: U.S. Department of Health and Human Services, Public Health Service.

Fiore, M. C., Jorenby, D. E., Schensky, A. E., Smith, S. S., Bauer, R. R., Baker, S. B., et al. (1995). Smoking status as the new vital sign: Effect on assessment and intervention in the patients who smoke. *Mayo Clinical Proceedings, 70*, 209–213.

Fisher, N. M., Pendergast, D. R., & Calkins, E. (1991). Muscle rehabilitation in impaired elderly nursing home residents. *Archives of Physical Medicine and Rehabilitation, 72*, 181–185.

Frisby, W., & Hoeber, L. (2002). Factors affecting the uptake of community recreation as health promotion for women on low incomes. *Canadian Journal of Public Health, 93*(2), 129–133.

Garr, R. (2003). Wine, health and political correctness. *Signal Mountain Post, 10*(1), 17.

Gaziano, J. M., Hennekens, C. H., Godfried, S. L., Sesso, H. D., Glynn, R. J., Breslow, G. L., et al. (1999). Type of alcoholic beverage and risk of myocardial infarction. *American Journal of Cardiology, 83*, 52–57.

Geesaman, B. J., Benson, E., Brewster, S. J., Kunkel, L. M., Blanche, H., Thomas, G., et al. (2003). Haplotype-based identification of a microsomal transfer protein marker associated with the human lifespan. *Proceedings of the National Academy of Sciences of the United States of America, 100*, 14115–14120.

Goldstein, M. G., Niaura, R., Willey-Lessne, C., DePue, J., Eaton, C., Rakowski, W., et al. (1997). Physicians counseling smokers: A population-based survey of patients' perceptions of health care provider–delivered smoking cessation interventions. *Archives of Internal Medicine, 157*, 1313–1319.

Gough, I. R., Furnival, C. M., Schilder, L., & Grove, W. (1983). Assessment of quality of life of patients with advanced cancer. *European Journal of Clinical Oncology, 19*, 1161–1165.

Grant, M., Ferrell, B., Schmidt, G. M., Fonbuena, P., Niland, J. C., & Forman, S. J. (1992). Measurement of quality of life in bone marrow transplantation survivors. *Quality of Life Research, 1*(6), 375–384.

GrønbÉk, M., Becker, U., Johansen, D., Gottschau, A., Schnohr, P., Hein, H. O., et al. (2000). Type of alcohol consumed and mortality from all causes, coronary heart disease, and cancer. *Annals of Internal Medicine, 133*, 411–419.

Hanestad, B. R. (1990). Errors of measurement affecting the reliability and validity of data acquired from self-assessed quality of life. *Scandinavian Journal of the Caring Sciences, 4*(1), 29–34.

Hawkes, K. (2003). Grandmothers and the evolution of human longevity. *American Journal of Human Biology, 15*, 380–400.

Hekimi, S., & Guarente, L. (2003). Genetics and the specificity of the aging process. *Science, 299*, 1351–1354.

Houde, S. C., & Melillo, K. D. (2002). Cardiovascular health and physical activity in older adults: An integrative review of research methodology and results. *Journal of Advanced Nursing, 38*(3), 219–234.

Hurdle, D. E. (2001). Social support: A critical factor in women's health and health promotion. *Health and Social Work, 26*(2), 72–79.

Joint Committee on Smoking and Health. (1995). Smoking and health: Physician responsibility; A statement of the Joint Committee on Smoking and Health. *Chest, 198*, 201–208.

King, A. C. (1991). Community intervention for promotion of physical activity and fitness. *Exercise and Sport Sciences Review, 19*, 211–259.

King, A. C. (2001). The coming of age of behavioral research in physical activity. *Annals of Behavioral Medicine, 23*, 227–228.

King, A. C., Haskell, W. L., Taylor, C. B., Kraemer, H. C., & DeBunk, R. F. (1991). Group versus home-based exercise training in healthy older men and women: A community-based clinical trial. *Journal of the American Medical Association, 266*, 1535–1542.

King, A. C., Rejeski, W. J., & Buchner, D. M. (1998). Physical activity interventions targeting older adults. A critical review and recommendations. *American Journal of Preventive Medicine, 15*, 316–333.

King, M. C., Marks, J. H., & Mandell, J. B. (2003). Breast and ovarian cancer risks due to inherited mutations in BRCA1 and BRCA2. *Science, 302*, 643–646.

Kirsch, I., Jungeblit, A., Jenkins, L., & Kolstad, A. (1993). *Adult literacy in America. U.S. National Adult Literacy Survey*. Princeton, NJ: Educational Testing Service.

Klein, S., Burke, L. E., Bray, G. A., Blair, S., Allison, D. B., Pi-Sunyer, X., et al. (2004). Clinical implications of obesity with specific focus on cardiovascular disease: A statement for professionals from the American Heart Association Council on Nutrition, Physical Activity, and Metabolism: Endorsed by the American College of Cardiology Foundation. *Circulation, 110*, 2952–2967.

Lahdenpera, M., Lummaa, V., Helle, S., Tremblay, M., & Russell, A. F. (2004). Fitness benefits of prolonged post-reproductive lifespan in women. *Nature, 428*, 178–181.

Lange-Collette, J. (2002). Promoting health among perimenopausal women through diet and exercise. *Journal of the American Academy of Nurse Practitioners, 14*(4), 172–177.

Lichtenstein, A. (2008). Modified MyPyramid for older adults. *Journal of Nutrition*, *138*(1), 5–11.

Lueckenotte, A. G. (2000). *Gerontologic nursing* (2nd ed.). New York: Mosby.

Mallet, L. (1992). Counseling in special populations: The elderly patient. *American Pharmacy, NS32*(10), 835–843.

Malveaux, J. O., Murphy, P. W., Arnold, C., Davis, T. C., Jackson, R. H., & Sentell, T., et al. (1996). Improving patient education for patients with low literacy skills. *American Family Physician, 53*(1), 205–211.

Marcus, B. H., Napolitano, M. A., King, A. C., Lewis, B. A., Whiteley, J. A., Albrecht, A., et al. (2007). Telephone versus print delivery of an individualized motivationally tailored physical activity intervention: Project STRIDE. *Health Psychology, 26*(4), 401–409.

Martin, G. M., Oshima, J., Gray, M. D., & Poot, M. (1999). What geriatricians should know about the Werner syndrome. *Journal of the American Geriatrics Society, 47*, 1136–1144.

Mattson, M. P., Chan, S. L., & Duan, W. (2002). Modification of brain aging and neurodegenerative disorders by genes, diet, and behavior. *Physiological Reviews, 82*(3), 637–672.

McMurdo, M. E., & Rennie, L. (1993). A controlled trial of exercise by residents of old people's homes. *Age and Ageing, 22*, 11–15.

Meister, K. A., Whelan, E. M., & Kava, R. (2000). The health effects of moderate alcohol intake in humans: An epidemiologic review. *Critical Reviews in Clinical Laboratory Sciences, 37*, 261–296.

Miller, R. A. (2002). Extending life: Scientific prospects and political obstacles. *Milbank Quarterly, 80*, 155–174.

Mirand, A. L., & Welte, J. W. (1996). Alcohol consumption among the elderly in a general population, Erie County, New York. *American Journal of Public Health, 86*, 978–984.

Mitchell, B. D., Hsueh, W. C., King, T. M., et al. (2001). Heritability of life span in the Old Order Amish. *American Journal of Medical Genetics, 102*, 346–352.

Nanada, C., Fanale, J., & Kronholm, P. (1990). The role of medication noncompliance and adverse reactions in hospitalizations of the elderly. *Archives of Internal Medicine, 150*, 841–846.

National Council on Patient Information and Education. (2007). *Enhancing prescription medicine adherence: A national action plan.* Retrieved June 23, 2008, from http://www.talkaboutrx.org/med_compliance.jsp

O'Connor, P. G., & Schottenfeld, R. S. (1998). Patients with alcohol problems. *New England Journal of Medicine, 338*, 592–602.

Oguma, Y., Sesso, H. D., Paffenbarger, R. S. Jr, & Lee, I.-M. (2002). Physical activity and all cause mortality in women: A review of the evidence. *British Journal of Sports Medicine, 36*, 162–172.

Organisation for Economic Co-operation and Development. (1998). Maintaining prosperity in an ageing society. *OECD Observer*. Retrieved June 25, 2008, from http://www.oecd.org/dataoecd/21/10/2430300.pdf

Ouwehand, C., de Ridder, D. T. D., & Bensing, J. M. (2007). A review of successful aging models: Proposing proactive coping as an important additional strategy. *Clinical Psychology Review*, *27*, 873–884.

Patterson, W. B. (1975). The quality of survival in response to treatment. *Journal of the American Medical Association, 233*(3), 280–281.

Perls, T. T., Wilmoth, J., Levenson, R., Drinkwater, M., Cohen, M., Bogan, H., et al. (2002). Life-long sustained mortality advantage of siblings of centenarians. *Proceedings of the National Academy of Sciences of the United States of America, 99*, 8442–8447.

Pletcher, S. D., Khazaeli, A. A., & Curtsinger, J. W. (2000). Why do life spans differ? Partitioning mean longevity differences in terms of age-specific mortality parameters. *Journals of Gerontology, Series A, 55*, B381–B389.

Prochaska, J., & Goldstein, M. G. (1991). Process of smoking cessation: Implications for clinicians. *Clinics in Chest Medicine, 12*, 727–735.

Pullen, C., & Walter, S. N. (2002). Midlife and older rural women's adherence to U.S. dietary guidelines across stages of change in healthy eating. *Public Health Nursing, 19*(3), 170–178.

Ravaglia, G., Forti, P., Lucicesare, A., Pisacane, N., Rietti, E., Bianchin, M., et al. (2008). Physical activity and dementia risk in the elderly: Findings from a prospective Italian study. *Neurology, 70*(19 Pt 2), 1786–1794.

Rehm, J., Greenfield, T. K., & Rogers, J. D. (2001). Average volume of alcohol consumption, patterns of drinking, and all-cause mortality: Results from the U.S. National Alcohol Survey. *American Journal of Epidemiology, 153*, 64–71.

Rigler, S. (2000). Alcoholism in the elderly. *American Family Physician, 61*, 1710–1716.

Rowe, J. W., & Kahn, R. L. (1998). *Successful aging*. New York: Pantheon/Random House.

Sauvage, L. R. Jr., Myklebust, B. M., Crow-Pan, J., Novak, S., Millington, P., Hoffman, M. D., et al. (1992). A clinical trial of strengthening and aerobic exercise to improve gait and balance in elderly male nursing home residents. *American Journal of Physical Medicine & Rehabilitation, 71*(6), 333–342.

Schnelle, J. F., MacRae, P. G., Ouslander, J. G., Simmons, S. F., & Nitta, M. (1995). Functional incidental training (FIT), mobility performance and incontinence care with nursing home residents. *Journal of the American Geriatrics Society, 43*, 1356–1362.

Schulte, J. N., & Yarasheski, K. E. (2001). Effects of resistance training on the rate of muscle protein synthesis in frail elderly people. *International Journal of Sport Nutrition and Exercise Metabolism, 11*, S111–S118.

Shikany, J. M., & White, G. L. (2002). Dietary guidelines for chronic disease prevention. *Southern Medical Journal, 93*(12), 1138–1151.

Smith, M. C. (1996). Predicting and detecting noncompliance. In M. C. Smith & A. I. Wertheimer (Eds.), *Social and behavioral aspects of pharmaceutical care* (pp. 323–350). New York: Pharmaceutical Products Press.

Smits, C. H. M., Deeg, B. J. H., Kriegsman, D. M. W., & Schmand, B. (1999). Cognitive functioning and health as determinants of mortality in an older population. *American Journal of Epidemiology, 150*, 878–986.

Swartzberg, J. E., Margen, S., & Editors of UC Berkeley Wellness Letter. (2001). *The complete home wellness handbook: Home remedies, prevention, self care*. New York: Rebus.

Task Force for Compliance. (1994). *Noncompliance with medications: An economic tragedy with important implications for health care reform*. Baltimore, MD: Author.

Terry, D. F., Wilcox, M., McCormick, M. A., Lawler, E., & Perls, T. T. (2003). Cardiovascular advantages among the offspring of centenarians. *Journals of Gerontology, Series A, 58*, M425–M431.

Thompson, L. V. (2002). Skeletal muscle adaptations with age, inactivity, and therapeutic physical activity. *Journal of Orthopaedic and Sports Physical Therapy, 32*(2), 44–57.

Van der Bij, A. K., Laurant, M., & Wensing, M. (2002). Effectiveness of physical activity interventions for older adults: A review. *American Journal of Preventive Medicine, 22*(2), 120–133.

Wilkins, S. (2001). Women with osteoporosis: Strategies for managing aging and chronic illness. *Journal of Women and Aging, 13*, 59–77.

World Health Organization. (1958). *The first ten years. The health organization*. Geneva: Author.

World Health Organization. (1994). *Statement developed by WHO Quality of Life Working Group*. Published in the WHO/Health Promotion Glossary 1998. WHO/HRP/HEP 98.1. Geneva: Author.

World Health Organization. (2002). *Active aging: A policy framework*. Geneva: Author.

World Health Organization & International Network for the Prevention of Elder Abuse. (2002). *Missing voices: Views of older persons on elder abuse*. Geneva: World Health Organization. Retrieved June 25, 2008, from http://www.who.int/ageing/projects/elder_abuse/missing_voices/en/

Young, D. R., & King, A. C. (1995). Exercise adherence: Determinants of physical activity and applications of health behavior change theories. *Medicine, Exercise, Nutrition and Health, 4*, 335–348.

Zuger, A. (2002, December 31). The case for drinking. *New York Times*, p. F1.

CHAPTER 23

The Gerontological Nurse as Manager and Leader

Dawna S. Fish, RN, BSN, COS-C
Kristen L. Mauk, PhD, RN, CRRN-A, GCNS-BC
Marilyn Ter Maat, MSN, CRRN-A, NEA, BC, FNGNA

LEARNING OBJECTIVES

At the end of this chapter, the reader will be able to:

- Identify characteristics of effective nurse managers.
- Contrast the roles of manager and leader.
- Compare various leadership styles and strategies.
- Discuss characteristics of assertive behavior.
- Describe the process of delegation, including how it is used in the management of unlicensed assistive personnel.
- Analyze the characteristics of the four major generations of nurses.
- Recognize the value of professional associations to the nurse manager and leader.
- Evaluate one's own strengths and weaknesses as a future leader or manager.

KEY TERMS

- Aggressive
- Assertive
- Authoritarian
- Charismatic leadership
- Delegation
- Democratic
- Intimidation
- Laissez-faire
- Leader
- Manager
- Multigenerational nursing
- Nonassertive
- Situational
- Transactional leadership
- Transformational leadership
- Unlicensed assistive personnel (UAP)

The nursing profession has changed significantly since the days of Florence Nightingale. Advances in nursing science have required nurses to expand their knowledge base and keep current on constant changes in the health care system. Exciting breakthroughs in patient care occur daily, and with those come greater responsibilities for professional nurses.

Nurse managers and leaders have additional challenges in caring for older adults with complex needs. As the number of elderly persons in the population increases, so will the number of caregivers who will need to be managed. Nurse leaders in gerontology "must be able to lead at the bedside, in clinical teams, and in management teams" (Mancino, 2005, p. 117). All geriatric nurses, whether they hold a formal **manager** position or not, need to develop good management skills.

In this chapter, the gerontological nurse as manager and the skills required for effective leadership will be discussed. Characteristics of successful managers and leaders, as well as the concepts of assertiveness and delegation, will also be presented.

Although the primary aim of gerontological nurse managers is to promote quality of patient care, this goal is accomplished more through facilitation in management than with bedside nursing. Nurse managers in settings involving older adults should focus on implementing, and assisting others to implement, best practices. Although this may seem obvious, education of health professionals and subsequent translation into practice in the care of older adults continue to demand attention.

When nurses move from a direct care position into management, their focus on patient care shifts to the quality, education, and experience of the staff they supervise, empowering others who provide the hands-on care to patients. Thus, the gerontological nurse manager is in a unique position to improve the quality, positive outcomes, and cost-effectiveness of patient care in a variety of settings. Those nurses who serve in assistant director or director of nursing positions in long-term care facilities, for example, use both managerial and leadership skills and have the potential to positively impact a broader population.

THE NURSE MANAGER

The University of Iowa (2005) defines the nurse manager's basic function and responsibility in this way:

> *The nurse manager provides clinical and managerial leadership to assure that all staff can identify the customers they serve; understand the aim of the work to serve those customers; and has the education, methods and resources to accomplish their performance objectives. Nurse managers develop and direct the planning, implementation, and evaluation of clinical and nursing services within area of responsibility. The area of responsibility might include clinic(s), unit(s), service(s), center(s) and/or program(s).*

Nurse managers are specialists who undertake a multitude of tasks including dealing with others on a daily basis, and ensuring quality nursing care, patient and family satisfaction, and staff retention, commitment, and contentment. Resident and patient satisfaction is one outcome measure that nurse managers use to determine positive progress. Weeks (2003) provided an example of the steps used on one unit to attain better patient satisfaction (see **Box 23-1**).

Recruitment and retention of reliable employees are an ongoing issue in long-term care. There is a direct relationship between fewer RN and nursing assistant hours and poorer quality of care in nursing homes (Arling, Kane, Mueller, Bershadsky, & Degenholtz, 2007; Harrington, Zimmerman, Karon,

BOX 23-1 Steps to Patient Satisfaction

1. Identify a clear objective.
2. Identify the right people.
3. Identify the right approach.
4. Walk the talk (leaders participating).
5. Role model politeness or PTAS (please, thank you, action, smiles).
6. Involve the entire team.
7. Recognize that little things mean a lot.
8. Convey compassion and pride in work.
9. Practice the satisfaction Cs:
   - Cheerfulness
   - Courtesy
   - Cleanliness
   - Call-lights
   - Coaching
   - Collaboration
   - Communication
   - Commitment
   - Confidentiality
   - Compassion

Source: Adapted from Weeks, S. K. (2003). Everyday steps to patient satisfaction. *Rehabilitation Nursing, 28*(4), 104.

Robinson, & Beutel, 2000). A high turnover rate among nurse's aides (40–100% in some facilities) is also associated with a decrease in patient care quality (Castle, 2008; Service Employees International Union, 2007).

Nurse managers can address issues such as staff turnover and job satisfaction by examining research results from studies that demonstrate success in addressing these problems. Using evidence-based practice in this way, nurse managers can create a working environment more likely to improve quality of care. Work settings that address concerns and stressors of caregivers, focus on positive communication and teamwork, reduce paperwork, ensure adequate staffing, and foster the employee's sense of belonging and investment in the organization have been shown to have positive results in staff retention, morale, and care quality (Arling et al., 2007; Cherry, Ashcraft, & Owen, 2007; Donoghue & Castle, 2006; Sikorska-Simmons, 2006).

With the restructuring of many health care systems, nurse managers have had to accept more responsibilities that have extended over broader areas. Nurse managers contribute to strategic planning of current and future goals of the workplace, whether in regards to a specific unit or the company in general. Management direction needs to be reasonable and nonthreatening. Being a competent nurse manager requires prioritizing, organization, and consistency in decisions and treatment of others. The dual degrees of MSN/MBA or MSN/JD being offered at many universities bear witness to the fact that not only are nurse leaders and managers in greater demand, but also the expectations for education have become increasingly higher for nurse leaders in the past decade.

BOX 23-2 Characteristics of Effective Nurse Managers

- Organized
- Consistent
- Fair
- Optimistic
- Goal-oriented
- Flexible
- Creative
- Resourceful
- Professional
- Standard-setter
- Trustworthy
- Honest
- Empowered
- Nonthreatening

Characteristics of Effective Nurse Managers

Several character traits of effective nurse managers are listed in **Box 23-2**. Certain qualities of a nurse manager may be considered essential in producing effective nursing care (Thompson, 2004). Some of these qualities will be discussed here.

Integrity

Integrity suggests honesty and trustworthiness, qualities that are evident to others over time. This is a quality most recognized as important for any nurse leader or manager (Carroll, 2005/2006). Integrity means that a person is dependable, punctual, fair, and consistent. Patients and families recognize integrity as an important value in society and certainly in health care. Persons of integrity make excellent managers because they earn the trust of others. The supervisors to whom they answer know that patients will be cared for appropriately and safely.

Nurse managers should treat all staff members equally. Staff members look at fairness with high regard (Marquis & Huston, 2003). Showing favoritism will develop a stressful and divided environment. At times, the nurse manager may have to make difficult decisions about staff discipline or termination. Such duties of the manager may be unpleasant but are necessary. Managers with integrity will take into account that each person is unique, displays specific individual skills, and contributes to the overall goals of the unit.

Professionalism

One important goal of nurse managers is to provide a professional, positive atmosphere within the workplace. Workers who feel valued and invested in the organization tend to report higher job satisfaction (Donoghue & Castle, 2006; Sikorska-Simmons, 2006). The nurse manager sets the tone for the unit or division and acts as a role model for others. Professionalism encompasses the person's manner of appearance, language, and behavior. The way a manager dresses, speaks, and even his or her posture can influence how receptive others will be to that manager (personal communication, Dawna Fish). A manager needs to maintain an image that displays confidence and competency. Nurse managers are responsible for maintaining an ethical standard and setting an expectation of the same standard for those they supervise.

Organization

Being organized, creativity, and flexibility are necessary traits. Every day, nurse managers and directors of nursing are faced with many new and complex situations. The function of organizing can be defined as relating people and things to each other in such a way that they are combined and interrelated into a unit capable of being directed toward organizational objectives (Longest, 1976). Health care delivery systems work best when an interdisciplinary team performs a variety of skills in a complex care environment. Based on the creative, flexible, and organizational skills of the nurse manager, those under his or her supervision will be affected negatively or positively. If the nurse manager keeps deadlines and meets staff expectations, then staff members will generally view this as a priority.

Being organized takes work and determination. Prioritization is essential. Starting each day with a prioritized list of tasks may help the manager stay on track. There will be days when those priorities will change several times to better meet the needs of patients and staff. Ask "How can I, as a nurse manager, complete my priorities today realistically and completely in the best interest of the patients or residents, families, and employees?"

Creativity

Creativity calls for imagination. Keeping staff involved and excited about work and changes requires the use of critical and creative thinking, yet it is a factor associated with higher job satisfaction in long-term care and assisted living settings (Cherry, Ashcraft, & Owen, 2007; Sikorska-Simmons, 2006). An initial role for nurse managers is to encourage the staff to offer their unique ideas and suggestions. Cultivating those suggestions is the responsibility of the manager.

Knowing how the staff perceives the milieu of the workplace and allowing them to express their ideas may help the manager to draw out some hidden gifts of the staff. Perhaps staff members would benefit from more input into scheduling. Indeed, some long-term care facilities allow the staff to make their own work schedules within the parameters and staffing needs set by the manager. Such practices promote a sense of ownership and control within the nursing team and increase job satisfaction. Better job satisfaction has been correlated with better patient or resident care (Harrington et al., 2000).

Flexibility

Daily dilemmas require flexibility. Many times a nurse manager's day will not go as planned; for example, a staff member may call in sick to work, may have a personal crisis, or may have car trouble. Those are unexpected situations that require not only flexibility, but also creativity and the ability to reorganize as needed. Nurse managers would benefit from having a backup plan to accommodate the unforeseen changes that inevitably happen in the health care environment.

Skills of Nurse Managers

Gerontological nurse managers will develop a skill set related to accomplishing the goals and objectives of the particular unit they service. Certain skills, such as those summarized in **Box 23-3**, will facilitate more positive outcomes.

Delegating

One skill that all nurses need to develop is that of **delegation**. Nurses do not work in isolation, but are dependent upon the smooth communication and activity of an interdisciplinary team. Charge nurses, nurse managers, nursing supervisors, and directors are all called upon daily to make decisions about those who help them achieve the

BOX 23-3 Skills of Nurse Managers

Team building

Maintaining balance in the workplace

Prioritizing

Setting realistic goals

Delegating

Multitasking

Decision making

Using excellent judgment

Empowering others

Facilitating change

desired outcomes for patient care. Delegation is one of the primary tools used by geriatric nurse managers to ensure the quality of patient care.

Delegation may be defined simply as giving authority to a specific person for a specific task. Delegation is both a managerial and a legal act, and a skill that must be learned and practiced. It involves more than just handing out patient assignments or duties to be performed. It also is not abdication of one's own responsibilities. Licensed nurses are still accountable for the well-being and safety of the patients entrusted to them. Thus, when a licensed nurse delegates duties to **unlicensed assistive personnel (UAP)**, such as nursing assistants or nurse technicians, the licensed nurse is still ultimately responsible for the quality of patient care. Kelly-Heidenthal stated, "inappropriate use of UAP in performing functions outside their scope of practice is a violation of the state nursing practice act and is a threat to patient safety. The RN has an increased scope of liability when tasks are delegated to UAP" (2004, p. 103). The nurse can delegate tasks such as bathing, feeding, and toileting to qualified and trained UAP. Although UAP can give supportive care, they cannot lawfully perform nursing duties such as assessment, treatment, or total patient care.

Delegation involves a problem-solving process. Decisions about how and when to delegate duties are complex and involve critical thinking skills on the part of the nurse manager or charge nurse. One study found that the group climate on a unit "was significantly associated with the head nurse's ability to delegate tasks and to make decisions with confidence" (Hern-Underwood, 1991, p. 4). How does one make decisions about delegating care or assigning patients?

The Delegation Process. Delegating is a process that, much like the nursing process or any other critical thinking process, involves several steps: assessment, planning, delegation, supervision, and evaluation (**Figure 23-1**).

The first step in the delegation process is assessment. The nurse manager should examine the situation with which he or she is charged and gather data. This involves more than just looking at a standard acuity form. Questions must be answered, such as: How many patients need to be cared for? What is their level of complexity? What nursing hours are required to provide safe and competent care? Are there any other factors that will add to the duties the staff will need to perform on this shift? Are there any admissions or discharges? Are any fire drills or other interruptions planned? Does any extra teaching need to be done with family members? Are there any patients whose condition has deteriorated and who might need extra nursing time? Remember that geriatric patients often present with subtle changes in health status that may become emergencies quickly if not properly treated.

After assessing the needs of the patients under her or his supervision, the nurse manager must assess the available staff. Another set of questions must be asked: Is the staffing adequate? Are there enough licensed professionals per patient based on acuity and other needs assessed? Are the available staff members able and competent to perform the assigned skills? How much supervision will the nursing assistants require? Are any float nurses or assistants assigned to the unit? If so, what is their background and experience? Will the RNs on the unit need to perform any additional duties for LPNs or nurse technicians who are working (such as taking and noting physicians' orders or starting IVs)? What is the scope of practice of the LPNs, nursing assistants, or nurse technicians on duty? The nurse manager must realize that each state and each

FIGURE **23-1** **The process of delegating.**

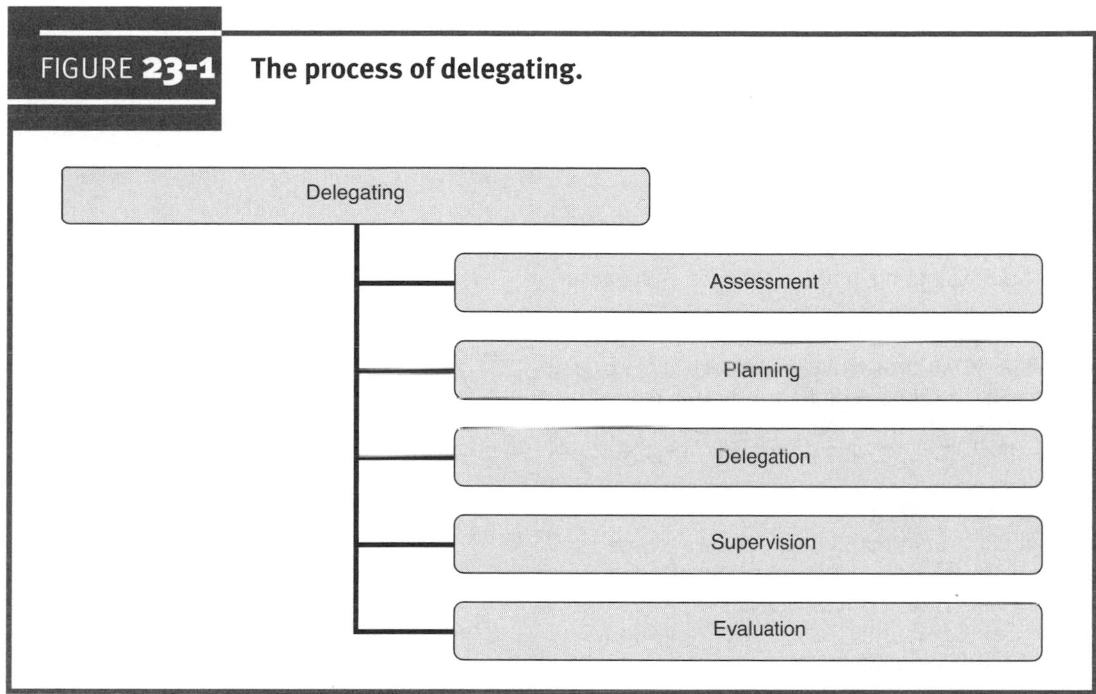

facility may have different skills that are acceptable under different job titles. How much supervision will the unlicensed staff require?

With the answers to these questions in mind, the nurse manager then plans staffing/patient assignments, keeping in mind the five rights of delegation (**Box 23-4**). Planning involves critical thinking in using the assessment data to make the best decision for quality patient care with the resources available.

Once planning is complete, the nurse manager delegates duties to each team member as determined by thorough assessment and planning. Instructions and assignments should be clear and in writing to minimize confusion about job assignments. UAPs should be provided with necessary information about patients in their care in the form of a brief report. Any assignments in addition to patient care, such as replenishing stock or cleaning, should be fairly and evenly distributed and given in writing.

Nurses should be provided with a written list of patients and their pertinent information. Reports should be given from shift to shift, either by tape recording or in person. Any additional information should be communicated in person during change of shift. Many units tape record reporting to the next shift to save time and free additional personnel to cover patient needs during shift change.

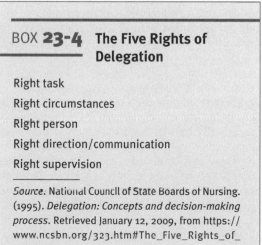

BOX **23-4** **The Five Rights of Delegation**

Right task

Right circumstances

Right person

Right direction/communication

Right supervision

Source. National Council of State Boards of Nursing. (1995). *Delegation: Concepts and decision-making process.* Retrieved January 12, 2009, from https://www.ncsbn.org/323.htm#The_Five_Rights_of_Delegation

Once assignments are delegated, the nurse manager is responsible for supervising both licensed personnel and UAP to ensure that duties are being carried out as expected. Although licensed personnel are responsible for their own actions or failure to act under their scope of practice, the nurse manager who delegates must be accountable for the correct performance of the tasks assigned to UAP. Supervision implies monitoring and evaluating, making changes or suggestions as necessary. The manager must be willing to adjust assignments as the need arises. Education and training of UAP while under the manager's supervision may be needed. UAP should feel comfortable enough with their nurse managers to inform them of any lack of preparation to carry out certain tasks, and of their ability to carry out the delegated assignment.

Last, the nurse manager evaluates the entire process of delegation (National Council of State Boards of Nursing, 1995). Evaluate the patient, the person carrying out the task, and how well it was accomplished. Provide feedback at the end of the shift as to how well quality of care was accomplished. This may be as informal as telling the staff they did a good job that day, or it may be necessary to do further teaching in areas of weakness where improvement is needed.

The delegation process is an important one for nurse managers. Without teamwork, quality of patient care cannot be accomplished. Delegating is one skill that all nurse managers need, and one that can be developed with practice and mentoring. **Case Study 23-1** gives an example of the delegation process.

Case Study 23-1

Ms. Brown is the night charge nurse for an inpatient geriatric rehabilitation unit with 30 beds in a small acute care hospital. She is making her night assignments and finds that she has herself, one LPN, and two CNAs to care for 28 patients with high acuity. Ms. Brown does not feel this staffing is adequate, because the evening charge nurse reported that one of the patients was receiving a blood transfusion and might need to be transferred to intensive care, and another patient was complaining of atypical shortness of breath, so tests were being run to determine the cause. The LPN is experienced, but one of the CNAs is still in orientation to the night shift and has little experience.

Questions:

1. What is Ms. Brown's best course of action?
2. If she feels she needs more help to provide quality care to her patients, whom should she contact?
3. What should she do if told no more help is available?
4. What is the most assertive response in this situation?
5. How should Ms. Brown divide assignments between herself and the LPN? Between the CNAs?
6. Is there a certain nursing model of care that might work better than another in this situation?
7. How would Ms. Brown apply the delegation process to this situation?

Team Building

Good team building is an essential skill needed by gerontological nurse managers. Caring for older patients is a multitask endeavor with an interdisciplinary team contributing to the safe delivery of quality patient care. Team members may include many levels of nursing staff as well as members from other disciplines such as therapy, medicine, dietary, social work, housekeeping, lab, and pharmacy. In upper management positions, nurse managers may have supervisory authority for those in other disciplines. Good teamwork involves contributing, analyzing, criticizing constructively, and accepting a common ground. Working together toward common goals promotes a sense of team solidarity.

The gerontological nurse manager promotes team building by enhancing each team member's skills and abilities, encouraging individuals to use their skills productively and confidently. Nurse managers need to know the strengths and weaknesses of each team member and demonstrate a concern and interest in each one as a unique individual. To create a motivating climate in the work environment, Marquis and Huston (2003) suggest the following additional strategies: make expectations clear, be fair and consistent, be a firm decision maker, provide experiences that promote employee growth, give positive rewards for desired behavior, and let employees have as much control and independence as possible within the limits of the organization. Creativity, research, and cooperation are all needed to foster each team member's best contributions to the team.

Goal Setting

A nurse manager sets goals and specific objectives to reach them. Goals are set individually and also collectively as a team or group. Goals should be measurable, realistic, time-limited, and mutually established. In today's society, facilities and companies usually set attainable goals that exceed the previous year's goals. Goals are victory builders. Factors including finances, retention of staff, morale of individuals, resources, and desire to achieve may influence goal attainment. The responsibility of the nurse manager is to set goals and objectives that are realistic and attainable. Staff nurses should be given clear directions as to what is required of them.

Short- and long-term goals should be delineated. Short-term goals could be hourly, daily, weekly, or monthly. Long-term goals are more detailed and may encompass yearly or even longer time spans. Realistic goals are easier to accept and achieve as a team. Goals can be altered based on the needs of the nurses or company, and being an effective manager requires sensitivity and flexibility to those needs.

Facilitating Change

Nurse managers participate in staff and corporate meetings of the local agency. Maintaining competency related to the current changes within the company and health care in general is a requirement for solid management. Implementing change may be a challenge. Changes may be instituted based on feedback from the interdisciplinary team members; however, change can make an individual feel uncomfortable and vulnerable. When comfort zones are challenged, the nurse manager should provide encouragement, clear direction, and specific expectations. Knowledgeable input about policies and procedures, staffing needs, and financial involvement need to be given on a regular basis. Meetings need to be held to problem solve, assess where the company is as a whole at that given time, and assess the needs of staff members and patients or clients.

As an example, a local health care agency may hold corporate meetings weekly. Individual department meetings are generally held once a month. Department issues are discussed and evaluated and changes are made. Think of these meetings like a chain reaction in the following steps—corporate meetings–department meetings–individual needs. Each is important and each has specific objectives, but ultimately the same goal is in the forefront—to make better and achieve more.

A group of researchers (Scalzi, Evans, Barstow, & Hostvedt, 2006) studying organizational culture change in nursing homes found that there were several key barriers to and enablers of change. Barriers included not involving staff nurses in the change activities, the perception of staff that the corporation and its regulations were most important, and a high turnover of administrators and staff. Positive enablers to change included having a key group of "change champions" (p. 368), having shared values and goals, gaining participation of residents and families, and empowering the facility to make decisions.

Change in the workplace, whether positive or negative, generally produces stress. Going outside of the established comfort zone brings uncomfortable feelings and emotions. But change often provides opportunities, which in turn should produce positive outcomes. How changes are implemented often determines how those changes are accepted. Providing clear direction with any changes will help to reduce the negative responses generally associated with change. "The leader/manager must attempt to view change positively and to impart this view to subordinates" (Marquis & Huston, 2003, p. 90). The stress resulting from change may be minimized by instituting changes gradually. How would you respond to the situation in **Case Study 23-2**?

Stress Management

The nurse manager's most difficult responsibilities are providing stress management and using those

Case Study 23-2

Ms. Casey, RN, BSN, is the unit manager of a geriatric medical floor in a large acute care hospital. The hospital is introducing a new computerized charting system that requires the staff to attend training to be approved to use it. All of her 44 staff members are required to attend a 4-hour training class within 1 month to prepare for the switch to computerized charting. Most of the nursing staff who have been working on this unit for years are resistant to the idea of a new charting system and wish to continue using the traditional paper and pencil means of charting. Ms. Casey hears many complaints about this change in policy and sees that it threatens morale.

Questions:

1. What are some practical ways that Ms. Casey can facilitate change to the new computerized charting system?
2. Can you think of any incentives that might help the staff be more open to this change in policy?
3. How might the resistance of the nursing staff to this change affect morale? Patient care?
4. Devise a plan for how Ms. Casey would be able to send each of her 44 nurses to attend computer class and continue to adequately staff her unit.
5. What problems can you foresee that might arise? Are there any resources that Ms. Casey could use to aid in this transition?

skills to manage her or his own stress as well. Stress has a tendency to filter down from one person to another. Each individual may perceive stress differently with different triggers that cause them stress. What one person may see as a negative connotation, another may see as positive. Attitude and individual behaviors determine how stress is managed. Stress may be defined as "any event that places a demand on the body, mentally or physically" (Gmelch, 1982, p. 5).

According to Gmelch in his book *Beyond Stress to Effective Management* (1982), the Chinese have two different definitions for stress. Two different symbols are used in their vocabulary, and they have completely opposite meanings. The first symbol describes danger, and the second symbol describes opportunity. Gerontological nurse managers experience both of these challenges in the workplace, but have the responsibility to choose which perspective should take priority. Which will provide the best outcome? Which will provide the greatest learning experience? Which will draw out the positive attitudes of staff members? Between these two descriptors, opportunity provides more imagination and advantage that could produce new skills and attitudes in staff members. The nurse manager must identify actions to develop a resolution and provide steps to restore energy, calmness, and a spirit of oneness. These steps enable the nurse manager and staff members to be ready for the next challenge with either greater confidence for resolution or trepidation to face yet another stressful situation. Stress is a realistic part of nursing management, but how stress is approached and defined will eventually determine the outcome of the situation.

A small study of nurse managers (Judkins, Reid, & Furlow, 2006) found that hardiness training could increase their abilities to cope with stress and improve workplace culture. Managers with higher levels of hardiness also were more committed to the organization and had a more positive attitude toward change. Higher job satisfaction has been associated with greater hardiness, so if such a coping mechanism can be taught to managers and filtered to staff, the potential to decrease burnout and frustration is great. In long-term care, the need to attract and retain staff is ever present, and exploring new methods of stress management is essential for both managers and staff.

Decision Making and Conflict Resolution

Nurse managers are expected to make intelligent, informed decisions when conflicts arise. Obtaining all of the vital information that explains the conflicts helps to avoid blame and judgment on the part of the manager. Skill is required to deal with conflict and determine a peaceful and fair resolution. Approaching problems in a timely manner and with confidence will assist the staff in realizing that the nurse manager is available and willing to help. How the nurse manager resolves conflict reveals character. Nurse "managers should expect employees to attempt to resolve conflicts among themselves" (Thompson, 2004, p. 64), though staff may require some education in this area. The offer of assistance and the attitude of approaching conflicts as important are necessary for resolution. The staff needs to have support and needs to have confidence that the manager is a resource for solving both minor and major conflicts. **Case Study 23-3** provides an example of a situation requiring both decision making and conflict resolution.

Expertise

Nurse managers should have specialized knowledge in the area of expertise of the job. This particularly helps in being able to relate to the staff and set realistic goals for quality of patient care. Someone who doesn't have a good perspective of what the staff deals with on a day-to-day basis will not understand fully how they feel and why they think the way they do. Nurse managers who have a solid nursing clinical background, which generally includes years of experience in different areas of expertise, may more easily earn the respect of the staff. Respect is difficult to earn if one does not have an equal or more extensive background, knowledge, or experience than the staff. Gerontological nurses wishing to enter into management positions may transition through various levels of increasing responsibility. **Figures 23-2** and **23-3** give examples of various levels of management in different settings. The benefit of mastering each consecutive level of management and leadership is that the nurse manager can readily identify the needs of her or his staff members as well as the needs of the patients she or he ultimately serves.

Case Study 23-3

Mr. Gonzalez, RN, is the charge nurse on the evening shift of the skilled care unit at a long-term care facility. The day shift nurses have complained to Mr. Gonzalez that the evening shift CNAs have not been showering the residents as scheduled. They tell him that family members of the residents have complained about poor hygiene of their loved ones.

Questions:

1. What is the first step Mr. Gonzalez should take in resolving this situation?
2. To which staff members does he need to speak?
3. What immediate steps must be put in place to remedy this situation?
4. If no action is taken by Mr. Gonzalez and the complaints are true, what could happen?
5. Who has responsibility in this situation for the quality of patient care?

Communication

One of the most important skills for nurse managers to master is good communication. By definition, communication is the passing of information and understanding from a sender to a receiver. Clearly, this definition does not restrict the concept to words alone, either written or spoken. Communication includes all methods by which meaning is conveyed from one person to another. Even silence can convey meaning and must be considered part of communicating (Twinarne & Boyd, 2002). Effective and correct communication is vital to meeting the everyday demands of the job.

Communication is often classified as verbal (the spoken or written word) and nonverbal (tone of voice, gestures, body language, inflection, and the like). Both are important independently and collectively. Congruence of these two forms of communication is usually displayed through similar words, facial expressions, and body language. Interpersonal relationships are developed among health professionals by way of active and healthy communication. "Through effective communication, nurses and other professionals develop collaborative relationships that enable them to provide well-coordinated, high-quality health care" (Oermann, 1997, p. 139).

The importance of simple and regular positive communication in the forms of a smile, or greeting a resident, staff member, or family member by name cannot be overemphasized. Such positive communication can change the atmosphere of a unit or facility (personal communication, Piper Bakrevski, February 28, 2008). Nurse managers should learn to talk with the staff, not at, about, or

FIGURE 23-2 Example of an organizational chart in a long-term care facility.

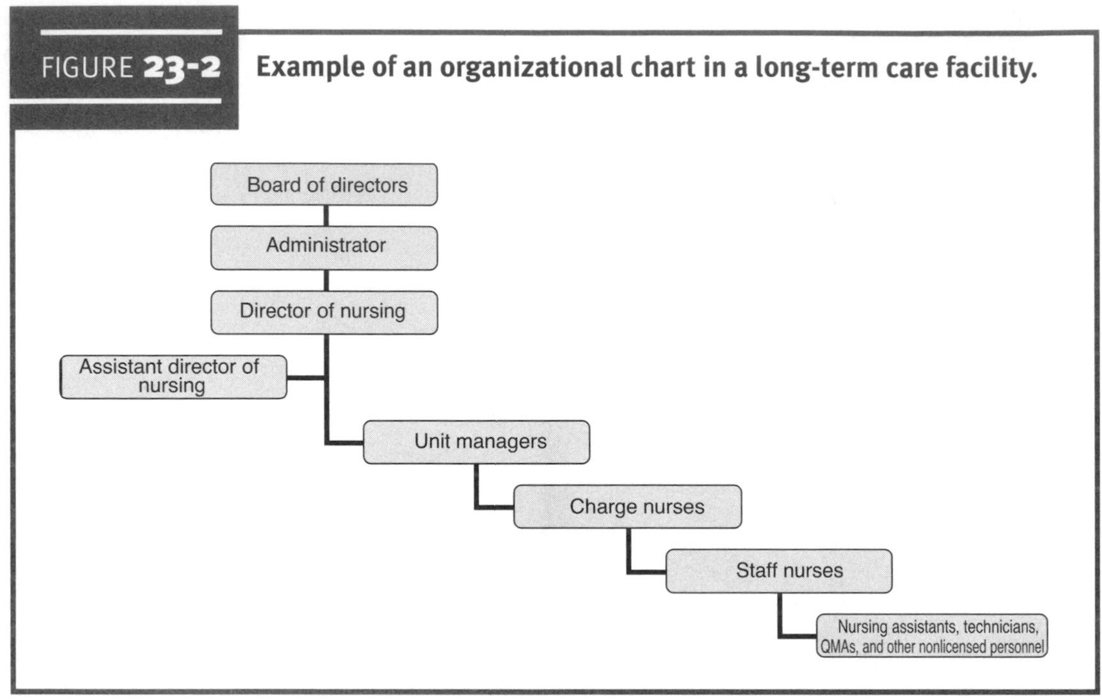

to them. Positive interactions develop mutual respect. Pointing out the wrong things people do or say is easy, but providing constructive criticism and encouragement is the ideal. Case Study 23-3 also gives an example of a dilemma requiring effective communication among a charge nurse, his staff, nursing assistants, and patient families.

According to Gloria York (2000) in her book *Supervisory Skills for Nurses*, there are several barriers that affect good communication. The first barrier is verbal skills. Vocal expression and inflection convey feelings such as anger, excitement, anxiety, self-confidence, or uncertainty as much as words. Attention must be paid not only to what is said, but to how a message is conveyed. Physical barriers such as noise, distance, lighting, and time constraints may also interfere with communication in the workplace. Perceptual filters such as life experience, personal social feelings, fears, stereotypes, and self-image can also influence two-way communication. Cultural mores may also pose a challenge for nurse managers. Cultural awareness and sensitivity are important aspects to consider in order to promote good communication between staff and management. Nurse managers who take a holistic approach to addressing issues within their control will pay additional attention to these aspects of communication.

Listening

Listening is an active part of communication. Listening is a skill that is learned and practiced, and one that has to be fine-tuned repeatedly. Many assessments can be made just through listening. The nurse manager needs to provide the individual with his or her undivided attention and good eye contact. The nurse manager must look and act interested. If incongruent nonverbals are displayed, the staff member may feel like the nurse manager doesn't care about his or her needs or personal well-being. Taking the uninterested look and action personally will produce increased lack of communication. The nurse manager must show outward support to prevent staff members from avoiding a future opportunity to communicate when the need arises. Establishing an open door policy will help to instill confidence that the nurse manager is welcoming input and has an attitude of "I am

FIGURE 23-3 **An example of logical progression of increasing management responsibilities in a hospital setting.**

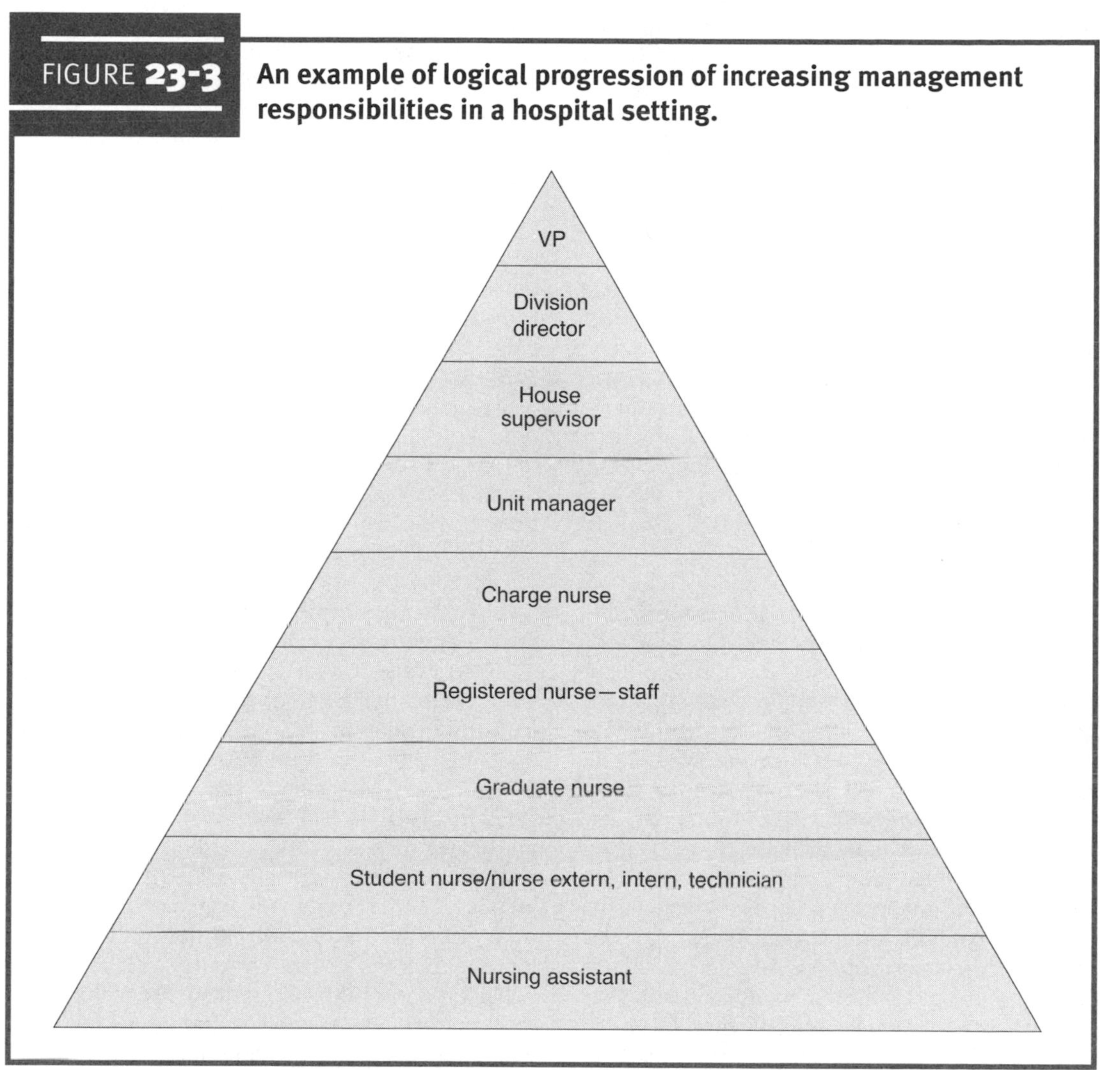

available." To show support with a simple gesture may be all it takes to provide support and reassurance to a staff member (personal communication, Dawna Fish, February 2008).

Staff nurses and UAP need to be allowed to display fears, hopes, and disappointments. With the demands of the fast-paced work arena of today, managers should be careful to remember those who are putting their hearts and minds into helping others each day. Many nursing assistants make around $9 per hour with poor benefits that are not enough to care for a family (Service Employees International Union, 2007). Being a nurse takes a tremendous amount of time, energy, sacrifice, skill, and dedication. As a nurse manager, it is challenging to turn these feelings of being overpowered into feelings of self worth and empowerment (Martin, 2004).

Regardless of what type of nurse one chooses to be, one thing remains the same: Nurses are specialized in health care and the ultimate goal is to enhance the wellness of persons through specific knowledge and skills. Despite differences in educational backgrounds, all nurses are important in what they do and how they accomplish the goals set before them. Each should be seen as worthy and with unique contributions to make to the profession.

Inspiring Trust

Inspiring trust is another management skill. Just as a therapeutic nurse–patient relationship requires trust, so does a positive manager–staff relationship. Working together and obtaining open, honest relationships help build trust. Trust takes time to earn. Staff members may need to learn to trust the judgment of the nurse manager. Communicating needs completely and discreetly, allowing room for improvement when errors occur, and practicing positive reinforcements are all tasks needed to build lasting trust.

Settings

Nurse managers practice in a variety of settings, each of which has descriptions and responsibilities related to the specific field of involvement. Gerontological nurse managers are found in acute care hospitals, rehabilitation facilities, nursing homes, assisted living, skilled nursing facilities, and home care. Within these settings, managers may hold a variety of positions, from management of staff to jobs in case management, care coordination, quality assurance, education, or research.

In a skilled nursing environment, for example, the nurse manager is responsible for overseeing the total care of the patients. Individuals involved in the daily care usually include nurses; social workers; physical, occupational, and speech therapists; nurse's aides; and dieticians. The nurse manager must know how and why individual caregivers are involved with the patient. Working in a skilled facility is challenging and requires organization, interest, and the ability to supervise others under the manager's jurisdiction. The manager or charge nurse is directly involved in the administration of medications, charting, fulfilling doctors' orders, performing daily treatments such as wound care, making sure the patient partakes in ordered therapies, and overseeing the aides' adequate performance of activities of daily living such as bathing, dressing, and grooming.

Nurse managers hold positions of authority regardless of the care setting. Whether acute care, hospital units, dialysis and rehabilitation centers, skilled or assisted living centers, or home care, the nurse manager displays learned skills and professional qualities, and focuses on goal achievement with an emphasis on quality patient care.

THE NURSE LEADER

Leadership interfaces with management, yet there are some distinctions between nurse **leaders** and managers. Warren Bennis (1989) conducted a study from which he drew 12 comparison distinctions between managers and leaders. These appear in **Table 23-1**.

A leader is a person who holds a position of authority, who influences people, and who has the ability to direct and guide others. "Leaders have the ability to take people to places they've never gone before . . . successful leaders enroll rather than sell people on their vision" (Evashwick & Riedel, 2004, p. 3).

Effective management requires leadership skills, and effective leadership requires management skills. However, leaders tend to be visionaries who focus on the larger picture and managers focus on the day-to-day operations. Managers are appointed, but leaders arise from within a group.

For nurses who wish to take active leadership roles in organizations or within the profession, additional demands are inherent. "Nurses who aspire to formal leadership roles require additional preparation to move into the administrative arenas. In addition to the clinical knowledge and skills, there are business, human resource, organizational behavior, and health care system issues that must be mastered. Leadership is a rewarding and challenging lifelong learning commitment" (Mancino, 2005, p. 117).

Characteristics of Nurse Leaders

In a survey of 137 women executives, including nurse executives, researchers found that six factors were identified as most important: personal integrity, strategic vision, teambuilding/communication, management and technical competency, people skills such as empowering others, and personal survival skills/attributes (see **Box 23-5**) (Carroll, 2005/2006; Carroll & Jowers, 2002). When compared with female leaders in other fields, nurse executives were found to value personal integrity

TABLE 23-1 Comparisons Between Managers and Leaders

Managers	Leaders
Administer	Innovate
Ask how and when	Ask what and why
Focus on systems	Focus on people
Do things right	Do the right things
Maintain	Develop
Rely on control	Inspire trust
Short-term perspective	Long-term perspective
Accept status quo	Challenge status quo
Have eye on the bottom line	Have eye on the horizon
Imitate	Originate
Classic "good soldiers"	Own person
A copy	The original

SOURCE: Bennis, W. (1989). *On becoming a leader.* New York: Addison-Wesley.

highest among all other traits. These results suggest that including the study of ethics in higher education would assist nurses in being more effective leaders.

In Britain, the NHS Hospital Trust piloted a new role called directorate senior nurse (DSN), and over a 1-year period engaged a facilitator to guide a small group of DSNs to develop systems of thinking related to leadership, strategic planning, and service planning and development. The results indicated that DSNs felt an improvement in self-awareness and self-esteem that led to increased collaboration and creativity within the workplace (Graham & Partlow, 2002). Certainly, models such as this suggest that nurse leaders may be mentored and trained to be more effective managers and role models.

Notable Quotes

"A leader takes people where they want to go. A great leader takes people where they don't necessarily want to go, but ought to be."

—Rosalynn Carter

Ponte et al. (2007) described eight characteristics of powerful nursing practice that could be used to help nurse leaders guide health care delivery. These researchers found that nurses who have a powerful nursing practice (p. 8):

- Acknowledge their unique role in the provision of patient- and family-centered care
- Commit to continuous learning through education, skill development, and evidence-based practice
- Demonstrate professional comportment and recognize the critical nature of presence
- Value collaboration and partner effectively with colleagues in nursing and other disciplines
- Actively position themselves to influence decisions and resource allocation
- Strive to develop an impeccable character; to be inspirational, compassionate, and have a credible, sought-after perspective
- Recognize that the role of the nurse leader is to pave the way for nurses' voices to be heard and to help novice nurses develop into powerful professionals

- Evaluate the power of nursing and the nursing department in the organization they enter by assessing the organization's mission and values and its commitment to enhancing the power of diverse perspectives

Leaders in gerontological nursing are those who are themselves empowered, and who have the skills and desire to also empower others toward a common goal (see Box 23-5). By recognizing the shared traits of nurse leaders, one can evaluate areas for improvement in the management area.

Leadership Strategies

Two types of leadership are notable: transactional and transformational. "Transactional leaders acted as caretakers who had no vision for the future and no overtly shared values, while excellent nurse leaders had transformational skills and qualities and were perceived to have them by staff" (Moiden, 2002, p. 20). **Transactional leadership** involves the system of "contingent reward and management by exception" (Moiden, 2002, p. 2) versus **transformational leadership** that emphasized "charisma, consideration, and intellectual stimulation" (Moiden, 2002, p. 20). Obviously, transformational leadership produces more positive results in gerontological nursing settings.

According to Marilyn Oermann, based on a study by Bennis and Nanus, transformational leadership involves four major strategies used by successful leaders: "(1) attention through vision, (2) meaning through communication, (3) trust through positioning, and (4) deployment of self" (Oermann, 1997, p. 257).

BOX 23-5 Attributes of Nurse Leaders

Personal integrity

- Holding ethical standards
- Trustworthiness
- Credibility

Strategic vision/action orientation

Team building/communication skills

Management and technical competencies

People skills

- Empowering others
- Networking
- Valuing diversity
- Collaboration

Personal attributes

- Political sensitivity
- Self-direction
- Self-reliance
- Courage
- Candor

Source: Carroll, T. (2005/2006). Leadership skills and attributes of women and nurse executives. *Nursing Administration Quarterly*, *29*(2), 146–154.

The first strategy enables the leader to see past the present. Based on past experiences, uncertainties, and evaluation of challenges, the leader is able to focus and strive onward toward the goals established and look beyond the difficulties that are faced. The leader understands the ever-present changes that exist and uses them to an advantage. Learning is the tool to attain growth and maturity.

The second strategy is based on using good communication techniques to inform and convince others of the same vision the leader has. Everyone has his or her own opinions, which should be expressed openly and with the respect of others. Leaders use this method to get across what is expected from others as well as personally. Achieving follow-through is much easier when others see the leader partake in the tasks with persistence, patience, and excitement. Nurse leaders must reassess when communication is not going well. Keeping focused and keeping the ultimate visions foremost but balanced need to be a priority.

The third strategy leaders use is trust through positioning (Oermann, 1997). In this strategy, leaders stand up for what they believe. People working with that leader know where he or she stands on issues of vision. The leader, on the other hand, needs to realize the factors that influence vision, whether from staff involvement or environmental factors.

The final strategy is called deployment of self. Learning is the key to success. With health care changes occurring daily, the nurse leader's responsibility is to educate herself or himself and others. Leaders do not see failure as the end (**Box 23-6**). Failure is an opportunity to learn and take what is learned to accomplish visions of growth. Leaders are willing to take risks to accomplish the end result. Leadership is an opportunity to provide a style of management that all benefit from. Great leaders not only possess a great vision with deep roots, but also are possessed by the greater vision (see **Notable Quotes**).

Charismatic style is also involved with transformational leadership (Conger & Kanungo, 1994). Leaders can bring unity to others regardless of turmoil and change. "Charismatic leaders are characterized by their determination to change the current state of affairs accompanied by an awareness of forces in the environment and their followers' needs" (Oermann, 1997, p. 258). There are three stages of **charismatic leadership** involving followers. In the first stage the leader is able to determine the conditions that cause change and recognize followers who will be able to manage those changes. In the second stage the leader encourages followers to partake in the vision and require clear details, direction, and an attitude of excitement toward change. The final stage is the ability and desire to go above and beyond what is expected to achieve the goals established. **Case Study 23-4** presents a thought-provoking situation of challenge to a nurse leader.

In the best-selling book *Good to Great* (2001), Jim Collins described five levels of a hierarchy of executive capabilities based on his extensive research on companies that went from good to great. Leaders at level 5 were key to moving a company to achieve well beyond its goals and aspirations. Level 5 leaders were those who "build enduring greatness through a paradoxical blend of person humility and professional will" (p. 20). Such leaders were found to be ambitious, but for the institution rather than

BOX 23-6 Research Highlights

Aims: To discover barriers and enablers to organizational change within nursing homes.

Methods: Researchers interviewed staff ($n = 64$) and families ($n = 14$) from three different nursing home facilities that were in the midst of organizational change to identify barriers and enablers to change.

Findings: Barriers identified were: excluding nurses from culture-change activities, perceived corporate emphasis on following rules and making money, and high staff turnover of both caregivers and administrators. Enablers to organizational change included those who promote staff empowerment.

Application to practice: The researchers recommended that all levels of staff, residents, and the community be involved in culture-change activities. Incentives and rewards should be congruent with the new values of the organization. Individual nursing homes should be empowered to make their own decisions at the facility level. Organizations should work with their corporate partners to be able to quickly implement recommended changes from research or data gathering.

Source: Scalzi, C. C., Evans, L. K., Barstow, A., & Hostvedt, K. (2006). Barriers and enablers to changing organizational culture in nursing homes. *Nursing Administration Quarterly*, *39*(4), 368–372.

Case Study 23-4

Mrs. Petty, RN, BSN, is the director of nursing (DON) for the assisted living portion of a for-profit health care facility. One of her jobs is to hire an assistant director of nursing, a new position created to help the DON with the growing number of residents in the facility.

Questions:

1. What qualifications should Mrs. Petty look for in an assistant director of nursing?
2. Describe the ideal candidate for this position. What types of experience, background, and education would be expected in this position?
3. Where does the ADON position fall in the organizational structure of this facility?
4. Where does the DON position fall in the organizational chart?

themselves, and were "modest and willful, humble and fearless" (p. 22).

Leadership Styles

Certain leadership styles have been widely recognized, including authoritarian or dictatorial, democratic, laissez-faire, and situational.

Authoritarian leadership involves the leader making the decisions with little input from the staff. This type of leadership rarely works well in the interdisciplinary care of older adults. Conversely, persons with a **democratic** leadership style welcome the input of staff and generally believe that their opinions and vote are important. This is the notion of the majority rules.

A **laissez-faire** leader is much more relaxed and tends to "go with the flow." Although this type of leadership might work if the employees are highly motivated and independently able to meet goals and objectives, it is generally considered not to be the ideal leadership style for most long-term nursing situations. One example where laissez-faire leadership might work temporarily is in the case of a faculty or small corporation where a few highly skilled individuals work toward a common goal without the need of a designated "leader" to motivate and inspire. Such challenges come from the group members to each other.

In contrast to these three styles, a person with a **situational** leadership style will choose the appropriate type of leadership depending on the situation. For example, perhaps democracy works in one situation where a decision does not have a direct negative impact on patients and allows for flexibility, but in another situation the leader needs to be more autocratic or dictatorial because of an immediate change that must be made in order to ensure patient safety and care. A good leader will be able to adjust and adapt to a variety of situations.

Assertive Behavior

In addition to the desirable characteristics previously discussed, **assertive** behaviors are associated with good nurse managers (Campbell, 2002). Assertiveness is preferred over **nonassertive**, **aggressive**, or **intimidating** behaviors.

Leadership requires assertive behavior. How the nurse leader displays assertiveness will determine how others respond to follow through and support. "Being assertive means being positive, direct, and genuine" (Twiname & Boyd, 2002, p. 49). Assertiveness is often associated with progressive and forward behavior. The nurse leader must act reasonably and without judgment. The old adage that "actions speak louder than words" may be a true statement. Nurse leaders hold themselves and others responsible for actions and reactions. Characteristics of assertive behavior appear in **Box 23-7**.

Body language is important in assertiveness. Eye contact is one of the first indications that show interest and true listening. Stating "I am truly interested in what is being said" begins the whole conversation in the right way. Posture, distance, and direct contact are expressions used in most conversations. "Over 65–90% of every conversation is interpreted through body language. We react more to what we think a person meant than to the words that are said" (Warfield, 2004, p. 1). Few individuals know how to read body language. The words used and the emphases placed on those words produce different interpretations. The body language used needs to match the words spoken.

BOX 23-7 Examples of Assertive Behavior

Standing up for one's rights no matter what the circumstances

Correcting the situation when one's rights are being violated

Seeking respect and understanding for one's feeling about a particular situation or circumstance

Interacting in a mature manner with those found to be offensive, defensive, aggressive, hostile, blaming, attacking, or otherwise unreceptive

Direct, upfront (not defensive or manipulative) behavior; those using assertive behavior confront problems, disagreement, or personal discomforts head on, and their intent is unmistakable to others

Verbal "I" statements, where individuals tell others how they feel about a situation, circumstance, or the behavior of others

Taking the risk of being misunderstood as being aggressive, abrasive, or attacking

Being able to protect one's rights while protecting and respecting the rights of others

Risk-taking behavior that is not ruled by fear of rejection or disapproval but is directed by the rational belief that "I deserve to stand up for my rights"

Rational thinking and the self-affirmation of personal worth, respect, and rights

A healthy style in which to conduct interpersonal relationships

Finding a "win-win" solution in handling problems between two individuals

Source: Messina, J. J., & Messina, C. M. (2005). *Improving assertive behavior.* Retrieved February 11, 2005, from http://www.coping.org/relations/assert.htm

Speaking effectively is also an art. Tone of voice is another form of nonverbal communication. Vocal volume should be at a normal conversational level and without edge, sharpness, or harshness.

The ideal posture when exercising assertiveness is standing or sitting straight at a comfortable distance from the other person (generally 2–4 feet away and outside the other person's personal space). Hand gestures are considered usual in normal conversation. Using relaxed nondirect contact provides for a comfortable conversation. If physical contact in the form of appropriate touch is used, soft minimal contact should be controlled and sensitive.

A final language skill in assertiveness is timing. Trying to talk to an individual when both parties are hurried or stressed will not facilitate proper communication and outcomes. The best time and place for a conversation are at a neutral site and a relaxed time.

Assertive behavior relies on the use of "I" statements and not "you" statements. This allows for no blame to be placed intentionally. Assertive responses are more likely to get individuals to change inappropriate attitudes or behaviors. Showing healthy and uplifting behaviors benefits all involved and provides good inward feelings about self. Good behaviors ultimately produce good, helpful outward actions.

Assertive behavior is essential in getting a job done in a time frame that may feel threatening due to the purposes and obligations that have been set. Assertive behavior is positive and allows the individuals to protect their ideas, motivations, and beliefs while at the same time being able to value and respect the ideas and contributions of others without being threatened.

PROVIDING LEADERSHIP AND MANAGEMENT IN A MULTIGENERATIONAL AGE

One of the important leadership functions for both the nurse manager and leader is facilitating the growth and development of nursing staff. This can be a difficult task in the presence of a **multigenerational nursing** workforce. This is uncharted territory for most nursing leaders. Working with four different generations that represent unique work habits and experiences adds richness and strength to an organization, but also brings particular challenges (Sherman, 2006). The four generations of professional registered nurses (RN) in today's workforce are described in the following sections.

Notable Quotes

"Surround yourself with the best people you can find, delegate authority, and don't interfere as long as the policy you've decided upon is being carried out."

—Ronald Reagan

The Veterans or Traditional Professional RNs (Born Pre-1945)

These nurses grew up in difficult times with life experiences during the Depression and World War II. Their strengths are notable: hard work, pride in doing a good job, working together, financially conservative, and cautious. Many of these nurses were trained in hospital-based diploma programs. Veteran nurses look to the past for what has worked and what hasn't worked. Seniority and organizational loyalty are important to these nurses. They see this as a lifetime career with one employer. They will be disheartened by lack of respect for their wisdom. Veteran nurses are comfortable with a one-on-one coaching style and formal instructions. Face-to-face or written communications will be more effective than using technology. Many of these nurses, even though they have begun transitioning to retirement, continue to work at some level (Kupperschmidt, 2006; Sherman, 2006).

The Baby Boomers (Born 1945–1964)

Baby boomers represent the largest percentage of the nursing workforce and hold many nursing leadership positions. They challenged and changed the values held by the veteran nurses. The strengths they bring are a sense of professionalism and view of nursing as a career. They have a strong work ethic and work defines who they are. These nurses have a great degree of loyalty to the organization. They can be workaholics, and burnout is often highest in this group. Baby boomers enjoy lifelong learning and want to be asked for their feedback. These nurses find public recognition for a job well done, along with professional award nominations, to be stimulating. Promotions are based on length of service that demonstrates loyalty from the organization to the employee. Baby boomers prefer open, direct, and less formal types of communication. They will use e-mail if they are familiar with the technology. Baby boomers will be eligible to retire beginning in 2010, and work will need to be redesigned to retain these nurses (Kupperschmidt, 2006; Sherman, 2006).

Generation X (Born 1964–1980)

This was the first generation in which both parents worked, and many were raised as "latch key" children. Generation X's nurses saw their parents laid off from work after sacrificing their time with their children to advance their careers. They learned to value work-life balance, and that there is no such thing as job security. Rather, they want career security. These nurses do not feel loyalty to the organization, but to themselves or to a team that will help them achieve their goals. They want to build their skills and experiences so that they can take them with them if they need to. Technology is an important part of their lives and they are able to work alone, which are strengths that they bring to the organization. This group wants feedback that is immediate and honest; they don't want it sandwiched between good things. Because of this, they are not good at work politics. Gen X nurses feel that career advancement should be based on merit, not seniority. They want rewards such as paid time off, cash awards, and increased marketability. This group does not value retirement benefits, because they tend to be mobile, and often will not work anywhere long enough to qualify. Generation X nurses prefer technology to be the main form of communication (Kupperschmidt, 2006; Sherman, 2006).

The Millennial or Net Generation (Born 1980–2000)

This is a group of nurses who were raised during a time of violence, terrorism, and drugs. They see multiculturalism as a way of life. Technology and cell phones also have been a way of life for them. Nursing is more an occupation than a profession. This group may have as many as 10 career changes (not job changes) in their lifetime. The strengths they bring are competence in technology and expectations of virtual teams who maintain collaboration partly through the use of technology. Millennial nurses expect coaching and mentoring. They are optimistic and goal oriented. They value flexible scheduling and immediate feedback. E-mails and chat rooms rather than long written documents are ways to communicate with this group. Rewards need to be tangible and intangible. The tangible rewards are ones that will help them with their busy lives, and the intangible rewards are working in teams, bosses they can relate to, and participation in decision making (Kupperschmidt, 2006; Sherman, 2006).

PROFESSIONAL ASSOCIATIONS

Knowledge about professional associations will assist in providing quality care to patients and offers the latest information in gerontology for staff and the community. There are many organizations for the gerontological nurse manager or leader. A few of the more common associations pertaining to this field are presented in this section.

All of the associations provide useful education and have Web sites that are easily accessed. Information provided by the associations ranges from certification exams, continuing education, standards of care, best practices, and political updates (important legislation impacting long-term care) to research and publications. The gerontological nurse manager or leader can use information from these individual Web sites to provide the latest information to staff, improve care for residents, and empower caregivers in a variety of settings.

National Gerontological Nursing Association (NGNA)

The National Gerontological Nursing Association (NGNA, http://ngna.org) was founded in 1984 and is dedicated to the clinical care of older adults across diverse care settings. It is the first and only nursing specialty organization dedicated to helping realize the full potential of gerontological nurses. The organization is composed of a growing, dynamic, and dedicated group of professionals who share ideas and information that improve the quality of nursing care for older adults. Members include clinicians, educators, and researchers with vastly different educational preparation, clinical roles, and interest in practice issues. A striking feature is the substantial number of certified gerontological clinical nurse specialists who select NGNA for membership. Members of the NGNA work in the following roles: staff nurse, clinical nurse specialist, manager, administrator, clinical educator, academic educator, nurse practitioner, and researcher. Membership benefits include:

- A subscription to *Geriatric Nursing* magazine
- Reduced rates to attend the annual NGNA convention and other educational offerings
- Bi-monthly newsletter: *SIGN (Supporting Innovations in Gerontological Nursing)*
- NGNA local chapter networking opportunities
- Research and education to promote professional development of gerontological nurses
- NGNA fellows program
- Discounted certification exams through a cooperative arrangement between NGNA and the American Nurses Credentialing Center (ANCC) for gerontological nurse, clinical specialist in gerontological nursing (CNS), and gerontological nurse practitioner (GNP)

National Association of Directors of Nursing Administration in Long Term Care (NADONA/LTC)

NADONA/LTC (http://www.nadona.org) is the largest educational organization committed exclusively to nursing and administration professionals in the long-term care and assisted living professions.

Membership is in both the United States and Canada. "NADONA has worked to establish professional relationships with the various disciplines in long term care, to promote quality of care and quality of life for long term care residents. NADONA has established Standards of Practice for DONs in long term care as well as providing a Certification System for DONs to enhance professional esteem for its members" (NADONA, 2007). Membership benefits include:

- Mentor system that allows directors to speak with a veteran director of nursing administration (DON)
- Education, including conferences, and other professional materials
- A quarterly journal, which provides CEs and has both clinical and newsworthy items
- Scholarships for all educational stages
- Director of Nursing certification program
- Both regional and national educational conferences offering CEs, clinical symposia, networking, relaxation, and fun

American Association of Nurse Executives (AANEX)

The American Association of Nurse Executives (http://www.aanex.org), formed in 2007, is a nonprofit professional organization dedicated to supporting nurse executives in long-term care. This organization provides accurate and timely information on:

- Leadership and management
- Survey, enforcement, and compliance strategies
- Clinical protocols and standards of practice
- Human resources information including preparing staff for success and retaining high quality staff
- Quality assessment and assurance processes
- Risk management
- Budgeting
- Oversight of the Resident Assessment Instrument/Minimum Data Set (RAI/MDS) process
- Assessment and care planning

Membership benefits include:

- Networking, including online discussion groups and state chapters
- Web site with FAQs
- Publications—*The ExecutiveQuarterly Newsletter*
- Certification

American Association for Long Term Care Nursing (AALTCN)

The American Association for Long Term Care Nursing (http://aaltcn.org) was formed in 2007 and promotes the importance of and advances excellence in practice for the entire nursing department of long-term care facilities. By addressing issues that affect the entire nursing team and promoting measures to foster unity in meeting shared goals, AALTCN removes fragmenting silos to promote working relationships that support a caring culture. AALTCN advocates for long-term care nursing staff with consumers, agencies, the business community, and other groups. AALTCN provides a strong voice in casting a positive image for long-term care nursing and ensuring that others understand the complexities and importance of this specialty. Membership (for the entire nursing department) benefits include:

- Subscription to *The LTC Nurse*, AALTCN's official publication, which contains current long-term care news and educational modules for the nursing department
- Access to relevant educational materials, including Train the Trainer and certificate program discounts at national and regional conferences, seminars, and other live educational programs
- Opportunities for networking and sharing of resources
- Scholarships: as a 501(c)(3) organization, contributions are sought to support movement up the career ladder for staff committed to long-term care nursing
- Representation on national committees and with national initiatives
- Web site job market to find and post job opportunities

American Association of Nurse Assessment Coordinators (AANAC)

The American Association of Nurse Assessment Coordinators (http://www.aanac.org) is a not-for-profit professional association that provides access to accurate and timely information on clinical assessment, regulatory requirements, reimbursement, computer automation, research, and the law. Membership benefits include:

- Networking opportunities with formal mentoring programs for Minimum Data Set/Prospective Payment System (MDS/PPS) neophytes
- Online question and answer service through the AANAC Web site
- Online discussion group
- Online seminars
- Easy access to recognized experts
- Management and inservice aids—forms and protocols
- Online archive of most frequently asked questions
- Reasonably priced conferences and continuing education
- Career recognition and development
- Newsletter and bulletins
- Membership certificate

American Health Care Association (AHCA)

The American Health Care Association (AHCA, http://ahcancal.org) is a not-for-profit group of state health organizations representing a variety of long-term care providers that care for more than one and a half million elderly and disabled individuals across the country (AHCA, 2009).

AHCA "represents the long term care community to the nation at large—to government, business leaders, and the general public. It also serves as a force for change within the long term care field, providing information, education, and administrative tools that enhance quality at every level" (AHCA, 2009, para. 2). The focus of the organization is to provide support for those affilates providing care to the frail elderly and disabled.

Membership benefits (through state affiliates only) include:

- Up-to-date news and publications including the *Provider* magazine
- Research and data on areas such as surveys, facility trend reports, and completed studies
- Legislative information including issue briefs and testimonies
- Conferences and educational offerings
- Quality improvement programs including Advancing Excellence in Nursing Homes and Radiating Excellence, which focuses on the assessment of specific leadership roles and competencies essential to nurse leaders
- Access to members-only sections of the Web site

American Association of Homes and Services for the Aging (AAHSA)

The American Association of Homes and Services for the Aging (http://www.aahsa.org) "is committed to advancing the vision of healthy, affordable, ethical long term care for America" (2007, para. 2). The association represents not-for-profit nursing homes, continuing care retirement communities, assisted living and senior housing facilities, and community service organizations. Every day, AAHSA's members serve 2 million older persons across the country.

AAHSA "serves its members by representing the concerns of not-for-profit organizations that serve the elderly through interaction with Congress and federal agencies. It also strives to enhance the professionalism of practitioners and facilities through the Certification Program for Retirement Housing Professionals, Continuing Care Accreditation Commission, conferences and programs, and publications representing current thinking in the long term care and retirement housing fields" (2007, para. 4). AAHSA also helps members with purchasing as groups and insurance programs.

Membership benefits vary based on the type—provider, business, or associate. Some of the benefits are:

- Publications such as *Future Age*, weekly newsletters, and other publications helpful to the consumer and the professional
- Advocacy, policy, and government
- The facts on aging services
- Consumer information
- Discounts on national and international conferences
- Access to members-only sections on the Web site.
- Other areas such as Center for Aging Services Technology, International Association of Homes and Services for the Aging

National Association of Health Care Assistants (NAHCA)

The National Association of Health Care Assistants (http://www.nahcacares.org/) began as the National

Association of Geriatric Nursing Assistants. This organization was started by former certified nursing assistants Lori Porter and Lisa Cantrell, both of whom later became senior managers and realized that nursing assistants are both the backbone and the heart and soul of the nursing home profession. The name was changed in 2006 to meet the growing needs of all health care assistants including those in nongeriatric facilities. NAHCA member benefits include:

- Association shirt
- *CNA Today* news magazine
- CNA resource center
- Educational opportunities—CNA Institute
- Membership pack
- NAHCA news
- *CNA Federal Regulation Handbook*
- Members' Assistance Program
- Accidental death and dismemberment (AD&D) insurance
- NAHCA Pharmacy Discount Program
- Uniform purchasing program
- Dell computer discount program
- Choice Hotels savings program
- CNA hall of fame
- CNA Retirement Foundation
- "Key to Quality" national annual CNA awards
- National annual convention and expo
- Scholarship program for higher education

American Medical Directors Association (AMDA)

The American Medical Directors Association (http://www.amda.com) is the professional association of medical directors and physicians practicing in the long-term care continuum. Many nurse leaders also belong to this organization to help deal with difficult clinical, administrative, and ethical issues in long-term care. Membership benefits include:

- Educational programs
- Print and online resources, including *Caring for the Ages*, *Journal of the American Medical Directors Association*, *AMDA Reports*, and *Health Policy Advisor*
- Exclusive member rates and members-only access
- State chapters
- AMDA Foundation Research Network Answers the Long-term Care Questions

American College of Health Care Administrators (ACHCA)

The American College of Health Care Administrators (http://www.achca.org) is a nonprofit membership organization that provides superior educational programming, certification in a variety of positions, and career development for its members. Membership benefits include:

- Peer2Peer network
- Education opportunities such as the annual convention and the ACHCA Winter Marketplace
- Self-study programs
- Various publications such as the *ACHCA Continuum* and *ACHCA E-News*
- Online university
- Professional development catalog
- Computer-based testing for certification

SUMMARY

In conclusion, both nurse managers and nurse leaders are needed in gerontological nursing. Although managers focus on direction of the details of a unit, leaders are visionaries who see the larger picture. Both must develop good communication skills and healthy interpersonal relationships. Specific strategies discussed in this chapter can be used to assist staff in feeling they are a part of a unit or organization, to foster recruitment and retention, and ultimately to result in better health outcomes for patients and residents. Developing sound management strategies requires the desire to change and maintain a constant state of self-reflection.

Nurse managers and leaders of today are faced with unique challenges related to multigenerational staffing patterns. Professional organizations can be excellent resources to provide support and information to those in management positions. Gerontological nurses should choose the most appropriate professional organization(s) to be active in, and as nursing leaders, also contribute to advancing the mission and services of their organization through scholarly activities and political activism.

BOX **23-8** **Web Exploration**

Check out the various links at the Long-term Care Nurse Leader Web site from University of Minnesota Center for Gerontological Nursing:

http://www.nursing.umn.edu/CGN/LTCNurseLeader/LeadershipResources/home.html

Critical Thinking Exercises

1. Examine the organizational chart of a facility where you work or have your clinical experiences. Analyze the hierarchical levels in comparison to the discussion of leadership roles in this chapter.
2. Follow a nurse manager around for a day. Make a list of duties that you observe and what skills seem important.
3. Map out your own personal strategic plan for your career goals. Set goals for 1 year, 5 years, and 10 years.
4. Make a list of your own strengths and weaknesses as a manager or leader. Determine which of your weaknesses you wish to improve upon and how you will accomplish this.
5. Think of a nurse whom you admire as a good role model of a leader or manager. Write down the qualities you have observed in this person. Compare them to the list in Table 23-1.

Personal **Reflections**

1. Where do you presently see yourself in the hierarchy of management in nursing? Where do you want to be in 5 years? Ten years? What is your ultimate goal related to advancement in your nursing career? Do you have a plan to accomplish this?
2. Is management an avenue you have considered? What are your personal strengths and weaknesses with regard to the qualities of leaders and managers discussed in this chapter?
3. Do you see yourself more as a leader or as a manager? What leadership styles fit your personality the best? How do you feel about delegating tasks to other nurses and UAPs? What skills do you feel you need to develop in order to be comfortable in a charge nurse position?
4. What nursing organizations do you belong to? Have you ever considered applying for a leadership position? Why or why not?

References

AAHSA (American Association of Homes and Services for the Aging). (2007). *About AAHSA: Vision, mission, and ideals.* Retrieved on December 22, 2007, from http://www.aahsa.org/about.aspx

AHCA (American Health Care Association). (2009). *About AHCA*. Retrieved January 13, 2009, from http://www.ahcancal.org/about_ahca/Pages/default.aspx

Arling, G., Kane, R. L., Mueller, C., Bershadsky, J., & Degenholtz, H. B. (2007). Nursing effort and quality of care for nursing home residents. *The Gerontologist, 47*(1), 672–682.

Bennis, W. (1989). *On becoming a leader*. New York: Addison-Wesley.

Campbell, S. (2002). *Great leaders grow deep roots: The six characteristics of exceptional leaders*. Retrieved January 22, 2005, from http://www.16types.com

Carroll, T. (2005/2006). Leadership skills and attributes of women and nurse executives. *Nursing Administration Quarterly, 29*(2), 146–154.

Carroll, T. L., & Jowers, D. L. (2002). *A comparison of leadership skills and attributes of women leaders and nurse executives: Implications for the education of nurse leaders*. Published abstract. 13th International Nursing Research Congress of Sigma Theta Tau International, Brisbane, Australia.

Castle, N. G. (2008). Nursing home caregiver staffing levels and quality of care: A literature review. *Journal of Applied Gerontology, 27*, 375-405.

Cherry, B., Ashcraft, A., & Owen, D. (2007). Perceptions of job satisfaction and the regulatory environment among nurse aides and charge nurses in long-term care. *Geriatric Nursing, 28*(3), 183–192.

Collins, J. (2001). *Good to great*. Boulder, CO: Collins.

Conger, J. A., & Kanungo, R. N. (1994). Charismatic leadership in organizations: Perceived behavioral attitudes and their measurement. *Journal of Organizational Behavior, 15*, 439–452.

Donoghue, C., & Castle, N. G. (2006). Voluntary and involuntary nursing turnover. *Research on Aging, 28*(4), 454–472.

Evashwick, C., & Riedel, J. (2004). *Managing long-term care*. Chicago, IL: Health Administration Press.

Gmelch, W. H. (1982). *Beyond stress to effective management*. New York: John Wiley & Sons.

Graham, I. W., & Partlow, C. M. (2002). *Professional development for nurse leadership*. Published abstract. 13th International Nursing Research Congress of Sigma Theta Tau International, Brisbane, Australia.

Harrington, C., Zimmerman, D., Karon, S. L., Robinson, J., & Beutel, P. (2000). Nursing home staffing and its relationship to deficiencies. *Journals of Gerontology Series B: Psychological Sciences and Social Sciences, 55*, S278–S287.

Hern-Underwood, M. J. (1991). *Group climate: A significant retention factor for nurse managers*. Published abstract. 31st Biennial Convention of Sigma Theta Tau International, Tampa, Florida.

Judkins, S., Reid, B., & Furlow, L. (2006). Hardiness training among nurse managers: Building a healthy work place. *Journal of Continuing Education in Nursing, 37*(5), 202–207.

Kelly-Heidenthal, P. (2004). *Essentials of nursing leadership and management*. Clifton Park, NY: Delmar.

Kupperschmidt, B. R. (2006). Addressing multi-generational conflict: Mutual respect and care-fronting as strategy. *Online Journal of Issues in Nursing, 11*(2). [Online]. Retrieved May 31, 2006, from http://www.nursingworld.org/ojin

Longest Jr., B. B. (1976). *Management practices for the health professional*. Reston, VA: Reston.

Mancino, D. J. (2005). Professional associations. In K. K. Chitty (Ed.), *Professional nursing: Concepts and challenges* (pp. 105–134). St. Louis, MO: Elsevier Saunders.

Marquis, B. L., & Huston, C. J. (2003). *Leadership roles and management functions in nursing*. Philadelphia: Lippincott.

Martin, C. A. (2004). Turn on the staying power. *Nursing Management, 35*(3), 22–26.

Messina, J. J., & Messina, C. M. (2005). *Improving assertive behavior*. Retrieved February 11, 2005, from http://www.coping.org/relations/assert.htm

Moiden, N. (2002). Evolution of leadership in nursing. *Journal of Nursing Administration, 9*(7), 20–25.

NADONA (National Association of Directors of Nursing Administration/Long Term Care) (2007). *About us*. Retrieved February 4, 2008, from http://www.nadona.org/aboutus.php

National Council of State Boards of Nursing. (1995). *Delegation: Concepts and decision-making process*. Retrieved February 11, 2005, from https://www.ncsbn.org/323.htm

Oermann, M. H. (1997). *Professional nursing practice*. Stamford, CT: Appleton and Lange.

Ponte, P. R., Glazer, G., Dann, E., McCollum, K., Gross, A., Tyrrell, R., et al. (2007). The power of professional nursing practice—An essential element of patient and family centered care. *The Online Journal of Issues in Nursing, A Scholarly Journal of The American Nurses Association, 12*(1), Manuscript 3. Available at http://www.nursingworld.org/ojin

Scalzi, C. C., Evans, L. K., Barstow, A., & Hostvedt, K. (2006). Barriers and enablers to changing organizational culture in nursing homes. *Nursing Administration Quarterly, 39*(4), 368–372.

Serbus, L. (2007). *Human resource consultant*. Sioux Falls, SD: Evangelical Lutheran Good Samaritan Society.

Service Employees International Union. (2007). *Workforce shortages*. Retrieved January 4, 2008, from http://www.seiu.org

Sherman, R. O. (2006). *Leading a multigenerational nursing workforce: Issues, challenges and strategies, 11*(2), Retrieved January 12, 2009, from http://www.nursingworld.org/MainMenuCategories/ANAMarketplace/ANAPeriodicals/OJIN/TableofContents/Volume112006/No2May06/tpc30_216074.aspx/

Sikorska-Simmons, E. (2006). Innovations in long-term care: Organizational culture and work-related attitudes among staff in assisted living. *Journal of Gerontological Nursing, 32*(2), 19–27.

Thompson, S. A. (2004). The top 10 qualities of a good nurse manager. *American Journal of Nursing, 104*(8), 64C–64D.

Twiname, B. G., & Boyd, S. M. (2002). *Student nurse handbook: Difficult concepts made easy.* Upper Saddle River, NJ: Prentice Hall.

University of Iowa. (2005). *Classification description*. Retrieved January 22, 2005, from http://www.uiowa.edu/hr/classcomp/psdesc/PD16.doc

Warfield, A. (2004). *Your body speaks volumes, but do you know what it is saying?* Retrieved October 26, 2005, from http://www.hodu.com/body-language.shtml

Weeks, S. K. (2003). Everyday steps to patient satisfaction. *Rehabilitation Nursing, 28*(4), 104.

York, G. (2000). *Supervisory skills for nurses*. Brockton, MA: Western Schools Press.

SECTION

12

MEMBER OF A PROFESSION

(Competency 30)

CHAPTER 24

End-of-Life Care

Patricia Warring, RN, MSN, ACHPN
Luana S. Krieger-Blake, MSW, LCSW

LEARNING OBJECTIVES

At the end of this chapter, the reader will be able to:

- Identify historical influences and attitudes toward death and dying.
- Recognize the choices of older adults and their families in directing their end-of-life care as well as the nurse's role in support/implementation of the patient's choice of care.
- Compare curative care, hospice care, and palliative care.
- Examine the goals/objectives of curative, palliative, and hospice care at end of life.
- Discuss the nurse's role at end of life using the preceding concepts of care.
- Describe the nurse's role as a member of an interdisciplinary team focused on end-of-life care.
- Identify the fundamentals of pain and other symptom management.
- Contrast several psychosocial, emotional, spiritual, and cultural issues that may affect end-of-life care.
- Describe some effects of grief and mourning on the elderly.
- Recognize several aspects of care contributing to a "good death."

KEY TERMS

- Addiction
- Advance directives
- Allow natural death (AND)
- Communicating bad news
- Complementary therapies
- Curative care
- Dependence
- Do not resuscitate (DNR)
- End of life
- Five Wishes
- Good death
- Grief
- Hope
- Hospice care
- Interdisciplinary group/team (IDG/IDT)
- Mourning
- Pain scales
- Palliative care
- SUPPORT study
- Symptom management
- Tolerance

Woody Allen once said, "It's not that I'm afraid to die, I just don't want to be there when it happens" (Allen, 1976).

Reality tells us that every person will die. Less than 10% will die suddenly; more than 90% will die after prolonged illness (Emanuel, von Gunten, & Ferris, 1999). The accumulation of experiences throughout a person's lifetime helps to clearly define the way he or she wishes to experience his or her own end of life. Familial and cultural factors, along with life events, often provide defining moments that influence a person's choices when facing the end of one's life and a death that will come sooner rather than later. Anthropologist Margaret Mead was quoted as saying, "When a person is born we rejoice, and when they're married we jubilate, but when they die we try to pretend nothing happened."

This chapter deals with the nurse's role in assisting a patient and family to identify the options for meeting end-of-life needs. It promotes the role of the nurse as a member of a team of professionals who focus on care and treatment of issues specific to the elderly as their health declines. It also offers practical assistance for nurses as they deal with various aspects of end-of-life care.

Historically, education about end-of-life issues and medical needs has been lacking. Initiatives including those by Last Acts and those encouraged by the Robert Wood Johnson Foundation such as Education in Palliative and End-of-Life Care (EPEC), End-of-Life Nursing Education Consortium (ELNEC), and Center to Advance Palliative Care (CAPC) are in place to address the need for additional information and research in this area.

One of the most demanding roles nurses undertake is that of caring for patients near the end of life. Nurses provide the most direct care for patients and families, and also help the family provide care that is competent, comprehensive, and compassionate. Therefore, nurses "must take the lead in integrating palliative and end-of-life care into the daily practice of every nurse, making it a core competency for all nurses who care for people with actual or potentially life-limiting illnesses. . . . Nurses must advocate for and deliver this quality care—regardless of specialty" (Rushton, Spencer, & Johanson, 2004, p. 34).

Caring for dying patients and their families can be particularly distressing for nursing students, because very little classroom or clinical time is spent in this area. It has been suggested that because of the inherent richness in working with these patients, clinical rotations should be structured appropriately to include end-of-life experiences (Allchin, 2006). Partnering with local hospices and/or palliative care programs to provide educational opportunities and hands-on care of the dying would benefit the student by providing a relevant life experience.

HISTORICAL ATTITUDES TOWARD DEATH AND DYING

With the advent of ever-increasing modern technology, especially following World War II, dying in the United States underwent a multitude of changes. In years past, Americans frequently lived in multigenerational homes, often in rural settings where living and dying experiences occurred commonly among the animals. Children were exposed to life and death issues as a matter of fact and grew to be adults having some experience of death before experiencing the death of someone close to them. As the ability to cure illnesses and to prolong life developed, technology took death to the hospital—to the sophistication of machines, antibiotics, chemotherapy, surgery, and such—and away from the comforts of home and family.

The role of nursing has changed along with the evolution of technology in administering end-of-life care in this country. For the most part, nurses shared the focus toward cure prevalent in the hospital setting. Training to care for the dying patient is often linked to the technical aspects of care and the physical preparation of the body after death (Krisman-Scott, 2003). A research and literature review performed by Benoliel for the period 1900–1960 revealed only 21 articles for nurses about caring for the dying patient. "There was little evidence that care of the dying was ever a major concern of nurses in this country" (Quint, 1967, p. 11).

As a result of the changes in our attitudes toward death and dying over time, some have said that the United States is a death-denying society. Kerry Crammer, MD, said: "In the Orient, dying is a requirement. In Europe, dying is inevitable. In America, dying appears to be an option" (Lewis, 2001, p. 24).

This death-denying attitude has created very expensive medical care. Spending on behalf of Medicare beneficiaries in their last year of life is five to six times as much as for other beneficiaries. Medicare expenditures are not distributed evenly across the last 12 months of life, but accelerate rapidly in the last few months, peaking at 20 times the amount for other beneficiaries in the last month of life as a result of inpatient hospital spending (Hogan et al., 2003).

Even though the expense of medical care at **end of life** is great, it does not necessarily follow that the needs of the elderly terminally ill are being met. The **SUPPORT study** (the Study to Understand Prognosis and Preferences for Outcomes and Risks of Treatment) conducted over the last decade reported that nurses often were the first to recognize the impending death of a patient (Sheehan & Schirm, 2003). It also revealed that our health care system does not meet either the needs of patients with advanced chronic illnesses or the needs of dying, terminally ill patients (Quaglietti, Blum, & Ellis, 2004). Nor does the care we have come to accept meet the *wishes* of many Americans who are terminally ill. The National Hospice Foundation's research reports that 80% of Americans say their wish is to die at home. Of the 2.4 million Americans who die each year, less than 25% actually die at home. Of the 1.3 million patients who received hospice care in 2006, nearly 75% died at home (National Hospice and Palliative Care Organization [NHPCO], 2007).

Recently, dying is beginning to be seen in a newer, more realistic light. Ira Byock, a leading palliative care physician and advocate for improving care at end of life, has linked dying to an ongoing potential for growth. "Dying represents more than a set of problems to be solved; it represents an extraordinary opportunity—an opportunity for review, for restitution, for amends, for exploration, for development, for insight. In short, it is an opportunity for growth" (Kinzbrunner, Weinreb, & Policzer, 2002, p. 259). Instead of growing up, growing old, and dying, Dr. Byock suggests we grow up, grow old, and grow on. "Growing on takes place for both the terminally ill aged and their families. And although patients and their families will universally find growth producing deaths as important and positive, it may not be easy. Indeed there are typically many obstacles that must be overcome if the process of death is to unfold in a productive manner" (McKinnon & Miller, 2002, pp. 259–260).

Nurses have the opportunity and ability to influence the process of death by virtue of their proximity to patients and families. Nurses spend more time with patients and their families at end of life than any other member of the health care team (Ferrell, Grant, & Virani, 1999). Families and patients look to the nurse for support, education, and guidance at this difficult time, yet little education is provided to prepare nurses for this unique type of care. Nurses face end-of-life situations in almost all practice settings, including hospitals, hospices, long-term care facilities, home care, prisons, and clinics, but many remain uncomfortable providing care. Because of the importance of end-of-life care, nursing education is beginning to focus on care at this stage of life (Hospice and Palliative Nurses Association [HPNA], 2004b).

The focus of care at end of life should center on *living* with terminal illness—with medical care, support, and interventions geared toward quality of life and comfort, rather than on prolonging suffering or the dying process—if that is what the patient wants. In determining the wishes of patients for end-of-life care, their physical, emotional, psychosocial, and spiritual needs must all be addressed. The cumulative nature of these aspects of a person's life will impact the choices they make at this important time.

COMMUNICATION ABOUT END OF LIFE

Talking About Death and Dying

Talking about death and dying is often difficult for both nurses and patients. If the nurse doesn't respond in a way that encourages discussion, that discussion will likely not take place, and death will become the "elephant in the room"—something unavoidable and yet taboo (Griffie, Nelson-Marten, & Muchka, 2004; see Box 24-1).

Perhaps the easiest method of learning about a person's preferences is for the caregiver to simply ask them! However, these conversations are often not held because of fear—the elderly person's fear of being perceived as giving up, the family's fear of not wanting the elderly person to think they are wished to be dead, or perhaps the care provider's fear of not knowing what to say or how to discuss bad news. The societal attitudes about denying death are

BOX 24-1 There's an Elephant in the Room

By Terry Kettering

There's an elephant in the room.
It is large and squatting, so it's hard to get around it.
Yet we squeeze by with, "How are you?" and, "I'm fine . . ."
And a thousand other forms of trivial chatter.
We talk about the weather,
We talk about work.
We talk about everything else . . .
Except the "elephant" in the room.
There's an elephant in the room.
We all know it is there,
We are thinking about the elephant
As we talk together.
It is constantly on our minds.
For, you see, it is a very big elephant.
It has hurt us all, but we do not talk about
The elephant in the room.
Oh, please, say her name.
Oh, please, say, "Barbara" again.
Oh, please, let's talk about
The elephant in the room.
For if we talk about her death,
Perhaps we can talk about her life.
Can I say, "Barbara" to you
And not have you look away?
For if I cannot,
Then you are leaving me alone—
In a room—
With an elephant!

Source: Reprinted with permission of Bereavement Publishing, Inc., (888) 604-4673, 4765 Carefree Circle, Colorado Springs, CO 80917.

certainly a factor in whether these conversations are held. The National Hospice Foundation Web site notes that most people would rather talk to their children about drugs and sex than to their elderly parents about terminal illness. There are resources designed to assist with these conversations, because not having the conversation may prohibit an individual from having the type of care they want, simply because they are not aware of the options.

Communicating Bad News

The Education in Palliative and End-of-Life Care (EPEC) Project, supported by the American Medical Association and the Robert Wood Johnson Foundation (Emanuel et al., 1999), as well as End-of-Life Nursing Education Consortium (ELNEC), views **communicating bad news** as an essential skill for physicians. It is also an essential skill for nurses and other interdisciplinary team members who interact with the patients and families.

EPEC Project Module 2 presents a six-step approach to communicating bad news (Emanuel et al., 1999):

1. *Get started:* Plan what to say, confirm medical facts, create a conducive environment, determine who else the patient would like present, and allocate adequate time.
2. *Find out what the patient knows:* Assess his or her ability to comprehend bad news.
3. *Find out how much the patient wants to know:* Recognize and support patient preference to decline information and to designate someone else to communicate on his or her behalf; accommodate cultural, religious, and socioeconomic influences.
4. *Share information:* Say it, then stop. Pause frequently, check for understanding, and use silence and body language; avoid vagueness, jargon, and euphemisms

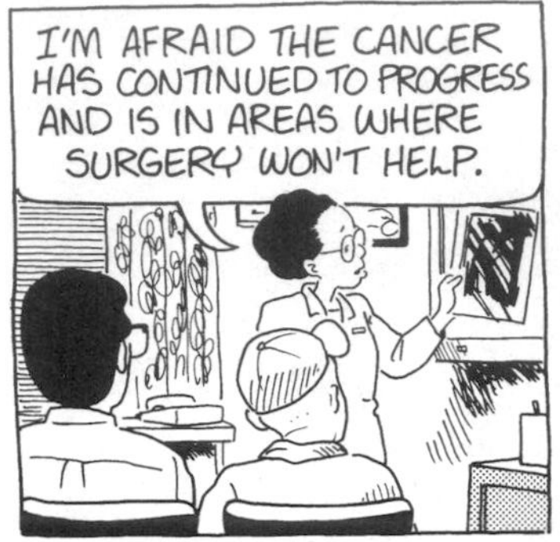

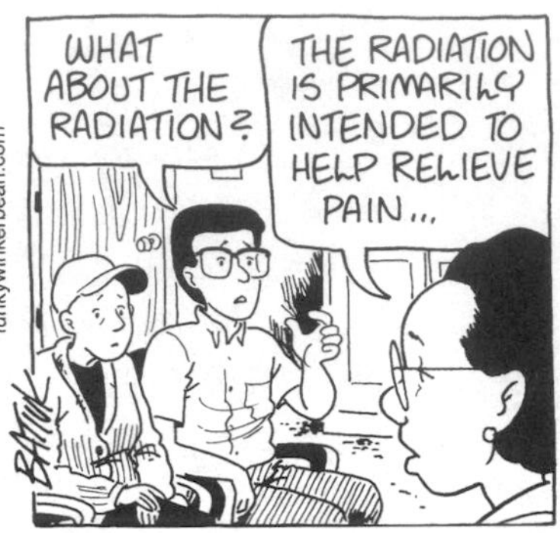

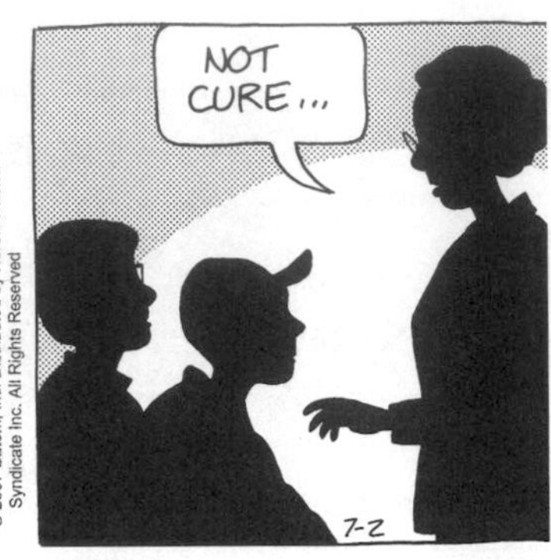

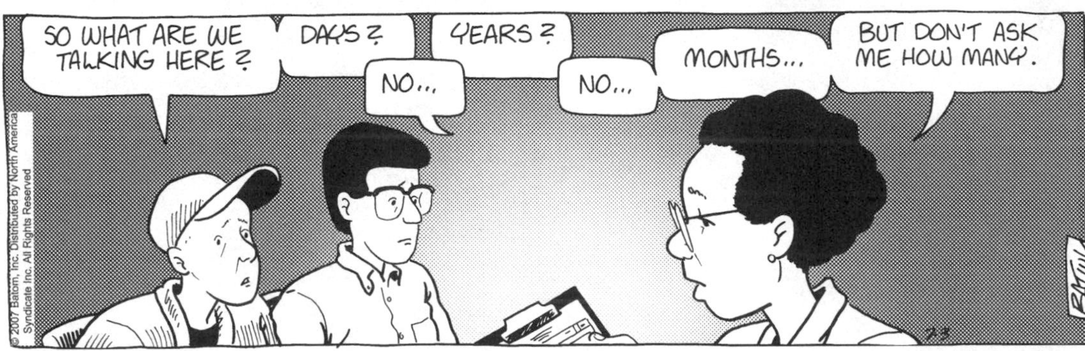

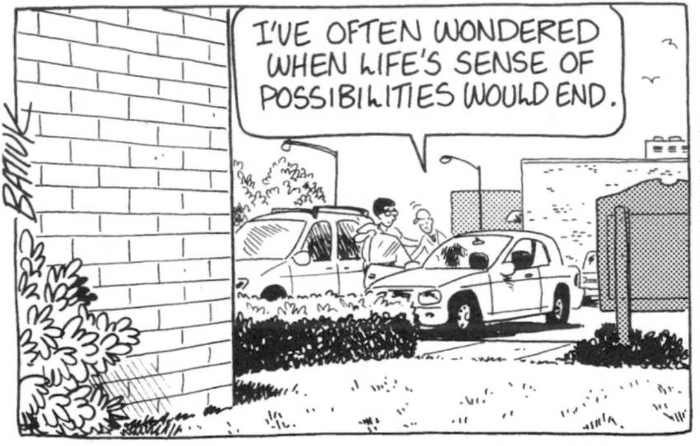

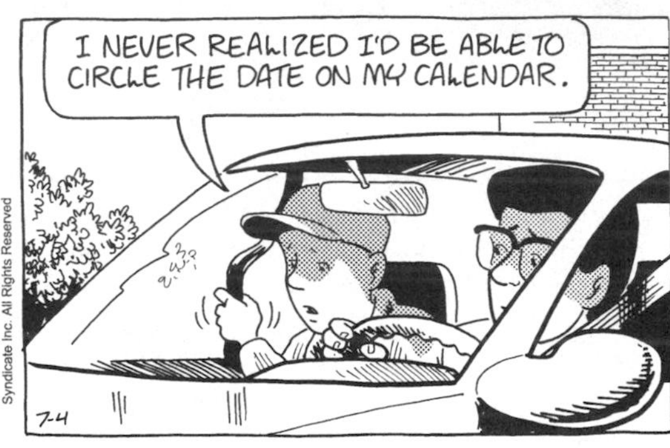

SOURCE: ©BATOM, INC. NORTH AMERICAN SYNDICATE

5. *Respond to feelings:* Expect affective, cognitive, and fight–flight responses; be prepared for strong emotions and a broad range of reactions. Give time to react; listen, and encourage description of feelings. Use nonverbal communication of touch and eye contact.
6. *Plan/follow up:* Provide additional tests, symptom treatment, and referrals as needed. Discuss potential sources of support; assess the safety of the patient and home supports before he or she leaves. Repeat the news at future visits.

Advance Directives

The Patient Self-Determination Act (PSDA), a federal law, requires health care providers to routinely provide information about **advance directives**. There are several nationally recognized advance directives to help an individual identify their personal wishes in a legal manner and to share that information with the people around them, including medical personnel. Durable power of attorney, living will declaration, appointment of health care representative, **do not resuscitate (DNR)**, and

BOX 24-2 Ten Self-Care Tips for the Nurse Caring for Patients at End of Life

1. Become educated . . . knowledge is power! Develop expertise in symptom management. It lessens anxiety in working with patients and their families.
2. Maintain professional boundaries and relationships with patients and families.
3. Utilize the other palliative care or hospice team members. Each has a perspective and expertise to add to the case. The nurse does not have to do it all.
4. Develop an interdisciplinary care team in your palliative or end-of-life care setting or facility.
5. Utilize all facility staff/team members in their respective roles.
6. Find and maintain balance in your personal life.
7. Locate and use appropriate support persons for debriefing during and after a difficult case.
8. Allow yourself and all team members to grieve the death of your patient.
9. Include the other members of the team (including CNAs, housekeeping, and other staff who knew the patient) in rituals or memorial activities following the death of your patient.
10. Practice good self-care in your personal and professional life. Eat, sleep, play, laugh, cry (. . . enough!!) . . . and wear comfortable shoes!

life-prolonging procedures declaration are all legally recognized documents for indicating one's health care wishes.

Additionally, **Five Wishes** (Towey, 2005) and **allow natural death (AND)** are two more recent options for stating end-of-life care wishes. Five Wishes is a movement that encourages people to provide more specific instructions than those offered by a living will, including one's wishes in five categories:

- The person chosen to make decisions when the individual can no longer make them for himself or herself—a durable power of attorney for health care
- The kind of treatment the person wants or doesn't want—a living will
- How comfortable the person wants to be
- How the person wants to be treated by others
- What the person wants his or her loved ones to know

The Five Wishes documents are legal in 40 states and can be used as attachments to other documents, showing intent in the remainder of states (Aging with Dignity, 2007).

An AND order is considered a more descriptive and positive order than a DNR. Its focus is on allowing death as nature takes its course at the end of an illness. DNR implies taking something away, or not doing something for the patient (i.e., resuscitation), and can be viewed as a harsh and insensitive statement of medical care that promotes a feeling of abandonment by patients and families alike. AND provides for comfort measures so that even with the withdrawal of artificially supplied nutrition and hydration, the dying process would occur as comfortably as possible (Meyer, 2001).

Advance directives can also be crafted for specific and personal concerns (e.g., for ongoing care for dependents or a pet). All advance directives should include a periodic review to ensure clarity and to reflect changing needs and concerns. All documents relating to health care should be discussed and shared with physicians, family members, or decision makers and placed in the medical records held by each of the patient's physicians (see **Case Study 24-1**).

BOX 24-3 Death and Dying: A Simulation Exercise

This is a very effective guided reflection, with the facilitator reading the scenario and the participants listening, actively taking part with their responses to the slips of paper and subsequent instructions. The element of surprise is effective if the participants do not know the scenario before beginning the exercise. This exercise often provokes emotional responses, which can then be discussed and processed to incorporate into the learning experience.

Supplies: One packet of 12 slips of paper for each participant

Writing utensil

Overhead transparency of questions for class or small group discussion (optional)

Instructions: Slips of paper can be premarked with the following four topics (three slips for each topic):

- A person who is very dear to you
- A thing you own that you regard as very special
- An activity in which you enjoy participating
- A personal attribute or role of which you are proud

Verbal instruction by facilitator:

Write one item per topic on each slip of paper.

Arrange the 12 slips of paper in front of you so that you can see all of them.

Get into a comfortable position; take a deep relaxing breath.

Listen without comment and follow the instructions given to you while I describe some happenings, some situations, and some people.

(Facilitator should develop the scenario carefully, allowing time for awakening all the senses.)

1. You are at your doctor's office; you hear the diagnosis—cancer.

   Please select and tear up three slips of paper.

   (Allow time [15–30 seconds] for selection and tearing . . . brief pause . . . facilitator or assistant may want to physically collect the papers and deposit them in a wastebasket for greater effect.)

2. You are back at home—who is there? Who do you want to be there? What do you say? What do you want to hear?

   Please tear up another three slips of paper.

   (Provide another appropriate-length pause. Collect and discard.)

3. It is now 2 months later. You are aware your symptoms are worsening and you are feeling weaker. Where are you? What is your lifestyle? What do you continue to do? What can you do?

   Tear up another two slips of paper.

   (Provide appropriate time between each phrase for reflection and for choices of paper to be discarded.)

BOX **24-3** continued

4. Now, it is 4 months later—you are undeniably ill. The pain has increased considerably. Where are you? Who stays with you? Who visits you? Who are the people you want around you?

   Tear up another two slips of paper (discard).

5. Six months have now passed, and you find that even the smallest activity of daily living takes most of your energy. How do you feel about yourself? Where are you? Who is with you?

   Turn over the last two slips of paper in front of you.

   I will take one of them at random.

   (Facilitator takes one of the remaining slips from each participant and tears and discards.)

6. Facilitator says only: Tear up your last slip of paper . . . you have died.

Discussion and Reflection:

May be discussed in small groups in the class setting.

Personal reflection:

- What issues arose for you from each scenario? Fears? Concerns?
- What were the easiest things to give up? Most difficult?
- What emotional reactions did you have with each scenario? (possibly denial, bargaining, depression, acceptance, avoidance, relief, comfort, anger, feelings of unfairness, sadness with remembered real-life scenarios)
- What did you think/feel/experience when one of the slips was randomly taken from you?
- Did you anticipate the content of the last scenario?
- What were your thoughts/feelings/reactions to tearing up the last slip of paper?

Reflection in reference to the elderly:

- What different issues would arise for the elderly population? Fears? Concerns? (e.g., caregiving issues, financial concerns, being alone, lack of support, physical limitations)
- Might an elderly person have a harder/easier time giving up things in the four categories on the slips of paper? Why/why not for each category?
- Would the emotional responses of an elderly person be different from your own for each scenario? Why/why not?

Source: First used by Hospice of Bloomington in April 1986, provided by Rev. Dick Lentz from St. Vincent's Hospice, Indianapolis, IN; adapted for use with VNA Hospice of Porter County; further adapted for use in this book.

OPTIONS FOR END-OF-LIFE CARE

Curative/Acute Care

Curative, life-prolonging, and acute care options focus on cure. Despite the findings of the SUPPORT study, there are those patients, families, and cultures who choose the life-prolonging focus of care of a hospital death (see **Case Study 24-2**). Many of these deaths will take place in an ICU setting, with tubes, vents, and devices to promote doing

Case Study 24-1

FAMILY DISAGREEMENT WITH ADVANCE DIRECTIVES

Mary is 78, just home from the acute care hospital and the rehab unit at a local extended care facility for treatment of a CVA. She has come home with a feeding tube, placed at the urging of the hospital staff when she was unable to take solid foods. Mary's daughter, Sue, is the POA/HCR (Power of attorney/Health care representative)—the only remaining child, because her sibling died 2 years prior. Mary was widowed about 10 years ago.

Sue had been distraught when she received the call from Mary's neighbor and found that her mother had called 9-1-1. When Sue arrived at the hospital, Mary was in the ER, and was subsequently transferred to ICU. Mary was minimally responsive and therefore unable to speak, nor able to make her needs and wishes known. IV nutrition and hydration were implemented. Although Mary had an advance directive, indicating no use of tubes, her daughter Sue acquiesced to the physician's statement that "Starving to death is an awful way to die. . . . I wouldn't want that for MY mother," and agreed to placement of a G-tube for feeding.

Mary survived and underwent a few weeks of rehabilitation therapy. She regained some abilities—but not the ability to speak or swallow without significant aspiration. Sue noted that Mary seemed very angry, sullen, and withdrawn. Sue was able to ascertain that Mary was very angry with her for the placement of the feeding tube against her wishes. Sue's attempts to explain the rationale for the placement did not make Mary any less angry. Sue was able to learn that Mary wanted the tube removed, and she contacted the primary physician to facilitate this. The physician contacted the visiting nurse agency seeking an evaluation of the situation, Mary's frame of mind, and requested objective assistance in helping determine a future plan of care for his patient.

Questions:

1. As the evaluating nurse, what information would you want to reference?
2. How would you attempt to obtain input from Mary?
3. How would you respond to Sue's strong statements of guilt for having had the tube placed in spite of Mary's advance directive?
4. What would you begin to look for in evaluating appropriateness for hospice care?

Suggested Actions/Responses

The evaluating nurse asked to see Mary's advance directive and found it to be the typical state-approved document, but with some additional clauses that Mary had deemed important as part of her instructions to her family. In actuality, Mary had indicated three specific provisions that mirrored her perceptions of quality of life—the ability to smoke a cigarette, the ability to pet her dog, and meaningful verbal communication.

The evaluating nurse communicated directly with Mary using statements/questions that she could acknowledge with a yes/no nod of the head. The nurse decided, with Mary's nodded approval, to use the provisions of her advance directive to evaluate Mary's quality of life and to generate discussion about her end-of-life wishes. Mary agreed that she was unable to communicate in a meaningful way with her family. Her little dog was placed on her lap, and she was unable to pet it or caress it behind its ears. Her daughter lit a cigarette for her, and she was unable to puff on it. The nurse confirmed with Mary that this was a fair assessment of her wishes.

The nurse asked if Mary wanted to hear about the hospice option, and with an affirmative nod in response, explained the goals of comfort and dignity as nature took its course with her remaining life. The nurse further explained how Mary's illness might progress without the feeding tube, and Mary nodded her understanding. Mary indicated she wanted hospice care and confirmed, in her daughter's presence and with her daughter's tearful apology for her hasty decision in the hospital, that hospice was her choice for end-of-life care.

For Personal Reflection

How could this uncomfortable scenario have been avoided for Mary and Sue?

Did Mary actually talk to her daughter about her wishes? Could Mary have taken Sue with her when she made the advance directive? Did Sue have a copy when she met Mary in the ER? Was there a family conference held to discuss options for care? Could the nurse taking care of Mary have helped Sue advocate by virtue of the advance directive when the physician pressed for tube placement?

everything possible to preserve life. It is important that judgments not be made about these choices, but to note that other choices exist as well. Options for non-life prolonging care at end of life are available and focus on comfort rather than cure.

Hospice Care

Hospice care provides one option for non-life-prolonging care and has the following philosophy:

> *Hospice provides care and support for persons in the last phases of incurable disease so they may live as fully and comfortably as possible. Hospice recognizes dying as part of the normal process of living, and focuses on maintaining the quality of remaining life. Hospice affirms life and neither hastens nor postpones death. Hospice exists in the hope and belief that through appropriate care, and the promotion of a caring community sensitive to their needs, patients and their families may be free to attain a degree of mental and spiritual preparation for death that is satisfactory to them. (NHPCO, 2004)*

Hospice care originated in order to provide comfort and dignity at end of life. Eligibility for hospice services is based on a life expectancy of 6 months or less, if an illness runs its normal course. Services are available as long as a patient is considered to be terminally ill, even though it may be longer than 6 months. Hospice utilizes a team approach to address the physical, emotional, social, and spiritual needs of the patient and family. Hospice care is discussed in more detail later in this chapter.

Palliative Care

Palliative care evolved from the hospice movement in the 1960s and 1970s. It has since become more mainstream as nurses and physicians embrace its philosophy of whole-person care for

Case Study 24-2

HOSPITAL DEATH

Despite studies showing the majority of people would prefer to die outside the hospital setting, there are those who find comfort in a more structured environment. Death in the hospital need not be a terrible or frightening event, as evidenced in this case study.

Jake is a 90-year-old man, diagnosed with end-stage dementia. He has been living in the home of his daughter and son-in-law, who are retired and in their 60s. His daughter is a power of attorney–health care representative. He has a living will in which he indicates an intentional nondecision about artificially supplied nutrition and hydration. In the past 2 years, he has become progressively weaker, unable to ambulate, unable to carry on a meaningful conversation, and increasingly incontinent of bowel and bladder. He was admitted to the hospital with dehydration and lethargy. A hydration IV has been started at 75 cc/hr. The physician has mentioned the possibility of a G-tube for feedings if the family so wishes. The CNA reports Jake moaned when she turned him during his bath, and he did not arouse when she attempted to feed him his breakfast.

You are the nurse caring for this patient. The daughter is in a quandary, stating, "I don't think Dad would want a tube in his stomach, but he never told me that for sure. My brother thinks we should do it so dad doesn't starve to death. I tried to feed him his oatmeal this morning, but he seemed to choke. He's been coughing when he eats for a couple of months now." Your physical assessment reveals crackles throughout the lung fields, respiratory rate of 44 breaths per minute, edema to lower extremities, decreased level of consciousness, an irregular apical pulse, and a blood pressure of 76/48.

Questions:

1. What active symptoms affect the decision making for Jake?
2. What quality-of-life issues might also be involved in the decision making?

(continued)

3. How would you help Jake's daughter understand the benefits and burdens of tube feedings?
4. How would your hospital-based team address the son's differing opinion?
5. What treatment would be appropriate for Jake's pain? His shortness of breath? The crackles in his lungs?

Suggested Actions/Responses

- Jake's symptoms clearly indicate an end-of-life process. You notify the physician of the family's quandary and request permission to set a family meeting for discussion of all the issues, including his terminal status.
- In answering the daughter's questions about G-tubes, you explain to her that sometimes a G-tube may be beneficial when the outcome is uncertain—for example, when there is potential for recovery as in a car accident or after a CVA. Dementia is a progressive disease, with little hope for improvement, and with an expectation of terminality at some point in time. When fluids are added to a failing body, the burdens may outweigh the benefits. These burdens might include increased congestion, edema, and nausea.
- The hospital social worker and/or chaplain might explore Jake's son's fears and feelings about Jake's end-of-life status. Quality-of-life issues might also be discussed in order to ascertain the importance of this family's cultural background in their decision making.
- Jake's nonverbal cues of pain must be addressed. Because dementia patients are often unable to report pain or its location, it is important for the nurse to observe behavior and treat appropriately. Because Jake is having difficulty swallowing, oral medications are not feasible. A low-dose opioid by IV or SQ route would be appropriate.
- The low-dose opioid initiated for pain would also help with his shortness of breath; supplemental oxygen may also be of benefit. Lowering or discontinuing the IV rate could improve the congestion and edema. The addition of hyoscine could also be helpful.

those persons with life-limiting illnesses who are not yet eligible for hospice support (Bretscher & Creagan, 1997).

Palliative care refers to the comprehensive management of the physical, psychological, social, spiritual, and existential needs of patients. It is especially suited to the care of people with incurable, progressive illnesses (Quaglietti et al., 2004). According to a 1997 task force, palliative care has become an area of special expertise within medicine, nursing, social work, pharmacy, chaplaincy, and other disciplines (Task Force on Palliative Care, 1997). The goal of palliative care is to achieve the best possible quality of life for patients and their families. Control of pain, of other symptoms, and of psychological, social, and spiritual problems is paramount (Storey, 1996).

The Choice of End-of-Life Care

It can be very difficult for a patient and family to choose one of these options for care. A practical suggestion that may help the patient and/or family in weighing the choices is to encourage a frank discussion with the physician, which would include several important questions: What is the expected outcome if I do treatment option #1? What is the expected outcome if I do treatment option #2? What is the expected outcome if I do neither of these, and choose comfort care? Weighing the answers to each of these questions may help the individual make an informed choice, based on the differences between the expected outcomes and the individual's own philosophy about how to experience his or her end of life (see **Figure 24-1**).

END-OF-LIFE HOSPICE CARE

Cicely Saunders, a nurse, social worker, and physician, started St. Christopher's Hospice in London in 1967. She incorporated a variety of team members to work together to help with the problems of care at end of life. The success of her type of care prompted expansion of hospice services to other parts of the world. Hospice care has existed in the United States since 1974 (Storey, 1996) (see **Case Study 24-3**).

The U.S. government, recognizing the cost-effectiveness of hospice care, incorporated hospice benefits into the Medicare program in 1983. Credentialing agencies require that hospices provide

Case Study 24-3

OPTIONS FOR END-OF-LIFE CARE

Hospice care is appropriate when the plan of care shifts from cure to comfort. This case study exemplifies this process.

Dee is a 72-year-old woman with advanced chronic obstructive pulmonary disease (COPD) with a history of congestive heart failure (CHF). She has been a patient with a home care agency, receiving nursing and physical therapy services for the past 6 weeks. Dee has been unable to maintain the rigors of physical therapy due to her poor lung status. She is oxygen and steroid dependent, and homebound. Dee is dependent on her husband, Jay, also age 72, for all aspects of her care. He is in need of a knee replacement, but is unable to meet this need due to his caregiving role. Until several years ago, Dee and Jay enjoyed socialization with friends and neighbors, going out to dinner, playing golf and cards, and attending her church on a regular basis. They have a supportive adult daughter who works, lives about 15 miles away, is attentive, and visits nearly every day. Their son lives out of state, calls frequently, and visits on occasion.

Dee voiced to her home care nurse the desire not to return to the hospital, "It doesn't do any good. I'm tired of living this way. Can't we do something at home?" In response to Dee's inquiry, the home care nurse indicates the possibility of hospice care at home because hospice is appropriate for any end-stage illness and because Dee's prognosis was determined to be 6 months or less by her attending physician (according to the National Hospice Organization's guidelines for noncancer diagnoses). For end-stage lung disease, these symptoms include dyspnea at rest, poor response to brochodilator therapy, and other debilitating symptoms such as decreased functional activity, fatigue, and cough. Dee has had multiple hospitalizations for these symptoms without significant improvement in her overall condition. Her appetite is fair to poor; constipation has been a problem; she is short of breath with any exertion; and has crackles to bilateral bases, with frequent complaints of mid-back pain. She has pedal edema; hands and feet are cyanotic. Her current medications include an ACE inhibitor, furosemide 40 mg qd, prednisone 5 mg qd, and O2 2 lpm/nc. Jay reports Dee is forgetful and cries "at the drop of a hat." Dee is admitted to hospice care at home.

Questions:

1. As the admitting nurse, what are your recommendations after this initial assessment?
2. Which team members should be a part of Dee's care plan?
3. How can we determine Dee's goals for her end of life?
4. Evaluate Dee's emotional status; how does it affect her daily functioning? How does it affect her relationship with her husband? How can other team members assist with these issues?
5. What impact do Dee's spiritual life/beliefs have on her condition and functional ability?
6. How might we offer Jay assistance in meeting the physical care needs of Dee?
7. What can be done for Dee's shortness of breath?
8. What should be done for Dee's complaint of constipation?
9. How might one address Dee's back pain?

Suggested Actions/Responses

- The easiest way to determine a patient/family's goals is simply to ask them! Dee is in physical distress, so that is foremost on her mind. Addressing her physical needs first will allow her to be able to identify and concentrate on other goals as her comfort is increased.
- Based on physical and psycho-social-spiritual assessment, Dee and Jay are offered the services of the whole hospice team. They know their individualized plan of care is under the direction of Dee's attending physician and managed by the interdisciplinary team, which includes the services of a hospice-skilled medical director. Although apparently overwhelmed by the admission process, Dee and Jay initially agreed to a nurse, social worker,

and home health aide (HHA), and decide to consider a volunteer and chaplain.

- The primary nurse first attends to physical symptoms, because that is often the overwhelming need. Dee's shortness of breath is her primary complaint; after consultation with the attending physician, the nurse received orders to initiate liquid morphine 5 mg q 4 h prn. The nurse instructed and demonstrated the use of morphine to Jay and Dee because he will be responsible for administration of medications.
- Depending on the underlying pathology of Dee's back pain, the liquid morphine may also help this complaint. An NSAID was ordered for possible bone pain.
- Adding opioids contributes to additional constipation, so a stool softener/laxative was ordered on a scheduled basis.
- Because ADLs are an increasing problem, and in light of Jay's knee pain, hospice can assist with the physical care needs by interventions of an HHA as needed. Stand-by assistance to full bed-bath is available depending on Dee's condition on a given day.
- The social worker often accompanies the admitting nurse for the admission process. This enables the family to be exposed to the "team" from the very beginning, as well as allowing the social worker to hear the patient/family "story" from the beginning, as an aid to assessment. Initial assessment reveals Dee is somewhat tearful in describing her physical decline and realization that her illness is life-ending. However, she is adamant about staying at home, avoiding rehospitalization, and voices several times that she is "tired, not able to fight this anymore. I want to be comfortable. I want Jay to have help."
- When Dee's symptoms indicated she was near death, and when Jay could no longer physically provide her care, she was transferred to the hospice center for the last week of her life. She received around-the-clock symptom management and physical care, allowing Jay to change roles from that of caregiver to husband.

all of the mandated services in order to be licensed and/or certified by Medicare and Medicaid and to be recognized by other insurers and some states. Reimbursement to provider agencies is contingent upon this certification (Centers for Medicare and Medicaid Services [CMS], 2004).

According to the CMS Conditions of Participation and standards, hospice services include, but are not limited to:

- Nursing services and coordination of care
- Physical therapy, occupational therapy, and speech-language pathology services
- Medical social services
- Home health aides and homemaker services
- Physician services/medical director
- Counseling services (dietary, pastoral, bereavement, and other)
- Short-term inpatient care
- Medical appliances and supplies
- Medications and biologicals

Hospice Team

The **interdisciplinary group or team (IDG/IDT)** provides or supervises the care and services offered by the hospice, including ongoing assessment of each patient/caregiver/family's needs. It is composed of (CMS, 2004):

- Doctor of medicine or osteopathy
- Registered nurse—coordinates the plan of care for each patient
- Social worker
- Pastoral or other counselor

Other team members who also are required include:

- Volunteers with training appropriate to their tasks—must contribute at least 5% of all staff hours
- Clergy/spiritual support and counseling
- Additional counseling (dietary, bereavement)

Complementary therapies are not required but are often provided to enhance the patient/family care with services such as massage, healing touch, music therapy, pet therapy, and others. Many of these additional therapies are provided by volunteers skilled in these particular areas.

FIGURE 24-1 Algorithm for choosing the proper end-of-life care provider.

Questions to Ask:

Is the hospice certified by Medicare?

Is the hospice certified by JCAHO or another recognized agency?

Does the hospice offer all levels of care: home care, continuous care, general inpatient care, respite care?

Does the hospice serve residents of long-term care facilities?

Is inpatient care provided in a dedicated unit manned by hospice-trained and employed staff?

Does the hospice allow the attending physician to continue to actively care for the patient?

Does the hospice have validated guidelines for pain and symptom management?

Does the hospice have an active bereavement program?

Is the program supported by a recognized funding agency or other recognized institution?

Does the program provide care in both inpatient and home care settings?

If not, does the program have relationships to ensure that care can be provided in both settings?

Is the staff of the program specially trained in palliative care?

Does the program allow the attending physician to continue to actively care for the patient?

Does the program have validated guidelines for pain and symptom management?

Does the program have an active bereavement program?

Choose a program that can assure YES answers to all or most questions.

SOURCE: Kinzbrunner, Weinreb, and Policzer, 20 Common Problems: End-of-life care. 2002. McGraw-Hill Publishers.

FOCUS ON SYMPTOMS

Among the nurse's primary responsibilities as a member of any interdisciplinary team is to coordinate the patient's care and to assist with **symptom management**. The remainder of this chapter will provide practical assistance with managing the variety of symptoms frequently encountered at end of life.

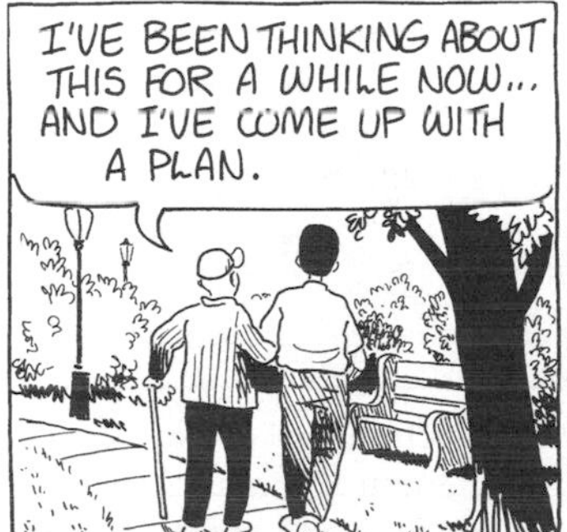
I'VE BEEN THINKING ABOUT THIS FOR A WHILE NOW... AND I'VE COME UP WITH A PLAN.

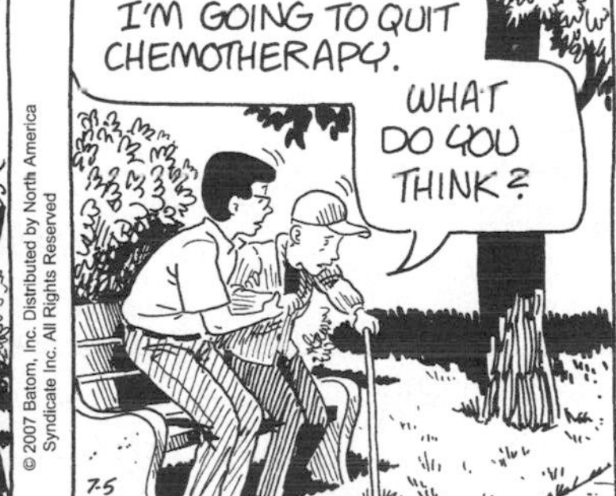
I'M GOING TO QUIT CHEMOTHERAPY.
WHAT DO YOU THINK?
7-5

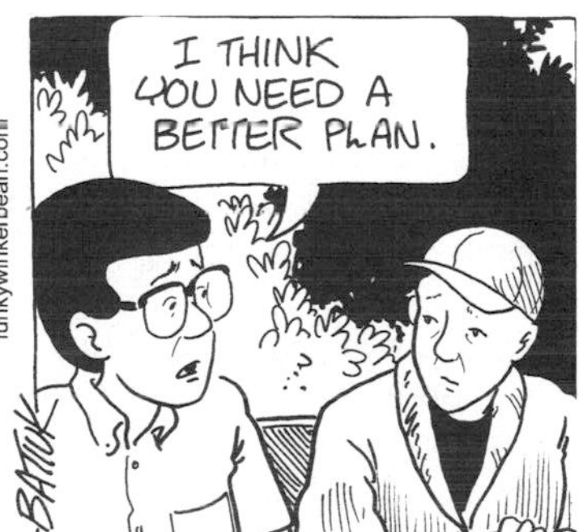
funkywinkerbean.com
I THINK YOU NEED A BETTER PLAN.
BATIUK

SOURCE: ©BATOM, INC. NORTH AMERICAN SYNDICATE

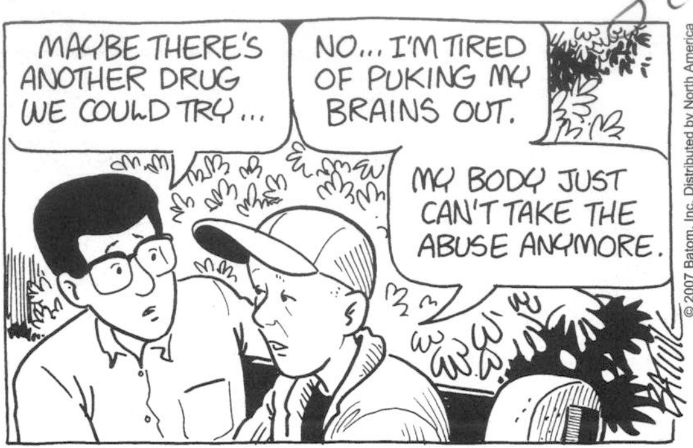

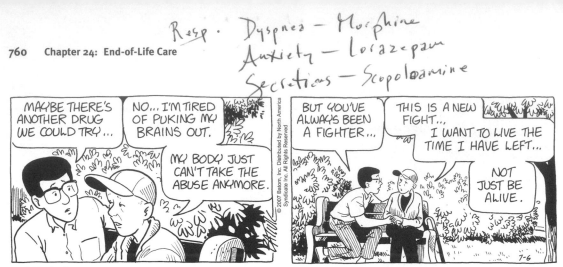

SOURCE: ©BATOM, INC. NORTH AMERICAN SYNDICATE

Physical, Nonpain Symptoms

Respiratory

Dyspnea means a distressing difficulty in breathing. It is a symptom, not a sign. A patient may have difficulty breathing and have no abnormal physical signs. Dyspnea, like pain, is whatever the patient perceives it to be. Episodic shortness of breath is sometimes due to hyperventilation. Any patient with dyspnea is prone to episodes of anxiety or panic. The goal of treatment for terminal dyspnea is to relieve the perception of breathlessness (Enck, 1992).

> **Notable Quotes**
>
> *"You matter because you are. You matter to the last moment of your life, and we will do all we can not only to help you die peacefully, but to live until you die."*
>
> —Cicely Saunders (1984, p. 33)

Opioid therapy is used to treat shortness of breath. Morphine reduces the inappropriate and excessive respiratory drive. A low dose is usually very effective—liquid morphine 2.5–5 mg PO every 4 hours is a good starting dose. It may also be given subcutaneously at one-third the oral dose if the patient is unable to swallow. It reduces inappropriate tachypnea (rapid breathing) and overventilation of the large airways (dead space). It does not cause CO_2 retention and can reduce cyanosis by slowing ventilation and making breathing more efficient. Morphine does not depress respirations when used judiciously and titrated appropriately. For patients who do not tolerate morphine, other opioids such as oxycodone and hydromorphone can be used (McKinnis, 2002).

Anxiety can be precipitated by the fear of suffocation, which worsens the perception of dyspnea, creating a vicious cycle. Anti-anxiety agents, such as lorazepam 0.5–2.0 mg every 4–6 hours PRN, will help with restlessness and thus often decrease respiratory effort. It can be given PO, SL, bucally, or rectally (McKinnis, 2002).

Oxygen may not be effective if hypoxemia is not the cause of dyspnea, but may have a placebo effect and decrease the individual's anxiety. O_2 should be started at 2 lpm/nc; increase to 4 lpm/nc if needed.

Other helpful and practical techniques might include:

- Head of the bed elevated 30–45 degrees
- Cool, humidified air
- Relaxation techniques
- Fan at bedside or ceiling fan

Excess secretions, resulting from fluid overload from artificial hydration or from increasing inability to swallow secretions, allow a buildup in large airways and cause a rattling sound. This rattle may be more distressing to the family at bedside than uncomfortable for the patient. Scopolamine TD or SQ or hyoscyamine SL may be helpful in treating this condition (McKinnis, 2002).

Gastrointestinal

Constipation results from a variety of causes for persons at end of life. Nonmedical causes include inactivity and decrease in food and fluid intake. Exercise contributes to bowel motility, but persons with

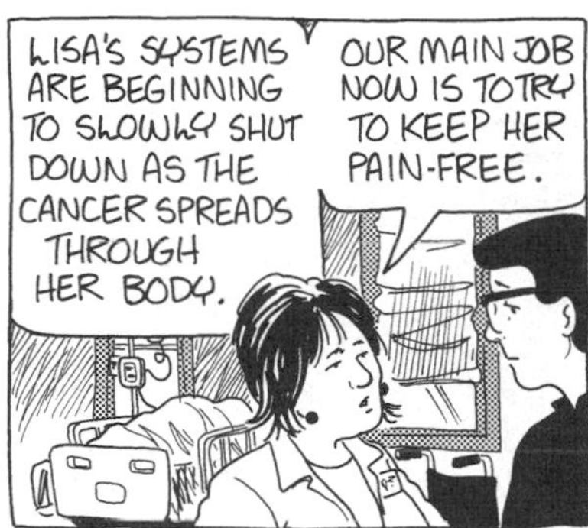

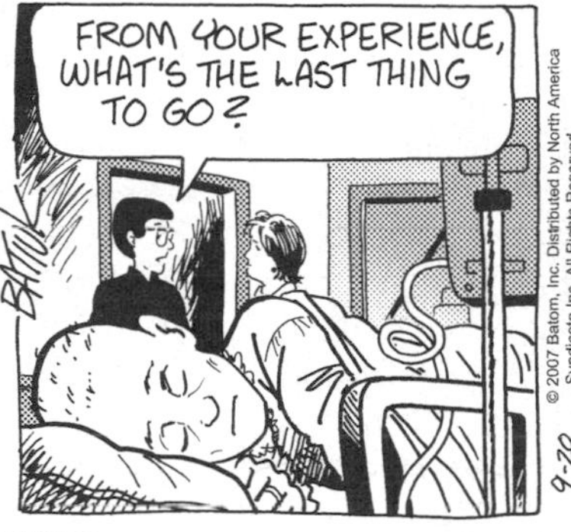

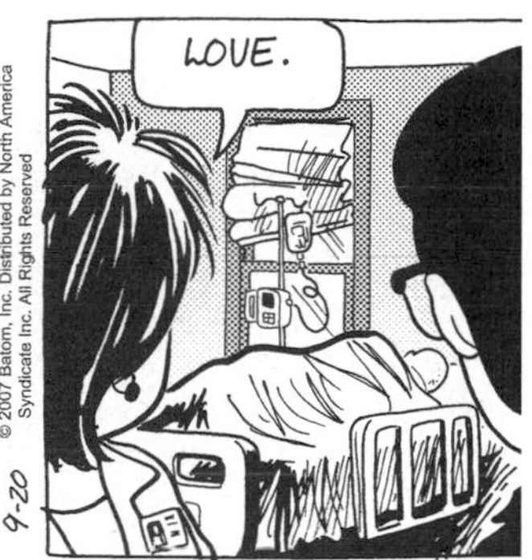

SOURCE: ©BATOM, INC. NORTH AMERICAN SYNDICATE

life-ending illnesses are often incapacitated by their disease processes. Medications used to control pain almost always have a constipating effect. Rather than withholding opioids, the constipating side effects of the medications must be treated. A combination softener/stimulant should be used, because use of a softener alone could lead to a soft impaction. Legend indicates that Dr. Cicely Saunders (mother of the modern hospice movement) gave a lecture in which every fourth slide read, "Nothing matters more than the bowels!" (Levi, 1991).

Nausea/vomiting, while common at end of life, may have multiple causes. Treatment of choice depends upon which of four areas of the brain are stimulated. One or more of these areas sends a message to the vomiting center located in the midbrain, causing emesis. For this reason, a combination of medications may be required to control nausea and vomiting. Storey (1986) lists the following four areas:

1. Cerebral cortex
   - Stimulated by overwhelming visual, sensory, or cognitive input
   - Anxiety—may control with lorazepam
   - Brain metastases (due to intracranial pressure)
   - May respond to dexamethasone
2. Vestibular apparatus
   - Inner ear responsible for motion sickness (e.g., infection or Meniere's disease)
   - May respond to cyclizine, meclizine, or hyoscine
3. Chemoreceptor trigger zone (CTZ) (most common causes of nausea are mediated by this route)
   - Triggered by uremia, hypercalcemia, chemotherapy, and certain drugs
   - Mild—may respond to hyoscine patch or promethazine
   - More severe—may respond to prochlorperazine suppository or a more potent CTZ antiemetic like haloperidol
4. Gastrointestinal tract
   - Caused by noxious material in stomach, peptic ulcers, severe constipation, or bowel obstruction
   - "Squashed stomach syndrome" or bowel obstruction—may respond to halperidol
   - Delayed gastric emptying—use metoclopramide

Anxiety and Delirium

Anxiety at end of life can be caused by a variety of factors. Loss of control, loss of self-esteem, and loss of independence can be very distressing to a person who has previously been autonomous. A change in environment for the dying person may add to the anxiety. These changes may be large—as in a family caregiver, a place of care, or meeting new professional staff—or small, such as a change of bed or medication. Treatment for anxiety includes relieving physical symptoms that may be present, such as pain or shortness of breath. The simple presence of someone the dying person trusts can be very reassuring. Anti-anxiety medications may also be used in conjunction with these interventions (Wright, 2002).

Delirium is a fluctuating cognitive disturbance, characterized by changes in mental status over a short period of time. It occurs in the last hours to days of life in a large percentage of dying patients.

Delirium is especially devastating to family and friends because it can stand in the way of meaningful conversations and good-byes. The most common physical causes may include dyspnea, pain, constipation, or urinary retention, all of which can be treated. Environmental comfort can be provided by reducing stimuli, reorientation if possible, familiar persons at bedside, and interdisciplinary team members providing emotional, social, and spiritual support. Music therapy, therapeutic/healing touch, and nonmedical nursing interventions should be considered. Anti-anxiety medications, used cautiously, may also be helpful.

Nutrition and Hydration

Declining appetite is a natural occurrence in the process of dying. This concept is one of the most difficult for caregivers to embrace, because our society tends to equate love with provision of food. When end of life nears, the body is less active and requires less nourishment. From the patient's perspective, food does not taste the same, so favorite foods may no longer provide comfort; appetite is easily satisfied by bites of food rather than regular portions. Caregivers should be encouraged to offer small amounts of a variety of foods. When a patient clenches his or her teeth to negate feeding attempts, it may be his or her way of exerting control.

The attempt to artificially hydrate may be detrimental to comfort, because the failing body may not be able to process the added fluids, contributing to fluid overload. In this case, thirst may be satisfied by providing small amounts of oral fluids, popsicles, or ice chips. Dry mouth may be successfully managed with meticulous mouth care (Kinzbrunner, 2002).

Physical, Pain Symptoms

Relevant Issues for the Elderly

Albert Schweitzer said, "We all must die. But if I can save him from days of torture, that is what I feel is my great and ever new privilege. Pain is a more terrible lord of mankind than even death itself."

Pain in the elderly is particularly problematic. "Unrelieved pain can contribute to unnecessary suffering, as evidenced by sleep disturbance, hopelessness, loss of control and impaired social interactions. Pain may actually hasten death by increasing physiological stress, decreasing mobility, contributing to pneumonia and thromboemboli" (HPNA, 2004a). Underreporting of pain is common, because the elderly learn to expect chronic pain and accept it as part of growing older. They may minimize pain to avoid diagnostic testing or to protect families or themselves against a poor prognosis. They may also use softening words, such as discomfort, soreness, or aching instead of the word "pain." In addition, health care providers may tend to underestimate and undertreat pain in this population, for fear of promoting **addiction** to pain medications.

Research has shown that approximately 25–50% of community-dwelling elders have significant chronic pain, and between 45% and 80% of nursing home residents have undertreated, substantial pain. The pain of those in nursing homes is generally "underappreciated, underreported and undertreated" (Ferrell, 1991, p. 2).

Additionally, McCaffery and Pasero (1999) identify that there are many misconceptions about pain in the elderly.

- Pain is a natural outcome of growing old.
- Pain perception or sensitivity decreases with age.
- If an elderly person does not report pain, he or she does not have pain.
- If an elderly patient appears to be asleep or otherwise distracted, he or she does not have pain.
- Potential side effects of opioids make them too dangerous to use to relieve pain in the elderly.
- Alzheimer patients and others with cognitive impairments do not have pain, and their reports of pain are most likely invalid.

It is important that nurses recognize the many facets of pain in older dying adults. The plan of care should be guided by consideration of physical, psychological, and social aspects of pain. This interdisciplinary plan should evolve over time, in response to the patient's changing needs (Gibson & Schroder, 2001).

To successfully treat pain, the nurse must be able to assess the pain of the individual. "Pain is whatever the experiencing person says it is, existing whenever he says it does" (McCaffery, 1968, p. 95). However, individuals may require assistance in describing their pain. A commonly used **pain scale** is shown in **Figure 24-2**.

Treatment of pain in the elderly is very effective when based on a basic understanding of origins of pain and a systematic approach to treatment. Different types of pain require different treatments (see **Case Study 24-4**). Sometimes a combination of pain medication and adjuvants (such as antidepressants or anticonvulsants) can be more therapeutic than each used alone.

Pharmacological interventions remain the first line of treatment for unrelieved pain. Opioids are needed when pain does not respond to nonopioids alone. Some clinicians and patients avoid opioids due to fear of addiction. Nurses need to be able to understand and explain to patients and families the differences among addiction, **tolerance**, and physical **dependence**. Fear of addiction should not be a factor in pain control. The findings of several studies have shown that addiction as a result of using opioids for pain relief occurs in less than 1% of patients (McCaffery & Pasero, 1999) (**Box 24-4**).

Pain is divided into two major physiological types—nociceptive and neuropathic. Nociceptive pain is further divided into two types, somatic and visceral.

Somatic nociceptive pain typically involves the following symptoms and treatments:

- Tissue injury resulting in stimulation of afferent nerve endings.
- The skeletal system, soft tissue, joints, skin, or connective tissue.
- The patient typically can localize the pain, may be able to point with finger to area; may describe as dull, aching, throbbing, or gnawing in nature.
- Best treated with NSAIDs or steroids, and partially responsive to opioid therapy; may require a combination.
- Examples: bone fracture, bone metastases, muscle strain.

Visceral nociceptive pain typically involves the following:

- Activation of nociceptors
- Internal organs
- Patient often unable to localize; may use an open hand to show area affected, because pain may be diffuse
- May describe as deep, aching, cramping, or sensation of pressure
- Very responsive to opioid therapy
- Examples: shoulder pain, secondary to lung or liver metastases

Neuropathic pain typically involves the following:

- Injury to peripheral nerves or central nervous system

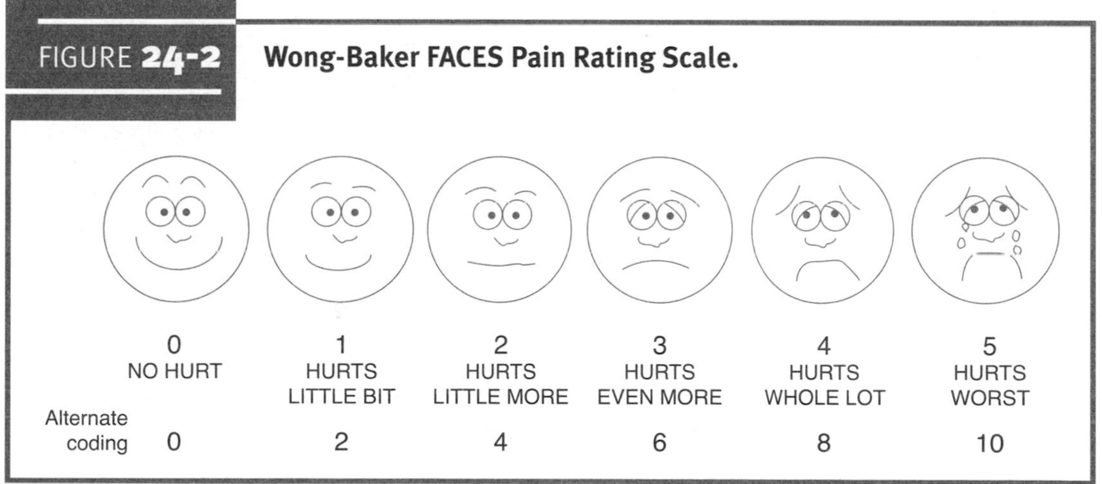

FIGURE 24-2 Wong-Baker FACES Pain Rating Scale.

SOURCE: From Wong, D. L., Hockenberry-Eaton, M., Wilson, D., Winkelstein, M. L., Schwartz, P.: Wong's Essentials of Pediatric Nursing, 6/e, St. Louis, 2001, p. 1301. Copyrighted by Mosby, Inc. Reprinted by permission.

Case Study 24-4

USE OF MEDICATIONS FOR TREATMENT OF PAIN

Jane is an 84-year-old woman, diagnosed with breast cancer 2 years ago, now with metastases to the bone and lung. She has refused any further active treatment (i.e., chemotherapy and radiation) and has asked her health care representative daughter Patty to help her talk to her oncologist about her wishes. After this discussion, the patient, daughter, and physician have agreed upon a hospice evaluation.

Upon evaluation and subsequent admission to hospice services, the patient's most pressing need was adequate pain control. Previously, she had tried scheduled Tylenol without relief—her pain rated at an 8 on a 0–10 scale. Her oncologist then prescribed hydrocodone 7.5/750 mg, 1–2 tabs q 4 hrs as needed, which lowered her pain acuity to a 6.

Questions:

1. As the admitting hospice nurse, you recognize that 8 on the pain scale greatly impairs Jane's quality of life. Using the WHO step approach, what would be your plan of intervention?
2. Knowing that Jane probably has two types of pain due to the metastases, what adjuvant might you consider for the bone pain?
3. Looking to the future, what other comfort issues might Jane face as her lung metastasis impacts her life?
4. How could you help Jane reach her goal of selected activities (e.g., shopping, lunch, church)?

Possible Solutions

The hospice nurse recognized that the maximum dose of Tylenol would be exceeded by the hydrocodone combination, and so short-acting morphine was initiated in place of hydrocodone. Using a conversion chart comparing the two medications, the nurse calculated the amount of morphine that could safely be given every 4 hours. Jane received "around the clock pain medication for her around the clock pain," to keep the pain from getting out of control. The starting dose was at a conservative starting point of 5 mg every 4 hours. The daughter was instructed to call hospice if the patient's pain was not managed at this dose. She was also educated that Jane may be sleepy for 24–48 hours until her body adjusted to the new medication, and this would be a temporary side effect and not an adverse reaction. The nurse made plans to visit daily until the pain was controlled.

Twenty-four hours later, Jane reported, "It's better; I'm at a 5 most of the time." Asking Jane about her acceptable level of pain, she indicated, "If I could just get it to a 2, I could do the things I would like to do." The dose was then taken to 10 mg q 4 hrs. After 48 hours, Jane reported, "You know, I think I could do a little shopping today and have some lunch with my daughter—of course she will have to drive." The hospice nurse then calculated the therapeutic amount of morphine used in 24 hours, which was 60 mg. The 60 mg was divided by 2, as long-acting morphine lasts for 12 hours. The therapeutic dose would be 30 mg of extended release morphine every 12 hours. A break-through dose of 10 mg (one-third of the 12-hour dose) immediate release morphine is available for prn use in case pain occurs between the 12-hour doses during Jane's shopping trip.

At this point, an adjuvant might be considered for bone pain—possibly decadron, 2–4 mg daily—because steroids are helpful for the inflammation of bone pain. At this time in Jane's life, steroids are appropriate for use, because her life expectancy is weeks or months rather than years, and long-term side effects are less of an issue.

If Jane experiences shortness of breath related to lung metastasis, the morphine and decadron are both helpful in alleviating this symptom.

A variety of interventions can improve the quality of Jane's life, allowing her the flexibility and freedom to continue some favorite activities.

BOX 24-4 Research Highlight—Suffering in Terminally Ill Dementia Patients

Aim: This study attempted to evaluate the suffering of terminally ill dementia patients over time, from admission to the hospital until death.

Method: The study included consecutive end-stage dementia patients who were dying in the hospital. Using the Mini Suffering State Examination (MSSE) scale, 71 patients in a 2-year period were evaluated weekly for level of suffering.

Findings: Using the MSSE scale, 63.4% of patients died with high levels of suffering, and 29.6% died with intermediate levels of suffering. The level of suffering actually increased during the hospital stay, which averaged about 38 days. Seven percent of patients died with a low level of suffering. The most significant aspects of suffering included restlessness, pressure sores, nutritional issues, and medical instability.

Application to practice: Despite traditional nursing and medical care, a significant portion of dying dementia patients experienced an increase in suffering as they approached death. New palliative measures need to be developed for dying dementia patients.

Source: Aminoff, B. Z., & Adunsky, A. (2004). Dying dementia patients: Too much suffering, too little palliation. *American Journal of Alzheimer's Disease and Other Dementias, 19*(4), 243–247.

BOX 24-5 Tolerance of and Physical Dependence on Opioids

Tolerance of opioids and physical dependence on opioids are not the same as addiction to opioids, but these three terms are often confused. Following are the definitions used by the American Pain Society (1992):

- Opioid *addiction* is psychologic dependence. It is "a pattern of compulsive drug use characterized by continued craving for an opioid and the need to use the opioid for effects other than pain relief" (McCaffery & Pasero, 1999, p. 50) or for nonmedical reasons. In other words, taking opioids for pain relief is not addiction, regardless of the dose or length of time on opioids.
- *Physical dependence* is the occurrence of withdrawal symptoms when the opioid is suddenly stopped or an antagonist such as naloxone (Narcan) is given. Withdrawal symptoms usually are easily suppressed by gradual withdrawal of the opioid.
- *Tolerance* is a decrease in one or more effects of the opioid (e.g., decreased analgesia, sedation, or respiratory depression). Tolerance to analgesia may be treated with increases in dose. However, disease progression, not tolerance to analgesia, appears to be the reason for most dose escalations. Thus, tolerance to analgesia poses very few clinical problems.

Source: Reprinted from Pain: Clinical Manual, 2/E, McCaffery and Pasero, p. 50. © 1999, with permission from Elsevier.

- May be described as shooting, stabbing, burning, or shock-like
- May be constant or intermittent
- Less responsive to opioids; responds best to anticonvulsants or tricyclic antidepressants
- Examples: herpes zoster or diabetic neuropathy (Weinreb, Kinzbrunner, & Clark, 2002).

Guidelines for Treatment of Pain in the Older Population

Older adults may experience many different types of pain, and often at the same time. Because they may have lived with pain over many years, older adults may be reluctant to report new pain. The nurse must use appropriate assessment skills to get an accurate picture of the person's pain.

- As in all patient populations, it is important to assess the type of pain being treated: somatic, visceral, neuropathic, or a combination. The type of pain determines the appropriate medication to use.
- A systematic approach should be utilized in the treatment of pain. The World Health Organization recommends a step approach (Lipman, 2006):
  - *Step 1:* Mild pain (1–3 on 0–10 scale, with 0 being no pain and 10 being the worst possible imaginable pain). Acetaminophen and NSAIDs are the recommended medications for this step. Acetaminophen should be dosed at 4,000 mg/day or less. An adjuvant may also be used.
  - *Step 2:* Moderate pain (4–6 on a 0–10 scale). Low-dose, short-acting opioids, in combination with acetaminophen and NSAIDs, are recommended in this step. Combination medications have a ceiling dose because of the nonopioid components of acetaminophen and NSAIDs. Opioid-naïve patients should be started at this level. If their pain is uncontrolled with this combination, they may require a move to step 3. Adjuvants may also be used.
  - *Step 3:* Severe pain (7–10 on a 0–10 scale). Opioids used at this step are not used in combination with Tylenol or NSAIDs, so there is no ceiling for dosing at this level. This allows for the use of higher doses of these opioids as the disease progresses. Nonopioids and adjuvants may also be used at this step.
- Oral medication is the route of choice and is well-tolerated in the geriatric population. However, other routes are acceptable when the patient is unable to swallow at the end of life. These routes may include sublingual, subcutaneous, intravenous, rectal, or topical, depending on the medication.
- To avoid possible adverse drug reactions, it is often recommended to prescribe half the dose usually prescribed to a younger person. However, even though the advice of "start low and go slow" is common, it may create the risk of undertreatment of pain. It is important to treat the individual and not the "geriatric population" (Perley & Dahlin, 2007).
- Special considerations for the geriatric population:
  - Acetaminophen is recommended for long-term use, because it is well tolerated in the older population. It is especially therapeutic for musculoskeletal pain, a common source of pain in the older adult. Doses higher than 4,000 mg per day should be avoided.
  - NSAIDs are also useful in the treatment of pain. Older adults with a history of ulcer disease or congestive heart failure are more vulnerable to the side effects of these medications, however. In the palliative setting, the risk-benefit ratio helps determine the plan of care, and if prognosis is days–weeks, a trial of NSAIDs is acceptable.
  - Opioids are an acceptable option for older persons with moderate to severe pain. It is best to start with a short half-life agonist (e.g., morphine, hydromorphone, oxycodone) because they are generally easier to titrate than the longer half-life agonists (e.g., fentanyl patch, methodone).
  - Morphine is considered the "gold standard" and is the most commonly used opioid due to its cost and various routes of administration. The elderly population may develop sedation or confusion due to the metabolites of morphine after several days of use. If this happens, it might be wise to change to another opioid. (Remember, however, the patient may be drowsy or sleepy because

their pain is controlled, and they are finally able to rest.) This side effect should subside in 48 hours. Assessment continues to be very important. Long-acting morphine should be used only after a several day trial of short-acting morphine. Morphine is also therapeutic in the treatment of shortness of breath.

- Opioids other than morphine may also be used (e.g., oxycodone, transdermal fentanyl) using the same principle of a short-acting trial before initiation of a long-acting formulation.
- Opioids are constipating, so implementing a concurrent bowel program is essential. A stimulant and stool softener combination is recommended at the onset of opioid therapy (Derby & O'Mahoney, 2006).

Loss and Grief

The elderly are confronted with a variety of losses in many aspects of their lives, not just with the death of a spouse, family members, or long-time friends. Loss of bodily function occurs as illness becomes more prevalent. Loss of support systems and family and friends occurs as companions die. Loss of independence is a factor as one's physical abilities wane, including loss of mobility, decision making, and access to various other support systems. Not only are the bodily functions lost, but the realization of never regaining these functions is particularly difficult. Primary losses are the loss of people close to them—spouses, children, parents, or siblings. Secondary losses are those resulting

BOX 24-6 Research Highlight: Hospice Patients Live Longer

Aim: Some health care providers perceive that symptom control in hospice patients, especially the use of opioids and sedatives, may cause patients to die sooner than they otherwise might. Some evidence has suggested, however, that the lives of some patients might be extended through the use of hospice care. This study evaluated the effect of hospice care on elevating the longevity of terminally ill patients.

Method: In this retrospective cohort study, an innovative prospective/retrospective case control method and Medicare administrative data were used to measure time until death starting from dates narrowly defined within the data. Multiple regression models were used to evaluate the difference of survival periods of terminal illness for patients using hospices and those who did not.

Findings: The survival period was significantly longer for the hospice cohort than for the nonhospice cohort for those patients with congestive heart failure, lung cancer, and pancreatic cancer, and longer—but not statistically significant—for those with colon cancer.

Application to practice: Hospice may, indeed, have a positive impact on patients' longevity, or at least not hasten death. For certain well-defined terminally ill populations, patients who choose hospice care live an average of 29 days longer than similar patients who do not choose hospice. This pattern persisted over four of the six disease categories studied. The findings are important in helping to dispel the myth that hospice care hastens a patient's death. Some factors that may contribute to this longevity may include avoidance of the risks of overtreatment, improved monitoring and treatment, and that the psychosocial supports inherent in hospice care may tend to prolong life. Additional research would clarify the applicability of these findings to other patients and diseases, but nurses can assure patients and families that the use of hospice is not associated with hastening death.

Source: Connor, S. R., Pyenson, B., Fitch, K., Spence, C., & Iwasaki, K. (2007). Comparing hospice and nonhospice patient survival among patients who die within a three year window. *Journal of Pain and Symptom Management*, *33* (3), 238–242.

BOX 24-7 Gone from My Sight: The Dying Experience

Summary of Guidelines for Impending Death

Recognizing that although each person approaches death in his or her own way, there are some identified patterns that assist in the recognition of end-stage status, noted in common language for ease of comprehension by patients and families.

One to three months:

- Withdrawal from the world and people
- Decreased food intake
- Increase in sleep
- Going inside of self
- Less communication

One to two weeks:

Mental changes:

- Disorientation
- Agitation
- Talking with the unseen
- Confusion
- Picking at clothes

Physical changes:

- Decreased blood pressure
- Pulse increase or decrease
- Color change (pale, bluish)
- Increased perspiration
- Respiration irregularities
- Congestion
- Sleeping but responding
- Complaints of body being tired and heavy
- Not eating, taking little fluid
- Body temperature hot/cold

Days or hours:

- Intensification of 1- to 2-week signs
- Surge of energy
- Decrease in blood pressure
- Eyes glassy/tearing/half open
- Irregular breathing
- Restlessness or no activity
- Purplish/blotchy knees, feet, hands
- Pulse weak and hard to find
- Decreased urine output
- May wet or stool the bed

Minutes:

- "Fish out of water" breathing
- Cannot be awakened

Source: Summary of Guidelines, pp. 12–23. Gone from My Sight: The Dying Experience, Barbara Karnes, RN, P.O. Box 189, Depoe Bay, OR, 97341. Copyright 1986.

from the primary loss—companionship, roles the deceased assumed in the relationship (e.g., bill payer, cook), and independence.

Although the terms *grief* and *mourning* are frequently used interchangeably, each does have a specific meaning. **Grief** is the natural and normal response to loss of any kind and is experienced psychologically, behaviorally, socially, and physically. It involves many changes over time (Rando, 1993). **Mourning** is the cultural and/or public display of grief through one's behaviors. These include accepting the reality of the loss, reacting to the separation and finding ways to channel the reactions, handling the unfinished business, and transferring the attachment to the deceased from physical presence to symbolic interaction. It seeks to accommodate the loss by integrating its realities into ongoing life (Rando, 1993). Alan Wolfelt (2001) distinguishes mourning as the shared social response to grief—grief gone public.

In this author's experience with hospice bereavement support, the practical application of this information suggests a concept that seems logical and is acceptable to people who are mourning: The goal of grieving is not to "get over it" as much of our society encourages, but rather to figure out how to go on living without the loved one actively present in one's life.

Wolfelt (2004) suggests the following mourner's reconciliation needs:

- Acknowledge/accept the reality of the death.
- Embrace the pain of the loss.
- Convert the relationship of the person who died from one of presence to one of memory.
- Develop a new self-identity.
- Search for meaning
- Receive ongoing support from others.

These present some challenges for the elderly because of the limits they may experience physically and emotionally, and due to chronic or other illnesses. However, it is still important to emphasize reasonable versus unreasonable expectations—grievous loss will produce strong grief, and mourners must be allowed to experience the full dimensions of their unique process.

There are patterns to grief that help describe and show progression in the mourning process, regardless of age. Knowing patterns exist is sometimes comforting, but individualized responses must be acknowledged and affirmed. A reasonable goal is to find a personal balance in each of the aspects of grief patterns—physical aspects such as eating and sleeping and emotional aspects such as tears and stoicism, to name a few—as the mourner attempts to incorporate the loss into his or her daily life patterns.

The mourning process has been characterized by stages or phases. Although it is tempting to consider it as a neat and tidy progression, the concept of overlapping, retrogressing, and recurring jumbles of feelings and responses is probably more realistic. Phases include the period of numbness occurring at the time of the loss, which provides some emotional protection for a brief time. The period of yearning for the loved one's return tends to deny the permanence of the loss for a time and may include feelings of anger about a variety of aspects of the loss (including, for example, anger at the medical profession, at the person who died, and/or at God). The phase of disorganization and despair is one of difficulty in functioning in the environment, in which the mourner begins to do the "figuring out" of how to function in each area of disarray. The phase of reorganized behavior is when one pulls life back together, and in which a new "normal" might be identified (Parkes & Bowlby in Worden, 1991).

A brief review of the risk factors for complicated mourning provides special insight into the vulnerabilities of the elderly, especially in light of the secondary losses noted earlier. According to Rando (1993), there are seven high-risk factors in two categories that might predispose a person to complicated mourning.

Factors associated with the specific death:

- Sudden, unexpected (traumatic, violent, random)
- Overly lengthy illness (multidimensional stresses including anger, ambivalence, guilt, problems obtaining health care)
- Loss of a child, including adult children
- Perception of the death as preventable (lack of closure, attempt to regain control, search for reasons and meaning)

Antecedent and subsequent variables:

- Markedly angry/ambivalent/dependent relationship
- Unaccommodated losses/stresses/mental health problems
- Perception of lack of social support

Mourners must be given the opportunity to process the aspects of their grief, but in a context that is helpful to them. Nurses, who are likely to frequently encounter grieving patients, can facilitate the mourning process by being aware of the aspects of grief and mourning, and by advocacy with the people who surround the mourner. Alan Wolfelt (2007a) suggests a Mourner's Bill of Rights to help mourners sift out the unacceptable advice they are often given. This includes the right to:

- Experience unique grief, without the pressure of "shoulds/shouldn'ts"

- Talk about grief, or be silent as needed
- Feel a multitude of emotions, without feeling judgment
- Tolerate physical and emotional limits, and fatigue
- Experience sudden surges of grief
- Use rituals
- Embrace spirituality, or not
- Search for meaning, recognizing some questions may not have answers
- Treasure memories; share them
- Move toward grief and heal; avoid people who are intolerant of your grief
- Recognize that "grief is a process, not an event"

Other ways nurses can help include active listening without judging the mourner; having compassion and allowing the expression of feelings without criticizing; allowing the mourner to identify his or her own feelings without saying, "I know how you feel"; and offering presence over time (Wolfelt, 2007b).

Frequently, when an elderly person experiences the death of a spouse of long standing, the life expectancy of the remaining spouse may be shortened because of the inability to reconcile the needs of mourning, the complications of grief, and the lack of physical and emotional reserves to make the additional investment into a reconfiguration of one's own future. It is also important to note the potential for difference in mourning styles between men and women, and among various cultural styles.

BOX 24-8 Psychosocial and Spiritual Opportunities Near the End of Life

The opportunity to . . .

- Reframe society's view of dying: grow on!
- Expand the definition of quality of life.
- Focus on the individual, not the disease.
- Address as a whole physical pain, psychosocial issues, and spiritual concerns
- Move through fear to peace.
- Move through confusion to meaning.
- Move through despair to hope.
- Move from isolation to community.
- Come to terms with the physical body.
- Move from loss to closure.
- Adjust to new roles.
- Get affairs in order.

Source: Kinzbrunner, Weinreb, and Policzer, 20 Common Problems: End-of-Life Care. 2002. McGraw-Hill Publishers.

Psychosocial, Emotional, and Spiritual Symptoms

Although we frequently attempt to distinguish among psychosocial, emotional, and spiritual issues, the reality is that the range and depth of being human make it nearly impossible to recognize where one aspect of being ends and another begins. It has been suggested to address these areas as a continuum, and to view the issues that arise in these aspects of our human functioning at end of life as opportunities, rather than as problems (McKinnon & Miller, 2002). "For those caring for the terminally ill, psychosocial and spiritual issues that in the past have been seen as problems can, with information and compassion, become opportunities—opportunities that will allow each of us to live fully until we say goodbye" (McKinnon & Miller, 2002, p. 273).

Some issues that arise must be viewed in a practical light, because addressing them might assist in providing resources for the dying elderly to promote quality of life and dignity.

Psychosocial Issues

When family members are the primary caregivers of the elderly, role changes are very common. Caregivers may resist providing increasing physical care, not wanting to recognize the decline or not wanting to diminish the dignity of the patient. The patient may resist it as well, resenting the need for the increased level of care because it demonstrates yet more limitations and inabilities in level of independence. Caregivers may not comprehend the emotional changes and resistance of their elder, and may become frustrated with the increasing tasks of care and with the emotional burdens of its constancy.

It may be helpful for caregivers to view the last year of a person's life as a reversal of the first year of life. This revised perspective helps the caregiver see that the person is not intentionally increasingly helpless, or necessarily giving up certain functions. Rather, he or she may be losing abilities in a reverse order of that in which infants gain abilities over the first year of life. These may affect the areas of mobility, activities of daily living, cognition, and personal care needs. As physical ability declines, people begin to withdraw from activities, which may further increase dependence on persons around them and their sense of isolation.

Notable Quotes

"One of the most surprising lessons our teachers (the dying) offer is that life doesn't end with the diagnosis of a life-challenging illness—that's when it truly begins . . . because when you acknowledge the reality of your death, you also have to acknowledge the reality of your life . . . that you have to live your life now. . . . The primary lesson the dying teach us is to live every day to its fullest."

Kubler-Ross & Kessler, 2000, p. 190

Having sufficient physical care—whether from family, paid caregiver resources, or in assisted living or long-term care facilities—is important for those facing end of life. What constitutes sufficient care may vary with the individual, but it is always an aspect of end-of-life care that will become more important as the person's physical abilities decline. Although some elderly enjoy this increased dependence, very independent individuals often find this increasing caregiver need to be one of the hardest aspects of treatment to accept.

Many patients and families have financial concerns. The concerns are greater, of course, for individuals or families with few resources, or with only some resources. Although subsidies for some services are available, many people may not have the ability to access them. The palliative care or hospice team may be helpful in linking the patient and family with appropriate financial resources. Nurses may also want to have basic information available for possible referrals when access to other team members is not available. There are agencies and individuals available to augment the family's ability to provide care. Most require private pay resources, but some are government sponsored in order to keep people in their homes a bit longer (e.g., some Medicaid-sponsored hours that provide in-home support are available in some states for those individuals who financially qualify).

Emotional Issues

A person's place in the life cycle affects their reaction to end-of-life circumstances. As an elderly person faces death, the individual looks back upon life and reflects upon its experiences. There is an attempt to emotionally integrate all the aspects of one's life, including determination of its meaning and acceptance of its uniqueness (Rando, 1984). It is an unfair exaggeration to imply that the elderly are all at peace with their coming death. Some are and some are not. The elderly do appear to see death as an important issue, one they often think about and plan for.

Caring intervention should continue to facilitate an appropriate death for the aged individual.

Anticipatory grief is a process of adjustment during the course of the terminal illness that is faced by the patient as well as by the family/caregivers. It usually begins at the time of diagnosis and can be caused by a variety of adjustments and secondary losses experienced by and required of the individual. These might include loss of control, independence, productivity, security, various abilities, predictability and consistency, future existence, pleasure, ability to complete plans and projects, significant others, meaning, dreams, and hopes for the future (Rando, 1984).

Persons who are facing end of life often encounter feelings of hopelessness. They may find comfort and be helped to adjust to their changing condition by recognizing a changing focus of **hope**. "A patient can hear a terminal diagnosis and still have hopes for the type of life remaining" (Rando, 1984, p. 270). When a person is confronted with the possibility of a life-ending illness, usually the first response is: "I hope it's nothing serious or that it can be easily treated without much disruption in my life." As treatment is not successful and as the illness progresses, one might hope that "my family and I will have the opportunity to get things done . . . have closure . . . see my granddaughter get married."

When getting better or prolonging life is not feasible, one is often confronted with giving up hope altogether. That is how some people feel when they choose hospice or palliative care. That is, in fact, what some physicians imply when they say, "There is nothing more that can be done for you." Hospice and palliative care personnel believe that hope can continue—but the focus of hope changes from that of getting better. One can hope for the appropriate help and support for themselves and their families through the transitions that end of life brings. They can hope that they will be provided with guidance and emotional comfort, and that their care will be provided with respect for their dignity through the dying process. They can hope that their passing will be comfortable and pain free. They can hope that their families will receive the appropriate support before and after their death. They can hope to be treated holistically—as an individual with unique needs, wishes, and desires.

Four powerful statements proposed by Ira Byock provide a clear path to emotional wellness throughout a lifetime. They also provide a format for resolving some personal, emotional, and/or spiritual issues at end of life. They are:

"Please forgive me. . . . I forgive you. . . . Thank you. . . . I love you" (Byock, 2004, p. 3).

Spiritual/Cultural Issues

Spiritual issues may or may not be related to the person's relationship to or lack of affiliation with an organized religion. Some may find great peace and comfort in a religion and its practices and rituals. Others are just as spiritual, without the link to religious ties and practices, perhaps finding comfort in nature or some other source.

Spiritual and cultural rituals may be important for some people at end of life. Nurses may be in a position to help patients and families to obtain access to the rituals that may be important as a person is nearing death. For some religions, this may

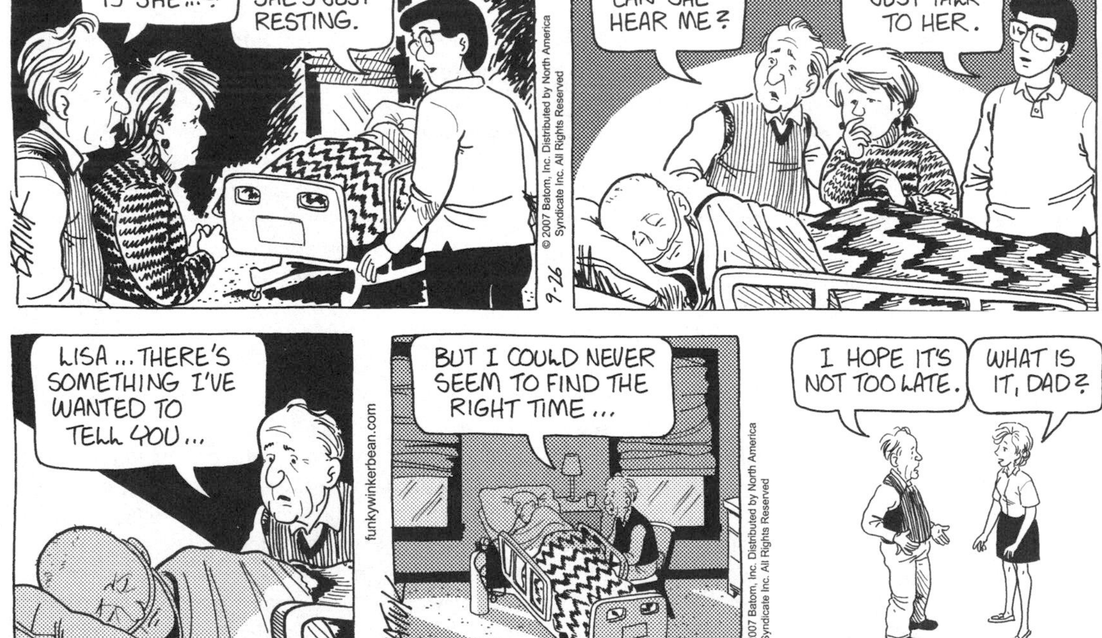
IS SHE...?
SHE'S JUST RESTING.
© 2007 Batom, Inc. Distributed by North America Syndicate Inc. All Rights Reserved
CAN SHE HEAR ME?
JUST TALK TO HER.
LISA ... THERE'S SOMETHING I'VE WANTED TO TELL YOU...
funkywinkerbean.com
BUT I COULD NEVER SEEM TO FIND THE RIGHT TIME ...
© 2007 Batom, Inc. Distributed by North America Syndicate Inc. All Rights Reserved
I HOPE IT'S NOT TOO LATE.
WHAT IS IT, DAD?

SOURCE: ©BATOM, INC. NORTH AMERICAN SYNDICATE

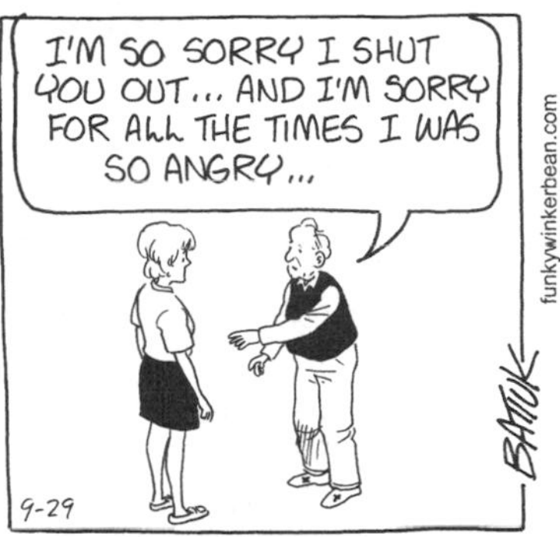
I'M SO SORRY I SHUT YOU OUT... AND I'M SORRY FOR ALL THE TIMES I WAS SO ANGRY...
9-29
BATIUK
funkywinkerbean.com

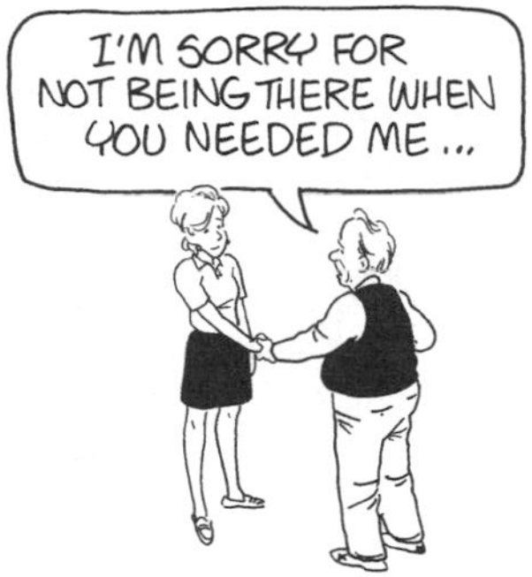
I'M SORRY FOR NOT BEING THERE WHEN YOU NEEDED ME...

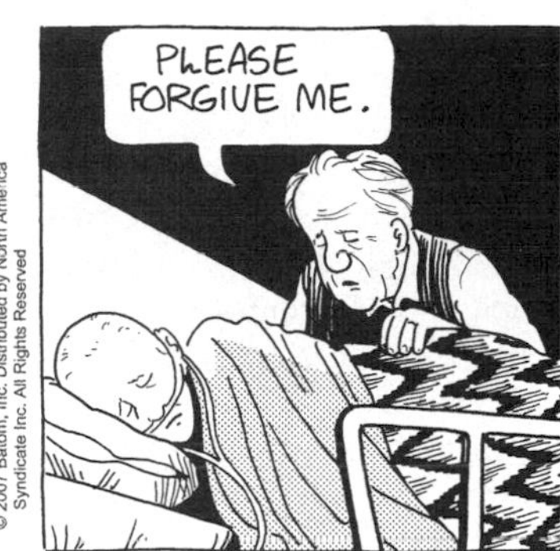
© 2007 Batom, Inc. Distributed by North America Syndicate Inc. All Rights Reserved
PLEASE FORGIVE ME.

SOURCE: ©BATOM, INC. NORTH AMERICAN SYNDICATE

BOX 24-9 Suggested Resources

Albom, M. (1997). *Tuesdays with Morrie: An old man, a young man, and life's greatest lesson*. New York: Doubleday.

Association for Death Education and Counseling (ADEC). *Promoting excellence in death education, bereavement counseling, and care of the dying*. Available at http://www.adec.org.

Callanan, M., & Kelley, P. (1992). *Final gifts: Understanding the special awareness, needs and communications of the dying*. New York: Poseidon Press.

Ferrell, B. R., & Coyle, N. (2001). *Textbook of palliative care nursing*. New York: Oxford University Press.

Hospice Foundation of America. Available at http://www.hospicefoundation.org.

Matzo, M. L., & Sherman, D. W. (2001). *Palliative care nursing: Quality care to the end of life*. New York: Springer.

National Hospice and Palliative Care. Available at http://www.nhpco.org.

Nuland, S. B. (1993). *How we die: Reflections on life's final chapter.* New York: Random House.

Project on Death in America. Open Society Institute. Available at http://www.soros.org/initiatives/pdia.

Smith, W. J. (2000). *The culture of death: The assault on medical ethics in America*. San Francisco: Encounter Books.

Toole, M. M. (2006). *Handbook for chaplains: Comfort my people*. New York: Paulist Press.

Webb, M. (1997). *The good death: The new American search to reshape the end-of-life*. New York: Bantam Books.

Wit. (2001). A movie made for HBO and a Pulitzer prize–winning play by Margaret Edson featuring a single-minded English professor, who in the face of imminent death learns the power and importance of simple acts of human kindness. Available for purchase at http://www.hbo.com/films/catalog/w.html.

mean obtaining appropriate clergy for confession, communion, and anointing. For others it may mean a more general ritual for commendation of the dying. For some cultures, certain foods, fasting, handling of the body, and placement in a certain position to facilitate burial may be important (Kirkwood, 1993) (see **Table 24-1**.) As in other aspects of individualized care, it is appropriate to ask the patient and/or family about these preferences.

To formalize this asking, several brief assessments have been developed for use by nurses to incorporate a spiritual component into their nursing plan of care. These are available for detailed review in *Spiritual Care in Nursing Practice* (Mauk & Schmidt, 2004). The assessments are easy to incorporate, using acronyms as reminders in obtaining the spiritual history content. The information obtained by the nurse may be useful for interventions with the patient and family by other members of the care team, regardless of the setting in which care is provided.

COMPONENTS OF PEACEFUL DYING

It may be possible to plan for a peaceful death, given the knowledge of having a terminal illness. "The key to peaceful dying is achieving the components of peaceful living during the time you have left" (Preston, 2000, p. 161). Some components are accomplished only by the individual, whereas others may require the assistance of family and medical providers, such as the following (Preston, 2000):

- Instilling good memories
- Uniting with family and medical staff
- Avoiding suffering, with relief of pain and other symptoms
- Maintaining alertness, control, privacy, dignity, and support
- Becoming spiritually ready
- Saying good-bye
- Dying quietly

A **good death** is possible and can be facilitated by the nurse who advocates for and works to ensure that the patients, families, and caregivers are free from avoidable distress and suffering, that the process is in accord with the wishes of the patient and family, and that it is consistent with clinical, cultural, and ethical standards (Dobbins, 2005).

POSTMORTEM CARE

Pronouncing Death

Pronouncing the death of a person varies from state to state and institution to institution. In some states, nurses may be able to pronounce the death, whereas in others this is not allowed. In inpatient settings, policies differ and the individual institutional policies are followed. In hospice home care, generally a nurse makes a visit, determines the lack of vital signs, and contacts the physician who has already agreed to sign the death certificate because the death has been anticipated. The funeral home or mortuary is contacted for removal of the body.

In pronouncing the death, it is customary to identify the patient and note the following (Berry & Griffie, 2006):

- General appearance of the body
- Lack of reaction to verbal or tactile stimulation
- Lack of pupillary light reflex (pupils fixed and dilated)

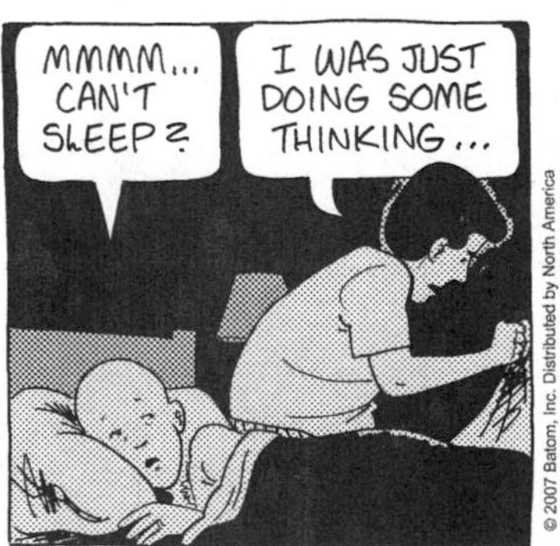
MMMM... CAN'T SLEEP?
I WAS JUST DOING SOME THINKING...

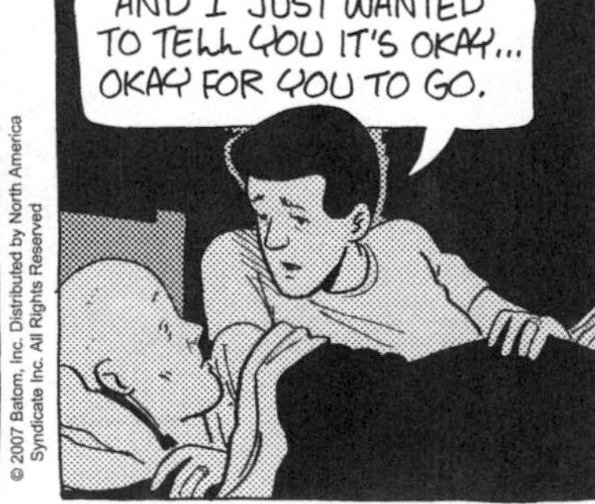
AND I JUST WANTED TO TELL YOU IT'S OKAY... OKAY FOR YOU TO GO.
© 2007 Batom, Inc. Distributed by North America Syndicate Inc. All Rights Reserved

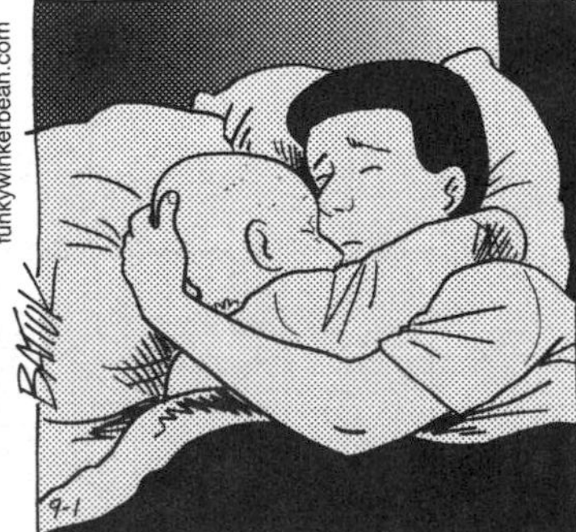

SOURCE: ©BATOM, INC. NORTH AMERICAN SYNDICATE

TABLE 24-1 Cultural and Religious Practices at End of Life

Religion	During Sickness	Dying/Death	After Death
Buddhism	Important to die in positive state of mind; organ permitted	Help die peacefully by encouraging forgiveness; position on right side, left hand on left thigh, legs stretched out; no special body preparations	Leave body alone as long as possible to avoid disturbing the consciousness during transition from death to new life.
Hinduism	Family does daily care; father/oldest son makes health decisions; same-sex caregiver due to modesty	Terminal diagnosis, dying information given to family, not the patient; family decides how much info to share with the patient	Body washed, usually by eldest son, then cremated.
Islam/Muslim	Prayer 5× day; clean area of any body waste, including person and sheets; can use pitcher and basin provided; use clean sheet to cover patient during prayer. Best efforts provided to maintain life; hardship is a test from Allah; can remove life support; natural death will allow person to accept the will of Allah	Body on its side, facing Mecca; friends and loved ones pray for mercy, forgiveness, and blessings of Allah	Person of same gender prepares body for burial; same day as death if possible; cremation forbidden.
Jehovah's Witness	No blood transfusions; organ transplants per individual conscience	Respectful care for dying person and family; respond to their individual needs	Generally follow traditional state mandates for burial or cremation.
Judaism	In serious illness, patient is not to be left alone—to be attended by family; doctor's duty to prolong life unless death is imminent and certain; cannot hasten death	Autopsy not permitted unless required by law; organ donation only after person declared dead (not at all by Orthodox)	Cremation forbidden; focus on deceased and funeral; mourning occurs in the home for 7 days after the funeral. Orthodox: extend arms alongside the body, fingers outstretched, tubing, body

TABLE 24-1 continued

Religion	During Sickness	Dying/Death	After Death
			fluids, sheets/blankets with blood are buried with the body; designated Orthodox Jew should clean the body. Someone stays with body, praying until body enters ground.
Christianity (general)	Respect and dignity for body; organ donation and autopsy allowed; if treatment is of no benefit or unreasonable burden, may forgo and allow natural death; decision up to patient/family	Open to pastoral care; some have a rite of anointing by a priest; some have service of commendation of the dying	Practices may vary by denomination, but commonly include a gathering with family and friends after the funeral or memorial service.
Orthodox Christianity	Fasting on certain days = no meat, milk, fish, eggs; no eating before communion; can use drugs to reduce pain/suffering; removing life supports done after prayer and discussion with family members, medical professional, and spiritual director; organ donation acceptable	Family encouraged to be at bedside; invite priest; Anointing of the Sick (Holy Unction)	Body buried in ground, w/coffin, grave liner, monument with image of the cross; cremation is not allowed.
Roman Catholicism	If possible, fast 1 hour before receiving Eucharist; moral obligation to use ordinary or proportionate means of preserving life (in judgment of patient)	Sacrament of Anointing of the Sick before surgery, for elderly in weakened condition, by a priest	May be cremated; cremains may be brought to funeral mass.

SOURCE: Table generated from Handbook for Chaplains, by Mary M. Toole. Copyright 2006 by Mary M. Toole Paulist Press, Inc, New York/Manwah, NJ. Reprinted by permission of Paulist Press, Inc. www.paulistpress.com

BOX 24-10 SPIRIT Model

S = Spiritual belief system (formal affiliation)
P = Personal spirituality (beliefs, practices, personal meaning)
I = Integration and involvement in a spiritual community
R = Ritualized practices and restrictions (encouraged or forbidden)
I = Implications for medical care (to include, or as barriers)
T = Terminal events planning (decision making, advance directives)

Source: Maugans, T. A. (1996). The SPIRITual History. *Archives of Family Medicine*, 5(1), 11–16.

BOX 24-11 HOPE Model

H = Sources of hope, meaning, comfort, strength, peace, love, and connection: What do you hold on to during difficult times?
O = Organized religion: Importance? Helpful and nonhelpful aspects?
P = Personal spirituality and practice: Relationship with God? Most helpful aspects of spiritual practices?
E = Effects on medical care and end-of-life issues: Has illness affected your ability to do the things that usually help you spiritually? Are there specific practices to be aware of in providing care? Can I help access resources helpful to you?

Source: Reproduced with permission from Spirituality and medical practice: using the HOPE questions as a practical tool for spiritual assessment. January 1, 2001, American Family Physician.

BOX 24-12 FICA Model

F = Faith or beliefs (What gives meaning to life?)
I = Importance and influence (Is faith important? How do beliefs influence behavior toward illness?)
C = Community (Is the spiritual or religious community supportive? How? Person or people important to you? People you love?)
A = Address (How would you like health care providers to address these issues in your health care?)

Source: Puchalski, C., & Romer, A. L. (2000). Taking a spiritual history allows clinicians to understand patients more fully. *Journal of Palliative Medicine*, 3(1), 129–131.

- Absent breathing and lung sounds
- Absent carotid and apical pulses (In some situations, listening for an apical pulse for a full minute is advisable)

Physical Care of the Body

Care of the body is an important nursing function. It is not surprising that families often recall the actions of the nurse after the death of their loved one. Careful and gentle handling of the body communicates care and concern on the part of the nurse. Rituals and customs should have been identified before the death, to now be incorporated into this care, reflecting the patient/family wishes.

Family members should be allowed to touch the body if they so desire and are comfortable with this action. They may wish to select special clothes for their loved one's transfer to the funeral home. If they choose to remain present through the postmortem care, they should be educated about the potential for some body changes. For example, there may be the sound of air escaping from the lungs when the body is turned (a sighing sound), and stool and urine may be present in a previously continent person, as the rectal and urinary bladder sphincters relax. Nursing care also includes the removal of drains, tubes, IVs, and any other devices. Family members may wish to participate in bathing and dressing the body; some may find comfort in the small details of "a favorite gown and the hair just right" (Berry & Griffie, 2006).

SUMMARY

When death approaches for the elderly patient, the role of the nurse changes along with the patient's changing condition. The role moves from a fix-it focus to that of presence—the ability to be with the patient and with his or her family. This presence involves the provision of comfort measures, lending a listening ear, providing a peaceful environment, and compassionately educating patient and family about the dying process.

Nurses caring for the dying also need to care for themselves.

The nurse's gratification does not come from curing, but rather from supporting the patient in a peaceful and dignified "good death."

BOX 24-13 Web Exploration

Explore the Web site for the Hospice Foundation of America at http://www.hospicefoundation.org and compare the contents with those at Ira Byock's Web site at http://www.dyingwell.com.

Critical Thinking Exercises

1. Visit a funeral home and talk with the funeral home director(s) about their experiences. What are the major components of their job? How do they feel they provide a service to the community?
2. Review your local newspaper and read the obituaries. What are the ages of the persons who have died? Are most of them older or younger?
3. Recall a funeral for a family member that you may have attended in the past. What were the components of the service? How did religious and cultural aspects play a part in the funeral or memorial service? The burial? The grieving and mourning? How did family and friends grieve? How did they remember the loved one?

Personal **Reflections**

1. This chapter has provided a large amount of information on caring for older adults at end of life. Which portions of the chapter were you the least familiar with? Are there areas of your nursing practice that you need to further develop in order to provide effective care to the dying? List a few of those areas in which you could improve your practice.
2. If an older family member who is close to you was recently given a terminal diagnosis, how would you respond? What questions would you ask of him or her? What actions, if any, would you take?
3. Do you have advance directives or a living will for yourself? Why or why not?
4. Have you ever been with a person when they died? What was that experience like for you?
5. After learning the material in this chapter, will you view any aspects of end of life differently?
6. Have you ever provided postmortem care for a patient? If so, what was the most difficult aspect of that experience?

References

Aging with Dignity. (2007). *Five wishes: 2007 edition*. Retrieved January 1, 2008, from http://www.agingwithdignity.org/fw2007.html

Allchin, L. (2006). Caring for the dying: Nursing student perspectives. *Journal of Hospice and Palliative Nursing, 8*(2), 112–115.

Allen, W. (1976). *Without feathers, death* [Play]. New York: Ballantine Books.

American Geriatrics Society Panel on Chronic Pain in Older Persons. (1998). The management of chronic pain in older persons. *Journal of the American Geriatrics Society, 46*, 635–651. In Ebner, M. K. (1999). Older adults living with chronic pain: An opportunity for improvement. *Journal of Nursing Care Quality, 13*(4), 1–7.

American Pain Society. (1992). *Principles of analgesic use in the treatment of acute pain and cancer pain* (3rd ed.). Skokie, IL: The Society.

Aminoff, B. Z., & Adunsky, A. (2004). Dying dementia patients: Too much suffering, too little palliation. *American Journal of Alzheimer's Disease and Other Dementias, 19*(4), 243–247.

Berry, P., & Griffie, J. (2006). Planning for the actual death. In B. R. Ferrell & N. Coyle (Eds.), *Textbook of palliative nursing* (pp. 561–577). New York: Oxford University Press.

Bretscher, M. E., & Creagan, E. T. (1997). Understanding suffering: What palliative medicine teaches us. *Mayo Clinic Proceedings, 72*, 785–787.

Byock, I. (2004). *The four things that matter most: A book about living*. New York: Free Press.

Centers for Medicare and Medicaid Services. (2004). Appendix M: Guidance to surveyors. *State Operations Manual*, standards 418.68, 418.68(a), 418.70(d). Washington, DC: Author.

Connor, S. R., Pyenson, B., Fitch, K., Spence, C., & Iwasaki, K. (2007). Comparing hospice and non-hospice patient survival among patients who die within a three-year window. *Journal of Pain and Symptom Management, 33*(3), 238–246.

Derby, S., & O'Mahoney, S. (2006). Elderly patients. In B. R. Ferrell & N. Coyle (Eds.), *Textbook of palliative nursing* (pp. 639–640, 646–647). New York: Oxford University Press.

Dobbins, E. H. (2005). Helping your patient to a "good death." *Nursing, 35*(2), 43–45. Retrieved January 16, 2008, from http://www.nursing2008.com

Emanuel, L. L., von Gunten, C. F., & Ferris, F. D. (1999). *Trainer's guide, module 2: Communicating bad news. The education for physicians on end-of-life care (EPEC) curriculum*. Princeton, NJ: Robert Wood Johnson Foundation.

Enck, R. E. (1992). The last few days. *American Journal of Hospice and Palliative Care, 9*(4), 11–13.

Ferrell, B. R. (1991). Pain in elderly people. *Journal of the American Geriatrics Society, 39*, 64–73. In Ebner, M. K. (1999). Older adults living with chronic pain:

An opportunity for improvement. *Journal of Nursing Care Quality, 13*(4), 1–7.

Ferrell, B. R., Grant, M., & Virani, R. (1999). Strengthening nursing education to improve end-of-life care. *Nursing Outlook, 47*, 252–256.

Gibson, M., & Schroder, C. (2001).The many faces of pain for older, dying adults. *American Journal of Hospice and Palliative Care, 18*(1), 19–25.

Griffie, J., Nelson-Marten, P., & Muchka, S. (2004). Acknowledging the "elephant": Communication in palliative care: Speaking the unspeakable when death is imminent. *American Journal of Nursing, 104*(1), 48–58.

Hogan, C., Lunney, J., Gabel , J., & Lynn, J. (2003). Medicare beneficiaries cost of care in the last year of life. *Health Affairs, 20*, 4.

Hospice and Palliative Nurses Association. (2004a). Pain. *Journal of Hospice and Palliative Nursing, 6*(1), 62–64.

Hospice and Palliative Nurses Association. (2004b). Value of the professional nurse in end-of-life care. *Journal of Hospice and Palliative Nursing, 6*(1), 65–66.

Karnes, B. (2001). *Gone from my sight: The dying experience* (pp. 12–13). Depoe Bay, OR: B. K. Books.

Kinzbrunner, B. M. (2002). Nutritional support and parenteral hydration. In B. M. Kinzbrunner, N. J. Weinreb, & J. S. Policzer (Eds.), *Twenty common problems in end-of-life care* (pp. 313–327). New York: McGraw-Hill.

Kinzbrunner, B. M., Weinreb, N. J., & Policzer, J. S. (2002). *20 common problems in end-of-life care*. New York: McGraw-Hill.

Kirkwood, N. A. (1993). *A hospital handbook on multiculturalism and religion: Practical guidelines for health care workers*. Harrisburg, PA: Morehouse.

Krisman-Scott, M. A. (2003). Origins of hospice in the United States: The care of the dying, 1945–1975. *Journal of Hospice and Palliative Nursing, 5*(4), 205–210.

Kubler-Ross, E., & Kessler, D. (2000). *Life lessons*. New York: Simon and Schuster.

Levi, M. H. (1991). Constipation and diarrhea in cancer patients. *Cancer Bulletin, 43*, 412–422. In Storey, P. (1996). *Primer of palliative care* (2nd ed., p. 52). Gainesville, FL: American Academy of Hospice and Palliative Medicine.

Lewis, L. (2001, July). Toward a good death in the nursing home: Pain management and hospice are key. *Caring for the Ages*, 24–26.

Lipman, A. G. (2006). Pharmacotherapy for pain control at end of life. In K. J. Doka (Ed.), *Pain management at the end of life: Bridging the gap between knowledge and practice* (pp. 156–158). Washington, DC: Hospice Foundation of America.

Mauk, K. L., & Schmidt, N. K. (2004). *Spiritual care in nursing practice*. Philadelphia: Lippincott Williams & Wilkins.

McCaffery, M. (1968). *Nursing practice theories related to cognition, bodily pain, and man-environment interactions*. Los Angeles: University of California at Los Angeles Student Store.

McCaffery, M., & Pasero, C. (1999). *Pain: Clinical manual* (2nd ed.). St. Louis: Mosby.

McKinnis, E. A. (2002). Dyspnea and other respiratory symptoms. In B. M. Kinzbrunner, N. J. Weinreb, & J. S. Policzer (Eds.), *Twenty common problems in end-of-life care* (pp. 147–162). New York: McGraw-Hill.

McKinnon, S. E., & Miller, B. (2002). Psychosocial and spiritual concerns. In B. M. Kinzbrunner, N. J. Weinreb, & J. S. Policzer (Eds.), *Twenty common problems in end-of-life care* (pp. 257–274). New York: McGraw-Hill.

Meyer, C. (2001). *Allow natural death—an alternative to DNR?* Hospice Patients Alliance. Retrieved December 17, 2007, from http://www.hospicepatients.org/and.html

National Hospice and Palliative Care Organization. (2004). *Keys to quality care*. Retrieved December 17, 2007, from http://www.nhpco.org/i4a/pages/index.cfm?pageid=3303

National Hospice and Palliative Care Organization. (2007). *NHPCO facts and figures: Hospice care in America*. Retrieved January 1, 2008, from http://www.caringinfo.org/userfiles/File/2009%20NHPCO%20Outreach%20Guide/National%20Hospice%20-%20Palliative%20Care%20Month%20Outreach/Media%20Outreach%20Documents/Background%20Documents%20-%20PDFs/NHPCO_Facts_and_Figures_Nov_2007.pdf

Perley, M. J., & Dahlin, C. (Eds.). (2007). *Core curriculum for the advanced practice hospice and palliative nurse*. Washington, DC: Hospice and Palliative Nurses Association.

Preston, T. A. (2000). *Final victory: Taking charge of the last stages of life, facing death on your own terms*. Roseville, CA: Prima.

Quaglietti, S., Blum, L., & Ellis, V. (2004). The role of the adult nurse practitioner in palliative care. *Journal of Hospice and Palliative Nursing, 6*(4), 209–213.

Quint, J. C. (1967). *The nurse and the dying patient*. New York: Macmillan.

Rando, T. A. (1984). *Grief, dying and death: Clinical interventions for caregivers*. Champaign, IL: Research Press.

Rando, T. A. (1993). *Treatment of complicated mourning*. Champaign, IL: Research Press.

Rushton, C. H., Spencer, K. L., & Johanson, W. (2004). Bringing end-of-life care out of the shadows. *Nursing Management, 35*(3), 34–40.

Saunders, C. (1984). On dying well. *Cambridge Review*, 49–52. In Storey, P. (Ed.), *Primer of palliative care*. Gainesville, FL: American Academy of Hospice and Palliative Medicine.

Sheehan, D. K., & Schirm, V. (2003). End of life care of older adults. *American Journal of Nursing, 103*(11), 48–57.

Storey, P. (1996). *Primer of palliative care* (2nd ed.). Gainesville, FL: American Academy of Hospice and Palliative Medicine.

Task Force on Palliative Care. (1997). *Last acts, care and caring at the end of life: Precepts of palliative care*. Chicago, IL: Stewart Communications.

Toole, M. M. (2006). *Handbook for chaplains: Comfort my people*. New York: Paulist Press.

Towey, J. (2005). *Five wishes: Questions and answers*. Retrieved January 22, 2008, from http://www.agingwithdignity.org/answers.html

Weinreb, N. J., Kinzbrunner, B., & Clark, M. (2002). Pain management. In B. M. Kinzbrunner, N. J. Weinreb, & J. S. Policzer (Eds.), *Twenty common problems in end-of-life care* (pp. 91–145). New York: McGraw-Hill.

Wolfelt, A. D. (2001). *Healing a teen's grieving heart: 100 practical ideas*. Ft. Collins, CO: Companion Press.

Wolfelt, A. D. (2004). *The understanding your grief support group guide*. Ft. Collins, CO: Companion Press.

Wolfelt, A. D. (2007a). *The mourner's bill of rights*. Retrieved January 13, 2008, from http://www.centerforloss.com/articles.php?file=mourners.php

Wolfelt, A. D. (2007b). *Helping others in grief*. Retrieved January 13, 2008, from http://www.centerforloss.com/grieve.php

Worden, J. W. (1991). *Grief counseling and grief therapy: A handbook for the mental health practitioner*. New York: Springer.

World Health Organization. (2008). *Pain relief and palliative care*. Retrieved January 27, 2008, from http://www.searo.who.int/LinkFiles/Publications_ch11.pdf

Wright, J. B. (2002). Depression and other common symptoms. In B. M. Kinzbrunner, N. J. Weinreb, & J. S. Policzer (Eds.), *Twenty common problems in end-of-life care* (pp. 221–240). New York: McGraw-Hill.

CHAPTER 25

Trends That Impact Gerontological Nursing

Kristen L. Mauk, PhD, RN, CRRN-A, GCNS-BC
James M. Mauk, BS, ChFC, CASL

LEARNING OBJECTIVES

At the end of this chapter, the reader will be able to:

- Identify current educational trends in gerontological nursing.
- Describe several settings and positions in which gerontological nurses may be employed.
- Define financial gerontology.
- Distinguish among the certification requirements for Chartered Advisor for Senior Living, Registered Financial Gerontologist, Certified Senior Advisor, and Certified Life Care Planner.
- Recognize the benefits of life care planning for the elderly with catastrophic injury or chronic illness.
- Analyze concepts related to community living designs for older adults.
- Explain the concept of long-term care insurance.
- Compare the concept of Green Houses with continuing care retirement communities.
- Discuss the role of the geriatric care manager.

KEY TERMS

- Advanced practice nurse
- Certified Life Care Planner (CLCP)
- Certified Senior Advisor (CSA)
- Chartered Advisor for Senior Living (CASL)
- Clinical nurse leader (CNL)
- Community living designs
- Continuing care retirement community (CCRC)
- Doctor of nursing practice (DNP)
- Financial gerontology
- Life care plan (LCP)
- Long-term care insurance
- Professional geriatric care manager (PGCM)
- Registered Financial Gerontologist (RFG)

Dozens of career options exist in the field of gerontological nursing. In addition to various job descriptions, gerontological nurses work in a variety of settings, from the community with well elderly to hospice with the dying, and every point in between along the continuum of care. A few unique possibilities in gerontological nursing will be discussed later in this chapter.

EDUCATIONAL TRENDS IN GERONTOLOGICAL NURSING

Opportunities in gerontological nursing are somewhat correlated with education level. The common settings for gerontological nursing practice were discussed in Chapter 1. Many levels of preparation are available for nurses in gerontology. First, as has been noted throughout this text, all nurses should receive special education in caring for older adults during their basic nursing preparation, whether at the LPN, RN associate degree, diploma RN, or RN BSN level. Postbaccalaureate nurses may choose a clinical nurse specialist (CNS) in gerontology or geriatric nurse practitioner (GNP) program. Online programs for graduate or post-master's study are becoming increasingly popular options that allow students to take courses online and complete clinical hours in their own geographic location. In addition, some programs offer a post-master's GNP certificate. The certifications in gerontology currently available from the American Association of Colleges of Nursing (AACN) are discussed in Chapter 1.

Some gerontological nurses with basic preparation find work in long-term care facilities such as nursing homes, assisted living, independent living centers, or adult day care, or in an acute care hospital. Nurses who obtain a BSN and continue to work in geriatrics often become unit managers, then assistant directors or directors of nursing in nursing homes or other long-term care settings. Many geriatric nurses work in home health care and hospice, those specialties that service many chronically ill and/or dying older adults.

For **advanced practice nurses**, opportunities for further career development are many, but often depend upon one's geographic location. Certainly larger teaching hospitals in big cities have many more positions for gerontological clinical nurse specialists and GNPs than smaller towns. Positions in education through county hospitals or religiously affiliated health care systems are generally available, though many CNSs and NPs have been known to carve their own niche, write their own job descriptions, and literally "make a job for themselves" by marketing their expertise in an area of need. Indeed there may be significant overlap in some clinical specialty areas that tend to serve a large elderly population, such as oncology or wound/ostomy nursing, creating even more job possibilities. One thing is certain, the advanced practice nurses of today and the future will need to be more business-minded to obtain their ideal desired position.

For nurses with doctoral-level education, careers as faculty members abound. The current faculty shortage is projected to continue. There is a tremendous need for certified and well-prepared faculty members in gerontological nursing to teach students who will care for the aging population. Nurses may obtain one of several doctorates that may be considered terminal degrees, though this varies with each university and school of nursing. The PhD (doctor of philosophy in nursing) and DNS (doctor of nursing science) are currently recognized as terminal nursing degrees by most universities. The PhD is a universal research degree recognized in most countries. This degree prepares the holder to design and conduct research, also mastering coursework in theory, statistics, and philosophy.

Some nursing faculty members hold an EdD, an educational doctorate, with coursework emphasizing curricular development and teaching. Most doctorally prepared gerontological nurses work in academic or research institutions, as authors, speakers, consultants, or private business owners. Those with the ND designation are found more often in collaborative practice with physicians in primary care settings, though some gerontological nurses have branched into rehabilitation and outpatient clinics that deal with older adults.

The **DNP (doctor of nursing practice)** is a clinical doctorate that is gaining more popularity in combination with obtaining certification as a nurse practitioner or other type of advanced practice nursing. It is not intended to prepare the nurse to be a researcher, but focuses on evidence-based clinical practice. There is no uniformity in the curricula when comparing DNP programs, although because the American Association of Colleges of Nursing (AACN, 2005) recommended that all programs conform to prepare advanced practice nurses at the doctoral level by 2015, some common threads in programs have emerged to include topics such as ethics, business, legal aspects, epidemiology, and evidence-based practice. Instead of a dissertation, DNP programs require a clinical project.

A minimum number of clinical hours for the DNP is also recommended, but incorporated in various ways throughout different curricula. The National Association of Clinical Nurse Specialists (NACNS) has identified some areas of concern with relation to requiring the DNP to practice as a clinical nurse specialist, and this organization stated that the DNP proposal from the AACN focused mainly on nurse practitioners (NACNS, 2005). Indeed, NPs have been the driving force behind the movement toward requiring a doctorate as the entry level into advanced practice. Critics of the DNP degree continue to voice concerns that include the limited input sought from affected parties, the lack of uniformity of curricula, many unanswered questions regarding critical issues, and the haste with which the AACN prepared and released the proposal (NACNS, 2005). Additionally, how a mandated practice doctorate will affect the numbers of future nurses taking the GNP certification exam is unclear, but remains a topic of discussion.

Recognition of the DNP varies. Although many programs recognize the DNP as a terminal nursing degree for purposes of promotion and/or tenure, some universities do not, and others place those with the DNP in a clinical track for promotion and tenure, distinguishing this from a research track. As of this writing, not all universities choose to recognize equality between the PhD and DNP degrees.

Another role in graduate education for nurses has emerged, taking on new meaning as nursing programs across the United States struggle to redefine themselves in terms of the AACN's position on the practice doctorate. This role is the **clinical nurse leader (CNL)**. The AACN (2007) defines the CNL thus:

> *The CNL is a leader in the health care delivery system across all settings in which health care is delivered, not just the acute care setting. The implementation of the CNL role, however, will vary across settings. The CNL role is not one of administration or management. The CNL functions within a microsystem and assumes accountability for healthcare outcomes for a specific group of clients within a unit or setting through the assimilation and application of research-based information to design, implement, and evaluate client plans of care. The CNL is a provider and a manager of care at the point of care to individuals and cohorts. The CNL designs, implements, and evaluates client care by coordinating, delegating and supervising the care provided by the health care team, including licensed nurses, technicians, and other health professionals. (p. 6)*

CNL students must complete 400–500 hours of clinical contact hours as part of their educational program, the vast majority of which are done in the CNL role mentored by a preceptor and guided by a faculty partner over a 10- to 15-week period of immersion. Common threads in the CNL program include critical thinking, clinical decision making, ethics, communication, health care systems, professional values, technology, and resource management (AACN, 2007). Graduates of a qualified CNL program will be eligible to sit for the CNL certification examination developed through the AACN.

Although the CNL role is conceptualized differently depending on the setting of practice, the definition cited previously suggests that gerontological nurses with CNL certification might, in the future, play a unique role in care coordination and team management in long-term care settings or case management organizations that provide services to older adults.

In addition to all of the educational opportunities in nursing, many colleges and universities offer majors, minors, certificates, or concentrations in gerontology that can be taken in addition to or even along with the nursing major. According to the Association for Gerontology in Higher Education (AGHE), "there are over 500 colleges and universities that offer more than 1,000 credit programs in aging" (AGHE, 2005) in some formal programs, and more than 1,000 additional schools offer some type of coursework in aging. For nurses wishing to specialize in gerontology from the beginning of their career, additional coursework in the field is recommended.

POTENTIAL OPPORTUNITIES IN GERONTOLOGICAL NURSING

The opportunities for nurses in geriatrics cover a wide variety of educational levels and settings for employment. All nurses working in acute care will care for older adults at some time, and evidence of this is provided through grants funded by the John A. Hartford Foundation to increase gerontological content in the nursing curriculum. The Hartford Foundation has provided millions of dollars in funding to promote education in both nursing and social work, particularly to prepare these health care professionals to give quality care to older adults. The AACN in cooperation with the Hartford Foundation gives annual awards to programs and individuals for their work in gerontological nursing.

Although many nurses will find their first jobs in acute care hospitals, nurses historically change positions throughout their careers. With the projected changes in the population distribution to a large older cohort of baby boomers, nurses are likely to see a dramatic shift in the types and numbers of non-hospital opportunities for career advancement.

The need for clinical nurse specialists in gerontology is likely to increase, as is the need for geriatric nurse practitioners. Because the baby boomer generation is known to be an autonomous, well-educated, informed consumer group, this population cohort is more likely to demand a higher level of education and expertise among care providers. As health-conscious and savvy researchers, baby boomers will want the highest quality care from those with the most expertise (and for the best value for their money). These trends point to advanced practice nurses as the most valuable professionals for the upcoming older generation.

Over the next decades, the health care system may experience unexpected shifts, such as more care being provided in the home by spouses and family members. Nurses may be called upon to train family members to care for loved ones in their home to a much greater extent than occurs today. On the other hand, though baby boomers may not wish to be cared for in institutions or long-term care facilities, their children are a generation that tends to be quite mobile and more focused on meeting their own life goals than perhaps taking care of elderly parents. If life expectancy continues at its current rate or even increases, baby boomers may be assisted in later life more often by their spouses, friends, church communities, and with assistive technology than ever before. The demand for better, higher quality, more personal and professional care in nursing homes may also increase if aging baby boomers can no longer be cared for in the home environment.

Indeed, there is a trend today for large churches or even groups of churches to come together to build and maintain their own retirement facilities with care ranging from independent living to assisted living, intermediate, skilled, Alzheimer's units, and rehabilitation. Nurses with faith-based backgrounds may find such new ventures challenging as they assist with development during the planning phase before even the first brick is laid. Certainly no such facilities would be possible without nurses, so such interesting ventures funded largely by donations and gifts from church members to care for their own elderly members present exciting possibilities for new nursing positions in both staff and management. Facilities such as these are often more open to the enterprising nurse who approaches them with his or her ideas for a new job position, such as a wellness coordinator or clinical nurse specialist to educate staff and focus on maintaining function and independence for older residents.

All these potential changes lead to the possibility that gerontological nurses of the future will need to be more highly educated and have a good business sense, excellent management skills, and greater flexibility in the workplace (**Case Study 25-1**).

Case Study 25-1

Norma is a 66-year-old married woman whose 87-year-old father has recently been diagnosed with early stage Alzheimer's disease (AD). With her father's progressive forgetfulness, Norma wishes to have him in a more supervised environment than she can provide, yet one in which he can still maintain his independence for as long as possible. A nearby long-term care facility offered an early AD unit, but Norma is concerned about exhausting her father's financial resources to pay for his care over what could be a long period of time.

Questions:

1. To what type of professional(s) could Norma go to for assistance with her concerns?
2. What new models of care/settings might be possible for Norma's father?
3. What role would a nurse consultant play in this situation?
4. Could a financial gerontologist be of assistance, or would a financial planner with a CASL designation be more likely to provide the information Norma needs?
5. Which of the professionals discussed in this chapter would you refer Norma to first?
6. What types of costs could she expect to incur for these types of services?
7. Would a professional geriatric case manager be helpful in this situation? Why or why not?

Nurses may be seen more often in collaborative practice to meet the growing needs of greater numbers of older adults. Advanced practice nurses will become more entrepreneurial, creating companies that specialize in educating businesses, churches, organizations, and private health care consumers about the aging process and how to stay healthy longer. Nurses will collaborate on a new level with other disciplines such as financial planners (**financial geronotology**) (Mauk & Mauk, 2006) and church leaders (parish nursing) to meet the various needs of the upcoming older health care consumer. All of these changes make gerontological nursing an exciting field to be in today! In this chapter, several emerging trends within other disciplines will be discussed in light of how the roles of nurses in gerontology are changing and expanding (**Case Study 25-2**).

LIFE CARE PLANNING

The concept of life care planning was first developed in the 1980s to meet a growing need for an informed document that presented actual estimated costs of care for persons who had experienced a catastrophic injury or accident. Many settlements for those persons in devastating accidents were made arbitrarily without actual calculation and consideration of the multitudes of factors influencing these costs, such as doctors' visits, equipment, medications, tests, cost of caregiving, and potential complications over a lifetime.

Definition

A **life care plan (LCP)** is a comprehensive document designed to help meet the long-term financial and health needs of a person who has experienced a catastrophic injury (Weed, 1999). For example, a person suffering paralysis from a complete spinal cord injury as a result of a car accident may have a lawyer who uses the services of a life care planner to determine as closely as possible the care needs of the person over many years of living with a disability. Armed with this information in court, and able to use the testimony of a life care planner, lawyers are more likely to obtain an equitable, reasonable, and necessary settlement for their clients.

Life care planners generally develop plans for insurance companies or lawyers representing individual clients, but the ultimate goal is to promote the best outcome for the person for whom the life care plan was written (**Case Study 25-3**).

The best life care planners have a nearly equal mix between work for insurance carriers and work for lawyers who present patients, thus maintaining a neutral and professional reputation for fairness. It is common for there to be much give and take in the discussion of arriving at a fair monetary settlement for the patient who has been the victim of a catastrophic accident. Life care planners research, analyze, compile, and present the facts in

Case Study 25-2

Terry is a nursing student who is finishing his BSN in an accelerated program. He has a previous degree in sports management and thinks he would like to combine a gerontological nursing focus with his prior experience and education. Terry enjoyed working with older adults in the community during his clinical experiences, and he has even thought about going on for further education as an advanced practice nurse with an emphasis in gerontology.

Questions:

1. Given Terry's first degree, what options should he consider for his first job out of the nursing program?
2. How could Terry combine his prior knowledge in sports management with his love of gerontology and his nursing knowledge?
3. What types of jobs might he apply for?
4. If Terry decided to go into business for himself, what marketable services could he offer? Who would be his target audience?
5. If Terry did go on for a master's degree, what types of programs should he look into to meet his long-term goals?
6. What types of advanced practice nursing programs might offer Terry greater opportunities to use his background in sports management as well as his desire to work in gerontology?
7. Should Terry explore the role of the PGCM? Why or why not?

Case Study 25-3

Mr. Lopez is an active 72-year-old man who recently sustained a complete C4 spinal cord injury as a result of a motorcycle accident. Mr. Lopez and his family are seeking damages from the insurance company of the person in the vehicle who hit Mr. Lopez while he was riding his motorcycle. Mr. Lopez exhibits quadriplegia, neurogenic bowel and bladder, spasticity, ongoing pain syndromes, and frequent respiratory infections. He is expected to need a great deal of care and rehabilitation. His rehabilitation nurse suggests the services of a life care planner to assist Mr. Lopez and his attorney in devising a plan to cover his expected costs over the rest of his lifetime.

Questions:

1. Is the use of a life care planner a good suggestion in the case of Mr. Lopez?
2. How might the expertise of a life care planner help Mr. Lopez in the long run?
3. What types of information would a life care planner ask for?
4. What information does the life care planner provide to the attorney, courts, and insurance companies?

a comprehensive, balanced document that details all of the expenses that a person with catastrophic injury may incur over his or her expected lifetime. Software programs are available that help manage the data obtained from various sources, including physicians, pharmacists, nurses, the patient, family, and other team members.

Certification

The **Certified Life Care Planner (CLCP)** designation may be earned through 128 continuing education hours, successful completion of a sample life care plan, and passing an examination (MediPro Seminars, 2004). **Table 25-1** gives an example of some of the topics for life care planning certification.

The CNLCP (Certified Nurse Life Care Planner) designation is offered by the American Association of Nurse Life Care Planners Certification Board. It is similar to the CLCP, but with additional requirements, and is definitely designed for registered nurses with case management experience (American Association of Nurse Life Care Planners, 2007). The strict prerequisites and large number of practice hours make this a more difficult credential to obtain than the CLCP. This certification demonstrates that the life care planner is a seasoned registered nurse. Conversely, the CLCP designation may be earned by any variety of professionals or nonprofessionals, including financial planners and lay persons who meet the criteria.

To recertify in either of these certifications requires a certain number of continuing education hours as well as practice hours and renewal fees within a certain number of years, as with most such designations.

Future Potential

Life care planning may be a concept that will be carried into the senior population. Not only are seniors living longer, but they continue participating in higher risk activities today than in generations past. The rate of catastrophic accidents formerly considered to be prevalent among younger adults may now be seen with older adults in activities such as motorcycle riding, horseback riding, skiing, and continuing to operate automobiles and other machinery well into late life. This also places older adults at risk of requiring the services of a life care planner at some time in their life.

Although originally designed for those with catastrophic illness or accident, the principles of life care planning could also easily be extrapolated for use with those seniors who have long-term chronic health problems. Although a good financial planner could provide a comprehensive financial life plan that takes health status into account, a life care planner could provide a more accurate and detailed projection of health care costs over a lifetime of disability or illness.

As the population ages, so does the incidence of chronic illnesses and disease. The demand for professionals in gerontology and rehabilitation is likely to grow quickly with the aging baby boomer group. Gerontological nurses are in a unique position to combine their knowledge in health care with some financial training to offer distinctive services to the older age group. A life care plan allows individuals

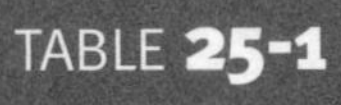

TABLE 25-1 **Examples of Topic Areas for the Life Care Planning Examinations**

- Life care planning principles
- Case management principles
- Medical interventions and complications associated with medical conditions:

  Traumatic brain injury, spinal cord injury, burns, amputations, common pediatric and neonatal disabilities, chronic pain, AIDS, cancer, orthopedic injuries, other complex disabilities, vocational tools
- Interdisciplinary team
- Legal/ethical issues
- Legislation
- Measurement and statistics
- Psychological issues
- Life care planning charts

to prepare for the likely impact of their health condition over their life span and to plan accordingly. "In the areas of finance, economics, and marketing, new trends are being seen that combine the expertise of financial planners with health care advisors and advocates for seniors" (Mauk & Mauk, 2006, p. 2). The baby boomer generation, as has been noted, is made up of conscious and conscientious health consumers who are informed, educated, thrifty, and autonomous. The life care planning market may be an area for exponential growth in the next decades.

FINANCIAL GERONTOLOGY

Financial gerontology is a growing subfield of financial planning. Financial gerontology is defined as "the intellectual intersection of two fields, gerontology and finance, each of which has practitioner and academic components" (Cutler, 2004, p. 29). Mauk and Mauk (2006) stated "financial gerontology combines the knowledge and skills associated with financial planning and asset management with expertise in meeting the unique needs of older adults" (p. 4). This emerging market presents excellent opportunities for gerontological nurses who also have an interest in finances and health care decision making. Three certifications will be discussed here: **Chartered Advisor for Senior Living (CASL)**, **Registered Financial Gerontologist (RFG)**, and **Certified Senior Advisor (CSA)**. Many graduate nursing programs are now offering dual degrees of Master of Business Administration (MBA) and Master of Science in Nursing (MSN). These educational trends support the idea that there is a growing need for health care professionals such as nurses to be educated beyond traditional health-related science.

Chartered Advisor for Senior Living (CASL)

The CASL (a designation obtainable from The American College) "is a financial service professional who is uniquely qualified to work with mature clients and those planning for retirement" (American College, 2005, p. 2). A person with a CASL certification assists older persons with retirement savings, pension and social security planning, health and long-term care issues, estate planning, and "managing life course transitions, family relationship and living arrangements" (American College, 2005, p. 3). This designation is appropriate for persons who work with older adults, including financial planners, case managers, accountants, attorneys, long-term care specialists, and nurses (**Case Study 25-4**).

Gerontological nurses, both at the basic preparation level and in advanced practice, already have

Case Study 25-4

George is a 56-year-old man preparing to retire from a career in private business. He notices that many of his friends, some much older than he, have made little or no plans for financial security after retirement. These friends often come to George for advice on finances, but he feels ill-prepared to give them an opinion on things related to the senior market and the possibilities for investments and retirement planning. After his retirement, George thinks he would like to have a small home business to advise seniors on financial matters, but he feels he would need additional training and does not wish to spend a lot of time or money "tinkering" with this business after retirement.

Questions:

1. Given George's situation, what options are available to him to increase his knowledge about financial advising for older adults?
2. What might be the best program to fit George's needs and goals?
3. Which programs are most costly?
4. Which programs require the most investment of George's time?
5. Does George even need a special credential to start his small business?
6. What are the benefits and disadvantages of George obtaining a designation or certification in one of the areas discussed in this chapter?

some basis of expertise through education and experience that would make obtaining this certification more meaningful. Although the content on aging would be familiar to most nurses, the financial aspect of the certification is challenging if one does not have an accounting or business background.

To earn the CASL designation, a person must successfully complete five courses that take approximately 60–80 hours of study each. After each course, the individual must pass a computerized exam. Maintenance of the certification is comparable to most nursing certifications, with continuing education credits required. A code of ethics must also be agreed to in writing prior to being granted the designation.

Registered Financial Gerontologist (RFG)

The Registered Financial Gerontologist (RFG) certification is a similar designation to the CASL, but is offered through the American Institute of Financial Gerontology and supported by the American Society on Aging (American Institute of Financial Gerontology, 2004). To earn this certification, individuals must complete six courses, a learning requirement, and a comprehensive examination. Course content is related to wealth span planning, ethics, and serving the older client. Compared to the CASL courses, the curriculum appears more suited to gerontologists than financial planners. This should be kept in mind when choosing the most appropriate designation for a nurse's career planning.

Certified Senior Advisor (CSA)

The Certified Senior Advisor (CSA) is a designation offered by the Society of Senior Advisors. There are currently 17,000 persons in the United States with this certification. The curriculum includes a large number of topics in aging, chronic illness, end of life, and long-term care as well as Medicaid and financial planning (Society of Certified Senior Advisors, 2005). It is a self-study program that takes 2–6 months to complete. To obtain the CSA, the person must also pass a secured, computerized, final comprehensive examination online that consists of 150 multiple choice questions within 3 hours (Society of Certified Senior Advisors, 2005).

TRENDS IN LONG-TERM CARE

Each of the certifications discussed in this chapter prepare persons to help the elderly with long-term care needs. Long-term care is "the broad range of medical, custodial, social, and other care services that assist people who have an impaired ability to live independently for an extended period" (Beam & O'Hare, 2003, p. 3). The National Council on Aging (2005) estimates that 6.4 million people over the age of 65 and 50% of those over age 85 will need long-term care. Thirteen million persons in the United States currently report having long-term health care needs. This number is expected to grow to 22 million in the next two decades (Chiappelli, Koepke, & Cherry, 2005). The nation spent $183 billion on long-term care services in 2003 (American Health Care Association & National Center for Assisted Living, 2005). In 2005, Medicaid spent nearly $95 billion on long-term care (Houser, Fox-Grage, & Gibson, 2006). Persons must pay for many long-term care expenses from their savings and assets, or spend down their financial assets before being eligible for Medicaid. This has prompted new sources of funding for future long-term health care needs.

Long-Term Care Insurance

Long-term care insurance is designed to cover individuals needing health care outside of the hospital, including diagnostics testing, rehabilitation, and custodial care. Reasons for purchasing long-term care insurance include worrying about being a burden to their family, staying financially independent, having more choices for care if needed (such as remaining in the home), preserving their assets, and providing peace of mind (United Seniors Health Council, 2005).

The cost of long-term care insurance premiums (at age 65) ranges from $1,000–$2,650 per year, depending upon a number of factors including health status and history. The average stay in a nursing home is 2 years. The average cost for a private room in a nursing home in 2003 was $181.24/day (National Council on Aging, 2005). This average cost had increased to $194/day by 2006 (over $70,000/year), though costs vary widely by geographic area (Gengler & Regnier, 2007). Assisted living facilities average $2,691/month for a one-bedroom unit (American Health Care Association & National Center for Assisted Living, 2005). Financial analysts predict that if nursing home care costs rise a bit faster than inflation, by 2026 a room in a nursing home could cost $177,000 per year (Gengler & Regnier, 2007); another source projected the cost to increase to $200,000 per year by 2030 (Beam & O'Hare, 2003).

Long-term care insurance can be purchased at any time, but premiums increase with age. In 2005, the annual premium for a low-option policy for a person who was age 65 was about $1,800, and increased to about $5,500 at age 79 (American Health Care Association & National Center for Assisted Living, 2005). Long-term care insurance may cover any one or all of the following types of care (Beam & O'Hare, 2003):

- Nursing home care
- Assisted living
- Hospice
- Home health
- Adult day care
- Respite
- Caregiver training
- Home health care coordinators

A comprehensive policy is probably the best option for anyone who anticipates the possibility of needing several levels of care throughout the life span. Depending on what the individual wishes to pay, benefits may be calculated daily with limits ranging generally from $50–$500 per day. Monthly benefits may vary greatly, from $1,000–$6,000 per month.

Nurses should be informed about the possibility of clients having or obtaining long-term care insurance. This is a question nurses should ask of any long-term care patient. Some persons without informed family members may not realize they have this type of coverage, and those with newly diagnosed conditions that will eventually require long-term care may benefit from earlier investment in this type of insurance. Only about 5 million people have long-term care insurance, but there are now 120 companies that offer this type of insurance (Beam & O'Hare, 2003). Ultimately, the decision to purchase long-term care insurance rests with the patient and family, but gerontological nurses should be prepared to answer basic questions about the benefits and disadvantages of purchasing such policies. Nurses who are interested in learning more about the financial planning aspects of gerontological care may wish to consider the benefits of additional certification in one of the related areas discussed in this chapter (**Boxes 25-1** and **25-2**). Also, the role of the geriatric care manager, discussed in the next section, may be expanded to include some aspects of other disciplines, as discussed in this chapter.

EMERGING MODELS OF CARE

A Shift to Different Living Facilities

One of the most significant changes in care for older adults is the shift away from nursing homes,

BOX 25-1 Web Links

Explore these links to learn more about some of the trends that affect gerontological nursing:

- American Association of Nurse Life Care Planners: http://www.aanlcp.org
- American Institute of Financial Gerontology: http://www.aifg.org
- Geriatric Nursing Education Consortium: http://www.aacn.nche.edu/gnec.htm
- National Association of Area Agencies on Aging: http://www.n4a.org
- National Association of Professional Geriatric Care Managers: http://www.caremanager.org
- National Gerontological Nursing Association: https://www.ngna.org/

BOX 25-2 Helpful Resources on Careers in Gerontology

AARP
601 E St. NW
Washington, DC 20049
(202) 434-2277
http://www.aarp.org

American Geriatrics Society
http://www.americangeriatrics.org

American Society on Aging (ASA)
833 Market St., Suite 511
San Francisco, CA 94103
(415) 974-9600
http://www.asaging.org

Association for Gerontology in Higher Education (AGHE), an educational unit of:
Gerontological Society of America
1030 15th Street NW, Suite 240
Washington, DC 20005-1503
(202) 289-9806 or fax (202) 289-9824
http://www.geron.org
http://www.aghe.org

John A. Hartford Foundation Institute for Geriatric Nursing
http://www.hartfordign.org

U.S. Administration on Aging
http://www.aoa.dhhs.gov

as they have been known traditionally. Some predict that the only nursing homes that will survive will be the excellent ones. The institutional look of the older nursing home that was modeled after the hospital, with long hallways and a sterile-looking environment, is becoming unacceptable to many older adults as a place to live out their final days. Newer long-term care facilities promote private rooms, residents' choices and control, and a more home-like environment that mirrors assisted living facilities of today.

Continuing care retirement communities (CCRCs) are the growing trend for older adults. Older adults of today are healthier than in the past and have less disability until advanced age. CCRCs have met the growing demand for services by promoting aging in place through offering various levels of care on a continuum that might include independent living, assisted living, skilled care, and home health services all on one campus. The trend will be to bring services to the CCRCs versus transferring persons to the next level of care on the continuum (for example, sending them to the "nursing home" when their care demands increased).

Another new concept is Green Houses, a movement to replace nursing homes with more home-like environments. Green Houses, started through the vision of a physician named Bill Thomas, consist of 10–12 residents in a home setting who enjoy private rooms and share a common living space (Lagnado, 2008). Instead of the institutional-like setting of many aging nursing homes, Green Houses are designed to provide a full range of care services, but in a friendly atmosphere that reminds one of home (see Chapter 11 for more information). Although there are currently 41 Green Houses in 10 states, the concept has met with resistance from some in the nursing-home system. There are many existing regulations within the elder care system that are barriers to the kind of care Dr. Thomas envisioned. The mindset of the traditional care model for older adults is slow to change.

Notable Quotes

"We should all be concerned about the future because we have to spend the rest of our lives there."

—C. F. Kettering

Geriatric Care Management

Another emerging trend in gerontological nursing is the role of the geriatric care manager. The **professional geriatric care manager (PGCM)** is a specialist who helps families care for older adults while encouraging as much independence as possible. Although PGCMs may come from a variety of backgrounds such as social work, psychology, sociology, geriatrics, and nursing, nurses have emerged as natural leaders in this growing field. The educational background of nurses as health promoters with strong background knowledge of the aging process make this role an excellent fit for nurses who seek a position that affords independence and autonomy while using their skills. Nurses with experience in home care, case management, gerontology, or rehabilitation may find this an exciting new area of practice.

According to the National Association for Professional Geriatric Care Managers (2008), a PGCM may perform the following services:

- Conduct assessments
- Develop care plans that address pertinent problems
- Arrange, interview for, and monitor in-home caregivers or other services
- Act as a consultant for caregivers who live near or far
- Review financial, health-related, or legal issues
- Provide referrals to other geriatric specialists
- Intervene in times of crisis
- Act as an advocate and/or liaison between families and service providers
- Keep the family informed of any problems
- Coordinate or oversee care
- Assist with transitions in living arrangements, including recommending the most appropriate settings and helping facilitate the move
- Provide education and links to resources
- Offer counseling and support
- Some PGCMs also offer guardianship, caregiving, and/or financial services

The current generation of older adults often has children who live in different geographic locations, making it unlikely for these children to care for their older parents. Geriatric care managers fill that gap between the care that family members wish to provide for their loved ones and the problem that distance creates in doing so. Adult children can employ the services of the PGCM to ensure that quality care is provided in their absence, and still be kept informed and part of the care process in this way. It is likely this will be a steadily growing trend as baby boomers age and wish to remain independent for as long as possible, but have children who are extremely mobile and may not have the financial resources or the motivation to care for their older parents at home. PGCMs of the future may facilitate the aging in place of older adults who wish to remain living in the community but who need additional resources and services.

COMMUNITY LIVING DESIGNS

Another fascinating trend related to gerontological nursing is the emergence of companies completely devoted to the strategic planning, engineering, architecture, building, and marketing of **community living designs** that are tailored to today's older adults. Older adults who choose to live in senior communities expect to have access to transportation and needed services such as health care, appropriate housing, and opportunities for socialization. Baby boomers are predicted to live in suburban communities versus urban or rural areas (Frey, 2007), so the need for age-appropriate and friendly retirement communities is projected to increase. Lehning, Chun, and Scharlach (2007) stated that:

> *An aging-friendly community has three primary characteristics: 1) age is not a significant barrier to the maintenance of life-long interests and activities; 2) supports and accommodations exist to enable individuals with age-related disabilities to meet basic health and social needs; and 3) opportunities exist for older adults to develop new sources of fulfillment and engagement. (p. 15)*

In spite of the need for such communities, shortfalls in public policy and lack of creativity in architecture have led to structural barriers related to best use of land, housing policies, transportation, and opportunities for involvement in the larger community (Lehning et al., 2007). There remains a general lack of concern and investment of suburban communities in providing housing for the aging portion of their citizens. This has created a gap in service that potentially can be filled by forward-thinking companies who recognize the plight of long-term care in this area and stand ready to assist.

One such example of a company developed to assist organizations with designing and building appropriate and age-friendly living spaces is Community Living Solutions (2008) of Neenah, Wisconsin. This company advertises its purpose as "enlightening your life and community with expert knowledge and sustainable solutions" (para. 1). With a unique team of professionals that includes engineers, architects, and other design experts, companies such as Community Living Solutions work with organizations such as **continuing care retirement communities (CCRCs)**, independent living facilities, and assisted living to design and build attractive, contemporary living areas within a fiscally responsible budget. The ideal team takes into consideration the mission and needs of the community and understands the unique limitations and desires of their older clientele. A great deal of thought and effort goes into designing an environment that will be attractive and functional for older adults, and marketable for the institution. Attention to details such as positioning of garden areas and windows to best use the space and sunlight is essential, and the savvy builder carefully plans all aspects of the environment with consideration to the older residents.

Community Living Solutions is an example of a creative team of professionals coming together to meet a need for older adult living situations. Its services are representative of what today's long-term care administrators and resident consumers have come to expect, including personal program and project development and management, market and financial analysis, operational and space programming, project budgeting and timelines, architectural design within the scope and mission of the organization, and construction management of the project through completion. Such full-service groups allow residents, staff, and administrators to develop a personal working relationship with the professional team and feel a sense of security and confidence when undertaking a major building project or renovation. Services such as these certainly seem to be the trend for the future in community living for seniors and will impact the environments in which nurses typically provide care for older adults.

SUMMARY

This is an exciting time to be a gerontological nurse. The specialty is continuing to grow, and the demand for health services will change and expand as the baby boomers begin to enter retirement age in 2011. There is more of an emphasis on gerontological nursing to be integrated in the baccalaureate curriculum. Many resources are accessible for nurses in this area that were unavailable even 10 years ago. Nurses should expect that within the next few decades, the need for gerontological nursing expertise will increase exponentially, and that nurses will be providing care in a variety of new settings. For advanced practice nurses and entrepreneurs, the specialty of gerontological nursing offers numerous opportunities to collaborate with those from other disciplines to address the needs of this growing and changing population.

Critical Thinking Exercises

1. Explore the suggested Web sites for this chapter in Box 25-2 and consider the various options for obtaining certifications related to gerontology and finances.
2. Find a law student or an attorney who would informally discuss with you the advantages and disadvantages of using a life care planner in obtaining the desired settlement for a person who sustained a catastrophic injury as the result of someone else's negligence.
3. Surf the World Wide Web for life care planners. Check out the educational background and experience of those offering these services. How many are nurses? What are their credentials? What are their Web sites like? Do they offer any other services?
4. Call an insurance company and inquire about long-term care insurance. What are the monthly premiums for a healthy 60-year-old versus a 75-year-old with diabetes? When does long-term health care insurance become a burden versus an asset?
5. Look at the Web site http://www.consultgerirn.com. What specific tools from this site might be helpful in answering questions from older adults about planning for the future?

Personal **Reflections**

1. Are any of the certifications discussed in this chapter new to you? Would you ever be interested in combining your nursing knowledge in gerontology with some type of financial planning?
2. What would it take for you to obtain a certification or designation in one of the areas discussed here? Is this something you might like to do in the future? If you were starting your own business and offering services to older adults, which of these certifications would be of most interest to you?
3. What do you think about long-term care insurance? Will you think about purchasing it when you are middle aged? Old aged? Why or why not?
4. What information from this chapter is useful to you as you think about working as a nurse with older adults?
5. If you were a board member of a CCRC and helping to plan a major renovation for existing senior living apartments in a large facility, what would be your major concerns for restructuring? for design? for health facilities? for dining areas? for recreational space? for aesthetics? for outside attractiveness? for marketing the new changes?

References

American Association of Colleges of Nursing. (2005). *The essentials of doctoral education for advanced nursing practice*. Washington, DC: Author.

American Association of Colleges of Nursing. (2007). *White paper on the education and role of the clinical nurse leader*. Washington, DC: Author.

American Association of Nurse Life Care Planners. (2007). *Initial board certification by exam*. Retrieved October 29, 2007, from http://www.aanlcp.org/cnlcpinitcertification.asp

American College. (2005). *Chartered advisor for senior living* [Brochure]. Bryn Mawr, PA: Author.

American Health Care Association and National Center for Assisted Living. (2005). *Paying for long term care*. Retrieved January 22, 2008, from http://www.longtermcareliving.com/pdf/how_to_pay.pdf

American Institute of Financial Gerontology. (2004). *Requirements and benefits of RFG designation*. Retrieved November 16, 2004, from http://www.aifg.org

Association for Gerontology in Higher Education. (2005). *How do you become a professional in aging?* Retrieved March 24, 2005, from http://www.careersinaging.com

Beam, B. T., & O'Hare, T. P. (2003). *Meeting the financial need of long-term care*. Bryn Mawr, PA: The American College.

Chiappelli, T., Koepke, C., & Cherry, K. (2005). *Planning for long-term care involves more than money*. Retrieved April 26, 2005, from http://www.financialpro.org

Community Living Solutions. (2008). *Community living solutions*. Retrieved January 22, 2008, from http://www.communitylivingsolutions.com

Cutler, N. E. (2004). Aging and finance 1991 to 2004. *Journal of Financial Service Professionals, 58*(1), 29–32.

Frey, W. H. (2007). *Mapping the growth of older America: Seniors and boomers in the early 21st century*. Washington, DC: Brookings Institution.

Genegler, A., & Regnier, P. (2007, November). Facing up to the costs of long-term care. *Money*, pp. 137–142.

Houser, A., Fox-Grage, W., & Gibson, M. J. (2006). *Across the states: Profiles of long-term care and independent living*. Retrieved January 7, 2008, from http://assets.aarp.org/rgcenter/health/d18763_2006_ats.pdf

Lagnado, L. (2008, June 24). Rising challenger takes on elder-care system. *Wall Street Journal*, pp. A1, A16.

Lehning, A., Chun, Y., & Scharlach, A. (2007). Structural barriers to developing "aging-friendly" communities. *Public Policy and Aging Report, 17*(3), 15–20.

Mauk, K. L., & Mauk, J. M. (2006). Financial gerontology and the rehabilitation nurse. *Rehabilitation Nursing, 31*(2), 58–62.

MediPro Seminars. (2004). *Life care planning (LCP) certificate program*. Retrieved November 16, 2004, from http://www.mediproseminars.com

National Association of Clinical Nurse Specialists. (2005). *White paper on the nursing practice doctorate*. Retrieved October 29, 2007, from http://www.nacns.org/nacns dnpwhitepaper2.pdf

Society of Certified Senior Advisors. (2005). *CSA: Certification*. Retrieved April 26, 2005, from http://www.society-csa.com

United Seniors Health Council, National Council on Aging. (2005). *Private long-term care insurance: To buy or not to buy?* Retrieved May 26, 2005, from http://www.ncoa.org

Weed, R. O. (1999). *Life care planning and case management handbook*. Boca Raton, FL: CRC Press.

Glossary

Chapter 1

Activities of daily living (ADLs): Include bathing, dressing, grooming, showering, and toileting activities.

Ageism: A negative attitude toward aging or older persons.

Assisted living facility: Level of care in which some assistance is available for certain activities of daily living; for those who are not completely independent and require some assistance with daily activities.

Certification: A type of credential earned through meeting specific requirements that validate one's expertise and knowledge in a specialty area.

Continuing care retirement community: A community that generally is housed in a common geographic area, is designed for older adults, and provides various levels of assistance for those who desire to age in place; often has independent and assisted living apartments with common areas that provide services such as meals, exercise rooms, and other services for older adults.

Core competencies: The essential skills and knowledge needed to provide quality care to older adults.

Financial gerontology: An emerging field that combines financial management, planning, and knowledge with special coursework and training in the unique needs of the elderly.

Geriatrics: Medical care of the aged.

Gerontological nursing: A specialty within nursing practice where the clients/patients/residents are older persons.

Gerontological rehabilitation nursing: Gerontological nursing care of older persons in which rehabilitation is emphasized; care for those with rehabilitation problems such as stroke, brain injury, neurological disorders, or orthopedic surgeries.

Gerontology: The study of aging or the aging process.

Geropharmacology: A specialty in medications and pharmacy of older adults.

Hospice: Provides holistic, comprehensive care to the terminally ill patient and his or her family through the dying and bereavement processes.

Independent living: A type of setting/housing in which the older adult performs all IADLs and ADLs independently or with minimal supervision.

Middle old: Those persons ages 75–84 years.

Old old: Those persons age 85 years or over; sometimes called the oldest old, the very old, or the frail elderly.

Rehabilitation: Care that promotes the maximum functional capacity of adults recovering from or adapting to a long-term or chronic condition.

Skilled care: Setting in which patients require less nursing care than in an acute hospital, but more than in other long-term settings; generally for those with higher acuity; may also be called skilled nursing facilities (SNFs); often found in long-term care facilities.

Social gerontology: A subfield of gerontology focused on the social aspects of aging.

Subacute care: For complex patients who require more intensive nursing care than the traditional nursing home can provide, but less than what's provided in an acute care hospital.

Unlicensed assistive personnel (UAP): Includes nursing assistants, nurse technicians, and other staff who do not have licenses to practice.

Young old: Those persons ages 65–74.

Chapter 2

Baby boomers: A large group of people born between 1946 and 1964, in the time after the Second World War.

Centenarian: Someone who is 100 years of age or older.

Chronic disease: A disease that is ongoing or recurring. Some types of cancer, as well as AIDS, have recently been designated as chronic diseases.

Cohort: A group of people with a similar characteristic, such as age or exposure to toxic chemicals, who are studied over time.

Demographic tidal wave: A term that describes the baby boomers; a large group about to "crash" into the resources of the United States.

Elderly: Usually described as those persons age 65 or over.

Foreign-born: Born outside of the United States; not a U.S. citizen at birth.

Graying of America: Similar to the aging of America, referring to the increase in numbers of older Americans.

Native-born: A U.S. citizen at birth.

Older adult: Someone age 65 or older.

Oldest old: Someone age 85+.

Pig in a python: Another descriptor of the baby boomers, as if they were a large lump inside a snake that is slowly moving along toward the tail; in other words, a bulge in population moving slowly through time.

Seniors: Those age 65+.

Chapter 3

Apoptosis: A process of programmed cell death marked by cell shrinkage.

Free radicals: Chemical species that arise from atoms as single unpaired electrons.

Immunomodulation: The effects of various chemical mediators, hormones, and drugs on the immune system.

Lipofuscin: An undegradable material that decreases lysosomal function; age pigment.

Melatonin: A hormone produced by the pineal gland that is linked to sleep and wake cycles.

Mitochondria: Parts of a cell that transform organic compounds into energy.

Nonstochastic theories of aging: Theories stating that a series of genetically programmed events occur to all organisms with aging.

Reactive oxygen species (ROS): Short-lived, highly reactive products of mitochondrial oxidative metabolism that destroy proteins, lipids, and nucleic acids.

Senescence: The process of growing old.

Stochastic theories of aging: Theories stating that random events occurring in one's life cause damage that accumulates with aging.

Telomerase: An enzyme that regulates chromosomal aging by its action on telomeres.

Telomere: Repeated sequences of DNA that protect the tips of the outermost appendages of the chromosome arms.

Chapter 4

Activities of daily living (ADLs): Basic tasks that one needs to perform in order to survive.

Agnosia: Failure to recognize or identify objects.

Agraphia: Inability to write.

Alzheimer's disease: A progressive neurodegenerative disease of the brain.

Anarthria: Complete inability to move the articulators for speech.

Anhedonia: Lack of interest or pleasure in activities that one used to enjoy.

Aphasia: An inability to express or understand the meaning of words due to damage in the language areas.

Apraxia: Impaired motor activities due to damage to the motor cortex.

Broca's area: An area in the brain in charge of speech production.

Cataracts: Clouding of the lens, which blocks light reflecting through the lens and can blur the image that is reflected onto the retina, resulting in hazy vision.

Chronic obstructive pulmonary disease: A condition characterized by blockage of airflow in the lungs.

Compensation: Making up for.

Conductive problems: Sound waves are blocked as they travel from the outer ear canal to the inner ear; thus, there is a decrease in hearing sensitivity.

Confabulation: Filling in words or memory gaps with information that is made up in order to compensate for memory loss.

Cortex: A large, wrinkly sheet of neurons that covers the brain.

Crystallized intelligence The accumulation of knowledge over the life span.

Delirium: An acute, reversible state of agitation and confusion.

Dementia: A decline in several mental abilities including memory.

Depression: A serious disorder that involves sadness, lack of interest, and other symptoms, such as hopelessness and decreased energy, for at least 2 weeks.

Diabetic retinopathy: As a long-term effect of diabetes, the blood vessels to the eyes grow weak and rupture, causing vision loss; may lead to blindness.

Disability: Physical impairment.

Disturbed executive functioning: Planning, organizing, sequencing, and abstracting problems due to frontal lobe damage.

Divided attention: The ability to attend to and analyze two stimuli presented simultaneously.

Dysarthria: Disturbed articulation.

Electroconvulsive therapy: The delivery of an electrical shock that causes electrical activity in the brain.

Electrolarynx: A voice box that produces sounds based on air vibrations.

Expressive (nonfluent) aphasia: Inability to produce language in either an oral or a written form, but relatively intact language comprehension.

Fine motor movement: Movement produced by the small muscle groups.

Fluid intelligence: The acquisition of new information.

Forebrain: A higher-order part of the brain.

Glaucoma: A collection of eye disorders characterized by a buildup of viscous fluid (aqueous humor) in the intraoccular cavity.

Gross motor movement: Movement produced by the large muscle groups.

Gustation: The senses of taste.

Hearing: Perception of auditory stimulation.

Hyperorality: The need to taste and orally examine objects small enough to be placed in the mouth.

Hypothermia: A condition in which an organism's temperature drops below that required for normal metabolism and bodily functions.

Information processing speed: The time it takes to analyze data.

Instrumental activities of daily living (IADLs): More complex tasks that include handling finances, preparing meals, or managing one's medications.

Iris: The colored part of the eye.

Irreversible dementia: Dementia that cannot be cured or reversed with medical or psychological treatment.

Language: The actual selection of words and the integration of words into sentences.

Laryngectomy: An operation used to treat patients with laryngeal or hypopharyngeal cancers.

Lens: Encased in a capsular-like bag and suspended within the eye.

Long-term memory: Large storage capacity for information for long periods of time or even indefinitely.

Macular degeneration: A condition in which neurons in the center part of the retina no longer function.

Mixed hearing loss: A mixture of both sensorineural and conductive hearing loss.

Movement: A change in place or position.

Olfaction: The senses of smell.

Ototoxic substances: Medications or poisons that damage the hearing process.

Parkinson's disease (PD): A chronic neurodegenerative condition characterized by impairment in the nerves that control movement.

Pitch: How high or low a tone sounds.

Presbycusis: Age-related hearing loss (Latin for "old man's hearing").

Presbyopia: A condition in which a person cannot focus as clearly when objects are up close (Latin for "old eyes").

Pressure ulcer: An area of skin that breaks down when a person stays in one position for too long without shifting weight.

Primary aging: The gradual and inevitable process of bodily deterioration that takes place throughout life.

Pseudodementias: Cognitive deficits that resemble dementia but are due to other factors, such as depression or medication use.

Pupil: The opening in the center of the iris.
Receptive (fluent) aphasia: Inability to comprehend spoken or written language, but intact expressive ability.
Retinal detachment: When the retina separates from the back of the eye and fills with vitreous fluid.
Reversible dementia: See *Pseudodementias*.
Sensorineural loss: Sound wave transmission is interrupted from the inner ear to the brain, most likely due to damage to the cochlea and/or auditory nerve.
Short-term memory: Modest capacity for storing information for a few seconds.
Somatosensory system: Provides information about a variety of skin sensations, including temperature, touch, or pain.
Speech: The primary form of communication with our environment; involves both articulation and pronunciation.
Sustained attention: The ability to focus cognitive activity on a stimulus.
Thalamus: A relay station in the center of the brain.
Timber: The quality of a sound.
Tinnitus: A condition in which a person experiences a persistent ringing, buzzing, humming, roaring, or other noise in the ears that only that person can hear.
Touch: One of the five senses; involves feeling or striking.
Velocity: Speed.
Verbal apraxia: A neurological disorder characterized by impairment in initiation, coordination, and sequencing of muscle movement, which results in difficulties executing mouth and speech movements.
Vision: The faculty of sight.
Visual acuity: The ability to identify objects by sight.
Visual illusions: Distorted perceptions of vision.
Wernicke's area: An area in the brain in charge of the meaning of language.

Chapter 5

Affective communication: More informal type of communication that focuses on how the health care provider is caring about the patient and his or her feelings or emotions.
Aphasia: Difficulty with the use of language.
Assistive technology: Any piece of equipment or technology that helps improve the function of individuals with functional limitations.
Augmentative and alternative communication (AAC): An integrated group of components or assistive devices and strategies that help individuals improve communication.
Communication: The act of giving and/or receiving information; can be verbal or nonverbal.
Dysarthria: Impairments in the muscles used in speech.
Instrumental communication: Task-focused type of communication related to assessing and solving problems.
Language: Symbols, sounds, and gestures used by a common group to share thoughts, ideas, and emotions.

Chapter 6

Acquired immunity: The branch of the immune system consisting of humoral immunity and cell-mediated immunity.
Actin: Protein within muscle that, together with myosin, is responsible for muscle contraction.
Adrenal cortex: The outer portion of the adrenal glands.
Adrenal glands: Paired glands located above the kidneys.
Adrenal medulla: The inner portion of the adrenal glands.
Adrenoceptors (α): Control vessel constriction.
Adrenoceptors (β): Trigger vessel dilation.
Adrenocorticotropic hormone (ACTH): Pituitary hormone stimulating the release of glucocorticoids and sex hormones from the adrenal cortex.
Aldosterone: A mineralocorticoid targeting the kidneys and regulating fluid–electrolyte balance.
Alveoli: Tiny, spongy air sacs that are the functional units of the lungs and the site of gas exchange.
Amino acid neurotransmitters: Glutamate is the major excitatory neurotransmitter and gamma-aminobutyric acid (GABA) is the major inhibitory neurotransmitter.
Andropause: Loss of androgen hormone such as testosterone in aging males.

Anemia: A disease characterized by a deficiency of erythrocytes.

Anorexia of aging: Age-related decline in food intake.

Antibodies: Antigen-attacking proteins of the immune system.

Antigen: Any foreign substance invading the body.

Apoptosis: Programmed cell death.

Arteries: Carry blood from the heart to the rest of the body or the lungs.

Atria: The two upper chambers of the heart; they receive blood from the venous system.

Autoimmunity: The immune system's attack of the body's own cells.

Autonomic nervous system: Part of the peripheral nervous system; contains the sympathetic and parasympathetic pathways.

B cells: Cells of the immune system that mature in the bone marrow and produce antibodies in response to antigen exposure.

Barorecepter: Sensory nerve ending in vessels that responds to pressure changes.

Baroreflex: Reflex stimulated by baroreceptor activity.

Basic multicellular unit (BMU): Temporary anatomic structure composed of osteoblasts, osteoclasts, vasculature, nerve supply, and connective tissue; responsible for bone modeling and remodeling.

Calcitonin: A hormone of the thyroid gland that stimulates increased uptake of calcium by bone-forming cells.

Cardiac output: The amount of blood pumped by the heart per minute.

Cartilaginous joints: Joints composed of two bones separated by a layer of cartilage.

Catecholamines: Hormones of the adrenal medulla released in response to sympathetic nervous system activity.

CD34$^+$ cells: The primary circulating progenitor stem cells.

Cell-mediated immunity: The branch of acquired immunity responsible for destroying intracellular antigens.

Chemoreceptors: Receptors related to the abilities to smell and taste.

Cholinergic neurons: Neurons that release the neurotransmitter acetylcholine, which plays a significant role in learning and memory in humans and animals.

Chronological aging: The process of physiological change caused only by the passage of time.

Clonal expansion: A process through which B and T cells of the immune system multiply to produce cellular clones.

Colon: Another term for the large intestine; extends from the small intestine to the rectum.

Complement system: A collection of proteins of the immune system involved in the destruction of antigens and initiation of the inflammatory response.

Cortical bone: The outer layer of bone; also known as compact bone.

Corticotropin-releasing hormone (CRH): Hypothalamic hormone that stimulates release of adrenocorticotropic hormone from the pituitary gland.

Cortisol: The primary glucocorticoid in the human body and a hormone regulating the stress response.

Cytokines: Chemical messengers of the immune, hematopoietic, and other physiological systems.

Dehydroepiandrosterone (DHEA): An adrenal sex hormone able to convert to a multitude of other hormones, primarily estrogen and testosterone.

Dermis: The intermediate layer of the skin.

Detrusor: Muscle in the bladder that assists with voiding.

Diaphragm: A sheet of muscle located across the bottom of the chest that aids in respiration through its contraction and relaxation.

Diastole: Relaxation of ventricles when filling with blood.

Dopaminergic system: Releases dopamine, affecting motor control.

Elastic recoil: A measure of the lungs' ability to expand and contract.

Epidermis: The thin, outermost layer of the skin.

Epinephrine: A catecholamine of the adrenal medulla that regulates the body's stress response; also known as adrenaline.

Erythrocytes: Red blood cells.

Esophagus: extends from the pharynx to the stomach.

Extrinsic aging: Aging due to chronic exposure to external factors such as smoking.

Fast-twitch fibers: Muscle fibers that provide short bursts of energy but fatigue easily; used in activities of high intensity and low endurance.

Follicle-Stimulating hormone: Hormone released from the pituitary that stimulates follicle production in females and sperm in males.

Forced expiratory volume (FEV): The amount of air that can be forcefully expelled in 1 second.

Free radicals: A molecule with an unpaired electron in the outer shell of electrons that remains unstable until paired with another molecule.

Gallbladder: A small sac located below the liver that stores the bile sent from the liver.

Gastrointestinal immunity: Antibodies in the intestine that block antigens and bacteria in addition to neutralizing toxins.

Glomerular filtration rate: Kidney filtration system for waste and toxins.

Glomeruli: Bundles of capillaries located in the kidneys.

Glucagon: A pancreatic hormone regulating blood glucose levels through stimulation of the release of stored glucose.

Glucocorticoids: Hormones of the adrenal cortex involved in both metabolic and anti-inflammatory functions.

Glucose tolerance: The ability to respond effectively to dramatic rises in blood glucose levels.

GLUT4: An insulin-mediated glucose transporter protein located within cytoplasmic vesicles.

Gonadotropin-releasing hormone (GnRH): Released by the hypothalamus and stimulates the synthesis and release of follicle-stimulating hormone (FSH) and luteinizing hormone (LH).

Growth hormone (GH): A pituitary hormone that stimulates amino acid uptake and synthesis of proteins.

Hematopoiesis: The process of blood cell production.

Homeostasis: The ability to maintain balance in the organ systems.

Hormones: Chemical messengers of the endocrine system.

Humoral immunity: The branch of acquired immunity mediated by antibodies and responsible for defending the body against extracellular antigens.

Hypogeusia: Age-related decline in taste.

Hypophysiotropic: Acting on the pituitary gland.

Hypothalamic-pituitary-adrenal (HPA) axis: Regulates glucocorticoid levels in the body and allows the body to respond to stressful conditions.

Immovable joints: Joints composed of collagen fibers that allow only minimal bone shifting; also known as fibrous joints.

Immunosenescence: Aging of the immune system.

Inflammatory response: Redness, swelling, and warmth produced in response to infection.

Inhibin B: Glycoprotein that suppresses FSH.

Innate immunity: The branch of the immune system with which a person is born and that is the body's first line of defense against invading antigens.

Insulin: A pancreatic hormone regulating blood glucose levels through stimulation of glucose uptake.

Insulin resistance: A resistance to the actions of insulin.

Islets of Langerhans: Glandular cells of the pancreas.

Keratinocytes: Cells of the epidermis that produce the protein keratin.

Killer T cells: T cells that directly attack and destroy infected cells within the body; also termed cytotoxic T cells.

Langerhans cells: Cells of the epidermis involved in immune response.

Leukocytes: White blood cells.

Lipofuscin: A brown pigment found in aging cells relating to oxidative mechanisms.

Liver: The largest gland in the body; secretes bile in the small intestine and screens blood from the stomach and intestines for toxins.

Luteinizing hormone (LH): A hormone released from the pituitary that stimulates ovulation and corpus luteum growth in females; stimulates testosterone production in males.

Macrophage: An immune cell that acts as a scavenger, engulfing foreign substances, dead cells, and other debris through phagocytosis.

Mechanoreceptors: Receptors related to the ability to touch.

Melanin: A pigment produced by melanocytes and essential to protecting the body against ultraviolet radiation.

Melanocytes: Cells located within the epidermis that produce melanin.

Melatonin: A pineal gland hormone that synchronizes internal body functions to a day–night cycle.

Menopause: Cessation of menstrual cycles within the aging female.

Mineralocorticoids: Hormones of the adrenal cortex involved in the regulation of extracellular mineral concentrations.

Monoaminergic system: Release of the neurotransmitters norepinephrine and serotonin.

Motor unit: The combination of a single nerve and all the muscle fibers it innervates.

Muscle quality: Strength generated per unit of muscle mass.

Muscle strength: The capacity of muscle to generate force.

Myocardial cells: Cells located in the heart, also known as cardiomyocytes.

Myofibril: A contractile filament that comprises skeletal muscle fibers; composed of actin and myosin proteins.

Myosin: Protein within muscle that, together with actin, is responsible for muscle contraction.

Natural killer (NK) cells: Cells of the immune system that attack and destroy infected cells.

Nephrons: Located in the kidneys; combination of the Bowman's capsule and renal tubule with the glomerulus.

Nerve cells: Neurons within the nervous system that transmit chemical and electrical signals.

Neurogenesis: Formation of new neurons.

Neurotransmitter: Chemical messengers located in synaptic vesicles in the neuron.

Nocturia: An increased number of fluid voids occurring at night.

Norepinephrine: A catecholamine of the adrenal medulla that regulates the stress response; also known as noradrenaline.

Olfaction: The ability to smell.

Osteoblast: Bone cell responsible for formation of new bone and repair of damaged or broken bone.

Osteoclast: Bone cell responsible for bone resorption.

Osteocyte: Dormant osteoblast embedded in bone matrix.

Pancreas: A gland located below the stomach and above the small intestine; secretes pancreatic fluid that neutralizes stomach acid and breaks down large nutrients.

Parathyroid gland: A group of cells located at the back of the thyroid gland that secretes parathyroid hormone.

Parathyroid hormone (PTH): A hormone of the parathyroid gland involved in promoting elevation of blood calcium levels.

Pharynx: Connects the oral cavity to the esophagus.

Photoaging: The process of change in skin structure and function resulting only from exposure to ultraviolet radiation.

Pineal gland: A small gland located deep in the brain that secretes melatonin.

Plaques: Made up of the amyloid β-peptide shown to be neurotoxic; occur outside of the neuronal cell and consist of gray matter with a protein core surrounded by abnormal neurites.

Plasma cell: An antibody-producing B cell.

Plasticity: The ability to form new neuronal connections onto available existing neurons.

Pluripotent stem cells: Cells possessing the ability to differentiate into cells of any other type.

Presbycusis: Age-related hearing loss that generally occurs at higher frequencies first.

Presbyopia: Age-related vision loss of objects at close range; known as farsightedness.

Replicative senescence: A phenomenon in which cells are able to undergo only a finite number of divisions.

Reproductive axis: Integration of the hypothalamus, pituitary, and gonad to control reproductive hormones.

Sarcomere: Muscle compartments containing actin and myosin.

Sarcopenia: Age-related loss of muscle mass.

Sarcoplasmic reticulum: A portion of the endoplasmic reticulum; membrane network in the cell cytoplasm in striated muscle fibers.

Skeletal muscle: Muscle under voluntary control; comprises the majority of all muscle mass and is also known as voluntary or striated muscle.

Slow-twitch fibers: Muscle fibers that contract steadily but are not easily fatigued; used in activities of low intensity and high endurance.

Stem cell progenitors: The progeny cells of pluripotent stem cells.

Subcutaneous layer: The innermost layer of the skin.

Suppressor T cells: T cells that suppress the immune response.

Synapses: Space between the dendrites on neurons where chemical signals via neurotransmitters are relayed to other neurons.

Synaptogenesis: Generation of new synapses.

Synovial fluid: Fluid secreted by the synovium that allows smooth, easy movement of the bones comprising a synovial joint.

Synovial joint: Joint connecting two bones containing smooth cartilage on their opposing ends.

Synovium: Synovial joint capsule membrane that secretes synovial fluid.

Systole: Contraction of the heart that forces blood into the aorta.

T cells: Cells of the immune system that mature in the thymus and play a critical role in cell-mediated immunity.

Tangles: Paired helical filaments and a few straight filaments that occur in the neuronal cell body; the main protein associated with neurofibrillary tangles is known as tau.

T-helper cells: T cells that regulate the immune system.

Thrombocytes: Blood platelets responsible for blood clotting.

Thyroid: A small, butterfly-shaped gland located in the lower front portion of the neck.

Thyroid-stimulating hormone (TSH): A pituitary hormone stimulating the synthesis and release of triiodothyronine and thyroxine.

Thyroxine (T4): A thyroid hormone involved in metabolic and thermal regulation.

Total lung capacity: The maximum volume to which the lungs can expand during the greatest inspiratory effort.

Trabecular bone: The inner portion of bone; also known as spongy bone.

Triiodothyronine (T3): A thyroid hormone involved in metabolic and thermal regulation.

Ureters: Tubes connecting the kidneys to the bladder.

Urethra: Canal that leads from the bladder out of the body.

Vasopressin: A pituitary hormone responsible for regulation of blood and osmotic pressure.

Ventilatory rate: The volume of air inspired in a normal breath multiplied by the frequency of breaths per minute; also known as the minute respiratory rate.

Ventricles: The two lower chambers of the heart; the left ventricle expels oxygen-rich blood into the aorta to be delivered to the entire body excluding the lungs, and the right ventricle expels oxygen-poor blood into pulmonary arteries traveling to the lungs for reoxygenation.

Vital capacity: The maximum amount of air that can be expelled from the lungs following a maximum inspiration.

Chapter 7

Agnosia: Loss of ability to understand auditory, visual, or other sensations.

Aphasia: Impaired ability to communicate.

Apraxia: Inability to perform purposeful movements.

Cataracts: A clouding of the lens of the eye, its capsule, or both.

Cerumen: Ear wax.

Dysphagia: Difficulty in swallowing.

Functional incontinence: The genitourinary tract is functioning and incontinence is due to immobility or cognitive limitations.

Glaucoma: An eye disease of increased intraocular pressure that can lead to blindness if not treated.

Ketones: Acetone bodies in the urine indicating inadequate management of diabetes mellitus.

Longevity: A long life.

Macular degeneration: Loss of central vision, associated with aging.

Osteoarthritis: Deterioration of joints and vertebrae as a consequence of wear and tear.

Osteoporosis: Reduction in bone mass leading to thin, weak bones.

Otosclerosis: Damage to the inner ear of unknown cause that leads to progressive deafness.

Overflow incontinence: Incontinence that occurs because the bladder has not been emptied and it has become overdistended.

Polydipsia: Excessive thirst.

Polyphagia: Excessive eating.

Polyuria: Excessive urination.

Presbycusis: Age-related progressive loss of hearing.

Presbyopia: Age-related loss of elasticity of the lens of the eye.

Stress incontinence: Leaking of urine occurs during activities that increase abdominal pressure, such as laughing, sneezing, and exercising.

Urge incontinence: Incontinence occurs because of an inability to delay urination.

Chapter 8

Absorption: Movement of drugs from the point of entry to the body into the bloodstream.

Activities of daily living (ADL): Self-care activities, including washing, bathing, grooming, dressing, toileting, eating, and mobility.

Adherence: Compliance with a prescribed medication regimen.

Adverse drug reaction (ADR): Any noxious or unintended reaction to a drug that is administered in standard doses by the proper route for the purpose of prophylaxis, diagnosis, or treatment.

Compliance: Taking the prescribed medication at the right time, in the right dose, by the right route, by the right person.

Distribution: Movement of a drug from plasma into the cells.

Drug–disease interaction: The worsening of a disease by a medication.

Drug–drug interaction: Alteration of the pharmacodynamics of Drug A when taken at the same time as Drug B.

Excretion: Elimination of a drug from the body after metabolism.

Food–drug interaction: Alteration in pharmacodynamics of a drug when taken with food or certain foods.

Function: The physiological activity of a body part.

Instrumental activities of daily living (IADLs): Higher level ADLs—preparing meals, shopping, managing money, using the telephone, and performing housework.

Metabolism: The process by which the body breaks down and converts medication into active chemical substances.

Peak blood level: Blood test done to measure the level of medication in the blood; drawn when the highest amount of medication in the bloodstream is expected to be present.

Pharmacodynamics: The time course and effect of drugs on cellular and organ function.

Pharmacokinetics: The time course by which the body absorbs, distributes, metabolizes, and excretes drugs.

Polypharmacy: The prescription, administration, or use of more medications than are clinically indicated in a given patient.

Random blood level: Blood test done to measure the level of medication in the blood; drawn without regard to the time of administration of the drug.

Trough blood level: Blood test done to measure the level of medication in the blood; drawn immediately before the next scheduled dose of medication.

Chapter 9

Adult learning theory: Developed by Malcolm Knowles, applies principles to enhance learning in adults over 18 years old who have completed mandatory public education.

Andragogy: Related to the teaching of adults.

Baby boomers: People born between the years 1946 and 1964, after World War II.

Cultural diversity: Ethnic, gender, racial, and socioeconomic variety in a situation, institution, or group; the coexistence of different ethnic, gender, racial, and socioeconomic groups within one social unit.

Gerogogy: Related to the teaching of older adults.

Health disparity: Differences in mortality and morbidity of illness based on culture and ethnic background.

Health literacy: The degree to which individuals have the capacity to obtain, process, and understand basic health information and services needed to make appropriate health decisions.

Lifelong learning: Learning that occurs throughout life, motivated by situational and developmental periods.

Social cognitive theory (SCT): States that behavior, cognitive factors, and the environment influence outcome expectations; outcome expectations are a person's beliefs that when he or she engages in a certain behavior, certain outcomes will result.

Theory of self-efficacy: The belief that one's actions influence outcomes; self-efficacy and outcome expectations affect behavior, motivation, thought patterns, and emotions.

Chapter 10

Basic activities of daily living (BADLs): Functions involved in maintaining personal physical care; bathing, toileting, dressing, feeding.

Frailty: General decline in the physical function of older adults.

Functional ability: Personal capacity to maintain activities of daily living.

Independence: Ability to care for oneself.

Instrumental activities of daily living (IADLs): Functions involved in maintaining a household; cleaning, cooking, shopping, paying bills, keeping appointments.

Living skills: Ability to meet the tasks of daily self-care.

Quality of life: Features that define a person's satisfaction with the circumstances of his or her life situation.

Restraints: Any device, material, or equipment attached or adjacent to the body that the individual cannot remove easily and that restricts freedom of movement or access to one's own body.

Chapter 11

Center for Science in the Public Interest: The nation's premier educational and advocacy organization for promoting better nutritional habits.

Exercise: Continuous physical activity.

Green House: An innovative and home-like alternative to nursing homes developed by the physician William Thomas and supported by the Robert Wood Johnson Foundation for the purpose of national replication.

Health contract/calendar: A behavior-changing tool that relies on the self-management capability of a client, after initial assistance is provided by a clinician or a health educator.

Healthy People initiatives: Ten-year initiatives led by the U.S. Public Health Service in an effort to reduce preventable death and disability for Americans.

Life review: A series of questions that help guide older adults in the task of recording their life stories; activity directors and others can help older adults on a one-on-one basis or by facilitating group experiences.

Medicare prevention: Free or partially reimbursed prevention interventions for eligible Medicare recipients.

Model health promotion programs: Programs that have received federal funding and foundation support to evaluate their effectiveness, and to encourage their replication.

MyPyramid: The 2005 revised Food Guide Pyramid with an associated Web site that provides an interactive food guidance system.

Nutrition: Source of nourishment; food.

Nutrition bull's-eye: An educational tool that helps clients differentiate specific foods and drinks on the basis of fat, sugar, sodium, and fiber.

Re-engagement: The likely alternative to retirement for a baby boom cohort blessed with longevity, education, health, and a positive attitude toward remaining engaged.

Surgeon General's Report on Physical Activity and Health: The 1996 government report that provides an outstanding review of the research on the effects of physical activity on people's health.

Chapter 12

Activities of daily living (ADLs): Activities performed in the course of daily life; they include bathing, dressing, transferring, walking, eating, and continence.

Adult protective services (APS) agency: A social service agency designed to investigate and intervene when complaints of elder abuse or neglect are reported. APS agencies are generally organized as a division of local county government social service agencies (Teaser, Dugar, Mendiondo, Abner, & Cecil, 2006).

Chronic Disease Self-Management program: A care model developed by Dr. Kate Lorig, at Stanford University, to facilitate self-management of chronic illnesses. Clients have been shown to benefit by improved self-efficacy when they are taught to improve symptom management, maintain functional ability, and adhere to their medication regimens (Lorig & Holman, 2000).

Contracting: A specific agreement between the nurse and client in which a behavior change is described and a plan for the change is committed to paper.

Dietary Approaches to Stop Hypertension (DASH) diet: A diet promoted by the U.S. Department of Health and Human Services that has been proven to be palatable and effective in lowering blood pressure. It is rich in potassium, magnesium, and calcium, and low in salt (U.S. Department of Health and Human Services, National Institute of Health, & National Heart, Lung, and Blood Institute, 2006).

Framingham Heart Study: A 50-year, longitudinal study of over 5,000 subjects designed to identify factors that cause and prevent cardiovascular disease (National Heart, Lung, and Blood Institute & Boston University, 2007).

Functional decline: Decreased ability to independently perform activities of independent living or instrumental activities of daily living, such as dressing, bathing, shopping, and bill paying.

Health promotion: Activities aimed at improving or enhancing health.

Health screening: Population-wide efforts to detect early disease.

Healthy People 2010: An initiative of the U.S. Department of Health and Human Services that set forth health care objectives designed to increase the quality and quantity of years of healthy life of Americans and to eliminate health disparities (Healthy People 2010, 2005).

Instrumental activities of daily living (IADLs): Activities related to independent living; they include meal preparation, money management, shopping, housework, and using a telephone.

Nutrition Screening Initiative: A multidisciplinary effort led by the American Academy of Family Physicians and the American Dietetic Association to promote the integration of nutrition screening and dietary interventions into health care for the elderly (American Academy of Family Physicians Clinical Care and Research, 2005).

Primary prevention: Activities designed to completely prevent a disease from occurring, such as immunization against pneumonia or influenza.

Secondary prevention: Efforts directed toward early detection and management of disease, such as the use of colonoscopy to detect small, cancerous polyps.

Tertiary prevention: Efforts used to manage clinical diseases in order to prevent them from progressing or to avoid complications of the disease, as is done when beta blockers are used to help remodel the heart in congestive heart failure.

U.S. Preventive Services Task Force (USPSTF): A task force convened by the U.S. Public Health Service to systematically review the evidence of effectiveness of clinical preventive services. Its mission is to evaluate the benefits of individual services and to create age-, gender-, and risk-based recommendations about services that should routinely be incorporated into primary medical care (USPSTF, 2004).

Chapter 13

Activities of daily living (ADLs): Include activities such as dressing, grooming, eating, toileting, and oral-facial hygiene.

Age-related macular degeneration (ARMD): A condition associated with aging in which the macula of the eye deteriorates, causing loss of central vision.

Alzheimer's disease (AD): A terminal neurological disorder characterized by deterioration of the brain leading to progressive forgetfulness and loss of independence.

Angina: Chest pain resulting from lack of oxygen to the heart muscle.

Atherosclerosis: Hardening and narrowing of the arteries to the heart from plaque buildup in vessel walls.

Benign paroxysmal positional vertigo (BPPV): One of the more common and treatable causes of dizziness in older adults resulting from otoconia being displaced in the ear canal.

Benign prostatic hyperplasia (BPH): Enlargement of the prostate gland that often occurs with advanced age.

Bone mineral density (BMD): Screening test for osteoporosis.

Cardiovascular disease (CVD): Includes hypertension, coronary heart disease, congestive heart failure, and stroke.

Cataracts: Clouding of the lens.

Cerebrovascular accident (CVA): Stroke; brain attack.

Chronic bronchitis: A type of COPD characterized by increased mucus production and scarring of bronchial tubes that obstructs airflow.

Chronic obstructive pulmonary disease (COPD): A group of diseases related to obstructed airflow in the lungs.

Congestive heart failure (CHF): A chronic deficiency in the heart's ability to pump blood to the body.

Continuous bladder irrigation (CBI): Used after a TURP to flush the bladder.

Corneal ulcers: Irritation of the cornea that may be caused by stroke, infection, fever, or trauma, and often results in scarring.

Coronary artery disease (CAD): Also called coronary heart disease or ischemic heart disease; results from atherosclerosis.

Coronary heart disease (CHD): Includes myocardial infarction, angina, and other conditions.

Cystectomy: Surgical removal of the bladder.

Delirium: Acute confusion characterized by cognitive perceptual disturbances of short duration.

Diabetic retinopathy: Impaired vision due to bleeding in the retina from ruptured vessels.

Diverticulitis: Inflammation of the intestinal diverticuli.

Dysphagia: Difficulty with eating or swallowing.

Emphysema: A type of COPD that causes irreversible lung damage and results in decreased gas exchange at the alveolar level related to loss of elasticity.

Erectile dysfunction (ED): Impotence.

Gastroesophageal reflux disease (GERD): When gastric acid and/or stomach contents come up into the esophagus.

Glaucoma: A group of degenerative eye diseases whereby vision is damaged by high intraocular pressure.

Gonioscopy: Tool to directly examine the eye.

Helicobacter pylori: A common bacterial contributor to symptoms of gastritis and peptic ulcers.

Hemiparesis: Weakness of one side of the body.

Hemiplegia: Paralysis of one side of the body.

Herpes zoster: The virus that causes chicken pox and shingles.

Histamine 2 (H_2) blockers: Medications used for the treatment of GERD.

Hypertension: Currently defined as a consistently elevated reading of 140/90 mm Hg.

Incontinence: Involuntary loss of stool or urine.

Instrumental activities of daily living (IADLs): Include such activities as shopping, using the telephone, and balancing the checkbook.

Intraocular pressure (IOP): The amount of pressure inside the eye; normal is 9–21 mm HG.

Mauk model for poststroke recovery: A theoretical model derived using grounded theory methods that suggests a common process for stroke recovery and rehabilitation.

Meniere's syndrome: A common cause of vertigo in the elderly characterized by dizziness and tinnitus.

Mini Mental State Examination (MMSE): A brief series of questions to help determine the presence of cognitive impairment.

Myocardial infarction (MI): Heart attack.

Osteoporosis: Demineralization of the bones; decreased bone density.

Otoconia: "Stones" in the ear canal that affect balance.

Parkinson's disease (PD): A neurological disorder characterized by lack of dopamine in the brain secondary to loss of neurons in the basal ganglia.

Peripheral artery disease (PAD): A problem with blood flow in the arteries due to blockage or narrowing.

Peripheral vascular disease (PVD): The most common form of peripheral artery disease.

Phantom limb pain: Pain in an absent/amputated extremity.

Proliferative retinopathy: The fourth and most advanced stage of diabetic retinopathy in which abnormal and fragile vessels develop to compensate for blocked blood flow to the retina; this leads to visual disturbances and often blindness.

Prostate-specific antigen (PSA): A screening test for prostate cancer.

Radical prostatectomy: Surgical removal of the prostate as a treatment for cancer.

Retinal detachment: Situation in which the retina becomes displaced due to trauma or illness and requires immediate medical attention to restore vision.

Scatter laser treatment: Treatment for diabetic retinopathy in which a laser burns abnormal vessels away from the retina to reduce further vision loss.

Stroke: An interruption of the blood supply to the brain.

Tinnitus: Ringing in the ears.

Tonometer: An instrument used to measure intraocular pressure.

t-PA (tissue plasminogen activator): Used to treat acute ischemic stroke.

Transient ischemic attack (TIA): Stroke symptoms that last from minutes to less than 24 hours with no residual effects.

Transurethral resection of the prostate (TURP): Surgical intervention for BPH.

Tuberculosis (TB): Disease caused by *Mycobacterium tuberculosis;* can affect any body part, but particularly the lungs.

Urostomy: Stoma through which urine passes into a receptacle on the outside of the body, used when the bladder has been removed.

Vitrectomy: Evacuation of the vitreous humor in order to remove blood that has leaked from damaged vessels in diabetic retinopathy.

Chapter 14

Adverse drug reaction (ADR): A detrimental response to a given medication that is undesired, unintended, or unexpected in recommended doses.

Bladder diary: A daily record of the time and volume of fluid intake, voiding, and incontinence episodes with associated activities.

Bladder training: An intervention that focuses on providing patients with the tools to delay urination and suppress urgency in order to establish more normal voiding intervals.

Braden Scale for Pressure Ulcer Risk Assessment: An instrument that determines the risk of pressure ulcer development.

Chemical restraint: The use of a psychopharmacological drug for the purpose of discipline or convenience, and that is not required to treat medical symptoms.

Deglutition: The act of swallowing in which a food or liquid bolus is transported from the mouth through the pharynx and esophagus into the stomach.

Delirium: Manifests as a disturbance in consciousness, or cognitive or perceptual change that develops over time, fluctuates during the course of the day, and is a physiological consequence of a medical condition or medication.

Dementia: A group of symptoms, accompanying disease, that manifests as memory loss, disorientation, changes in mood or personality, and difficulties in abstract thinking, task performance, and language use.

Dependent continence: Requires the assistance (physical help, cues, or supervision) of another person to maintain continence.

Depression: A disorder that includes changes in feelings or mood, described as feeling sad, hopeless, pessimistic, or "blue," lasting most of the day, with loss of interest in pleasurable activities.

Drug–drug interaction: An interaction that occurs when two or more drugs are taken concurrently.

Dysphagia: Problems with swallowing.

Established incontinence: Incontinence that persists beyond resolution of acute causes or is longstanding.

Extrinsic risk factors for falls: Environmental hazards and challenges that cause or contribute to falls.

Fall: An event that results in a person unintentionally coming to rest on the ground or lower surface.

Functional urinary incontinence: Incontinence that results from factors external to the lower urinary tract such as cognitive impairments, physical disabilities, and environmental barriers.

Generalized anxiety disorder (GAD): Characterized by persistent, excessive worry with fluctuating severity of symptoms that include restlessness, irritability, sleep disturbance, fatigue, and impaired concentration.

Independent continence: Continence or control that is based on the competence of the individual and does not require the assistance of others.

Insomnia: Difficulty falling asleep or staying asleep.

Intrinsic risk factors for falls: Changes associated with aging and with physical functioning needed to maintain balance.

Medication error: Taking the wrong medicine, or the wrong dose at the wrong time or for the wrong purpose.

Mixed urinary incontinence: The existence of urge and stress urinary incontinence symptoms at the same time.

Nocturia: The awakening from sleep to urinate more than once during the night.

Nonadherance: A person's unwillingness to follow the instructions given for a medication or treatment.

Nonrapid eye movement (NREM) sleep: Part of the sleep cycle that does not include rapid eye movement.

Overflow urinary incontinence: Urine leakage that occurs when the bladder is overdistended.

Panic disorder: Characterized by an autonomic arousal that includes tachycardia, difficulties breathing, diaphoresis, light-headedness, trembling, and severe weakness.

Partial continence: Situations in which a caregiver's assistance is sometimes needed to maintain continence, but is not required all the time.

Pelvic muscle rehabilitation: An exercise program designed to increase the strength, tone, and control of the pelvic floor muscles to facilitate a person's ability to voluntarily control the flow of urine and suppress urgency.

Pharmacodynamics: The biochemical or physiological interactions of drugs or "what the drugs do to the body."

Pharmacokinetics: The absorption, distribution, metabolism, and excretion of a drug or "what the body does to the drug."

Physical restraint: Any physical or mechanical device that involuntarily restrains a patient as a means of controlling physical activity.

Polypharmacy: The act of taking many medications concurrently.

Pressure ulcer: A lesion caused by unrelieved pressure with damage to the underlying tissue.

Pressure Ulcer Scale for Healing (PUSH): A tool that provides a consistent method of recording the healing of a pressure ulcer or the effectiveness of treatment.

Prompted voiding (PV): A scheduled intervention aimed at helping the individual recognize and act effectively on the sensation of the need to void.

Rapid eye movement (REM) sleep: Part of the sleep cycle, characterized by rapid eye movements and that is associated with deeper, more quality sleep.

Recurrent falls: More than two falls in a 6-month period.

Restless leg syndrome: A disorder in which a person experiences periodic leg movements during sleep.

Sleep apnea: A sleep disorder characterized by cessation of breathing.

Social continence: Situations in which continence cannot be achieved, but urine leakage is contained to maintain dignity and comfort.

Stress urinary incontinence: The involuntary loss of urine during activities that increase intra-abdominal pressure, such as lifting, coughing, or sneezing.

Total urinary incontinence: Complete involuntary loss of urine; may be from mixed causes.

Transient incontinence: Incontinence caused by the onset of an acute problem that once successfully treated will result in resolution of the UI.

Urge suppression techniques: Strategies that help control bladder contractions and therefore minimize or resolve urgency.

Urge urinary incontinence: Associated with a strong, abrupt desire to void and the inability to inhibit leakage before reaching the toilet.

Urinary incontinence (UI): The involuntary leakage of urine.

Chapter 15

Acetylcholine: A neurotransmitter that plays an important role in learning and memory.

Agnosia: Loss of ability to recognize common objects in the environment.

Alzheimer's disease: The most common type of dementia.

Anticholinergic: Medications that block acetylcholine and can cause or worsen confusion.

Aphasia: Loss of the ability to use language.

Apolipoprotein E: A protein that carries cholesterol in blood and that appears to play some role in brain function. Variants of this gene are associated with the development of Alzheimer's disease.

Apraxia: Loss of capacity to do simple movements (e.g., brush one's teeth), unrelated to the physical ability to perform.

Beta-amyloid plaques: Deposits found in the spaces between nerve cells in the brain that are made of beta amyloid.

Cholinesterase: An enzyme that degrades acetylcholine.

Cholinesterase inhibitor: A medication that inhibits cholinesterase and indirectly increases acetylcholine. Used as a treatment for Alzheimer's disease.

Delirium: Acute confusion caused by physiological illness.

Dementia: A broad term referring to the symptoms associated with a progressive decline in cognitive function to the extent that it interferes with daily life and activities.

Depression: A mood disorder, common in persons with dementia.

Executive function: Higher level function of the cerebral cortex supporting abstraction, planning, sequencing, and decision making ability.

Hallucinations: False sensory beliefs, such as seeing, hearing, feeling, tasting, or smelling things that others do not.

Neurofibrillary tangles: Collections of twisted tau found in the cell bodies of neurons; a symptom of Alzheimer's disease.

Neurotransmitter: A chemical messenger between neurons.

Paranoia: False beliefs that others are conspiring against oneself; unfounded mistrust of others.

Chapter 16

Assistive device: "Any item, piece of equipment, or product system, whether acquired commercially off the shelf, modified, or customized, that is used to increase, maintain, or improve functional capabilities of individuals with disabilities" (U.S. Congress, 1988).

Assistive technology: Technological tools used to access education, employment, recreation, or communication, enabling someone to live as independently as possible.

Augmentative and alternative communication (AAC): All forms of communication that enhance or supplement speech and writing, either temporarily or permanently or that involve the use of personalized methods or devices to aid a person's ability to communicate.

Emergency response system (ERS): A device that evaluates self-care and/or physiologic parameters and allows a person at high risk (for example, an older person who lives alone and has a health problem) to get immediate help in the event of an emergency.

Environmental controls: Electronic systems that allow individuals to control lights, heating and cooling, and just about any electrical piece of equipment, such as curtains, garage doors, and gates, from a remote location.

Internet: A vast collection of resources that includes people, information, and multimedia and is best characterized as the biggest labyrinth of computer networks on earth.

Nursing informatics: A blending of computer, information, and nursing science designed to assist in the management and processing of nursing data, information, and knowledge to support the practice of nursing and the delivery of nursing care.

World Wide Web: A system of clients (Web browsers or software applications used to locate and display Web pages) and servers that use the Internet for data exchange.

Chapter 17

Advance directive: Legal document that records decisions regarding life-saving or life-sustaining care and actions to be taken in a situation where the patient is no longer able to provide informed consent.

Advocacy: The act or process of pleading the case of another.

Autonomy: Referring to self-governance or self-directing freedom; being in charge of one's own being; having moral independence.

Beneficence: Doing or producing good.

Codes of ethics: Codes of moral reasoning used by members of a profession to direct the moral behavior of their work.

Competence: Having the capacity to function or respond; having requisite or adequate abilities or qualities to perform a task or respond to a situation. Mental competence is evaluated to determine whether a person has adequate capacity to make informed decisions.

Confidentiality: Being entrusted with confidences. Maintaining confidentiality is required to protect the right of privacy.

Conflict: Occurs when a choice must be made between two equal choices.

Conflict of interest: Conflict that arises from competing loyalties and opportunities. This may include conflicts between the nurse's value system and choices made by the patients, their families, other health care team members, the organization, or the insurance company, or when incentive systems or other financial gains create conflict between professional integrity and self-interest.

Cost-benefit analysis: A strategy used in decision making regarding the advantages and disadvantages of financial situations.

Dilemma: Occurs when it appears there are no acceptable choices. To qualify as a dilemma, there must be active engagement in the situation that forces an evaluation of and need for choices. Actions are uncertain because alternatives are equally unattractive.

Ethics of care: Ethical principles applied to health care situations.

Failure to rescue: Neglecting to take action or to recognize a preventable complication.

Fidelity: The state of being faithful and loyal, referring to allegiance to another.

Fiduciary responsibility: An ethical obligation to good stewardship of both the patient's and the organization's funds.

Informed consent: Consent that has been granted, not assumed, following an educational process that facilitates the weighing of benefits, risks, and available options.

Justice: Conformity to principles of what is right and fair; establishment of rights following rules of equity.

Moral dilemma: Arises when two or more moral principles apply that support mutually inconsistent actions.

Moral distress: Occurs when someone wants to do the right thing but is limited by the constraints of the organization or society.

Moral principles: Those values, ethics, beliefs, and positions that guide behavior and thought.

Moral uncertainty: The confusion surrounding situations in which a person is uncertain what the moral problem is or which moral principles or values apply to it.

Nonmaleficence: Not committing harm or evil.

Paternalism: Using authority to regulate the behaviors of others; directing and controlling the behaviors of others because they either are not trusted to have good judgment or are believed to be incapable of making the best decision.

Patient rights: Rights to which patients are entitled; usually defined or described by the organization charged with providing care or protecting patients.

Quality of life: An individual's perception about the value and benefits of life.

Reciprocity: Referring to a mutual exchange of privileges, such as the ability to be true to one's self while respecting and supporting the values and views of another.

Sanctity of life: The belief that all life is of value and that this value is not based on how functional or effective a person's life is, but rather that all have a right to life.

Values: Beliefs and attitudes that reflect a person's thoughts and culture.

Veracity: To tell the truth.

Chapter 18

Acculturation: To adopt the perceived practices of the culture in which one resides.

Culture: Beliefs, values, customs, and traditions that are socially transmitted by a population of people. They are constantly changing and are individual.

Diversity: Differences between persons, whether ethnic, religious, or cultural.

Dyspareunia: Painful intercourse.

Erectile dysfunction (ED): The inability to attain or maintain an erection sufficient for intercourse.

Ethnicity: Identification with a particular religious, racial, national, or cultural group.

Heritage: A person's ethnic origin, nationality, religion, and culture.

Human sexual response: Three phases: excitement, plateau, and orgasm.

Nationality: The geographic location of the person's birth (or the country with which he or she identifies).

Race: Genetic differences having to do with skin and eye color, blood type, and other physical characteristics.

Racism: Discrimination against a person based on race or ethnicity.

Religion: An organized set of beliefs or ways of worship; often associated with a church or denomination.

Sexuality: The total experience of being a sexual being; more than sexual intercourse.

Spirituality: A feeling of connectedness with something higher than oneself, whether it be God, nature, or another being.

Chapter 19

Acute care: Short-term, episodic care.

Assisted living: Living arrangement that provides minimal assistance with activities of daily living and personal care services such as meals and housekeeping.

Copayment: The amount of money one pays to a care provider in addition to what the insurance pays.

Deductible: The amount of money one pays to a care provider before the insurance benefits are activated.

Delayed retirement credit (DRC): Additional money one can earn in addition to full Social Security benefits if one works past age 65.

Home care: Services provided in the home of a home-bound person; may include skilled nursing, therapy, and home health aides.

Life expectancy: How long one can expect to live based on statistical probability; usually calculated at birth and at age 65.

Long-term care: A variety of services to help persons with personal or health care needs over a period of time; usually custodial care in a nursing home type facility.

Medicaid: Title XIX of the Social Security Act; a welfare program.

Medicare: Title XVIII of the Social Security Act; an insurance program.

Minimum Data Set (MDS): Standardized data on resident health and outcomes; used as a quality indicator in nursing homes.

Mortality: Death.

Nursing home: A facility that provides daily help for residents with physical or other problems who are unable to live on their own.

Outcome and Assessment Information Set (OASIS): Standardized information assessing client health and functional status in home care; used as a quality indicator.

Prospective payment system (PPS): System whereby payment to the health care provider is determined before services are used; established to contain cost, particularly in the Medicare system.

Social Security: A federal program that provides financial assistance to the elderly and disabled; federal "old age" pension program.

Chapter 20

Acute care for elders (ACE) unit: A specialized hospital-based unit providing interdisciplinary acute care for older adults.

Geriatric assessment interdisciplinary team (GAIT): An interdisciplinary training model developed in Maryland as an elective for students from various health care disciplines.

Geriatric assessment team (GAT): An interdisciplinary team of professionals specializing in assessment of the elderly.

Geriatric evaluation and management (GEM): Defined inpatient units or services where the elderly are assessed and treated.

Geriatric interdisciplinary team training (GITT): An organized training program for professionals of various disciplines focused on learning about working in teams and the use of teams in gerontology.

Interdisciplinary team: A team in which members of various disciplines interact, collaborate, and work together for common goals.

Intradisciplinary team: A team in which members are within a discipline but members may be at different levels of preparation.

Multidisciplinary team: A team made up of members of various disciplines.

Palliative and hospice care team: A team whose focus is comfort and/or end of life care.

Chapter 21

Acupuncture: Insertion of very thin needles at pathways of meridians in the body to increase the flow of vital energy (qi).

Ayurveda: Traditional medical system of India.

Biofeedback: Use of feedback from a machine to control target functions in the body with the mind; eventually the machine feedback is eliminated.

Biologically based practices: Use of those substances found in nature such as botanicals, vitamins, and minerals.

Chiropractic practice: Manipulation of the skeletal system by trained practitioners to put the body back in balance.

Dosha: Energy in the Ayurvedic medical system.

Guided imagery: Use of imagery to elicit responses in the body.

Homeopathy: Medical system that follows the natural law of "like cures like."

Massage therapy: Manipulation of soft tissues in the body by kneading or other techniques.

Meditation: A conscious process used to produce the relaxation response.

Mind-body medicine: Use of the powers of the mind to alter physical states in the body.

Music therapy: Use of music to enhance physical and psychological well-being.

Naturopathic medicine: A variety of healing practices that support the body to heal itself.

Pet-assisted therapy: Use of animals to decrease stress and increase feelings of well-being.

Prayer: A conversation with a higher being.

Putative energy field: Vital energy that cannot be measured.

Qi (chi): Vital energy in traditional Chinese medicine.

Reiki: Holistic Japanese technique of stress reduction in which life force energy is transferred to the client through the practitioner's hands.

Sound energy therapy: Use of sound frequencies to facilitate healing.

Therapeutic (healing) touch: Movement of the practitioner's hands over a patient's body to balance its energy fields.

Traditional Chinese medicine: The medical system that balances the opposing forces of yin and yang.

Veritable energy field: Energy that can be measured.

Yang: One half of the principle of opposites; it represents the bright, active, upward, hot, male force in traditional Chinese medicine.

Yin: One half of the principle of opposites; it represents the cold, dark, weak, female force in traditional Chinese medicine.

Chapter 22

Active aging: A program with suggestions from the WHO about how to remain independent and active while aging.

Activity: The state of being active.

Autonomy: A person's right to choose and make independent decisions.

Determinants of health: Behavioral, social, and physical environments; personal, economic, and social service systems.

Food Guide Pyramid for Older Adults: Updated food pyramid that depicts the need for older adults to engage in physical activity, drink plenty of fluids, and consume adequate vitamins, as well as have an adequate, balanced diet.

Health related quality of life (HRQOL): A term the CDC has focused on measuring by using an instrument that assesses the number of healthy days an individuals has in a given month.

Independence: A person's ability to direct or carry out his or her own decisions and act autonomously.

Quality of life: How a person rates his or her life as satisfactory or not; best done on a continuum.

Chapter 23

Aggressive: Using intimidation tactics to achieve personal goals.

Assertive: Behavior in which persons are able to defend and protect their own opinions, values, and beliefs and still respect those of others.

Authoritarian: A leadership style in which the leader dictates the behavior of others.

Charismatic leadership: Leading by enthusiasm, empowerment, and motivation of others.

Delegation: The process of assessing, planning, delegating, supervising, and evaluating assigned tasks or duties.

Democratic: A leadership style in which the staff has a voice, a vote, and an opinion, and the majority generally rules.

Intimidation: Using threats, force, or coercion to manipulate the behavior of others.

Laissez-faire: "Laid back" leadership style in which the leader allows others to determine the direction and goals of the group.

Leader: A visionary person with the ability to motivate others to accomplish goals for the greater good.

Manager: A day-to-day coordinator and organizer of activities or care.

Multigenerational nurses: Refers to the four generations of nurses practicing in the workforce today.

Nonassertive: Passive behavior shown by not standing up for one's rights or beliefs.

Situational: Flexible leadership in which the leadership style is chosen based on context and the needs of the group.

Transactional leadership: Leading by an inconsistent system of rewards and consequences.

Transformational leadership: Leading by example, encouragement, and empowerment of the staff.

Unlicensed assistive personnel (UAP): Staff without licenses, such as nursing assistants.

Chapter 24

Addiction: Compulsive psychological dependence on and use of a habit-forming substance, characterized by continued craving and well-defined physiological symptoms upon withdrawal; not considered to be an issue when using opioids for end-of-life and palliative care.

Advance directives: Spoken and written instructions about future medical care and treatment; legal documents outlining a person's wishes for future medical treatments to be (or not to be) provided at some time in the future, at a time when the individual is not able to verbalize or make his or her wishes known. These include a living will, durable power of attorney for health care, and life-prolonging procedures documents; they are only in effect if the individual is unable to make his or her wishes known.

Allow natural death (AND): Used as an advance directive in some locations instead of a DNR (do not resuscitate) order; promotes a more positive approach to consideration of a person's wishes at end of life.

Analgesic ladder: World Health Organization suggestions for implementing increasing strengths/types of pain medications based on increasing symptoms.

Communicating bad news: Module 2 of Education in Palliative and End-of-Life Care (EPEC). This training for medical personnel promotes honest and compassionate discussion about end-of-life care and options for treating life-ending illnesses.

Complementary therapies: Interventions used in collaboration with conventional health care interventions that promote comfort or healing.

Curative care: Medical care focused on healing/cure of disease.

Dependence: Physical response to use of opioids, characterized by withdrawal symptoms when the opioid is stopped.

Do not resuscitate (DNR): A physician's written order instructing health care providers not to attempt cardiopulmonary resuscitation (CPR) in case of cardiac or respiratory arrest.

End of life: Last stages of living; in this context usually caused by a terminal illness.

Five Wishes: An alternative advance directive that gives additional information and explanation about a person's wishes for end-of-life care; not legally recognized in all states.

Good death: Death free from avoidable distress and suffering, according to patient/family wishes, consistent with clinical, cultural, and ethical standards.

Grief: A natural and normal reaction to a loss of any kind.

Hope: To expect with confidence.

Hospice care: A program to deliver palliative care to individuals in the final stages of a terminal illness; additionally provides personal support and care to the patient, and supports to the patient's family/caregivers while the patient is dying; provides bereavement support after the patient's death.

Interdisciplinary group/team (IDG/IDT): Professional staff and volunteers who focus on physical, emotional, psychological, social, and spiritual aspects of a person in designing and/or implementing holistic care; common in hospice and palliative care and other care settings.

Mourning: The outward demonstration of a person's grief responses to a loss.

Pain scales: Measurement options by which medical personnel can translate a person's self-assessment of pain for appropriate intervention decisions.

Palliative care: Concept of care designed to promote comfort and holistic management of symptoms at any stage of illness or disease.

SUPPORT study: The Study to Understand Prognoses and Preferences for Outcomes and Risks of Treatment; it revealed deficiencies in care and treatment of the terminally ill in U.S. medical practices.

Symptom management: Focus on promotion of comfort and alleviation of a variety of symptoms.

Tolerance: Decrease in one or more effects of an opioid, usually due to disease progression; may be treated with increased doses with few clinical problems in the terminally ill.

Chapter 25

Advanced practice nurse (APN): A nurse with expertise in a certain area who holds a master's degree or higher; four major types are nurse practitioner, clinical nurse specialist, nurse midwife, and nurse anesthetist.

Certified Life Care Planner (CLCP): A person meeting the requirements for certification and who holds certification to develop life care plans.

Certified Senior Advisor (CSA): A designation offered by the Society of Senior Advisors to persons completing a course of study that prepares them to advise seniors in matters of finance and planning.

Chartered Advisor for Senior Living (CASL): A certified professional who assists older persons with retirement savings, pension and social security planning, health and long-term care issues, and estate planning.

Community living designs: Concept that focuses on designing, building, engineering, and marketing to older adults, especially in senior living communities.

Continuing care retirement community (CCRC): A community living setting or situation designed for older adults that offers a continuum of care.

Doctor of nursing practice (DNP): The most recent clinical doctorate that looks to be the entry level into advanced practice beginning in 2015.

Financial gerontology: Combines the knowledge and skills associated with financial planning and asset management with expertise in meeting the unique needs of older adults.

Life care plan (LCP): A comprehensive document designed to help meet the long-term financial and health needs of a person who has experienced a catastrophic injury.

Long-term care insurance: Insurance designed to cover individuals needing health care outside of the hospital, including diagnostics testing, rehabilitation, or custodial care.

Professional geriatric care manager (PGCM): A professional who specializes in helping families care for older adults.

Registered Financial Gerontologist (RFG): A person certified to provide services related to comprehensive financial planning with older adults and whose studies emphasized knowledge of the aging process.

INDEX

Note: page numbers followed by b, f, or t denote boxes, figures, or tables respectively

B

E

F

H

M

Q

R

S

U

W

Y

Z